The Oxford Handbook of Eye Movements

The Oxford Handbook of Eye Movements

Edited by

Simon P. Liversedge

School of Psychology, University of Southampton,
Southampton, UK

Iain D. Gilchrist

School of Experimental Psychology,
University of Bristol, Bristol, UK

Stefan Everling

University of Western Ontario,
London, Ontario, Canada

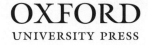

OXFORD
UNIVERSITY PRESS

OXFORD
UNIVERSITY PRESS

Great Clarendon Street, Oxford, OX2 6DP,
United Kingdom

Oxford University Press is a department of the University of Oxford.
It furthers the University's objective of excellence in research, scholarship,
and education by publishing worldwide. Oxford is a registered trade mark of
Oxford University Press in the UK and in certain other countries

Chapters 1–5 © Oxford University Press, 2011
Chapter 6 © Elsevier, 2009
Chapters 7–54 © Oxford University Press, 2011

The moral rights of the authors have been asserted

First Edition published in 2011
First published in paperback 2013
Impression: 2

British Library Cataloguing in Publication Data
Data available

Library of Congress Cataloging in Publication Data
Data available

ISBN 978–0–19–953978–9
ISBN 978–0–19–968343–7 (pbk)

Printed and bound on acid-free paper by
CPI Group (UK) Ltd, Croydon, CR0 4YY

Preface

The measurement of eye movements as an experimental method in the field of psychology is increasing at an exponential rate. For example, thirty years ago it was possible to count the number of eye movement laboratories in Psychology Departments in the UK on the fingers of one (or maybe two) hands. Today, the majority of Psychology Departments have some form of eye tracking device that is used in research. Indeed, there are many such devices in research departments associated with disciplines other than psychology (e.g., Computer Science, Engineering, etc). It is fair to say that eye movement methodology is now firmly established as a core tool in the experimentalist's armoury. To those who conduct eye movement research, this exponential growth is not at all surprising given the very tight relationship between eye movements and many aspects of human cognitive processing. This is most obvious when considering complex visual cognitive processes (e.g., reading, problem solving etc.) in which higher order, abstract mental representations directly influence oculomotor behaviour. More recently, however, researchers have started to establish that eye movements are vital for, and informative of, a much greater breadth of human psychological processes (e.g. shared social attention, interpersonal communication, etc.). In addition the eyes have a simple, well-defined repertoire of movements controlled by oculomotor neurons inside the cranium that are accessible to electrophysiological techniques. By recording from these and other neurons in alert animals, it has been possible to reveal many of the details of the motor and premotor circuitry that controls eye movements. This has resulted in a considerable understanding of motor control in general and in the pathophysiology of many visual and eye movement disorders. The saccadic circuitry is now understood at a level that allows us to investigate the neural basis of higher cognitive processes, including target selection, working memory, and response suppression. Without question, the field continues to expand, and this expansion has occurred as a consequence of how useful the methodology has been in furthering research, and how measurement techniques have improved and become simpler to use.

This rapid expansion in the field of eye movement research has two distinct consequences. First, researchers who haven't previously recorded eye movements as part of their research are increasingly doing so, and second it is becoming increasingly difficult for established researchers in the area to keep abreast of progress or discoveries in other areas of eye movement research. As a result of these perceived needs we felt it was timely to produce a handbook comprised of chapters by experts that are representative of the main areas of research in the field. The current volume, the Oxford Handbook on Eye Movements, is the product of that decision. When we set out to produce the Handbook, we had a clear set of objectives in mind. It needed to provide wide-ranging coverage, coverage that is representative of the breadth of the field at the moment. The chapters needed to be written by leading experts in the field. The content of the chapters needed to be up to date and informative both to other experts working in different areas of the field, and to advanced undergraduate and postgraduate students with an interest in eye movements. In summary, the Handbook needed to represent a snapshot of the current state of the field, a cross section of the work that is currently underway in the eye movement community.

In contributing a chapter, authors were tasked with providing a concise, to the point, high quality review of one or more particular issues that are currently of theoretical significance. All of the chapters were peer reviewed and thorough revisions were carried out on the basis of the reviews. The result, in our view, is a series of pieces of high quality writing delivered by individuals who maintain a very high profile in the field. The Handbook is a blend of both methodologically motivated content and theoretical analysis. The Handbook represents a significant, broad based, theoretical volume comprised of individual chapters focused on research that shares a common methodology.

The Handbook is structured around seven broad themes. In Part 1, we have two chapters offering overviews of eye movements in different species and of the history of eye movement research and five chapters that introduce different types of eye movements. Part 2 delivers a series of 14 chapters in which the anatomy and neural mechanisms underlying oculomotor control are discussed in detail. Part 3 contains six chapters detailing the relationship between eye movements and attention, and in Part 4 there are seven chapters that consider eye movements in relation to visual cognitive processing. In Part 5, five chapters cover aspects of development and pathology, and eye movements in special populations. In Parts 6 and 7 (eight and seven chapters respectively), the topic of reading is addressed, with Part 6 covering issues of oculomotor control in relation to reading, and the latter dealing with eye movements and their relationship to issues associated with linguistic processing. In total, the Handbook contains 54 Chapters that deliver a comprehensive coverage of the field. Inevitably there are areas of research which we have not included. In most cases this was to avoid producing a handbook that was simply too big. One example would be the limited coverage of eye movement research in an applied context (e.g., sports, engineering, ergonomics). The other obvious omission is the exclusion of a broad coverage of the neurology of eye movements.

Producing a volume of this magnitude would not be possible without the support of a dedicated team. The Editors are extremely grateful to Gwen Gordon who provided a tremendous amount of editorial assistance throughout. We would also like to thank Pippa Smith and Kathryn Smith who also assisted with editorial duties. The team at Oxford University Press have provided excellent support from the very beginning to the end of this project, and we are extremely grateful for their help and patience. Particularly, we would like to thank Martin Baum, Charlotte Green, Carol Maxwell and Priya Sagayaraj. We are also very grateful to Gerry Altmann who came up with the word cloud design for the front cover. We would also like to thank all the contributors to the volume – without them the Handbook would not have been possible. When we initially approached potential contributors to the volume, we were curious to see what the uptake to our invitation would be – to what extent would colleagues in the field not only be responsive to our request to contribute, but also take their task earnestly? It was a great pleasure to us that we had an overwhelmingly positive response to our invitation, and we were delighted that all of the authors delivered such high quality chapters. We are also grateful to the authors for taking the peer review process seriously both by acting as reviewers and responding carefully and diligently to the reviews of their own work. We know that this process has contributed significantly to the quality of the finalised chapters. Again, we are very grateful to the authors for making the effort to write such good chapters. Finally, it is likely that we have managed to forget to thank a number of people who have helped along the way, and to those people, we apologise.

In summary, we believe that together we have produced an Oxford Handbook on Eye Movements that is a high quality comprehensive volume. We anticipate that it will be used as a text by undergraduate and postgraduate students, and eye movement researchers alike to obtain synopses of specific topics currently under investigation in the eye movement community. We hope that you enjoy reading it.

Simon P. Liversedge
Iain D. Gilchrist
Stefan Everling

Contents

Part 3: Saccades and attention

Part 4: Visual cognition and eye movements

Part 5: Eye movement pathology and development

Part 6: Eye movement control during reading

List of Contributors

Gerry T.M. Altmann
Department of Psychology,
University of York, UK

Richard Amlôt
Department of Psychology, Royal Holloway,
University of London, UK

Dora E. Angelaki
Department of Neurobiology,
Washington University Medical School, USA

Thierry Baccino
University of Paris 8,
Cité des sciences et de l'industrie de la Villette,
France

Xuejun Bai
Academy of Psychology and Behavior,
Tianjin Normal University, P.R. China

Dana H. Ballard
Department of Computer Science,
University of Texas at Austin, USA

Graham R. Barnes
Faculty of Life Sciences,
University of Manchester, UK

Michele A. Basso
Department of Neuroscience,
University of Wisconsin, USA

Melissa R. Beck
Department of Psychology,
Louisiana State University, USA

Valerie Benson
School of Psychology,
University of Southampton, UK

Hazel I. Blythe
School of Psychology,
University of Southampton, UK

Bruce Bridgeman
Psychology Department,
University of California, Santa Cruz, USA

James R. Brockmole
Department of Psychology,
University of Notre Dame, USA

Brett A. Clementz
Departments of Psychology and
Neuroscience, Bio-Imaging Research Center,
University of Georgia, USA

Charles Clifton, Jr
Department of Psychology,
University of Massachusetts Amherst, USA

Jeremiah Y. Cohen
Department of Psychology,
Vanderbilt University, USA

Lawrence K. Cormack
Center for Perceptual Systems and
Department of Psychology,
The University of Texas at Austin, USA

Brian D. Corneil
Departments of Physiology & Pharmacology,
and Psychology,
University of Western Ontario, Canada

J. Douglas Crawford
Department of Psychology,
York University, Canada

Kathleen E. Cullen
Department of Physiology,
McGill University, Canada

Clayton E. Curtis
Psychology & Neural Science,
New York University, USA

Rick Dale
Cognitive and Information Sciences,
University of California, Merced, USA

C. Distler
Faculty of Biology and Biotechnology,
Ruhr University, Germany

Michael C. Dorris
Centre for Neuroscience Studies,
Queen's University, Canada

Denis Drieghe
School of Psychology, University of
Southampton, UK

Ralf Engbert
Department of Psychology,
University of Potsdam, Germany

Stefan Everling
University of Western Ontario,
London, Ontario, Canada

Ruth Filik
School of Psychology,
University of Nottingham, UK

Sue Fletcher-Watson
Moray House School of Education,
University of Edinburgh, UK

Neeraj J. Gandhi
Department of Otolaryngology,
University of Pittsburgh, USA

Wilson S. Geisler
Center for Perceptual Systems and
Department of Psychology,
The University of Texas at Austin, USA

Iain D. Gilchrist
School of Experimental Psychology,
University of Bristol, UK

Chris Harris
SensoriMotor Laboratory,
School of Psychology,
University of Plymouth, UK

Mary M. Hayhoe
Center for Perceptual Systems and
Department of Psychology,
The University of Texas at Austin, USA

John M. Henderson
Department of Psychology,
University of South Carolina, USA

Bernhard J.M. Hess
Department of Neurology,
University Hospital Zurich, Switzerland

Matthew D. Hilchey
Department of Psychology,
Dalhousie University, Canada

K.-P. Hoffmann
Faculty of Biology and Biotechnology,
Ruhr University, Germany

Jukka Hyönä
Department of Psychology,
University of Turku, Finland

Kevin Johnston
Centre for Neuroscience Studies,
Queen's University, Canada

Holly S.S.L. Joseph
Department of Experimental Psychology,
University of Oxford, UK

Barbara J. Juhasz
Department of Psychology,
Wesleyan University, USA

Husam A. Katnani
Department of Bioengineering,
University of Pittsburgh, USA

Julie A. Kirkby
Department of Psychology,
Bournemouth University, UK

Raymond M. Klein
Department of Psychology,
Dalhousie University, Canada

Reinhold Kliegl
Department of Psychology,
University of Potsdam, Germany

Eliana M. Klier
Department of Anatomy and Neurobiology,
Washington University School of Medicine,
USA

Helene Kreysa
Cognitive Interaction Technology
Center of Excellence,
Bielefeld University, Germany

Árni Kristjánsson
Department of Psychology,
University of Iceland, Iceland

Jun Kunimatsu
Department of Physiology,
Hokkaido University School of Medicine,
Japan

Michael F. Land
School of Life Sciences,
University of Sussex, UK

Simon P. Liversedge
School of Psychology,
University of Southampton, UK

Casimir J.H. Ludwig
School of Experimental Psychology,
University of Bristol, UK

Beatriz Luna
Laboratory of Neurocognitive Development,
Western Psychiatric Institute and Clinic,
University of Pittsburgh Medical Center,
University of Pittsburgh, USA

Stephen L. Macknik
Barrow Neurological Institute,
Phoenix, USA

Safraaz Mahamed
Department of Neuroscience,
University of Wisconsin, USA

Susana Martinez-Conde
Laboratory of Visual Neuroscience,
Division of Neurobiology,
Barrow Neurological Institute, Phoenix, USA

Michi Matsukura
Department of Psychology,
University of Iowa, USA

Jennifer E. McDowell
Departments of Psychology and
Neuroscience, Bio-Imaging Research Center,
University of Georgia, USA

Douglas P. Munoz
Centre for Neuroscience Studies,
Queen's University, Canada

René M. Müri
Perception and Eye Movement Laboratory,
Department of Neurology,
University of Bern, Switzerland

Thomas Nyffeler
Perception and Eye Movement Laboratory,
Department of Neurology,
University of Bern, Switzerland

Martin Paré
Centre for Neuroscience Studies,
Queen's University, Canada

Kevin B. Paterson
School of Psychology,
University of Leicester, UK

Matthew S. Peterson
Department of Psychology,
George Mason University, USA

Martin J. Pickering
Department of Psychology,
University of Edinburgh, UK

Alexander Pollatsek
Department of Psychology,
University of Massachusetts

Keith Rayner
Department of Psychology,
University of California, San Diego, USA

Erik D. Reichle
Department of Psychology,
University of Pittsburgh, USA

Eyal M. Reingold
Department of Psychology,
University of Toronto, Canada

Antje Sauermann
Department of Linguistics,
University of Potsdam, Germany

Jeffrey D. Schall
Department of Psychology,
Vanderbilt University, USA

Heather Sheridan
Department of Psychology,
University of Toronto, Canada

Michael J. Spivey
Cognitive and Information Sciences,
University of California, Merced, USA

Adrian Staub
Department of Psychology,
University of Massachusetts Amherst, USA

Petroc Sumner
School of Psychology,
Cardiff University, UK

John A. Sweeney
Department of Psychiatry and Pediatrics,
University of Texas Southwestern,
Dallas, USA

Masaki Tanaka
Department of Physiology,
Hokkaido University School of Medicine, Japan

Benjamin W. Tatler
School of Psychology,
University of Dundee, UK

Peter Thier
Department of Cognitive Neurology,
Hertie-Institute for Clinical Brain Research,
University of Tübingen, Germany

Marion R. Van Horn
Department of Physiology,
McGill University, Canada

Katerina Velanova
Laboratory of Neurocognitive Development,
Western Psychiatric Institute and
Clinic, University of Pittsburgh Medical Center,
University of Pittsburgh, USA

Françoise Vitu
Laboratoire de Psychologie Cognitive,
CNRS UMR 6146, Université de Provence,
Marseille, France

Corinne R. Vokoun
Department of Neuroscience,
University of Wisconsin, USA

Nicholas J. Wade
School of Psychology,
University of Dundee, UK

Robin Walker
Department of Psychology, Royal Holloway,
University of London, UK

Tessa Warren
Learning Research and Development
Center and Departments of Psychology
and Linguistics,
University of Pittsburgh, USA

Brian J. White
Centre for Neuroscience Studies,
Queen's University, Canada

Sarah J. White
School of Psychology,
University of Leicester, UK

Guoli Yan
Academy of Psychology and Behavior,
Tianjin Normal University, P.R. China

Chuanli Zang
Academy of Psychology and Behavior,
Tianjin Normal University, P.R. China

List of Abbreviations

2D	two-dimensional
3D	three-dimensional
AC	attentional capture
ACC	anterior cingulate cortex
ADHD	attention deficit hyperactivity disorder
AES	ectosylvian sulcus
AFC	alternative forced choice
AoA	age of acquisition
AOS	accessory optic system
APB	2-amino-4-phosphonobutyric acid
AS	Asperger's syndrome
ASD	autism spectrum disorder
BCI	brain–computer interface
BG	basal ganglia
BN	burst neuron
BOLD	blood oxygen-level dependent
BSS	blind source separation
BTN	burst-tonic neuron
CCN	central caudal nucleus
CDF	cumulative distribution function
CEF	cingulate eye field
CF	climbing fibre
cFN	caudal fastigial nucleus
CL	central lateral
CM	central median
CMAd	dorsal cingulate motor area
CMAr	rostral cingulate motor areas
CMAv	ventral cingulate motor areas
cMRF	central mesencephalic reticular formation

CNV	contingent negative variation
DA	dopamine
dLLBN	dorsal excitatory burst neuron
DLPFC	dorsolateral prefrontal cortex
DLPN	dorsolateral pontine nucleus
DPF	dorsal paraflocculus
dSC	deep layers of the superior colliculus
DTI	diffusion tensor imaging
dTMS	double-pulse transcranial magnetic stimulation
DTN	dorsal terminal nucleus
EBN	excitatory burst neuron
EFRP	eye fixation-related potential
EFT	embedded figures test
EH	eye-head
eLLBN	excitatory long-lead burst neuron
EMG	electromyography
EOG	electro-oculography
ERP	event-related potential
FEF	frontal eye field
fMRI	functional magnetic resonance imaging
FR	floccular region
FTN	flocculus target neuron
GABA	gamma-aminobutyric acid
GBS	gamma-band synchronization
GC	granule cell
GFS	general flash suppression
GP	globus pallidus
GPe	globus pallidus external
GPi	globus pallidus internal
HCI	human–computer interface
hOKR	horizontal optokinetic reflex
IBN	inhibitory burst neuron
ICA	independent component analysis
iGBR	induced gamma-band response
IML	internal medullary lamina
INC	interstitial nucleus of Cajal
INS	infantile nystagmus syndrome
IOR	inhibition of return
IOVP	inverted optimal viewing position
IPSP	inhibitory postsynaptic potential
ISI	interstimulus interval

ISL	intended saccade length
IVN	inferior (or descending) vestibular nucleus
LD	lateral dorsal
LFP	local field potential
LGN	lateral geniculate nucleus
LIP	lateral intraparietal
LLBN	long-lead burst neuron
LP	levator palpebrae
LTD	long-term depression
LTM	long-term memory
LTN	lateral terminal nucleus
LVN	lateral vestibular nucleus
MD	mediodorsal
MEG	magnetoencephalography
mhOKR	monocular horizontal optokinetic reflex
MLF	medial longitudinal fasciculus
mOKR	monocular optokinetic reflex
MRF	mesencephalic reticular formation
MST	medial superior temporal
MT	middle temporal
MTN	medial terminal nucleus
MVN	medial vestibular nucleus
nBOR	nucleus of the basal optic root
nLM	nucleus lentiformis mesencephali
NOT	nucleus of the optic tract
nPH	nucleus prepositus hypoglossi
NR	near response
NRTP	nucleus reticularis tegmentis pontis
OCD	obsessive–compulsive disorder
OKN	optokinetic nystagmus
OKR	optokinetic reflex
OO	orbicularis oculi
OPN	omnipause neuron
OVP	optimal viewing position
PAN	phasically active neuron
PCN	paracentral nucleus
PDF	probability density function
PET	positron emission tomography
Pf	parafascicular
PFC	prefrontal cortex
PG	processing gradient

PLP	preferred landing position
PPC	posterior parietal cortex
PPN	pedunculopontine nucleus
PPRF	paramedian pontine reticular formation
PSP	progressive supranuclear palsy
PSS	posterior suprasylvian
PVP	vestibular pause neuron
PVP	preferred viewing position
RB	range bias
RCP	rectus capitis posterior
RDE	remote distractor effect
RDK	random dot kinetogram
RF	receptive field
riMLF	rostral interstitial nucleus of the medial longitudinal fasciculus
RIP	raphe interpositus
ROI	region of interest
RT	response time
rTMS	repetitive transcranial magnetic stimulation
RVOR	rotational vestibulo-ocular reflex
SAI	stratum album intermediale
SAP	stratum album profundum
SAS	sequential attention shifts
SBN	saccadic burst neuron
SC	superior colliculus
SCi	intermediate layer of the superior colliculus
SCs	superficial layer of the superior colliculus
SEF	supplementary eye field
SGI	stratum griseum intermediale
SGP	stratum griseum profundum
SGS	stratum griseum superficiale
SIF	saccade initiation failure
SMA	supplementary motor area
SNc	substantia nigra pars compacta
SNr	substantia nigra pars reticulata
SO	stratum opticum
SOA	stimulus onset asynchrony
SOA	supraoculomotor nucleus
SPR	self-paced reading
SRE	saccadic range error
SRT	saccadic reaction time
SSRT	stop signal reaction time

STC	sensory trigeminal complex
STM	short-term memory
STN	subthalamic nucleus
SVN	superior vestibular nucleus
SWM	spatial working memory
SZ	stratum zonale
TAN	tonically active neuron
TD	typically-developed/developing
TMS	transcranial magnetic stimulation
TVOR	translational vestibulo-ocular reflex
VA	ventroanterior
VL	ventrolateral
VLPFC	ventrolateral prefrontal cortex
VN	vestibular nucleus
VOR	vestibulo-ocular reflex
VPL	ventral posterolateral
VPM	ventral posteromedial
VTA	ventral tegmental area
WCC	weak central coherence
WM	working memory

PART 1

The eye movement repertoire

CHAPTER 1

Oculomotor behaviour in vertebrates and invertebrates

Michael F. Land

Abstract

Humans use a 'saccade and fixate' strategy when viewing the world, with information gathered during stabilized fixations, and saccades used to shift gaze direction as rapidly as possible. This strategy is shared by nearly all vertebrates, whether or not their eyes possess foveas. Remarkably, the same combination is found in many invertebrates with eyes that resolve well. Cephalopod molluscs, decapod crustaceans, and most insects stabilize their eyes, head, or body against rotation while in motion, and also make fast gaze-shifting saccades. Praying mantids, like primates, are also capable of smooth tracking. Other invertebrates have eyes in which the retina is a long narrow strip, and these make scanning movements at right angles to the strip. These include heteropod sea-snails, certain copepods, jumping spiders, mantis shrimps, and some water beetle larvae. Scanning speeds are always just slow enough for resolution not to be compromised.

Humans and other primates

To begin this chapter I will summarize the human eye movement repertoire, and use it as a basis for comparing the eye movement of other animals. Humans and higher primates have four kinds of eye movements. *Saccades* are the fast eye movements that redirect gaze. They can have a wide variety of amplitudes and for a given size have a defined duration and peak velocity. They occur up to four times a second and while in progress subjects are effectively blind. Between saccades gaze is held almost stationary (fixation) by slow *stabilizing movements*. These are brought about by two reflexes: the vestibulo-ocular reflex (VOR) in which the semicircular canals measure head velocity, and cause the eye muscles to move the eyes in the head at an equal and opposite velocity (see also Cullen and Van Horn, Chapter 9, this volume); and the optokinetic reflex (OKN) in which wide-field image velocity signals from retinal ganglion cells are fed back to the eye muscles to null out any residual slip of the image across the retina (see also Distler and Hoffman, Chapter 4, this volume). For small targets *smooth pursuit* is possible up to speeds of about $15°s^{-1}$. At higher velocities pursuit starts to lag the target, and the tracking becomes interspersed with catch-up saccades which take over completely above $100°s^{-1}$ (see also Barnes, Chapter 7, this volume). When a target moves towards or away from the viewer it is tracked by *vergence* movements in which the eyes converge or diverge, in contrast to all other eye movements which are conjugate, i.e. the eyes move in the same direction.

Other vertebrates

Mammals

Mammalian voluntary saccades are always conjugate, unlike other vertebrates where they are, to varying degrees, independent in the two eyes. Spontaneous saccades are most prominent in primates, and are associated with the deployment of the fovea to fixate new targets. Other mammals do not have a deep fovea, although they may have 'areas' or 'visual streaks' with a somewhat elevated ganglion cell density, and hence increased functional acuity. Spontaneous saccades are also seen in carnivores such as cats and dogs, but are much less obvious in ungulates. Horses and cows, for example, will face and track an object of interest with their heads, whilst the laterally directed eyes perform a typical counter-rotation, interspersed with resetting saccades, as the head rotates. The eyes are simply retaining a fixed relationship with the surroundings, rather than being directed at targets. Similarly, many non-predators, such as rabbits and most rodents, make few if any spontaneous saccades when stationary but vigilant.

Birds

Birds have large eyes, light heads, and flexible necks, and typically move their eyes by moving their heads. This leads to the very characteristic pattern of head saccades seen when birds are foraging or watching out for predators. Most birds do have eye movements of limited extent (typically about 20°), but the main function of these is to 'sharpen up' the head saccades (Wallman and Letelier, 1993). The head starts to move but the eye initially counter-rotates (VOR); the eye then moves rapidly to a new position, before counter-rotating again as the head catches up. This ensures that the gaze change is extremely rapid, and stable fixations last longer than they would without the eye movements. Pursuit movements, made by the head, are seen in some birds, particularly predators. Although they can appear smooth, they actually consist of a succession of small saccadic head movements. It is not clear whether eye movements are ever involved in pursuit: they are certainly not available in owls, where the eyes are so large that eye movements are impossible. Most birds have two foveas in each eye: a central fovea directed anterolaterally and a temporal fovea directed forwards. The temporal foveas of the two eyes are used binocularly, for example, when pecking at food. The size of the binocular field is typically about 20°, but may be as much as 50° in owls. Many sea-birds have a visual streak, supplementing or replacing the foveas, and corresponding to the location of the horizon and the region of sea below it. Another characteristic behaviour, particularly of ground feeding birds, is the pattern of translational head saccades (head-bobbing). When the bird walks forward the neck moves the head backwards. It is then thrust rapidly forwards before moving backwards again at about the same speed as the forward locomotion. The result is that the head is stabilized in space for much of the time, presumably permitting an unblurred view of nearby objects to the side. Birds in flight do not head-bob, except when landing. They do, however, make head saccades and maintain rotationally stable fixations (Eckmeier et al., 2008).

Reptiles

Many reptiles sit for long periods without making spontaneous eye movements, although most are capable of them, and they certainly have the usual vestibular and visual stabilizing reflexes. Lizards make monocular saccades to fixate new targets. These are particularly obvious in chameleons, in which independent saccadic eye movements are used to survey the surroundings with the well-developed foveas. Once an insect prey has been located the chameleon turns towards it, rotates the two eyes forward, fixates the prey binocularly, and catches it with a ballistic extension of the tongue. The distance of the prey is determined not by triangulation but by focus (Harkness, 1977). A typical lizard has about 40° of eye movement, but in chameleons the turret-like eyes can be rotated through 180° horizontally and 90° vertically. Although chameleons give the impression that they are surveying the two halves of the visual world simultaneously and independently, their attention is only directed to one side at a time. While one eye is actively 'looking', the other is actually defocused (Ott et al., 1998). Attention switches between eyes at approximately 1-s intervals.

Amphibia

According to Walls (1942) no amphibian is known to perform any eye movements other than retraction and elevation. This is probably an overstatement: some tree frogs with visible slit pupils can be seen to counter-rotate their eyes when the head rotates, but in general frogs and toads make no spontaneous eye movements. Their strategy seems to be to let the stationary world go blank (as it does with humans when the image is stabilized) so that they only see motion, which is likely to be caused by either potential prey or a predator. During prey capture the head and body rotate to align the prey with the tongue.

Fish

The majority of fish do not have a fovea and do not have eye movements that target particular objects. The typical pattern of eye movements that accompany locomotion is for the eyes to make a saccade in the direction of an upcoming turn, and then for the eyes to counter-rotate as the turn

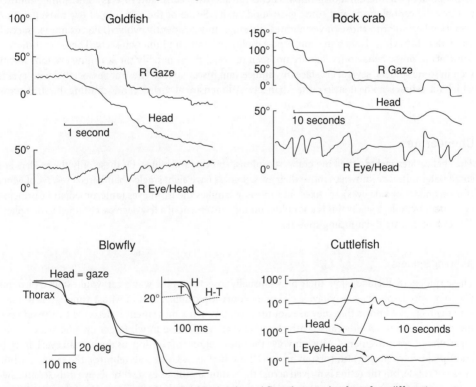

Fig. 1.1 Examples of independently evolved 'saccade and fixate' strategies from four different animal groups. Goldfish turning; redrawn from Easter et al. (1974). Reproduced with permission from *Journal of Experimental Biology*, Paul, H., Nalbach, H-O., & Varjú, D., Eye movements in the rock crab Pachygrapsus marmoratus walking along straight and curved paths, 1990, **154**, pp. 81-97. jeb. biologists.org. Blowfly in flight, inset shows the contribution of the neck (H-T); Reprinted by permission from Macmillan Publishers Ltd: *Nature*, C. Schilstra and J.H. van Hateren, Stabilizing gaze in flying blowflies, **395**(6703), copyright (1998). Cuttlefish (gaze not shown); Reproduced with permission from *Journal of Experimental Biology*, Land, M.F. Scanning eye movements in a heteropod mollusc, 1982, **96**, pp. 427-430. jeb.biologists.org All records are in the horizontal (yaw) plane.

is made (Fig. 1.1). The saccades made by the two eyes are not usually synchronized, as they would be in mammals. As Walls (1962) points out, this behaviour represents the origin of the saccade and fixate strategy in vertebrates: '. . . the ancient and original function of the eye muscles was not really to move the eye, but rather to hold it still with respect to the environment . . .' Rotational movements around the optic axis, tending to keep the dorsoventral axis of the eye aligned with gravity, are particularly noticeable when a fish tilts the body up or down, indicating the importance of the oblique muscles. Predating fish bring the whole body into line with the prey. Some fish do have an area, or even a fovea, located in the temporal retina which can be actively directed forward during prey capture. Such fish often have a pear-shaped pupil with an open space nasal to the lens to permit a forward view for the temporal retina. Fixation may then be monocular or binocular. Sea horses (*Hippocampus*) and their relatives are unusual in having a well-developed fovea near the centre of each retina, and their eye movements are very similar to those of chameleons. The turret-like eyes make saccades several times a second, apparently quite independently in the two eyes.

Invertebrates

Eye movements are seen in those invertebrate groups that have well-developed vision. These include arthropods of the three major groups (chelicerates, crustaceans, and insects), and some molluscs, notably the cephalopods and some gastropod snails. Some of the patterns of eye movement are remarkably similar to those of vertebrates, although independently evolved. For example, 'saccade and fixate' behaviour is seen in cephalopod molluscs, crabs, and many insects. There are, however, some oculomotor behaviours that are not seen in vertebrates, notably the scanning eye movements seen in some spiders, several crustaceans, and certain insect larvae. These are associated with eyes in which the retina is a linear strip rather than a two-dimensional surface, and scanning the strip across the field of view provides the second dimension (Fig. 1.2).

Chelicerates

The chelicerates include the king crabs, scorpions, spiders, and mites. Of these only the spiders and some water mites are known to move their eyes. Spiders have eight single-chambered eyes, six of which (the secondary or side eyes) are fixed, but in some families the front eyes (anteromedian or principal eyes) are moveable. Usually this is a simple scanning movement of a few degrees, confined to one plane. The exceptions are the jumping spiders.

Jumping spiders

These spiders (Salticidae) stalk their prey—usually insects—in the way a cat would stalk a bird, but like many predators they also have a elaborate courtship display, part of whose function is to make sure the recipient knows that they are not for eating. When a movement is detected by the side eyes the spider turns to face its cause with the principal eyes. These much larger eyes have a complex repertoire of eye movements, which involve the same degrees of freedom as the human eye: left–right and up–down rotations and torsion around the visual axis. Unlike vertebrates, the eye as a whole does not rotate, but the retina is moved across the stationary image by a set of six eye muscles attached to the eye tube. Each muscle is innervated by a single axon (Land, 1969). The principal eye retinae are elongated vertical structures, with the receptors arranged in four layers, the deepest of which is about 200 cells high by five cells wide. When the animal is at rest the retinae make spontaneous excursions of up to 50°, mostly in the horizontal plane, and these are mostly but not exclusively conjugate. However, if a moving object is detected in the field of view of the (fixed) anterolateral eyes the high-resolution central regions of the principal retinae are directed to it with a conjugate saccade. If the target continues to move both retinae will track it smoothly. Thereafter the retinae will usually scan the target using a stereotyped pattern of movements in which they oscillate laterally across the target with a frequency of 0.5–1 Hz, while at the same time making 50° torsional movements around the eye's axis at a much slower frequency, between 0.2 and 0.07 Hz. (Fig. 1.2).

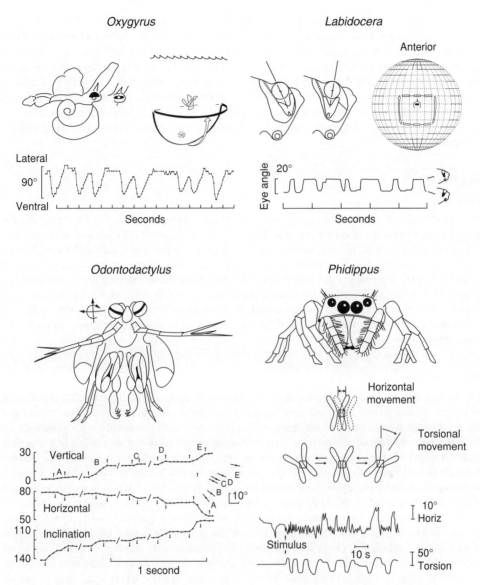

Fig. 1.2 Examples of animals with scanning eyes. *Oxygyrus* is a planktonic sea-snail. Views of the eye when pointing downwards and laterally. The insert on the right shows the quadrant covered in an upward scan. Below is a record of eight scans over an 18-s period. Reproduced with permission from *Journal of Experimental Biology*, Land, M.F., The functions of eye and body movements in Labidocera and other copepods, 1988, **140**, pp. 381-391. jeb.biologists.org *Labidocera* is a copepod crustacean. View of head from the side showing the eye-cup in two positions. Extended field of view above the animal is shown on right. Below is a record of scans made over 5 s. Reproduced with permission from, *Journal of Experimental Biology*, Land, M.F. Movements of the retinae of jumping spiders in response to visual stimuli, 1969, **51**, pp. 471-483. jeb.biologists.org *Odontodactylus* is a mantis shrimp (stomatopod crustacean). Animal from the front showing resting orientation of the mid-bands of the eyes. Below is a record of five scanning movements showing complex motion around three axes; orientation of mid-band shown on right. With kind permission from Springer Science+Business Media: *Journal of Comparative Physiology A*, The eye-movements of the mantis shrimp *Odontodactylus scyllarus* (Crustacea: Stomatopoda), **167**(2), 1990, M.F. Land. *Phidippus* is a jumping spider (Salticidae). View from the front showing principal and anterolateral eyes, and angles made by the legs. Below is a diagram and recording of the movements of the retinae of the principal eyes when scanning a recently presented square target. After Land (1969).

These scanning eye movements almost certainly represent a procedure for determining the identity of the target. Experiments by the ethologist Oscar Drees in the 1950s had established that the key feature that determines whether a male jumping spider will make a courtship display in front of a picture of another spider is the presence of legs. Jumping spider legs typically make angles of about 30° with the vertical axis of the body (many salticids also have body markings making similar angles), and it seems that it is these linear contours that the scanning procedure is designed to pick up. If an object of appropriate size lacks appropriate contours then it is treated as potential prey and stalked. Colour markings, including ultraviolet, are also involved in identifying conspecifics.

Crustacea

Daphnia

In spite of having a single cyclopean eye with only 22 ommatidia, the water flea *Daphnia pulex* has an impressive repertoire of eye movements. There are 'flicks' made to brief flashes of light, sustained 'fixations' to light stimuli of long duration, and 'tracking' movements to moving light stimuli made at about half the speed of the stimulus itself (Consi et al., 1990). There is a region of the eye, 80° dorsal to its axis, described as the 'null region' from which eye movements are not evoked, and it is proposed that flick and fixation movements rotate the eye so that a stimulus is brought into this region, and is then tracked when it strays outside the boundaries of this zone. Since *Daphnia* lives on suspended food particles the main role of the eyes is likely to be to orient the animal to the down-welling light while swimming.

Copepods

Most copepods are small filter-feeding crustaceans with insignificant tripartite 'nauplius' eyes. However in a few groups these eyes have become larger and more specialized. The most famous of these is *Copilia*, studied by Sigmund Exner in the 1890s. Here two elements of the nauplius eye have become large and separated, and have each developed an optical system consisting of a large lens situated anteriorly in the body which throws an image onto a smaller second lens some distance behind the first, rather as in a pair of binoculars. Immediately behind the second lens is a small group of three to seven receptors. The second lens and receptors move laterally in the body, through about 15° with respect to the first lens, thereby scanning its image. These spontaneous scans are in opposite directions in the two eyes and occur spontaneously at rates of 0.5–5 Hz. They can also be evoked by moving a stripe pattern in front of the animal (Downing, 1972). Female *Copilia* are predatory (only females have scanning eyes) so presumably this arrangement facilitates prey capture. However, as the field of view of the retina is only about 3° wide, extended by the scans of the two eyes to a line perhaps 30° long, the amount of sea scrutinized is still very small. One suggestion is that *Copilia* feeds during periods of planktonic vertical migration, and this vertical motion of potential prey through *Copilia*'s scan line effectively provides a second dimension to its field of view.

Another copepod with a scanning system is *Labidocera*. It is a member of a family, the Pontellidae, in which several species have well-developed visual systems (see Land and Nilsson, 2002). In *Labidocera* the males have an enlarged pair of upward-pointing eyes, with spherical lenses, which cast images onto a pair of conjoined retinae. Each retina consists of five vertically oriented flat receptors which together make a line subtending 40° laterally by less than 5° anteroposteriorly. The line of receptors is moved by a pair of muscles which pull the eye cups backwards, and by elastic ligaments that pull them forwards (Fig. 1.2). The maximum excursion is about 40°, meaning that a scan causes the receptor line to scan through a 40° by 40° square of the sea above the animal at a speed of about 220°s^{-1} (Land, 1988). Females have much reduced eyes, which leads one to suspect that the male's eyes are used in mate finding. Both sexes are elongated and deep blue in colour, which suggests that they might make detectable targets for such a scanning mechanism.

Stomatopods

The mantis shrimps are an order of large malacostracan crustaceans that mainly inhabit coral reefs. They are fearsome predators with a unique visual system. Each of the two mobile compound eyes has three parts, an upper and lower hemisphere of fairly conventional apposition construction, separated by a narrow mid-band which, in most genera, has six rows of ommatidia. Four of these rows subserve colour vision, with a system involving a total of 12 visual pigments arranged in three tiers of receptors in each row. The other two rows are responsible for polarization vision (Cronin and Marshall, 2004). The field of view of the mid-band is about 180° by 5°, and so represents a linear strip embedded in a normal two-dimensional eye. Not surprisingly the eye movements, which are always independent, are quite remarkable. The eyes make fast saccades to target new objects, they can track objects saccadically, and show typical slow optokinetic behaviour in a rotating drum. In addition they make low amplitude (~12°) slow (~40°s^{-1}) rotations that usually also involve some torsion (Land et al., 1990). These movements are mostly at right angles to the mid-band, and are interpreted as scanning movements that allow the mid-band to analyse objects for their colour and polarization content (Fig. 1.2). It is worth noting that reef-living mantis shrimps are themselves highly coloured, with particular body regions that reflect both linear and circularly polarized light (Chiou et al., 2008).

Decapod crustaceans

The shrimps, lobsters, crayfish, and crabs all have mobile eyes, and show strong optokinetic responses, although none either target or track objects with the eyes alone. Crabs have been best studied, and their saccade and fixate behaviour is remarkably similar to that of lower vertebrates (Fig. 1.1). The compound eyes are fixed on eyestalks, which are supplied with muscles that can rotate them about all three axes (yaw, pitch, and tilt) with respect to the body carapace. When walking, the eyes are stabilized about all of these axes. A crab can change direction either by rotating, or by changing the direction of translation; crabs typically walk sideways, although not exclusively (Paul et al., 1990). Rotation of gaze is prevented by the OKR, supplemented by information from the statocysts and leg proprioceptors. From time to time saccades in the opposite direction interrupt these stabilizing rotations, just as they do in fish. There is little or no compensation for translational changes. The fiddler crabs (*Uca*) keep their eyes exactly aligned with the horizon, using a combination of a statocyst response to gravity and the sight of the horizon itself. (*Uca* eyes have a region of high vertical acuity corresponding to a strip around the horizon—effectively a visual streak—but no corresponding specialization in the horizontal plane). This behaviour is important because these crabs determine if a moving object is likely to be a predator by whether or not it intersects the horizon. If it does, then it must be bigger than the crab; if it does not, then it is probably another crab (Zeil and Hemmi, 2006).

Insects

Insects have eyes that are a fixed part of the head, and so their eye movements are essentially neck movements, much as in birds. In some flying insects, notably hoverflies, the whole body can function as the vehicle for redirecting gaze and in that case some flight manoeuvres can be thought of as eye movements.

Mantids

Praying mantids have long attracted attention because of their creepily familiar way of peering attentively at other animate objects. Mantids have a forward-pointing region of high acuity in each eye in which the inter-ommatidial angle is about 0.6°, as opposed to 2° in the periphery. Moving targets seen in the periphery are brought to this acute zone (analogous to a fovea) with saccadic neck movements that can reach 560°s^{-1}.

Rossel (1980) filmed the tracking behaviour evoked by moving a live cockroach across the mantid's field of view. Against a plain background tracking was smooth, with an overall gain of 0.95 when the target was in the 20° zone around the fixation centre, but fell to zero at 30° from the centre.

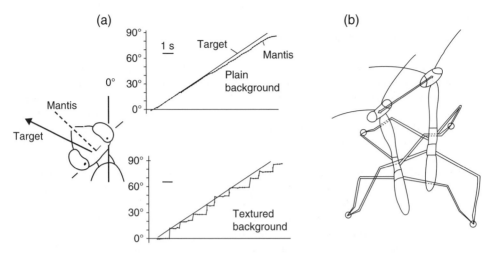

Fig. 1.3 a) Praying mantis tracking a stimulus (live cockroach) smoothly against a plain background, and saccadically against a textured background. With kind permission from Springer Science+Business Media: *Journal of Comparative Physiology A*, Foveal fixation and tracking in the praying mantis, **139**(4), 1980, Samuel Rossel. b) Young mantis 'peering' before jumping. Note that the head does not rotate in space as it is moved laterally by the body. With kind permission from Springer Science+Business Media: *Journal of Comparative Physiology A*, Motion and vision: why animals move their eyes, **185**(4), 1999, M.F. Land.

Interestingly, against a textured background tracking consisted entirely of 10–20° saccades, evoked when the target moved outside the fixation zone (Fig 1.3a). In normal settings tracking is exclusively saccadic. It seems that smooth tracking is normally prevented by the powerful optokinetic response, and that the saccadic mechanism overcomes this. However, the velocity input responsible for smooth tracking does show up during saccadic tracking, as these saccades do have a velocity as well as a position component.

Mantids and locusts have another interesting oculomotor behaviour. When about to jump from one stem to another they precede the jump by 'peering' (Fig. 1.3b). The whole body rotates so that the head is swung from side to side by up to a centimetre. The head, however, does not rotate, because retinal slip detected in the lateral parts of the eye causes the neck to counter-rotate the head (Collett, 1978). This means that in the forward direction the eyes see a pure lateral translational flow-field, allowing unambiguous measurement of distance.

Dragonflies

Dragonflies have a pronounced high resolution crescent (fovea) across the top of their compound eyes. This region points upwards and forwards, and is used to detect insect prey passing overhead. Some dragonflies catch prey while cruising, others detect prey from a perched position from which they dart up to make the capture from below. *Eurythemis simplicicollis*, a percher, captures prey by taking an interception course, aiming ahead of the prey's current position. The head first targets the prey with a neck saccade which centres it on the middle of the fovea. Then as the dragonfly takes off the fovea maintains fixation while the body is manoeuvred into the interception course, which in general will not be in line with the head. Capture flights are nearly always successful and rarely last longer than 200ms (Olberg et al., 2007).

Cruising dragonflies also use a flight manoeuvre—motion camouflage—which makes them appear stationary on the retina of their prey, or a conspecific during a territorial confrontation, even though they are engaged in active pursuit. This involves moving in such a way that as the prey moves forward the bearing of the predator remains constant. In the simplest case this could involve flying at the same speed on a parallel track, although there are other more complex strategies (Mizutani et al., 2003).

Blowflies

When making turns in flight, blowflies and houseflies make rapid saccade-like turns of the head and body at rates of up to 10 per second. Using a remarkable system of two search coils, Schilstra and van Hateren (1998) managed to record both thorax and head movements during flight around all three axes of rotation. Their main findings were that both thorax and body make fast turns, but the head movement is augmented by neck movements and so moves faster. A 25° turn takes the thorax about 45ms to complete, but the head-in-space (i.e. gaze) change is made in about 20ms. When the thorax starts to yaw the head first counter-rotates, then moves rapidly in the same direction as the thorax, then counter-rotates again at the end of the turn (Fig. 1.1). The strategy is very similar to the eye-in-head saccades of vertebrates, and the function is the same: to keep motion blur to a minimum. The yaw saccades are accompanied by roll of the thorax of 10° or more, which is counteracted by the neck so that the amount of roll experienced by the head is only 1–2°. Changes in pitch are minimal. The principal mechanism involved in stabilizing gaze is the haltere system. These are gyroscopic sensors on the thorax that are functionally analogous to the vertebrate semicircular canals, although anatomically homologous to the hind wings of other insects. Male flies also chase conspecifics in flight, so have a visual pursuit mechanism, but the relative movements of head and body during such chases have not been investigated.

Hoverflies

These are perhaps the most agile of all insects, with an astonishing ability to control flight direction and speed. The larger species can often be seen in sunlit woodland making sudden interception flights from stationary hovering positions in mid-air. The small hoverfly *Syritta pipiens* is sexually dimorphic, with the male possessing a region of enlarged facets and increased acuity (~0.6°) in the frontodorsal region of each eyes; in the rest of the male eye, and the whole of the female eye, interommatidial angles are about 1.5°. Males do not chase females, but shadow them at a distance of about 10 cm, until they land on a flower, at which point the males pounce. At this distance the male is invisible to the female by virtue of her lower resolution. The female's flight consists of saccadic turns of the whole body, with periods of straight flight between them. Unlike blowflies, the neck does not rotate the head separately, at least in the yaw plane. The males have a similar mode of flight, but when they see a female they track her by rotating the body smoothly, keeping her image within about 5° of the body axis, and maintaining a nearly constant distance at the same time (Fig. 1.4). If the female moves fast they can also track her with a series of saccades. Thus the flight path of the male can be regarded as both a series of flight manoeuvres and as eye movements. Think of a primate eye with wings (Collett and Land, 1975).

Hymenoptera

When bees and wasps leave their nests, or find a new source of food, they typically make a reconnaissance flight consisting of a series of increasing arcs centred on the nest or feeder. According to Zeil et al. (2007) they are setting up series of boundary 'snapshots' which define a V-shaped flight corridor leading to the nest, and on their return use these views to locate the centre of this corridor. During these arcing flights ground-nesting wasps (*Cerceris*) make a series of head saccades interspersed with stabilizing movements which, as in blowflies, serve to keep gaze direction temporarily constant (Fig. 1.4). The saccades are always made towards the nest, and tend to keep its location on the retina in a roughly constant location to one side or the other of the head axis during each arc.

Water beetle larvae

The larvae of certain water beetles have six single-chambered ocelli on each side of the head. Two of these are large, tubular, and very unusual. In *Thermonectus marmoratus* the retinae consist of a horizontal row of receptors organized in two tiers, somewhat reminiscent of the principal eyes of

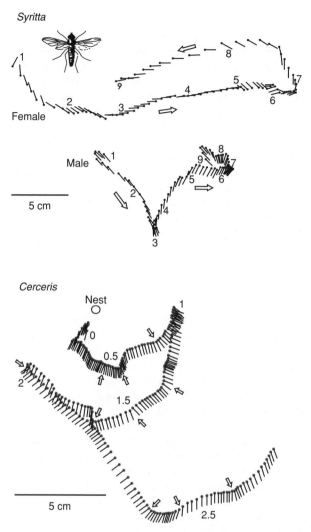

Fig. 1.4 *Syritta* is a small hoverfly. The figure shows a single video record of the body axes of a pair of flies, seen from above. The flight of the female is essentially saccadic, with long periods in which the body orientation does not change, punctuated by rapid turns. The male, who is shadowing her at a constant distance of about 10 cm, rotates smoothly, maintaining her image within 5° of his body axis. Corresponding times are numbered every 0.4 s. With kind permission from Springer Science+Business Media: *Journal of Comparative Physiology A*, Visual control of flight behaviour in the hoverfly *Syritta pipiens* L., **99**(1), 1975, T.S. Collett. *Cerceris* is a small ground-nesting wasp. The record shows that it makes a series of expanding arcs as it backs away from the nest. The lines attached to the head show the orientation of the head axis, and indicate that, like the hoverfly, the head direction changes saccadically (arrows), with intervening periods of flight in which there is no change in orientation. Times in seconds. Redrawn and modified with kind permission from Cold Spring Harbor Laboratory Press: *Inverterbrate Neurobiology*, p. 389 figure 3b, 2007, North and Greenspan.

jumping spiders. These forward-pointing eyes have horizontal fields of view 30° and 50° wide, but the vertical field is only a few degrees high. The eyes themselves are not mobile, but during the approach to prey the neck and thorax move the head and eyes up and down through up to 50°, thereby greatly extending the fields of view of the linear retinae (Buschbeck et al., 2007).

Molluscs

Cephalopods

The cuttlefish, octopuses, and squid all have large lens eyes which show remarkable evolutionary convergence with those of fish. They also have a very similar range of eye movements. Collewijn (1970) used a search-coil technique to measure optokinetic nystagmus in the cuttlefish *Sepia officinalis*, both when restrained in a rotating striped drum and when swimming freely. Movement of the stripes at speeds between 0.035 and $35°s^{-1}$ evoked a typical nystagmus, with fast and slow phases of about 10° amplitude. The fast phases were slower than in vertebrates, with a maximum speed of about $60°s^{-1}$. When rotated in the dark a transient nystagmus was also seen indicating that the statocysts also contribute to eye stabilization. This stabilization is not perfect: the maximum gain during the slow phases of nystagmus was rarely more than 0.5. Free swimming cuttlefish show a similar pattern of eye movement to fish, making saccades into each turn and stabilizing, at least partially, during its progress (Fig. 1.1).

Sepia and *Octopus* also fixate their prey (prawns and crabs) before they strike. The presence of prey in the field of view of one eye evokes a body turn towards it, and an eye movement that tends to bring the prey's image towards the posterior region of the retina. This typically involves a forward shift of the optic axis by about 27.5°, from 80° lateral to the body axis down to 52.5°. The contralateral eye also rotates forward, resulting in the prey being seen binocularly. In *Octopus* attacks are predominantly monocular (Hanlon and Messenger, 1996).

Heteropod gastropods

Most gastropod snails have eyes of some sort, and they move their heads from side to side as they move forward, so in some sense they can be said to have eye movements. However, there is no obvious organization to these movements, and in general the eyes are not independently mobile. There is, however, one superfamily, the Heteropoda, whose members do have well-developed vision. These marine snails are active predators in the plankton, and have large paired eyes with long narrow retinae, which are often tiered. *Oxygyrus* has a retina 400 receptors long and three receptors wide. The eyes scan an arc of about 90° at right angles to the long axis of the retina, through the dark quadrant beneath the snail (Fig. 1.2), and the assumption is that they are looking for planktonic prey illuminated by the light from above (Land, 1982).

Conclusions and future directions

The ubiquity of the saccade and fixate strategy, in animals from widely separated evolutionary backgrounds (Fig. 1.1), argues strongly that this behaviour solves a problem common to all animals with good vision. This problem stems from the fact that photoreceptors are slow: it takes a mammalian cone about 20ms to respond fully to a change in brightness, and about half this for a fly photoreceptor. This means that motion blur—the loss of high spatial frequency information—is an inevitable consequence of an unstabilized image. As a general rule, blur starts to set in if the rate of image movement exceeds one receptor acceptance angle per receptor response time. For humans this is about one degree per second. The better the resolution of an eye (i.e. the smaller the receptor acceptance angle) the greater the need for precise stabilization. Thus far, Walls' (1962) remark, quoted earlier, that the main function of eye movements is to stabilize gaze with respect to the surroundings, seems to hold across much of the animal kingdom. It seems, however, that avoidance of motion blur is not the only reason for image stabilization. Hoverflies and crabs stabilize gaze with much more precision than blur alone requires. Other possibilities are, first, the prevention of rotation during locomotion so that the translational flow field can be used for distance judgements (Fig. 1.4), and, second, the need for a stationary background image to allow the better detection of other moving objects (Land, 1999).

In a mobile animal an image fixed to the surroundings cannot be maintained for long, because when the animal turns the eyes would hit their back stops, and so there is a need for movements that return the eyes to a central position. To avoid loss of vision these must take up as little time as possible, hence saccadic eye movements. In some groups, from praying mantids to primates, saccades have taken on the additional role of centring specialized high-resolution retinal regions onto parts of the image requiring detailed scrutiny.

As we have seen there are also a number of animals that do not use a saccade and fixate strategy, but instead make scanning movements in which the retina is moved systematically and continuously across the image of the surroundings. These include the animals in Fig. 1.2, and the larvae of some water beetles. All these animals have essentially one-dimensional retinae, and the scanning strategy is a way of providing a two-dimensional field of view. (*Copilia*, with an almost point-like field of view, is an even more extreme case of dimensional reduction.) At first sight it would seem that scanning eyes would compromise their ability to detect detail by violating the blur rule mentioned above. This is not the case. In all the known examples the speed of scanning is at or below the 'one acceptance angle per response time' limit (Land, 1999). Thus scanning with a one-dimensional retina is a viable (and parsimonious) alternative to more conventional two-dimensional viewing.

While we now have a fairly good idea of the range of eye movement types across the animal kingdom, we have much less knowledge of how sequences of eye movements are used strategically to obtain the information an animal needs to pursue its behavioural goals. Human eye movement studies have made some advances in this direction (see Land and Tatler, 2009), and from some insect studies it is becoming clear that extended sequences of gaze movements are also important, for example, in obtaining landmark patterns for homing (*Cerceris*, Fig. 1.4). Future developments in the field are likely to lie in this direction.

References

Buschbeck, E., Sbita, S., and Morgan, R. (2007). Scanning behavior by larvae of the predaceous diving beetle *Thermonectus marmoratus* (Coleoptera: Dytiscidae) enlarges visual field prior to prey capture. *Journal of Comparative Physiology A*, **193**, 973–982.

Chiou, T-H., Kleinlogel, S., Cronin, T., Caldwell, R., Siddiqi, A., Goldizen, A., and Marshall, J. (2009). Circular polarization vision in a stomatopod crustacean. *Current Biology*, **18**, 429–434.

Collett, T.S. (1978). Peering: a locust behaviour pattern for obtaining motion parallax information. *Journal of Experimental Biology*, **76**, 237–241.

Collett, T.S. and Land, M.F. (1975). Visual control of flight behaviour in the hoverfly *Syritta pipiens* L. *Journal of Comparative Physiology*, **99**, 1–66.

Collewijn, H. (1970). Oculomotor reactions in the cuttlefish *Sepia officinalis*. *Journal of Experimental Biology*, **52**, 369–384.

Consi, T.R., Passani, M.B., and Macagno, E.R. (1990). Eye movements in *Daphnia magna*. Regions of the eye are specialized for different behaviors. *Journal of Comparative Physiology A*, **166**, 411–420.

Cronin, T.S. and Marshall, J. (2004). The unique world of mantis shrimps. In F.R. Prete (ed.) *Complex worlds from simpler nervous systems* (pp. 239–269). Cambridge MA: MIT Press.

Downing, A.C. (1972). Optical scanning in the lateral eyes of the copepod *Copilia*. *Perception*, **1**, 247–261.

Easter, S.S., Johns, P.R., and Heckenlively, D. (1974). Horizontal compensatory eye movements in goldfish (*Carrassius auratus*). I. The normal animal. *Journal of Comparative Physiology*, **92**, 23–35.

Eckmeier, D., Geurten, B.R.H., Kress, D., Mertes, M., Kern, R., Egelhaaf, M., *et al.* (2008). Gaze strategy in the free flying zebra finch (*Taeniopygia guttata*). *PLoS ONE*, **3**(12), e3956. doi:10.1371.

Hanlon, R.T. and Messenger, J.B. (1996). *Cephalopod behaviour*. Cambridge: Cambridge University Press.

Harkness, L. (1977). Chameleons use accommodation cues to judge distance. *Nature*, **267**, 346–349.

Land, M.F. (1969). Movements of the retinae of jumping spiders in response to visual stimuli. *Journal of Experimental Biology*, **51**, 471–483.

Land, M.F. (1982). Scanning eye movements in a heteropod mollusc. *Journal of Experimental Biology*, **96**, 427–430.

Land, M.F. (1988). The functions of eye and body movements in *Labidocera* and other copepods. *Journal of Experimental Biology*, **140**, 381–391.

Land, M.F. (1999). Motion and vision: why animal move their eyes. *Journal of Comparative Physiology A*, **185**, 341–352.

Land, M.F. and Nilsson, D-E. (2002). *Animal eyes*. Oxford: Oxford University Press.

Land, M.F. and Tatler, B.W. (2009). *Looking and acting: Vision and eye movements in natural behaviour*. Oxford: Oxford University Press.

Land, M.F, Marshall, N.J., Brownless, D., and Cronin, T. (1990). The eye movements of the mantis shrimp *Odontodactylus scyllarus* (Crustacea: Stomatopoda). *Journal of Comparative Physiology A*, **167**, 155–166.

Mizutani, A., Chahl, J.S., and Srinivasan, M.V. (2003). Motion camouflage in dragonflies. *Nature*, **423**, 604.

Olberg, R.M., Seaman, R.C., Coats, M.I., and Henry, A.F. (2007). Eye movements and target fixation during dragonfly prey-interception flights. *Journal of Comparative Physiology A*, **193**, 685–693.

Ott, M., Schaeffel, F., and Kirmse, W. (1998). Binocular vision and accommodation in prey-catching chameleons. *Journal of Comparative Physiology A*, **182**, 319–330.

Paul, H., Nalbach, H-O., and Varjú, D. (1990). Eye movements in the rock crab *Pachygrapsus marmoratus* walking along straight and curved paths. *Journal of Experimental Biology*, **154**, 81–97.

Rossel, S. (1980) Foveal fixation and tracking in the praying mantis. *Journal of Comparative Physiology A*, **139**, 307–331.

Schilstra, C. and van Hateran, J.H. (1998). Stabilizing gaze in flying blowflies. *Nature*, **395**, 654.

Wallman, J. and Letelier, J-C. (1993). Eye movements, head movements and gaze stabilization in birds. In Zeigler, H.P. and Bischof, H-J. (eds.) *Vision, brain and behavior in birds* (pp. 245–263). Cambridge, MA: MIT Press.

Walls, G.L. (1942) *The vertebrate eye and its adaptive radiation*. Bloomington Hills, MI: Cranbrook Institute. Reprinted (1967) New York: Hafner.

Walls, G.L. (1962). The evolutionary history of eye movements. *Vision Research*, **2**, 69–80.

Zeil, J. and Hemmi, J.M. (2006). The visual ecology of fiddler crabs. *Journal of Comparative Physiology A*, **192**, 1–25.

Zeil, J., Boeddeker, N., Hemmi, J.M., and Stürzl, W. (2007). Going wild: towards an ecology of visual information processing. In North, G. and Greenspan, R.J. (eds.) *Invertebrate neurobiology* (pp. 381–403). New York: Cold Spring Harbor Laboratory Press.

CHAPTER 2

Origins and applications of eye movement research

Nicholas J. Wade and Benjamin W. Tatler

Abstract

Research on oculomotor behaviour is examined historically. The first phase involved describing phenomena associated with eye movements; these typically concerned normal and abnormal binocular coordination and vertigo. Such descriptions became more refined, although attention was confined more to the directions the eyes adopted rather than their dynamics. Afterimages were the principal means by which the characteristics of eye movements were determined prior to the application of photographic methods in the early twentieth century. Many types of eye tracking devices are now available, and oculomotor behaviour provides insights into many perceptual and cognitive processes.

Introduction

The widespread modern application of indices of oculomotor behaviour might suggest a long historical concern with them, but such is not the case. Even descriptions of eye movement patterns, let alone their measurement, reflect relatively recent developments rather than long-standing interests. The aim of this chapter is to trace the emergence of scientific interest in and the experimental measurement of eye movements and to survey the areas in which they were and are applied.

In examining the origins of eye movement research it is instructive to place them within a general framework of discovery and development of naturally occurring phenomena. Such a framework illuminates the phases through which the studies of phenomena pass. The first phase is a description of the phenomenon, which is followed by attempts to measure it in some way. Measurement enables the characteristics of the phenomenon to be determined and incorporated within extant theory. Finally, the phenomenon is accepted and utilized to gain more insights into wider aspects of behaviour (see Table 2.1). In many cases, the phenomena have been described in antiquity, and no clear origin can be determined. In others, there is an obvious break with the past and a phenomenon is described and investigated for the first time. Both of these features apply to the unfolding understanding of eye movements.

Not all aspects of behaviour that are universal, like eye movements, have warranted description unless their normal functions are disrupted by disease or accident. This has certainly been the case for oculomotor behaviour. Moreover, description does not occur in a vacuum; it requires some context, be it philosophical, medical, or psychological. Scientific descriptions are a modern preoccupation, and so the

Table 2.1 A natural history of perceptual phenomena indicating the phases through which their investigation can pass

Origins	
Description	Phenomenology
Confirmation	Refining observations
Measurement	Applying extant technology then developing new techniques
Applications	
Interpretation	Within existing psychological concepts
Integration	Links with underlying physiology
Exploitation	Phenomena used to test particular theoretical ideas

search for the origins of accounts of eye movements must delve into pre-scientific periods. We will examine this heritage under the headings given in Table 2.1. The first phase of understanding any phenomenon is an adequate description of it. This can occur independently of theory, but the phenomena are rarely free from the psychological spirit of the times. The latter often intrude on the phenomenology so that a clear description remains difficult to extract. Not only do eye movements have many components but some of these are also dynamic, and difficult to detect without the aid of specially devised instruments. However, there needs first to be a phenomenon for which the instruments can assist in recording. The history of eye movement research provides a delightful discourse between description and measurement, between the subjective reports of effects and their objective measurement. In addition, the study of eye movements has, perforce, addressed the integration of vision and action. This integration is not restricted to the functions served by eye movements, but the clues to the patterns of eye movements usually derived from examining visual phenomena (see Tatler and Wade, 2003; Wade, 2007a, 2010; Wade and Tatler, 2005; Wade et al., 2003). Moreover, the descriptions of oculomotor behaviour are based on the sense that is observing its own actions: eyes observing eye movements. One of the intriguing aspects of the history we are about to examine is that subjective impressions of their motor aspects were often taken as evidence of their occurrence rather than observing the eyes of others. Feeling if the eyes had moved in the orbit was used as an index of whether the eyes had moved; this becomes particularly significant in the context of vertigo.

Origins

The eyes move in order to locate objects of interest in the region of greatest visual resolution—the fovea. They are moved by muscles attached to the eyeball and the socket. Knowledge about the range of movements was available to early anatomists, like Galen in the second century:

> Since there are four movements of the eyes, one directing them in toward the nose, another out toward the small corner, one raising them up toward the brows, and another drawing them down toward the cheeks, it was reasonable that the same number of muscles should be formed to control the movements. . . . Since it was better that the eye should also rotate, Nature made two other muscles [*obliqui, superior* and *inferior*] that are placed obliquely, one at each eyelid, extending from above and below toward the small corner of the eye, so that by means of them we turn and roll our eyes just as readily in every direction.
>
> (May, 1968, p. 483.)

Thus, the three axes around which the eye can rotate were clearly described, but the emphasis was on the direction the eye would take following a rotation rather than the rotations themselves.

Description

Initially, phenomena are described in a general way, often incorporating elements of the putative cause. The phenomenology is thereafter refined, and perhaps subdivisions of the phenomena are introduced. Eye movements present particular challenges in this regard because of their dynamic component. Descriptions of gaze direction preceded those of movement. Many of the phrases in our language concerning the eyes reflect a greater appreciation of their static than their dynamic aspects. Indeed, the directions of the eyes are potent cues in social intercourse—we use terms like seeing 'eye to eye' with someone, honesty is determined by 'looking someone straight in the eye', or doubt is cast on someone's integrity if they have a 'shifty look'.

Amongst the oldest descriptions of eye directions are those related to binocular alignment. We are exceedingly sensitive to detecting deviations in the eyes of those who have squints. It is the binocular features of eye movements that were amongst the first aspects that were subjected to scrutiny. In large part this was because a consequence of squinting is the disruption of binocular single vision, and this has been an overarching issue in the study of vision (see Wade, 1998). On the other hand, throughout the long descriptive history of studies of eye movements a vital characteristic of them remained hidden from view, both in ourselves and in our observations of others. The rapid discontinuous nature of eye movements is a relatively recent discovery, as are the small involuntary movements that accompany fixation. For most of recorded history, the eyes were thought to glide over scenes to alight on objects of interest, which they would fix with unmoved accuracy.

Binocular eye movements

One of the most distinctive features of eye movements is also related to their binocularity—they tend to move together. Such conjoint motion is not always in the same direction, as was noted by Aristotle over 2000 years ago (Ross, 1927). He distinguished between version (movements in the same direction) and convergence eye movements. He also commented that there were certain movements that were not possible, namely, divergence beyond the straight ahead, and movements of one eye upward and the other downward. A similar description was given by Ptolemy several centuries later, but he did appreciate the function eye movements served: they resulted in corresponding visual pyramids for the two eyes (A.M. Smith, 1996). Aristotle believed that there was a single source of control for the movements of both eyes, although he did not make such a clear statement as the eleventh-century scholar, Ibn al-Haytham (or Alhazen): 'When both eyes are observed as they perceive visible objects, and their actions and movements are examined, their respective actions and movements will be found to be always identical' (Sabra, 1989. p. 229).

This later became called the law of equal innervation (see Howard, 2002). Thus, Ibn al-Haytham proposed that the two eyes acted together in order to achieve single vision, and that the movements of the eyes were coordinated to this end. It appears that he supported the proposal by observing the eyes of another person while they were inspecting an object. Robert Smith (1738, 2004) introduced a simple demonstration of corresponding eye movements—the closed eye follows the movements of the open one, as can be ascertained by lightly placing a finger over the closed lid. He elaborated on the analysis of binocular single vision by recourse to the stimulation of corresponding points in the two eyes, and he related the misalignment of the two eyes to double vision. Smith integrated several strands of interest in binocular vision: singleness of vision with two eyes was considered to be a consequence of stimulating corresponding points on the two retinas; distinct vision was restricted to the central region of the retina; both eyes moved in unison to retain correspondence; this could be demonstrated by feeling the movements of the closed eye; double vision occurs when one eye is moved out of alignment with the other. Such squinting can be induced artificially (by displacing one open eye with the finger) and it also occurs naturally.

Ophthalmology has a longer recorded history than optics: several surviving papyri dating from the second millennium B.C. describe disorders of the eye and treatments of them. For example, the Ebers papyrus described dimness of sight and strabismus (see Bryan, 1930). A millennium later, there were specialists in diseases of the eye practising in Egypt. An illustration of a cataract operation of the type that was probably performed almost 2000 years ago was redrawn by Thorwald (1962), and written records indicate that such operations had been conducted a thousand years earlier (see Magnus, 1901). Greek medicine profited greatly from these earlier endeavours, and added to them.

Neither Egyptian nor Greek ophthalmology was free from the mystical and metaphysical, and observation was frequently subservient to philosophical doctrine.

Strabismus, squint, or distortion of the eyes, was recorded in antiquity, but its reported association with problems of binocular vision are more recent (see Duke-Elder and Wybar, 1973; Hirschberg, 1899; van Noorden, 1996; Shastid, 1917). The eye specialists in Babylonia, Mesopotamia, and Egypt must have had a working knowledge of ocular anatomy in order to carry out the operations they are known to have performed. However, the records that have survived (such as the Ebers papyrus) relate mainly to the fees they charged and the penalties they suffered for faulty operations rather than the conditions they cured. Their skills and understanding would have been passed on to Greek physicians, who both developed and recorded them. Many Greek texts, through their translations, have been transmitted to us, but any illustrations that they might have included have not survived. Aristotle described many features of perception, including strabismus and the ensuing diplopia: 'Why do objects appear double to those whose eyes are distorted? Is it because the movement does not reach the same point on each of the eyes?' (Ross, 1927, p. 958b). This reflected Aristotle's belief that the eyes operated as a unit rather than independently.

In addition to his description of the extraocular muscles, Galen also recorded that deviations of the eyes in strabismus were always nasal or temporal. However, he did state that those with strabismus rarely make errors in object recognition. Corrections for the deviation of an eye were advocated by many, like Paulus Ægineta in the seventh century. He recommended the use of a mask for children, which had small apertures so that the eyes would need to align themselves appropriately to see objects. A similar scheme was introduced and illustrated by Ambroise Paré in the sixteenth century. More elaborate masks were prescribed by Georg Bartisch (1583). They indicate that he was aware of convergent and divergent squint and he recognized that strabismus was more amenable to correction in children than in adults. From the eighteenth century attention was directed to the manner in which those with strabismus saw objects singly. There were many possible causes of squint, most of which were enumerated by Porterfield (1759). The overriding historical concern with squinting has been with its medical treatment, rather than its relevance to theories of vision or eye movements. It was in this medical context that Erasmus Darwin (1778) investigated squinting in a young child who had alternating dominance.

Porterfield is an important figure in the early descriptive phase of research on eye movements (see Wade, 2000, 2007b). Prior to publication of his influential *Treatise on the eye* (Porterfield, 1759), he wrote two long articles in 1737 and 1738; one was on external and the other was on internal motions of the eye. In the course of the latter, Porterfield coined the term accommodation for the changes in focus of the eye for different distances. He also examined an aphakic patient, in whom the lens in one eye had been removed, and demonstrated that the lens is involved in accommodation. However, it is his analysis of eye movements during scanning a scene and reading that are of greater interest here. Porterfield's studies started, as had earlier ones, from an understanding that distinct vision was limited to a small region of the visual field—around the point of fixation. This did not correspond with our visual experience of the scene, and he described this paradox eloquently:

> In viewing any large Body, we are ready to imagine that we see at the same Time all its Parts equally distinct and clear: But this is a vulgar Error, and we are led into it from the quick and almost continual Motion of the Eye, whereby it is successively directed towards all the Parts of the Object in an Instant of Time.
>
> (Porterfield, 1737, pp. 185–186.)

Porterfield applied this understanding of the requirement for rapid eye movements to reading itself, although his analysis was logical rather than psychological:

> Thus in viewing any Word, such as MEDICINE, if the Eye be directed to the first Letter M, and keep itself fixed thereon for observing it accurately, the other Letters will not appear clear or distinct ... Hence it is that to view any Object, and thence to receive the strongest and most lively Impressions, it is always necessary

we turn our Eyes directly towards it, that its Picture may fall precisely upon this most delicate and sensible Part of the Organ, which is naturally in the *Axis* of the Eye.

(Porterfield, 1737, pp. 184–185, original capitals and italics.)

Porterfield did not provide empirical support for the ideas he developed. He also appreciated the historical background in which his researchers were placed. Moreover, he applied his understanding of eye movements to a wide range of phenomena, including visual vertigo. It was from vertigo that the first signs of discontinuous eye movements derived: the fast and slow phases of nystagmus were demonstrated with the aid of afterimages.

Confirming phenomenology

Visual motion of the world following body rotation was described in antiquity. Perhaps the fullest accounts were given by Theophrastus (see Sharples, 2003); he described the conditions that can induce dizziness, including rotation of the body, but he did not relate these to movements of the eyes. Porterfield (1759) did add an eye movement dimension to it but he denied their existence following rotation—because he was not aware of feeling his eyes moving. That is, the index of eye movement he used was the conscious experience of it. He proposed that the post-rotational visual motion was an illusion in which the stationary eye is believed to be moving. In modern terminology he was suggesting that it was the signals for eye movements, rather than the eye movements themselves, that generated the visual motion following body rotation.

Porterfield's description stimulated others to examine vertigo and to provide interpretations of it, some of which involved eye movements. The most systematic studies were carried out by William Charles Wells in the late eighteenth century. They were reported in his monograph concerned with binocular single vision (Wells, 1792). The text of the book has been reprinted in Wade (2003a). The characteristics of eye movements following rotation were clearly described: he formed an afterimage (which acted as a stabilized image) before rotation so that its apparent motion could be compared to that of an unstabilized image when rotation ceased. The direction of the consequent slow separation of the two images and their rapid return (nystagmus) was dependent on the orientation of the head and the direction of body rotation. In the course of a few pages Wells laid the foundations for understanding both eye movements and visual vertigo (which he referred to as giddiness). Thus, Wells used afterimages to provide an index of how the eyes move by comparing them with real images. He confirmed his observations by looking at the eyes of another person who had rotated. By these means he cast doubt on evidence derived from subjective impressions of how the eyes were moving. In addition to his clear accounts of dynamic eye movements, Wells (1794a) rejected alternative interpretations of visual vertigo and even provided evidence of torsional nystagmus (Wells, 1794b).

Jan Evangelista Purkinje (1820, 1825) essentially repeated Wells's experiments, but was ignorant of them. Indeed, Purkinje's experiments were inferior to those by Wells, but both adopted interpretations of visual vertigo in terms of eye movements. Purkinje added a novel method for studying vertigo and eye movements—galvanic or electrical stimulation of the ears. Stimulating the sense organs with electricity from a voltaic pile was widely applied in the nineteenth century (see Wade, 2003b). The technique was amplified by Eduard Hitzig (1871). He examined eye and head movements during galvanic stimulation of the ears and likened nystagmus to a fisherman's float drifting slowly downstream and then being snatched back. The 1870s was the decade of added interest in eye movement research because of its assistance in determining semicircular canal function. Post-rotational eye movements were measured and related to the hydrodynamic theory, which was proposed independently by Ernst Mach, Josef Breuer, and Alexander Crum Brown.

Breuer (1874) provided a similar description of post-rotational nystagmus to Wells, but he was able to relate the pattern of eye movements to the function of the semicircular canals. Breuer argued that during rotation the eyes lag behind the head in order to maintain a steady retinal image; then they make rapid jerky motions in the direction of head rotation. The eye movements reduce in amplitude and can stop with rotation at constant angular velocity. When the body rotation ceases the

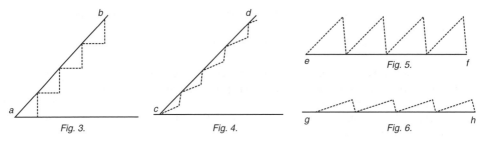

Fig. 2.1 Schematic diagrams by Crum Brown (1878) of eye movements during and after body rotation: 'When a real rotation of the body takes place the eyes do not at first perfectly follow the movement of the head. While the head moves uniformly the eyes move by jerks. Thus, in the diagram, Fig. 3, where the abscissæ indicate time and the ordinate the angle described, the straight line *a b* represents the continuous rotatory motion of the head and the dotted line the continuous motion of the eye. Here it will be seen that the eye looks in a fixed direction for a short time, represented by one of the horizontal portions of the dotted line *a b*, and then very quickly follows the motion of the head, remains fixed for a short time, and so on. After the rotation has continued for some time the motion of the eye gradually changes to that represented by the dotted line *c d* in Fig. 4. The eye now never remains fixed, but moves for a short time more slowly than the head, then quickly makes up to it, then falls behind, and so on. At last the discontinuity of the motion of the eye disappears, and the eye and the head move together. If now the rotation of the head be stopped (of course the body stops also) the discontinuous movements of the eyeballs recommence. They may now be represented by the dotted line in Fig. 5. The intermittent motion of the eyes gradually becomes less, passing through a condition such as that shown by the dotted line in Fig. 6, and at last ceases.' (Crum Brown, 1878, p. 658).

eyes rotate in the same direction as prior head rotation, and the visual world appears to move in the opposite direction interspersed with rapid returns. He also stated, like Wells, that there is no visual awareness during these rapid returns. This is a clear reference to saccadic suppression, although he did not use the term saccade.

Afterimages were also employed by Mach (1873, 1875), who rediscovered Wells's method for examining post-rotational eye movements. In addition to observing an afterimage, he applied the time-honoured technique of placing a finger by the side of the eye, and also using pressure figures as stabilized retinal images. However, perhaps the clearest descriptions of eye movements during and following body rotation were given by Crum Brown (1878), who provided diagrams of the steady head and jerky eye movements (Fig. 2.1). Wells's account of the dynamics of eye movements following rotation was beautifully refined by Crum Brown, although no reference was made to Wells. Like most other historians of the vestibular system, Crum Brown championed Purkinje as the founder of experimental research linking eye movements to vestibular stimulation (see Wade, 2003b).

In the early twentieth century, two aspects of eye movements and vertigo attracted attention. The first was the use of post-rotational nystagmus as a clinical index of vestibular function. These characteristics of nystagmus were defined more precisely by Robert Bárány (1906, 1913), who was awarded the Nobel Prize in 1914 for his vestibular researches. Indeed, the rotating chair is now called the Bárány chair. He also refined the method of stimulating the semicircular canals with warm and cold water so that the eye movements they induce could be easily observed. The second aspect was the use of post-rotational eye movements as a screening test for aviators.

Aircraft flight placed demands on the vestibular receptors that were beyond the normal range. Only the human centrifuge had subjected the human frame to similar forces. It had been devised by Erasmus Darwin as a treatment for insanity (Wade et al., 2005), it was adopted as an instrument for generating vertigo, and now it was applied to simulating the pressures of aircraft flight. Griffith (1920) examined eye movements with aircraft pilots following body rotation. Initially aviators were selected on the basis of their vestibular sensitivity, as determined by tests on a Bárány chair.

However, seasoned pilots were not so susceptible to vertigo, and he argued that they had habituated to the repeated rotations to which they had been exposed. In order to examine habituation more rigorously, Griffith tested students on repetitive rotations in a modified Bárány chair. They were exposed to 10 rotations of 20 seconds, alternating in direction, per session and they were tested over many days. Measures of the duration of apparent motion and the number and duration of nystagmic eye movements were recorded after the body was stopped:

> We have found that, as turning is repeated from day to day, the duration of after-nystagmus, the number of ocular movements made, and the duration of the apparent movement rapidly decrease. The major part of this decrease occurs within the first few days. The decrease takes place not only from day to day but also within a period of trials on any single day.
>
> (Griffith, 1920, p. 46.)

The topic of vestibular habituation attracted Raymond Dodge (1923) and he sought to determine how the eyes moved during and after rotation. The problem of adaptation to rotation is a general one, and it is relevant to the relative immunity to motion sickness of those, like seafarers, who are regularly exposed to the conditions which can induce it. As he remarked: 'The very existence of habituation to rotation was vigorously denied during the war by those who were responsible for the revolving chair tests for prospective aviators' (Dodge, 1923, p. 15). Dodge had previously measured eye movements during reading and was noted for the ingenuity of the recording instruments he made. Recording eye movements during rotation provided a particular challenge (Dodge, 1930). In examining the possibilities he had noticed that the convexity of the cornea was visible as a moving bulge beneath the eyelid. Dodge (1921) mounted a mirror over the closed eyelid and was able to record eye movements by the reflections from it. With it he was able to confirm the results of Griffith: without the possibility of visual fixation, after-nystagmus declines with repeated rotations. In the next section it will become evident that Dodge was a pioneer of recording eye movements generally, and during reading in particular. It is of interest to note that following his developments in these novel areas he engaged in examining eye movements following body rotation—the problem tackled by previous pioneers over a century earlier. Indeed, Dodge shared with Purkinje a willingness to engage in heroic experiments. When Purkinje gained access to a rotating chair he noted the effects of being rotated for one hour in it. Dodge similarly subjected himself to a gruelling regime: 'The experiment consisted of a six-day training period during which the subject (myself) was rotated in the same direction one hundred and fourteen times each day at as nearly uniform speed as possible' (Dodge, 1923, p. 16). The amplitude of post-rotational nystagmus decreased from day to day throughout the experiment. Any feelings of dizziness also disappeared with prolonged practice, and the experience was said to be soothing.

Visual vertigo and nystagmus are usually examined following rotation of the body around a vertical axis, whereas torsion results from lateral rotation around the roll axis. The extent of torsion is much smaller than that of lateral nystagmus, and in the eighteenth and nineteenth centuries there was much debate about whether it occurred at all. Galen had described the oblique muscles that could produce eye rolling or ocular torsion, but evidence of its occurrence was to wait many centuries. The problem related to reconciling the anatomy of the eye muscles with the difficulty of observing small rotations of the eye around the optic axis. The early attempts to measure ocular torsion are described in Wade (2007a).

Eye movements during reading

Understanding the ways the eyes move when reading was derived from some of those who had examined eye torsion and binocular coordination, particularly Hermann Helmholtz and Ewald Hering in the second half of the nineteenth century. One of the great advantages that Helmholtz (1867) bestowed on eye movement research was the introduction of the bite bar for controlling head position. Hering devised an improved version of Helmholtz's bite bar and he was much more concerned with binocular than monocular eye movements (Hering, 1879a, 1942).

However, Hering's work on binocular eye movements seems to have diverted interest from his brief but insightful experiments on eye movements during reading (Hering, 1879b). He employed after-images to study eye movements, but in a radically different way from that applied by Mach (1875) and Breuer (1874) in the context of vertigo. Hering accepted that the movements between real images and afterimages reflected the movements of the eyes, and used this as a source of evidence to support a novel method of measurement. He used two rubber tubes, rather like a miniature stethoscope, placed on the eyelids to listen to the sounds of the ocular muscles. With this technique he observed: 'Throughout one's observations, one hears quite short, dull clapping sounds, which follow each other at irregular intervals' (Hering, 1879b, p. 145). He found that these 'clapping' sounds were evident when observers read lines of text but disappeared if they were instructed to fixate a stationary target. The sounds were attributed to contractions of the oculomotor muscles accompanying eye movements. Hering provided evidence for this conclusion by comparing the occurrences of clapping sounds with the movements of an afterimage: 'every clapping sound corresponds to a displacement of the afterimage' (Hering, 1879b, p. 145). Thus, Hering described the discontinuity of eye movements and recognized the class of rotations that we now refer to as saccadic. He was amongst the first to offer a description of the discontinuity of eye movements outside the context of vestibulo-ocular reflexes.

Hering's experiment is significant not only because he compared afterimage movement to the sounds of muscular movements, but also because he applied the technique to reading: 'One can observe the clapping sounds very clearly during reading. Although the eyes appear to glide steadily along the line, the clapping sounds disclose the jerky movement of the eyeball' (1879b, p. 146). Hering's report of his experiments was published in the same year as Louis-Émile Javal (1839–1909) gave a brief description of 'saccades' during reading. Javal is generally considered to have instigated research in eye movements during reading. Statements to this effect can be found in Huey (1908), Vernon (1931), and Woodworth (1938) and they have been repeated many times since (see Wade et al., 2003).

In fact, Javal said virtually nothing about eye movements in his eight essays on the physiology of reading (see Wade and Tatler, 2005, 2009), and saccades were only mentioned in passing in the final article. Moreover, he was not referring to his own work:

> Following the research of M. Lamare in our laboratory, the eye makes several saccades during the passage over each line, about one for every 15–18 letters of text. It is probable that in myopes the eye reacts with a rapid change in accommodation with every one of these saccades.
>
> (Javal, 1879, p. 252).

Javal tried, unsuccessfully, to attach a pointer to the eye so that eye movements could be recorded on a smoked drum. He also tried, with a similar lack of success, to measure the deflections of light from a mirror attached to the eye. Throughout, his concern was with distinguishing between horizontal and vertical eye movements. It was Lamare who observed and recorded the jerky or saccadic movements during reading in 1879. However, Lamare did not describe his experiments until 13 years later. He tried various methods, including observing the eyes of another person, but:

> The method that gives the best results is one by which the movements are heard via a drum with an ebonite membrane in the centre and to which a small tube is attached; the tube is in contact with the conjunctiva or eyelid and is connected to both ears by rubber tubes . . . The apparatus yields distinctive sounds which an assistant can count and add, and note for each line. The return movement of the eyes to the beginning of a line gives a longer and louder noise that is easy to recognise; one counts the number of *saccades* from the start of the line to be able to *note* the number of divisions that occur in a line.
>
> (Lamare, 1892, p. 357, original italics.)

Lamare's intricate technique for recording eye movements was clearly described by Javal's successor as director of the ophthalmological laboratory at the Sorbonne, Marius Hans Erik Tscherning: he did not mention Javal in the context of his brief description of saccadic eye movements in his *Optique physiologique* (1898); the book was translated into English 2 years later. He noted:

> The eyes are, therefore, in perpetual motion which is made by jerks: they fix a point, make a movement, fix another point, and so forth. While reading, the eyes move also by jerks, four or five for each line of an ordinary book. *Lamare* constructed a small instrument, formed by a point which is supported on the eye across the upper eyelid, and which is fastened to the ears of the observer by rubber tubes. With this instrument each movement of the eye causes a sound to be heard. We hear four or five sounds during the reading of one line, and a louder sound when we begin to read a new line.
>
> (Tscherning, 1900, p. 299.)

Hering (1879b) remarked that he had known about the muscle sounds for some years and the technique he employed was very similar to that described by Lamare 13 years later; they should both be accorded the credit for demonstrating the discontinuity of eye movements in reading. It is of interest to note that Tscherning's (1898) book in French used the word 'saccades' which was translated as 'jerks' in the English edition (Tscherning, 1900). As the nineteenth century ended and the twentieth began there was a proliferation of eye tracking technologies. Huey (1898, 1900) and Delabarre (1898) developed eye trackers that used a lever attached to an eye cup to record movements of the eyes on the surface of a smoked drum. Lever devices were limited by their mechanics; they applied additional force to the eye and their inertia resulted in considerable overshoots in the eye movement traces recorded (Fig. 2.2). Alternative devices were developed rapidly in which direct attachment between eye and recording surface was not required. Orschansky (1899) attempted to record light reflected from a mirror attached to the surface of an eye-cup and variants of this principle were used throughout the twentieth century. An alternative to recorded light reflected from an eye-cup, or other attachment on the surface of the eye, was to record light reflected directly from the surface of the eye itself. The key figure in the development of such devices was Dodge (Dodge, 1903, 1904; Dodge and Cline, 1901). Photographic devices that required no attachment on the eye were more comfortable for the participants and many of the modern eye trackers are based on this principle.

After Dodge's development of the photographic eye tracker there followed something of a revolution in eye movement research and a proliferation of new experiments in this field (see Taylor, 1937). Other researchers developed similar convenient and effective eye trackers and research extended beyond the domain of reading. Researchers began to consider whether the newly described saccade-and-fixate strategy applied to tasks other than reading, and it was soon realized that this was the case.

Dodge (1916) suggested that the term 'saccade' should be used by writers in English 'to denote the rapid eye movements for which we have only the arbitrary name of "type I". I am not sure with whom the term originated, but it seems worth adopting' (1916, pp. 422–423). Vestibular researchers in Britain had recognized the discontinuity of eye movements for some time, and Crum Brown (1878) both described and illustrated them (see Fig. 2.1). However, it was not until Crum Brown's (1895a, 1895b) general consideration of eye and head movements that writers in English used the term 'jerk' to describe these eye movements. Importantly, Crum Brown recognized that such discontinuous eye movements were not confined to post-rotational nystagmus, and despite what we might feel, our eyes always move by these jerks as we look around the world.

In psychological terms, saccades have generally been given less consideration than fixations. One area in which this did not apply was in the saccadic eye movements that occur periodically during sleep. Despite the fact that sleep was surveyed by one of the prominent figures in early eye movement research (Purkinje, 1846), the discovery of patterns of eye movements during different stages of sleep is relatively recent. Aserinsky and Kleitman (1953) reported that the eyes moved rapidly at certain periods during sleep. This could be observed directly by the movements of the eyes beneath the eyelids, but it could be recorded more precisely by electro-oculography and there were also correlated changes in the electroencephalogram. The related discovery that dreams were more likely to be

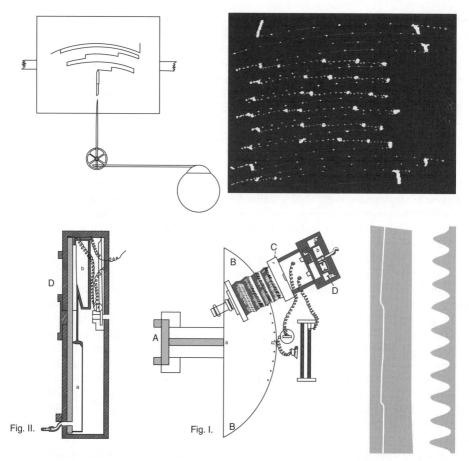

Fig. 2.2 Upper left, Huey's (1898) technique for recording eye movement during reading. A lever was attached to a plaster eye-cup and moved a pen over a rotating smoked drum. The initial records shown are for calibration across the lines, followed by jerks and pauses during reading. Upper right, a record of eye movements during reading using the lever device (from Huey, 1900). The tracing on the smoked drum was photographed and then engraved. 'The curve shows the movements of the eye in reading six lines, preceded and followed by two free movements of the eye each way, in which it was swept from one end of the line to the other, the beginning and end alone being fixated' (Huey, 1900, p. 290). Lower left, the photographic apparatus used by Dodge and Cline (1901) to record eye movements. Lower right, their first published trace of an eye movement (from Dodge and Cline, 1901).

reported when people were awoken during rapid eye movement (REM) sleep led to an explosion of research (see Jouvet, 2001). However, the interests were not directed to the eye movements themselves but rather to their application as an index of dreaming.

The early work by Dodge and his contemporaries was followed by a divergence in research focus. We have seen the path taken by those interested in fixations above, and that this has arguably dominated recent eye movement research. However, the research in the middle part of the twentieth century was dominated by an interest in saccades themselves, and in determining the physiological mechanisms involved in their control (Becker, 1991; Robinson, 1973, 1975) and in their abnormalities (Leigh and Zee, 2006). Applications of models to reading have been reviewed by Radach et al. (2007). These aspects of saccades are treated in detail elsewhere in the book.

Applications

The proliferation of eye tracking devices at the end of the nineteenth century went hand-in-hand with a rapid evolution of ideas about the link between fixations, saccades, perception, and cognition. An immediate application of the recognition of saccades and fixations was to consider how our apparently smooth and continuous visual experience could be reconciled with an eye movement strategy that was anything but smooth and continuous. Thus, some of the early interest in this newly recognized strategy centred on visual perception at the time of the saccade.

Interpreting eye movements

Prior to the widespread recognition of the saccade-and-fixate oculomotor strategy, it was widely believed that eye movements were continuous, with the eye making uninterrupted sweeps across the scene. Thus, both eye movements and visual perception were considered to be continuous, a notion that intuitively fitted the apparent continuity of visual experience. Javal expressed such sentiments, suggesting that in reading 'gaze glides along a line slightly higher than the centre of the characters' (Javal, 1878, p. 251). It is not surprising therefore that as reports of discontinuous eye movements in reading began to proliferate in the late nineteenth century, one of the earliest concerns in interpreting this work was to try to reconcile these reports with the widely held view that eye movements and perception were both continuous. It represents a similar contrast to that which was obtained for visual vertigo: the eyes did not feel as though they were undergoing fast and slow phases as this did not seem to correspond to the characteristics of perception.

Cattell (1900a) initially remained a firm proponent of the notion that the eyes moved in continuous sweeps, and went as far as dismissing the idea of saccades and fixations and finding alternative explanations for the new reports of saccades during reading. These views were based on the introspective experience of viewing a static grating while moving the eyes compared with viewing a moving grating while keeping the eyes still:

> When black and white surfaces are moved across the retina with the color wheel at the rate of fifty white stimuli per second, a gray is seen. When, however, the eye moves so that the line of sight passes over black and white surfaces at the same rate, there is no fusion whatever, the surfaces being seen distinctly side by side. No fusion occurs even when 1000 stimuli per second fall upon each retinal element.
>
> (Cattell, 1900a, p. 325.)

Not only did Cattell propose continuous perception during rapid rotations of the eyes, but also he clearly doubted the recent evidence for the saccade-and-fixate strategy, preferring the previous position that eye movements were indeed continuous. As is evident from the quotation above, Cattell was clearly confident of his reasoning with respect to viewing a grating:

> The only other possible explanation seems to be that the moving eye makes a series of jumps, seeing at each stop a distinct field, or that the distinctiveness of the field is an illusion, being really a memory image. But these suggestions are invalid. It can readily be observed that the eye does move continuously over the field.
>
> (Cattell, 1900a, p. 328.)

Of course the objective measurements of saccades in reading that were already being reported, did not fit neatly with Cattell's views and so he proposed an alternative interpretation of why saccades and fixations might be seen in reading:

> In reading a line of printed text the eyes do stop as they sweep over the page. This, however, is not because there is any blurring of the letters with the moving eyes, but owing to the limited amount that can be simultaneously perceived and the time it takes to perceive it.
>
> (Cattell, 1900a, pp. 328–329.)

In the same year as Cattell's clear arguments against the new measurements of saccades and fixations, Dodge presented an alternative exploration of the possibility of perception within eye movements. This paper built on earlier observations made during his time with Benno Erdmann in which they conducted experiments concerning vision during reading (Erdmann and Dodge, 1898). They had been using mirrors to observe subjects' eye movements whilst reading text. When looking into the mirrors themselves Erdmann and Dodge both found it impossible to see their own rapid eye movements. This simple observation cast serious doubt on the idea that perception continued during saccades. Critically, Dodge appreciated the errors and pitfalls of self-observation when describing eye movements and perception, in the same way that Wells had distrusted Porterfield's recourse to subjective experience over 100 years earlier. Consequently, Dodge employed the use of an assistant to observe his eye movements, or to be observed:

> It will be clear that when the eye moves as rapidly as possible from one fixation point to the other nothing new is seen; but it will seem that, when the eye moves more slowly, the entire line is seen very distinctly. If the observer takes the precaution to have some one watch his eyes, as recommended, he will find that what in self-observation passes for slow movements of the eyes is in reality broken by one or more clearly defined full stops.
>
> (Dodge, 1900, p. 457.)

In the light of Dodge's work, Cattell was forced to concede his position and this marked perhaps the first theoretical shift that arose from the measurement of eye movements:

> Professor Dodge finds that there is fusion when objects are exposed only when the eye is moving. It would follow from this that the hypothesis discussed in my paper, but there rejected, must be accepted or at least considered. That is, that there is clear vision only in the pauses of movement, there being no peripheral perceptions while the eye is moving and the apparent distinctiveness of the field of view being an illusion.
>
> (Cattell, 1900b, pp. 507–508.)

While it was this exchange in 1900 that can be seen to change the subsequent theoretical interpretation of eye movements, earlier researchers had expressed similar views about the suspension of perception during post-rotational vision (Wells, 1794b). For example, Crum Brown recognized both the pitfalls of introspection, and the lack of perception during fast ballistic phases of eye movement:

> We fancy that we can move our eyes uniformly, that by a continuous motion like that of a telescope we can move our eyes along the sky-line in the landscape or the cornice of a room, but we are wrong in this. However determinedly we try to do so, what actually happens is, that our eyes move like the seconds hand of a watch, a jerk and a little pause, another jerk and so on; only our eyes are not so regular, the jerks are sometimes of greater, sometimes of less, angular amount, and the pauses vary in duration, although, unless we make an effort, they are always short. During the jerks we practically do not see at all, so that we have before us not a moving panorama, but a series of fixed pictures of the same fixed things, which succeed one another rapidly.
>
> (Crum Brown, 1895, pp. 4–5.)

The early work concerned with voluntary eye movements, as in reading, did not take note of the previous research on eye movements in the context of visual vertigo. The existence of fast ballistic movements in which perception was suspended was stated with clarity and economy first by Wells, and later by Mach, Breuer, and Crum Brown. Rather, researchers at the end of the nineteenth century painstakingly rediscovered the manner in which the eyes moved. With this rediscovery came a proliferation of new avenues of research that would place saccades and fixations at the heart of many aspects of vision research and psychology to the present day. In this context, Dodge was not only a key figure in the interpretation of early work on eye movements, but he also pioneered new recording techniques that would form the basis of eye movement devices to the present day: he developed a method for photographically recording eye movements (Dodge and Cline, 1901; figure 2). Dodge's observations and studies of visual perception during and between eye movements have been of central importance in understanding visual processing of text. Eye movements can also allow insights into the neuropathology underlying disorders (Diefendorf and Dodge, 1908). Common to all areas of research in which eye movements are studied, crucial insights into their normal functions and implications can be gained from eye movement dysfunction (see Carpenter, 1991; Duke-Elder and Wybar, 1973; Leigh and Zee, 2006; von Noorden, 1996).

Following the theoretical shift to understanding that saccades and fixations were distinct perceptual events, a similar division of interest in the research that followed can be seen. Some researchers chose to focus on the mechanisms of the saccades themselves, whereas others placed primary importance on the fixations and the processes that occur within a fixation.

Fixations

Soon after the discovery of saccades and fixations during reading, both Stratton and Judd considered whether the places that the eyes were brought to rest might correlate with the perceptual experience of illusions. Stratton (1902) employed a photographic technique to examine eye movements when viewing simple geometrical patterns. This was an important new direction for eye movement research and served to highlight the importance of saccades outside the context of reading. Like Cattell, he was surprised by the discontinuity of eye movements recorded:

> The eye darts from point to point, interrupting its rapid motion by instants of rest. And the path by which the eye passes from one to another of these of these resting places does not seem to depend very nicely upon the exact form of the line observed.
>
> (Stratton, 1902, p. 343.)

Stratton's work is significant because it attempted to bridge the gap between visual phenomena (illusions), cognition (aesthetic judgements), and the underlying mechanisms (eye movements and fixations). Moreover, his studies signify a shift of emphasis in approaches to understanding the link between eye movement behaviour and perception. Where his predecessors had primarily considered perception with respect to the movements of the eyes, Stratton's work shows a transition from this approach to an emphasis upon the locations selected for fixation.

The transition is most evident in Stratton's (1906) article exploring the relationship between eye movements and perception when viewing simple patterns and line illusions. He placed emphasis not only on the movements of the eyes but on the locations at which the eyes paused for fixations:

> [O]ne is struck by the almost grotesque unlikeness between the outline observed and the action of the eye in observing it. For the most part the eye moves irregularly over the figure, seeking certain points of vantage from which the best view of important features may be obtained. And these positions are marked by the eye's momentary resting there.
>
> (Stratton, 1906, p. 94.)

Despite this shift of emphasis in the direction of fixations, Stratton was unable to reconcile viewing behaviour with the aesthetic experience:

> The sources of our enjoyment of symmetry, therefore, are not to be discovered in the form of the eye's behaviour. A figure which has for us a satisfying balance may be brought to the mind by most unbalanced ocular motions.
>
> (Stratton, 1906, p. 95.)

It is clear from Stratton's closing remarks in his article on eye movements and symmetry that he appreciated the gulf between perception and cognition and that he was aware that his work was defining new questions in vision that would be addressed in the future.

Charles Judd also worked on geometric illusions and was interested, like Stratton, in whether the experience of illusions correlated with the placement of fixations. Judd was impressed by the work of Dodge and Stratton, but felt that the eye trackers used by both were somewhat limited in the range of tasks to which they could be applied: Dodge's eye tracker was designed for recording movements only along a straight line (as occurs in reading) and Stratton's lacked temporal resolution and required a dark room in which the photographic plate was exposed during experimental recording. Judd developed a 'kinetoscopic' eye tracker in which a small fleck of Chinese white, which had been affixed to the cornea, was photographed; eye movements could thus be discerned in two dimensions, and did not require a dark room (Judd, et al., 1905). While Judd's eye tracker offered specific advantages over previous photographic devices, it was still somewhat limited in its temporal resolution, typically operating at about eight to nine frames per second (in comparison to Dodge's 100-Hz Photochronograph). One impressive feature of Judd's eye tracker was that it allowed binocular recordings to be taken.

Judd's interest in interpreting the results of the studies on illusions was in addressing the relationship between movement and perception (Judd, 1905). He sought to use his results to dismiss the notion that perceptions might arise directly from movements themselves. His alternative interpretation stressed the importance of visual information from the retina both in forming perceptions and in coordinating the movements:

> When the eye moves toward a point and the movement does not at first suffice to bring the point in question on the fovea, the retinal sensations which record the failure to reach the desired goal will be a much more powerful stimulus to new action than will any possible muscle sensation.
>
> (Judd, 1905, p. 218)

This again places emphasis on the locations fixated rather than on the saccades themselves. While much of Judd's discussion of his eye movement studies focused upon the discussion of their relation to theories of movement sensation, he did also notice that the pattern of fixations was likely to be influenced by the instructions given to the observers during the experiments. The recognition that fixation locations were not entirely selected by the stimulus being viewed echoed the opinion expressed by Stratton at the same time, but it was not investigated in any great depth by either Judd or Stratton.

It is the question of what drives the selection of particular locations upon which to fixate that was eventually to assume unrivalled prominence in both eye movement and attention research late in the twentieth century. Perhaps the key figure in the emergence of this area of research was Guy Buswell. While Buswell's (1937) research on reading is probably his most renowned work, it was from his study of eye movements when viewing pictures that one of his major contributions to eye movement research arises. The latter work was published in his impressive monograph *How people look at pictures* (Buswell, 1935). He reported eye movement data recorded from 200 participants each viewing multiple pictures, such that his data comprised almost 2000 eye movement records each containing a large number of fixations. This volume of eye movement data is impressive by modern standards, but particularly so given the technology at the time and the need to transform manually the horizontal and vertical position of the eye indicated in the eye movement records into precise locations on the pictures viewed. This work was the first to explore systematically eye movements of observers while viewing complex pictures, rather than text or simple geometrical patterns, and represented somewhat of a revolution in eye movement research. Using complex images and scenes has become a central aspect of modern eye movement research and is an important part of understanding eye movements in everyday vision. It is interesting to note that while Buswell's work is heralded as a key study in eye movement research, the character of the eye movements themselves was not the topic of much consideration: rather it was about the placement of the fixations between them.

Buswell's monograph explored a wide range of issues regarding the eye movements made while viewing pictures, including some surprisingly modern concerns: he looked at the overall distribution of fixations on pictures; he compared the first few fixations on a painting to the last few; he compared the durations of fixations made early in viewing to those made near the end of viewing; he looked at how fixation duration changed with viewing time; he compared the consistency between different observers when viewing the same picture; and he looked at the influence of instructions given to observers upon their eye movements when viewing a picture. Buswell made density plots of where all participants fixated when viewing pictures and showed that not all locations and objects in pictures are fixated, with particular 'centers of interest' where fixations are concentrated. He also appreciated that there could be quite large individual differences in where people fixate when viewing pictures.

The issue of individual differences in the patterns of fixations was explored in detail in a section at the end of the second chapter. The differences that were present in the locations fixated by individuals when viewing each image were also reflected in the durations of the fixations, with a large variation between observers in their average fixation duration on each picture. Buswell's investigation of individual differences extended to exploring differences between artistically trained individuals and those without training, between children and adults, and between Western and Oriental participants. In all cases, differences between the groups were small: 'The average differences between the groups were so much less than the individual differences within each group that the results cannot be considered significant' (Buswell, 1935, p. 131). Differences were found in the eye movement data that emerged over the course of viewing a picture for some time. The regions fixated in the picture were more consistent between observers for the first few fixations than for the last few on each picture. He also found that fixation duration increased over the course of viewing a picture for some time.

Buswell devoted a chapter of the book to looking at the influence of the characteristics of the picture upon where is fixated. This work is very reminiscent of that conducted some years earlier by Stratton although he did not cite Stratton's work. In places Buswell appeared to argue that eye movements do tend to follow contours in pictures. This is contrary to Stratton's suggestion that eye movements do not seem to be particularly influenced by the form of the figure being viewed. However, other aspects of Buswell's data suggested less concordance between eye movements and the characteristics of the picture. When he showed participants more basic designs and patterns he found that:

> The effect of different types of design in carrying the eye swiftly from one place to another is apparently much less than is assumed in the literature of art... The writer should emphasize that the data from eye movements are not to be considered as evidence either positively or negatively for any type of artistic interpretation.
>
> (Buswell, 1935, p. 115.)

Like Stratton, Buswell felt that the pattern of eye movements was insufficient to explain our visual experience and so highlighted the need to appeal to cognitive explanations of vision.

Perhaps the most often overlooked aspect of Buswell's work was his investigation of how different instructions given to observers prior to viewing an image can influence the locations selected for fixation during viewing. For example, when presented with a picture of the Tribune Tower in Chicago, eye movements were first recorded while the participant viewed the picture 'without any special directions being given. After that record was secured, the subject was told to look at the picture again to see if he could find a person looking out of one of the windows of the tower' (Buswell, 1935, p. 136). Very different eye movement records were obtained in these two situations, demonstrating that cognitive factors such as the viewer's task can have a strong effect upon how a picture is inspected. Such descriptions of influences played by high level factors upon eye movements are not typically associated with Buswell, but rather it is Yarbus (1967) who is generally regarded to be the first to have offered such an observation.

Not only was Buswell's work significant in the topics that it addressed and issues it raised, but it also demonstrated that more realistic scenes could provide a wealth of insights into eye movement behaviour. Subsequently, eye movement research has diverged somewhat into two rather different approaches: one places emphasis upon experimental control and elegant simplicity in eye movement paradigms (for an excellent review of much of this work see Findlay and Gilchrist, 2003); the other places emphasis upon the realism of scene stimuli and ecological validity of experimentation (e.g. Land and Tatler, 2009). It is upon this latter direction in research that we will concentrate in the remainder of this chapter. In this respect, recent reviews have emphasized the importance of using photographs of real scenes (Henderson, 2003), or real-world environments themselves (Hayhoe and Ballard, 2005; Land and Tatler, 2009) to understand oculomotor behaviour. This move toward ever more realistic stimuli is mirrored in work both on the factors that underlie fixation placement and in studies of visual memory across saccades.

The question of the factors underlying fixation placement was revived by Alfred Yarbus in his work during the 1950s and 1960s, translated into English in 1967 (Tatler et al., 2010). Within this work, Yarbus conducted an experiment where a single observer was shown the same painting (Repin's *An Unexpected Visitor*) seven times, but with a different question asked before each viewing (Fig. 2.3). This elegant experiment confirmed Buswell's earlier observation that the instructions given to an observer can radically change the places that the observer fixates. Yarbus's demonstration has become a classic in eye movement research and is frequently cited as an unequivocal demonstration that high-level factors can over-shadow any low-level, stimulus-driven guidance of attention.

It is interesting that despite the seminal works of Buswell and Yarbus, which both demonstrated the importance of high-level factors in selecting where to fixate, investigation of eye movements when viewing images of complex scenes was dominated by the notion of low-level attentional guidance in the late twentieth century. After findings in psychophysics and visual search experiments demonstrated that simple visual features such as orientation, colour, and luminance contrast can automatically capture attention, it was perhaps natural to assume that this principle could be extended to more complex scenes. Koch and colleagues proposed a model of complex scene viewing based upon low-level feature guidance (Itti and Koch, 2000; Itti et al., 1998; Koch and Ullman, 1985). This model has had a profound influence on recent studies, with a large literature devoted to evaluating it. Apparent support for this model was drawn from consistent and robust statistical differences between the low-level feature content at locations selected for fixation and at control locations (e.g. Mannan et al., 1997; Parkhurst et al., 2002; Reinagel and Zador, 1999). However, more recent research has tended to criticize the basic tenet of the model, finding that while significant, the magnitude of the differences in feature content between fixation and control locations is small (e.g. Einhäuser et al., 2008a; Nyström and Holmqvist, 2008; Tatler et al., 2005a); and disappears both for larger amplitude saccades (Tatler et al., 2006), and when cognitive tasks, like those employed by Buswell and Yarbus, are given to the observer (e.g. Einhäuser et al., 2008b; Foulsham and Underwood, 2008; Henderson et al., 2007). It has recently been suggested that not only is the association between features and fixation weak, but may be an artefact of a natural tendency for humans to fixate near the centre of the screen of a computer monitor, coupled with a tendency for photographers to place objects of interest, which are often visually conspicuous, at the centre of the image (Tatler, 2007). Thus over 70 years after Buswell eloquently observed it, consensus has returned to favouring top-down interpretations in explaining how people look at pictures.

After an early flurry of interest in the consequences of saccades upon our perceptual experience of seeing by researchers such as Cattell, Dodge, and Stratton, this question assumed a less prominent position in eye movement research for some time. During the 1970s interest was revived both within and outside the context of reading. Using the newly-developed method of changing stimuli in a manner that is time-locked to the occurrence of saccades (McConkie and Rayner, 1975) the question of how information from each fixation is 'stitched' together by the brain to give rise to a coherent visual experience could be studied with greater precision. This gaze-contingent-display-change technique has had a profound impact on eye movement research. Initially, it was assumed that the retinal images from successive fixations must be fused to create a complete and coherent representation, and McConkie and Rayner (1976) described an 'integrative visual buffer' that served this purpose. However, gaze-contingent experiments by other authors were used to question this assumption (e.g. McConkie and Zola, 1979; O'Regan and Lévy-Schoen, 1983). When Grimes (1996) showed that large changes made to complex images would often go unnoticed if timed to coincide with a saccade, opinion in the area changed profoundly, rejecting the notion of transsaccadic integration in favour of sparse representation (Rensink, 2000), or, in extreme cases, suggesting that visual representations were never constructed (O'Regan and Noe, 2001). Subsequent transsaccadic integration work relating the number or duration of fixations on objects to what is recalled about those objects

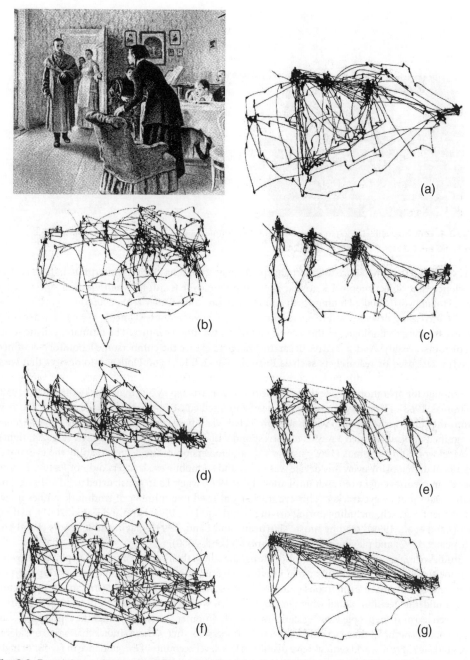

Fig. 2.3 Examining a picture with different questions in mind (*An Unexpected Visitor* by Repin). Each record lasts 3 minutes. a) Free examination. b) Estimate the material circumstances of the family in the picture. c) Give the ages of the people. d) Surmise what the family had been doing before the arrival of the 'unexpected visitor'. e) Remember the clothes worn by the people. f) Remember the position of the people and objects in the room. g) Estimate how long the 'unexpected visitor' had been away from the family. Reprinted from: Springer and Plenum Press, *Eye movements and vision* (trans. B. Haigh), 1967, Yarbus, A.L., with kind permission from Springer Science+Business Media B.V.

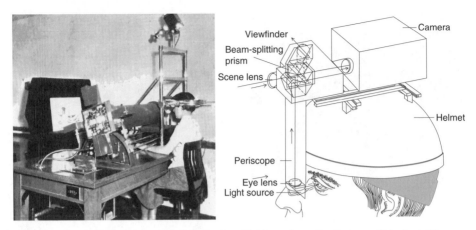

Fig. 2.4 Left: Buswell's bench-mounted eye tracker. Right: a schematic diagram of Mackworth's portable eye tracker.

has suggested that the failure to detect abrupt changes should not be over-interpreted: there is clear evidence that object memories appear to accumulate over fixations when viewing static scenes (e.g. Hollingworth, 2006; Hollingworth and Henderson, 2002; Tatler et al., 2005b).

The increasing drive toward realistic stimuli in eye movement experiments placed new demands on eye tracking technologies in the second half of the twentieth century. The ultimate realistic scene is, of course, reality! And so a drive began to emerge to evolve the cumbersome laboratory-confined eye trackers used by researchers such as Buswell (Fig. 2.4, left) and Dodge, into devices that were portable enough to use during less constrained behaviour. The first such eye tracker that was portable enough for operation outside the laboratory was constructed by Norman Mackworth in the 1950s (Thomas, 1968). His device consisted of a head-mounted ciné camera which made a film of the view from the subject's head, onto which was projected, via a periscope, an image of the corneal reflex magnified optically in such a way as to correspond with the direction the visual axis (Fig. 2.4, right).

Mackworth and Thomas (1962) used a TV camera version of the device to study the eye movements of drivers. However, this device was bulky and so mobile eye trackers did not feature prominently in eye movement research until after about 1990, when Land constructed a video-based and lightweight mobile eye tracker. This eye tracker was used in a number of landmark studies in eye movement research, including during driving (Land and Lee, 1994; Land and Tatler, 2001), making tea (Land et al., 1999), reading music (Furneaux and Land, 1999), playing table tennis (Land and Furneaux, 1997) and playing cricket (Land and McLeod, 2000).

Studies of eye movements in real-world settings are still in their relative infancy. Despite the growing call for studying eye movements when viewing real scenes, it is photographic images displayed on computer screens that are often considered 'real scenes'. Most of what we have learnt about what factors might underlie decisions about where to fixate or what we might remember from fixation to fixation has been learnt from people viewing static images on computer screens. Whether these principles scale up to our operation in the real world has yet to be understood fully. Those studies that have considered eye guidance in real-world settings have dismissed low-level accounts of eye guidance in favour of high-level task-based explanations (e.g. Pelz and Canosa, 2001; Rothkopf et al., 2007; Sprague et al., 2007). Similarly, what we remember during complex tasks seems sparser than recent studies of static scene viewing have suggested (see Hayhoe, 2008). It is interesting to note that the two questions that dominated early eye movement research—the perceptual consequences of saccades and fixations, and what factors underlie fixation placement—continue to play a prominent role in contemporary studies.

Involuntary eye movements during fixation

While much of the research effort since Dodge can be categorized as primarily focusing on fixations or on saccades, a third and less consistent area of interest has been in the importance of miniature movements within fixations. It has long been recognized that even when apparently fixating stably, the eye is rarely truly still. For example, Mariotte stated that 'the *Eyes* are always in motion, and very hard to be fixt in one place, though it be desired' (1683, p. 266) and Darwin (1786) amplified this with regard to forming afterimages:

> When we look long and attentively at any object, the eye cannot always be kept entirely motionless; hence, on inspecting a circular area of red silk placed on white paper, a lucid crescent or edge is seen to librate on one side or the other of the red circle.
>
> (p. 341.)

Indeed instability seems important for ongoing perception: Troxler (1804) showed perceptual fading during fixations. While Troxler's observations have become associated almost exclusively with peripheral fading, he also reported central fading after prolonged fixation and with binocular vision (Brewster, 1818).

Given the popular metaphor of the eye as a camera, adopted since the time of Kepler (see Wade, 2007c; Wade and Finger, 2001), the notion that fixations were not stable and that this instability was necessary to avoid perceptual fading, seemed to present problems. The eye-camera analogy made an unstable detecting device (the eye) an oddity, and suggested that it would interfere with visual resolution. Would not acuity be better if the eye was stationary? Jurin (1738) suggested that differences in measured visual resolution with different stimuli could be a consequence of 'instability of the eye', but it remained difficult to measure minor movements. This puzzle was revitalized in the 1950s when technology had advanced sufficiently to measure the miniature eye movements that occur within fixations. Importantly, technological advances allowed not only the measurement of these miniature movements, but also the presentation of stimuli that were stabilized with respect to these movements. Three research groups were very active in the development of this area: Ditchburn and Ginsborg at Reading University, Riggs and Ratliff at Brown University, and Barlow at Cambridge University.

Ratliff and Riggs (1950) employed an optical lever system and photography to record the involuntary motions of the eye during fixation. They found small rapid motions of about 17.5 s of arc at 30–70 Hz, slow motions of irregular frequency and extent, slow drifts and rapid jerks. Barlow (1952) placed a droplet of mercury on the cornea and photographed the eye during motion and fixation; the instabilities during fixation were small but measurable. He confirmed his photographic measurements by comparing them with afterimages. At about the same time, Ratliff specifically investigated the effects of the instabilities on visual acuity:

> Involuntary drifts of the visual axis during the presentation of the test object are clearly detrimental to monocular acuity. Relatively large amounts of the minute rapid tremor during presentation of the test object are a hindrance to monocular acuity. These findings are compatible with the assumption that acuity, as measured by a typical grating test object, depends upon simultaneous differential responses of adjacent receptors. They are not in agreement with the assumption that the small involuntary eye movements contribute to visual acuity by providing temporal variations in the stimulation of each receptor as it is exposed to various parts of the retinal image.
>
> (Ratliff, 1952, p. 171.)

Two of the initial systems employed to stabilize images on the retina are shown in Fig. 2.5 (upper left and right). Both used contact lenses on the eye with small mirrors attached to them from which images could be reflected. Broadly similar results were reported by both groups. Ditchburn and Ginsborg (1952) used a disc subtending 1° separated into halves vertically. Luminance differences between the two parts were visible initially but disappeared after 2 or 3 s; the diffuse disc remained visible with occasional reappearances of the bipartite disc. Riggs and colleagues (1953) conducted more systematic experiments with line stimuli in a circular annulus; they found that the line faded and then disappeared all together. They also examined the effects of the involuntary eye movements on visual acuity. With very brief presentations (less than 0.1 s) acuity was superior with a stabilized image.

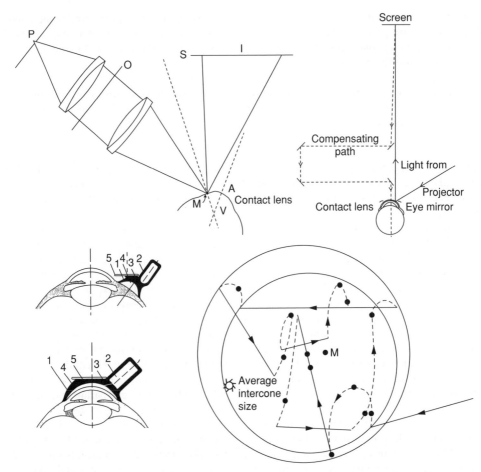

Fig. 2.5 Upper left, the optical system employed by Ditchburn and Ginsborg (1952) for stabilizing an image on the retina. Upper right, that used by Riggs et al. (1953). Lower left, two of the rubber eye cups designed and used by Yarbus (1967) to record eye movements. Reprinted from: Springer and Plenum Press, *Eye movements and vision* (trans. B. Haigh), 1967, Yarbus, A.L., with kind permission from Springer Science+Business Media B.V. Lower right, involuntary eye movements during fixation; the high-frequency tremor is superimposed on the slow drifts (dashed lines), with intermittent microsaccades. Reproduced from Dichtburn, R.W., *Eye-Movements and visual perception*, 1973, with permission from Oxford University Press.

Their succinct conclusion was 'that eye movements are bad for acuity but good for overcoming the loss of vision due to uniform stimulation of the retinal receptors' (Riggs et al., 1953, p. 501).

Yarbus developed a fuller-fitting contact lens which retained its position by suction (see Fig. 2.5, lower left); the studies were published in Russian from the mid-1950s, and are summarized in Yarbus (1967). With his optical system he found that 'in any test field, unchanging and stationary with respect to the retina, all visible differences disappear after 1-3 sec, and do not reappear in these conditions' (Yarbus, 1967, p. 59). The source of the differences between the various studies was examined by Barlow (1963). He used a full fitting contact and a suction cap after the manner of Yarbus in order to compare their possible slippage; an afterimage was used as a perfectly stabilized target. The suction cap was more stable than the full-fitting contact lens, but neither was free from some slippage. His conclusion was that 'Good-quality images stabilized as well as possible . . . "blur" and lose contrast rapidly: detail and texture cease to be visible, and do not reappear' (Barlow, 1963, p. 50).

Higgins and Stultz (1953) examined the minute involuntary tremor motions of the eye by photographing a blood vessel in the sclera: the tremors occurred with a frequency of 50 Hz and an average amplitude of 1.2 min of arc. Rapid technical advances were made thereafter (see Ditchburn, 1973), and attention was directed to the pattern characteristics of disappearances (see Pritchard, 1958, 1961). They resulted in a more accurate understanding of the involuntary eye movements, which have three components: high-frequency tremor, slow drifts, and micro-saccades (see Fig. 2.5, lower right).

Miniature movements during saccades did not feature prominently in research toward the end of the twentieth century, and Kowler and Steinman (1980) argued that they did not serve a useful purpose for vision. However, over the last few years interest in microsaccades has been rekindled (see Engbert, 2006). One interesting recent interpretation of microsaccades is as an indicator of covert attention (Engbert and Kliegl, 2003; Laubrock et al., 2005). In simple attentional cuing tasks, microsaccade direction appears to indicate the cued direction, particularly for exogenous cues. It would appear that microsaccades are now assuming an increasingly prominent role in studies of visual perception (Collewijn and Kowler, 2008; Martinez-Conde, 2006).

Conclusion

Several paradoxes are posed by investigations of eye movements when considered in an historical context. They are a fundamental feature of our exploration of the world. We are aware that our own eyes move and we can readily detect movements in the eyes of those we observe. This awareness was, however, partial. Throughout the long descriptive history of studies of eye movements a vital characteristic of them remained hidden from view, both in ourselves and in our observations of others. The rapid discontinuous nature of eye movements is a relatively recent discovery, as are the small involuntary movements that accompany fixation. For most of recorded history, the eyes were thought to glide over scenes to alight on objects of interest, which they would fix with unmoved accuracy.

Another paradox is that initial knowledge about eye movements derived from generating stimuli that did not move with respect to the eye when the eye moved. The first of these was the afterimage which, since the late eighteenth century, has been applied to determining the ways the eyes moved. More complex photographic recording devices appeared a century later, and the assistance of computers was incorporated three-quarters of a century later still. Nonetheless, the insights derived from the skilful use of afterimages have tended to be overlooked in the histories of eye movements. One of the reasons that less attention has been paid to studies using afterimages is that they became tainted with other 'subjective' measures of eye movements as opposed to the 'objective' recording methods of the twentieth century. A second factor was that the early studies were concerned with vertigo, which resulted in involuntary movements of the eyes. Moreover, histories of vertigo have been similarly blind to the early studies of it employing afterimages.

These points apply particularly to the experiments conducted by Wells (1792, 1794a, 1794b), both in the context of voluntary and involuntary eye movements. In the case of voluntary eye movements, Wells demonstrated that afterimages appeared to move with active eye movements whereas they appeared stationary when the eye was moved passively (by finger pressure). This procedure of comparing the consequences of passive eye movements on the apparent motion of real images and afterimages became one of the critical tests of afference versus efference, of inflow versus outflow. That is, whether the signals for compensating for the retinal consequences of an eye movement originated in the ocular musculature or in the signals sent to contract them. Thus, the essential aspects of visual stability during eye movements were examined using afterimages, and the procedure was repeated throughout the nineteenth century. There was nothing novel about afterimages themselves at that time. Wells produced them by the time-honoured technique of viewing a bright stimulus (like a candle flame) for many seconds; the afterimage remained visible for long enough for him to examine its apparent movement under a range of conditions. One of these was vertigo generated by rotating the body around a vertical axis.

Wells's work was forgotten, but the techniques he pioneered were rediscovered by those scientists puzzling over the mechanisms of vestibular function. Mach, Breuer, and Crum Brown all employed

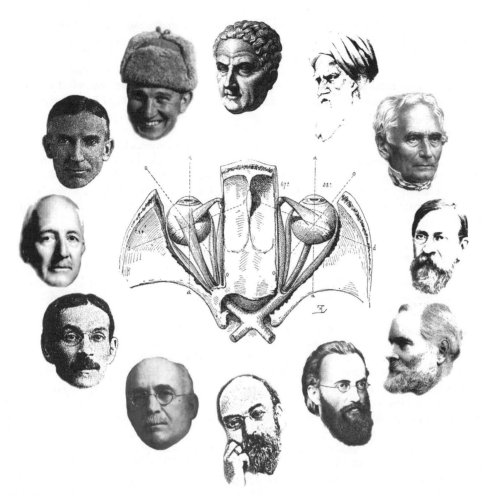

Fig. 2.6 *Rotation of eye movement researchers* by Nicholas Wade and Benjamin Tatler. The portraits (clockwise from the top) are of Galen, Ibn al-Haytham, Purkinje, Mach, Crum Brown, Hering, Javal, Dodge, Huey, Stratton, Buswell and Yarbus. It is to be noted that we have been unable to locate portraits of Porterfield and Wells, who should also be included in this array of luminaries. The central diagram of the eye and its musculature is from Landolt, published in 1879, the year in which Hering described the discontinuous movements of the eyes during reading.

afterimages to measure the movements of the eyes after body rotation. They were able to link vertigo with their hydrodynamic theory of semicircular canal activity. Crum Brown forged the link between eye movements during vertigo and normal scanning of scenes; again afterimages were the tool used to demonstrate how scanning proceeds via a sequence of rapid movements interspersed with brief stationary pauses.

Afterimages had been enlisted to attempt to examine eye movements during reading by Javal but the contrast between the printed letters and paper made the afterimage difficult to discern. Novel methods were required and he was instrumental in trying some, but with little success. Javal's student, Lamare (1892), developed an indirect method that was more successful and yielded interesting and unexpected results. Lamare's technique was to use a tube placed over the eyelid, from which sounds could be heard by the observer whenever the eyes moved. Using this technique, Lamare observed that, contrary to expectation and introspection, eye movements during reading were discontinuous. A very similar acoustic technique had been employed by Hering (1879b) to observe eye movements. However, Hering's technique had the added advantage of comparing the sounds thought to arise from eye movements to the movement of afterimages. Thus, Hering was able to confirm that the sounds coincided with movements of the afterimage and were therefore likely to be associated with eye movements. Some pioneers of eye movement research are represented in Fig. 2.6. Unfortunately, three of the significant figures mentioned above (Porterfield, Wells, and Lamare) are not shown because we have been unable to find portraits of them; perhaps none were made.

The objective eye trackers developed in the late nineteenth and early twentieth centuries allowed crucial new insights into the true nature of eye movements (see Venezky, 1977). Researchers were unanimously surprised by what they found; eye movements were not as smooth and continuous as they subjectively appeared. With these new devices for measuring eye movements so began a proliferation of interest in their nature. The technological advancements allowed new questions to be addressed and indeed identified new and unexpected questions in the psychology and physiology of eye movements and their relation to cognition and visual experience. Eye tracking technology continues to evolve, and with it so do the range of questions that can be addressed. Increasingly, the eyes are measured when inspecting objects in three-dimensional space and it is probable that these applications will have the most profound influence on our understanding of this most integrated aspect of active vision (see Findlay and Gilchrist, 2003; Land and Tatler, 2009; Tatler, 2009).

References

Aserinsky, E. and Kleitman, N. (1953). Regularly occurring periods of eye motility, and concomitant phenomena, during sleep. *Science*, 118, 273–274.

Bárány, R. (1906). Untersuchungen über den vom Vestibularapparat des Ohres reflektorisch ausgelösten rhythmischen Nystagmus und seine Begleiterscheinungen. *Monatsschrift für Ohrenheilkunde*, 40, 193–297.

Bárány, R. (1913). Der Schwindel und seine Beziehungen zum Bogengangapparat des inneren Ohres. Bogengangapparat und Kleinhirn. (Historische Darstellung. Eigene Untersuchungen.) *Naturwissenschaften*, 1, 396–401.

Barlow, H.B. (1952). Eye movements during fixation. *Journal of Physiology*, 116, 290–306.

Barlow, H.B. (1963). Slippage of contact lenses and other artefacts in relation to fading and regeneration of supposedly stable retinal images. *Quarterly Journal of Experimental Psychology*, 15, 36–51.

Bartisch, G. (1583). *ΟΦΘΑΛΜΟΔΟΥΛΕΙΑ. Das ist, Augendienst*. Dresden: Stockel.

Becker, W. (1991). Saccades. In R.H.S. Carpenter (ed.) *Vision and visual dysfunction. Vol. 8. Eye movements* (pp. 95–137). London: Macmillan.

Breuer, J. (1874). Über die Function der Bogengänge des Ohrlabyrinthes. *Wiener medizinisches Jahrbuch*, 4, 72–124.

Brewster, D. (1818). On a singular affection of the eye in the healthy state, in consequence of which it loses the power of seeing objects within the sphere of distinct vision. *Annals of Philosophy*, 11, 151.

Bryan, C.P. (1930). *The Papyrus Ebers*. London: Geoffrey Bles.

Buswell, G.T. (1935). *How people look at pictures: a study of the psychology of perception in art*. Chicago, IL: University of Chicago Press.

Buswell, G.T. (1937). *How adults read*. Chicago, IL: University of Chicago Press.

Carpenter, R.H.S. (ed.) (1991). *Vision and visual dysfunction. Vol. 8. Eye movements*. London: Macmillan.

Cattell, J.M. (1900a). On relations of time and space in vision. *Psychological Review*, 7, 325–343.

Cattell, J.M. (1900b). Vision with the moving eye. *Psychological Review*, 7, 507–508.

Collewijn, H. and Kowler, E. (2008). The significance of microsaccades for vision and oculomotor control. *Journal of Vision*, 8, 1–21.

Crum Brown, A. (1878). Cyon's researches on the ear. II. *Nature*, 18, 657–659.

Crum Brown, A. (1895a). The relation between the movements of the eyes and the movements of the head. *Nature*, 52, 184–188.

Crum Brown, A. (1895b). *The relation between the movements of the eyes and the movements of the head*. London: Henry Frowde.

Darwin, E. (1778). A new case in squinting. *Philosophical Transactions of the Royal Society*, 68, 86–96.

Darwin, R.W. (1786). New experiments on the ocular spectra of light and colours. *Philosophical Transactions of the Royal Society*, 76, 313–348.

Delabarre, E.B. (1898). A method of recording eye movements. *American Journal of Psychology*, 9, 572–574

Diefendorf, A.R. and Dodge, R. (1908). An experimental study of the ocular reactions of the insane from photographic records. *Brain*, 31, 451–489.

Ditchburn, R.W. (1973). *Eye-movements and visual perception*. Oxford: Clarendon Press.

Ditchburn, R.W. and Ginsborg, B.L. (1952). Vision with a stabilized retinal image. *Nature*, 170, 36–37.

Dodge, R. (1900). Visual perception during eye movement. *Psychological Review*, 7, 454–465.

Dodge, R. (1903). Five types of eye movement in the horizontal meridian plane of the field of regard. *American Journal of Physiology*, 8, 307–329.

Dodge, R. (1904). The participation of eye movements and the visual perception of motion. *Psychological Review*, **11**, 1–14.

Dodge, R. (1916). Visual motor functions. *Psychological Bulletin*, **13**, 421–427.

Dodge, R. (1921). A mirror-recorder for photographing the compensatory movements of the closed eyes. *Journal of Experimental Psychology*, **4**, 165–174.

Dodge, R. (1923). Habituation to rotation. *Journal of Experimental Psychology*, **6**, 1–35.

Dodge, R. (1930). Raymond Dodge. In C. Murchison (ed.) *A history of psychology in autobiography*, Vol. 1 (pp. 99–121). Worcester, MA: Clark University Press.

Dodge, R. and Cline, T.S. (1901). The angle velocity of eye movements. *Psychological Review*, **8**, 145–157.

Duke-Elder, S. and Wybar, K. (1973). *System of ophthalmology. Vol. 6. Ocular motility and strabismus*. London: Kimpton.

Einhauser, W., Spain, M., and Perona, P. (2008a). Objects predict fixations better than early saliency. *Journal of Vision*, **8(14)**, 18: 11–26.

Einhauser, W., Rutishauser, U., and Koch, C. (2008b). Task-demands can immediately reverse the effects of sensory-driven saliency in complex visual stimuli. *Journal of Vision*, **8**(2), 2: 1–19.

Engbert, R. (2006). Microsaccades: a microcosm for research on oculomotor control, attention, and visual perception. *Visual Perception, Part 1, Fundamentals of Vision: Low and Mid-Level Processes in Perception*, **154**, 177–192.

Engbert, R. and Kliegl, R. (2003). Microsaccades uncover the orientation of covert attention. *Vision Research*, **43**(9), 1035–1045.

Erdmann, B. and Dodge, R. (1898). *Psychologische Untersuchungen über das Lesen auf experimenteller Grundlage*. Halle: Niemeyer.

Findlay, J.M. and Gilchrist, I.D. (2003). *Active vision: the psychology of looking and seeing*. Oxford: Oxford University Press.

Foulsham, T. and Underwood, G. (2008). What can saliency models predict about eye movements? Spatial and sequential aspects of fixations during encoding and recognition. *Journal of Vision*, **8**(2), 6: 1–17.

Furneaux, S. and Land, M.F. (1999). The effects of skill on the eye-hand span during musical sight- reading. *Proceedings of the Royal Society of London Series B-Biological Sciences*, **266**(1436), 2435–2440.

Griffith, C.R. (1920). The organic effects of repeated bodily rotation. *Journal of experimental Psychology*, **3**, 15–47.

Grimes, J. (1996). On the failure to detect changes in scenes across saccades. In K. Atkins (ed.) *Perception: Vancouver studies in cognitive science*, Vol. 2 (pp. 89–110). New York: Oxford University Press.

Hayhoe, M.M. (2008). Visual memory in motor planning and action. In J.R. Brockmole (ed.) *The visual world in memory* (pp. 117–139). Hove: Psychology Press.

Hayhoe, M. and Ballard, D.H. (2005). Eye movements in natural behavior. *Trends in Cognitive Sciences*, **9**, 188–193.

Helmholtz, H. (1867). *Handbuch der physiologischen Optik. In Allgemeine Encyklopädie der Physik*. Vol. 9. (ed. G. Karsten). Leipzig: Voss.

Henderson, J.M. (2003). Human gaze control in real-world scene perception. *Trends in Cognitive Sciences*, **7**, 498–504.

Henderson, J.M., Brockmole, J.R., Castelhano, M.S., and Mack, M.L. (2007). Visual saliency does not account for eye movements during search in real-world scenes. In R.P.G. van Gompel, M.H. Fischer, W.S. Murray and R.L. Hill (eds.) *Eye movements: A window on mind and brain* (pp. 537–562). Oxford: Elsevier.

Hering, E. (1879a). Der Raumsinn und die Bewegungen des Auges. In L. Hermann (ed.) *Handbuch der Physiologie*, Vol. 3, Part 1 *Physiologie des Gesichtssinnes* (pp. 343–601). Leipzig: Vogel.

Hering, E. (1879b). Über Muskelgeräusche des Auges. *Sitzberichte der kaiserlichen Akademie der Wissenschaften in Wien. Mathematisch-naturwissenschaftliche Klasse*, **79**, 137–154.

Hering, E. (1942). *Spatial sense and movements of the eye* (trans. C.A. Radde). Baltimore, MD: The American Academy of Optometry.

Higgins, G.C. and Stultz, K.F. (1953). Frequency and amplitude of ocular tremor. *Journal of the Optical Society of America*, **43**, 1136–1140.

Hirschberg, J. (1899). Geschichte der Augenheilkunde. In A.C. Graefe and T. Saemisch (eds.) *Handbuch der gesamten Augenheilkunde*, Vol. 12. Leipzig: Engelmann.

Hitzig, E. (1871). Ueber die beim Galvanisiren des Kopfes entstehenden Störungen der Muskelinnervation und der Vorstellung vom Verhalten im Raume. *Archiv für Anatomie, Physiologie und wissenschaftliche Medicin*, 716–771.

Hollingworth, A. (2006). Scene and position specificity in visual memory for objects. *Journal of Experimental Psychology-Learning Memory and Cognition*, **32**, 58–69.

Hollingworth, A. and Henderson, J.M. (2002). Accurate visual memory for previously attended objects in natural scenes. *Journal of Experimental Psychology-Human Perception and Performance*, **28**, 113–136.

Howard, I.P. (2002). *Seeing in depth. Vol. 1. Basic mechanisms*. Toronto: Porteous.

Huey, E.B. (1898). Preliminary experiments in the physiology and psychology of reading. *American Journal of Psychology*, **9**, 575–586.

Huey, E.B. (1900). On the psychology and physiology of reading. I. *American Journal of Psychology*, **11**, 283–302.

Huey, E.B. (1908). *The psychology and pedagogy of reading*. New York: Macmillan.

Itti, L. and Koch, C. (2000). A saliency-based search mechanism for overt and covert shifts of visual attention. *Vision Research*, **40**, 1489–1506.

Itti, L., Koch, C., and Niebur, E. (1998). A model of saliency-based visual attention for rapid scene analysis. *IEEE Transactions on Pattern Analysis and Machine Intelligence*, **20**, 1254–1259.

Javal, L.É. (1878). Essai sur la physiologie de la lecture. *Annales d'Oculistique*, **80**,240–274.

Javal, L.É. (1879). Essai sur la physiologie de la lecture. *Annales d'Oculistique*, **82**, 242–253.

Jouvet, M. (2001). *The paradox of sleep: the story of dreaming* (trans. L. Garey). Cambridge, MA: MIT Press.

Judd, C.H. (1905). Movement and consciousness. *Psychological Monographs*, **7**, 199–226.

Judd, C.H., McAllister, C.N., and Steele, W.M. (1905). General introduction to a series of studies of eye movements by means of kinetoscopic photographs. *Psychological Monographs*, **7**, 1–16.

Jurin, J. (1738). An essay on distinct and indistinct vision. In R. Smith (ed.) *A compleat system of opticks in four books*. (pp. 115–171). Cambridge: Published by the author.

Koch, C. and Ullman, S. (1985). Shifts in selective visual-attention - towards the underlying neural circuitry. *Human Neurobiology*, **4**, 219–227.

Kowler, E. and Steinman, R.M. (1980). Small saccades serve no useful purpose – reply. *Vision Research*, **20**, 273–276.

Lamare, M. (1892). Des mouvements des yeux dans la lecture. *Bulletins et Mémoires de la Société Française d'Ophthalmologie*, **10**, 354–364.

Land, M.F. and Furneaux, S. (1997). The knowledge base of the oculomotor system. *Philosophical Transactions of the Royal Society of London Series B-Biological Sciences*, **352**, 1231–1239.

Land, M.F. and Lee, D.N. (1994). Where we look when we steer. *Nature*, **369**, 742–744.

Land, M.F. and McLeod, P. (2000). From eye movements to actions: how batsmen hit the ball. *Nature Neuroscience*, **3**, 1340–1345.

Land, M.F. and Tatler, B.W. (2001). Steering with the head: The visual strategy of a racing driver. *Current Biology*, **11**, 1215–1220.

Land, M.F. and Tatler, B.W. (2009). *Looking and acting: vision and eye movements in natural behaviour*. Oxford: Oxford University Press.

Land, M.F., Mennie, N., and Rusted, J. (1999). The roles of vision and eye movements in the control of activities of daily living. *Perception*, **28**, 1311–1328.

Laubrock, J., Engbert, R., and Kliegl, R. (2005). Microsaccade dynamics during covert attention. *Vision Research*, **45**, 721–730.

Leigh, R.J. and Zee, D.S. (2006). *The neurology of eye movements* (4th edn). New York: Oxford University Press.

Mach, E. (1873). Physikalische Versuche über den Gleichgewichtssinn des Menschen. *Sitzungsberichte der Wiener Akademie der Wissenschaften*, **68**, 124–140.

Mach, E. (1875). *Grundlinien der Lehre von den Bewegungsempfindungen*. Leipzig: Engelmann.

Mackworth, N.H. and Thomas, E.L. (1962). Head-mounted eye-movement camera. *Journal of the Optical Society of America*, **52**, 713–716.

Magnus, H. (1901). *Die Augenheilkunde der Alten*. Breslau: Kern.

Mariotte, E. 1683. An account of two letters of Mr Perrault and Mr Mariotte, concerning vision. *Philosophical Transactions of the Royal Society*, **13**, 266–267.

Mannan, S.K., Ruddock, K.H., and Wooding, D.S. (1997). Fixation sequences made during visual examination of briefly presented 2D images. *Spatial Vision*, **11**, 157–178.

Martinez-Conde, S. (2006). Fixational eye movements in normal and pathological vision. *Visual Perception, Part 1, Fundamentals of Vision: Low and Mid-Level Processes in Perception*, **154**, 151–176.

May, M.T. (1968). *Galen On the usefulness of the parts of the body*. Ithaca, NY: Cornell University Press.

McConkie, G.W. and Rayner, K. (1975). The span of the effective stimulus during a fixation in reading. *Perception and Psychophysics*, **17**, 578–586.

McConkie, G.W. and Rayner, K. (1976). Identifying the span of the effective stimulus in reading: literature review and theories of reading. In H. Singer and R.B. Ruddell (eds.) *Theoretical Models and Processes of Reading* (pp. 137–162). Newark, NJ: International Reading Association.

McConkie, G.W. and Zola, D. (1979). Is visual information integrated across successive fixations in reading? *Perception and Psychophysics*, **25**, 221–224.

Nyström, M. and Holmqvist, K. (2008). Semantic override of low-level features in image viewing–both initially and overall. *Journal of Eye Movement Research*, **2**(2), **2**, 1–11

Orschansky, J. (1898). Eine Methode die Augenbewegungen direct zu untersuchen. *Zentralblatt für Physiologie*, **12**, 785.

O'Regan, J.K. and Lévy-Schoen, A. (1983). Integrating visual information from successive fixations - does trans-saccadic fusion exist? *Vision Research*, **23**, 765–768.

O'Regan, J.K. and Noë, A. (2001). A sensorimotor account of vision and visual consciousness. *Behavioral and Brain Sciences*, **24**, 939–973; discussion 973–1031.

Parkhurst, D.J., Law, K., and Niebur, E. (2002). Modeling the role of salience in the allocation of overt visual attention. *Vision Research*, **42**, 107–123.

Pelz, J.B. and Canosa, R. (2001). Oculomotor behavior and perceptual strategies in complex tasks. *Vision Research*, **41**, 3587–3596.

Porterfield, W. (1737). An essay concerning the motions of our eyes. Part I. Of their external motions. *Edinburgh Medical Essays and Observations*, **3**, 160–263.

Porterfield, W. (1738). An essay concerning the motions of our eyes. Part II. Of their internal motions. *Edinburgh Medical Essays and Observations*, **4**, 124–294.

Porterfield, W. (1759). *A treatise on the eye, the manner and phænomena of vision.* Vol. 2. Edinburgh: Hamilton and Balfour.

Pritchard, R.M. (1958). Visual illusions viewed as stabilized retinal images. *Quarterly Journal of Experimental Psychology,* **10,** 77–81.

Pritchard, R.M. (1961). Stabilized images on the retina. *Scientific American,* **204**(5), 1–8.

Purkinje, J. (1820). Beyträge zur näheren Kenntniss des Schwindels aus heautognostischen Daten. *Medicinische Jahrbücher des kaiserlich-königlichen öesterreichischen Staates,* **6,** 79–125.

Purkinje, J. (1825). *Beobachtungen und Versuche zur Physiologie der Sinne. Neue Beiträge zur Kenntniss des Sehens in subjectiver Hinsicht.* Berlin: Reimer.

Purkinje, J. (1846). Wachen, Schlaf, Traum und verwandte Zustände. In R. Wagner (ed.) *Handwörterbuch der Physiologie.* Vol. 3. (pp. 412–480). Braunschweig: Vieweg.

Radach, R., Reilly, R., and Inhoff, A. (2007). Models of oculomotor control in reading: toward a theoretical foundation of current debates. In R.P.G. van Gompel, M.H. Fischer, W.S. Murray, and R.L. Hill (eds.) *Eye movements: A window on mind and brain* (pp. 237–269). Oxford: Elsevier.

Ratliff, F. (1952). The role of physiological nystagmus in monocular acuity. *Journal of Experimental Psychology,* **43,** 163–172.

Ratliff, F. and Riggs, L.A. (1950). Involuntary motions of the eye during monocular fixation. *Journal of Experimental Psychology,* **40,** 687–701.

Reinagel, P. and Zador, A.M. (1999). Natural scene statistics at the centre of gaze. *Network-Computation in Neural Systems,* **10,** 341–350.

Rensink, R.A. (2000). The dynamic representation of scenes. *Visual Cognition,* **7,** 17–42.

Riggs, L.A., Ratliff, F., Cornsweet, J.C., and Cornsweet, T.N. (1953). The disappearance of steadily fixated visual test objects. *Journal of the Optical Society of America,* **43,** 495–501.

Robinson, D.A. (1973). Models of the saccadic eye movement control system. *Biological Cybernetics,* **14,** 71–83.

Robinson, D.A. (1975). Oculomotor control signals. In F. Lennerstrand, and P. Bach-y-Rita (eds.) *Basic mechanisms of ocular motility and their clinical implications* (pp. 337–374). Oxford: Pergamon Press.

Ross, W.D. (ed.) (1927). *The works of Aristotle.* Vol. 7. Oxford: Clarendon.

Rothkopf, C.A., Ballard, D.H., and Hayhoe, M.M. (2007). Task and context determine where you look. *Journal of Vision,* **7**(14): 1–20.

Sabra, A.I. (1989). (Trans. and ed.) *The Optics of Ibn Al-Haytham. Books I-III. On direct vision.* London: The Warburg Institute.

Sharples, R.W. (2003). On dizziness. In W.W. Fortenbaugh, R.W.Sharples, and M.G. Sollenberger (eds.) *Theophrastus of Eresus on sweat, on dizziness, and on fatigue* (pp. 169–250). Leiden: Brill.

Shastid, T.H. (1917). History of ophthalmology. In C.A. Wood (ed.) *The American encyclopedia and dictionary of ophthalmology,* Vol. 11 (pp. 8524–8904). Chicago, IL: Cleveland Press.

Smith, A.M. (1996). *Ptolemy's theory of visual perception: An English translation of the* Optics *with introduction and commentary.* Philadelphia, PA: The American Philosophical Society.

Smith, R. (1738). *A compleat system of opticks in four books.* Cambridge: Published by the author.

Smith, R. (2004). *A compleat system of opticks in four books.* Bristol: Thoemmes Continuum.

Sprague, N., Ballard, D.H., and Robinson, A. (2007). Modeling embodied visual behaviors. *ACM Transactions on Applied Perception,* **4**(2), 1–23.

Stratton, G.M. (1902). Eye-movements and the aesthetics of visual form. *Philosophische Studien,* **20,** 336–359.

Stratton, G.M. (1906). Symmetry, linear illusions and the movements of the eye. *Psychological Review,* **13,** 82–96.

Tatler, B.W. (2007). The central fixation bias in scene viewing: selecting an optimal viewing position independently of motor biases and image feature distributions. *Journal of Vision,* **7**(14), 1–17.

Tatler, B.W. (2009). *Eye guidance in natural scenes.* Hove: Psychology Press.

Tatler B.W. and Wade N.J. (2003). On nystagmus, saccades, and fixations. *Perception,* **32,** 167–184.

Tatler, B.W., Baddeley, R.J., and Gilchrist, I.D. (2005a). Visual correlates of fixation selection: effects of scale and time. *Vision Research,* **45,** 643–659.

Tatler, B.W., Gilchrist, I.D., and Land, M.F. (2005b). Visual memory for objects in natural scenes: From fixations to object files. *Quarterly Journal of Experimental Psychology Section A-Human Experimental Psychology,* **58,** 931–960.

Tatler, B.W., Baddeley, R.J., and Vincent, B.T. (2006). The long and the short of it: spatial statistics at fixation vary with saccade amplitude and task. *Vision Research,* **46,** 1857–1862.

Tatler, B.W., Wade, N.J., Kwan, H., Findlay, J.M., and Velichkovsky, B.M. (2010). Yarbus, eye movements, and vision. *i-Perception,* **1**(1), 7–27.

Taylor, E.A. (1937). *Controlled reading.* Chicago, IL: University of Chicago Press.

Thomas, E.L. (1968). Movements of the eye. *Scientific American,* **219**(2), 88–95.

Thorwald, J. (1962). *Science and secrets of early medicine* (trans. R. and C. Winston). London: Thames and Hudson.

Troxler, D. (1804). Ueber das Verschwinden gegebener Gegenstände innerhalb unseres Gesichtskreises. *Ophthalmologische Bibliothek,* **2,** 1–53.

Tscherning, M. (1898). *Optique physiologique.* Paris: Carré and Naud.

Tscherning, M. (1900). *Physiologic optics* (trans. C. Weiland). Philadelphia, PA: Keystone.

Venezky, R.L. (1977). Research on reading processes. A historical perspective. *American Psychologist,* **32,** 339–345.

Vernon, M.D. (1931). *The experimental study of reading*. Cambridge: Cambridge University Press.

von Noorden, G.K. (1996). *Binocular vision and ocular motility* (5th edn.). St Louis, MO: Mosby.

Wade, N.J. (1998). *A natural history of vision*. Cambridge, MA: MIT Press.

Wade, N.J. (2000). William Charles Wells (1757–1817) and vestibular research before Purkinje and Flourens. *Journal of Vestibular Research*, **10**, 127–137.

Wade, N.J. (2003a) *Destined for distinguished oblivion: The scientific vision of William Charles Wells (1757–1817)*. New York: Kluwer/Plenum.

Wade, N.J. (2003b). The search for a sixth sense: The cases for vestibular, muscle, and temperature senses. *Journal of the History of the Neurosciences*, **12**, 175–202.

Wade, N.J. (2005). The original spin doctors–the meeting of perception and insanity. *Perception*, **34**, 253–260.

Wade, N.J. (2007a). Scanning the seen: vision and the origins of eye movement research. In R.P.G. van Gompel, M.H, Fischer, W.S. Murray, and R.L. Hill (eds.) *Eye movements: A window on mind and brain* (pp. 31–61). Oxford: Elsevier.

Wade, N.J. (2007b). The vision of William Porterfield. In H. Whitaker, C.U.M. Smith, and S. Finger (eds.) *Brain, mind, and medicine: Essays in 18th century neuroscience* (pp. 163–176). New York: Springer.

Wade, N.J. (2007c). Image, eye and retina. *Journal of the Optical Society of America A*, **24**, 1229–1249.

Wade, N.J. (2010). Pioneers of eye movement research. *iPerception*, **1**(2), 33–68.

Wade, N.J. and Finger, S. (2001). The eye as an optical instrument. From *camera obscura* to Helmholtz's perspective. *Perception*, **30**, 1157–1177.

Wade, N.J. and Tatler, B.W. (2005). *The moving tablet of the eye: the origins of modern eye movement research*. Oxford: Oxford University Press.

Wade, N.J. and Tatler, B.W. (2009). Did Javal measure eye movements during reading? *Journal of Eye Movement Research*, **2**(5), 1–7.

Wade, N.J., Tatler, B.W., and Heller, D. (2003). Dodge-ing the issue: Dodge, Javal, Hering, and the measurement of saccades in eye movement research. *Perception*, **32**, 793–804.

Wade, N.J., Norrsell, U., and Presly, A. (2005). Cox's chair: 'a moral and a medical mean in the treatment of maniacs'. *History of Psychiatry*, **16**, 73–88.

Wells, W.C. (1792). *An essay upon single vision with two eyes: together with experiments and observations on several other subjects in optics*. London: Cadell.

Wells, W.C. (1794a). Reply to Dr Darwin on vision. *The Gentleman's Magazine and Historical Chronicle*, **64**, 794–797.

Wells, W.C. (1794b). Reply to Dr Darwin on vision. *The Gentleman's Magazine and Historical Chronicle*, **64**, 905–907.

Woodworth, R.S. (1938). *Experimental psychology*. New York: Holt.

Yarbus, A.L. (1967). *Eye movements and vision* (trans. B. Haigh). New York: Plenum Press.

CHAPTER 3

Vestibular response

Bernhard J.M. Hess

Abstract

This chapter deals with vestibular mechanisms in motor control of eye movements with a focus on all three rotational degrees of freedom of movements. After a short overview in the first section, we address in the following the problem of inertial motion detection and kinematic restrictions, which are essential for an understanding of the spatiotemporal organization of the vestibulo-ocular reflexes (VOR). In the last two sections, finally, we discuss the issue of optimal retinal image stabilization and gain modulations by target proximity in both the rotational and translational VOR.

Introduction

Orientation and navigation in space rely on a close interaction of vision with vestibular signals from sensors in the inner ear that provide information about self-motion in space. These sensors function by the principle of inertia of motion that allows hair cells in the otolith organs to detect head orientation relative to gravity and linear translations of the head by sensing the shear of the otoconial membrane whereas the ampullary hair cells in the cupulae selectively detect rotatory head movements by the inertial motion of the endolymph in the semicircular canals (Wilson and Melville, Jones, 1979, see also Cullen and Van Horn, Chapter 9, this volume). The vestibular information is used by the brain in the oculomotor system for retinal image stabilization at rest and during locomotion.

Reflexive eye movements driven by otolith activity appear relatively early in the ontogenesis and evolution of vertebrates, whereas the semicircular canal-born ocular reflexes emerged later and become functional only after the canal lumina have reached a critical size in the development (Lambert et al., 2008; Muller, 1999; Rabbit, 1999). Otolith-driven eye and neck reflexes are fundamental mechanisms controlling the orientation of the eyes and head relative to gravity. Similar orientation reflexes can be found throughout the vertebrates and also exist in invertebrates (Wells, 1963). In lateral-eyed species that benefit from an almost panoramic visual field, these reflexes pin the visual streak (Hughes, 1971), an area of high receptor density along the horizontal retinal meridian, to the physical horizon. Traces of otolith-born orientation reflexes are preserved in primates.

One of the challenges that the brain faced while developing more skilled locomotor activity was the integration of otolith and semicircular canal-born afferent signals into an inertial navigation channel that enables motor control in a feedforward manner. Such information can be used to support the more delayed available afferent visual information for retinal image stabilization at short latency. Since most head movements result in combined rotations and translations of the eyes, vestibular mechanisms of retinal image stabilization must rely on such integrated information of head-in-space motion, backed up by proprioceptive information of extravestibular origin. The primordial *static otolith-ocular reflexes*, also called *tilt (or tilt-linear) vestibulo-ocular reflexes* (VORs) by some authors, are amongst the first observed vestibular eye movements (Hunter, 1786; Nagel, 1868). From a functional perspective, two classes of dynamic VORs are usually distinguished: *translational or sometimes also called linear (or translational-linear) VORs* in response to head translations (linear accelerations), and *rotational VORs* in response to head rotations. Natural head movements can rarely be sorted out in terms of translations and rotations as they most often consist of a mixture of rotational and translational components.

Vestibulo-ocular reflexes: a short overview

The main function of the VOR is to stabilize the retinal image by maintaining ocular orientation and gaze stabile in space. Changes in head orientation relative to gravity elicit otolith-ocular reflexes at low frequencies that control the ocular orientation relative to the physical space by counter-rolling the eyes about the same axis as the head. In the rabbit, these *static* or *quasi-static otolith-ocular reflexes* have been reported to have a gain of up to 0.6 (Baarsma and Collewijn, 1975; Fleisch, 1922; Van der Hoeve and de Kleijn, 1922, but see also: Maruta et al., 2001). With increasing frequency, the gain decreases rapidly and large phase lags develop. A functional effect is practically absent above 1 Hz, which qualifies these reflexes as orientation reflexes, excluding any functional capability of retinal image stabilization for near targets. During rapid locomotion, rabbits are unable to focus on nearby objects, having clear vision only of the farther environment. An orientation function of otolith-ocular reflexes is also preserved in primates, although the functional requirements of frontally placed eyes and forward oriented visual fields with large binocular overlap are different. When tilting the head about the roll axis (for axis definitions see Fig. 3.1A), the frontally oriented eyes counter-roll about the same axis with a gain of about 0.1 (Collewijn et al., 1985; Seidman et al., 1995a). However, contrary to lateral-eyed species like the rabbit, primates have developed foveal vision and powerful head-independent saccadic eye movements by which they scan the visual environment (Collewijn, 1977; Yarbus, 1976). Since the fovea is a disk-like structure with no preferred direction, the brain might have recurred to means independent of vision for establishing a link between ocular orientation and gravity. Indeed, the low-frequency otolith-ocular reflexes, sometimes also called tilt-linear VORs in primates to distinguish them from translational-linear VORs, mediate a consistent, head-tilt dependent relation between the orientation of each eye's rotation axes and the direction of gravity (Crawford et al., 1991; Haslwanter et al., 1992; Hess and Angelaki, 1997a, 2003). A similar gravity-dependent spatial organization of fast phases of vestibulo-ocular eye movements has been recognized in response to dynamic head and body reorientations relative to gravity (Hess and Angelaki, 1997a, 1997b, 1999). These gravity-dependent spatial properties are imprinted on all visually guided eye movements. In near vision, the oculomotor control can override these orientation reflexes when they interfere with binocular fixation of close targets (Misslisch et al., 2001).

Although the vestibular organs operate like inertial detectors of linear and angular head acceleration, the afferent information from these organs does not unambiguously tell the brain how the head rotates in space (compare the rotation in the earth horizontal plane with that about a tilted plane in Fig. 3.2C, D). Nevertheless, the semicircular canal signals are perfectly sufficient for generating oculomotor commands that compensate rotational disturbances of the head at short latency. The operation of the semicircular canals resembles integrating angular accelerometers by providing head angular velocity information over a frequency range from about 0.1–5 Hz (Wilson and Melvill Jones, 1979).

From the viewpoint of oculomotor control, retinal image stabilization requires two functionally different reactions that closely overlap in time: One is issuing a rapid motor command proportional to head velocity that counter rotates the eye at shortest latency to compensate disturbances of head position. The other slightly delayed action is generating position commands that keep the new ocular orientation stable. In the rotational VOR, the velocity commands are fed forward from the semicircular canals with little modifications to the extraocular muscles via short parallel transmission lines that consist of just three synaptic relays (3-neuronal arc: Lorente de No, 1935; Szentágothai, 1950). Accordingly, reflexive eye movements can be observed within less than 10 ms (Aw et al., 1996;

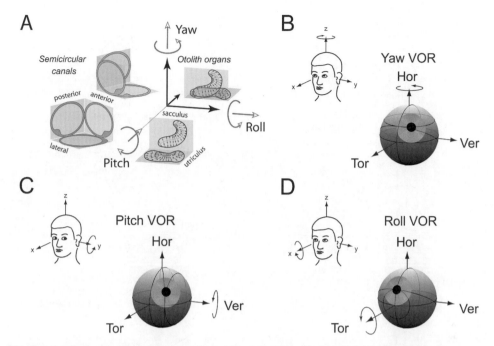

Fig. 3.1 Overview of vestibular sensors controlling eye position through VORs. A) Mirror-symmetric arrangement of the semicircular canal pairs (right–left lateral, anterior, posterior) and their ampullae housing the sensory hair cells; otolith organs with fan-like arranged polarizations of hair cells. B), C), and D) Yaw, pitch and roll VORs elicited by rotations of the head about a head-vertical (z-), lateral (y-) and forward (x-) pointing axis. For perfect compensation of the head rotation, the eye would have to counter-rotate such that the pupil follows a small circle path in a plane orthogonal to the head rotation axis.

Collewijn and Smeets, 2000; Johnston and Sharpe, 1994; Tabak and Collewijn, 1994; reviews: Fuchs, 1981; Precht, 1978; Straka and Dieringer, 2004). Without additional processing, a step-like change in head velocity should generate an eye velocity that reaches rapidly a peak and subsequently follows an exponential time course with a single time constant according to (Robinson, 1986):

$$dE/dt = gain\,\Omega_{head}e^{-t/T_{VOR}}$$

This simple picture requires, however, important modifications. In the first place, the experimentally determined time constants do not reflect the dynamics of the semicircular canals but are about three times as long (15–20 s) as those of the afferent velocity signals (in primates ~6 s) and, secondly, the description of the time course is more complex, requiring at least two exponentials (Buettner et al., 1978; Waespe and Henn, 1977). As a consequence, the VOR velocity often shows a plateau after a step-like change in head velocity before starting to decay (Fig. 3.3B). Both phenomena can be explained by the action of a central network that conjointly processes proprioceptive visual and vestibular self-motion signals, operating parallel to the short 3-neuron arc transmission lines, a phenomenon that has been termed velocity storage (Cohen et al., 1977, Raphan et al., 1977, 1979; Robinson, 1977). Subsequent studies of this phenomenon have revealed that the 'stored' velocity signals represent in fact not only a temporally but also a spatially transformed signal: the head angular velocity that is encoded by the semicircular canals in head-fixed coordinates appears here as a signal transformed into gravity-centred coordinates (Angelaki and Hess, 1994, 1995; Merfeld and Young, 1995; Merfeld et al., 1991; Raphan and Cohen, 1988; Raphan and Sturm, 1991). It is now generally agreed that the originally termed velocity storage network is in fact an inertial vestibular motion centre (discussed in more detail below), which is well

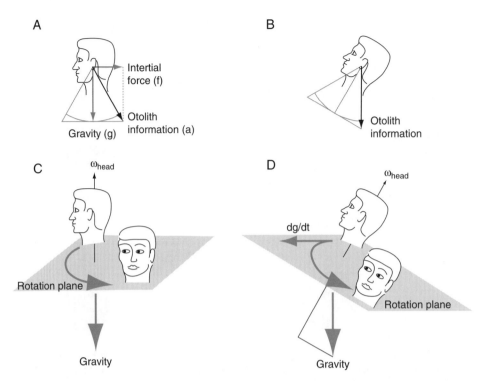

Fig. 3.2 A) If the head undergoes a forward translation, the otoliths of the inner ear experience in addition to the gravitational force (**g**) an inertial force (**f**). At any point in time, the afferent information from the otoliths (**a**) corresponds to the linear sum of these two acceleration components: **a** = **g** + **f**. B) From the total otolith afferent information alone it is a priori not possible to distinguish translation (in A: **a** = **g** + **f**) from tilt (in B: **a** = **g**, **f** =0). C) and D) The afferent information of the semicircular canals is independent of the orientation of the rotation plane relative to gravity. However, the afferent information from the otolith organs tells the brain that d**g**/dt =0 in C, whereas d**g**/dt = ω_{head} x **g** ≠ 0 in D with ω_{head}: angular velocity of the head (detected by the semicircular canals). Bold letters represent vectors; ' ' stands for cross vector product.

developed in subhuman primates, whose role in the human vestibulo-oculomotor system, however, is less clear.

The second important modification comes from the observation that eye velocity commands in all eye movements, not just those of vestibular origin, need to be supplemented by eye position signals that hold the eyes in its new orientation (Robinson, 1981; Seung, 1996; Skavenski and Robinson, 1973). Extensive research has been devoted to determine how and where in the brainstem and cerebellum this integration occurs (Aksay et al., 2007; Cannon and Robinson, 1987; Cheron and Godaux, 1987; Crawford et al., 1991, 2003; see also Thier, Chapter 10, this volume). For a long time, the prevailing, hardly questioned concept was that eye position holding signals can be obtained by mathematical integration of eye velocity commands. In the VOR, where the angular head velocity signals originate directly from the peripheral sense organs, it seems straightforward to integrate these signals by feeding them through a network of cascading, reverberating collaterals with positive and/or negative feedback, parallel to the direct 3-neuron arc connections to the motoneurons (Pastor et al., 1994). While this is true in two dimensions, it does not hold, however, in three dimensions, a mathematical fact that has first been pointed out in a seminal study by Tweed and Vilis (1987). The implementation of these mathematical principles in the oculomotor system considering all rotational degrees of freedom of eye movements is a hard problem that still waits to be resolved (Quaia and Optican, 1998, Raphan, 1998; Smith and Crawford, 1998; Tchelidze and

Hess, 2008; for recent reviews: Angelaki and Hess, 2004; Miller, 2007; see also Angelaki, Chapter 8, this volume).

The rotational VORs discussed so far, together with the primordial static otolith-ocular reflexes, are perfectly adequate for supporting the more slowly reacting visual mechanisms in retinal image stabilization and spatial orientation (Fig. 3.3). While this is true for far vision, retinal image stabilization of objects of regard in the near visual surround requires not only a refinement of the rotational VOR but also calls for additional rapid stabilization mechanisms. First and foremost, near vision requires individual control of each eye to appropriately converge the gaze lines for binocular fixation of

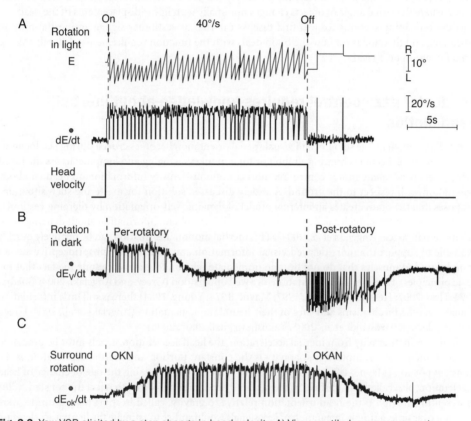

Fig. 3.3 Yaw VOR elicited by a step change in head velocity. A) Visuo-vestibular eye movements to rotation of the animal against a stationary visual surround. Sawtooth-like eye position trace (E) consisting of slow phase movements (to the right), interrupted by much faster quick phases, also called nystagmus. Note the rapid rise in horizontal eye velocity (dE/dt) towards steady-state at the onset followed by an abrupt drop at the offset of rotation, closely matching the head velocity profile (40°/s). The noisy slow phase velocity trace is interrupted by fast spikes with opposite polarity, representing the (clipped) velocities of the quick phases that reposition the eye in the orbita. B) Rotation in the dark showing the vestibulo-ocular response (dE$_V$/dt) to the same head velocity stimulus as in (A). Note the plateau-like eye velocity during the per-rotatory phase at rotation onset, and a similar decay at the end of rotation. B) Visuo-ocular (= optokinetic) response (dE$_{ok}$/dt), evoked by rotation of the visual surround about the stationary animal. Same stimulus velocity profile as in (A) and (B). Note slow rise and fall at the beginning and stop of visual surround rotation. Comparison of the visuo-vestibular response in A with the responses in (B) and (C) reveals that the ocular rotation in the light is the linear sum of the vestibulo-ocular response in the dark and the optokinetic response in the light. Unpublished recording from a brown rat (DA-HAN strain).

near objects. Thus, vestibular stabilization reactions have to be individually adjusted for each eye. Second, the rotational VORs can provide perfect image stabilization only if the fixation plane is far away relative to the distance of the eyes from the actual head rotation axis. Third, if the head is subject to translational disturbances, for example up-down oscillations during running or jumping, the rapid linear displacements of the eyes induce retinal image shifts across the fovea of close but not of targets far away. The low-frequency 'static' otolith ocular reflexes that have evolved for helping to maintain visual spatial orientation are not well suited for dealing with these problems. Thus, there is need for otolith-mediated reflexes that specifically deal with stabilizing the foveal image of objects in the near visual surround, close to the current fixation plane. In contrast to the rotational VORs these 'new' reflexes, called *translational VORs* can only selectively stabilize the retinal image and play no role in far vision, where the visual angle of objects changes minimally with linear displacements of the head.

In the remaining sections we will first discuss the role of vestibular signals in inertial motion processing and then focus on how the brain deals with the function requirements of stabilizing the retinal image in near vision.

Vestibular gaze control requires knowledge about inertial head motion

Controlling retinal image stability and visual spatial orientation becomes crucial during fast locomotion, e.g. when a cheetah is hunting a rabbit or for a monkey swinging and jumping across the forest canopy, where adequate motor control requires continuous sensory information on head and body orientation with respect to the ground. A widely discussed solution for mastering such situations proposes that the brain creates an internal model of dynamic self-orientation by merging vestibular inputs from both the semicircular canals and the otoliths to obtain information about dynamic head orientation in space (Angelaki et al., 2004). This inertial motion information can be relatively quickly available to support the more delayed visual information and adjust other proprioceptive signals from joints and muscles that do not bear an immediate relation to gravity. Despite the fact that the basic principles of the inertial computations are well understood (Green and Angelaki, 2004; Guedry, 1974; Hess, 2007; Hess and Angelaki, 1997; Mayne, 1974; Young, 1984) there is still little information available on the mechanisms and sites of their neural implementation (Angelaki et al., 2004; Green and Angelaki, 2003; Shaikh et al., 2005; Yakusheva et al., 2007, 2008).

To discriminate gravity from inertial acceleration, the head acceleration signals must be processed based on the prior assumption that gravity is the constant portion and inertial acceleration is the transient portion (Mayne, 1974). This goal can be achieved by processing the rate of change of head acceleration, also called jerk, instead of the net head acceleration in order to reject the constant value representing gravity. If the head orientation relative to gravity, called in short head attitude, were constant over time, a simple integration of jerk signals would suffice to estimate the inertial acceleration of the head up to three free integration constants (formally one has : linear acceleration = $\int da=a+c$ where da: increment in net acceleration over the time interval dt, c: vector of three integration constants). In general, however, motor control of head attitude is challenged also by rotational disturbances such that the rate of change of net head acceleration (net jerk) includes a vector term that is due to the rate of change of gravity (gravitational jerk). But because gravity is everywhere constant, the only way it could contribute to the overall rate of change of acceleration is by a change in head attitude. During evolution, the brain has probably internalized this possibility, which in fact corresponds to establish a forward model relating changes in head attitude to a rate of change in gravity as follows:

$$dg/dt = -\omega_{head}(t) \times g(t)$$

In this equation, the vector ω_{head} represents the head angular velocity with its three components along the roll, pitch and yaw axes (Fig. 3.1A), which is detected by the semicircular canals and 'x' denotes the cross vector product. Thus, if the head rotates, say from nose up towards left ear down, the rate of change of the gravitational force vector, $d\mathbf{g}/dt$, points initially towards the left ear. Obviously, only head velocity components orthogonal to gravity can change head attitude (compare Fig. 3.2C and D). Starting from an initial head attitude, the brain would need to continuously integrate the angular velocity signals from the semicircular canals to be able to keep track of head orientation. Formally, this process is captured by the following approximate solution to the above equation:

$$\mathbf{g}(t) \cong \mathbf{g}_0 + \varphi(t) \times \mathbf{g}_0$$

where $\mathbf{g}_0$ is the initial head attitude at time t =0, i.e. before motion onset, and $\varphi(t) = \int_0^t \omega(s)ds$ is the integral over the angular velocity information (ω) from the semicircular canals. Because of the cross vector product in this first order solution (i.e. the second term on the right hand side), only head angular velocity components about an earth horizontal axis (i.e. orthogonal to $\mathbf{g}_0$) are involved (Green and Angelaki, 2003, 2004). Interestingly, evidence for this type of integration of head angular velocity information has recently been provided from neural recordings in the cerebellum (Yakusheva et al., 2007, 2008). For larger tilts, it is questionable whether the brain proceeds along this line because in the first place large head tilts are less common in everyday human activity and second the computational burden heavily increases as higher order terms in angular velocity have to be included (the complete solution writes:

$$\mathbf{g}(t) = (1/k!) \sum_{k=0}^{\infty} \Phi^k \mathbf{g}_0 \text{, with } \Phi(t) = \int_0^t \Omega(s)ds \text{ and } \Omega = [\omega_{ik}] \text{ with } w_{ik} = -w_{ik}, i,k=1...3).$$

It should also be stressed that, beside the availability of veridical head angular velocity information, an accurate estimate of initial head attitude (i.e. the vector $\mathbf{g}_0$) is crucial for making this strategy work.

Otolith afferent signals encode not only information about the net head acceleration but to some extent also the rate of change of head acceleration or combinations of both (Fernandez and Goldberg, 1976a, 1976b, 1976c). The reasons for this are not clear, although they might be related to an economic way of solving the inertial motion encoding problem (Hess, 1992). In this context, the forward problem of inertial motion encoding can be formulated as follows (Fig. 3.2A):

$$d\mathbf{a}/dt = d/dt(\mathbf{g}+\mathbf{f}) = -w_{head} \times \mathbf{g} + d\mathbf{f}/dt$$

(see Fig. 3.2A–C for a geometric interpretation of the vectors $\mathbf{g}$, $\mathbf{f}$, and ω_{head}). If the brain has access to veridical information about head angular velocity (e.g. based on semicircular canal afferent information), the inverse encoding model, namely the representation of inertial head acceleration as a function of head angular velocity and orientation relative to gravity can be estimated by a mathematical integration. One of the difficulties of implementing this approach lies again in the determination of the initial values, which specify the initial accelerations along each of the three spatial directions (also called integration constants). A number of models have addressed these and related problems in various contexts while experimental verifications are unfortunately still in their infancy (Green and Angelaki, 2003, 2004; Green et al., 2005; Laurens and Angelaki, 2011; Merfeld, 1995; Merfeld et al., 1993, Mergner and Glasauer, 1999, Zupan et al., 2002).

Another intriguing aspect that has barely received due attention is related to the problem of the reference frame, in which inertial signals might be encoded. The above discussed equations can be rewritten in the following equivalent form (Angelaki et al., 1999; Hess and Angelaki, 1997; Viéville and Faugeras, 1990):

$$d\mathbf{f}/dt + w_{head} \times \mathbf{f} = d\mathbf{a}/dt + w_{head} \times \mathbf{a}$$

Although the solution to this differential equation can explicitly be written down in terms of the input signals on the right hand side, i.e. the net head acceleration ($\mathbf{a}$) and the rate of change of acceleration ($d\mathbf{a}/dt$), a physiological implementation of these equations is not straightforward for the following reasons (Hess, 2007): first of all, the otolith afferent inflow to the brain carries information encoded in some gravity-centred reference frame (i.e. a Cartesian reference frame with one axis parallel to gravity). As a consequence, the inertial acceleration on the output side, $\mathbf{f}$, as well as the head angular velocity, ω_{head}, must be encoded in the same coordinates. Since the velocity signals that the brain has at hand from the semicircular canals are necessarily encoded in head-fixed rather than gravity-centred coordinates there is an additional transformation step necessary before the inertial head acceleration can be estimated based on the afferent inflow. The brain thus requires angular velocity information about the head rotation relative to the physical surround in order to be able to compute head attitude. In turn it requires accurate head attitude information to compute head angular velocity relative to the physical space. Thus, it appears that the required neural computations have to be conceived as a self-tuning process, comparable to the technique of bootstrapping, which is bound to rely on extravestibular information. From this viewpoint, it is not surprising that structures of the cerebellum that are related to or involved in inertial vestibular processing not only receive vestibular and visual but also heavy neck proprioceptive input (Manzoni et al., 1998, 1999; Precht et al., 1976; Shaikh et al., 2004).

Because of the mathematical integrations involved, an implementation of the outlined computations has to depend strongly on feedback processing, which would manifest itself in the low-frequency domain of the VOR due to the long time constants. It has long been known that the VOR shows not only a sharp onset in response to a step-like change in rotational head velocity but also a rather sluggish after-response when the head comes to an abrupt halt in the dark (Fig. 3.3B). This after-response outlasts by a factor of three or more the low frequency response dynamics of the semicircular canal afferents, and has therefore been characterized as a 'velocity storage' network (Cohen et al., 1977; Raphan et al., 1977, 1979). Neural activity in the vestibular nuclei of the brainstem also reflects this low frequency dynamics, which is shared by vestibular and optokinetic signals (Dai et al., 1991; Waespe and Henn, 1977, 1978). Sites of inertial vestibular processing are the vestibular nuclei in the brainstem and mid line areas in the cerebellum including the cerebellar nodulus and uvula (Yakusheva et al., 2007, 2008).

Kinematic restrictions interfere with optimal retinal image stabilization

In contrast to vestibular eye movements, saccades or smooth pursuit eye movements during tracking of a moving object (e.g. a swallow in the sky) are subject to particular kinematic restrictions. These visually-guided eye movements follow a law, called Listing's law after the German mathematician and physicist Johann Benedikt Listing (1808–1882) that imposes certain restrictions (see also Angelaki, Chapter 8, and Crawford and Klier, Chapter 18, this volume). The law states that the angular velocity at which the eye moves during a saccade or tracks a moving object depends in a particular way on eye position: it always lies in a plane that rotates relative to *primary position* in the same direction as the gaze line, but only by half the angle (Tweed and Vilis, 1990; von Helmholtz, 1867). In simple terms, primary eye position can be defined as the unique eye position in head upright position such that in far viewing any horizontal and vertical redirection of gaze, respectively, keeps the horizontal and vertical retinal meridian invariant relative to the physical space (for a more technical definition see, e.g. Tweed and Vilis, 1990).

The angular velocity of an optimal rotational VOR should not underlay any such kinematic restrictions. For example, during any of the cardinal rotational VORs (see Fig. 3.1B, C) the angular eye velocity should stay parallel to the head angular velocity. Ideally, the compensatory eye movements during yaw and pitch head rotations should follow great circles through primary position, because these circles describe torsion-free positions that comply with Listing's law. This is, however, clearly not possible for the roll VOR (Fig. 3.1C), which has to brake the kinematic restrictions imposed by Listing's law. But even the yaw and pitch vestibulo-ocular responses cannot always comply with Listing's law. Consider for example what happens if the observer looks away from primary position, say to the left and up while a rotational disturbance of the head about the yaw axis challenges retinal image stability (Fig. 3.1B). In this case, the compensatory eye movement has to occur along the small circular path through the desired initial fixation position, entailing a change in the torsion in proportion to the deviation from the torsion-free great circle (Fig. 3.1B). Such changes in torsional eye position violate Listing's law. A similar argument holds for compensatory movements during pitch movements if the desired fixation position happens to be in a secondary horizontal or in a tertiary position (Fig. 3.1C). During yaw VOR, the required torsional deviations increase linearly with vertical gaze eccentricity, and so does the associated torsional eye velocity. To move the eye along the small circles (Fig. 3.1B, C) the oculomotor system must continuously update its torsional orientation, which implies integration of the underlying torsional velocity in the mathematical sense. If the yaw movement is followed by a pitch movement or vice versa, the required changes in ocular torsion can accumulate (Tchelidze and Hess, 2007).

To characterize this crucial condition for an optimal performance, it is instructive to consider the gain of the torsional velocity-to-position integration, which can conveniently be defined by the ratio of the observed change in ocular torsion, abbreviated by ΔE^*_{tor}, and the change in torsion during optimal performance, abbreviated by ΔE_{tor}:

$$k = \Delta E^*_{tor} / \Delta E_{tor}$$

The required change in torsion during optimal performance is illustrated by the small circles in Fig. 3.1B–D. For example in the yaw VOR, it corresponds to the difference that would be obtained by rotating the eye about the roll axis from a corresponding position on the great circle to its current position on the small circle. The torsional position gain provides a direct measure of how much the actual VOR deviates from its optimal performance. How is it related to the angular velocity of the eye? If the torsional position gain is less than unity, the gaze can not move along the optimal path, which implies the emergence of a torsional angular velocity component. As a consequence, the over-all angular eye velocity tilts in the yaw (in case of pitch VOR) or in the pitch plane (in case of yaw VOR). Although these torsional velocity components increase approximately linearly with vertical or horizontal gaze eccentricity it affects the peak main angular velocity component only little. Nevertheless, since the eye does now no longer rotate about the same axis and speed as the head, the VOR becomes less than optimal. In both the yaw and pitch VOR, the angular eye velocity will always tilt in the same direction as the gaze line with respect to primary gaze direction if the torsional velocity-to-position integration is reduced.

Studies in subhuman primates have shown that they use an optimal stabilization strategy in both yaw and pitch VOR. Thus, independent of gaze direction, the axis of angular eye velocity always aligns with the head rotation axis (as illustrated in Fig. 3.1B, C) with the benefit of stabilizing the entire retinal image against rotational disturbances of the head. In humans this seems not to be the case, at least under laboratory conditions: during sinusoidal head oscillations, tilts of the resulting angular eye velocity corresponding to a torsional gain of as little as about 0.5 have been reported (Misslisch et al., 1994). Interestingly, transient responses of head thrusts elicited at high head accelerations in yaw are closer to optimal and show little dependence on vertical gaze during the first 40–50 ms (Thurtell et al., 1999).

In contrast to yaw and pitch, optimal image stabilization in the roll VOR must always occur about an axis, the roll axis, which is incompatible with Listing's law, because in this case the eye has to change torsional position irrespective of current gaze direction (Fig. 3.1D). Experimental studies in subhuman primates have shown that the axis alignment in the roll VOR closely correlates with the actual reflex gain: the reflex response to roll head oscillations is nearly optimal with minimal axis tilt when the reflex gain is high, whereas at lower gains the axis tilt increases as a function of eccentric gaze in the direction predicted by Listing's law (Misslisch and Hess, 2000). A similar correlation has been reported in humans, although over a more limited gain range (Tweed and Misslisch, 2001). As already mentioned, humans appear to use a suboptimal strategy even during yaw and pitch head rotations, where the axes tilts correlate well with the observed low roll reflex gain around 0.5 (Collewijn et al., 1985; Crawford and Vilis, 1991; Leigh et al., 1989; Schmid-Priscoveanu et al., 2000; Seidman et al., 1995a,b; Tweed et al., 1994). This reflex gain reflects in fact the low torsional velocity-to-position integration gain rather than a reduced velocity gain (Tchelidze and Hess, 2008).

Modulation of the vestibulo-ocular reflexes by target proximity

The computational demands on the brain to stabilize the retinal image of far objects are relatively simple because both eyes can be controlled in conjugacy, and there are no effects of motion parallax.

The weight of the various factors that determine otherwise the computational load in near viewing increases proportional to target proximity. For both linear and rotational disturbances, the gain of compensatory reflex movements depends on target eccentricity as well as the distance of each eye to the target of interest. Accordingly, the smaller the distance the more disturbing are small inadvertent movements of the head. Motion parallax becomes dominant in near viewing: Small linear head displacements lead increasingly to blur of retinal image if not counteracted.

The impact of these proximity effects is summarized in the diagrams illustrated in Fig. 3.4 for horizontal eye movements. In the first place, near targets need to be binocularly foveated to avoid double vision, which requires individual oculomotor commands to the two eyes to control the vergence angle. The vergence angle depends inversely on the eye-to-target distance, which can readily be appreciated for targets in the mid-sagittal plane, where each eye shares half of the angle. The functional relation for vergence shows a hyperbolic dependence on target distance:

$$v = 2\sin^{-1}(\Delta/d_{ET}) \cong 2\Delta/d_{ET}$$

with d_{ET} = length of the eye-to-target vector (Fig. 3.4A: see direction vectors $\mathbf{r}_{ET}$ and $\mathbf{l}_{ET}$) and Δ = half the interocular distance.

A similar dependence on target distance should set the gain of the VOR of each eye when expressed as a function of the location of the head rotation axis and the eye-to-target distance of either eye to the target (Fig. 3.4A). Designing the position vectors from the location of the head rotation axis and the right eye to the target by $\mathbf{r}_{AT}$ and $\mathbf{r}_{ET}$, respectively, and the corresponding distances by d_{AT} and d_{ET}, we can write the relation between the velocity of the right eye and head velocity as follows:

$$d\vartheta_R/dt = -q_R G_\infty \, d\eta_H/dt$$

where G_∞ is the gain for far viewing (optimally $G_\infty = 1$) and

$$q_R = (d_{AT}/d_{ET})\hat{r}_{AT} \hat{\mathit{r}}_{ET}$$

is a modulation factor that depends (1) on the direction vector $\mathbf{r}_{AT}$ and its length d_{AT} ($\hat{r}_{AT} = \mathbf{r}_{AT}/d_{AT}$, unit direction vector) and (2) on the direction vector $\mathbf{r}_{ET}$ and its length d_{ET} ($\hat{r}_{ET} = \mathbf{r}_{ET}/d_{ET}$, unit direction vector). Both eye velocity, $d\vartheta_R/dt$, and head velocity, $d\eta_H/dt$, are in the horizontal plane. The gain modulation factor q_R captures the influence of both target distance (by the quotient d_{AT}/d_{ET}) and target eccentricity (by the angle ε_{AE} subtended by the axis-to-target vector $\mathbf{r}_{AT}$ and the eye-to-target vector $\mathbf{r}_{ET}$, obtained from the dot product: $\hat{r}_{AT} \hat{\mathit{r}}_{ET} = \cos(\varepsilon_{AE})$) . This near-target-gain modulation, expressed here in a compact geometric way for ease of interpretation, is equivalent to a previously published formulation by Hine and Thorne (1987). A corresponding equation has been given in the position domain by Viirre et al. (1986). Clearly, for targets far away, the q-factors (i.e. q_R for the right and q_L for the left eye) are normally close to one for either eye, because of the normally relatively small axis-to-eye distance during natural head motion. In near vision, several important requirements for retinal image stability of a fixation target can be derived from this relation, most of which have been experimentally examined in terms of a potential preattentive vestibular contributions (Crane and Demer, 1997, 1998; Crane et al., 1997; Hine and Thorn, 1987; Paige et al., 1998; Snyder and King, 1992; Viirre and Demer, 1996a, 1996b; Viirre et al., 1986). The described relation suggests in the first place that the overall optimal gain (i.e. gain $q_R G_\infty$) must have a component that increases inversely to the target distance, except for cases where the axis of the (passive) head rotation is located at the level of or in front of the eye in consideration. This conclusion derives from the quotient d_{AT}/d_{ET}, which in the case of a linear alignment of rotation axis, eye and target location (in this order) can be parsed as follows:

$$d_{AT}/d_{ET} = (d_{AE}+d_{ET})/d_{ET} = d_{AE}/d_{ET} +1$$

where d_{AE} is the distance between the location of the rotation axis and the eye. It shows the postulated $1/d_{ET}$ dependence, provided that the axis-to-eye distance d_{AE} is constant (Fig. 3.4B). During natural yaw or pitch head motions, the rotation axes are approximately 0.1m behind the eyes. For a more

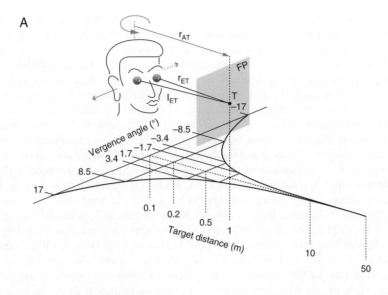

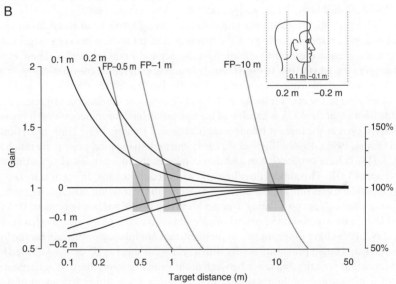

Fig. 3.4 Effects of target proximity on retinal image stabilization. A) Fixation of close targets requires (1) individual adjustments of the reflex gain for each eye and (2) modulation and maintenance of vergence that increases with reciprocal target distance (*solid black curves*). r_{AT}: axis-to-target direction vector; r_{ET}: right eye-to-target direction vector; l_{ET}: left eye-to-target direction vector. B) In the optimal rotational VOR, the reflex gain of each eye must be modulated as a function of target distance, depending on the relative location of the head rotation axis (solid black curves). Simulations for five different axis locations (see inset). For comparison, the dependence of motion parallax on target proximity for three different fixation planes is also shown (solid grey curves). Parameters: interocular distance = 0.06 m; all target located straight ahead in the mid-sagittal plane.

comprehensive description of the multi-joint head-neck system, see Medendorp and colleagues (1998). Based on this simple approximation, a dependence on viewing distance should become effective at distances of about 0.5 m and less. In contrast to the effects of motion parallax, which strongly depend on the actual fixation plane, retinal slip of the target image can only be minimized by controlling the gain of the reflex, for the gain curves asymptotically approach unity (Fig. 3.4B).

For rotation axes located in front of the eyes, the optimal overall gain for stabilizing retinal images can vary between large negative values and unity depending on the location of the target. For example, if the target is straight ahead at double the eye-to-axis distance the gain needs to be down modulated by a $q = 0.5$ because the eye has to move half as far as the head, and it decreases further towards zero as the target approaches the location of the rotation axis (see example curves labelled '0', '−0.1m' and '−0.2m' in Fig. 3.4B). If the target comes even closer towards the observer, the eye velocity has to switch direction compared to the normal VOR. Formally, this 'negative' gain condition as it could be called in short is hidden in the dot product $\hat{r}_{AT}\,\hat{g}_{ET}$ between the axis-to-target and the eye-to-target vectors (Fig. 3.4A): if these vectors point into opposite directions then the cosine of the subtended angle is negative. At about half the distance between the observer's eye and the axis the required gain reaches −1 and decreases to more negative values closer up. The required polarity switch for stable fixation of these targets can cause confusion in experimental tests because the actual or even the intended fixation target of a proband has to be taken into account (Barr et al., 1976).

Finally, also the eccentricity of the target relative to the eye matters, as described by the angle ε_{AE}. It results in a down modulation of the effectively required gain for a compensatory response. Although the influence of this parameter is limited because the angles fall usually within a range of ±30°, where the cosine modulates only between 1 and 0.87, it nevertheless shows that the required gains for the eyes can differ by 10% or more. For optimal depth vision the oculomotor control must exert individual control of the two eyes at coordinated but generally different gains, which modulate the VOR (Misslisch and Hess, 2002; Snyder et al., 1992; Viirre et al., 1986).

Hine and Thorn (1987) studied near target fixation using active head rotations or oscillations and found high gain responses following the theoretical gain function between target distances of 0.22–1.80 m that extended earlier observations of Biguer and Prablanc (1981). These experiments could not answer what was the role of the fixation light and of extraretinal cues to distance, in particular vergence. A number of subsequent experimental studies have tested the effect of eccentric rotations posterior or anterior to the eyes on the gain of the VOR as well as the effect of target distance. While there is little doubt that the VOR is capable of the optimal behaviour in near vision if provided with visual feedback even at the highest frequencies (Crane and Demer, 1997; Hine and Thorne, 1987; Viirre and Demer, 1996a, 1996b; Viirre et al., 1986), the underlying mechanisms are much less clear. Buizza et al. (1981) have proposed a model that combines the independently operating rotational and translational VOR. This model does however not account for the different translations of the otolith organs and the eyes due to their different distances to the rotation axis. An elegant mathematical solution of this problem postulating a 'target locator network' has been proposed by Viirre et al. (1986) but little is known about the neural implementation of the postulated mechanisms. Snyder and King (1992, 1996) have shown in rhesus monkeys that modulation of the gain for the location of the rotation axis and target proximity occurs with a delay of as short as 20–30 ms, followed by further adjustments attributed to the difference between otolith and eye translation. In agreement with this report, transient responses of the rotational VOR in humans are also independent of both target distance and rotational eccentricity during the first 30–50ms. Whether there is a gain correction for the position of the otoliths relative to the eyes remains unresolved (Crane and Demer, 1998; Crane et al., 1997). Taken together it appears that interaction of otolith and semicircular canal signals alone cannot fully account for the process of gain modulation that accommodates for axis eccentricity and target location effects before visual feedback becomes effective.

From a slightly different viewpoint, eccentric axis rotations have been extensively used to investigate whether semicircular canal and otolith signals in the VOR combine linearly (Anastasopoulos et al., 1996; Bronstein and Gresty, 1991; Crane and Demer, 1997; Crane et al., 1997; Fuhry et al., 2002; Gresty et al., 1987; Merfeld, 1996; Sargent and Paige, 1991; Seidman et al., 2002; Telford et al., 1996, 1998). In the facing nose-out rotation paradigm, the tangential and angular accelerations of the head activate the otolith organs and the semicircular canals in synergy, both generating rightward eye movements during a rotation of the head to the left. In the facing nose-in rotation paradigm, however, the phase of translation and rotation is reversed (a fact that is of course independent of relative target locations): while the head rotates to the one side it translates to the other side. Thus, in contrast to natural head movements, the activation of the otolith organs (by the tangential accelera-tion) and of the semicircular canals (by the angular acceleration) are now no longer in synergy. In terms of fixation tasks, this experimental paradigm is complicated by the fact that the required polarity of compensatory eye movements now depends on the location of the target relative to the observer (including effects of target eccentricity relative to straight ahead) as well as relative to the location of the rotation axis as outlined previously. Since these confounding effects are difficult to control experimentally they may be part of the reasons why such studies have provided conflicting evidence as to whether otolith-canal interaction is linear or not. However this issue of linearity will be resolved, it is clear that optimal gaze stability requires non-linear processing to fully account for the intricate geometric effects of rotation and translation of the eyes with respect to close targets.

Translational vestibulo-ocular reflexes

Linear displacements of head lead to an apparent shift of objects of regard, called motion parallax, by changing the observer's vantage point. Although motion parallax can enhance depth vision at low frequencies of head movements it ultimately jeopardizes retinal image stability if the linear displace-ments of the head occur at high frequency. To stabilize the retinal image, the brain could use otolith signals selectively at high frequencies to generate compensatory eye movements. For this, it has to resolve the inherent ambiguity of otolith information as discussed earlier: if the underlying motion of the otoconia in the otolith organs is caused by inertial forces the afferents signal a translation of the head, requiring different eye movements than if the motion is caused by gravity indicating a change in head orientation. In terms of retinal image stabilization, this discrimination is of crucial importance. For example, to compensate a quick forward displacement of the head, the horizontal position of each eye needs to be adjusted to maintain fixation on the object of regard. If it is a head tilt, an adjustment of the vertical eye positions is appropriate instead (Fig. 3.2A, B). Presently two main hypotheses are discussed as to how the brain might solve this tilt-translation discrimination problem. One is the frequency-segregation hypothesis, which proposes that the brain uses frequency filters to interpret low frequency otolith information as head-tilt signal and high frequency informa-tion as head-translation signal (Paige and Tomko, 1991a; Telford et al., 1997). The other hypothesis is that the brain reconstructs head-in-space orientation by using information from both the otolith organs and semicircular canals as outlined earlier.

But apart from this tilt-translation discrimination problem, how are the translational VORs generated? First of all, there is general agreement that these reflexes are responses to centrally esti-mated translational velocity signals rather than straight forward integration of otolith acceleration signals. Thus, after the brain has decided, whether the acceleration information carried by the otolith afferent inflow indicates a translation in space rather than a head tilt, further central process-ing is required for deriving translational head velocity. This is in stark contrast to the rotational VORs, where a mathematical-like integration of head angular accelerations is established by the hydrodynamics of the semicircular canals, at least across a frequency range covering most natural head movements. Studies in primates have shown that estimation of head-in-space translation veloc-ity is no longer possible if the afferent input from the semicircular canals is deficient or missing, indicating that the translational VOR is in fact a multisensory response (Angelaki et al., 1999; Green and Angelaki, 2003, 2004; Shaikh et al., 2005). How and where the integration of signals proportional to head acceleration that activate the otolith organs takes place is still not known (for a recent review see Angelaki, 2004).

Apart from the high-pass filter dynamics, the response dynamics of the translational VORs is char-acterized by two parameters, both related to foveal vision, which again contrasts these reflexes with the much simpler organized rotational VOR (Angelaki et al., 2003). The most important one is *target proximity* (Angelaki and McHenry, 1999; McHenry and Angelaki, 2000; Schwarz et al., 1989; Schwarz and Miles, 1991; Miles, 1993; Paige, 1989; Telford et al., 1998). As the effect of motion parallax disap-pears with increasing viewing distance the translational reflex gain becomes minimal and vice versa. In contrast to rotations, target proximity challenges visual acuity during translations much more dramatically, requiring appropriate modulation of the reflex gain at the shortest latencies (Angelaki and McHenry, 1999; Gianna et al., 1995; Zhou et al., 2002) (Fig. 3.4B). To stabilize the retinal image of an object at 1m distance against a lateral head displacement that reaches 1 m/s, the eyes have to counter rotate with a velocity profile reaching 1 rad/s (= 57.3°/s). Objects in front of the fixation plane are quickly out of focus since the retinal image slip velocity becomes too large (e.g. 100% larger for objects moving at the same velocity but at a distance of 0.5 m; see solid grey curve crossing the unity gain line at 1 m in Fig. 3.4B) whereas the image of objects further away blur because the eye moves too fast. The depth range centred around the observer's fixation plane, where the retinal image remains stabile, is thus much narrower in the case of translations compared to rotations (see shaded areas in Fig. 3.4B).

The second major function parameter that the translational VORs need to account for, apart from the slightly differing viewing distance for each eye, is *target eccentricity* (Angelaki et al., 2000; McHenry and Angelaki 2000, 2003; Paige and Tomko, 1991a, 1991b). During a head displacement, say by moving one step sidewards or forwards, both distance and eccentricity of fixation targets generally change with respect to the eyes, challenging fixation stability. Although there are strong visual mechanisms that help stabilizing the retinal image, they are typically not fast enough to counteract high frequency-small amplitude disturbances of head position due to the relative long processing delays. Here, the afferent inflow from the otolith receptors carries, on a population basis, graded magnitude and directional information of head acceleration, covering a large angular range at very short latencies. This information is optimally suited for estimating changes in the direction and magnitude of head velocity. A number of studies have shown that the functional interplay of these two geometric factors in the translational VOR can be summarized by the relation

$$d\vartheta/dt = (v_H/d)\sin(\alpha_H - \vartheta)$$

(α_H: heading direction, ϑ direction angle of gaze relative to the observer's mid sagittal plane; Angelaki and Hess, 2001; Hess and Angelaki, 2003; Paige, 1991; Paige and Tomko, 1991; Schwarz and Miles, 1989). The angular velocity described by this equation is in general different for each eye, reflecting their different vantage points. Thus, unless the observer looks at objects far ahead, the angles of the gaze lines of the right and the left eye differ when foveating an object of regard. On this basis, otolith-ocular reflexes are automatically involved in the early control of the vergence of the eyes (Busettini et al., 1991; Schwarz and Miles, 1991). The gain and sensitivity of both rotational and translational reflexes are not only modulated by absolute target distance, but also by target eccentricity. In the case of translation, this modulation depends on the translation direction ('heading direction') relative to the gaze line foveating the target. An important feature is the switch in the polarity of the velocity of each eye when the gaze line crosses the direction of heading. More specifically, when the observer changes fixation from one object of regard on one side to another one on the other side relative the direction of heading (e.g. during running), the velocity for keeping track of the new fixation object must switch sign. Conversely, depending on the direction of disturbance, the reflex must switch polarity in order to help retinal image stabilization. This property is reflected in the equation by the sine of the angle subtended by the heading direction and the gaze line. It captures the visual consequences of fore-aft translation on vision. The resulting pattern of optic flow on the retinae consists of flow lines that emanate to the right and the left of a neutral point with increasing speed. The location of the neutral point is in the direction, where the gaze line coincides with the heading direction (i.e. the directions where $\alpha_H = \vartheta_R$ for the right eye and $\alpha_H = \vartheta_L$ for the left eye). As a consequence, the retinal image can only locally be stabilized against a translational disturbance in for-aft direction (for recent reviews see: Angelaki and Hess, 2005; Miles, 1993, 1998).

Most experimental studies of the translational VOR have used one of two prototypical paradigms, which have qualitatively different visual consequences for the observer: One paradigm consists of transient or sinusoidal translations from side to side. In this case version eye movements are called for to compensate the visual consequences of translation because the heading direction is orthogonal to the frontally oriented visual field (assuming the observer keeps the head immobile). The two eyes will approximately move conjugately, which is reflected in the above geometric description by the fact that the sin $(\alpha_H - \vartheta)$ stays close to one without changing polarity (e.g. sin $(\pi/3) = 0.87$ for $\vartheta \pm 30°$). The other more interesting paradigm is fore-aft translation. In this case, the retinal images of the two eyes expand as the observer moves forward and contract as he moves backward relative to a stabile focus not too far from the axis of translation. The appropriate horizontal eye movements to this optic flow pattern are vergence and divergence movements since all potential fixation objects move now towards or away from the observer. In the formal description presented above, these properties are captured in the translational VOR by the fact that the sine varies closely around zero (i.e. $|\sin(\alpha_H - \vartheta)| = |-\sin(\vartheta)| \leq 0.5$ for $\vartheta \leq \pm 30°$). Since the sine changes with a slope of unity around zero the required modulation with gaze angle is significantly stronger during fore-aft than during side-to-side translations and, most importantly, the modulations have different signs because of the required vergence of the eyes for fixating close targets. For stabilization of a fused binocular image, the eyes must therefore move disconjugately at significantly different velocities, implying that otolith-born signals must be differentially processed for each eye (Snyder et al., 1992). The described functional description of the sensitivity of fore-aft translational VOR has received experimental support by a number of studies in both humans and subhuman primates (Angelaki and Hess, 2001; Hess and Angelaki, 2003; McHenry and Angelaki, 2000; Paige and Tomko, 1991; Seidman et al., 1999).

Although a dependence on inverse viewing distance has been widely documented in both human and subhuman primates the functional dependence has been found to be typically undercompensatory (Schwarz and Miles, 1991; Telford et al., 1997). This observation suggests that the brain's estimation of absolute target distance is possibly impaired under the typical laboratory conditions (usually presentation of a single fixation target in an otherwise dark room; the target typically extinguishes shortly before motion onset to isolate the vestibular input). Disparity and efference copies from motor signals that control vergence are cues that the brain could use for absolute depth estimates (Bishop, 1989; Blohm et al., 2008; DeAngelis et al., 1998) but based on available experimental evidence it is not clear whether these cues are used in the translational VOR at all (Busettini et al., 1991; Snyder et al., 1992; Wei et al., 2003). More natural activations of the vestibular organs by combining translation with rotations have been found to improve the brain's target distance estimation, as evidenced in the translational VOR (Wei and Angelaki, 2004). Also active head movements have been shown to improve retinal image stability (Crane and Demer, 1997; Medendorp et al., 2002; Moore et al., 1999).

Taken together, the properties of the translational VORs reveal a highly developed and sophisticated machinery, which is optimally adapted to anticipate the visual consequences of translational head displacements. Since these reflexes occur at very short latency (Angelaki and McHenry, 1999; Schwarz et al., 1989) they can prepare the grounds for the slower but more powerful visual stabilization mechanisms (Busettini et al., 1997; Masson et al., 1997; for reviews see: Angelaki and Hess, 2005; Miles, 1998).

Acknowledgement

Supported by the Betty and David Koetser Foundation for Brain Research.

References

Anastasopoulos, D., Gianna, C.C., Bronstein, A.M., and Gresty, M.A. (1996). Interaction of linear and angular vestibulo-ocular reflexes of human subjects in response to transient motion. *Experimental Brain Research*, 110, 465–472.

Angelaki, D.E. (2004). Eyes on target: what neurons must do for the vestibulo-ocular reflex during linear motion. *Journal of Neurophysiology*, 92, 20–35.

Angelaki, D.E. and Hess B.J.M. (1994). Inertial representation of angular motion in the vestibular system of rhesus monkeys. I. Vestibuloocular reflex. *Journal of Neurophysiology*, 71, 1222–1249.

Angelaki, D.E. and Hess B.J.M. (1995). Inertial representation of angular motion in the vestibular system of rhesus monkeys. II. Otolith-controlled transformation that depends on an intact cerebellar nodulus. *Journal of Neurophysiology* 73, 1729–1751.

Angelaki, D.E. and Hess B.J.M. (2001). Direction of heading and vestibular control of binocular eye movements *Vision Research*, 41, 3215–3228.

Angelaki, D.E. and Hess B.J.M. (2004). Control of eye orientation: where does the brain's role end and the muscle's begin? *European Journal of Neuroscience*, 19, 1–10.

Angelaki, D.E. and Hess B.J.M. (2005). Self-motion induced eye movements: effects on visual acuity and navigation. *Nature Reviews*, 6, 966–976.

Angelaki, D.E. and McHenry M.Q. (1999). Short-latency primate vestibulo-ocular responses during translation. *Journal of Neurophysiology*, 82, 1651–1654.

Angelaki, D.E., McHenry M.Q., Dickman J.D., Newlands S.D., and Hess B.J.M. (1999). Computation of inertial motion: neural stategies to resolve ambiguous otolith information. *Journal of Neuroscience*, 19, 316–327.

Angelaki, D.E., McHenry M.Q., and Hess B.J.M. (2000). Primate translational vestibulo-ocular reflexes. I. High-frequency dynamics and three-dimensional properties during lateral motion.*Journal of Neurophysiology*, 83, 1637–1647.

Angelaki, D.E., Zhou H.H., Wei M. (2003). Foveal versus full-field visual stabilization strategies for translational and rotational head movements. *Journal of Neuroscience*, 23, 1104–1108.

Angelaki, D.E., Shaikh A.G., Green A.M., and Dickman J.D. (2004). Neurons compute internal models of the physical laws of motion. *Nature*, 430, 560–564.

Aksay E., Olasagastri I., Mensh B.D., Baker R., Goldman M.S., and Tank D.W. (2007). Functional dissection of circuitry in a neural integrator. *Nature Neuroscience*, 10, 494–505.

Aw S.T., Haslwanter T., Halmagyi G.M., Curthoys I.S., Yavor R.A., and Todd M.J. (1996). Three-dimensional vector analysis of the human vestibuloocular reflex in response to high-acceleration head rotations. I. Responses in normal subjects. *Journal of Neurophysiology*, 76, 4009–4020.

Baarsma E.A. and Collewijn H. (1975). Eye movements due to linear accelerations in the rabbit. *Journal of Physiology*, 245, 227–247.

Barr C.C., Schultheis L.W., and Robinson D.A. (1976). Voluntary, non-visual control of the human vestibulo-ocular reflex. *Acta Otolaryngologica*, 81, 365–375.

Biguer B. and Prablanc C. (1981). Modulation of the vestibulo-ocular reflex in eye-head coordination as a function of target distance in man. In A.F. Fuchs and W. Becker (eds.) *Progress in Oculomotor Research* (pp. 525–530). New York: Elsevier.

Bishop P.O. (1989). Vertical disparity, egocentric distance and stereoscopic depth constancy: A new interpretation. *Proceedings of the Royal Society of London B; Biological Sciences*, 237, 445–469.

Blohm G., Khan A.Z., Ren L., Schreiber K.M., and Crawford J.D. (2008). Depth estimation from retinal disparity requires eye and head orientation signals. *Journal of Vision*, 8, 3.1–23.

Bronstein, A.M. and Gresty, M.A. (1991). Compensatory eye movements in the presence of conflicting canal and otolith signals. *Experimental Brain Research*, 85, 697–700.

Buettner U.W., Büttner U., and Henn V. (1978). Transfer characteristics of neurons in vestibular nuclei of the alert monkey. *Journal of Neurophysiology*, 41, 1614–1628.

Buizza A., Avanzini P., and Schmid R. (1981). Visual-vestibular interaction during angular and linear body acceleration: modeling and simulation. In L. Fedina, B. Kanyar, B. Kocsis, and M. Kollai (eds.) *Mathematical and computational methods in physiology* (pp.13–19). Oxford: Pergamon.

Busettini, C., Miles, F.A., and Schwarz, .U (1991).Ocular responses to translation and their dependence on viewing distance. II. Motion of the scene. *Journal of Neurophysiology*, 66, 865–878.

Busettini C., Masson G.S., and Miles F.A. (1997). Radial optic flow induces vergence eye movements with ultra-short latencies. *Nature*, 390, 512–515.

Cannon S.C. and Robinson D.A. (1987). Loss of the neural integrator of the oculomotor system from brain stem lesions in monkey. *Journal of Neurophysiology* 57, 1383–1409.

Cheron G. and Godaux E. (1987). Disabling of the oculomotor neural integrator by kainic acid injections in the prepositus-vestibular complex of the cat. *Journal of Physiology* 394, 267–290.

Collewijn H. (1977). Eye- and head movements in freely moving rabbits. *Journal of Physiology*, 266, 471–498.

Cohen B., Matsuo V., and Raphan T. (1977). Quantitative analysis of the velocity characteristics of optokinetic nystagmus and optokinetic after-nystagmus. *Journal of Physiology*, 270, 321–344.

Collewijn H. and Smeets J.B. (2000). Early components of the human vestibulo-ocular response to head rotation: latency and gain. *Journal of Neurophysiology*, 84, 376–389.

Collewijn H., Van der Steen J., Ferman L., and Jansen T.C. (1985). Human ocular counterroll: assessment of static and dynamic properties from electromagnetic scleral coil recordings. *Experimental Brain Research*, 59, 185–196.

Crane B.T., and Demer J.L. (1997). Human gaze stabilization during natural activities: translation, rotation, magnification, and target distance effects. *Journal of Neurophysiology*, 78, 2129–2144.

Crane B.T., and Demer J.L. (1998). Human horizontal vestibulo-ocular reflex initiation: effects of acceleration, target distance, and unilateral differentation. *Journal of Neurophysiology*, 80, 1151–1166.

Crane B.T., Viirre E.S., and Demer J.L. (1997). The human horizontal vestibulo-ocular reflex during combined linear and angular acceleration. *Experimental Brain Research*, 114, 304–320. Erratum in: *Experimental Brain Research*, 1997, 117, 178.

Crawford J.D. and Vilis T. (1991). Axes of eye rotation and Listing's law during rotations of the head. *Journal of Neurophysiology*, 65, 407–423.

Crawford J.D. Cadera W., and Vilis T. (1991). Generation of torsional and vertical eye position signals by the interstitial nucleus of Cajal. *Science*, **252**, 1551–1553.

Crawford J.D., Tweed D.B., and Vilis T. (2003). Static ocular counterroll is implemented through the 3-D neural integrator. *Journal of Neurophysiology*, **90**, 2777–2784.

Dai M.J., Raphan T., and Cohen B. (1991). Spatial orientation of the vestibular system: dependence of optokinetic after-nystagmus on gravity. *Journal of Neurophysiology*, **66**, 1422–1439.

DeAngelis G.C., Cumming B.G., and Newsome W.T. (1998). Cortical area MT and the perception of stereoscopic depth. *Nature*, **394**, 677–680.

Fernández C. and Goldberg J.M. (1976a). Physiology of peripheral neurons innervating otolith organs of the squirrel monkey. I. Response to static tilts and to long-duration centrifugal force. *Journal of Neurophysiology*, **39**, 970–984.

Fernández C. and Goldberg J.M. (1976b). Physiology of peripheral neurons innervating otolith organs of the squirrel monkey. II. Directional selectivity and force-response relations. *Journal of Neurophysiology*, **39**, 985–995.

Fernández C. and Goldberg J.M. (1976c). Physiology of peripheral neurons innervating otolith organs of the squirrel monkey. III. Response dynamics. *Journal of Neurophysiology*, **39**, 996–1008.

Fleisch A. (1922). Tonische Labyrinthreflexe auf die Augenstellung. *Pflügers Archiv für die gesamte Physiologie des Menschen und der Thiere*, **194**, 554–573.

Fuchs A. (1981) Eye-Head Coordination. In A.L. Towe, E.S. Luschei (eds.) *Handbook of Behavioral Neurobiology, Vol. 5: Motor coordination* (pp. 303–366). New York: Plenum Press.

Fuhry L., Nedvidek J., Haburcakova C., and Büttner U. (2002). Non-linear interaction of angular and translational vestibulo-ocular reflex during eccentric rotation in the monkey. *Experimental Brain Research*, **143**, 303–317.

Gianna C.C., Gresty M.A., and Bronstein A.M. (1995). Influence of target distance and acceleration level on eye movements evoked by lateral acceleration steps. *Acta Otolaryngologica Supplement 520*, Pt **1**, 65–67.

Green A.M. and Angelaki D.E. (2003). Resolution of sensory ambiguities for gaze stabilization requires a second neural integrator. *Journal of Neuroscience*, **23**, 9265–9275.

Green A.M. and Angelaki D.E. (2004). An integrative neural network for detecting inertial motion and head orientation. *Journal of Neurophysiology*, **92**, 905–925.

Green A.M., Shaikh A.G., and Angelaki D.E. (2005). Sensory vestibular contributions to constructing internal models of self-motion. *Journal of Neural Engineering*, **2**, S 164–179.

Gresty M.A., Bronstein A.M., and Barratt H. (1987). Eye movement responses to combined linear and angular head movement. *Experimental Brain Research*, **65**, 377–384.

Guedry F.E. (1974). Psychophysics of vestibular sensation. In H.H. Kornhuber (ed.) *Handbook of Sensory Physiology: The Vestibular System: Part 2. Psychophysics, Applied Aspects and General Interpretation* (pp. 3–154). Berlin: Springer-Verlag.

Haslwanter T., Straumann D., Hess B.J.M., and Henn V. (1992). Static roll and pitch in the monkey: shift and rotation of Listing's plane. *Vision Research*, **32**, 1341–1348.

Hess B.J.M. (1992). Three-dimensional head angular velocity detection from otolith signals. *Biological Cybernetics*, **67**, 323–333.

Hess B.J.M. (2007). Sensorimotor transformations in spatial orientation relative to gravity. In F.W. Mast and L. Jäncke (eds.) *Spatial processing in navigation, imagery and perception* (pp. 281–300). Berlin: Springer-Verlag.

Hess B.J.M. and Angelaki D.E. (1997a). Inertial vestibular coding of motion: concepts and evidence. *Current Opinion in Neurobiology*, **7**, 860–866.

Hess B.J.M. and Angelaki D.E. (1997b). Kinematic principles of primate rotational vestibulo-ocular reflex. I. Spatial organization of fast phase velocity axes. *Journal of Neurophysiology*, **78**, 2193–2202.

Hess B.J.M. and Angelaki D.E. (1999). Oculomotor control of primary eye position discriminates between translation and tilt. *Journal of Neurophysiology*, **81**, 394–398.

Hess B.J.M. and Angelaki D.E. (2003) Gravity modulates Listing's plane orientation during both pursuit and saccades. *Journal of Neurophysiology*, **90**, 1340–1345.

Hine T. and Thorn F. (1987).Compensatory eye movements during active head rotation for near targets: effects of imagination, rapid head oscillation and vergence. *Vision Research*, **27**, 1639–1657.

Hughes A. (1971). Topopgraphical relationships between the anatomy and physiology of the rabbit visual system. *Documenta Ophthalmologica*, **30**, 33–159.

Hunter J. (1786). *Observations on certain parts of the animal oeconomy*. London.

Johnston J.L. and Sharpe J.A. (1994). The initial vestibulo-ocular reflex and its visual enhancement and cancellation in humans. *Experimental Brain Research*, **99**, 302–308.

Lambert F.M., Beck J.C., Baker R., and Straka H. (2008). Semicircular canal size determines the developmental onset of angular vestibulo-ocular reflexes in larval Xenopus. *Journal of Neuroscience*, **28**, 8086–8095.

Laurens J. and Angelaki D.E. (2011). The functional significance of velocity storage and its dependence on gravity. *Experimental Brain Research*, **210**, 407–422.

Leigh, R.J., Maas, E.F., Grossman, G.E., and Robinson, D.A. (1989). Visual cancellation of the torsional vestibulo-ocular reflex in humans. *Experimental Brain Research*, **75**, 221–226.

Lorente de Nó R. (1935). The synaptic delay of motoneurons. *American Journal of Physiology*, **111**, 272–282.

Manzoni D., Pompeiano O., and Andre P. (1998). Convergence of directional vestibular and neck signals on cerebellar purkinje cells. *Pflügers Archiv*, **435**, 617–30.

Manzoni D., Pompeiano O., Bruschini L., and Andre P. (1999). Neck input modifies the reference frame for coding labyrinthine signals in the cerebellar vermis: a cellular analysis. *Neuroscience*, **93**, 1095–1107.

Maruta J., Simpson J.I., Raphan T., and Cohen B. (2001). Orienting otolith-ocular reflexes in the rabbit during static and dynamic tilts and off-vertical axis rotation. *Vision*, **41**, 3255–3270.

Masson G.S., Busettini C., and Miles F.A. (1997). Vergence eye movements in response to binocular disparity without depth perception. *Nature*, **389**, 283–286.

Mayne R. (1974) A systems concept of the vestibular organs. In H.H. Kornhuber (ed.) *Handbook of Sensory Physiology: Vestibular System* (pp. 493–580). New York: Springer-Verlag.

Merfeld, D.M. (1996). Vestibulo-ocular reflex of the squirrel monkey during eccentric rotation with centripetal acceleration along the naso-occipital axis. *Brain Research Bulletin*, **40**, 303–309.

McHenry M.Q. and Angelaki D.E. (2000). Primate translational vestibuloocular reflexes. II. Version and vergence responses to fore-aft motion. *Journal of Neurophysiology*, **83**, 1648–1661.

Medendorp W.P., Melis B.J., Gielen C.C., and Van Gisbergen J.A. (1998). Off-centric rotation axes in natural head movements: implications for vestibular reafference and kinematic redundancy. *Journal of Neurophysiology*, **79**, 2025–2039.

Medendorp W.P., Van Gisbergen J.A., and Gielen C.C. (2002). Human gaze stabilization during active head translations. *Journal of Neurophysiology*, **87**, 295–304.

Merfeld D.M. (1995). Modeling the vestibulo-ocular reflex of the squirrel monkey during eccentric rotation and roll tilt. *Experimental Brain Research*, **106**,123–134.

Merfeld D.M. and Young L.R. (1995). The vestibulo-ocular reflex of the squirrel monkey during eccentric rotation and roll tilt. *Experimental Brain Research*, **106**, 111–122.

Merfeld D.M., Young L.R., Tomko D.L., and Paige G.D. (1991). Spatial orientation of the VOR to combined vestibular stimuli in squirrel monkey. *Acta Otolaryngologica Supplement*, **481**, 287–292.

Merfeld D.M., Young L.R., Paige G.D., and Tomko D.L. (1993). Three dimensional eye movements of squirrel monkeys following postrotatory tilt. *Journal of Vestibular Research*, **3**, 123–139.

Mergner T. and Glasauer S. (1999) A simple model of vestibular canal-otolith signal fusion. *Annals of the New York Academy of Science*, **871**, 430–434.

Miller, J.M. (2007). Understanding and misunderstanding extraocular muscle pulleys. *Journal of Vision*, **30**, 10.1–15.

Miles F.A. (1993). The sensing of rotational and translational optic flow by the primate optokinetic system. *Reviews of Oculomotor Research*, **5**, 393–403.

Miles F.A. (1998). The neural processing of 3D visual information: Evidence from eye movements. *European Journal of Neuroscience* **10**, 811–822.

Misslisch H. and Hess B.J.M. (2000). Three-dimensional vestibuloocular reflex of the monkey: optimal retinal image stabilization versus Listing's law. *Journal of Neurophysiology* **83**, 3264–3276.

Misslisch H. and Hess B.J.M. (2002). Combined influence of vergence and eye position on three-dimensional vestibulo-ocular reflex in the monkey. *Journal of Neurophysiology*, **88**, 2368–2376.

Misslisch H., Tweed D., and Hess B.J.M. (2001). Stereopsis outweighs gravity in the control of the eyes. *Journal of Neuroscience*, **21**, RC126.

Muller M. (1999). Size limitations in semicircular canal duct systems. *Journal of Theoretical Biology*, **198**, 405–437.

Misslisch H., and Tweed D. (2001). Neural and mechanical factors in eye control. *Journal of Neurophysiology*, **86**, 1877–1883.

Misslisch H., Tweed D., Fetter M., Sievering D., and Koenig E. (1994). Rotational kinematics of the human vestibuloocular reflex. III. Listing's law. *Journal of Neurophysiology*, **72**, 2490–2502.

Moore S.T., Hirasaki E., Cohen B., and Raphan T. (1999). Effect of viewing distance on the generation of vertical eye movements during locomotion. *Experimental Brain Research*, **129**, 347–361.

Nagel A. (1868). Über das Vorkommen von wahren Rollungen des Auges um die Gesichtslinie (On the occurrence of true rolling of the eye about the line of sight). *Archiv für Ophthalmologie*, **14**, 228–246.

Pastor A.M., De la Cruz R.R., and Baker R. (1994). Eye position and eye velocity integrators reside in separate brainstem nuclei. *Proceedings of the National Academy of Sciences U S A*, **91**, 807–811.

Paige G.D. (1989). The influence of target distance on eye movement responses during vertical linear motion. *Experimental Brain Research*, **77**, 585–593.

Paige G.D. (1991). Linear vestibulo-ocular reflex (LVOR) and modulation by vergence. *Acta Otolaryngologica Supplement*, **481**, 282–286.

Paige G.D., Telford L., Seidman S.H., and Barnes G.R. (1998). Human vestibuloocular reflex and its interactions with vision and fixation distance during linear and angular head movement. *Journal of Neurophysiology*, **80**, 2391–2404.

Paige G.D. and Tomko D.L. (1991). Eye movement responses to linear head motion in the squirrel monkey. I. Basic characteristics. *Journal of Neurophysiology*, **65**, 1170–1182.

Pastor A.M., De la Cruz R.R., and Baker R. (1994). Eye position and eye velocity integrators reside in separate brainstem nuclei. *Proceedings of the National Academy of Sciences U S A*, **91**, 807–811.

Precht, W. (1978). *Neuronal Operations in the Vestibular System. Studies of Brain Function, Vol. 2*. Berlin: Springer-Verlag.

Precht, W., Simpson, J.I., and Llinás, R. (1976). Responses of Purkinje cells in rabbit nodulus and uvula to natural vestibular and visual stimuli. *Pflügers Archiv European Journal of Physiology*, **367**, 1–6.

Quaia C. and Optican L.M. (1998). Commutative saccadic generator is sufficient to control a 3-D ocular plant with pulleys. *Journal of Neurophysiology*, **79**, 3197–3215.

Rabbitt R.D. (1999). Directional coding of three-dimensional movements by the semicircular canals. *Biological Cybernetics*, **80**, 417–431.

Raphan, T. (1998). Modeling control of eye orientation in three dimensions I. Role of muscle pulleys in determining saccadic trajectory. *Journal of Neurophysiology*, **79**, 2653–2667.

Raphan T. and Cohen B. (1988). Organization principles of velocity storage in three dimensions: effects of gravity on cross-coupling of optokinetic after-nystagmus. *Annals of the New York Academy of Science*, **545**, 74–92.

Raphan T. and Sturm D. (1991). Modeling the spatiotemporal organization of velocity storage in the vestibuloocular reflex by optokinetic studies. *Journal of Neurophysiology*, **66**, 1410–1421.

Raphan T., Matsuo V., and Cohen B. (1977). A velocity storage mechanism responsible for optokinetic nystagmus (OKN), optokinetic after-nystagmus (OKAN) and vestibular nystagmus. In R. Baker and A. Berthoz (eds.) *Control of gaze by brain stem neurons* (pp. 37–47). Amsterdam: Elsevier.

Raphan T., Matsuo V., and Cohen B. (1979). Velocity storage in the vestibulo-ocular reflex arc (VOR). *Experimental Brain Research*, **35**, 229–248.

Robinson D.A. (1977). Vestibular and optokinetic symbiosis: an example of explaining by modeling. In R. Baker and A. Berthoz (eds.) *Control of gaze by brain stem neurons* (pp 49–58). Amsterdam: Elsevier.

Robinson D.A. (1981). The use of control systems analysis in the neurophysiology of eye movements. *Annual Review in Neuroscience* **4**, 463–503.

Robinson D.A. (1986). The systems approach to the oculomotor system. *Vision Research* **26**, 92–99.

Schmid-Priscoveanu, A., Straumann, D., and Kori, A.A. (2000). Torsional vestibulo-ocular reflex during whole-body oscillation in the upright and the supine position. I. Responses in healthy human subjects. *Experimental Brain Research*, **134**, 212–219.

Schwarz U., Bussettini C., and Miles F.A.(1989). Ocular responses to translation are inversely proportional to viewing distance. *Science*, **245**, 1394–1396.

Schwarz U. and Miles F.A. (1991). Ocular responses to translation and their dependence on viewing angle. *Journal of Neurophysiology*, **66**, 851–864.

Sargent E.W. and Paige G.D. (1991). The primate vestibulo-ocular reflex during combined linear and angular head motion. *Experimental Brain Research*, **87**, 75–84.

Seidman S.H., Leigh R.J., Tomsak R.L., Grant M.P., and Dell'Osso L.F. (1995a). Dynamic properties of the human vestibulo-ocular reflex during head rotations in roll. *Vision Research*, **35**, 679–689.

Seidman S.H., Telford L., and Paige G.D. (1995b). Vertical, horizontal, and torsional eye movement responses to head roll in the squirrel monkey. *Experimental Brain Research*, **104**, 218–226.

Seidman S.H., Paige G.D., and Tomko, D.L. (1999). Adaptive plasticity in the naso-occipital linear vestibulo-ocular reflex. *Experimental Brain Research*, **125**, 485–494

Seidman S.H., Paige G.D., Tomlinson R.D., and Schmitt N. (2002). Linearity of canal-otolith interaction during eccentric rotation in humans. *Experimental Brain Research*, **147**, 29–37.

Seung H.S. (1996). How the brain keeps the eyes still. *Proceedings of the National Academy of Sciences USA*, 93, 13339–13344.

Shaikh A.G., Meng H., and Angelaki D.E. (2004). Multiple reference frames for motion in the primate cerebellum. *Journal of Neuroscience*, **24**, 4491–4497.

Shaikh A.G., Green A.M., Ghasia F.F., Newlands S.D., Dickman J.D., and Angelaki D.E. (2005). Sensory convergence solves a motion ambiguity problem. *Current Biology*, **15**, 1657–1662.

Skavenski A.A. and Robinson D.A. (1973). Role of abducens neurons in vestibulooocular reflex. *Journal of Neurophysiology*, **36**, 724–738.

Smith M.A. and Crawford J.D. (1998). Neural control of rotational kinematics within realistic vestibuloocular coordinate systems. *Journal of Neurophysiology*, **80**, 2295–2315.

Snyder L.H. and King W.M. (1992). Effect of viewing distance and location of the axis of head rotation on the monkey's vestibuloocular reflex. I. Eye movement responses. *Journal of Neurophysiology*, **67**, 861–874.

Snyder L.H. and King W.M. (1996). Behavior and physiology of the macaque vestibulo-ocular reflex response to sudden off-axis rotation: computing eye translation. *Brain Research Bulletin*, **40**, 293–301; discussion 302.

Snyder L.H., Lawrence D.M., and King W.M. (1992). Changes in vestibulo-ocular reflex (VOR) anticipate changes in vergence angle in monkey. *Vision Research*, **32**, 569–575.

Straka H. and Dieringer N. (2004). Basic organization principles of the VOR: lessons from frogs. *Progress in Neurobiology*, **73**, 259–309.

Szentágothai J. (1950). The elementary vestibulo-ocular reflex arc. *Journal of Neurophysiology*, **13**, 395–407.

Tabak S. and Collewijn H. (1994). Human vestibulo-ocular responses to rapid, helmet-driven head movements. *Experimental Brain Research*, **102**, 367–378.

Tchelidze T. and Hess B.J.M. (2008). Noncommutative control in the rotational vestibulo-ocular reflex. *Journal of Neurophysiology*, **99**, 96–111.

Thurtell M.J., Black R.A., Halmagyi G.M., Curthoys I.S., and Aw S.T. (1999). Vertical eye position-dependence of the human vestibuloocular reflex during passive and active yaw head rotations. *Journal of Neurophysiology*, **81**, 2415–2428.

Telford L., Seidman S.H., and Paige G.D. (1996). Canal-otolith interactions driving vertical and horizontal eye movements in the squirrel monkey. *Experimental Brain Research*, **109**, 407–418.

Telford L., Seidman S.H., and Paige G.D. (1997). Dynamics of squirrel monkey linear vestibuloocular reflex and interactions with fixation distance. *Journal of Neurophysiology*, **78**, 1775–1790.

Telford L., Seidman S.H., and Paige G.D. (1998). Canal-otolith interactions in the squirrel monkey vestibulo-ocular reflex and the influence of fixation distance. *Experimental Brain Research*, **118**, 115–125.

Tweed D. and Vilis T. (1987). Implications of rotational kinematics for the oculomotor system in three dimensions. *Journal of Neurophysiology*, **58**, 832–849.

Tweed D. and Vilis T. (1990). Geometric relations of eye position and velocity vectors during saccades. *Vision Research*, **30**, 111–127.

Tweed D., Sievering D., Misslisch H., Fetter M., Zee D., and Koenig E. (1994). Rotational kinematics of the human vestibuloocular reflex. I. Gain matrices. *Journal of Neurophysiology*, **72**, 2467–2479.

Van der Hoeve J. and De Kleijn A. (1917). Tonische Labyrinthreflexe auf die Augen. *Pflügers Archiv für die gesamte Physiologie des Menschen und der Thiere*, **169**, 241–262.

Viéville T., and Faugeras O.D. (1990). Cooperation of the inertial and visual systems. In T.C. Henderson (ed.) *Traditional and non-traditional robotic sensors* (pp. 339–350). New York: Springer-Verlag.

Viirre E.S. and Demer J.L. (1996a). The vestibulo-ocular reflex during horizontal axis eccentric rotation and near target fixation. *Annals of the New York Academy of Science*, **781**, 706–708.

Viirre E.S., and Demer J.L. (1996b). The human vertical vestibulo-ocular reflex during combined linear and angular acceleration with near-target fixation. *Experimental Brain Research*, **112**, 313–324.

Viirre E., Tweed D., Milner K., and Vilis T. (1986). A reexamination of the gain of the vestibuloocular reflex. *Journal of Neurophysiology*, **56**, 439–450.

von Helmholtz, H. (1867). *Handbuch der Physiologischen Optik*. Leipzig: Leopold Voss. English translation from the 3rd German edition (Hamburg and Leipzig: Leopold Voss, 1909): *Helmholtz's Treatise on Physiological Optics*, J.P.C. Southall (ed), Optical Society of America, 3 vols, 1924.

Waespe W., and Henn V. (1977). Neuronal activity in the vestibular nuclei of the alert monkey during vestibular and optokinetic stimulation. *Experimental Brain Research*, **27**, 523–538.

Waespe W., and Henn V. (1978). Conflicting visual-vestibular stimulation and vestibular nucleus activity in alert monkeys. *Experimental Brain Research*, **33**, 203–211.

Wei M., and Angelaki D.E. (2004). Viewing distance dependence of the vestibulo-ocular reflex during translation: extra-otolith influences. *Vision Research*, **44**, 933–942.

Wei M., DeAngelis G.C., and Angelaki D.E. (2003). Do visual cues contribute to the neural estimate of viewing distance used by the oculomotor system? *Journal of Neuroscience*, **23**, 8340–8350.

Wilson V.J., and Melville-Jones G (1979). *Mammalian Vestibular Physiology*, New York: Plenum Press.

Wells M.J. (1963). The orientation of Octopus. *Ergebnisse der Biologie* **26**, 40–54.

Yakusheva T.A., Shaikh A.G., Green A.M., Blazquez P.M., Dickman J.D., and Angelaki D.E. (2007). Purkinje cells in posterior cerebellar vermis encode motion in an inertial reference frame. *Neuron*, **54**, 973–985.

Yakusheva T., Blazquez P.M., and Angelaki D.E. (2008). Frequency-selective coding of translation and tilt in macaque cerebellar nodulus and uvula. *Journal of Neuroscience*, **28**, 9997–10009.

Yarbus A.L. (1976). *Eye movements and vision*. New York: Plenum Press

Young L.R. (1984). Perception of body in space: Mechanisms. In I. Darian-Smith (ed.) *Handbook of physiology: The nervous system, Volume III. Sensory Processes, Part 1* (pp. 1023–1066), Bethesda, MD: American Physiological Society.

Zhou H.H., Wei M., and Angelaki D.E. (2002). Motor scaling by viewing distance of early visual motion signals during smooth pursuit. *Journal of Neurophysiology*, **88**, 2880–2885.

Zupan L.H., Merfeld D.M., and Darlot C. (2002). Using sensory weighting to model the influence of canal, otolith and visual cues on spatial orientation and eye movements. *Biological Cybernetics*, **86**, 209–230.

CHAPTER 4

The optokinetic reflex

C. Distler and K.-P. Hoffmann

Abstract

The present chapter describes the structures in the visual system relevant for the optokinetic reflex (OKR), their evolution and functional significance, as well as the neuronal substrate in vertebrates. After a phylogenetic overview of representative vertebrates investigated so far, the OKR in mammals will be described to characterize ontogenetic changes as well as certain pathologies. This will emphasize the importance of this basic reflex for judging developmental stage, damage after acquired lesions or maldevelopment, and for diagnosis of neurological disorders.

The optokinetic nystagmus has been noted by physicians for centuries (for review see Bender and Shanzer, 1983). In 1825, Purkinje described how optokinetic nystagmus is elicited by watching a unidirectionally moving scene, e.g. a cavalry parade, but only since 1907 has the optokinetic nystagmus been systematically investigated when Barany introduced the rotating striped cylinder or drum in front of the subject to elicit repetitive to and fro eye movements. Today the optokinetic reflex (OKR) is recognized as a basic mechanism to stabilize the image of the world on the retina during self-motion or in a moving environment. A stable image is a prerequisite for the visual analysis of fine detail in the world. To achieve this, the moving scene or object is pursued covertly by slow eye movements (slow phase of the OKR) which are interrupted by saccades (fast phase of the OKR). Importantly, the saccades shift the movements of the eyes (Schlagfeld) against the direction of the stimulus in mammals but rarely in other vertebrates. Lesions of the frontal eye field abolished this behaviour in rats (Bähring et al., 1994).

During the slow phase the difference between stimulus velocity and eye velocity (retinal slip) serves as an error signal to drive this compensatory circuit. In general, the underlying neuronal pathway is well understood in most vertebrates. Therefore, for decades the OKR has served as a model system to study the evolution, ontogeny, and pathology of the visual system. In this chapter first the current knowledge about the OKR and its underlying neural substrate in fish, amphibians, reptiles, and birds will be summarized. Then the OKR in mammals, which is probably best understood, is considered, notably, its neural substrate, the ontogeny, and also the pathology of the OKR and what can be learned from it will be elaborated.

Phylogeny of the optokinetic reflex

In most vertebrates, certainly in those with yoked eye movements, horizontal OKR (hOKR) is symmetrical during binocular vision, i.e. stimulus movement in clockwise and counterclockwise directions are equally effective in eliciting optokinetic eye movements. During monocular stimulation, however, hOKR often is highly asymmetrical, i.e. mostly only temporonasal stimulation seen by the viewing eye will elicit hOKR (Fig. 4.1). Monocular hOKR (mhOKR) varies between species, and

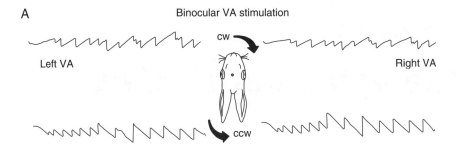

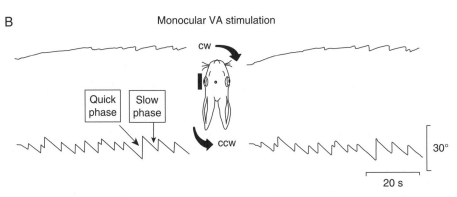

Fig. 4.1 Eye position recordings of both eyes from rabbit during binocular (A) and monocular (B) viewing of stimuli moving horizontally (vertical axis VA) at 2°/s in clockwise (CW) and counterclockwise (CCW) direction showing the typical see-saw pattern of optokinetic nystagmus with slow phase eye-movements in stimulus direction and quick phase resetting saccades. Whereas during binocular stimulation OKR responses are equal in both directions (symmetrical eye movements of both eyes as shown in (A)) closing of the left eye leads to an asymmetric response only to clockwise stimulation with stimulus movement from temporal to nasal for the seeing eye (B). Note that the closed eye moves conjugately in amplitude and frequency which is a specific trait of mammals. Reprinted from *Journal of Neurophysiology*, **69**, Tan, H.S., van der Stehen, J., Simpson, J.I., and Collewijn, H., Three-dimensional organization of optokietic responses in the rabbit, pp. 303–317, fig 2, © 1993 The American Physiological Society, used with permission.

various hypotheses have been put forward to explain these species-specific differences. Tauber and Atkin (1968) proposed that retinal specializations as foveae might be responsible for symmetric mhOKR. By contrast, Fukuda and Tokita (1957) suggested that the presence of ipsilaterally projecting retinofugal fibres might predetermine symmetry of hOKR. According to Ter Braak (1936), frontal eyed animals with large binocular visual overlap have a more symmetric mhOKR. Other authors suggested a correlation with lifestyle (Dieringer et al., 1992; Fritsches and Marshall, 2002). As summarized by Masseck and Hoffmann (2009), none of these hypotheses alone seems to hold true for all vertebrates. Figure 4.2 summarizes the ability of various vertebrates to match stimulus movement at various frequencies by slow phase eye movements.

In *sharks* (class Chondrichthyes), no data are available about optokinetic eye movements probably due to their undulating permanent swimming behaviour (Harris, 1965). Under laboratory conditions, no OKR could be elicited during binocular or monocular viewing in the spotted dogfish (*Scyliorhinus canicula*) (Masseck and Hoffmann, 2008). The neuronal visuomotor substrate for gaze stabilization probably is represented by neurons in the pretectal corpus geniculatum laterale (not homologous to the mammalian lateral geniculate!). About 35% of these neurons were selective for certain stimulus directions, and all directional preferences were equally represented. Another 10% were axis-selective,

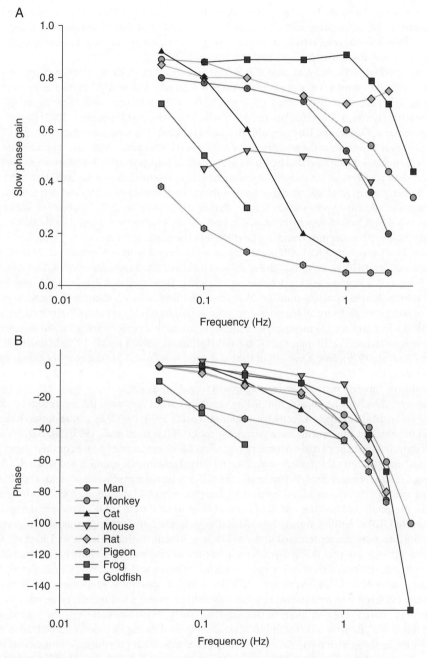

Fig. 4.2 Quality of optokinetic eye movements in various vertebrates presented in BODE plots. A) Slow phase gain (ordinate) in response to sinusoidal optokinetic stimulation at various frequencies. B) Phase shift (ordinate) between stimulus and slow phase eye movement during sinusoidal optokinetic stimulation (frequency (Hz)) (abscissa). Plots are based on data from the literature (cat: Godaux and Vanderkelen, 1984; frog: Dieringer and Precht, 1982; goldfish: Beck et al., 2004; human: Pola et al., 1987, 1993; Yasui and Young, 1984; monkey: Boyle et al., 1985; mouse: Van Alphen et al., 2002; pigeon: Gioanni, 1988; rat: Hess et al., 1985).

i.e. for stimulation along the horizontal, vertical, or oblique axes, respectively. The remaining neurons were found to be just motion sensitive. Notably, the activity of direction-selective neurons was elevated above spontaneous activity strongly during stimulation in the preferred but also although weakly in the null-direction (Masseck and Hoffmann, 2008).

In *teleosts* (class Osteichthyes), mhOKR is highly diverse. In goldfish, rainbow trout, sea bass (*Serranus cabrilla*), sandlance, and pipefish mhOKR is largely symmetrical at least at low stimulus velocities, whereas in zebrafish, butterfly fish, perch (*Perca fluviatilis*), and pike (*Esox lucius*) mhOKR is asymmetric (Easter, 1972; Fritsches and Marshall, 2002; Klar and Hoffmann, 2002; Rinner et al., 2005; Hoffmann, Kunkel and Klar, unpublished observations). The visuomotor interface for OKR in teleosts has been identified as the area praetectalis (Klar and Hoffmann, 2002; Masseck and Hoffmann, 2009). This nucleus is characterized by a high prevalence of direction-selective neurons. As in sharks, all directional preferences for stimulus movement are represented in one nucleus. In trout and in goldfish neuronal activity is elevated during stimulation in preferred direction and decreases moderately or not at all below spontaneous activity during stimulation in null-direction. Lesions in this nucleus in goldfish lead to deficits in mOKR in horizontal as well as in vertical directions, whereas a vertical optokinetic nystagmus could not be elicited in the rainbow trout.

Amphibians (class Amphibia) stabilize their gaze by body and head movements rather than by eye movements. Nevertheless, even though eye movements have low amplitudes mhOKR is asymmetrical in frogs and salamanders (e.g. Cochran et al., 1984; Dieringer and Precht, 1982; Manteuffel, 1984). Within the neuronal substrate for OKR, in amphibians, as in all other tetrapods, the representation of horizontal and vertical stimulus directions is now largely sorted into different nuclei. In the pretectal nucleus lentiformis mesencephali (nLM) neurons that prefer horizontal movements with largely temporonasal direction prevail (Katte and Hoffmann, 1980; Li et al., 1996; Manteuffel, 1984; but see Fite et al., 1979). In the nucleus of the basal optic root (nBOR) in the accessory optic system, vertical and other directions are represented (Lazar, 1983; Montgomery et al., 1982). Lesions of the basal optic root abolish vertical head nystagmus in frogs (Lazar, 1983).

In *reptiles* (class Reptilia), again, mhOKR is variable. Turtles can move their eyes independently, and show variable but largely asymmetric responses (Ariel, 1990, 1997). By contrast, the chameleon also has unyoked eye movements but a symmetric mhOKR (Gioanni et al., 1993; Ott, 2001). Various geckos show complete or partial asymmetry regardless of the presence of a fovea or their lifestyle, i.e. being nocturnal or diurnal (Masseck et al., 2008). Diurnal and foveate agamids and iguanids (*Pogona vitticeps, Cyclura cornuta*) display symmetric mhOKR, nocturnal and afoveate scincids and alligators (*Scincus scincus, Caiman crocodilus*) have an asymmetric mhOKR (Wachholz, 2008). As in amphibians, the pretectal nLM and the nBOR of the accessory optic system (AOS) represent the neuronal substrate for OKR in reptiles. Again, the nLM codes predominantly for temporonasal directions. The remaining directions are represented in the nBOR (e.g. Rosenberg and Ariel, 1990; Fan et al., 1995).

In *birds* (class Aves), mhOKR is asymmetrical but not as much as would have been expected from the lateral eye position of most of the species studied (Conley and Fite, 1980; Gioanni et al., 1981; Wallman and Pettigrew, 1985; Wallman and Velez, 1985). Importantly, gain of gaze stabilization by combined eye-head movements increases significantly, especially to high stimulus velocity when pigeons are put in a flying condition (Gioanni and Sansonetti, 1999) demonstrating the context specificity of this 'reflex'. Barn owls are the only birds studied so far showing an almost symmetrical mhOKR. Intriguingly, in young barn owls mhOKR is asymmetrical with lower gain during nasotemporal stimulation. This asymmetry disappears with age first for lower velocities (<10°/s) and last for middle range velocities (40°/s) (Wagner et al., 1993). This is very similar to the development of OKR in infant primates as will be described later (see section 'Development of the optokinetic reflex in mammals').

Again, nBOR neurons predominantly prefer vertical stimulus movements but units with nasotemporal preference also exist (Burns and Wallman, 1981; Gioanni et al., 1983b; 1984; Morgan and Frost, 1981; Wylie and Frost, 1990). The pretectal nLM predominantly contains neurons with temporonasal preferred directions, and lesions of this nucleus affect mainly hOKR (Gioanni et al., 1983a; Winterson and Brauth, 1985; Xiao et al., 2001).

Based on their location in the brain, their neuronal connections, their neuronal response properties, and their function as ascertained by lesions, the nLM of lower tetrapods has been homologized with the pretectal nucleus of the optic tract (NOT) of mammals, whereas the nBOR proper seems to correspond to the medial terminal nucleus (MTN), and the dorsal part of the nBOR to the lateral terminal nucleus (LTN) of the AOS in mammals (McKenna and Wallman, 1985).

The optokinetic reflex in mammals

The hypothesis that symmetry of mhOKR is linked to the position of the eyes in the head, i.e. frontal versus lateral, and by that to the size of a binocular field of viewing holds really only true for mammals (e.g. rat: Hess et al., 1985; rabbit: Collewijn, 1969; cat: Schweigart and Hoffmann, 1988; ferret: Hein et al., 1990; monkey: Pasik and Pasik, 1975).

In mammals the neuronal substrate for OKR has been most thoroughly investigated. The visuomotor interface in the neuronal circuit subserving the horizontal OKR is the pretectal nucleus of the optic tract and the dorsal terminal nucleus (NOT-DTN) of the accessory optic system, and for vertical OKR the lateral and medial terminal nuclei of the AOS. Retinal slip neurons in these nuclei are characterized by strongly direction selective responses to ipsiversive (NOT-DTN) or vertical (LTN, MTN) stimulation. Figure 4.3 demonstrates the direction selective responses of an LTN neuron (Mustari and Fuchs, 1989), and of a population of NOT-DTN neurons in macaques (Hoffmann and Distler, 1989). During stimulation to the left the neuronal activity in the left NOT-DTN is elevated above, during stimulation to the right, its activity is suppressed below spontaneous activity, and vice versa. Comparing the activity in the left and the right nucleus would thus increase the possible neuronal modulation depth and thereby the driving force for the OKR in a push–pull fashion (Hoffmann, 1982). The ipsiversive push was demonstrated by elevating the activity in one nucleus by electrical stimulation, e.g. stimulating the left NOT-DTN will elicit slow phases to the left (e.g. Kato et al., 1988; Hoffmann and Fischer, 2001; Ilg et al., 1993; Schiff et al., 1988). The contraversive pull was demonstrated by inactivating one nucleus by electrolytic lesions or muscimol injections, e.g. inactivating the right NOT-DTN will also cause slow phases to the left (Hoffmann and Fischer, 2001). This result is further demonstrated by the polar plots in Fig. 4.4. Whereas OKR in intact cats can be elicited equally well in upward and horizontal directions and somewhat diminished in downward direction, OKR towards the left hemifield was almost completely lost after inactivation of the left NOT-DTN (Hoffmann and Fischer, 2001). These accessory optic nuclei transmit the visual information via their projections to the inferior olive, the nucleus praepositus hypoglossi, the nucleus reticularis tegmenti pontis, and the dorsolateral pontine nucleus to the cerebellum and to oculomotor structures (for reviews see Simpson et al., 1988; Giolli et al., 2006) (Fig. 4.5).

The NOT and nuclei of the AOS receive direct input from ON-direction selective retinal ganglion cells (Buhl and Peichl, 1986; Dann and Buhl, 1987; Grasse et al., 1990; Hoffmann and Stone, 1985; Knapp et al., 1988; Kogo et al., 1998; Oyster et al., 1972, 1980; Rosenberg and Ariel, 1991; Yonehara et al., 2009).

The origin of retinal direction selectivity has fascinated scientists for decades but is still not fully understood. It is evident, however, that cholinergic and GABAergic starburst amacrine cells play a crucial role. Starburst amacrine cells are characterized by a radially symmetric dendritic tree that exerts directionally selective GABAergic inhibition on direction selective retinal ganglion cells (Fried et al., 2002; Lee and Zhou, 2006; Taylor and Vaney, 2002). Intriguingly, two-photon microscopy calcium imaging has shown that individual starburst dendrites are direction selective for stimulus movement from their soma to the tip of the dendrites. This direction selectivity is independent of inhibitory networks and likely depends on voltage gated channels and dendritic voltage gradients (Euler et al., 2002; Hausselt et al., 2007; Lee and Zhou, 2006). Furthermore, asymmetric distribution of cation-chloride cotransporters and by that of the chloride equilibrium potential seems to play a crucial role in the generation of direction selectivity in starburst dendrites and retinal

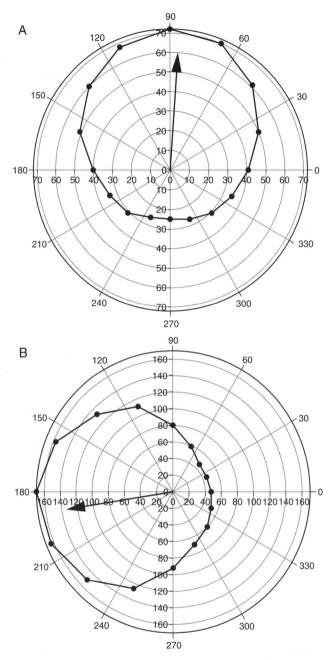

Fig. 4.3 Polar plots of the preferred directions of a representative LTN neuron (A) and a population of neurons in the left NOT-DTN in macaques. LTN neurons clearly prefer vertical stimulus movements, NOT-DTN neurons (B) prefer ipsiversive horizontal movement, in this case to the left. Data were taken and redrawn from Mustari and Fuchs (1989) and Hoffmann and Distler (1989).

ganglion cells (Gavrikov et al., 2003, 2006). In addition to asymmetric input–output relationships on starburst dendrites, a spatially offset lateral inhibition between neighbouring starburst amacrines (Fried et al., 2005; Lee and Zhou, 2006), local postsynaptic signal processing in the ganglion cells seems to be critical (Gavrikov et al., 2003, 2006; Oesch et al., 2005; for review see Zhou and Lee, 2008) for the generation of retinal direction selectivity. That these retinal circuits indeed play a crucial role

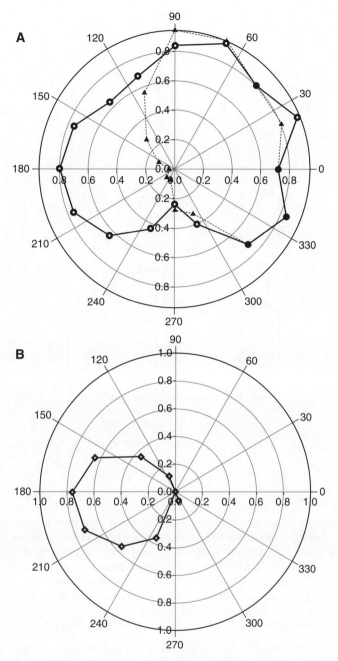

Fig. 4.4 A) Polar plots of slow phase gain of cat OKR during visual stimulation in 16 different directions. Intact cats respond to horizontal and upward directions equally well, to downward motion slightly less (open circles, continuous line). After inactivation of the left NOT-DTN horizontal optokinetic responses are limited to movements to the right, i.e. away from the lesioned side (triangles, dotted line). B) Polar plot demonstrating the difference between control condition and condition after left NOT deactivation. The tuning of the 'missing gain' to the left is very reminiscent to the directional tuning of the now deactivated neurons in the left NOT-DTN (Fig. 4.3B). Reprinted from *Vision Research*, **41** (25–26), Klaus-Peter Hoffmann and Wolfgang H. Fischer, Directional effect of inactivation of the nucleus of the optic tract on optokinetic nystagmus in the cat, pp. 3389–3398, © 2001, with permission from Elsevier.

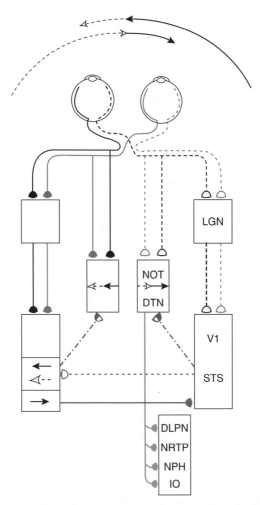

Fig. 4.5 Neuronal substrate for the processing of visual information for the horizontal optokinetic reflex in primates. Visual information reaches the NOT-DTN directly via retinofugal projections and indirectly via the lateral geniculate nucleus (LGN) and visual cortical areas (V1, motion sensitive areas in the superior temporal sulcus STS). Retinal slip cells in turn project to the inferior olive (IO), the nucleus reticularis tegmenti pontis (NRTP), the nucleus praepositus hypoglossi (NPH), and the dorsolateral pontine nucleus (DLPN). Black lines and symbols represent projections from the left eye, grey lines and symbols projections from the right eye. Binocular projections are shown by broken lines with dots. Continuous lines and filled symbols indicate information from the right hemifield, broken lines and open symbols information from the left hemifield.

for the optokinetic system has conclusively been demonstrated by ablation experiments in sauropsids and mammals. Selective destruction of starburst amacrine cells leads to a loss of direction selectivity in retinal ganglion cells and visuomotor neurons in the brain as well as to a loss of OKR (chicken: Reymond and Morgan, 1990; Yang and Morgan, 1990; mouse: Yoshida et al., 2001; rabbit: Amthor et al., 2002). Cholinergic amacrine cells have been described in reptile but not in amphibian retinae (Nguyen and Grzywacz, 2000; Nguyen et al., 2000; Vigh et al., 2000). However, to date, the role of cholinergic amacrine cells for the optokinetic system has not been ascertained in these animals. Blockage of retinal ON-channels with 2-amino-4-phosphonobutyric acid (APB) leads to a loss of direction selectivity in the nBOR, and to a loss of OKR in turtles (Ariel and Rosenberg, 1991). In rabbit, the eye injected with APB can no longer drive OKR (Knapp et al., 1988). In cat, APB causes a significant reduction in OKR gain over the whole velocity range tested and in both temporonasal and nasotemporal directions but no loss of OKR indicating that an additional input to the NOT-DTN has to supplement the retinal information (Hoffmann, 1986). Indeed, APB injection in cats with cortical lesions leads to a complete loss of OKR driven through the injected eye (Knapp et al., 1988). Retinal input to the NOT-DTN in non-primate mammals originates exclusively or predominantly from the contralateral eye. By contrast, in primates the retina projects bilaterally to the NOT-DTN (Kourouyan and Horton, 1997; Telkes et al., 2000).

In addition to the retinal input, NOT-DTN, MTN, and LTN also receive input from various cortical areas in all mammals studied so far. Projections from striate cortex have been demonstrated electrophysiologically, anatomically, and/or by lesion studies in rat (Schmidt et al., 1993; Shintani et al., 1999), guinea pig (Lui et al., 1994), ferret (Klauer et al., 1990), cat (Grasse et al., 1984; Kawamura et al., 1974; Tusa et al., 1989; Wood et al., 1973), and primates (Hoffmann et al., 1991). Additional and probably functionally more important inputs from extrastriate cortical areas, especially from motion analysing areas have been described in ferret (Distler et al., 2006; Hupfeld et al., 2007), cat (Berson and Graybiel, 1980; Marcotte and Updyke, 1982), and monkey (Distler and Hoffmann, 2001; Distler et al., 2002; Hoffmann et al., 1991, 2002, 2009; Leichnetz, 1982; Lui et al., 1995; Shook et al., 1990). What is the functional role of this cortical input? In frontal eyed mammals that normally have a symmetrical mhOKR cortical lesions lead to directional deficits in mhOKR during stimulation towards the lesioned side (Duersteler and Wurtz, 1988; Heide et al., 1996; Hupfeld et al., 2007; Lynch and McLaren, 1983; Thurston et al., 1988; Wood et al., 1973; Zee et al., 1987) as well as during vertical OKR (Grasse and Cynader, 1988) especially at higher stimulus velocities. These deficits, i.e. reduced symmetry and reduced range of effective stimulus velocities are paralleled by reduced binocularity and a response deficit during high velocity visual stimulation in the NOT-DTN and LTN, respectively (Grasse et al., 1984). Similar albeit quantitatively weaker deficits are seen in animal models with reduced cortical binocularity, i.e. strabismic cats and monkeys (Cynader and Harris, 1980; Cynader and Hoffmann, 1981; Distler, 1996; Distler and Hoffmann, 1996; Hoffmann et al., 1996; Sparks et al., 1986) and monocularly deprived animals (Hoffmann et al., 1998; Markner and Hoffmann, 1985). These data indicate that the cortical input mediates the response to high stimulus velocities via binocular projection neurons to the pretectum and accessory optic system thus promoting symmetric mhOKR also at high stimulus velocities (Fig. 4.5). However, they do not explain why lesions of an area that as an entity represents all possible directions of movements, e.g. monkey area MT, should lead to optokinetic deficits in only one particular horizontal direction. It turned out that MT and MST neurons identified by antidromic electrical stimulation to project to the NOT-DTN had the same preferred direction as their target cells in the NOT-DTN, i.e. as a population they preferred ipsiversive movement over all other directions. By contrast, MT and MST neurons projecting to the dorsolateral pontine nucleus (DLPN) had no common preferred direction on the population level thus reflecting the fact that neurons in the DLPN are direction selective but with preferences for all directions (Hoffmann et al., 2002, 2009; Thier et al., 1988). These data clearly indicate that it is the loss of a specific neuronal population, i.e. cortical neurons with ipsiversive preferred directions projecting to the NOT-DTN that causes the directional optokinetic deficits after cortical lesions.

One dilemma remains. The data described above are valid for mammals with frontal eyes that show symmetrical mhOKR. But what is the function of the cortical input to the NOT-DTN in lateral-eyed mammals, such as the rat? The rat has an asymmetric mhOKR. Cortical lesions have no effect on mhOKR (Harvey et al., 1997; but see Prusky et al., 2008). Nevertheless, areas 17, 18, and 18a do project to retinal slip cells in the NOT-DTN (Schmidt et al., 1993; Shintani et al., 1999). About half of these neurons receive both retinal and cortical input, and most retinal slip cells with cortical input are binocular. Either a proportion of 45% of retinal slip cells with cortical input is not sufficient to drive a symmetric mhOKR, or the function of the cortical projection in the rat has yet to be elucidated. It is also possible that the quality of this cortical input that arises from striate and early prestriate areas differs from cortical projections from extrastriate areas, especially motion sensitive regions. In ferret, cat, and monkey, but not so far in rat and guinea pig, specialized motion sensitive areas have been described.

In ferret and cat, cortical lesions of areas 17 and 18 that spare the motion sensitive areas do not affect OKR (Hupfeld et al., 2007; Tusa et al., 1989). In monkey, the projection to the NOT-DTN arising from V1 is much weaker than that from MT and MST (Hoffmann et al., 1991). Thus, it is feasible that only input from specialized motion sensitive cortical areas provides relevant information for gaze stabilization to the NOT-DTN and the subcortical pathway for optokinesis in toto.

Anatomical investigations indicate that humans have an accessory optic system very similar to that of other mammals (Fredericks et al., 1988). Deep-brain stimulation in the pretectum performed for epileptic treatment elicited nystagmus, and the localization of the stimulating electrode suggested that this resulted from stimulation of the pretectal complex including the NOT-DTN (Taylor et al., 2000). Recently, functional imaging studies revealed the subcortical and cortical areas involved in hOKR and vertical OKR, respectively, in humans (Bense et al., 2006a, 2006b).

Development of the optokinetic reflex in mammals

Much can be learned by analysing oculomotor behaviour during ontogeny. Van Hof-Van Duin described in 1978 that OKR in kittens can only be elicited from postnatal day P19. At that time, mhOKR is completely asymmetric, i.e. nasotemporal stimulation does not elicit hOKR. The first nasotemporal reaction occurs at about 4 weeks of age and matures until symmetry is reached between 3 and 6 months of age. Only a limited range of stimulus velocities drives OKR in young kittens and this only broadens gradually during development (Malach et al., 1981; Van Hof-Van Duin, 1978). In an electrophysiological approach the visual response properties of retinal slip cells in the NOT-DTN in kittens ranging from postnatal day P18–48 were analysed. Already in P18–23 kittens, retinal slip cells were direction selective for ipsiversive stimulus movement. However, they responded only to a very limited range of stimulus velocities, the overall neuronal activity was rather low, and most cells were exclusively driven by stimuli presented to the contralateral eye. In P27–33 kittens, the ipsilateral eye's influence upon retinal slip cells had suddenly significantly increased, and the neurons now responded also to higher stimulus velocities. During further development, the neurons became more and more binocular, and additionally responded to very low stimulus velocities (Distler and Hoffmann, 1993). Thus, the development of response properties of retinal slip cells mirrors optokinetic behaviour. But what is the cause for the abrupt changes in response properties and OKR? It is probably the maturation of the cortical input to the NOT-DTN which first becomes functional at 4 weeks of age and matures thereafter (Distler et al., 1993; Schoppmann, 1985).

Developmental studies in human infants indicate that mhOKR is largely asymmetric in early childhood and becomes symmetrical during the first few weeks to months of life depending on the method and paradigms used in the measurements (Atkinson, 1979; Naegele and Held, 1982; Roy et al., 1989). As the neuronal substrate for this development cannot be studied directly in humans, macaque monkeys are an appropriate model species. In a first approach the postnatal maturation of the dorsal cortical pathway for motion analysis was analysed using the 2-deoxy-glucose method to determine at what stage the metabolic activity of the cortical areas for motion analysis becomes adult-like assuming that at this stage the efferent projections and response properties should also be functioning. At 3 months of age the glucose utilization in these areas was indistinguishable from adults (Distler et al., 1996). In a second approach, longitudinal behavioural experiments using electro-oculography investigated whether the metabolic data were matched by sudden changes in mhOKR. Unexpectedly, mhOKR could be elicited both in temporonasal and, although weaker and less reliably, in nasotemporal direction already at postnatal day 3 (P3). The maturation of symmetry of mhOKR clearly depended on the stimulus velocity. At low stimulus velocities (10–20°/s) mhOKR was largely symmetrical at 2–5 weeks of age, at medium velocities (40°/s) symmetry was reached at about 14 weeks of age, and at high velocities (80–120°/s) symmetry was reached later than 5 months of age (Distler et al., 1999). Thus, there was no close correlation between metabolic maturation of cortical areas for motion analysis and behaviour. Therefore, recently, the visual response properties of retinal slip cells in the NOT-DTN of infant macaques ranging from 1–8 weeks of age were analysed. Surprisingly, retinal slip cells at P7 were already binocular, i.e. they could be driven from both eyes but predominantly from the contralateral eye. During further development, the influence of the ipsilateral eye increased until in adulthood the majority of retinal slip cells were equally activated by both eyes. Retinal slip cells at P7 were already direction selective for ipsiversive stimulus movement. Quantitatively, this property was adult-like at P14. Retinal slip cells in infant macaques responded to a broad range of stimulus velocity (2–50°/s) but with lower neuronal modulation, i.e. smaller difference between the activity during preferred and non-preferred stimulation than in adults. In adulthood, the effective velocity range in contrast to very young animals also includes velocities lower than 1°/s (Distler and Hoffmann, 2003, 2008; Hoffmann and Distler, 1989). Obviously, there is a strong correlation between the maturation of response properties of retinal slip cells and OKR development, exemplified by the effective velocity range, and binocularity in the NOT-DTN and symmetry of mhOKR at certain velocities. However, where does the binocularity in the NOT-DTN come from? As mentioned earlier, there is a bilateral retinal projection to NOT-DTN present at birth (Kourouyan and Horton, 1997). To follow the development of the cortical projection to the NOT-DTN, areas V1 and MT were electrically stimulated while recording from NOT-DTN neurons. At P7, electrical stimulation of V1 was not successful. However, starting at P14 retinal slip cells could be orthodromically activated from V1 and from MT. Activation from MT was more reliable, stronger (i.e. more spikes elicited per pulse), and more successful (i.e. more retinal slip cells were activated). The results strengthen the hypothesis that the cortical projections from motion sensitive cortical areas are functionally more relevant than projections from V1. However, the question whether the early binocularity in the NOT-DTN originates from the bilateral retinal input or whether it is mediated via cortical areas remains unresolved. Lesion studies in children where one cortical hemisphere had to be removed before 10 months of age show that hOKR is bidirectional but asymmetric during both monocular and binocular viewing. However, hOKR towards the lesioned side becomes progressively weaker and is finally lost completely (Morrone et al., 1999). These data then indicate that in primates the retinal input to the NOT-DTN imprints the subcortical optokinetic system as has been suggested for other mammals (Hoffmann et al., 1995). Later on, the maturing cortical input takes control and the retinal input could lose its functional influence almost completely. Thus, cortical lesions at 1 year or older severely reduce or abolish OKN towards the lesioned side in humans.

Pathology of the optokinetic reflex: the case of spontaneous nystagmus

Spontaneous nystagmus is a prevalent and rather unspecific symptom in a number of neurological disorders, e.g. it can be associated with migraine, amblyopia, cataract, misrouting of retinofugal axons, strabismus, deprivation, and albinism (e.g. Abadi and Pascal, 1994; Collewijn et al., 1985; Cheong et al., 1992; Dieterich and Brandt, 1999; Guyer and Lessell, 1986; Jeong et al., 2008; McCarty et al., 1992; Schor and Westall, 1984; Simon et al., 1984; St John et al., 1984).

In a non-human primate model short-term (for the first 25–55 days of life) binocular deprivation by lid-suture that impairs motion and form perception as well as sensory fusion led to strabismus, spontaneous nystagmus, and asymmetric mhOKR (Tusa et al., 2001). By contrast, alternating monocular occlusion by opaque contact lenses caused strabismus but did not affect mhOKR or caused nystagmus. Infant macaques reared in strobe light developed nystagmus but no strabismus (Tusa et al., 2002). What is the reason for these defects? Early binocular deprivation causes several alterations in the response properties of NOT-DTN neurons that are the more pronounced the longer the deprivation lasts. Binocularity was reduced or completely lost so that NOT-DTN neurons were mainly or exclusively activated from the contralateral eye. In about half of the NOT-DTN neurons direction preference was inversed, i.e. they preferred contraversive stimulation. Nevertheless, electrical stimulation elicited ipsiversive slow phase optokinetic reaction. During latent nystagmus NOT-DTN neurons discharged during contraversive visual motion (Mustari et al., 2001). In monkeys raised with alternating monocular occlusion binocularity in V1 and consequently stereoacuity was severely impaired whereas binocularity in motion sensitive area MT and in the NOT-DTN was intact. By contrast, latent nystagmus was associated with a loss of binocularity in MT as well as in the NOT-DTN (Mustari et al., 2008; Tusa et al., 2002).

Pathology of the optokinetic reflex: the case of albinism

Oculocutaneous albinism is a mutation affecting the enzyme tyrosinase in the tyrosine metabolism. As a consequence, no melanin is formed in the skin and iris of the eye. This condition can be found in all vertebrates and invertebrates. Because of the ready availability of pigmented and albino conspecifics the neuronal consequences of albinism have been studied most thoroughly in rats, rabbits, and ferrets. It is probably the loss of DOPA, a metabolite of the tyrosine metabolism in the retinal pigment epithelium cells caused by the lack or malfunction of tyrosinase that causes alterations in the spatiotemporal maturation of the retina during ontogeny and by that an alteration of the retinofugal decussation so that an abnormal contralateral projection from the temporal retina develops (Jeffery, 1997).

Altogether, mhOKR is highly variable in albinos within and across species. The range includes normal, asymmetric, inverted, or lacking OKR in humans, an inverted mhOKR in rabbit, and a complete lack of OKR in rat and ferret (Collewijn et al., 1978, 1985; Demer and Zee, 1984; Hahnenberger, 1977; Hoffmann et al., 2004; Precht and Cazin, 1979; St John et al., 1984; but see Sirkin et al., 1985). In rabbit, the inverted mhOKR in the frontal visual field is mirrored by a reversal of direction selectivity in the frontal part of the receptive fields of NOT-DTN neurons (Winterson and Collewijn, 1981). In rat and ferret the almost complete lack of OKR is mirrored by a complete loss of direction selectivity in the NOT-DTN (Precht and Cazin, 1979; Lannou et al., 1982; Hoffmann et al., 2004). However, as shown by retrograde transport from and antidromic stimulation in the inferior olive the retinal slip cells in the NOT-DTN of albino ferrets are present (Hoffmann et al., 2004; Telkes et al., 2001). Unilateral muscimol injections into the NOT-DTN that inactivate all neurons with $GABA_A$ and $GABA_C$ receptors cause a spontaneous nystagmus with the slow phase directed away from the injected hemisphere in albino and pigmented ferrets indicating that the part of the optokinetic pathway downstream from the NOT-DTN is intact (Hoffmann et al., 2004). So what is wrong with the NOT-DTN? Three hypotheses were investigated to explain the loss of direction selectivity. First, is the retinal input to the NOT-DTN direction selective? Immunohistochemical results indicate that ON-starburst amacrine cells are reduced in albino rats but not ferrets (Blaszczyk et al., 2004). Recent *in vitro* recordings of retinal ganglion cells retrogradely labelled by tracer injections into the MTN showed that response properties of albino rat ganglion cells do not differ from those in pigmented retinae (Krause and Hoffmann, in prep.).

Second, is the projection pattern of direction-selective ganglion cells specific? If retinal cells with horizontal preferred direction would project to the NOT-DTN as well as to the LTN and MTN and vice versa this would result in an unspecific sum of inputs which could still be direction specific in the retina but, the target cells would be non-direction selective. Dual tracer injections into the NOT-DTN and into the MTN of albino and wild type ferrets revealed that only in albinos, double labelled cells occurred (1–18% of the smaller population of labelled cells), i.e. there were ganglion cells with bifurcating axons that reached both the NOT-DTN and the MTN (Distler et al., 2009).

Third, is the cortical input to the NOT-DTN functional? Orthodromic electrical stimulation in area 17 of albino and pigmented ferrets indicates that the cortical input to the NOT-DTN is significantly reduced: the success rate in pigmented ferrets amounts to 96%, in albinos only to 63% (Hoffmann et al., unpublished observations). Recently a motion-specific area in the posterior suprasylvian (PSS) cortex of the ferret was identified that is characterized by a high prevalence of direction selective neurons and projects to the NOT-DTN (Distler et al., 2006; Philipp et al., 2006). The incidence of direction selective neurons in the PSS of albino ferrets was significantly lower (72%) than in pigmented ferrets (90%).

Taken together, none of the three hypotheses alone can completely explain the loss of direction selectivity in the albino NOT-DTN. However, new evidence from patch clamp studies in acute rat brain slices indicates that at least part of the problem may lie in the NOT-DTN itself. Reversal potentials for $GABA_A$ mediated currents are more positive in albino than in pigmented NOT-DTN cells. No such difference was seen in the superior colliculus indicating the specificity of the effect for the optokinetic system. This altered reversal potential is probably due to an accumulation of intracellular chloride caused by an abnormal activity of the chloride inward cotransporter NKCC2 (Krause and Hoffmann, 2009). Thus, in addition to altered retinal and cortical inputs to the NOT-DTN changes in local inhibition within the NOT-DTN could contribute to the loss of direction selectivity in the albino NOT-DTN which then would explain the lack of the optokinetic reaction.

Final notes

The optokinetic reflex is one of the most thoroughly studied behaviours in the animal kingdom. Its neuronal substrate has been elucidated in a number of invertebrates and vertebrates which allows us to extrapolate the understanding of the circuitry, development, and pathology to humans. Because it is so easy to elicit and quantify optokinetic reactions they were and will be in the future very useful and popular to study the adaptation of vision to lifestyle, to follow the ontogeny, and to screen genetic or pathological disorders of vision.

References

Abadi, R.V. and Pascal, E. (1994). Periodic alternating nystagmus in humans with albinism. *Investigative Ophthalmology and Visual Sciences*, **35**, 4080–4086.

Amthor, F.R., Keyser, K.T., and Dmitrieva, N.A. (2002). Effects of the destruction of starburst-cholinergic amacrine cells by the toxin AF64A on rabbit retinal directional selectivity. *Visual Neuroscience*, **19**, 495–509.

Ariel, M. (1990). Independent eye movements in the turtle. *Visual Neuroscience*, **5**, 29–41.

Ariel, M. (1997). Open loop optokinetic response in the turtle. *Vision Research*, **37**, 925–933.

Ariel, M., and Rosenberg, A.F. (1991). Effects of synaptic drugs on turtle optokinetic nystagmus and the spike responses in the basal optic nucleus. *Visual Neuroscience*, **7**, 431–440.

Atkinson, J. (1979). Development of optokinetic nystagmus in the human infant and monkey infant: an analogue to development in kittens. In R.D. Freeman (ed.) *Developmental Neurobiology of Vision* (pp. 277–287). New York: Plenum.

Bähring, R., Meier, R.K., and Dieringer, N. (1994). Unilateral ablation of the frontal eye field of the rat affects the beating field of ocular nystagmus. *Experimental Brain Research*, **98**, 391–400.

Bárány, R. (1907). Die Untersuchung der reflektorischen vestibulären und optischen Augenbewegungen und ihre Bedeutung für die topische Diagnostik der Augenmuskellähmungen. *Münchner Medizinische Wochenschrift*, **54**, 1072–1075.

Beck, J.C., Gilland, E., Tank, D.W., and Baker, R. (2004). Quantifying the ontogeny of optokinetic and vestibuloocular behaviors in zebrafish, medaka, and goldfish. *Journal of Neurophysiology*, **92**, 3546–3561.

Bender, M.B. and Shanzer, S. (1983). History of optokinetic nystagmus. *Neuro-ophthalmology*, **3**, 73–88.

Bense, S., Janusch, B., Schlindwein, P., Bauermann, T., Vucurevic, G., Brandt, T., *et al.* (2006a). Direction-dependent visual cortex activation during horizontal optokinetic stimulation (fMRI study). *Human Brain Mapping*, **27**, 296–305.

Bense, S., Janusch, B., Vucurevic, G., Bauermann, T., Schlindwein, P., Brandt, T., *et al.* (2006b). Brainstem and cerebellar fMRI-activation during horizontal and vertical optokinetic stimulation. *Experimental Brain Research*, **174**, 312–323.

Berson, D.M. and Graybiel, A.M. (1980). Some cortical and subcortical fiber projections to the accessory optic nuclei in the cat. *Neuroscience*, **5**, 2203–2217.

Blaszczyk, W.M., Telkes, I., and Distler, C. (2004). GABA-immunoreactive starburst amacrine cells in pigmented and albino rats. *European Journal of Neuroscience*, **20**, 3195–3198.

Boyle, R., Buettner, U., and Markert, G. (1985). Vestibular nuclei activity and eye movements in the alert monkey during sinusoidal optokinetic stimulation. *Experimental Brain Research*, **57**, 362–369.

Buhl, E.H. and Peichl, L. (1986). Morphology of rabbit retinal ganglion cells projecting to the medial terminal nucleus of the accessory optic system. *Journal of Comparative Neurology*, **253**, 163–174.

Burns, S. and Wallman, J. (1981). Relation of single unit properties to the oculomotor function of the nucleus of the basal optic root (accessory optic system) in chickens. *Experimental Brain Research*, **42**, 171–180.

Cheong, P.Y.Y., King, R.A., and Bateman, J.B. (1992). Oculocutaneous albinism: variable expressivity of nystagmus in a sibship. *Journal of Pediatric Ophthalmology and Strabismus*, **29**, 185–188.

Cochran, S.L., Dieringer, N., and Precht, W. (1984). Basic optokinetic ocular reflex pathways in the frog. *Journal of Neuroscience*, **4**, 43–57.

Collewijn, H. (1969). Optokinetic eye movements in the rabbit: input-output relations. *Vision Research*, **9**, 117–132.

Collewijn, H., Winterson, B.J., and Dubois, M.F. (1978). Optokinetic eye movements in albino rabbits: inversion in anterior visual field. *Science*, **199**, 1351–1353.

Collewijn, H., Apkarian, P., and Spekreijse, H. (1985). The oculomotor behaviour of human albinos. *Brain*, **108**, 1–18.

Conley, M. and Fite, K.V. (1980). Optokinetic nystagmus in the domestic pigeon. Effects of foveal lesions. *Brain, Behaviour, Evolution*, **17**, 89–102.

Cynader, M. and Harris, L. (1980). Eye movements in strabismic cats. *Nature*, **286**, 64–65.

Cynader, M. and Hoffmann, K.-P. (1981). Strabismus disrupts binocular convergence in cat nucleus of the optic tract. *Developmental Brain Research*, **1**, 132–136.

Dann, J.F. and Buhl E.H. (1987). Retinal ganglion cells projecting to the accessory optic system in the rat. *Journal of Comparative Neurology*, **262**, 141–158.

Demer, J.L. and Zee, D.S. (1984). Vestibulo-ocular and optokinetic deficits in albinos with congenital nystagmus. *Investigative Ophthalmology and Visual Sciences*, **25**, 739–745.

Dieterich, M. and Brandt, T. (1999). Episodic vertigo related to migraine (90 cases): vestibular migraine? *Journal of Neurology*, **246**, 883–892.

Dieringer, N. and Precht, W. (1982). Compensatory head and eye movements in the frog and their contribution to stabilization of gaze. *Experimental Brain Research*, **47**, 394–406.

Dieringer, N., Reichenberger, I., and Graf, W. (1992). Differences in optokinetic and vestibular ocular reflex performance in teleost and their relationship to different life styles. *Brain Behaviour Evolution*, **39**, 289–304.

Distler, C. (1996). Neuronal basis of optokinetic reflex pathology in naturally strabismic monkeys. *Strabismus*, **4**, 111–126.

Distler, C. and Hoffmann, K.-P. (1993). Visual receptive field properties in kitten pretectal nucleus of the optic tract and dorsal terminal nucleus of the accessory optic tract. *Journal of Neurophysiology*, **70**, 814–827.

Distler, C. and Hoffmann, K.-P. (1996). Retinal slip neurons in the nucleus of the optic tract and dorsal terminal nucleus in cats with congenital strabismus. *Journal of Neurophysiology*, **75**, 1483–1494.

Distler, C. and Hoffmann, K.-P. (2001). Cortical input to the nucleus of the optic tract and dorsal terminal nucleus (NOT-DTN) in macaques: a retrograde tracing study. *Cerebral Cortex*, **11**, 572–580.

Distler, C. and Hoffmann, K.-P. (2003). Development of the optokinetic response in macaques. A comparison with cat and man. *Annals of the New York Academy of Science*, **1004**, 10–18.

Distler, C. and Hoffmann, K.-P. (2008). Private lines of cortical visual information to the nucleus of the optic tract and dorsolateral pontine nucleus. *Progress in Brain Research*, **171**, 363–268.

Distler, C., Bachevalier, J., Kennedy, C., Mishkin, M., and Ungerleider, L.G. (1996). Functional development of the corticocortical pathway for motion analysis in the macaque monkey: a ^{14}C-2-deoxyglucose study. *Cerebral Cortex*, **6**, 184–195.

Distler, C., Vital-Durand, F., Korte, R., Korbmacher, H., and Hoffmann, K.-P. (1999). Development of the optokinetic system in macaque monkeys. *Vision Research*, **39**, 3909–3919.

Distler, C., Mustari, M.J., and Hoffmann, K.-P. (2002). Cortical projections to the nucleus of the optic tract and dorsal terminal nucleus and to the dorsolateral pontine nucleus in macaques: a dual retrograde tracing study. *Journal of Comparative Neurology*, **444**, 144–158.

Distler, C., Korbmacher, H., and Hoffmann, K.-P. (2006). Neuronal connections of motion sensitive area PSS of the ferret (*Mustela putorius furo*). *FENS Forum Abstracts*, **3**, A216.4.

Distler, C., Korbmacher, H., and Hoffmann, K.-P. (2009). Retinal projections to the accessory optic system in pigmented and albino ferrets (*Mustela putorius furo*). *Experimental Brain Research*, **199**, 333–343.

Duersteler, M.R. and Wurtz, R. H. (1988). Pursuit and optokinetic deficits following chemical lesions of cortical areas MT and MST. *Journal of Neurophysiology*, **60**, 940–965.

Easter, S.S. Jr (1972). Pursuit eye movements in goldfish (*Carassius auratus*). *Vision Research*, **12**, 673–688.

Euler, T., Detwiler, P.B., and Denk, W. (2002). Directionally selective calcium signals in dendrites of starburst amacrine cells. *Nature*, **418**, 845–852.

Fan, T.X, Weber, A.E., Pickard, G.E., Faber, K.M., and Ariel, M. (1995). Visual responses and connectivity in the turtle pretectum. *Journal of Neurophysiology*, **73**, 2507–2521.

Fite, K.V., Reiner, A., and Hunt, S.P. (1979). Optokinetic nystagmus and the accessory optic system of pigeon and turtle. *Brain Behaviour Evolution*, **16**, 192–202.

Fredericks, C.A., Giolli, R.A., Blanks, R.H., and Sadun, A.A. (1988). The human accessory optic system. *Brain Research*, **454**, 116–122.

Fried, S.I., Munch, T.A., and Werblin, F.S. (2002). Mechanisms and circuitry underlying directional selectivity in the retina. *Nature*, **420**, 411–414.

Fried, S.I., Munch, T.A., and Werblin, F.S. (2005). Directional selectivity is formed at multiple levels by laterally offset inhibition in the rabbit retina. *Neuron*, **46**, 117–127.

Fritsches, K.A. and. Marshall, N.J. (2002). Independent and conjugate eye movements during optokinesis in teleost fish. *Journal of Experimental Biology*, **205**, 1241–1252.

Fukuda, T. and Tokita, T. (1957). Über die Beziehung der Richtung der optischen Reize zu den Reflextypen der Augen- und Skelettmuskeln. *Acta Otolaryngology*, **48**, 415–424.

Gavrikov, K.E., Dmitriev, A.V., Keyser, K.T., and Mangel, S.C. (2003). Cation-chloride cotransporters mediate neuronal computation in the retina. *Proceedings of the National Academy of Science USA*, **100**, 16047–16052.

Gavrikov, K.E., Nilson, J.E., Dmitriev, A.V., Zucker, C.L., and Mangel, S.C. (2006). Dendritic compartmentalization of chloride cotransporters underlies directional responses of starburst amacrine cells in retina. *Proceedings of the National Academy of Science USA*, **103**, 18793–18798.

Gioanni, H. (1988). Stabilizing gaze reflexes in the pigeon (*Columba livia*). 1. Horizontal and vertical optokinetic eye (OKN) and head (OCR) reflexes. *Experimental Brain Research*, **69**, 567–582.

Gioanni, H. and Sansonetti, A,. (1999). Characteristics of slow and fast phases of the optocollic reflex (OCR) in head free pigeons (*Columba livia*): influence of flight behaviour. *European Journal of Neuroscience*, **11**, 155–166.

Gioanni, H., Rey, J., Villalobos, J., Bouyer, J.J., and Gioanni, Y. (1981). Optokinetic nystagmus in the pigeon (Columba livia). I. Study in monocular and binocular vision. *Experimental Brain Research*, **44**, 362–370.

Gioanni, H., Rey, J., Villalobos, J., Richard, D., and Dalbera, A. (1983a) Optokinetic nystagmus in the pigeon (*Columba livia*). II. Role of the pretectal nucleus of the accessory optic system (AOS). *Experimental Brain Research*, **50**, 237–247.

Gioanni, H., Villalobos, J., Rey, J., Richard, D., and Dalbera, A. (1983b). Optokinetic nystagmus in the pigeon (*Columba livia*). III. Role of the nucleus ectomamillaris (nEM): Interactions in the accessory optic system (AOS). *Experimental Brain Research*, **50**, 248–258.

Gioanni, H., Rey, J., Villalobos, J., and Dalbera, A. (1984). Single unit activity in the nucleus of the basal optic root (nBOR) during optokinetic, vestibular and visuo-vestibular stimulations in the alert pigeon (Columba livia). *Experimental Brain Research*, **57**, 49–60.

Gioanni, H., Bennis, M., and Sansonetti, A. (1993). Visual and vestibular reflexes that stabilize gaze in the chameleon. *Visual Neuroscience*, **10**, 947–956.

Giolli, R.A., Blanks, R.H.I., and Lui, F. (2006). The accessory optic system: basic organization with an update on connectivity, neurochemistry, and function. *Progress in Brain Research*, **151**, 407–440.

Godaux, E., and Vanderkelen, B. (1984). Vestibulo-ocular reflex, optokinetic response and their interaction in the cerebellectomized cat. *Journal of Physiology*, **346**, 155–170.

Grasse, K.L. and Cynader, M.S. (1988). The effect of visual cortex lesions on vertical optokinetic nystagmus in the cat. *Brain Research*, **455**, 385–389.

Grasse, K.L., Cynader, M.S., and Douglas, R.M. (1984). Alterations in response properties in the lateral and dorsal terminal nuclei of the cat accessory optic system following visual cortical lesions. *Experimental Brain Research*, **55**, 69–80.

Grasse, K.L., Ariel, M., and Smith, I.D. (1990). Direction-selective responses of units in the dorsal terminal nucleus of cat following intravitreal injections of bicuculline. *Visual Neuroscience*, **4**, 605–617.

Guyer, D.R. and Lessell, S. (1986). Periodic alternating nystagmus associated with albinism. *Journal of Clinical Neuro-Ophthalmology*, **6**, 82–85.

Hahnenberger, R.W. (1977). Differences in optokinetic nystagmus between albino and pigmented rabbits. *Experimental Eye research*, **25**, 9–17.

Harris, A.J., (1965). Eye movements of the dogfish Squalus acanthias. *Journal of Experimental Biology*, **43**, 107–130.

Harvey, R.J., De'Sperati, C., and, Strata, P. (1997). The early phase of horizontal optokinetic responses in the pigmented rat and the effects of lesions of the visual cortex. *Vision Research*, **37**, 1615–1625.

Hausselt, S.E., Euler, T., Detwiler, P.B., and Denk, W. (2007). A dendrite-autonomous mechanism for direction selectivity in retinal starburst amacrine cells. *PLoS Biology*, **5**, 1474–1493.

Heide, W., Kurzidim, K., and Kömpf, D. (1996). Deficits of smooth pursuit eye movements after frontal and parietal lesions. *Brain*, **119**, 1951–1969.

Hein, A., Courjon, J.H., Flandrin, J.M., and Arzi, M.(1990). Optokinetic nystagmus in the ferret: including selected comparisons with the cat. *Experimental Brain Research*, **79**, 623–632.

Hess, B.J., Precht, W., Reber, A., and Cazin, L. (1985). Horizontal optokinetic ocular nystagmus in the pigmented rat. *Neuroscience*, **15**, 97–107.

Hoffmann, K.-P. (1982) Cortical versus subcortical contributions to the optokinetic reflex in the cat. In G. Lennerstrand (ed.) *Functional Basis of Ocular Motility Disorders* (pp. 303–310). Oxford, New York: Pergamon Press.

Hoffmann, K.-P. (1986). Visual inputs relevant for the optokinetic nystagmus in mammals. *Progress in Brain Research*, **64**, 75–84.

Hoffmann, K.-P. and Distler, C. (1989). Quantitative analysis of visual receptive fields of neurons in the nucleus of the optic tract and dorsal terminal nucleus of the accessory optic tract in macaque monkeys. *Journal of Neurophysiology*, **62**, 416–428.

Hoffmann, K.-P. and Fischer, W.H. (2001). Directional effect of inactivation of the nucleus of the optic tract on optokinetic nystagmus in the cat. *Vision Research*, **41**, 3389–3398.

Hoffmann, K.-P. and Stone, J. (1985). Retinal input to the nucleus of the optic tract of the cat assessed by antidromic activation of ganglion cells. *Experimental Brain Research*, **59**, 395–403.

Hoffmann, K.-P., Distler, C., and Erickson, R. (1991). Functional projections from striate cortex and superior temporal sulcus to the nucleus of the optic tract (NOT) and dorsal terminal nucleus of the accessory optic tract (DTN) of macaque monkeys. *Journal of Comparative Neurology*, **313**, 707–724.

Hoffmann, K.-P., Distler, C., Mark, R.F., Marotte, L.R., Henry, G.H., and Ibbotson, M.R. (1995). Neural and behavioral effects of early eye rotation on the optokinetic system in the wallaby, *Macropus eugenii*. *Journal of Neurophysiology*, **73**, 727–735.

Hoffmann, K.-P., Distler, C., and Markner, C. (1996). Optokinetic nystagmus in cats with congenital strabismus. *Journal of Neurophysiology*, **75**, 1495–1502.

Hoffmann, K.-P., Distler, C., and Grüsser, O.J. (1998). Optokinetic reflex in squirrel monkeys after long-term monocular deprivation. *European Journal of Neuroscience*, **10**, 1136–1144.

Hoffmann, K.-P., Bremmer, F., Thiele, A., and Distler, C. (2002). Directional asymmetry of neurons in cortical areas MT and MST projecting to the NOT-DTN in macaques. *Journal of Neurophysiology*, **87**, 2113–2123.

Hoffmann, K.-P., Bremmer, F., and Distler, C. (2009). Visual response properties of neurons in cortical areas MT and MST projecting to the dorsolateral pontine nucleus or the nucleus of the optic tract in macaque monkeys. *European Journal of Neuroscience*, **29**, 411–423.

Hupfeld, D., Distler, C., and Hoffmann, K.-P. (2007). Deficits of visual motion perception and optokinetic nystagmus after posterior suprasylvian lesions in the ferret (*Mustela putorius furo*). *Experimental Brain Research*, **182**, 509–523.

Ilg, U.J., Bremmer, F., and Hoffmann, K.-P. (1993). Optokinetic und pursuit system: a case report. *Behavioural Brain Research*, **57**, 21–29.

Jeffery, G. (1997). The albino retina: an abnormality that provides insight into normal retinal development. *Trends in Neuroscience*, **20**, 165–169.

Jeong, S.H., Oh, Y.M., Hwang, J.M., Kim, J.S. (2008). Emergence of diplopia and oscillopsia due to Heimann-Bielschowsky phenomenon after cataract surgery. *British Journal of Ophthalmology*, **92**,1402.

Kato, I., Harada, K., Hasegawa, T. and, Ikarashi, T. (1988). Role of the nucleus of the optic tract of monkeys in optokinetic nystagmus and optokinetic after-nystagmus. *Brain Research*, **474**, 16–26.

Katte, O., and Hoffmann, K.-P. (1980) Direction specific neurons in the pretectum of the frog (Rana esculenta). *Journal of Comparative Physiology*, **140**, 53–57.

Kawamura, S., Sprague, J.M., and Niimi, K. (1974). Corticofugal projections from the visual cortices to the thalamus, pretectum und superior colliculus in the cat. *Journal of Comparative Neurology*, **158**, 339–362.

Klar, M., and Hoffmann, K.-P. (2002). Visual direction-selective neurons in the pretectum of the rainbow trout. *Brain Research Bulletin*, **57**, 431–433.

Klauer, S., Sengpiel, F., and Hoffmann, K.-P. (1990). Visual response properties and afferents of nucleus of the optic tract in the ferret. *Experimental Brain Research*, **83**, 178–189.

Knapp, A.G., Ariel, M., and Robinson, F.R. (1988). Analysis of vertebrate eye movements following intravitreal drug injections. I. Blockade of retinal ON-cells by 2-amino-4-phosphonobutyrate eliminates optokinetic nystagmus. *Journal of Neurophysiology*, **60**, 1010–1021.

Kogo, N., Rubio, D.M., and Ariel, M. (1998). Direction tuning of individual retinal inputs to the turtle accessory optic system. *Journal of Neuroscience*, **18**, 2673–2684.

Kourouyan, H.D. and Horton, J.C. (1997). Transneuronal retinal input to the primate Edinger-Westphal nucleus. *Journal of Comparative Neurology*, **381**, 68–80.

Krause, M. and Hoffmann, K.-P. (2009). Shift of chloride reversal potential in neurons of the accessory optic system in albinotic rats. *Experimental Brain Research*, **199**, 345–353.

Lannou, J., Cazin, L., Precht, W., and Toupet, M. (1982). Optokinetic, vestibular, and optokinetic-vestibular responses in albino and pigmented rats. *Pflueger's Archive*, **393**, 42–44.

Lázár, G. (1983). Transection of the basal optic root in the frog abolishes vertical optokinetic head nystagmus. *Neuroscience Letters*, **43**, 7–11.

Lee, S. and Zhou, Z.J. (2006). The synaptic mechanism of direction selectivity in distal processes of starburst amacrine cells. *Neuron*, **51**, 787–799.

Leichnetz, G.R. (1982). Connections between the frontal eye field and pretectum of the monkey: an anterograde/retrograde study using HRP gel and TMB neurohistochemistry. *Journal of Comparative Neurology*, **207**, 394–402.

Li, Z., Fite, K.V., Montgomery, N.M., and Wang, S.R. (1996). Single unit responses to whole field visual stimulation in the pretectum of *Rana pipiens*. *Neuroscience Letters*, **218**, 193–197.

Lui, F., Giolli, R.A., Blanks, R.H., and Tom, E.M. (1994). Pattern of striate cortical projections to the pretectal complex in the guinea pig. *Journal of Comparative Neurology*, **344**, 598–609.

Lui, F., Gredory, K.M., Blanks, R.H.I., and Giolli, R.A. (1995). Projectioms from visual areas of the cerebral cortex to pretectal nuclear complex, terminal accessory optic nuclei, and superior colliculus in macaque monkey. *Journal of Comparative Neurology*, **363**, 439–460.

Lynch, J.C. and McLaren, J.W. (1983). Optokinetic nystagmus deficits following parieto-occipital cortex lesions in monkeys. *Experimental Brain Research*, **49**, 125–130.

Malach, R., Strong, N., and Van Sluyters, R.C. (1981). Analysis of monocular optokinetic nystagmus in normal and visually deprived kittens. *Brain Research*, **210**, 367–372.

Manteuffel, G. (1984). Electrophysiology and anatomy of direction selective pretectal units in *Salamandra salamandra*. *Experimental Brain Research*, **54**, 415–425.

Marcotte, R.R. and Updyke, B.V. (1982). Cortical visual areas of the cat project differentially onto the nuclei of the accessory optic system. *Brain Research*, **242**, 205–217.

Markner, C. and Hoffmann, K.-P. (1985). Variability in the effects of monocular deprivation on the optokinetic reflex of the non-deprived eye in the cat. *Experimental Brain Research*, **61**, 117–127.

Masseck, O.A. and Hoffmann, K.-P. (2008) Responses to moving visual stimuli in pretectal neurons of the small-spotted dogfish (*Scyliorhinus canicula*). *Journal of Neurophysiology*, **99**, 200–207.

Masseck, O.A., Röll, B., Hoffmann, K.-P. (2008). The optokinetic reaction in foveate and afoveate geckos. *Vision Research*, **48**, 765–772.

Masseck, O.M. and Hoffmann, K.-P. (2009). Comparative neurobiology of the optokinetic reflex. *Annals of the New York Academy of Sciences*, **1164**, 430–439.

McCarty, J.W., Demer, J.L., Hovis, L.A., and Nuwer, M.R. (1992). Ocular motility abnomalies in developmental misdirection of the optic chiasm. *American Journal of Ophthalmology*, 113, 86–95.

McKenna, O.C. and Wallman, J. (1985). Accessory optic system and pretectum of birds: comparisons with those of other vertebrates. *Brain Behaviour Evolution*, 26, 91–116.

Montgomery, N., Fite, K.V., Taylor, M., and Bengston, L. (1982). Neural correlates of optokinetic nystagmus in the mesencephalon of *Rana pipiens*: a functional analysis. *Brain Behaviour Evolution*, 21, 137–150.

Morgan, B. and Frost, B.J. (1981). Visual response characteristics of neurons in nucleus of basal optic root of pigeons. *Experimental Brain Research*, 42, 181–188.

Morrone, M.C., Atkinson, J., Cioni, G., Braddick, O.J., and Fiorentini, S. (1999). Developmental changes in optokinetic mechanisms in the absence of unilateral cortical control. *Neuroreport*, 10, 2723–2729.

Mustari, M.J. and Fuchs, A.F. (1989). Response properties of single units in the lateral terminal nucleus of the accessory optic system in the behaving primate. *Journal of Neurophysiology*, 61, 1207–1220.

Mustari, M.J., Tusa, R.J., Burrows A.F., Fuchs, A.F., and Livingston, C.A. (2001). Gaze-stabilizing deficits and latent nystagmus in monkeys with brief, early-onset visual deprivation: role of the pretectal NOT. *Journal of Neurophysiology*, 86, 662–675.

Mustari, M.J., Ono, S., and Vitorello, K.C. (2008). How disturbed visual processing early in life leads to disorders of gaze-holding and smooth pursuit. *Progress in Brain Research*, 171, 487–495.

Naegele, J.R. and Held, R. (1982). The postnatal development of monocular optokinetic nystagmus in infants. *Vision Research*, 22, 341–346.

Nguyen, L.T., and Grzywacz, N.M. (2000). Colocalization of choline acetyltransferase and gamma-aminobutyric acid in the developing and adult turtle retinas. *Journal of Comparative Neurology*, 420, 527–538.

Nguyen, L.T., De Juan, J., Mejia, M., and Grzywacz, N.M. (2000). Localization of choline acetyltransferase in the developing and adult turtle retinas. *Journal of Comparative Neurology*, 420, 512–526.

Oesch, N., Euler, T., and Taylor, W.R. (2005). Direction selective dendritic action potentials in rabbit retina. *Neuron*, 47, 739–750.

Ott, M. (2001). Chamaeleons have independent eye movements but synchronize both eyes during saccadic prey tracking. *Experimental Brain Research*, 139, 173–179.

Oyster, C.W., Takahashi, E., and Collewijn, H. (1972). Direction-selective retinal ganglion cells and control of optokinetic nystagmus in the rabbit. *Vision Research*, 12, 183–193.

Oyster, C.W., Simpson, J.I., Takahashi, E.S., and Soodak, R.E. (1980). Retinal ganglion cells projecting to the rabbit accessory optic system. *Journal of Comparative Neurology*, 190, 40–61.

Pasik, P. and Pasik, T. (1975). A comparison between two types of visually-evoked nystagmus in the monkey. *Acta Otolaryngology Supplement*, 330, 30–37.

Philipp, R., Distler, C., and Hoffmann, K.-P. (2006). A motion-sensitive area in ferret extrastriate visual cortex: an analysis in pigmented and albino animals. *Cerebral Cortex*, 16, 779–790.

Pola, J., Wyatt, H.J., and Lustgarten, M. (1987). Suppression of OKN without retinal error signals: effects of attentional mode and stimulus frequency. *Society for Neuroscience Abstracts*, 13, 391.

Pola, J. and Wyatt, H.J. (1993). The role of attention and cognitive processes. In: F.A. Miles and J. Wallman (eds.) Visual motion and its role in the stabilization of gaze (pp. 371–392). Amsterdam: Elsevier.

Precht, W. and Cazin, L. (1979). Functional deficits in the optokinetic system of albino rats. *Experimental Brain Research*, 37, 183–186.

Prusky, G.T., Silver, B.D., Tchetter, W.W., Alam, N.M., and Douglas, R.M. (2008). Experience-dependent plasticity from eye opening enables lasting, visual cortex-dependent enhancement of motion vision. *Journal of Neuroscience*, 28, 9817–9827.

Purkinje, J.E. (1825). *Beobachtungen und Versuche zur Physiologie der Sinne. Neue Beiträge zur Kenntnis des Sehens in subjektiver Hinsicht. Vol. 2*. Berlin: Reimer.

Reymond, E. and Morgan, I.G. (1990). Destruction of cholinergic amacrine cells in the retina abolishes optomotor responses in chickens. *Proceedings of the Australian Neuroscience Association*, 1, 122.

Rinner, O., Rick, J.M., and Neuhauss, S.C.F. (2005). Contrast sensitivity, spatial and temporal tuning of the larval zebrafish optokinetic response. *Investigative Ophthalmology and Visual Sciences*, 46, 137–142.

Rosenberg, A.F. and Ariel, M. (1990). Visual response properties of neurons in turtle basal optic nucleus *in vitro*. *Journal of Neurophysiology*, 63, 1033–1045.

Rosenberg, A.F., and Ariel, M. (1991). Electrophysiological evidence for a direct projection of direction-selective retinal ganglion cells to the turtle's accessory optic system. *Journal of Neurophysiology*, 65, 1022–1033.

Roy, M.S., Lachapelle, P., and Leporé, F. (1989). Maturation of the optokinetic nystagmus as a function of the speed of stimulation in fullterm and preterm infants. *Clinical Vision Sciences*, 4, 357–366.

Schiff, D., Cohen, B., and Raphan, T. (1988). Nystagmus induced by stimulation of the nucleus of the optic tract in the monkey. *Experimental Brain Research*, 70, 1–14.

Schmidt, M., Zhang, H.Y., and Hoffmann, K.-P. (1993). OKN-related neurons in the rat nucleus of the optic tract and dorsal terminal nucleus of the accessory optic system receive a direct cortical input. *Journal of Comparative Neurology*, 330, 147–157.

Schoppmann, A. (1985). Functional and developmental analysis of visual corticopretectal pathway in the cat: a neuroanatomical and electrophysiological study. *Experimental Brain Research*, **60**, 363–374.

Schor, C.M. and Westall, C. (1984). Visual and vestibular sources of fixation instability in amblyopia. *Investigative Ophthalmology and Visual Sciences*, **25**, 729–738.

Schweigart, G. and Hoffmann, K.-P. (1988). Optokinetic eye and head movements in the unrestrained cat. *Behavioural Brain Research*, **31**, 121–130.

Shintani, T., Hoshino, K., Meguro, R., Kaiya, T., and Norita, M. (1999). A light and electron microscopic analysis of the convergent retinal and visual cortical projections to the nucleus of the optic tract (NOT) in the pigmented rat. *Neurobiology*, **7**, 445–460.

Shook, B.L., Schlag-Rey, M., and Schlag, J. (1990). Primate supplementary eye field: I. Comparative aspects of mesencephalic and pontine connections. *Journal of Comparative Neurology*, **301**, 618–642.

Simon, J.W., Kandel, G.L., Krohel, G.B., and Nelsen, P.T. (1984). Albinotic characteristics in congenital nystagmus. *American Journal of Ophthalmology*, **97**, 320–327.

Simpson, J.I., Giolli, R.A., and Blanks, R.H.I. (1988). The pretectal nuclear complex and the accessory optic system. In J. Büttner-Ennever (ed.) *Neuroanatomy of the oculomotor system* (pp. 335–363). Amsterdam: Elsevier.

Sirkin, D.W., Hess, B.J., and Precht, W. (1985). Optokinetic nystagmus in albino rats depends on stimulus pattern. *Experimental Brain Research*, **61**, 218–221.

Sparks, D.L., Mays, L.E., Gurski, M.R., and Hickey, T.L. (1986). Long- and short-term monocular deprivation in the rhesus monkey: effects on visual fields and optokinetic nystagmus. *Journal of Neuroscience*, **6**, 1771–1780.

St John, R.S., Fisk, J.D., Timney, B., and Goodale, M.A. (1984). Eye movements in human albinos. *American Journal of Optometry and Physiological Optics*, **61**, 377–385.

Tan, H.S., van der Stehen, J., Simpson, J.I., and Collewijn, H. (1993). Three-dimensional organization of optokinetic responses in the rabbit. *Journal of Neurophysiology*, **69**, 303–317.

Tauber, E.S. and Atkin, A. (1968). Optomotor responses to monocular stimulation: relation to visual system organization. *Science*, **160**, 1365–1367.

Taylor, R.B., Wennberg, R.A., Lozano, A.M., and Sharpe, J.A. (2000). Central nystagmus induced by deep-brain stimulation for epilepsy. *Epilepsia*, **41**, 1637–1641.

Taylor, W.R. and Vaney, D.I. (2002). Diverse synaptic mechanisms generate direction selectivity in the rabbit retina. *Journal of Neuroscience*, **22**, 7712–7720.

Telkes, I., Distler, C. and Hoffmann, K.-P. (2000). Retinal ganglion cells projecting to the nucleus of the optic tract and dorsal terminal nucleus of the accessory optic system in macaque monkeys. *European Journal of Neuroscience*, **12**, 2367–2375.

Telkes, I., Garipis, N., and Hoffmann, K.-P. (2001). Morphological changes in the neuronal substrate for the optokinetic reflex in albino ferrets. *Experimental Brain Research*, **140**, 345–356.

Ter Braak, J.W. (1936). Untersuchung über optokinetischen Nystagmus. *Archives Netherland Physiology*, **21**, 309–376.

Thier, P., Koehler, W., and Buettner, U.W. (1988). Neuronal activity in the dorsolateral pontine nucleus of the alert monkey modulated by visual stimuli and eye movements. *Experimental Brain Research*, **70**, 496–512.

Thurston, S.E., Leigh, R.J., Crawford, T, Thompson, A., and Kennard, C. (1988). Two distinct deficits of visual tracking caused by unilateral lesions of cerebral cortex in humans. *Annals of Neurology*, **23**, 266–273.

Tusa, R.J., Demer, J.L., and Herdman, S.J. (1989). Cortical areas involved in OKN and VOR in cats: cortical lesions. *Journal of Neuroscience*, **9**, 1163–1178.

Tusa, R.J., Mustari, M.J., Burrows A.F., and Fuchs, A.F. (2001). Gaze-stabilizing deficits and latent nystagmus in monkeys with brief, early-onset visual deprivation: eye movement recordings. *Journal of Neurophysiology*, **86**, 651–661.

Tusa, R.J., Mustari, M.J., Das, V.E., and Boothe, R.G. (2002). Animal models for visual deprivation-induced strabismus and nystagmus. *Annals of the New York Academy of Science*, **956**, 346–360.

Van Hof-Van Duin, J. (1978). Direction preference of optokinetic responses in monocularly tested normal kittens and light deprived cats. *Archives Italiennes Biologiques*, **116**, 471–477.

Van Alphen, A.M., Schepers, T., Luo, C., and De Zeeuw, C.I. (2002). Motor performance and motor learning in Lurcher mice. *Annals of the New York Academy of Sciences*, **978**, 413–424.

Vigh, J., Bánvölgyi, T., and Wilhelm, M. (2000). Amacrine cells of the anuran retina: morphology, chemical neuroanatomy, and physiology. *Microscopy Research and Technique*, **50**, 373–383.

Wachholz, S. (2008). Vergleichende Untersuchungen der Augenbewegungen bei Reptilien. Diploma thesis, Ruhr-University Bochum.

Wagner, H., Nalbach, H. and Pappe, I. (1993). Optokinetic responses in barn owls. *Society for Neuroscience Abstracts*, **19**, Part 1, 345.

Wallman, J. and Pettigrew, J.D. (1985). Conjugate and disjunctive saccades in two avian species with contrasting oculomotor strategies. *Journal of Neuroscience*, **5**, 1418–1428.

Wallman, J. and Velez, J. (1985). Directional asymmetries of optokinetic nystagmus: developmental changes and relation to the accessory optic system and to the vestibular system. *Journal of Neuroscience*, **5**, 317–329.

Winterson, B.J. and Brauth, S.E. (1985). Direction selective single units in the nucleus lentiformis mesencephali of the pigeon (*Columba livia*). *Experimental Brain Research*, **60**, 215–226.

Winterson, B.J. and Collewijn H. (1981). Inversion of direction selectivity to anterior fields in neurons of the nucleus of the optic tract in rabbits with ocular albinism. *Brain Research*, **220**, 31–49.

Wood, C.C., Spear, P.D., and Braun, J.J. (1973). Direction specific deficits in horizontal optokinetic nystagmus following removal of the visual cortex in the cat. *Brain Research*, **60**, 231–237.

Wylie, D.R. and Frost, B.J. (1990). The visual response properties of neurons in the nucleus of the basal optic root of the pigeon: a quantitative analysis. *Experimental Brain Research*, **82**, 327–336.

Xiao, Q., Cao, P., Gu, Y., and Wang, S.R. (2001). Visual responses of neurons in the pretectal nucleus lentiformis mesencephali to moving patterns within and beyond receptive fields in pigeons. *Brain Behaviour Evolution*, **57**, 80–86.

Yang, G. and Morgan, I.G. (1990). Destruction of cholinergic amacrine cells in the retina silences directionally selective units in the nucleus of the basal optic root of chicken. *Proceedings of the Australian Neuroscience Association*, **1**, 142.

Yasui, S. and Young, L.R. (1984). On the predictive control of foveal eye tracking and slow phases of optokinetic and vestibular nystagmus. *Journal of Physiology*, **347**, 17–33.

Yonehara, K., Ishikane, H., Sakuta, H., Shintani, T., Nakamura-Yonehara, K., Kamiji, N.L., *et al.* (2009). Identification of retinal ganglion cells and their projections involved in central transmission of information about upward and downward image motion. *PLoS One*, **4**, e4320.

Yoshida, K., Watanabe, D., Ishikane, H., Tachibana, M., Pastan, I., and Nakanishi, S. (2001). A key role of starburst amacrine cells in originating retinal direction selectivity and optokinetic eye movement. *Neuron*, **30**, 771–780.

Zee, D.S., Tusa, R.J., Herdman, S.J., Butler, P.H., and Gucer, G., (1987). Effects of occipital lobectomy upon eye movements in primate. *Journal of Neurophysiology*, **58**, 883–907.

Zhou, Z.J., and Lee, S. (2008). Synaptic physiology of direction selectivity in the retina. *Journal of Physiology*, **586**, 4371–4376.

CHAPTER 5

Saccades

Iain D. Gilchrist

Abstract

Saccades are fast ballistic movements of the eye. A saccade is followed by a fixation—a period of time when the eye is relatively stationary and useful visual information is gathered. Because visual acuity decreases rapidly away from the current direction of gaze, saccades are required to point the eye at regions of interest. Saccadic sampling and the rapid fall of visual ability define the temporal and spatial structure of the input to the visual system. During a fixation, peripheral vision is used to determine the location for the next fixation. In a scene that contains multiple possible targets, selecting the target for the next saccade involves an interplay between the visual properties of locations in the environment and the goal of the observer.

Introduction

One of the fundamental observations from eye movement research is that for humans, and other animals, the eyes move in a limited number of distinctive ways (see Land, Chapter 1, this volume). There are two primary functions of this repertoire. Eye movements occur either to stabilize all, or part, of the retinal image or they can point the primary axis of the eye—the fovea—to a region of 'interest' (Walls 1962). The vestibulo-ocular reflex moves the eye to compensate for head movements (see also Hess, Chapter 3, this volume) and so maintains retinal stability. Smooth pursuit eye movements (see Barnes, Chapter 7, this volume) allow the observer to track a visual target and so keep the target stable on the retina, even if this is at the expense of an equal and opposite movement of the background. This chapter is concerned with saccadic eye movements where the eye jumps rapidly to point the eye at a new location. The saccadic response is one of a class of eye-movement responses to point the fovea to a region of 'interest'. Vergence eye movements are another example of this class of eye movement. During a vergence response the two eyes move disjunctively to point the fovea at an object in a different depth plane. For both saccades and vergence, the need to look directly at objects or regions of interest is driven by the dramatic changes in visual ability at locations further away from the fovea. The extent of this acuity advantage in the fovea is much larger than is obvious from introspection. If we want to know how well we can see something then the reflex is to move the eyes rapidly to fixate it. Unfortunately, like the person who opens the refrigerator door to check if the light is always on, this saccade then moves the high acuity part of vision to point directly at the object of interest. For a single isolated letter presented at varying eccentricities away from the fovea, the ability to correctly identify the letter falls in a linear manner from 100% at 3° to 50% at 10°. When the letter to be identified is flanked by two other letters, performance is already at around 80% at just 1° and drops to 35% by 3° (Bouma, 1970). For stimuli of this sort, recognition is effectively impossible without foveation. It is no surprise then that saccadic eye movements occur so frequently and across such a wide range of tasks.

Why do humans make saccades?

The characteristic of the orienting response generated in humans is a by-product of the apparatus available for moving the eye. Saccades are generated by the six extraocular muscles and the eyeball is relatively light and mobile. As a result, the metabolic costs of making very frequent and fast movements are low and are balanced by the benefits that result from minimizing the time spent during saccades, and maximizing the number of locations that benefit from fixating. The study of a single case, A.I., suggests that saccadic sampling of the visual environment may be a more fundamental property of the visual system than this simple cost–benefit explanation suggests. A.I. was a young adult who as a result of extraocular muscular fibrosis was unable to move her eyes and it is likely that this had been the case since birth. Despite this deficit, A.I. was able to read and carry out most everyday tasks unaided. She achieved this through making saccade-like movements of her head. The amplitude and fixation duration of the head movements that she made during reading were strikingly similar to the eye movements of controls (Gilchrist et al., 1997). She showed 'eye saccade-like' behaviour in a range of standard saccade tasks during her head movements (Gilchrist et al., 1998). She also showed similar saccade and fixation behaviour to control participants during the more naturalist task of making a cup of tea in a kitchen (Land et al., 2002). During her development, A.I.'s brain had the opportunity to develop alternative sampling strategies to compensate for the lack of eye-based saccades (see Land, Chapter 1, this volume for alternatives from across the animal kingdom). Instead she has developed a system of saccadic sampling that is surprising similar to saccadic eye movements. There are significant costs associated with moving the head rather than the eyes, not least of which is the additional time lost during the slower head movements. This rigid reliance on saccade-like behaviour suggests that saccadic sampling is a more integral part of vision. The concentration of visual ability in the fovea and the use of saccadic sampling may structure the visual input in a way that is optimal for the visual system.

The characteristics of saccades

The term saccade derives from the French word for 'jerk' or 'twitch' which neatly captures the behaviour of the eye (see Wade and Tatler, Chapter 2, this volume; Wade and Tatler, 2005). Saccades are fast jerky movements of the eye that are typically followed by a *fixation* which is a period of time during which the eye is stationary. The eyes move in a *conjunctive* way: the movements in each eye have the same amplitude and direction. Saccadic eye movements are stereotypical in a number of respects. Across individuals, saccades tend to have a characteristic temporal profile. The eye is initially stable and then quickly accelerates up to a peak velocity followed by a rapid deceleration and then a quick return to stability. All of this is achieved in a relatively short timescale. For example, the 12° saccade illustrated in Fig. 5.1 has a duration of about 50 ms and, within that period, reaches a peak velocity of close to 400°/s. The peak velocity of a saccade is closely related to the amplitude. When plotted on log-log axis, there is a very tight linear relationship between peak velocity and amplitude. A similar close relationship exists between saccade duration and amplitude. This relationship has been termed the *main sequence* (Bahill et al., 1975a) as an analogy to the closely constrained relationship between the stellar colour and the brightness of dwarf stars in astronomy. The main sequence probably represents the behaviour of a system that is optimally trading off the accuracy and the duration of the movement (Harris and Wolpert, 2006).

Saccades can have a very wide range of amplitudes. In normal viewing situations most saccades have an amplitude of less than 15°, after which the head becomes involved in the movement to redirect the eye (see Corneil, Chapter 16, this volume; Bahill et al., 1975b).

Even during a fixation the eyes are not completely still. There are three types of miniature movements during fixation: *tremor*, *drift*, and *microsaccades* (Carpenter, 1988). All three types of movement reduce neural adaptation and so prevent fading of the visual image (see Martinez-Conde and Macknik, Chapter 6, this volume; Martinez-Conde et al., 2004). Recent research has demonstrated an interaction between covert attention and the generation of microsaccades suggesting that they are not simply under low-level control (Engbert and Kliegl, 2003).

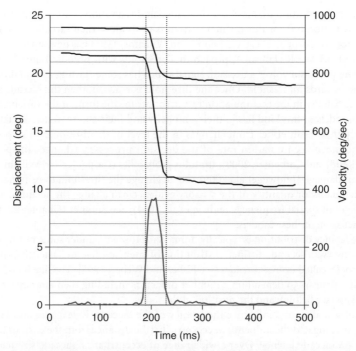

Fig. 5.1 An example saccade moving the eye about 12° down and to the right. The upper black line shows vertical eye displacement and the lower black line shows horizontal eye displacement. The grey line shows the velocity profile of the saccade with the vertical dotted lines marking the beginning and end of the movement.

Saccades do not always have simple linear trajectories. Specifically, oblique saccades tend to deviate towards the horizontal (e.g. Smit and Van Gisbergen, 1990). Although these effects are small they appear to be systematic both within and between participants. The vast majority of curved saccades curve only in one direction. However, a small proportion has a double curve (Ludwig and Gilchrist, 2002). Saccade trajectories to a target can be affected by the presence of a distractor. The distractor in these experiments is typically some distance away from the target and so the landing position of the saccade is unaffected by the distractor. However, for shorter latency saccades (less than about 200 ms) the saccade tends to curve towards the distractor and for longer latency saccades it tends to curve away from the distractor. These effects tend to be very small (measured in units of a 60th of a degree or minutes of arc) but remain consistent when compared to the trajectories of saccades observed when no distractor was present (McSorley et al., 2006).

Saccade latency

The saccade latency is the time taken to initiate a saccade. When a saccade is generated as part of a sequence of saccades or *scanpath* then this measure corresponds to the intersaccade interval. In most experimental studies of the saccadic response, the saccade latency is taken to be the duration between the event that is being responded to—for example, a peripheral visual flash—and the onset of the movement. One of the key characteristics of saccade latencies is their very wide variability. This takes two forms. The average saccade latency is substantially affected by the nature of the stimulus to be responded to and can range from as little as 100 ms to as much as 1000 ms. This type of variability is discussed in more detail below. Even if the stimulus is constant and the response is constant, latency is very variable at a trial-by-trial level.

The distribution of individual saccade latencies has a distinctive form. The distribution is skewed, with a long tail for longer latency saccades. A simple transformation of latency to the reciprocal of latency leads to a distribution that is close to a Gaussian distribution (see Carpenter and Williams, 1995). One way to account for this distinct pattern is to think of each saccade as being the result of a decision process. Carpenter (e.g. Carpenter and Williams, 1995) has developed a specific model of this kind, called LATER (Linear Approach to Thresholds with Ergodic Rate) for saccadic eye movements. The process involves a decision signal which has some starting level and then accumulates over time towards a threshold. Once the threshold is reached, then the saccade is generated. Trial-by-trial variability in the accumulation rate accounts for the form of the variability in latency. The power of models of this kind lies in their simplicity and their ability to disassociate changes in saccade latency that result either from changes in the level of the threshold to respond, or from changes in the mean accumulation rate of the decision processes. Changes in speed-accuracy instructions (Reddi and Carpenter, 2000), stimulus probability (Carpenter and Williams, 1995), and unilateral brain damage (Ludwig et al., 2009) can all change the threshold to respond. In contrast, changes in the quality or quantity of the sensory evidence can change the accumulation rate, for example, changes in spatial frequency (Ludwig et al., 2004). See Sumner (Chapter 22, this volume) for a fuller discussion of these models.

The saccade latency distribution is typically unimodal. However, under some testing conditions it is possible to observe a second, distinct, distribution of latencies that are faster than normal; these saccades have been called *express saccades* (see Fisher and Weber, 1993). The likelihood of observing express saccades appears to depend on a number of factors including then amount of practice, the presence of a gap (see below), and the position of the target.

A number of visual factors influence the latency of the saccade. Kalesnykas and Hallett (1994) systematically investigated the influence of eccentricity (the distance from the current fixation point to the target) on saccade latency. Over a wide range of eccentricities, saccade size had little or no effect on saccade latency. However, for small saccades that were less than about 1° of visual angle, there was evidence of an increase in saccade latency. In addition, for large saccades greater then about 15° there was also evidence of an increase in saccade latency. Stimulus properties appear to have a larger influence on saccade latency than eccentricity. Saccades are slower with decreased intensity (Kalesnykas and Hallett, 1994) and slower with decreased contrast and increased spatial frequency of the target (Ludwig et al., 2004).

Events at the currently fixated location can also affect the latency of a saccade. In a simple saccadic task, if the currently fixated item disappears before the new target appears, then the saccade latency is reduced—this is known as the gap effect. The gap effect was first described by Saslow (1967) and subsequent work has demonstrated that the effect is probably the result of two processes. The first is a general warning or alerting component. This is because the offset of the fixation point predicts, in time, the onset of the target. The second component is variously called *fixation release* or *fixation disengagement* and appears to speed ocular motor orienting by releasing the fixation system (see Forbes and Klein, 1996).

Events away from the current fixation point can also influence the latency of the saccade. The *remote distractor effect* describes the increase in saccade latency that results when the target for the saccade is presented concurrently with a distractor (see Walker et al., 1997). The effect occurs even when the direction of the target is known beforehand and the distractor is presented in the opposite direction. This suggests that the remote distractor effect is not simply a result of a confusion between the target or distractor but instead represents a low-level interference in saccade programming.

Saccades are not always directed to a specific target, for example, they may be exploratory. Under these conditions the saccade isn't target elicited, but rather is internally generated. Both antisaccade and memory-guided saccade paradigms have been used to investigate the properties of such saccades. In the antisaccade task (see Munoz and Everling, 2004) participants are instructed to generate a saccade away from a target when it appears. Despite the simplicity of the task, most human participants make a small proportion of errors. One model for the antisaccade task is that there is a competition between the correct voluntary saccade and a stimulus driven saccade towards the target. On some trials the stimulus driven saccade 'wins' this competition and an incorrect saccade towards the target will result. The latency of these errors tend to be short (about 150 ms) compared to the latency of the correct voluntary saccades in this task (about 300 ms). The increase in latency for voluntary saccades in the antisaccade task is also found in memory-guided saccade tasks (White et al., 1994) suggesting that voluntary saccades do, in general, have longer latencies.

Immediately before the onset of the saccade, the ocular-motor system enters a period of no return when it is committed to a given movement even when the saccade target either changes or moves. This period is referred to as the *dead-time*. For visually-guided saccades the dead-time has been studied using the double-step paradigm (Becker and Jürgens, 1979). In this paradigm, the observer is asked to follow a target dot with their eyes. On some trials the dot moves to a second location. If the target moves close in time to the execution of the saccade, then the saccade is directed to the first location regardless of the spatial shift. In contrast, if the target moves in a longer interval before the execution of the saccade, then the saccade is successfully directed to the second target. In between these two times there is a relatively rapid transition between a saccade being directed to the first or second location, including a reliable tendency to find some saccades that are directed to the midpoint between the two locations. These data are used to estimate the duration of the dead-time and the figure of about 80 ms is often quoted (see Ludwig et al., 2007). However, despite this it has been known for a while that the dead-time depends on the distance between the two locations (e.g. Becker and Jürgens 1979). Recent work by Ludwig and colleagues (2007) has shown that the dead time is not influenced by a gap manipulation and has demonstrated that variations in dead time can be captured by accumulator models similar to LATER.

In summary, the saccade latency can be thought of as a composite of the time to process the visual stimulus, the accumulation of a decision process, and the final motor execution.

Saccade landing position

In simple laboratory conditions, saccades tend to be hypometric—they fall slightly short of the intended target. As a result, orienting saccades are often followed by a small corrective saccade (see Carpenter, 1988). However, in more naturalistic tasks, such as making a cup of tea (Land et al., 1999), very large saccades that accurately land on the apparent target have been observed.

Saccades generated to extended regions of space, such as a line drawing of a shape, are accurately directed to the middle of the shape. This suggests that the edge information has been combined into a shape description for the programming of the saccade (He and Kowler, 1991). The remote distractor effect describes the increase in saccade latency to a target that occurs when a distractor is present. The increase in latency only occurs when the distractor is some distance away from the target (greater than 20° off the target axis; Walker et al., 1997). When the distractor is placed close to the target there is no longer an increase in the saccade latency but the distractor affects the landing position of the saccade instead. The saccade tends to land somewhere between the target and the distractor (Findlay, 1982). This effect has been called the *global effect*. The global effect occurs with a range of stimuli including items that have opposite contrast polarity (e.g. a black item and a white item on a grey background). This suggests that the global effect doesn't simply result from a process of the blurring of neighbouring items together (Findlay et al., 1993).

The original studies of the global effect focused on the effect of a single distractor on the landing position of a target-directed saccade. Subsequent studies in which participants have to saccade to a target embedded in distracters have revealed more about the effect of other items on saccade landing position. Findlay (1997) asked participants to saccade to the red target among green distractors. The stimuli were arranged on the circumference of a circle centred around the initial fixation point and the dependent measure was the number of first saccades that were correctly directed to the target. On some trials, two red targets were present side-by-side and Findlay (1997) found that the first saccade often landed in between the two targets in a manner that closely mirrored the global effect. In addition, on some trials, two targets were presented but with a green distractor in between them. Again, saccades were often directed between the two possible targets but also avoided the intervening distractor. This suggests that there was active inhibition of the distractor locations. When this task is made slightly harder, by using an orientation defined target (i.e. searching for a vertical target amongst horizontal distracters) then participants make an increased number of errors (Gilchrist et al., 1999). These errors show an interesting set of characteristics. First, the majority of errors are directed at a distractor item, rather than between items. Second, the errors are more likely to be directed towards an item that is closer to the target, rather than further away, and this effect is present across almost the whole area of the display (Gilchrist et al., 1999). This demonstrates that visual information that is really quite far away can have an impact on saccade landing position. So far, the focus has been on the effects on the first saccade landing position to a target amongst distractors. Zelinsky et al. (1997) investigated how landing positions changed in a sequence of saccade to find a target. In this task, participants searched for a target object amongst distractor objects. Zelinsky et al. (1997) found that the first saccade tended to be directed to a group of objects in the display and that subsequent saccades progressively target smaller groups. This suggested that the scale of visual analysis changes as the search process progressed.

The accurate programming of saccade landing position requires a process that responds to consistent landing position errors (McLaughlin, 1967). This process of *saccade adaptation* is important because it allows the system to make accurate motor responses despite changes in the system over time that can have a number of origins including growth, damage, and fatigue of the musculature and optical distortions due to changes in the eye, or even the wearing of spectacles (Optican, 1985). Experimentally this process can be studied by asking participants to generate a saccade to a target and, during the saccade, moving the target a consistent amount either toward or away from fixation. As a result of the target movement, the saccade will either land short of the target or overshoot it. Over a series of trials participants will begin to generate saccades that adapt to this shift and are once again target directed.

Saccade sequences

Saccades do not happen in isolation. Each saccade is preceded by a fixation and in turn that fixation is followed by a saccade and so on. Figure 5.2 illustrates such a saccade sequence while one observer viewed a picture. These saccade sequences are often referred to as *scanpaths*. This term carried with it a good deal of theoretical baggage and is linked to Scanpath Theory which was proposed by Norton and Stark (1971). Norton and Stark suggested that the sequence of eye movements generated to a given picture would be the same and that the sequence would play an important role in accessing the visual memory of that picture. Subsequent work has shown that scanpaths are not as deterministic as this theory suggests.

Most models of saccade generation (e.g. Findlay and Walker, 1999) assume that each saccade is programmed separately during the preceding fixation. However a number of experimental studies suggest that some parallel programming of saccades does occur. There are two kinds of evidence that support the idea of parallel programming of saccades. The first kind of evidence is based on experiments in which fixation durations are observed that are very short, specifically with a duration at, or below, the dead time. The argument is that a saccade that follows such short fixation durations cannot be the result of visual processing of the display, but instead must have been planned before the execution of the proceeding saccade. For example, it has long been known that second saccades in the double-step paradigm can have short latencies of less than 100 ms (Becker and Jürgens, 1979). The second kind of evidence that supports the suggestion for parallel programming of saccades relies on saccade contingent changes in the display. For example, McPeek et al. (2000) had participants carry out a search task in which they had to generate a saccade to a target presented with distractors. On some trials the participant's first saccade was erroneously directed to a distractor. When this occurred, the target position was switched during the saccade so that the participant would now generate a saccade towards the target. Following this first saccade, participants sometimes generated a second saccade to the old target position. This suggests that they had detected the target location before the execution of the first saccade and pre-programmed the second saccade to the old target location. The parallel programming of saccades, particularly during search, is one explanation

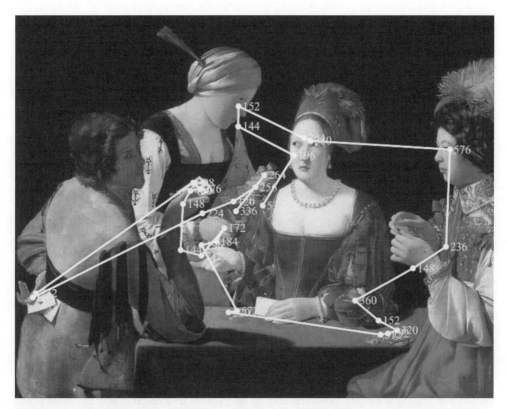

Fig. 5.2 An example sequence of saccades and fixations made during picture scanning. The dots indicate a location where a fixation has occurred and the fixation duration (in ms) is shown to the right of each fixation. The individual fixations are linked to indicate the order of fixation.

for why the accumulator models of saccade latency like LATER (Carpenter and Williams, 1995) do not prove a good description of the latency distribution of the saccades generated as part of a sequence during visual search (Van Loon et al., 2002).

Saccade target selection

The generation of a saccade to a new location results in a large processing advantage at the newly fixated location. In the majority of situations the target for the next saccade has to be selected using the more limited visual information that is available from peripheral vision. Two things are occurring during the fixation: processing the fixated location with the fovea and selecting the spatial location for the next fixation using peripheral visual information.

In the literature the distinction is often drawn between 'top-down' and 'bottom-up' factors that determine which location within space is selected for the next fixation. A 'bottom-up' signal is one that arises from the visual input and attracts the eyes to that location regardless of the task currently being carried out. For example, a sudden visual onset may result in the eyes fixating that location regardless of the task (Ludwig and Gilchrist, 2002; Theeuwes et al., 1998). A number of models of visual salience have been developed to explain how visual factors may guide the eyes to one location rather than another (e.g. Itti and Koch 2000; Navalpakkam and Itti, 2005). Which location is fixated is also determined by the task of the participant, this 'top-down' control allows the eyes to be directed to locations that are task relevant regardless of their visual salience. In a now classic study, Yarbus (1967) showed that when participants viewed pictures the locations that were fixated strongly depended on the task the participants were being asked to carry out. In this case the visual information in the picture remained constant across conditions so any differences between conditions must have been due to task-related or top-up factors. Stimulus and task-related factors combine to determine the target for the next saccade to ensure that the selection of the next saccade is determined by both the salience and relevance of the information at that location (see Schall and Cohen, Chapter 19, this volume; see Fecteau and Munoz, 2006).

Saccades and visual stability

The generation of a saccade has a profound effect on visual processing. Within a period of less than 50 ms the visual input to the retina is radically changed as the fovea and periphery are redirected to a new location in the environment. The movement of the eye leads to smearing of the image on the retina and backward masking reduces the ability to report visual information from the fixation before the saccade. One of the consequences of the high velocity of the eyeball during a saccade is that there is considerable distortion and additional displacement of the lens within the eye. Careful measurement of this phenomenon suggests that the distortion would result in as much as a 0.5° displacement of the retinal image. For larger saccades, lens stability may not occur for some 50 ms after the eyeball is stationary with a resulting instability of the retinal image (Deubel and Bridgeman, 1995). Over and above these effects there is evidence that vision is actively suppressed in the period of time around the generation of the saccade (see Ross et al., 2001). The reduction in sensitivity occurs before the onset of the saccade thereby ruling out explanations that claim that the suppression is simply a result or consequence of the movement itself. In addition, the suppression appears to be restricted to the visual magnocellular pathway which is tuned to lower spatial frequencies and higher temporal frequencies (Burr et al., 1994). Together these processes reduce the visual input around the time of the saccade which provides an explanation of why humans do not perceive strong motion as a result of a saccade. However, they do not provide an account of why the visual world appears stable. The question still remains how the visual system is structured to accommodate the radical change in visual input that is a consequence of a saccade (see Bridgeman, Chapter 28, this volume; Findlay and Gilchrist, 2003).

Conclusions

Saccades move the eye in a fast ballistic manner to point the fovea at a region of interest in the scene. In the interval preceding a saccade—the fixation—two processes occur simultaneously. Visual information at the currently fixated location is being processed while processing of information from the scene outside the currently fixated location is occurring to identify possible locations for the next fixation. The saccade target selection process is always based on degraded visual information because visual ability falls off so dramatically away from the currently fixated location. These two processes determine both when a saccade occurs—the saccade latency—and where the next saccade is directed.

This chapter has viewed the generation of saccadic eye movements in isolation. When participants are standing still and viewing a static image such as a painting (e.g. Fig. 5.2), the large movements of the eyes are exclusively saccadic. However, in more naturalistic settings the participant is moving, the environment is moving, and so are objects within that environment. As a result, in these dynamic situations, the types of eye movements discussed at the beginning of this chapter—saccades, smooth pursuit, vergence, vestibulo-ocular reflex—must act together in order to deliver visual stability and orient the fovea to regions of interest. In the case of saccades and pursuit, investigating the inter-relationship between these types of movements has revealed a closer functional and neural association between them than had previously been assumed (e.g. Krauzlis, 2004). How the different types of eye movements interact and how they are coordinated to function in a dynamic mobile world is a major challenge for further research in this area.

References

Bahill, A.T., Clark, M.R., and Stark L. (1975a). The main sequence, a tool for studying human eye movements. *Mathematical Biosciences*, **24**,191–204.

Bahill, A.T., Adler, D., and Stark, L. (1975b). Most naturally occurring human saccades have magnitudes of 15 degrees or less. *Investigative Ophthalmology*, **14**, 468–469.

Becker, W. and Jürgens, R. (1979). An analysis of the saccadic system by means of double step stimuli. *Vision Research*, **19**, 967–983.

Bouma, H. (1970). Interaction effects in parafoveal letter recognition. *Nature*, **226**, 177–178.

Burr, D.C., Morrone, M.C., and Ross, J. (1994). Selective suppression of the magnocellular visual pathway during saccadic eye movements. *Nature* **371**, 511–513.

Carpenter, R.H.S. and Williams, M.L.L. (1995). Neural computation of log likelihood in control of saccadic eye movements. *Nature*, **377**, 59–62.

Carpenter, R.H.S. (1988). *Movements of the Eyes* (2nd edn.). London: Pion.

Deubel H. and Bridgeman, B. (1995). Fourth Purkinje image signals reveal eye-lens deviations and retinal image distortions during saccades. *Vision Research*, **35**, 529–538.

Engbert, R. and Kliegl, R. (2003). Microsaccades uncover the orientation of covert attention. *Vision Research*, **43**, 1035–1045.

Fecteau, J.H. and Munoz, D.P. (2006) Salience, relevance, and spiking neurons: a priority map governs target selection. *Trends in Cognitive Science*, **10**, 382–390.

Findlay, J.M. and Gilchrist I.D. (2003). *Active vision: The psychology of looking and seeing.* Oxford University Press, Oxford.

Findlay, J.M. and Walker, R. (1999). A model of saccade generation based on parallel processing and competitive inhibition. *Behavioral and Brain Sciences* **22**, 661–674.

Findlay, J.M. (1982). Global visual processing for saccadic eye movements. *Vision Research*, **22**, 1033–1045.

Findlay, J.M. (1997). Saccade target selection during visual search. *Vision Research* **37**, 617–631.

Findlay, J.M., Brogan, D., and Wenban-Smith, M.G. (1993). The visual signal for saccadic eye movements emphasizes visual boundaries. *Perception and Psychophysics*, **53**, 633–641.

Fischer, B. and Weber, H. (1993). Express saccades and visual-attention. *Behavioral and Brain Sciences*, **16**, 553–567.

Forbes, K. and Klein, R. (1996). The magnitude of the fixation offset effect with endogenously and exogenously controlled saccade. *Journal of Cognitive Neuroscience*, **8**, 344–352.

Gilchrist, I.D., Brown, V., and Findlay, J.M. (1997). Saccades without eye movements. *Nature* **390**, 130–131.

Gilchrist, I.D., Brown, V., Findlay, J.M., and Clarke, M.P. (1998). Using the eye movement system to control the head. *Proceeding of the Royal Society: Biological Sciences*, **265**, 1831–1836.

Gilchrist, I.D., Heywood, C.A., and Findlay, J.M. (1999). Saccade selection in visual search: evidence for spatial frequency specific between-item interactions. *Vision Research*, **39**, 1373–1383.

Harris, C.M. and Wolpert, D.M. (2006). The main sequence of saccades optimizes speed-accuracy trade-off. *Biological Cybernetics*, **95**, 21–29.

He, P. and Kowler, E. (1991). Saccadic localization of eccentric forms. *Journal of the Optical Society of America, A*, **8**, 440–449.

Itti, L. and Koch, C. (2000). A saliency-based search mechanism for overt and covert shifts of visual attention, *Vision Research*, **40**, 1489–1506.

Kalesnykas, R.P. and Hallett, P.E. (1994). Retinal eccentricity and the latency of eye saccades. *Vision Research*, **34**, 517–531.

Krauzlis, R.J. (2004). Recasting the smooth pursuit eye movement system. *Journal of Neurophysiology*, **91**, 591–603.

Land, M.F., Furneaux, S.M., and Gilchrist, I.D. (2002). The organisation of visually mediated actions in a subject without eye movements. *Neurocase*, **8**, 80–87.

Land, M.F., Mennie, N., and Rusted, J. (1999). The roles of vision and eye movements in the control of activities of daily living. *Perception*, **28**, 1311–1328.

Ludwig, C.J.H. and Gilchrist, I.D. (2002). Measuring saccade curvature: A curve fitting approach. *Behavior Research Methods, Instruments, and Computers*, **34**, 618–624.

Ludwig, C.J.H., Butler, S.H., Rossit, S., Harvery, M., and Gilchrist, I.D. (2009). Modelling contralesional movement slowing after unilateral brain damage. *Neuroscience Letters*, **452**, 1–4.

Ludwig, C.J.H., Gilchrist, I.D., and McSorley, E. (2004). The influence of spatial frequency and contrast on saccade latencies. *Vision Research*, **44**, 2597–2604.

Ludwig, C.J.H. and Gilchrist, I.D. (2002). Stimulus-driven and goal-driven control over visual selection. *Journal of Experimental Psychology: Human Perception and Performance*, **28**, 902–912.

Ludwig, C.J.H., Mildinhall, J.W., and Gilchrist, I.D. (2007). A population coding account for systematic variation in saccadic dead time. *Journal of Neurophysiology*, **97**, 795–805.

Martinez-Conde, S. Macknik, S.L., and Hubel, D.H. (2004). The role of fixational eye movements in visual perception. Nature *Reviews Neuroscience*, **5**, 229–240.

McLaughlin, S.C. (1967). Parametric adjustment in saccadic eye movements. *Perception & Psychophysics*, **2**, 359–362.

McPeek, R.M., Skavenski, A.A., and Nakayama, K. (2000). Concurrent processing of saccades in visual search. *Vision Research*, **40**, 2499–2516.

McSorley, E., Haggard, P., and Walker, R. (2006). Time-course of oculomotor inhibition revealed by saccade trajectory modulation. *Journal of Neurophysiology*, **96**, 1420–1424.

Munoz, D.P. and Everling, S. (2004). Look away: The anti-saccade task and the voluntary control of eye movement. *Nature Reviews Neuroscience* **5**, 218–228.

Navalpakkam, V. and Itti, L. (2005). Modeling the influence of task on attention. *Vision Research*, **45**, 205–231.

Norton, D. and Stark, L.W. (1971). Scanpaths in saccadic eye movements while viewing and recognizing patterns. *Vision Research*, **11**, 929–942.

Optican L.M. (1985). Adaptive properties of the saccadic system. *Reviews of Oculomotor Research*, **1**, 71–79.

Reddi, B.A.J. and Carpenter, R.H.S. (2000). The influence of urgency on decision time. *Nature Neuroscience*, **3**, 827–830.

Ross, J., Morrone, M.C., Goldberg, M.E., and Burr, D.C. (2001). Changes in visual perception at the time of saccades. *Trends in Neurosciences*, **24**, 113–121.

Saslow, M.G. (1967). Effects of components of displacement-step stimuli upon latency of saccadic eye movement. *Journal of the Optical Society of America*, **57**, 1024–1029.

Smit, A.C. and Van Gisbergen, J.A.M. (1990). An analysis of curvature in fast and slow human saccades. *Experimental Brain Research*, **81**, 335–345.

Theeuwes, J., Kramer, A.F., Hahn, S., and Irwin, D.E. (1998). Our eyes do not always go where we want them to go: capture of the eyes by new objects. *Psychological Science*, **9**, 379–385.

Van Loon, E.M., Hooge, I.T.C., and Van den Berg, A.V. (2002). The timing of sequences of saccades in visual search *Proceedings of The Royal Society of London Series B-Biological Sciences*, **269**, 1571–1579.

Wade, N.J. and Tatler, B.W. (2005). *The moving tablet of the eye: The origins of modern eye movement research*. New York: Oxford University Press.

Walker, R., Deubel, H., Schneider, W.X., and Findlay, J. (1997). The effect of remote distractors on saccade programming: Evidence for an extended fixation zone. *Journal of Neurophysiology*, **78**, 1108–1119.

Walls, G.L. (1962). The evolutionary history of eye movements. *Vision Research*, **2**, 69–80.

White, J.M., Sparks, D.L., and Stanford, T.R. (1994). Saccades to remembered target locations: an analysis of systematic and variable errors. *Vision Research*, **34**, 79–92.

Yarbus, A.L. (1967). *Eye Movements and Vision*. New York: Plenum Press.

Zelinsky, G.J., Rao, R.P.N., Hayhoe, M.M., and Ballard, D.H. (1997). Eye movements reveal the spatiotemporal dynamics of visual search. *Psychological Science*, **8**, 448–453.

CHAPTER 6

Microsaccades[1]

Susana Martinez-Conde and Stephen L. Macknik

Abstract

Microsaccades are the largest and fastest of the fixational eye movements (i.e. the involuntary eye movements produced during attempted visual fixation). In recent years, the study of microsaccades has experienced a very rapid growth as a focus of visual and oculomotor research. Here we review the latest findings in microsaccade research, paying special attention to the perceptual, cognitive, and physiological effects of microsaccades and their interactions.

As you read this, your eyes are rapidly flicking from left to right in small hops, bringing each word sequentially into focus. When you stare at a person's face, your eyes similarly dart here and there, resting momentarily on one eye, the other eye, nose, mouth, and other features. With a little intro- spection, you can detect this frequent flexing of your eye muscles as you scan a page, face, or scene (Fig. 6.1A). But these eye movements, called saccades, are just a small part of the daily workout our eye muscles get. Our eyes *never* stop moving, even when they are apparently settled, say, on a person's nose or a mountaintop on the horizon. When the eyes fixate on something, as they do for 80% of our waking hours (Martinez-Conde, 2006; Otero-Millan et al., 2008), they still jump and jiggle imper- ceptibly in ways that turn out to be essential for seeing (Fig. 6.1B). If we halt these miniature motions while fixating our gaze, a static scene will simply fade from view (Fig. 6.1C).

Neural adaptation and visual fading

That the eyes move constantly has been known for centuries. In 1860 Hermann von Helmholtz pointed out that keeping one's eyes motionless was a difficult proposition and suggested that 'wandering of the gaze' prevented retinal fatigue (Helmholtz, 1985).

Animal nervous systems may have evolved to detect changes in the environment, because spotting differences promotes survival. Motion in the visual field may indicate that a predator is approaching or that prey is escaping. Such changes prompt visual neurons to respond with neural impulses. Unchanging objects do not generally pose a threat, so animal brains—and visual systems—did not evolve to notice them. Frogs are an extreme case. Just like *Tyrannosaurus rex* in *Jurassic Park*, frogs are blind to static objects. A fly sitting still on the wall will be invisible to a frog, but once the fly is aloft, the frog will immediately detect it and capture it with its tongue. Decades ago, Jerome Lettvin and colleagues classically stated that 'The frog does not seem to see or, at any rate, is not concerned with the detail of stationary parts of the world around him. He will starve to death surrounded by

---

[1] Portions of this chapter reprinted from Susana Martinez-Conde, Stephen L. Macknik, Xoana G. Troncoso, and David H. Hubel, Microsaccades: a neurophysiological analysis, pp. 463-475, Copyright (2009), with permission from Elsevier.

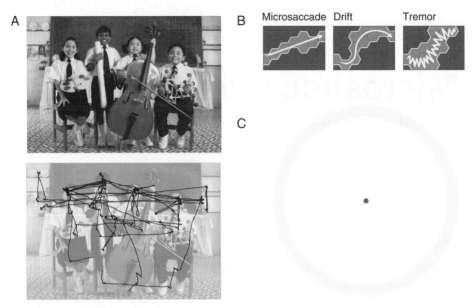

Fig. 6.1 Fixational eye movements and visual fading. A) An observer views a picture (top) while eye positions are monitored (bottom). The eyes jump, seem to fixate or rest momentarily, producing a small dot on the trace, then jump to a new region of interest. The large jumps in eye position illustrated here are called saccades. However, even during fixation, or 'rest' times, eyes are never still, but continuously produce fixational eye movements: drifts, tremor, and microsaccades. Modified from (Otero-Millan et al., 2008), with permission. Copyright held by Association for Research in Vision and Ophthalmology (ARVO). B) Cartoon representation of fixational eye movements in humans and primates. Microsaccades (straight and fast movements), drifts (curvy slow movements) and tremor (oscillations superimposed on drifts) transport the visual image across the retinal photoreceptor mosaic. Modified from (Martinez-Conde and Macknik, 2007), with permission. Copyright held by Jen Christiansen. C) Troxler fading. In 1804 Swiss philosopher Ignaz Paul Vital Troxler discovered that deliberately fixating on something causes surrounding stationary images to fade away. To elicit this experience, stare at the central dot while paying attention to the surrounding pale ring. The ring soon vanishes, and the central dot appears set against a white background. Move your eyes, and it pops back into view. Modified by permission from Macmillan Publishers Ltd: *Nature Reviews Neuroscience*, The role of fixational eye movements in visual perception, Susana Martinez-Conde, Stephen L. Macknik and David H. Hubel, **5**(3), copyright 2004.

food if it is not moving' (Lettvin et al., 1968). Frogs cannot see unmoving objects because an unchanging stimulus leads to 'neural adaptation'. That is, under constant stimulation, visual neurons adjust their gain as to gradually stop responding. Neural adaptation saves energy but also limits sensory perception. Primate neurons also adapt to sameness. However, the primate visual system does much better than a frog's at detecting unmoving objects, because primate eyes create their own motion. Fixational eye movements, the microscopic and unnoticed motions of the eye that we make when we fix our gaze between larger eye movements, shift the entire visual scene across the retina, prodding visual neurons into action and counteracting neural adaptation. They thus prevent stationary objects from fading away.

Fixational eye movements are perhaps the least understood of all eye movement types, despite their critical importance to normal vision. In 1804, Ignaz Paul Vital Troxler reported that precisely fixating one's gaze on an object of interest causes stationary images in the surrounding region to fade away (Troxler, 1804) (Fig. 6.1C). Thus, even a small reduction in the rate and size of fixational eye movements greatly impairs our vision. Totally ceasing all eye movements, however, can only be done in the laboratory. In the early 1950s, several groups achieved this stilling effect, demonstrating that in the absence of fixational eye movements observers become functionally blind to stationary objects during fixation (Ditchburn and Ginsborg, 1952; Riggs and Ratliff, 1952; Yarbus, 1967). Around the same time, three different types of fixational eye movements were characterized (Carpenter, 1988) (Fig. 6.1B).

Microsaccades are the small saccades that subjects produce when attempting to fixate their gaze on a visual target. They are the largest and fastest of the fixational eye movements. *Drifts* are slow meandering motions that occur between the fast, linear microsaccades. *Tremor* is a tiny, very fast (~90 Hz) oscillation superimposed on drifts. Tremor is the smallest type of fixational eye movement, its motion no bigger than the width of one photoreceptor. See table 1 from Martinez-Conde et al. (2009) for microsaccade parameters according to recent publications (2004–2009) and tables 1–3 from Martinez-Conde et al. (2004) for the characteristics of microsaccades, drift, and tremor according to studies published in 2004 and earlier.

Microsaccades contribute to maintaining visibility during fixation by shifting the retinal image in a fashion that overcomes adaptation, thus generating neural responses to stationary stimuli in visual neurons (Martinez-Conde et al., 2000, 2004, 2006). Recent discoveries have shown that microsaccades are critically related to many aspects of visual perception (Herrington et al., 2009; Laubrock et al., 2008; Martinez-Conde et al., 2006; Troncoso et al., 2008a, 2008b; van Dam and van Ee, 2006), attention and cognition (Engbert and Kliegl, 2003; Galfano et al., 2004; Hafed and Clark, 2002; Otero-Millan et al., 2008; Valsecchi et al., 2007), and thus potentially very important to neurological and ophthalmic disease (Martinez-Conde, 2006; Serra et al., 2008). The last decade of research has seen a very rapid increase in the numbers of papers dedicated to microsaccades, with the highest rise just in the last few years (Rolfs, 2009) (Fig. 6.2). Once considered a mere nervous tic (Kowler and Steinman, 1980), microsaccades are today a central and fast-growing topic of interest in the visual, oculomotor, and cognitive neurosciences: a field of inquiry that spans the perceptual effects of microsaccades, the neural responses they evoke, and their oculomotor generation mechanisms.

The physical and functional properties of microsaccades

Even though microsaccades are the largest and fastest fixational eye movement, they are relatively small in amplitude, carrying the retinal image across a range of several dozen to several hundred photoreceptor widths (Martinez-Conde et al., 2004). Such small amplitudes complicate objective microsaccade characterization; thus it is important to define the properties that microsaccades have in common with other types of eye movements, as well as those features that set them apart.

Microsaccades in monkeys are similar to those in humans (Martinez-Conde et al., 2000; Steinman et al., 1973) (see also Fig. 6.3 and tables 3 and 4 of Martinez-Conde et al. (2004)) for a comparison of the published characteristics of microsaccades in humans and primates), and they have been described in other foveate vertebrates as well (Martinez-Conde and Macknik, 2008). Importantly, microsaccades and saccades share many physical and functional characteristics, a fact that suggests that both eye movements have a common oculomotor origin (Hafed et al., 2009; Otero-Millan et al., 2008; Rolfs et al., 2008a; Zuber et al., 1965). The shared properties of microsaccades and saccades are summarized in the following list (modified and updated from Rolfs et al. (2008a)):

1. Microsaccades and saccades are generally binocular, conjugate movements, with comparable amplitudes and directions in both eyes (Ditchburn and Ginsborg, 1953; Krauskopf et al., 1960; Lord, 1951).

2. Microsaccades and saccades follow the main sequence. That is, microsaccade/saccade peak velocities are parametrically related to microsaccade/saccade amplitudes (Otero-Millan et al., 2008; Zuber et al., 1965) (see Fig. 6.6A later in this chapter), as are microsaccade/saccade durations (Bahill et al., 1975; Boghen et al., 1974; Garbutt et al., 2001; Troncoso et al., 2008a).

3. Visual perception thresholds are elevated during saccades and microsaccades, a phenomenon called 'saccadic/microsaccadic suppression' (Beeler, 1967; Herrington et al., 2009; Latour, 1962; Volkmann, 1962; Volkmann et al., 1968; Zuber and Stark, 1966; Zuber et al., 1964).

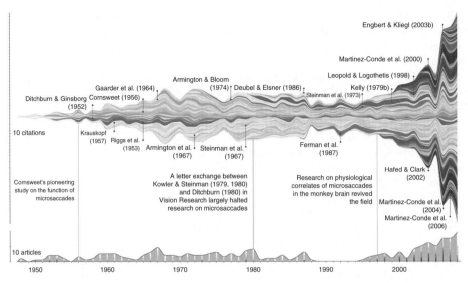

Fig. 6.2 (Also see Plate 1.) Impact of microsaccade research. The stacked graph at the top shows the impact of articles related to the function of microsaccades across time, from 1948 to 2008. Each stripe represents one of 253 articles for which data were available at the Web of Science. The height of the stripe shows the number of references to this article in a given year. Hence, the silhouette of the graph shows the overall impact of the field (685 citations in 2008). Stripe colours encode two dimensions: the age of an article (the warmer, the more recent) and its normalized impact (citations per year; the more saturated, the higher the impact; full saturation for >12 citations per year). The wiggle for each single stripe in the graph is minimized following the procedure proposed by Byron and Wattenberg (2008), ensuring best legibility. As time progresses, newer publications were evenly added at the rims, resulting in an inside-out (rather than bottom-to-top) layout and making the old literature the core of the graph. Labels highlight a selection of articles; both most cited and most neglected ones. The histogram at the bottom shows the number of items published in a given year; each dot is one article (same colour as in top panel). Modified from *Vision Research*, **49**(20), Martin Rolfs, Microsaccades: Small steps on a long way, 2415–2441. Copyright (2009), with permission from Elsevier.

4. Intersaccadic intervals during reading are comparable to intermicrosaccadic intervals during fixation of a single letter (Cunitz and Steinman, 1969).

5. Saccade and microsaccade rates can be reduced intentionally, as well as during specific tasks (Bridgeman and Palca, 1980; Fiorentini and Ercoles, 1966; Steinman et al., 1967; Winterson and Collewijn, 1976).

6. Voluntary saccades can be as small as fixational microsaccades (Haddad and Steinman, 1973).

7. Saccades and microsaccades have been linked to shifts in covert attention (i.e. attention directed to other stimuli than those on the centre of gaze; see section 'Attentional and cognitive modulation of microsaccades' for further references and discussion).

Recent research has moreover demonstrated strong interactions in the generation of saccades and microsaccades:

1. Microsaccade rates and amplitudes decrease before the launch of a saccade (Rolfs et al., 2006, 2008b).

2. Microsaccades occurring up to several hundred milliseconds before the saccadic 'go signal' delay the launch of the saccade (Rolfs et al., 2006, 2008b).

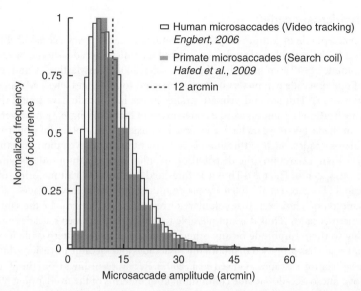

Fig. 6.3 Microsaccade amplitude against normalized frequency of occurrence in humans and primates. The data plots from two recent studies have been superimposed (Engbert, 2006; Hafed et al., 2009). Microsaccade amplitudes are comparable for humans and primates, irrespective of the eye-tracking method used (video tracking vs. magnetic search coil). Many of the microsaccades detected are considerably larger than 12 arcmin (an arbitrary amplitude threshold used in early studies of microsaccade characterization). One should note that prolonged visual fixation typically results in larger microsaccades than those depicted in this figure (data not shown; see figure 3B of (Otero-Millan et al., 2008), or figure 1E of Troncoso et al., 2008a)). Modified from *Progress in Brain Research*, **154**(1), Ralf Engbert, Copyright (2006), with permission from Elsevier; *Trends in Neurosciences*, **32**(9), Susana Martinez-Conde, Stephen L. Macknik, Xoana G. Troncoso, and David H. Hubel, Microsaccades: a neurophysiological analysis, Copyright (2009), with permission from Elsevier; and *Science*, Ziad M. Hafed, Laurent Goffart, and Richard J. Krauzlis, A neural mechanism for microsaccade generation in the primate superior colliculus, copyright 2009. Reprinted with permission from AAAS.

3. Intersaccadic intervals are equivalent for all pair-wise combinations of saccades and micro-saccades, during both fixation and free-viewing/visual search tasks (Otero-Millan et al., 2008). Thus the dichotomy between saccades and microsaccades proposed by previous studies may be fundamentally arbitrary.

The superior colliculus (SC) is a retinotopically organized structure involved in generating and controlling voluntary saccades (see also White and Munoz, Chapter 11, this volume). Current evidence overwhelmingly points towards a key role of the SC in microsaccade production. This idea has been explored in behavioural and computational studies (Otero-Millan et al., 2008; Rolfs et al., 2006, 2008a, 2008b), but has received direct confirmation only recently, through inactivation and electrophysiological studies in the primate SC (Hafed et al., 2009) (see section 'Brain mechanisms of microsaccade generation' for further discussion).

The term microsaccade was coined by Zuber et al. (1964). Throughout this review we use the term microsaccade because it has become the standard phrase to designate the saccades that occur during attempted fixation, thus we consider microsaccade a synonym to fixational saccade. We moreover propose that microsaccades should be defined operationally, as those *saccades that are produced while attempting to fixate* (Martinez-Conde, 2006; Otero-Millan et al., 2008), *irrespective of their amplitude*. That said, we acknowledge that an upper degree of 1° is reasonable, as a general rule, for practical experimental purposes (as it is the case with most of the studies reviewed here).

How big is a microsaccade?

Establishing an acceptable maximum amplitude for microsaccades poses a considerable challenge. In the 1960s and 1970s, a number of studies considered that microsaccades should have an arbitrary maximum amplitude of ~12 arcmin (Collewijn and Kowler, 2008) (see Martinez-Conde et al. (2004)) for a full list of microsaccade parameters in studies previous to 2004, and Otero-Millan et al. (2008) for further discussion). Human and primate studies in the last decade have found that saccades produced during fixation (i.e. microsaccades) often exceed 12 arcmin (Fig. 6.3), however. Thus studies conducted in the last 5–10 years have converged on using 1° as a practical upper threshold to characterize microsaccades. Such 1° threshold is convenient because (even though many microsaccades are larger than 12 arcmin) the distribution of microsaccade amplitudes asymptotes as it approaches 1° (also seen in Fig. 6.3). Thus a 1° threshold captures the vast majority (over 90%) of fixational saccades (Troncoso et al., 2008b) while excluding most voluntary saccades.

It is important to note, however, that voluntary or refixation saccades can be the same amplitude as fixational microsaccades. Thus it is not possible to distinguish between saccades and microsaccades according to their amplitude or any other physical parameter (Otero-Millan et al., 2008). Indeed, a recent study has proposed that both microsaccades and saccadic intrusions during fixation are referred to as 'fixation saccades' (Gowen et al., 2007). Recent recordings from the SC also support the existence of a microsaccade-saccade continuum, both in terms of the overlapping physical characteristics of microsaccades and saccades, and their generation mechanisms (Hafed et al., 2009).

Visual responses to microsaccades

Microsaccades play a critical role in maintaining visibility during fixation; thus the neural activity evoked by microsaccades throughout the visual system can help us to identify the neural codes of visibility. Visual responses to microsaccades are the neural responses to changes in visual inputs evoked by microsaccadic displacements of the retina (Fig. 6.4). Such responses have been measured in the lateral geniculate nucleus (LGN) (Fig. 6.4A), area V1 (Fig. 6.4B–D) and several areas of the extrastriate cortex of awake monkeys. Despite some discrepancies across studies, presumably caused by a combination of differences in eye movement recording systems, microsaccade characterization algorithms, visual stimuli, and behavioural tasks employed, there is general agreement that microsaccades primarily modulate neural activity in visual areas through retinal motion. That is, microsaccades primarily generate neural responses by displacing the receptive fields (RFs) of visual neurons over otherwise stationary stimuli (Martinez-Conde, 2006; Martinez-Conde et al., 2000, 2002) (Fig. 6.4) or even moving stimuli (Bair and O'Keefe, 1998a,b). See Martinez-Conde (2006) and Martinez-Conde et al. (2004) for reviews, and section 'Microsaccades as an optimal sampling strategy' for further discussion. Donner and Hemilä (2007) modelled the effects of microsaccades on the responses of primate retinal neurons, using physiologically realistic parameters. The results suggested that microsaccades may significantly enhance sensitivity to edges, 're-sharpen' the image, and improve spatial resolution. The results of this study support the prediction that microsaccades first generate neural activity in retinal neurons, perhaps as early as the photoreceptor level. This retinal activity may then be transmitted to subsequent levels in the visual hierarchy (Martinez-Conde et al., 2000, 2002, 2004).

Microsaccades could help to disambiguate latency and contrast in visual perception (Martinez-Conde et al., 2000, 2004). Changes in contrast can be encoded as changes in the latency of neuronal responses (Albrecht and Hamilton, 1982; Gawne et al., 1996). But how can latency information be used as a code for contrast, without the brain first knowing the timing of events? Because the brain 'knows' when a microsaccade is generated, differential latencies in visual responses might be used by the visual system to indicate differences in contrast and salience.

Microsaccades may also enhance spatial summation (i.e. the combination of two or more inputs arriving simultaneously through different synapses within a neuron's dendritic tree) by synchronizing the activity of neurons with neighbouring RFs. By generating bursts (i.e. clusters) of spikes in visual neurons, microsaccades may also enhance temporal summation (i.e. the combination of two

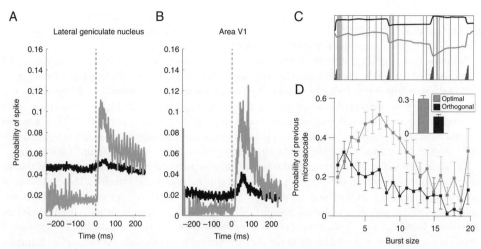

Fig. 6.4 Neural responses to microsaccades. A) Neural responses to microsaccades compared to neural responses to flashes in the LGN (n=57 neurons). B) Neural responses to microsaccades compared to flashes in area V1 (n=6 neurons). (A, B) The grey and black curves plot the same exact data, re-aligned to two different kinds of trigger events: flash onsets (grey) or microsaccade onsets (black). In each area, neuronal responses to flashes are larger than—but in the same order of magnitude as—responses to microsaccades. See section 'Microsaccades as an optimal sampling strategy' for further details. The oscillatory peaks on (A) (grey trace) were produced by the LGN cells following the flicker associated with the refresh rate of the monitor (74 Hz). Modified from *Trends in Neurosciences*, **32**(9), Susana Martinez-Conde, Stephen L. Macknik, Xoana G. Troncoso, and David H. Hubel, Microsaccades: a neurophysiological analysis, Copyright (2009), with permission from Elsevier. C) Relationship between microsaccades and bursts of spikes in area V1. The black and grey traces represent horizontal and vertical eye positions, respectively. The triangles at the bottom indicate occurrence of a microsaccade (the height of the triangles represents microsaccade amplitude). The vertical lines represent the spikes of a single V1 neuron. Microsaccades tend to be followed by a rapid burst of spikes. Modified by permission from Macmillan Publishers Ltd: *Nature Neuroscience*, Microsaccadic eye movements and firing of single cells in the striate cortex of macaque monkeys Susana Martinez-Conde, Stephen L. Macknik and David H. Hubel, **3**(3), copyright 2000. D) The size (number of spikes) of bursts following microsaccades in area V1 depends on the type of visual stimulation presented on the neuron's receptive field. Optimal stimuli (in this case, optimally oriented bars of light) lead to longer bursts; non-optimal stimuli (bars of light with orientations that are orthogonal to the optimal) lead to shorter bursts. Modified from Martinez-Conde, S., Macknik, S.L., & Hubel, D.H. (2002). The function of bursts of spikes during visual fixation in the awake primate lateral geniculate nucleus and primary visual cortex. *Proceedings of the National Academy of Sciences U S A*, **99**(21), 13920–13925. Copyright (2002) National Academy of Sciences, U.S.A.

or more inputs arriving non-simultaneously through the same or different synapses within a neuron's dendritic tree) of responses in neurons with neighbouring RFs (Martinez-Conde et al., 2004).

To date, most studies addressing the effects of microsaccades on visual physiology have been concerned with the responses of individual neurons. However, recent research has begun to tackle the physiological effects of microsaccades on neuronal populations. Synchronous neural oscillation has been described as a signature of perceptual processes associated with object representation, attention, memory and consciousness. A recent study has found microsaccades to modulate both neuronal activity and visually induced gamma-band (30–100 Hz) synchronization (GBS) in primate areas V1 and V4. Microsaccade-induced perturbations in GBS were moreover correlated with variability in behavioural response speed (Bosman et al., 2009). These results are consistent with those of an earlier study showing synchronization of neural activity due to fixational eye movements in the turtle retina (Greschner et al., 2002). Future research should further explore the modulation of synchronous activity by microsaccades along the primate visual pathway.

Yuval-Greenberg et al. (2008, 2009) have also recently pointed out that some commonly accepted measures of GBS might be contaminated by microsaccades in an unexpected fashion (see Melloni et al., 2009) for a counterpoint, and also the response by Yuval-Greenberg et al. (2009). Yuval-Greenberg et al. found that the scalp-measured induced gamma-band EEG response (iGBR) largely results from small muscle artefacts associated with microsaccade production (Yuval-Greenberg et al., 2008). Thus, whereas gamma-band activity might indeed play a role in brain processing (and might be modulated by microsaccades, as discussed above), care must be taken in the design and interpretation of future iGBR studies.

The study of microsaccade-driven neural activity may be pushed further in the near future, thanks to recent improvements in eye-tracking technology during functional imaging. The explosion of microsaccade studies over the last decade has had much to do with the recent availability of fast and reliable eye-tracking systems that allow non-invasive microsaccade measurements in human subjects (Martinez-Conde et al., 2004). Progress has been hampered due to the technical limitations of obtaining non-invasive measures of brain activity during microsaccade recordings in humans, however. Recent research has succeeded in measuring the BOLD (blood oxygen-level dependent) signal correlates of microsaccades in human visual cortex, via high-speed (1000-Hz sampling) infrared eye-tracking during functional magnetic resonance imaging (fMRI). This line of enquiry should be encouraged, as it will provide a much needed measure of the neural activity triggered by microsaccades throughout the human visual system, ideally in correlation with perceptual measures. Further, it raises the possibility that many past fMRI results may have been arisen due to uncontrolled microsaccades, thus forcing a re-evaluation of past functional imaging data (Tse et al., 2007). Indeed, a large amount of physiological and psychophysical visual research to date has been carried out while human and primate subjects were engaged in tasks involving visual fixation. Thus understanding the precise physiological and perceptual contributions of microsaccades may be critical to the interpretation of previous and future research in visual neuroscience.

Perceptual consequences of microsaccades

For many decades, the fixational eye movement field debated whether microsaccades might preserve vision by preventing visual fading. No studies had directly correlated microsaccades (or any other fixational eye movement) to visual perception, however. Thus by 1980 the field arrived at an impasse (Ditchburn, 1980; Kowler and Steinman, 1980). Over two decades later, a direct link between microsaccade production and visual perception was finally demonstrated. To establish the correlation between microsaccades and visibility, Martinez-Conde et al. conducted a behavioural experiment in which human subjects fixated a small spot, and simultaneously reported the visibility of a visual target, via button press (Martinez-Conde et al., 2006). Martinez-Conde et al. found that increased microsaccade production during fixation resulted in enhanced visibility for peripheral (9° and 6° of eccentricity) and parafoveal (3° eccentricity) visual targets. Conversely, decreased microsaccade production led to periods of visual fading. Head-restraint (or lack thereof) did not significantly change microsaccade dynamics (thus indicating that microsaccades are a natural oculomotor behaviour, rather than a laboratory artefact), or alter the link between microsaccade production and perceptual transitions (Martinez-Conde et al., 2006). These results established a potential causal relationship between microsaccades and target visibility during fixation, and corroborated predictions from physiological studies in which microsaccades were found to increase spiking rates in V1 and LGN neurons (Martinez-Conde et al., 2004) (Fig. 6.4A,B). Engbert and Mergenthaler (2006) moreover found that microsaccades were triggered when retinal image slip was low, further supporting the role of microsaccades in counteracting neural adaptation and visual fading. One should note that the fact that microsaccades counteract adaptation does not exclude their potential involvement in fixation correction. Engbert and Kliegl (2004) suggested that microsaccades counteract receptor adaptation on a short timescale and correct fixation errors on a longer timescale.

Microsaccade production has been subsequently linked to target visibility in other visual fading paradigms, such as the filling-in of artificial scotomas (Troncoso et al., 2008a) (Fig. 6.5) and motion-induced blindness (Hsieh and Tse, 2009), and also to perceptual transitions in other visual phenomena, such as binocular rivalry (van Dam and van Ee, 2006) and illusory motion (perceived speed as well as subjective direction (Laubrock et al., 2008; Troncoso et al., 2008b)).

Cui et al. (2009) recently showed that target visibility state modulates the rate and direction of microsaccades during 'general flash suppression' (GFS), a paradigm developed by (Wilke et al., 2003) in which a salient monocular target disappears following the sudden presentation of a binocular surrounding pattern. Cui et al. concluded that microsaccade production was affected by the percept, but that the target visibility/disappearance was not caused by changes in microsaccade rates. One should note that the Cui et al. findings do not contradict those of the above studies linking microsaccade production to target visibility during visual fading (Martinez-Conde et al., 2006), filling-in (Troncoso et al., 2008a), motion-induced blindness (Hsieh and Tse, 2009), or to perceptual alternations in other visual phenomena (Laubrock et al., 2008; Troncoso et al., 2008b; van Dam and van Ee, 2006). In all the above studies the percept changed (i.e. it undulated between two different states across time) even though the stimulus on the screen remained constant. In contrast, the Cui et al. study involved a physical change in the stimulus (the onset of the surround), which triggered the target's disappearance. Converging lines of research have shown stimulus visibility to be strongly related to transient bursts of neural activity (see section 'Microsaccades as an optimal sampling strategy' for more details). These neural transients may be triggered by sudden changes in the visual stimulus (as in the Cui et al. study), or in the case of an unchanging stimulus, by sudden eye movements such as microsaccades. Thus fluctuations in microsaccade production should not necessarily have the same effect on GFS (Cui et al., 2009) as they have on perceptual alternations taking place with unchanging stimuli (Hsieh and Tse, 2009; Laubrock et al., 2008; Martinez-Conde et al., 2006; Troncoso et al., 2008a, 2008b; van Dam and van Ee, 2006).

Perceptual suppression during large saccades is known to exist (Bridgeman and Macknik, 1995; Macknik et al., 1991; Ross et al., 2001; Wurtz, 1968, 1969), but the existence of microsaccadic suppression has been more controversial. Some studies have reported elevation of visual thresholds

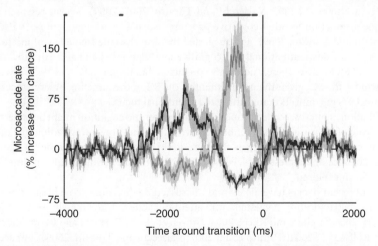

Fig. 6.5 Microsaccades counteract visual fading and filling-in. Microsaccade rates before transitions towards visibility ('unfilled' scotomas; grey) versus fading ('filled-in' scotomas; black). The horizontal line indicates average rate of microsaccades during the session. Shaded areas indicate SEM between subjects (n=6). The dots at the top indicate the bins where the 'unfilled' averages are significantly different from the 'filled-in' averages (one-sample one-tailed paired t-test, ≤0.05). Modified from Troncoso et al., 2008a. Copyright held by Association for Research in Vision and Ophthalmology (ARVO).

(Beeler, 1967; Ditchburn, 1955), but others have found little or no threshold elevation during micro-saccades (Krauskopf, 1966; Sperling, 1990). Recent results by Herrington et al. (2009) may represent a neural correlate of microsaccadic suppression. The authors recorded microsaccades and neural responses in areas middle temporal (MT), lateral intraparietal (LIP) and ventral intraparietal (VIP) while monkeys performed motion detection tasks. Microsaccades randomly occurring near the time of the test-stimulus onset decreased detection performance and suppressed neural activity, contributing to the correlation between neural activity and detection behaviour for all three brain areas investigated (microsaccades accounted for about one-fifth of the correlation). These findings could have important implications for future research aimed to determine the neuronal populations underlying perceptual decisions in behaving primates (who make microsaccades during the experiments).

Future research should determine how increases and decreases in visibility triggered by microsaccades may relate to different points in a microsaccade's lifetime. For instance, decreases in visibility may occur while a microsaccade is in flight, whereas enhanced visibility due to microsaccades could be driven by the microsaccade termination (i.e. the microsaccade's 'landing').

Attentional and cognitive modulation of microsaccades

Recent reports have shown a link between microsaccades and cognitive processes such as attention. This association is not altogether surprising, given the known considerable overlap between the neural systems contributing to the control of attention and the control of eye movements (Corbetta et al., 1998). Several studies have thus addressed the effects of shifts in spatial attention on microsaccade production. Hafed and Clark proposed that microsaccades occur due to the subliminal activation of the oculomotor system by covert attention (Hafed and Clark, 2002). Since then, the field has come to the consensus that microsaccade *rates* are modulated by both endogenous (top-down: attention is directed voluntarily, by top-down mechanisms) and exogenous (bottom-up: attention is automatically drawn to a stimulus in a reflexive or bottom-up manner) attentional shifts, with a transient rate drop in microsaccade production around 100–200 ms after cue onset, usually followed by a temporary enhancement about 300–400 ms after cue onset (Cui et al., 2009; Engbert and Kliegl, 2003; Hafed and Clark, 2002; Laubrock et al., 2005; Rolfs et al., 2004; Troncoso et al., 2008b; Tse et al., 2004; Turatto et al., 2007; Valsecchi and Turatto, 2007, 2009). Recent research has linked microsaccade production to other cognitive processes, such as working memory (Valsecchi et al., 2007; Valsecchi and Turatto, 2009), and suggested that the absolute frequency of microsaccades is also sensitive to top-down attentional and cognitive modulations (Betta and Turatto, 2006; Otero-Millan et al., 2008). Many of these studies have predicted that the neural circuitry controlling microsaccades includes the SC, given the involvement of the SC in the targeting of large saccades, which presumably occurs in connection to shifting the attentional focus.

The modulation of microsaccade production by attention and cognition might be (at least partially) related to a role of microsaccades in enhancing visibility and preventing fading during cognitive tasks. That is, cognitive processes such as attention could modulate microsaccade generation so as to dynamically enhance or suppress low-level visual information at various points in time. This possibility is thus far unexplored.

A number of recent papers have also found microsaccade directions to be biased towards and/or away from the spatial location suggested by an attentional cue (approximately 200 ms following the cue) (Engbert, 2006; Engbert and Kliegl, 2003; Gowen et al., 2007; Hafed and Clark, 2002; Laubrock et al., 2007; Rolfs et al., 2004; Turatto et al., 2007; Valsecchi and Turatto, 2009) (but see Horowitz et al. (2007a, 2007b; Tse et al. (2004) for a counterpoint). Some of the apparent disagreement across studies may be explained by the engagement of endogenous versus exogenous attention in different experimental tasks. Central informative cues (i.e. cues presented at fixation) that engage endogenous attention may produce microsaccade biases towards the peripheral location suggested by the cue (Engbert and Kliegl, 2003; Gowen et al., 2007; Hafed and Clark, 2002). In contrast, salient peripheral cues (visual or auditory, informative or uninformative) that engage exogenous attention may result in microsaccade biases opposite to the cue (Gowen et al., 2007; Laubrock et al., 2005; Rolfs et al., 2005).

The observation of microsaccade biases opposite to salient and abrupt peripheral events is consistent with inhibition of return, the phenomenon by which a stimulus presented at a recently attended location evokes a weaker reaction than a stimulus appearing at a location not yet attended (Betta et al., 2007; Galfano et al., 2004; Kliegl et al., 2009; Turatto et al., 2007).

A related topic of ongoing debate is whether biases in microsaccade directions indicate shifts in covert attention (Engbert and Kliegl, 2003; Hafed and Clark, 2002; Laubrock et al., 2007) and/or motor programming (Betta et al., 2007; Betta and Turatto, 2006; Horowitz et al., 2007a; Rolfs et al., 2006).

Brain mechanisms of microsaccade generation

Experimental evidence concerning the neurobiological origins of microsaccades has been sparse until very recently, constituting a major gap in our physiological understanding of these eye movements. Whereas the relationship between circuits controlling saccadic accuracy and fixation targeting is well documented (Goffart et al., 2004, 2006; Hafed et al., 2008; Munoz and Wurtz, 1993; Quinet and Goffart, 2007), few neurophysiological studies have aimed to determine the specific pathways responsible for the generation of microsaccades during fixation. Except for a handful of studies, most of the literature addressing the oculomotor mechanisms of microsaccade generation is only 2–3 years old. The studies by Van Gisbergen and colleagues in the late 1970s and early 1980s are worth noting. These authors found that putative motoneurons in the primate abducens nucleus and burst neurons in the nearby pontomedullary reticular formation (downstream of the SC) were active during saccades and microsaccades (Van Gisbergen et al., 1981; Van Gisbergen and Robinson, 1977). For decades, this was the main neurophysiological evidence of a common oculomotor mechanism underlying the generation of saccades and microsaccades.

In recent years, mounting behavioural evidence has moreover identified the SC as a key structure in the generation of both saccades and microsaccades (see previous section 'Microsaccade dynamics', and also White and Munoz, Chapter 11, this volume for further details). Recent physiological data support these predictions. Hafed and colleagues (Hafed et al., 2009) recorded from the rostral pole of the SC (which represents foveal goal locations) and found that individual neurons had particular preferences for a range of microsaccade amplitudes and locations (Fig. 6.6B). Further, the population data indicated a continuous representation of saccade amplitudes and directions throughout the SC, down to the smallest microsaccades. Neuronal activity during microsaccades sometimes extended to small voluntary saccades, consistent with previous studies suggesting a microsaccade/saccade continuum (Otero-Millan et al., 2008; Zuber et al., 1965). Neurons active during both microsaccades and voluntary saccades usually preferred voluntary saccades smaller than 5°. Conversely, neurons that were active during large voluntary saccades (~10° in amplitude; more caudal in the SC map) were not active during microsaccades. Importantly, the inactivation of the rostral SC led to reduced microsaccade rates, thus demonstrating the causal role of the rostral SC in microsaccade generation (Hafed et al., 2009) (Fig. 6.6C). These results, together with the earlier observations that premotor neurons in the brainstem reticular formation are active during microsaccades (Van Gisbergen et al., 1981; Van Gisbergen and Robinson, 1977), demonstrate that voluntary saccades and fixational microsaccades share the same neural mechanisms (Otero-Millan et al., 2008).

A computational model based on the SC data could also explain how covert attention shifts may bias microsaccade directions during fixation. In this model, attending a peripheral location caused the average locus of SC activity to slightly shift towards the peripheral site, leading to a higher probability of microsaccade directions towards the attended location (Hafed et al., 2009). Hafed and colleagues concluded that microsaccade occurrence depends on the variability of SC activity representing salient goal locations, and suggested that such a mechanism may also explain the link between changes in microsaccade rates and changes in visibility found by (Martinez-Conde et al., 2006) (Fig. 6.5; see section 'Perceptual consequences of microsaccades').

The recent SC experiments are an important milestone in establishing the neural mechanisms leading to microsaccade generation. Further research should be aimed at identifying the complete oculomotor pathway, as well as the specific circuitry involved at each neural stage.

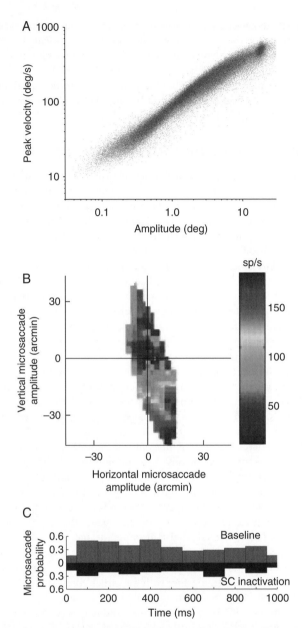

Fig. 6.6 (Also see Plate 2.) Microsaccade generation mechanisms. A) Microsaccades follow the saccadic main sequence, suggesting a common generator for microsaccades and saccades. Saccades and microsaccades recorded during free-viewing (blue) follow the same main sequence as those produced during fixation (red). (Note: some blue dots are obscured by the superimposed red dots.) N = 159,874 saccades and microsaccades combined for 8 subjects. From Otero-Millan et al. (2008). Copyright held by Association for Research in Vision and Ophthalmology (ARVO). B) Peak discharge of a SC neuron during microsaccades, plotted as a function of their horizontal and vertical amplitudes. The neuron preferred microsaccades directed to the lower right quadrant. C) Microsaccade probability during one second of fixation before (grey) and after (black) SC inactivation. Inactivation reduced microsaccade production. (B, C) From *Science*, Z.M. Hafed, L. Goffart, and R.J. Krauzlis, A neural mechanism for microsaccade generation in the primate superior colliculus, copyright 2009. Reprinted with permission from AAAS.

Microsaccades as an optimal sampling strategy

Eye movements are critical to normal vision: if all eye movements are counteracted, visual perception rapidly fades due to adaptation. Thus human eyes, as well as the eyes of other foveate vertebrates (Martinez-Conde and Macknik, 2008), are in continuous motion, with saccades and microsaccades abruptly shifting the retinal image at intervals ranging from once every several seconds to several times per second (Martinez-Conde et al., 2008). Saccades and microsaccades have comparable spatiotemporal characteristics across many varied visual tasks and viewing conditions (Otero-Millan et al., 2008). Here we discuss how the spatiotemporal dynamics of saccades and microsaccades may reflect an optimal sampling strategy by which the brain discretely acquires visual information.

Gilchrist et al. (1997) observed that a patient who was unable to make eye movements (except for small-amplitude drifts) produced head saccades that were comparable in many of their characteristics to eye saccades in normal observers. Such similar characteristics included the saccadic amplitudes, the duration of the intersaccadic intervals, the length of intervening fixations, and the range of visual scanning during the exploration of pictures, although the peak velocities of head saccades were slower than those of regular eye saccades). Such head saccades enabled the patient to read at normal speed and even perform complicated visuomotor tasks, such as making a cup of tea, with no problems. Although microsaccades were not tested per se, the authors concluded that 'saccadic movements, of the head or the eye, form the optimal sampling method for the brain' (as compared, for example, to smooth scanning of the visual scene) (Gilchrist et al., 1997, 1998; Land et al., 2002).

The idea that saccades and microsaccades discretely sample visual information is further supported by physiological studies comparing neuronal responses to saccades/microsaccades to responses triggered by instantaneous events, such as blinks and flashes (Fig. 6.4A,B). Gawne and Martin measured the responses of neurons in V1, V2, V3V/VP, and V4V to the onsets and terminations of visual stimuli elicited by flashes, blinks, and saccades. Although a minority of neurons presented responses that varied as a function of the neural event, most of them showed similar responses regardless of condition, suggesting that the neural circuitry underlying visual perception responds to different transient events in a similar manner (Gawne and Martin, 2002).

Martinez-Conde et al. (2002) compared the transient responses to microsaccade onsets versus those generated by visual flash onsets in 54 neurons of the LGN (n=48) and V1 (n=6). A periodic flashing bar (ON for 1 second; OFF for 1 second) was presented over the RF of a neuron while the monkey fixated a small cross. Responses to microsaccades that occurred while the flashing bar was ON were directly compared to responses to flash onsets that occurred while the monkey produced microsaccades. The effectiveness of each microsaccade thus depended on the relative positions of the bar and the RF at the time of the microsaccade onset. Likewise, the effectiveness of each flash depended on the relative positions of the bar and the RF at the flash onset: due to microsaccades, sometimes the flashing bar turned ON exactly on top of the RF, and sometimes it was displaced with respect to the RF centre. Thus any spatial shifts between the bar and the RF due to eye movements were equivalent across the microsaccade and flash response conditions. This experimental design permitted the direct statistical comparison of microsaccade- and flash-triggered responses, in the same neurons and at the same time. Neural responses to flashes were stronger than, but in the same order of magnitude as, responses to microsaccades, perhaps due to the relative abruptness of flashes with respect to microsaccades (Fig. 6.4A,B). Firing modulations caused by microsaccades could thus be equated to those caused by the 're-appearance' or 're-flashing' of the visual stimulus, albeit with a weaker neuronal response.

Bursting activity is a ubiquitous phenomenon in sensory systems (Krahe and Gabbiani, 2004). Transient responses evoked by microsaccades in primate visual neurons often take the form of bursts of spikes (Martinez-Conde et al., 2000, 2002, 2004) (Fig. 6.4C,D). These may or may not be accompanied by sustained firing during intersaccadic periods (Kagan et al., 2008). Bursty firing effectively indicates the presence of previous microsaccades in the awake primate, suggesting that this type of neural activity may be highly conducive to sustaining a visible image during fixation (Martinez-Conde, 2006; Martinez-Conde et al., 2000, 2002). In agreement with this idea, recent research has shown that microsaccades counteract perceptual fading during fixation (Martinez-Conde et al., 2006;

Troncoso et al., 2008a), and may lead to more efficient sampling of spatial detail (Donner and Hemilä, 2007). Further, the suppression of transient bursts of activity has been related to perceptual suppression during blinks (Gawne and Martin, 2000) and to decreased target visibility in visual masking (the phenomenon in which a visual target is rendered invisible by changing the context in which the target is presented, without actually modifying the physical properties of the target itself. That is, the target becomes less visible due solely to its spatial and/or temporal context) (Macknik and Livingstone, 1998; Macknik and Martinez-Conde, 2004; Macknik et al., 2000). Other studies suggest that V1 neurons produce stronger responses to transient than to drifting stimuli. Such neural transients may underlie the behaviour of cortical neurons as coincidence detectors (Shelley et al., 2002; Williams and Shapley, 2007).

Perceptual experiments have also shown that slow gradual changes (which presumably result in sustained neural firing) are difficult to detect, even in the absence of interruptions or distractions (Simons et al., 2000). These results further support the notion that discrete temporal sampling may be an optimal strategy for visual perception. By discrete sampling we refer to the periodic or aperiodic time-limited measurement of continuous-time varying data.

Discrete temporal sampling may be optimal across a number of sensory systems. Sniffs in rodent olfaction discretely sample sensory information every 200–300 ms and thus are similar in their temporal dynamics to primate saccades (Otero-Millan et al., 2008; Uchida et al., 2006) and microsaccades (Otero-Millan et al., 2008). A similar mode of discrete sampling may also be at play when objects are recognized through tactile information, for instance when subjects use their fingertips to identify an object with their eyes closed, or when blind individuals read Braille script. Uchida et al. (2006) suggested that discrete sensory sampling may be evolutionarily advantageous as it could speed up information processing (i.e. limiting the processing of low-level information to short chunks could facilitate the rapid construction of global perceptual images). Thorpe at al. (1996) showed that the visual processing required to determine the gist of a briefly flashed natural scene can be achieved in 150 ms. This interval could not be shortened even after extensive training; thus there may be a limitation on the number of neural stages and speed involved in the processing of visual information (Fabre-Thorpe et al., 2001). The generation of a saccade every 200–300 seconds could provide multiple individual high-acuity snapshots of a visual scene (Uchida et al., 2006) (intersaccadic intervals are equivalent for saccades and microsaccades (Otero-Millan et al., 2008)). But because of the limitations in visual processing speed stated above, faster rates of saccade/microsaccade production might not significantly improve vision.

Finally, microsaccades may not be randomly produced in time, but triggered dynamically as a function of low retinal slip (Engbert and Mergenthaler, 2006). Future research should thus investigate whether microsaccades dynamically displace retinal images with a temporal structure that serves to overcome adaptation within a discrete sampling framework.

Outstanding questions and directions for future research

The study of microsaccades is one of the fastest growing fields in contemporary neuroscience. Some important gaps remain to be addressed that would benefit from directed research efforts, however. Here we point out several areas of interest that are not discussed elsewhere in this chapter, alongside with some of the most promising current research directions.

Effect of microsaccades in central vision

Microsaccades have been linked to enhanced visibility of peripheral and parafoveal stimuli (Martinez-Conde et al., 2006) and they generate visual responses in RFs at all eccentricities (Martinez-Conde et al., 2002). The foveal image change resulting from a microsaccade may also determine percept dominance in binocular rivalry (van Dam and van Ee, 2006). The perceptual impact of microsaccades in foveal vision has not been directly investigated, however. Because foveal vision is sustained in the absence of microsaccades, it has been argued that the perceptual role of microsaccades solely concerns the visual periphery. However, the fact that drifts and/or tremor can maintain foveal vision on their own does not rule out the possibility that microsaccades also have a role. Thus if one were to eliminate drifts and tremor, microsaccades alone might sustain foveal vision during fixation (Martinez-Conde et al., 2004). Future research should determine the perceptual consequences of the interaction between microsaccade amplitudes and receptive field sizes at varying retinal eccentricities, including those in the foveal range.

Effects of microsaccades in various visual phenomena

Microsaccade dynamics are related to perceptual transitions in visual fading (Martinez-Conde et al., 2006), filling-in (Troncoso et al., 2008a), illusory motion (Laubrock et al., 2008; Troncoso et al., 2008b) and binocular rivalry (van Dam and van Ee, 2006). Many other visual illusions are attenuated or even disappear when the observer fixates carefully and thus suppresses microsaccades. Therefore microsaccades may drive (completely or partially) the generation of such illusory percepts (Martinez-Conde, 2006). Future research should determine the perceptual effects that are modulated by microsaccades, and relate them to the underlying neural circuits.

Neural correlates of microsaccadic suppression

The world remains perceptually stable during microsaccades, despite the fact that they cause sizable retinal motion that should be easily resolvable. Some studies have reported elevation of visual thresholds during microsaccades (i.e. microsaccadic suppression), but the neural correlates of this perceptual phenomenon are not well understood (Martinez-Conde et al., 2004) (but see Herrington et al. (2009)). Further, it is not known how perceptual suppression during microsaccades may interact temporally with the visibility enhancement also due to microsaccades (Martinez-Conde et al., 2006; Troncoso et al., 2008a).

Neural consequences of the attentional modulation of microsaccades

In the last few years, numerous studies have addressed how microsaccade rates and/or directions are modulated by attention in a variety of tasks. The physiological consequences of such attentional modulation remain fundamentally unexplored, however. Further, although the neural effects of increased attention versus increased microsaccade production can be separated (Chen et al., 2008), it is possible that some neural and perceptual effects currently attributed to attention are—at least partially—due to dynamic changes in microsaccade production during attentional tasks. Future experiments should trace the neural pathways by which attention, cognition, and microsaccades may interact.

Extraretinal modulation of neural responses by microsaccades

Microsaccades generate neural responses in visual neurons by displacing their RFs over otherwise stationary stimuli. But such clear-cut retino-geniculate-cortical responses may be accompanied by less evident extraretinal modulations. Some recent studies suggest that microsaccade-driven extraretinal modulations are present in a minority of neurons in area V1, but the evidence is conflicting as to the sign of such modulations (inhibitory, excitatory, or both) and their timing with respect to the primary retinal responses generated by microsaccades (Martinez-Conde et al., 2004). Different groups have found a) suppression of firing associated with microsaccade onsets in a marginal percentage of V1 neurons (Martinez-Conde et al., 2000), b) suppression of firing after microsaccades in about a third of V1 neurons (Leopold and Logothetis, 1998) (although this group later stated that microsaccades increase activity in area V1 (Moutoussis et al., 2005)), and c) weak suppression of firing after microsaccade onset followed by stronger enhancement 100–200 ms later in a third of V1 neurons (Kagan et al., 2008). In every study, the apparent extraretinal responses were much smaller than the neural responses due to straightforward retinal activation. Future research should ascertain the potential extraretinal modulations contributed by microsaccades throughout the visual pathway, determine their neural origins (i.e. corollary discharge from oculomotor centres of the brain, top-down attentional feedback, etc.), and determine their perceptual consequences (for instance, as the neural correlate of perceptual suppression during microsaccades).

Microsaccades in visual and neural pathologies

Insufficient fixational eye movements lead to neural adaptation and fading, whereas excessive eye motion produces blurring and unstable vision during fixation (Martinez-Conde, 2006). This delicate balance is a very common achievement in everyday vision. Even when we explore or search a visual scene, we fixate our gaze (in between large exploratory saccades) for 80% of the time (Martinez-Conde, 2006; Otero-Millan et al., 2008). Yet few studies have focused on pathological fixational eye movements as a sign of, or a contributor to, visual or neural disease (Serra et al., 2008) (see also Martinez-Conde (2006) for a recent review). Future research should assess the possible impairment of microsaccades and other fixational eye movements in central and peripheral pathologies, and the potential implications for treatment and/or early diagnosis.

Acknowledgements

We thank Jorge Otero-Millan and Hector Rieiro for scientific discussion and help with the figures, and Isabel Gomez-Caraballo, Manuel Ledo, and Andrew Danielson for technical assistance. This work was funded by grants from the National Science Foundation (awards 0643306 and 0852636 to SMC), the Arizona Biomedical Research Commission (award 07-102 to SMC), the Dana Foundation Program in Brain and Immuno-Imaging to SMC, and the Barrow Neurological Foundation to SMC and SLM.

References

Albrecht, D.G. and Hamilton, D.B. (1982). Striate cortex of monkey and cat: contrast response function. *Journal of Neurophysiology*, **48**, 217–237.

Bahill, A.T., Clark, M.R., and Stark, L. (1975). The main sequence, a tool for studying human eye movements. *Mathematical Biosciences*, **24**, 191–204.

Bair, W. and O'Keefe, L.P. (1998). The influence of fixational eye movements on the response of neurons in area MT of the macaque. *Visual Neuroscience*, **15**(4), 779–786.

Beeler, G.W. (1967). Visual threshold changes resulting from spontaneous saccadic eye movements. *Vision Research*, **7**, 769–775.

Betta, E. and Turatto, M. (2006). Are you ready? I can tell by looking at your microsaccades. *Neuroreport*, **17**(10), 1001–1004.

Betta, E., Galfano, G., and Turatto, M. (2007). Microsaccadic response during inhibition of return in a target-target paradigm. *Vision Research*, **47**(3), 428–436.

Boghen, D., Troost, B.T., Daroff, R.B., Dell'Osso, L.F., and Birkett, J.E. (1974). Velocity characteristics of normal human saccades. *Investigative Ophthalmology & Visual Science*, **13**(8), 619–623.

Bosman, C.A., Womelsdorf, T., Desimone, R., and Fries, P. (2009). A microsaccadic rhythm modulates gamma-band synchronization and behavior. *Journal of Neuroscience*, **29**(30), 9471–9480.

Bridgeman, B. and Palca, J. (1980). The role of microsaccades in high acuity observational tasks. *Vision Research*, **20**(9), 813–817.

Carpenter, R.H.S. (ed.) (1988). *Movements of the Eyes* (2nd edn.). London: Pion Ltd.

Chen, Y., Martinez-Conde, S., Macknik, S.L., Bereshpolova, Y., Swadlow, H.A., and Alonso, J.M. (2008). Task difficulty modulates the activity of specific neuronal populations in primary visual cortex. *Nature Neuroscience*, **11**(8), 974–982.

Collewijn, H. and Kowler, E. (2008). The significance of microsaccades for vision and oculomotor control. *Journal of Vision*, **8**(14), 20 21–21.

Corbetta, M., Akbudak, E., Conturo, T.E., Snyder, A.Z., Ollinger, J.M., Drury, H.A., *et al.* (1998). A common network of functional areas for attention and eye movements. *Neuron*, **21**(4), 761–773.

Cui, J., Wilke, M., Logothetis, N.K., Leopold, D.A., and Liang, H. (2009). Visibility states modulate microsaccade rate and direction. *Vision Research*, **49**(2), 228–236.

Cunitz, R.J. and Steinman, R.M. (1969). Comparison of saccadic eye movements during fixation and reading. *Vision Research*, **9**(6), 683–693.

Ditchburn, R.W. (1955). Eye-movements in relation to retinal action. *Optica Acta (London)*, **1**(4), 171–176.

Ditchburn, R.W. (1980). The function of small saccades. *Vision Research*, **20**(3), 271–272.

Ditchburn, R.W. and Ginsborg, B.L. (1952). Vision with a stabilized retinal image. *Nature*, **170**, 36–37.

Ditchburn, R.W. and Ginsborg, B.L. (1953). Involuntary eye movements during fixation. *Journal of Physiology*, **119**(1), 1–17.

Donner, K. and Hemilä, S. (2007). Modelling the effect of microsaccades on retinal responses to stationary contrast patterns. *Vision Research*, **47**(9), 1166–1177.

Engbert, R. (2006). Microsaccades: A microcosm for research on oculomotor control, attention, and visual perception. *Progress in Brain Research*, **154**, 177–192.

Engbert, R. and Kliegl, R. (2003). Microsaccades uncover the orientation of covert attention. *Vision Research*, **43**(9), 1035–1045.

Engbert, R. and Kliegl, R. (2004). Microsaccades keep the eyes' balance during fixation. *Psychological Science*, **15**(6), 431–436.

Engbert, R. and Mergenthaler, K. (2006). Microsaccades are triggered by low retinal image slip. *Proceeding of the National Academy of Sciences U S A*, **103**(18), 7192–7197.

Fabre-Thorpe, M., Delorme, A., Marlot, C., and Thorpe, S. (2001). A limit to the speed of processing in ultra-rapid visual categorization of novel natural scenes. *Journal of Cognitive Neuroscience*, **13**(2), 171–180.

Fiorentini, A. and Ercoles, A.M. (1966). Involuntary eye movements during attempted monocular fixation. *Atti della Fondazione Giorgio Ronchi*, **21**, 199–217.

Galfano, G., Betta, E., and Turatto, M. (2004). Inhibition of return in microsaccades. *Experimental Brain Research*, **159**(3), 400–404.

Garbutt, S., Harwood, M.R., and Harris, C.M. (2001). Comparison of the main sequence of reflexive saccades and the quick phases of optokinetic nystagmus. *British Journal of Ophthalmology*, **85**(12), 1477–1483.

Gawne, T.J., and Martin, J.M. (2000). Activity of primate V1 cortical neurons during blinks. *Journal of Neurophysiology*, **84**(5), 2691–2694.

Gawne, T.J., and Martin, J.M. (2002). Responses of primate visual cortical neurons to stimuli presented by flash, saccade, blink, and external darkening. *Journal of Neurophysiology*, **88**(5), 2178–2186.

Gawne, T.J., Kjaer, T.W., and Richmond, B.J. (1996). Latency: another potential code for feature binding in striate cortex. *Journal of Neurophysiology*, **76**(2), 1356–1360.

Gilchrist, I.D., Brown, V., and Findlay, J.M. (1997). Saccades without eye movements. *Nature*, **390**(6656), 130–131.

Gilchrist, I.D., Brown, V., Findlay, J.M., and Clarke, M.P. (1998). Using the eye-movement system to control the head. *Proceedings of the Royal Society of London Series B Biological Sciences*, **265**(1408), 1831–1836.

Goffart, L., Chen, L.L., and Sparks, D.L. (2004). Deficits in saccades and fixation during muscimol inactivation of the caudal fastigial nucleus in the rhesus monkey. *Journal of Neurophysiology*, **92**(6), 3351–3367.

Goffart, L., Quinet, J., Chavane, F., and Masson, G.S. (2006). Influence of background illumination on fixation and visually guided saccades in the rhesus monkey. *Vision Research*, **46**(1–2), 149–162.

Gowen, E., Abadi, R.V., Poliakoff, E., Hansen, P.C., and Miall, R.C. (2007). Modulation of saccadic intrusions by exogenous and endogenous attention. *Brain Research*, **1141**, 154–167.

Greschner, M., Bongard, M., Rujan, P., and Ammermuller, J. (2002). Retinal ganglion cell synchronization by fixational eye movements improves feature stimation. *Nature Neuroscience*, **5**(4), 341–347.

Haddad, G.M. and Steinman, R.M. (1973). The smallest voluntary saccade: implications for fixation. *Vision Research*, **13**(6), 1075–1086.

Hafed, Z.M. and Clark, J.J. (2002). Microsaccades as an overt measure of covert attention shifts. *Vision Research*, **42**(22), 2533–2545.

Hafed, Z.M., Goffart, L., and Krauzlis, R.J. (2008). Superior colliculus inactivation causes stable offsets in eye position during tracking. *Journal of Neuroscience*, **28**(32), 8124–8137.

Hafed, Z.M., Goffart, L., and Krauzlis, R. (2009). A neural mechanism for microsaccade generation in the primate superior colliculus. *Science*, **323**, 940–994.

Helmholtz, H. von (1985). *Helmholtz's Treatise on Physiological Optics* (trans. J.P.C. Southall. Translated from 3rd German Edition ed. Vol. 2). Birmingham, AL: Gryphon Editions, Ltd.

Herrington, T.M., Masse, N.Y., Hachmeh, K.J., Smith, J.E., Assad, J.A., and Cook, E.P. (2009). The effect of microsaccades on the correlation between neural activity and behavior in middle temporal, ventral intraparietal, and lateral intraparietal areas. *Journal of Neuroscience*, **29**(18), 5793–5805.

Horowitz, T.S., Fine, E.M., Fencsik, D.E., Yurgenson, S., and Wolfe, J.M. (2007a). Fixational eye movements are not an index of covert attention. *Psychological Science*, **18**(4), 356–363.

Horowitz, T.S., Fine, E.M., Fencsik, D.E., Yurgenson, S., and Wolfe, J. M. (2007b). Microsaccades and attention: does a weak correlation make an index? Reply to Laubrock, Engbert, Rolfs, and Kliegl (2007). *Psychological Science*, **18**(4), 367–368.

Hsieh, P.J. and Tse, P.U. (2009). Microsaccade rate varies with subjective visibility during motion-induced blindness. *PLoS ONE*, **4**(4), e5163.

Kagan, I., Gur, M., and Snodderly, D.M. (2008). Saccades and drifts differentially modulate neuronal activity in V1: effects of retinal image motion, position, and extraretinal influences. *Journal of Vision*, **8**(14), 19.11–25.

Kliegl, R., Rolfs, M., Laubrock, J., and Engbert, R. (2009). Microsaccadic modulation of response times in spatial attention tasks. *Psychological Research*, **73**(2), 136–146.

Kowler, E. and Steinman, R.M. (1980). Small saccades serve no useful purpose: reply to a letter by R.W. Ditchburn. *Vision Research*, **20**(3), 273–276.

Krahe, R. and Gabbiani, F. (2004). Burst firing in sensory systems. *Nature Reviews. Neuroscience*, **5**(1), 13–23.

Krauskopf, J. (1966). Lack of inhibition during involuntary saccades. *American Journal of Psychology*, **79**, 73–81.

Krauskopf, J., Cornsweet, T.N., and Riggs, L.A. (1960). Analysis of eye movements during monocular and binocular fixation. *Journal of the Optical Society of America*, **50**, 572–578.

Land, M.F., Furneaux, S.M., and Gilchrist, I.D. (2002). The organization of visually mediated actions in a subject without eye movements. *Neurocase*, **8**(1–2), 80–87.

Latour, P.L. (1962). Letter to the Editor: Visual threshold during eye movements. *Vision Researchearch*, **2**, 261–262.

Laubrock, J., Engbert, K., and Kliegl, R. (2008). Fixational eye movements predict the perceived direction of ambiguous apparent motion. *Journal of Vision*, **8**(14), 13.1–17.

Laubrock, J., Engbert, R., and Kliegl, R. (2005). Microsaccade dynamics during covert attention. *Vision Research*, **45**(6), 721–730.

Laubrock, J., Engbert, R., Rolfs, M., and Kliegl, R. (2007). Microsaccades are an index of covert attention: commentary on Horowitz, Fine, Fencsik, Yurgenson, and Wolfe (2007). *Psychological Science*, **18**(4), 364–366; discussion 367–368.

Leopold, D.A., and Logothetis, N.K. (1998). Microsaccades differentially modulate neural activity in the striate and extrastriate visual cortex. *Experimental Brain Research*, **123**(3), 341–345.

Lettvin, J.Y., Maturana, H.R., MsCulloch, W.S., and Pitts, W.H. (1968). What the frog's eye tells the frog's brain. In W.C. Corning and M. Balaban (eds.) *The mind: biological approaches to its functions* (pp. 233–258). London: John Wiley and Sons Inc.

Lord, M.P. (1951). Measurement of binocular eye movements of subjects in the sitting position. *British Journal of Ophthalmology*, **35**, 21–30.

Macknik, S.L., and Livingstone, M.S. (1998). Neuronal correlates of visibility and invisibility in the primate visual system. *Nature Neuroscience*, **1**(2), 144–149.

Macknik, S.L., and Martinez-Conde, S. (2004). The spatial and temporal effects of lateral inhibitory networks and their relevance to the visibility of spatiotemporal edges. *Neurocomputing*, **58–60**, 775–782.

Macknik, S.L., Fisher, B.D., and Bridgeman, B. (1991). Flicker distorts visual space constancy. *Vision Research,* **31**(12), 2057–2064.

Macknik, S.L., Martinez-Conde, S., and Haglund, M.M. (2000). The role of spatiotemporal edges in visibility and visual masking. *Proceedings of the National Academy of Sciences of the U S A*, **97**(13), 7556–7560.

Martinez-Conde, S. (2006). Fixational eye movements in normal and pathological vision. *Progress in Brain Research*, **154**, 151–176.

Martinez-Conde, S., and Macknik, S.L. (2007). Windows on the mind. *Scientific American*, **297**, 56–63.

Martinez-Conde, S., and Macknik, S.L. (2008). Fixational eye movements across vertebrates: comparative dynamics, physiology, and perception. *Journal of Vision*, **8**(14), 28.21–16.

Martinez-Conde, S., Macknik, S.L., and Hubel, D.H. (2000). Microsaccadic eye movements and firing of single cells in the striate cortex of macaque monkeys. *Nature Neuroscience*, **3**(3), 251–258.

Martinez-Conde, S., Macknik, S.L., and Hubel, D.H. (2002). The function of bursts of spikes during visual fixation in the awake primate lateral geniculate nucleus and primary visual cortex. *Proceedings of the National Academy of Sciences of the U S A*, **99**(21), 13920–13925.

Martinez-Conde, S., Macknik, S.L., and Hubel, D.H. (2004). The role of fixational eye movements in visual perception. *Nature Reviews. Neuroscience*, **5**, 229–240.

Martinez-Conde, S., Macknik, S.L., Troncoso, X., and Dyar, T.A. (2006). Microsaccades counteract visual fading during fixation. *Neuron*, **49**, 297–305.

Martinez-Conde, S., Krauzlis, R., Miller, J., Morrone, C., Williams, W., and Kowler, E. (2008). Eye movements and the perception of a clear and stable visual world. *Journal of Vision*, **8**(14), **i**, 1.

Martinez-Conde, S., Macknik, S.L., Troncoso, X.G., and Hubel, D H. (2009). Microsaccades: a neurophysiological analysis. *Trends in Neurosciences*, **32**(9), 463–475.

Melloni, L., Schwiedrzik, C.M., Wibral, M., Rodriguez, E., and Singer, W. (2009). Response to: Yuval-Greenberg et al., 'Transient Induced Gamma-Band Response in EEG as a Manifestation of Miniature Saccades.' Neuron 58, 429–441. *Neuron*, **62** (1), 8–10.

Moutoussis, K., Keliris, G., Kourtzi, Z., and Logothetis, N. (2005). A binocular rivalry study of motion perception in the human brain. *Vision Research*, **45**(17), 2231–2243.

Munoz, D.P., and Wurtz, R.H. (1993). Fixation cells in monkey superior colliculus. I. Characteristics of cell discharge. *Journal of Neurophysiology*, **70**, 559–575.

Otero-Millan, J., Troncoso, X., Macknik, S.L., Serrano-Pedraza, I., and Martinez-Conde, S. (2008). Saccades and microsaccades during visual fixation, exploration and search: foundations for a common saccadic generator. *Journal of Vision*, **8**(14), 21.1–18.

Quinet, J. and Goffart, L. (2007). Head-unrestrained gaze shifts after muscimol injection in the caudal fastigial nucleus of the monkey. *Journal of Neurophysiology*, **98**(6), 3269–3283.

Riggs, L.A., and Ratliff, F. (1952). The effects of counteracting the normal movements of the eye. *Journal of the Optical Society of America*, **42**, 872–873.

Rolfs, M. (2009). Microsaccades: Small steps on a long way. *Vision Research*, **49**(20), 2415–2441.

Rolfs, M., Engbert, R., and Kliegl, R. (2004). Microsaccade orientation supports attentional enhancement opposite a peripheral cue: commentary on Tse, Sheinberg, and Logothetis (2003). *Psychological Science*, **15**, 431–436.

Rolfs, M., Engbert, R., and Kliegl, R. (2005). Crossmodal coupling of oculomotor control and spatial attention in vision and audition. *Experimental Brain Research*, **166**(3–4), 427–439.

Rolfs, M., Laubrock, J., and Kliegl, R. (2006). Shortening and prolongation of saccade latencies following microsaccades. *Experimental Brain Research*, **169**(3), 369–376.

Rolfs, M., Kliegl, R., and Engbert, K. (2008a). Toward a model of microsaccade generation: The case of microsaccadic inhibition. *Journal of Vision*, **8**(11), 1–23.

Rolfs, M., Laubrock, J., and Kliegl, R. (2008b). Microsaccade-induced prolongation of saccadic latencies depends on microsaccade amplitude. *Journal of Eye Movement Research*, **1**(3), 1.1–8.

Ross, J., Morrone, M.C., Goldberg, M.E., and Burr, D.C. (2001). Changes in visual perception at the time of saccades. [see comments]. *Trends in Neurosciences*, **24**(2), 113–121.

Serra, A., Liao, K., Martinez-Conde, S., Optican, L.M., and Leigh, R.J. (2008). Suppression of saccadic intrusions in hereditary ataxia by memantine. *Neurology*, **70**(10), 810–812.

Shelley, M., McLaughlin, D., Shapley, R., and Wielaard, J. (2002). States of high conductance in a large-scale model of the visual cortex. *Journal of Computational Neuroscience*, **13**(2), 93–109.

Simons, D.J., Franconeri, S.L., and Reimer, R.L. (2000). Change blindness in the absence of a visual disruption. *Perception*, **29**(10), 1143–1154.

Sperling, G. (1990). Comparison of perception in the moving and stationary eye. In E. Kowler (ed.), *Eye movements and their role in visual and cognitive processes* (pp. 307–351). Amsterdam: Elsevier.

Steinman, R.M., Cunitz, R.J., Timberlake, G.T., and Herman, M. (1967). Voluntary control of microsaccades during maintained monocular fixation. *Science*, **155**(769), 1577–1579.

Steinman, R.M., Haddad, G.M., Skavenski, A.A., and Wyman, D. (1973). Miniature eye movement. *Science*, **181**(102), 810–819.

Thorpe, S., Fize, D., and Marlot, C. (1996). Speed of processing in the human visual system. *Nature*, **381**(6582), 520–522.

Troncoso, X., Macknik, S.L., and Martinez-Conde, S. (2008a). Microsaccades counteract perceptual filling-in. *Journal of Vision*, **8**(14), 15.1–9.

Troncoso, X., Macknik, S.L., Otero-Millan, J., and Martinez-Conde, S. (2008b). Microsaccades drive illusory motion in the Enigma illusion. *Proceedings of the National Academy of Sciences U S A*, **105**, 16033–16038.

Troxler, I.P.V. (1804). Ueber das Verschwinden gegebener Gegenstande innerhalb unseres Gesichtskreises. In K. Himly and J.A. Schmidt (eds.), *Ophthalmologische Bibliothek* (Vol. II. 2, pp. 1–53). Jena: Springer.

Tse, P.U., Baumgartner, F., and Greenlee, M. (2007). *fMRI BOLD signal reveals neural correlates of microsaccades*. Paper presented at the Vision Sciences Society, Sarasota, FL.

Tse, P.U., Sheinberg, D.S., and Logothetis, N.K. (2004). The distribution of microsaccade directions need not reveal the location of attention. *Psychological Science*, **15**(10), 708–710.

Turatto, M., Valsecchi, M., Tame, L., and Betta, E. (2007). Microsaccades distinguish between global and local visual processing. *Neuroreport*, **18**(10), 1015–1018.

Uchida, N., Kepecs, A., and Mainen, Z.F. (2006). Seeing at a glance, smelling in a whiff: rapid forms of perceptual decision making. *Nature Reviews. Neuroscience*, **7**(6), 485–491.

Valsecchi, M., Betta, E., and Turatto, M. (2007). Visual oddballs induce prolonged microsaccadic inhibition. *Experimental Brain Research*, **177**(2), 196–208.

Valsecchi, M. and Turatto, M. (2007). Microsaccadic response to visual events that are invisible to the superior colliculus. *Behavioral Neuroscience*, **121**(4), 786–793.

Valsecchi, M. and Turatto, M. (2009). Microsaccadic responses in a bimodal oddball task. *Psychologicaal Research*, **73**(1), 23–33.

van Dam, L.C. and van Ee, R. (2006). Retinal image shifts, but not eye movements per se, cause alternations in awareness during binocular rivalry. *Journal of Vision*, **6**(11), 1172–1179.

Van Gisbergen, J.A., Robinson, D.A., and Gielen, S. (1981). A quantitative analysis of generation of saccadic eye movements by burst neurons. *Journal of Neurophysiology*, **45**(3), 417–442.

Van Gisbergen, J.A.M. and Robinson, D.A. (1977). Generation of micro and macrosaccades by burst neurons in the monkey. In R. Baker and A. Berthoz (eds.) *Control of gaze by brain stem neurons* (301–308). New York: Elsevier/North-Holland.

Volkmann, F.C. (1962). Vision during voluntary saccadic eye movements. *Journal of the Optical Society of America*, **52**, 571–578.

Volkmann, F.C., Schick, A.M., and Riggs, L.A. (1968). Time course of visual inhibition during voluntary saccades. *Journal of the Optical Society of America*, **58**(4), 562–569.

Wilke, M., Logothetis, N.K., and Leopold, D.A. (2003). Generalized flash suppression of salient visual targets. *Neuron*, **39**(6), 1043–1052.

Williams, P.E. and Shapley, R.M. (2007). A dynamic nonlinearity and spatial phase specificity in macaque V1 neurons. *Journal of Neuroscience*, **27**(21), 5706–5718.

Winterson, B.J. and Collewijn, H. (1976). Microsaccades during finely guided visuomotor tasks. *Vision Research*, **16**(12), 1387–1390.

Wurtz, R.H. (1968). Visual cortex neurons: response to stimuli during rapid eye movements. *Science*, **162**, 1148–1150.

Wurtz, R.H. (1969). Comparison of effects of eye movements and stimulus movements on striate cortex neurons of the monkey. *Journal of Neurophysiology*, **32**, 987–994.

Yarbus, A.L. (1967). *Eye Movements and Vision* (trans. B. Haigh). New York: Plenum Press.

Yuval-Greenberg, S., Tomer, O. Keren, A.S., Nelken, I., Deouell, L.Y. (2008). Transient induced gamma-band response in EEG as a manifestation of miniature saccades. *Neuron*, **58** (3), 429–441.

Yuval-Greenberg, S., Keren, A. S., Tomer, O., Nelken, I., and Deouell, L.Y. (2009). Response to Letter: Melloni et al., 'Transient Induced Gamma-Band Response in EEG as a Manifestation of Miniature Saccades.' *Neuron*, **58**, 429–441. *Neuron*, **62**(1), 10–12.

Zuber, B.L., Crider, A., and Stark, L. (1964). Saccadic suppression associated with microsaccades. *Quarterly Progress Report*, **74**, 244–249.

Zuber, B.L. and Stark, L. (1966). Saccadic suppression: elevation of visual threshold associated with saccadic eye movements. *Experimental Neurology*, **16**(1), 65–79.

Zuber, B.L., Stark, L., and Cook, G. (1965). Microsaccades and the velocity-amplitude relationship for saccadic eye movements. *Science*, **150**(702), 1459–1460.

CHAPTER 7

Ocular pursuit movements

Graham R. Barnes

Abstract

Ocular pursuit movements allow moving objects to be tracked with a combination of smooth movements and saccades. The principal objective is to maintain smooth eye velocity close to object velocity, thus minimizing retinal image motion and maintaining acuity. Saccadic movements serve to realign the image if it falls outside the fovea, the area of highest acuity. Pursuit is initially driven by visual feedback when responding to unexpected object motion. However, internal (extraretinal) mechanisms rapidly take over and sustain pursuit if object velocity is constant. If object motion is periodic, delays in visual motion processing create potential response delays, but these are countered by predictive processes, probably also operating through internal, efference copy mechanisms using short-term memory to store motion information from prior stimulation.

Introduction

Ocular pursuit movements allow moving objects to be tracked with a combination of smooth movements and saccades. The principal objective is to maintain smooth eye velocity close to object velocity, thus minimizing retinal image motion and maintaining acuity. Saccadic movements serve to realign the image if it falls outside the fovea, the area of highest acuity. Pursuit movements are often portrayed as voluntary but their basis lies in processes that sense retinal motion and can induce eye movements without active participation. The factor distinguishing pursuit from such reflexive movements is the ability to select and track a single object when presented with multiple stimuli. The selective process requires attention, which appears to raise the gain for the selected object and/or suppress that associated with other stimuli, the resulting competition often reducing pursuit velocity. Although pursuit is essentially a feedback process, delays in motion processing create problems of stability and speed of response. This is countered by predictive processes, probably operating through internal efference copy (extraretinal) mechanisms using short-term memory to store velocity and timing information from prior stimulation. In response to constant velocity motion, the initial response is visually driven, but extraretinal mechanisms rapidly take over and sustain pursuit. The same extraretinal mechanisms may also be responsible for generating anticipatory smooth pursuit movements when past experience creates expectancy of impending object motion. Similar, but more complex, processes appear to operate during periodic pursuit, where partial trajectory information is stored and released in anticipation of expected future motion, thus minimizing phase errors associated with motion processing delays.

Motion stimuli used to investigate pursuit

Ramp and step-ramp stimuli

Smooth pursuit initiation

The simplest way to examine pursuit is by considering the response to the unexpected movement of a target that suddenly starts to move at constant velocity (a ramp motion stimulus) (Robinson, 1965). Fig. 7.1A shows typical eye displacement responses to ramp stimuli of varying velocity. There is normally a reaction time of approximately 100–130 ms before smooth movements start, although much shorter latencies of 70–100 ms have been recorded (Lisberger and Westbrook, 1985; Lisberger et al., 1987; Miles and Kawano, 1986). The latency is probably composed of a visuomotor processing delay of approximately 70 ms in humans coupled with an initial decision-making delay of 30 ms

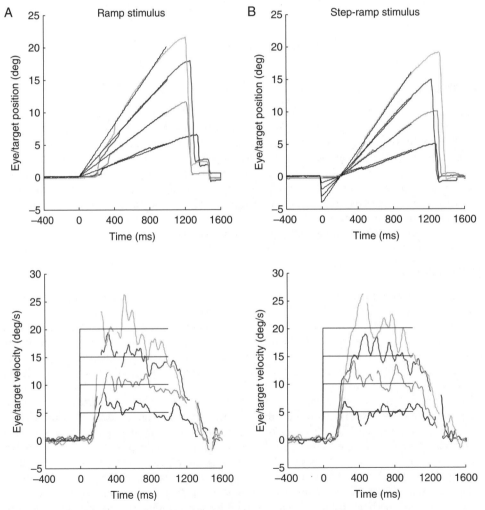

Fig. 7.1 (Also see Plate 3.) A) Typical eye position (upper) and smooth eye velocity (lower) responses to ramp target motion stimuli with velocity of 5 (blue), 10 (green), 15 (red) or 20 (cyan)°/s. B) Typical eye position (upper) and eye velocity (lower traces) in response to step-ramp stimuli with velocity of 5-20°/s. Gaps in smooth eye velocity traces represent occurrence of saccades.
Reprinted from *Brain and Cognition*, **68**(3), G.R. Barnes, Cognitive processes involved in smooth pursuit eye movements, copyright (2008), with permission from Elsevier.

(Wyatt and Pola, 1987). In contrast, the first saccade occurs after approximately 240 ms (Fig. 7.1A) and realigns the image close to the fovea. Actual eye displacement prior to the first saccade is often small and difficult to measure. When eye displacement is differentiated it is evident that eye velocity does not suddenly change to equal target velocity, but accelerates prior to the first saccade. However, after the saccade, eye velocity often jumps to a higher level (Lisberger, 1998) a feature referred to as post-saccadic enhancement. To eliminate the initial saccade or, at least, to ensure that it occurs later in the response, many investigators use the so-called step-ramp stimulus (Rashbass, 1961). The target first jumps to one side and then makes a ramp in the opposite direction, crossing over the starting point (Fig. 7.1B). This step-ramp stimulus often elicits a smooth movement without any saccade if the step size is such that the target crosses back over the origin in approximately 200 ms. Eye move-ment normally starts somewhat later than for a simple ramp at approximately 130–150 ms after the step, and may be ahead of the target motion as it crosses the midline so that a reverse saccade has to be made. Although this stimulus appears to indicate that the system is responsive only to the velocity of the target, since there is often no evidence of a response to the step, careful examination of the initial response shows that there is a small transient reversal of eye velocity in the direction of the step (Carl and Gellman, 1987). Once under way, the first 100 ms of the smooth response is often referred to as the open-loop phase, since the delay in visual processing dictates that within this time period the retinal velocity error is not changed by the movement of the eye. Detailed examination of the step-ramp response has shown two distinct phases. In the initial 20–30 ms eye acceleration shows some increase with target velocity but not with starting position of the target motion (Lisberger and Westbrook, 1985), whereas, in the period 60–80 ms after onset there is a much greater modula-tion of eye acceleration by target velocity and a strong dependence on eccentricity of starting position. Peak eye velocity is normally attained at a time that typically increases from approximately 220–330 ms after response onset as target velocity increases from 5–30°/s (Robinson et al., 1986).

Smooth pursuit maintenance

Following initial response onset eye velocity frequently overshoots target velocity and may oscillate at a frequency of 3–4 Hz in humans (Fig. 7.1B). Oscillations normally die away within one or two cycles and eye velocity settles to an average that is close to target velocity. Gain (the ratio of eye velocity to target velocity) is normally in the range 0.9–1.0 for target velocities <20°/s. Meyer et al. (1985) showed that gain could remain as high as 0.9 up to approximately 90°/s, but declines at higher veloc-ity. If gain falls substantially below unity, corrective saccades are made to realign the target image on the fovea.

Smooth pursuit termination

If pursuit were a straightforward linear feedback system, the response evoked by termination of a ramp stimulus should be the inverse of that at initiation; eye velocity should thus oscillate when reaching zero velocity (i.e. in the transition from pursuit to fixation). However, when target motion ceases unexpectedly, following a latency of approximately 100 ms, eye velocity simply decays to zero with a time constant of approximately 100 ms (Pola and Wyatt, 1997; Robinson et al., 1986) without evidence of overshoot. This was taken as evidence that fixation does not represent pursuit at zero velocity; rather, the simple decay of eye velocity represents the disengagement of pursuit (Robinson et al. 1986). Subsequent evidence shows that the absence of overshoot actually depends on the subject's expectation; when there is uncertainty about whether the target will stop or continue in motion, overshoot is observed (as in Fig. 7.1B), but not when termination is expected, even if timing of termination is randomized (Krauzlis and Miles, 1996b).

Periodic stimuli

If humans are instructed to follow the sinusoidal motion of a small target in the horizontal plane with head fixed, the eye movement is composed of both smooth and saccadic components (Fig. 7.2).

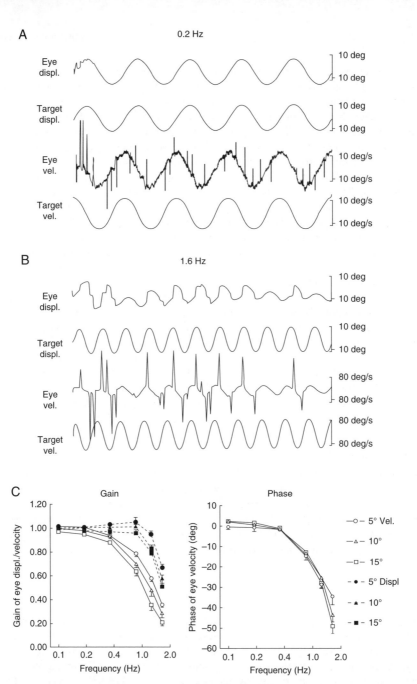

Fig. 7.2 Smooth pursuit eye movements evoked when tracking a target moving sinusoidally (peak displacement ±10°) at frequencies of 0.2 Hz (A) and 1.6 Hz (B). Spikes on the eye velocity trace represent catch-up saccadic movements which, at the lower frequency, are of very small amplitude and velocity and are almost undetectable on the eye displacement. Gain and phase characteristics of the pursuit response are shown in (C) for target frequencies between 0.1 and 1.6 Hz. Common symbols represent responses to target motion stimuli in which peak target displacement was held constant throughout the frequency range. Peak displacements were ± 5, 10, and 15° as indicated. Broken lines represent the ratio of overall eye displacement, (i.e. including any saccadic components), to target displacement, whereas solid lines represent the ratio of smooth eye velocity to target velocity. Eye displacement phase (not shown) is similar to eye velocity phase. Mean of 20 subjects (controls used in various experiments, e.g. Waterston et al. (1992)) + 1 SEM. Reprinted from *Brain and Cognition*, **68**(3), G.R. Barnes, Cognitive processes involved in smooth pursuit eye movements, copyright (2008), with permission from Elsevier.

At low frequencies (<0.4 Hz) the movement is almost wholly smooth and eye velocity closely matches target velocity. At higher frequencies eye velocity does not match target velocity so adequately, but small catch-up saccades re-align the target image on the fovea. Overall performance of the pursuit system is best described by consideration of two measures: a) total eye displacement, i.e. the combination of smooth and saccadic movements and b) the smooth eye velocity alone that remains after removal of the saccadic components. In response to a sinusoidal stimulus smooth eye velocity gain (the ratio of peak eye velocity to target velocity) breaks down at frequencies between 0.5 and 3 Hz (Fig. 7.2C). In contrast, the saccadic system maintains total eye displacement gain close to unity up to frequencies of 1 Hz. The phase of eye displacement is very similar to that of eye velocity, being close to zero for frequencies up to approximately 0.8 Hz, but progressively lagging behind the target at higher frequencies. This breakdown in gain and phase with frequency must ultimately be associated with the low-pass filter within the system that is responsible for the exponential decay of eye velocity in the termination of the step-ramp response (Fig. 7.1B). However, the pursuit reflex is also subject to velocity saturation, which causes gain to decrease as target velocity increases. The effects of velocity and frequency limitations combine above 1 Hz, so that increasing the amplitude of target displacement (and thus its velocity) causes greater gain decrease at any particular frequency (Barnes, 1993; Lisberger et al., 1981; Waterston et al., 1992; Wyatt and Pola, 1983). Although phase lag increases at high frequencies its magnitude is less than expected for a linear feedback system. Thus, a typical phase lag of 10° at 1.0 Hz is equivalent to a response delay of 30 ms, far less than the minimum onset latency of 70 ms. This is evidence of prediction, which is discussed later (see section 'Predictive processes in pursuit').

Triangular waveform stimuli, in which the target executes constant velocity movement that changes direction at regular intervals, are also used to test pursuit. Such stimuli are useful at low frequencies, since lengthy periods of constant velocity can be attained. However, the smooth eye movement system cannot change direction as rapidly as the stimulus (because of the high frequency filtering property noted above) and eye velocity thus becomes 'rounded' at these times. Importantly, the deceleration associated with this rounding starts well before the stimulus direction change, a clear example of prediction.

Randomized stimuli

In a bid to defeat prediction, various attempts have been made to use random or pseudo-random target motion stimuli to examine pursuit. Early investigators (Michael and Melvill Jones, 1966; St-Cyr and Fender, 1969) had shown that an effective pseudo-random stimulus could be generated by mixing together a number of harmonically unrelated sinusoidal waveforms. These studies showed that overall eye displacement (i.e. smooth + saccadic) responses exhibited larger phase errors than simple sinusoids and that gain and phase were modified by stimulus bandwidth. Subsequent experiments (Barnes et al., 1987) indicated that the critical factor determining pursuit efficacy was not the randomness of the stimulus but the frequency of the highest frequency component. If all frequencies within a stimulus were less than approximately 0.4 Hz, eye movements were quite smooth with high levels (>0.9) of eye velocity gain. In contrast, as the highest frequency increased above 0.4 Hz there was a progressive reduction in the gain of the lower frequencies, but not the highest frequency.

The role of retinal and extraretinal mechanisms in pursuit

Ocular pursuit is an example of a negative feedback control system and models based on control theory have been used very successfully to describe the dynamic characteristics. If all components in a control system are linear there are well defined relationships between input and output that can be extracted. In the simplest representation of the system (Fig. 7.3A), in which only velocity feedback is considered, the relationship between eye velocity (E) and target velocity (T) can be defined as:

$$G_{CL} = E/T = K/(1+K)$$

where G_{CL} represents measured (closed-loop) gain and K is the gain of the internal feedforward path (often referred to as open-loop gain) between the retina and extraocular muscles. Although this is a

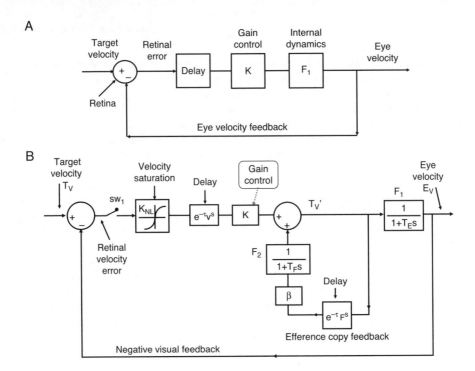

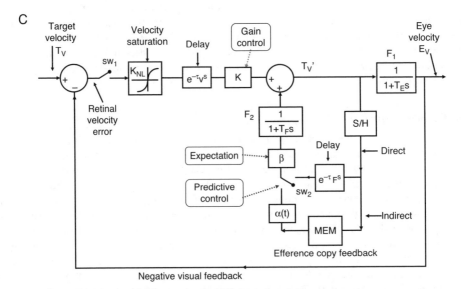

Fig. 7.3 A) Model of ocular pursuit with visual feedback alone. B) Simplified efference copy model incorporating positive feedback of an internal representation of eye velocity, with gain β (<1) and $T_F = T_E$. C) More detailed model in which there is extraretinal input from either a direct efference copy loop or an indirect (predictive) loop. Gain β is dependent on expectation of continued target movement (see Barnes and Collins, 2008b). During constant velocity pursuit maintenance, switch sw_2 allows the direct loop to operate as in B; when target motion is variable but predictable, sw_2 allows feedback via a short term memory (MEM) in the indirect pathway that holds velocity information captured from previous samples and generates anticipatory pursuit. The input to both direct and indirect pathways comes from sampling and holding a copy of the internally reconstructed target velocity estimate (T_V') in module S/H. The direct loop can thus sustain eye velocity even if visual input is withdrawn (Barnes and Collins, 2009a, 2009b). The gain ($\alpha(t)$) represents the ability to modulate the output of MEM as a function of time to allow more complex motion trajectories to be produced in anticipation of expected target motion (i.e. it forms a dynamic memory). From Barnes and Collins (2008b).

gross simplification, it emphasizes that closed loop gain bears a complex relationship to open loop gain: if K=1, G_{CL} is only 0.5, whereas K must be increased tenfold to increase G_{CL} to approximately 0.9, a typical level for pursuit closed loop gain. It is possible to artificially open this loop by summating a carefully recorded and calibrated eye movement signal with the drive signal controlling the target. This useful technique has been widely used to investigate open-loop characteristics. An alternative is to examine only the first 100 ms of the pursuit response, which can be considered open-loop as noted earlier. Provided that prediction is minimized by randomizing direction, timing and speed of successive trials, this allows the relationship between visual stimulus and pursuit response to be investigated without the complications imposed by feedback. Most models of pursuit have focussed on non-predictive responses to ramp or step-ramp stimuli. Such models simulate the rapid rise of eye velocity combined with the high levels of closed-loop gain achieved. These two requirements cannot be met by simple negative feedback without the system exhibiting unstable oscillation because of time delays associated with visual motion processing; although some oscillation is observed (Fig. 7.1), it is generally of small amplitude. The most widely accepted way in which stability is thought to be achieved is through summation of an efference copy of eye movement with the retinal velocity error signal, as represented in Fig. 7.3B. The resultant signal may be regarded as an internal reconstruction of target velocity (T_V' in Fig. 7.3B) (Deno et al., 1995; Krauzlis and Lisberger, 1994a; Krauzlis and Miles, 1996b; Robinson et al., 1986; Yasui and Young, 1975).

An important generic feature of these models is that if efference copy feedback gain is exactly unity the whole loop can sustain the response if the stimulus is cut off. This fits with an important observation; during pursuit of a target that unexpectedly disappears, smooth eye movements do not simply stop but can be sustained (Becker and Fuchs, 1985), albeit at a lower level. This occlusion paradigm has been used frequently to reveal features of the internal (or extraretinal) drive mechanisms for pursuit.

Recent evidence has called into question the validity of this simple efference copy model. Although target occlusion experiments lead to a decrease in eye velocity, there is often a recovery of eye velocity prior to expected target reappearance (Becker and Fuchs, 1985; Bennett and Barnes, 2003). Indeed, eye velocity can increase above the level attained prior to target disappearance if initial target exposure is very brief (100–150 ms) (Barnes and Collins, 2008a, 2008b) or if target velocity is expected to increase at the end of the occlusion (Bennett and Barnes, 2004). Such behaviour cannot be easily explained by simple efference copy models (Fig. 7.3B), which can only sustain eye velocity at the level prior to disappearance. Rather, it suggests that the efference copy signal can be captured and maintained in a specific sample and hold mechanism (S/H) as indicated in Fig. 7.3C. Ideally, any model of pursuit should also be able to explain the property of prediction discussed above. The direct efference copy pathway is incapable of emulating this behaviour. In fact, to the contrary; although it achieves stability, it introduces unrealistically large phase errors if used to simulate sinusoidal responses. However, it is possible to demonstrate a modification of this basic principle that does allow prediction using the indirect pathway in Fig. 7.3C and this will be discussed in the section 'Modelling predictive pursuit behaviour'.

Interaction of saccades with smooth pursuit

Positional errors that occur during pursuit are mostly corrected by saccades, which rapidly realign the object's image on the fovea. This not only reduces positional error but also allows the greatest level of visual feedback gain to be achieved by centring the target over the foveal area, which is more sensitive to image motion than the peripheral retina (Dubois and Collewijn, 1979). In fact, saccades do not simply correct for current retinal error, they allow future changes to be taken into account as a result of sensitivity to pre-saccadic velocity error (de Brouwer et al., 2002). The saccadic component of pursuit is thus essential and should be considered as an integral part of pursuit (see Orban de Xivry and Lefevre 2007). In fact, even if the target temporarily disappears, the saccadic system appears to have access to an estimate of the hidden target trajectory. Thus, even though smooth eye velocity may be reduced during extinction, a representation of target velocity is retained that can be integrated to predict the future target trajectory, which then forms a positional reference for saccadic corrections (Bennett et al., 2006; Collins and Barnes, 2006; Orban de Xivry et al., 2006).

Gain control—active versus passive mechanisms

Evidence indicates that the gain of pursuit is not fixed, but may be under volitional control. Several experiments have shown clear differences in the magnitude of responses evoked by active pursuit as opposed to passive stimulation, in which subjects simply stare at the moving target without actively pursuing it. This is well known for large moving patterns (optokinesis), but even a small stimulus, when presented in the absence of other visual cues, can induce reflexive eye movements (Barnes and Hill, 1984; Pola and Wyatt, 1985). Notably, important features of the response, such as the frequency-dependent characteristics, non-linear velocity dependence and prediction, appear very similar during passive stimulation and active pursuit (see Barnes 1993). Active pursuit, therefore, may simply involve the potentiation of visual motion information by increasing the gain of visual feedback. However, gain control has now been revealed to be more subtle than a simple two-level process implied by the foregoing arguments. Schwartz and Lisberger (1994) showed in monkey that when a high frequency (5 Hz) single cycle perturbation is superimposed on constant velocity target motion the eye velocity gain associated with the perturbation increases with target velocity. Experiments by Churchland et al. (2002) confirmed this effect in humans; gain increased approximately twofold as target velocity increased from 0°/s (fixation) through 5°/s to 10°/s. However, this is not confirmed by all experiments (Das et al., 1995). It is also evident that pursuit gain can be adaptively modified by repeated exposure to target motion changes that occur for brief periods (approximately 150 ms) close to normal pursuit latency (Fukushima et al., 1996).

Pursuit in the presence of a background

Since the motion of any visual stimulus across the retina has the potential to evoke eye movement it ought to be more difficult to track a target against a structured rather than a blank background. As the eye moves across the background, the induced optokinetic drive should slow pursuit eye movement. Such interactions can be demonstrated, although eye velocity normally decreases by only 10–20% (Barnes and Crombie, 1985; Collewijn and Tamminga, 1984; Worfolk and Barnes, 1992). This may be because active pursuit of the target raises the gain associated with that target, as indicated above, which then allows it to override the influence of the background. In support of this conclusion the background has an increasing influence on eye movement if visual feedback for the selected pursuit target is degraded (Barnes and Crombie, 1985; Worfolk and Barnes, 1992). Although this type of interaction explains some behaviour there are clearly other mechanisms. Thus, Keller and Kahn (1986) demonstrated that a stationary background that is present before pursuit onset reduces initial eye acceleration and increases the latency of pursuit, and others have obtained similar results (Kimmig et al., 1992). Interestingly, stationary backgrounds have no influence on ramp pursuit termination (Mohrmann and Thier, 1995). More recently this problem has been probed by introducing a brief transient perturbation of the background (Lindner et al., 2001; Schwarz and Ilg, 1999; Suehiro et al., 1999). These studies showed that when the background was initially stationary but then perturbed in the same direction as the pursuit target there was a much greater influence on eye velocity than when perturbation was oppositely directed. Subsequent studies (Lindner and Ilg, 2006), using target extinction, suggest that this asymmetry is present even when the target is not visible. This may indicate that intention to drive pursuit in a particular direction leads to suppression of background optokinetic influence in the opposite direction, but not in the same direction.

The effects of distractors, gaps, and the role of attention

Pursuit against structured backgrounds is one example of the need to selectively attend to a particular motion stimulus. Another common example occurs when other small objects are present that may act as distractors. Ferrera and Lisberger (1995, 1997) investigated how the initial pursuit response was affected by the presence of a second target (a distractor) moving in another direction.

They showed that the initial open-loop response was a vector average of responses that would be made to each of the stimuli separately. After this initial period a saccade was made to one of the targets and post-saccadic eye velocity was then in the direction of the selected target, reflecting a winner-take-all response. If the distractor moved in the opposite direction there was an increase in latency of the pursuit response (Lisberger and Ferrera, 1997). Knox and Bekkour (2004), showed that increased latency also occurred with a stationary distractor, but its effect was diminished as it was moved further into the periphery. An issue probably allied to the influence of distractors is the fact that removal of a fixation cue prior to the onset of target motion can also modify pursuit initiation. Experiments have shown that leaving a blank gap of up to 400 ms between fixation extinction and motion onset decreases pursuit latency (Krauzlis and Miles, 1996a; Merrison and Carpenter, 1995). The gap may act as a warning cue, triggering early release of fixation and redirection of attention to the pursuit target.

As well as affecting pursuit initiation, attention also plays a part during pursuit maintenance. Embedding a task requiring attention within the pursuit target has been found to improve pursuit performance (Shagass et al., 1976; Sweeney et al., 1994), whereas secondary tasks frequently impair pursuit (Hutton and Tegally, 2005; Kerzel et al., 2008; Lipton et al., 1980). A critical factor is that different levels of attention are probably required at different stages of pursuit, least attention being required in the maintenance phase (Chen et al., 2002). As shown recently (Kerzel et al., 2008), the mere presence of distractors has little influence unless they are attended to and their retinal motion conflicts with that of the pursuit target. Van Donkelaar and Drew (2002) have attempted to define where attention is directed during pursuit by assessing responses to a secondary cue appearing ahead of or behind the moving target. They conclude that the locus of attention is slightly (<2°) ahead of the moving target.

Although the aim of pursuit is normally to maintain the target image close to the fovea, it is possible to pursue extrafoveal targets when, for example, tracking the hidden (and therefore imagined), part of an incomplete figure (Steinbach, 1976). This is probably achieved through activation of velocity sensors in the peripheral retina, which however, are less sensitive than those in the fovea (Dubois and Collewijn, 1979). Thus, when subjects direct attention to and pursue the mid-point between two peripherally located targets, smooth eye velocity progressively decreases with increasing eccentricity (Barnes and Hill, 1984; Collewijn and Tamminga, 1986; Pola and Wyatt, 1985).

Pursuit of apparent motion stimuli

Apparent motion of an object can be induced by intermittent illumination of discrete, spatially separated targets if they are illuminated sequentially at short intervals (Morgan and Turnbull, 1978). Even stroboscopic illumination of a complete set of stationary targets can evoke smooth pursuit if the pursuit is seeded by the initial motion of a real target that then disappears (Behrens and Grüsser, 1979; Heywood, 1973; van der Steen et al., 1983). Barnes and Asselman (1992) quantified the changes in smooth eye velocity with increasing intervals and demonstrated a gradual decrease rather than a sudden transition associated with the changed perception; smooth movements were still evident for intervals of 960 ms even though there was no perception of continuous motion.

Other forms of apparent motion have also been used in attempts to link perception of motion with pursuit. Boman and Hotson (1989) used the technique of presenting an array of four discs with corners removed so as to give a Kanizsa-style illusory inner square. This illusory square jumped to left and right alternately, yielding an apparent motion and inducing some smooth anticipatory eye movements. Madelain and Krauzlis (2003) used a similar illusory square presentation arranged in a linear array. In successive 66-ms intervals the blank corners were rotated 90°, so that the illusory square moved from one frame to the next. Because the perception of motion could be bidirectional, they were able to ask the subjects to voluntarily reverse the direction of motion and could then examine the association between the timing of perceptual reversal and actual pursuit reversal. Perceptual reversal occurred approximately 50 ms earlier than motor reversal. The association between motion perception and pursuit has been the focus of many other studies, both at the behavioural and neurophysiological level (Beutter and Stone, 2000; Stone and Krauzlis, 2003); generally, there is a close link between the two. However, studies in which illusory target motion is caused by pursuit against a moving background suggest target motion perception is based more on the difference between target and background motions, whereas pursuit is governed by the average of the two (Schweigart et al., 2003; Spering and Gegenfurtner, 2007). Importantly, maintenance of a stable visual world during pursuit probably relies on comparison of retinal and extraretinal pursuit components, the latter requiring continual calibration, as shown by Haarmeier et al. (2001).

Local versus global motion effects in pursuit

In the real world, moving objects are likely to be complex, having edges with varying orientations to the global object motion. This is of interest because visual motion sensing is carried out by neurons with small receptive fields that view objects as if through an array of apertures. Each neuron senses motion orthogonal to edges within its receptive field and the direction of motion of the whole object can only be determined at what are called terminators, such as corners. Recently, experiments have specifically addressed the question of how the transition from processing local motion cues provided by edges to global object motion might influence pursuit. Pack and Born (2001) showed in monkey that during initiation of pursuit of a simple bar that moved horizontally but was tilted with respect to the horizontal there was a small vertical component of eye movement that reflected the early stage of local motion processing but which decayed in approximately 150 ms. Masson and Stone (2002), using human subjects, examined pursuit of more complex targets formed by a combination of lines in the shape of squares and elongated diamonds that could be tilted with respect to motion direction. They found that initial eye movement was biased in the direction of a vectored average of the motions of individual line segments and that alignment with the direction of global motion took approximately 90 ms. The general methods employed in these experiments provide a powerful way of examining the evolution of motion processing.

Predictive processes in pursuit

Prediction in pursuit is evident in two ways: a) when a tracked target temporarily disappears, smooth eye movement, whether constant velocity (Becker and Fuchs, 1985) or sinusoidal (Whittaker and Eaholtz, 1982), may continue for a short period; b) when the subject tracks a regular periodic waveform phase errors are smaller than when tracking a more irregular or randomized waveform. The improved performance with periodic stimuli is most probably associated with temporary storage of motion information that is then used to predict future motion (Barnes and Asselman, 1991). Deno et al. (1995) termed this long-term prediction. A second aspect of prediction depends on extraction of motion information from the moving object (what Deno et al. (1995) termed short-term prediction), allowing some on-line prediction of future motion.

Evidence for short-term prediction

Short-term prediction implies the use of immediately preceding motion history to predict future motion by extrapolation over a period sufficient to overcome time delays (i.e. approximately 200 ms). This can be accomplished most straightforwardly by using higher derivatives, such as acceleration, to predict future velocity. The strongest direct evidence for acceleration sensitivity was obtained by Krauzlis and Lisberger (1994a, 1994b). They examined the response to a step-ramp stimulus in which the initial 125 ms of the ramp was either an abrupt change in velocity (i.e. infinite acceleration) or a more gradual acceleration towards target velocity. They found differences in initial eye acceleration evoked by these two stimuli and extracted the specific component associated with acceleration. The effect was small and saturated for accelerations greater than approximately $100°/s^2$, but it suggests that acceleration sensitivity is present at the input to the system. Subsequently, Watamaniuk and Heinen (2003) addressed the question by examining the initial response to target motion stimuli that accelerated at rates up to $30°/s^2$. They found that sensitivity to acceleration was very poor at this early stage of the response. Recently, Bennett et al. (2007) have shown that up to

500 ms may be required to develop such sensitivity. Subjects were initially given a combination of constant velocity and either acceleration or deceleration up to $16°/s^2$. The target was exposed for an initial period of 200, 500, or 800 ms and then extinguished for a period of 800 ms before reappearing along its initial trajectory. Smooth eye movement during extinction was modulated in proportion to target acceleration only when initial exposure was greater than 200 ms.

Evidence for use of a short-term store in long-term prediction

The perseveration of eye velocity observed when the target temporarily disappears provides evidence for velocity memory (Becker and Fuchs, 1985). It led to the development of models in which an internal positive feedback loop might provide such a memory. However, such a simple system can only preserve a given level of velocity and cannot sustain continuation of sinusoidal movement, for example (Whittaker and Eaholtz, 1982). If information about target motion could be stored more permanently it should be possible to use it to initiate an appropriate pursuit response simultaneously with target motion onset and thus overcome visuomotor processing delays. However, most individuals are unable to initiate smooth eye movements of more than approximately 5°/s in the absence of target motion (Barnes et al., 1987; Kao and Morrow, 1994). Kowler and Steinman (1979a, 1979b) demonstrated that low velocity (<2°/s) anticipatory smooth movements can occur prior to target onset, but since prediction of sinusoidal stimuli can occur with much higher velocity stimuli, it was unclear how these anticipatory movements might contribute to prediction. Barnes and Asselman (1991) showed that much higher velocities of anticipatory smooth pursuit could be evoked by repeated, brief presentation of constant velocity stimuli. As shown in Fig. 7.4A, during the first presentation, smooth movement did not start until after the target had been extinguished and peak velocity was very low. But in subsequent presentations anticipatory smooth movements started to occur, building up to a steady state within three to four presentations. This build up of the response led to the hypothesis that the visual motion feedback available in the initial presentation might be used to form an internal store of pre-motor drive that could then be released as a predictive estimate of the required eye velocity. In this way, the release of relatively high velocity anticipatory smooth movements might be facilitated, when in normal circumstances, this would not be possible. This was supported by the observation that when the target unexpectedly failed to appear, a predictive velocity estimate of appropriately scaled velocity was initiated in the complete absence of the moving target (Fig. 7.4A). Moreover, this response occurred at a time that was correlated with the timing of the previous stimuli, suggesting that timing information had also been stored. It could not be sustained, however, and started to decay approximately 150 ms after the time of expected target appearance. Attempts to generate further smooth movements were normally unsuccessful, thus reinforcing previous findings that smooth movements cannot be sustained in the absence of a moving target. Subsequent experiments (Barnes et al., 1997) revealed that subjects could generate appropriately scaled anticipatory smooth movements after simply viewing the target motion without actively pursuing it. In fact, Poliakoff et al. (2005) showed that it is possible to store motion information for two separate targets with differing speed whilst fixating and subsequently make an appropriately scaled anticipatory response to either.

The importance of timing in prediction

Clearly, if stored motion information is to be used effectively for prediction it must be released at the right time to minimize velocity error. When tracking periodic motion, timing is probably extracted from the stimulus itself (Barnes and Asselman, 1991). However, independent cues can also be used to control timing when stimuli are aperiodic. Boman and Hotson (1988), for example, found that extinction of the fixation target at a fixed time (400 or 800 ms) before target motion onset enhanced anticipatory pursuit and Barnes and Donelan (1999) showed similar effects when other cues (visual, auditory, or tactile) were used. Even if cue time is variable, anticipatory movements are still evoked but with timing that is influenced by cue time distribution (Badler and Heinen, 2006; de Hemptinne et al., 2006; de Hemptinne et al., 2007).

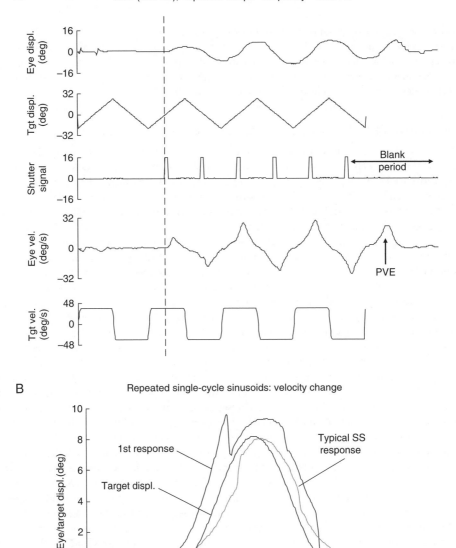

Fig. 7.4 A) Eye movements evoked by intermittent presentation of a target moving alternately to left and right at constant velocity (±36°/s). The underlying target motion stimulus was a triangular waveform of frequency 0.39 Hz. The target was exposed for a duration of 120 ms (indicated by the shutter signal) every half-cycle as it passed through centre. Fast phase components removed from eye velocity signal. PVE, predictive velocity estimate made when expected target fails to appear. Reprinted from *Brain and Cognition*, **68**(3), G.R. Barnes, Cognitive processes involved in smooth pursuit eye movements, copyright (2008), with permission from Elsevier. B). Catch trial response from experiment in which repeated single-cycle sinusoidal target motion stimuli were presented, each preceded by an audio warning cue. The first response represents the inappropriate response to an unexpected decrease in peak target velocity (reduced from 80°/s to 32°/s). Subject makes anticipatory response that has higher velocity than actual target velocity throughout much of cycle and must make corrective saccades to realign eye with target. Grey trace shows more typical response to the new, reduced target velocity. Reprinted from *Journal of Neurophysiology*, **84**, Barnes, G.R., Barnes, D.M., and Chakraborti, S.R., Ocular pursuit responses to repeated, single-cycle sinusoids reveal behaviour compatible with predictive pursuit, pp. 2340, fig 13, © 2000, The American Physiological Society, used with permission.

Timing is also important in response termination; for repeated ramp stimuli of fixed duration eye velocity starts to decrease in anticipation of ramp termination (Boman and Hotson, 1988; Kowler and McKee, 1987; Robinson et al., 1986). Randomization of ramp duration does not eliminate this (Collins and Barnes, 2009). Krauzlis and Miles (1996b) showed that the dynamics of pursuit offset are significantly affected by the subject's experience. If the target always stops, eye velocity gradually declines over the ramp duration, but if it sometimes continues at a different velocity or reverses direction, eye velocity continues unchanged for approximately 80 ms and then reacts to the changed motion. When ramp stimuli of identical duration are repeated, programming of response termination becomes so consolidated that an unexpected increase in duration results in inappropriate eye deceleration lasting for more than 400 ms (Barnes et al., 2005). Such predictive timing probably underlies the anticipatory reversals observed during tracking of triangular waveforms (Boman and Hotson, 1992). It probably also plays a dominant part during sinusoidal stimulation (van den Berg, 1988), particularly for higher frequency stimuli (>0.5 Hz) where there is insufficient time to detect target deceleration, i.e. to use short-term prediction.

The role of expectation and mismatch detection in predictive pursuit

Although regularly timed cues can be used to initiate anticipatory pursuit movements, they only occur if associated with expectation of future target motion (Kowler, 1989; Barnes et al, 1997). Past-history also affects timing, but the expectation created by cognitive cues probably outweighs the effects of past-history (Kowler 1989). Jarrett and Barnes (2002) showed that symbolic cues indicating speed and direction of forthcoming stimuli can be used not only to appropriately direct the eye, but also to volitionally scale anticipatory velocity prior to randomized stimuli. As well as being important for anticipatory response initiation, expectation is also necessary to sustain the internal drive for pursuit when the target is extinguished. If the target regularly reappears after extinction eye velocity is sustained during extinction. However, if experience indicates that the target usually does not reappear, eye velocity is not sustained, but decays towards zero (Barnes and Collins, 2008; Becker and Fuchs, 1985; Bennett and Barnes, 2003; Mitrani and Dimitrov, 1978) despite attempts to continue following the unseen target.

This dependence on expectation is probably part of a system that allows mismatch between prediction and sensory feedback to be detected, which is essential if false predictions are to be minimized. The effect is evident in Fig. 7.4; failure of the target to appear when expected leads to response termination at the time that visual feedback would have been expected. It might appear that this causes the temporary store of motion information to discharge. However, if subjects are given further timing cues but know that the target will not appear until a certain number of cues have elapsed, anticipatory movements can be revived, suggesting that the memory has not been lost (Barnes et al. 1997). Expectation thus appears to gate the output of the internally generated anticipatory response.

Dynamic characteristics of anticipatory smooth pursuit responses

When anticipatory movements are initiated they have a characteristic velocity profile (Barnes and Asselman, 1991; Kao and Morrow, 1994); eye movement is initiated approximately 200–300 ms before target onset and gradually increases in velocity, reaching approximately 30% of target velocity at motion onset. From approximately 70 ms after onset the response is potentially affected by visual feedback and it becomes difficult to determine how the internally driven component develops thereafter. Collins and Barnes (2006) have shown that when a repeated target motion is occluded for the initial 500 ms, more prolonged anticipatory eye movements lasting up to 600 ms may be revealed. Comparing these responses with those from a similar paradigm in which the early part of a randomized step-ramp stimulus was occluded reveals that anticipatory smooth pursuit has similar temporal development to the extraretinal component of reactive pursuit (Barnes and Collins, 2008), indicating that both may be generated by the same mechanism.

Although the continuation of anticipatory movement is difficult to observe under normal circumstances, it can be revealed by image stabilization. Barnes et al. (1995) used a regular intermittent presentation paradigm in which the image was stabilized on the fovea during a dark period between presentations, following several cycles of normal closed-loop stimulation. At the first stabilized presentation an anticipatory movement was already underway and, when the target appeared, its movement was controlled by the movement of the eye. Subjects could then continue generating alternating smooth eye movements repeatedly every time the target reappeared. The response in the stabilized mode can probably be continued because the mismatch detection system registers no velocity error.

Predictive pursuit of sinusoidal target motion

The major evidence for prediction comes from responses to periodic target motion and the role of anticipatory movements is not immediately apparent. However, there is evidence that anticipatory movements may be associated with the response of mechanisms that learn and reproduce time-varying velocity trajectories (Barnes et al., 2000). Repeated target motion stimuli comprising a single cycle of sinusoidal motion were presented at irregular intervals, but preceded by a regularly timed cue. Fixation was maintained between presentations. Eye velocity lagged well behind the target in the first presentation of each sequence of sinusoids but within two or three presentations anticipatory movements emerged and phase error was significantly reduced and comparable to those for responses to continuous sinusoidal waveforms of corresponding frequency. As confirmed by catch trials, subjects were effectively generating an internal drive that mimicked the sinusoidal waveform, releasing it in anticipation of actual stimulus presentation (Fig. 7.4B).

The ability to store information about the velocity and frequency of sinusoidal motion and then to mimic that motion has also been demonstrated using image stabilization. Attempts to do so are not always successful, since it is difficult to control both frequency and velocity of eye movement (van den Berg and Collweijn, 1987). When Barnes et al. (1995) used a modulated sound cue to indicate frequency, subjects could successfully generate sinusoid-like smooth movements across a range of velocities and frequencies. Altogether, these results suggest an ability to store velocity trajectories and volitionally control their output so as to predict future periodic motion, even for pursuit in two dimensions (Orban de Xivry et al., 2008).

Modelling predictive pursuit behaviour

In order to simulate the features of predictive pursuit discussed above the efference copy model requires additional features, notably the inclusion of a second internal loop, the indirect pathway (Fig. 7.3C). The indirect pathway holds sampled premotor drive that has been captured from prior stimulation in a form of working memory (MEM). This enables motion information to be retained, even during fixation, and thereby allows appropriately scaled anticipatory movements to be released in advance of future target movement if there is a firm expectation of target appearance. The release of this output from MEM is dependent on timing derived from external cues or cues derived from the motion itself if periodic. Results of experiments with complex sequences of motion suggest that multiple levels of velocity may be retained in this pathway (Barnes and Schmid, 2002). The manner in which this is accomplished is possibly through the temporary storage of gain levels within an adaptive network (schematically represented by the function $\alpha(t)$ in Fig. 7.3C). An important feature of the model is that output from the direct and indirect loops is gated by expectation and may be switched by a mechanism detecting mismatch between the predictive velocity and current visual feedback.

Conclusions

The findings discussed here emphasize the important role that cognitive processing plays in the initiation and maintenance of ocular pursuit. Although the basic information needed to drive pursuit is ultimately extracted from visual input, cognitive control exerts a strong influence over the manner in which that information is used to control the eye. Cognitive factors of most significance are attention, selection, expectation, working memory, prediction, and mismatch detection. Selective attention is required to track a specific moving object and to ignore or suppress motion information from other sources. Attention varies in different phases of pursuit and, in the steady-state, the locus of attention probably lies slightly ahead of the target. Prediction also plays an important part in normal pursuit. It is evident that extraretinal components derived from sampling and temporarily storing target motion information take over a large part of response generation in steady-state predictable conditions. In fact, pursuit is clearly a system in which the initial response may be driven by visual feedback, but the sustained response operates on the basis of predicting future movement and using visual feedback to monitor mismatch so as to check that the prediction is correct. Systems models have formed an important aid to understanding how the pursuit system operates, but no model that does not attempt to include prediction as well as response initiation can adequately represent the system, since prediction is ever-present. Finally, it is important to emphasize that the saccadic contribution to ocular pursuit is not insignificant; it corrects for inadequacies in the smooth movement, even in the absence of the target.

References

Badler, J.B. and Heinen, S.J. (2006). Anticipatory movement timing using prediction and external cues. *Journal of Neuroscience*, **26**(17), 4519–4525.

Barnes, G.R. (1993). Visual-vestibular interaction in the control of head and eye movement: the role of visual feedback and predictive mechanisms. *Progress in Neurobiology*, **41**, 435–472.

Barnes, G.R. (2008). Cognitive processes involved in smooth pursuit eye movements. *Brain and Cognition* **68**, 309–326.

Barnes, G.R. and Asselman, P.T. (1991). The mechanism of prediction in human smooth pursuit eye movements. *Journal of Physiology (London)*, **439**, 439–461.

Barnes, G.R. and Asselman, P.T. (1992). Pursuit of intermittently illuminated moving targets in the human. *Journal of Physiology (London)*, **445**, 617–637.

Barnes, G.R. and Collins, C.J.S. (2008a). The influence of briefly presented randomised target motion on the extra-retinal component of ocular pursuit. *Journal of Neurophysiology*, **99**, 831–842.

Barnes, G.R. and Collins, C.J.S. (2008b). Evidence for a link between the extra-retinal component of random-onset pursuit and the anticipatory pursuit of predictable object motion. *Journal of Neurophysiology*, **100**, 1135–1146.

Barnes, G.R. and Crombie, J.W. (1985). The interaction of conflicting retinal motion stimuli in oculomotor control. *Experimental Brain Research*, **59**, 548–558.

Barnes, G.R. and Donelan, A.S. (1999). The remembered pursuit task: evidence for segregation of timing and velocity storage in predictive oculomotor control. *Experimental Brain Research*, **129**(57), 57–67.

Barnes, G.R. and Hill, T. (1984). The influence of display characteristics on active pursuit and passively induced eye movements. *Experimental Brain Research*, **56**, 438–447.

Barnes, G.R. and Schmid, A.M. (2002). Sequence learning in human ocular smooth pursuit. *Experimental Brain Research*, **144**, 322–335.

Barnes, G.R., Donnelly, S.F., and Eason, R.D. (1987). Predictive velocity estimation in the pursuit reflex response to pseudo-random and step displacement stimuli in man. *Journal of Physiology (London)*, **389**, 111–136.

Barnes, G.R., Goodbody, S.J., and Collins, S. (1995). Volitional control of anticipatory ocular pursuit responses under stabilized image conditions in humans. *Experimental Brain Research*, **106**, 301–317.

Barnes, G.R., Grealy, M.A., and Collins, S. (1997). Volitional control of anticipatory ocular smooth pursuit after viewing, but not pursuing, a moving target: evidence for a re-afferent velocity store. *Experimental Brain Research*, **116**, 445–455.

Barnes, G.R., Barnes, D.M., and Chakraborti, S.R. (2000). Ocular pursuit responses to repeated, single-cycle sinusoids reveal behavior compatible with predictive pursuit. *Journal of Neurophysiology*, **84**, 2340–2355.

Barnes, G.R., Collins, C.J.S., and Arnold, L.R. (2005). Predicting the duration of ocular pursuit in humans. *Experimental Brain Research*, **160**, 10–21.

Becker, W. and Fuchs, A.F. (1985). Prediction in the oculomotor system: smooth pursuit during transient disappearance of a visual target. *Experimental Brain Research*, **57**, 562–575.

Behrens, F. and Grüsser, O.J. (1979). Smooth pursuit eye movements and optokinetic nystagmus elicited by intermittently illuminated stationary patterns. *Experimental Brain Research*, **37**, 317–336.

Bennett, S.J. and Barnes, G.R. (2003). Human ocular pursuit during the transient disappearance of a moving target. *Journal of Neurophysiology*, **90**, 2504–2520.

Bennett, S.J., and Barnes, G.R. (2004). Predictive smooth ocular pursuit during the transient disappearance of a visual target. *Journal of Neurophysiology*, **92**, 578–590.

Bennett, S.J., and Barnes, G.R., (2006). Combined smooth and saccadic ocular pursuit during the transient occlusion of a moving visual object. *Experimental Brain Research*, **168**, 313–321.

Bennett, S.J., Orban de Xivry, J.J., Barnes, G.R., and Lefevre, P. (2007). Target acceleration can be extracted and represented within the predictive drive to ocular pursuit. *Journal of Neurophysiology*, **98**, 1405–1414.

Beutter, B.R. and Stone, L.S. (2000). Motion coherence affects human perception and pursuit similarly. *Visual Neuroscience*, **17**(1), 139–153.

Boman, D.K. and Hotson, J.R. (1988). Stimulus conditions that enhance anticipatory slow eye movements. *Vision Research*, **28**, 1157–1165.

Boman, D.K. and Hotson, J.R. (1989). Motion perception prominence alters anticipatory slow eye movements. *Experimental Brain Research*, **74**, 555–562.

Carl, J.R. and Gellman, R.S. (1987). Human smooth pursuit: stimulus-dependent responses. *Journal of Neurophysiology*, **57**, 1446–1463.

Chen, Y., Holzman, P.S., and Nakayama, K. (2002). Visual and cognitive control of attention in smooth pursuit. *Progress in Brain Research*, **140**, 255–265.

Churchland, A.K. and Lisberger, S.G. (2002). Gain control in human smooth-pursuit eye movements. *Journal of Neurophysiology*, **87**(6), 2936–2945.

Collewijn, H. and Tamminga, E.P. (1984). Human smooth and saccadic eye movements during voluntary pursuit of different target motions on different backgrounds. *Journal of Physiology (London)*, **351**, 217–250.

Collewijn, H. and Tamminga, E.P. (1986). Human fixation and pursuit in normal open-loop conditions: effects of central and peripheral retinal targets. *Journal of Physiology (London)*, **379**, 109–129.

Collins, C.J.S. and Barnes, G.R. (2006). The occluded onset pursuit paradigm: prolonging anticipatory smooth pursuit in the absence of visual feedback. *Experimental Brain Research*, **175**, 11–20.

Collins, C.J.S. and Barnes, G.R. (2009). Predicting the unpredictable: weighted averaging of past stimulus timing facilitates ocular pursuit of randomly timed stimuli. *Journal of Neuroscience*, **29**(42), 13302–13314.

Das, V.E., Leigh, R.J., Thomas, C.W., Averbuch-Heller, L., Zivotofsky, A.Z., Discenna, A.O., et al. (1995). Modulation of high-frequency vestibuloocular reflex during visual tracking in humans. *Journal of Neurophysiology*, **74**(2), 624–632.

de Brouwer, S., Missal, M., Barnes, G.R., and Lefevre, P. (2002). Quantitative analysis of catch-up saccades during sustained pursuit. *Journal of Neurophysiology*, **87**, 1772–1780.

de Hemptinne, C., Lefevre, P., and Missal, M. (2006). Influence of cognitive expectation on the initiation of anticipatory and visual pursuit eye movements in the Rhesus monkey. *Journal of Neurophysiology*, **95**, 3770–3782.

de Hemptinne, C., Nozaradan, S., Duvivier, Q., Lefevre, P., and Missal, M. (2007). How do primates anticipate uncertain future events? *Journal of Neuroscience*, **27**(16), 4334–4341.

Deno, D.C., Crandall, W.F., Sherman, K., and Keller, E.L. (1995). Characterization of prediction in the primate visual smooth pursuit system. *BioSystems*, **34**, 107–128.

Dubois, M.F.W. and Collewijn, H. (1979). Optokinetic reactions in man elicited by localized retinal motion stimuli. *Vision Research*, **19**, 1105–1115.

Ferrera, V.P. and Lisberger, S.G. (1995). Attention and target selection for smooth pursuit eye movements. *Journal of Neuroscience*, **15**, 7472–7484.

Fukushima, K., Tanaka, M., Suzuki, Y., Fukushima, J., and Yoshida, T. (1996). Adaptive changes in human smooth pursuit eye movement. *Neuroscience Research*, **25**, 391–398.

Haarmeier, T., Bunjes, F., Lindner, A., Berret, E., and Thier, P. (2001). Optimizing visual motion perception during eye movements. *Neuron*, **32**, 527–535.

Heywood, S. (1973). Pursuing stationary dots: Smooth eye movements and apparent movements. *Perception*, **2**, 181–195.

Hutton, S.B. and Tegally, D. (2005). The effects of dividing attention on smooth pursuit eye tracking. *Experimental Brain Research*, **163**(3), 306–313.

Jarrett, C.B. and Barnes, G.R. (2002). Volitional scaling of anticipatory ocular pursuit velocity using precues. *Cognitive Brain Research*, **14**, 383–388.

Kao, G.W. and Morrow, M.J. (1994). The relationship of anticipatory smooth eye movement to smooth pursuit initiation. *Vision Research*, **34**(22), 3027–3036.

Keller, E.L. and Khan, N.S. (1986). Smooth-pursuit initiation in the presence of a textured background in monkey. *Vision Research*, **26**, 943–955.

Kerzel, D., Souto, D., and Ziegler, N.E. (2008). Effects of attention shifts to stationary objects during steady-state smooth pursuit eye movements. *Vision Research*, **48**, 958–969.

Kimmig, H.G., Miles, F.A., and Schwarz, U. (1992). Effects of stationary textured backgrounds on the initiation of pursuit eye movements in monkeys. *Journal of Neurophysiology*, **68**(6), 2147–2164.

Knox, P.C. and Bekkour, T. (2004). Spatial mapping of the remote distractor effect on smooth pursuit initiation. *Experimental Brain Research*, **154**(4), 494–503.

Kowler, E. (1989). Cognitive expectations, not habits, control anticipatory smooth oculomotor pursuit. *Vision Research*, **29**(9), 1049–1057.

Kowler, E. and McKee, S.P. (1987). Sensitivity of smooth eye movement to small differences in target velocity. *Vision Research*, **27**, 993–1015.

Kowler, E. and Steinman, R.M. (1979a). The effect of expectations on slow oculomotor control – I. Periodic target steps. *Vision Research*, **19**, 619–632.

Kowler, E. and Steinman, R.M. (1979b). The effect of expectations on slow oculomotor control – II. Single target displacements. *Vision Research*, **19**, 633–646.

Krauzlis, R.J. and Lisberger, S.G. (1994a). A model of visually-guided smooth pursuit eye movements based on behavioral observations. *Journal of Computational Neuroscience*, **1**, 265–283.

Krauzlis, R.J. and Lisberger, S.G. (1994b). Simple spike responses of gaze velocity Purkinje cells in the floccular lobe of the monkey during the onset and offset of pursuit eye movements. *Journal of Neurophysiology*, **72**(4), 2045–2050.

Krauzlis, R.J. and Miles, F.A. (1996a). Decreases in the latency of smooth pursuit and saccadic eye movements produced by the 'gap paradigm' in the monkey. *Vision Research*, **36**(13), 1973–1985.

Krauzlis, R.J. and Miles, F.A. (1996b). Transitions between pursuit eye movements and fixation in the monkey: Dependence on context. *Journal of Neurophysiology*, **76**, 1622–1638.

Lindner, A. and Ilg, U.J. (2006). Suppression of optokinesis during smooth pursuit eye movements revisited: the role of extra-retinal information. *Vision Research*, **46**(6–7), 761–767.

Lindner, A., Schwarz, U., and Ilg, U.J. (2001). Cancellation of self-induced retinal image motion during smooth pursuit eye movements. *Vision Research*, **41**, 1685–1694.

Lipton, R.B., Frost, L.A., and Holzman, P.S. (1980). Smooth pursuit eye movements, schizophrenia, and distraction. *Perceptual & Motor Skills*, **50**(1), 159–167.

Lisberger, S.G. (1998). Postsaccadic enhancement of initiation of smooth pursuit eye movements in monkeys. *Journal of Neurophysiology*, **79**, 1918–1930.

Lisberger, S.G. and Ferrera, V.P. (1997). Vector averaging for smooth pursuit eye movements initiated by two moving targets in monkeys. *Journal of Neuroscience*, **17**, 7490–7502.

Lisberger, S.G. and Westbrook, L.E. (1985). Properties of visual inputs that initiate horizontal smooth pursuit eye movements in monkeys. *Journal of Neuroscience*, **6**, 1662–1673.

Lisberger, S.G., Evinger, C., Johanson, G.W., and Fuchs, A.F. (1981). Relationship between eye acceleration and retinal image velocity during foveal smooth pursuit in man and monkey. *Journal of Neurophysiology*, **46**, 229–249.

Lisberger, S.G., Morris, E.J., and Tychsen, L. (1987). Visual motion processing and sensory-motor integration for smooth pursuit eye movements. *Annual Review of Neuroscience*, **10**, 97–129.

Madelain, L. and Krauzlis, R.J. (2003). Pursuit of the ineffable: perceptual and motor reversals during the tracking of apparent motion. *Journal of Vision*, **3**(11), 642–653.

Masson, G.S. and Stone, L.S. (2002). From following edges to pursuing objects. *Journal of Neurophysiology*, **88**(5), 2869–2873.

Merrison, A.F.A. and Carpenter, R.H. (1995). 'Express' smooth pursuit. *Vision Research*, **35**(10), 1459–1462.

Meyer, C.H., Lasker, A.G., and Robinson, D.A. (1985). The upper limit of human smooth pursuit velocity. *Vision Research*, **25**, 561–563.

Michael, J.A. and Melvill Jones, G. (1966). Dependence of visual tracking capability upon stimulus predictability. *Vision Research*, **6**, 707–716.

Miles, F.A. and Kawano, K. (1986). Short-latency ocular following responses of monkey III plasticity. *Journal of Neurophysiology*, **56**, 1381–1396.

Mitrani, L. and Dimitrov, G. (1978). Pursuit eye movements of a disappearing moving target. *Vision Research*, **18**, 537–539.

Mohrmann, H. and Thier, P. (1995). The influence of structured visual backgrounds on smooth-pursuit initiation, steady-state pursuit and smooth-pursuit termination. *Biological Cybernetics*, **73**(1), 83–93.

Morgan, M.J. and Turnbull, D.F. (1978). Smooth eye tracking and the perception of motion in the absence of real movement. *Vision Research*, **18**, 1053–1059.

Orban de Xivry, J.J., and Lefevre, P. (2007). Saccades and pursuit: two outcomes of a single sensorimotor process. *Journal of Physiology*, **584**(Pt 1), 11–23.

Orban de Xivry, J.J., Bennett, S. J., Lefevre, P.P., and Barnes, G.R. (2006). Evidence for synergy between saccades and smooth pursuit during transient target disappearance. *Journal of Neurophysiology*, **95**, 418–427.

Orban de Xivry, J.-J., Missal, M., and Lefèvre, P. (2008). A dynamic representation of target motion drives predictive smooth pursuit during target blanking. *Journal of Vision*, **8**(15), 6.1–13.

Pack, C.C. and Born, R.T. (2001). Temporal dynamics of a neural solution to the aperture problem in visual area MT of macaque brain. *Nature*, **409**(6823), 1040–1042.

Pola, J. and Wyatt, H.J. (1985). Active and passive smooth eye movements: Effects of stimulus size and location. *Vision Research*, **25**, 1063–1076.

Pola, J. and Wyatt, H.J. (1997). Offset dynamics of human smooth pursuit eye movements: effects of target presence and subject attention. *Vision Research*, **39**, 2767–2775.

Poliakoff, E., Collins, C.J.S., and Barnes, G.R. (2005). Attention and selection for predictive smooth pursuit eye movements. *Cognitive Brain Research*, **25**(3), 688–700.

Rashbass, C. (1961). The relationship between saccadic and smooth tracking eye movements. *Journal of Physiology (London)*, **159**, 326–338.

Robinson, D.A. (1965). The mechanics of human smooth pursuit eye movements. *Journal of Physiology (London)*, **180**, 569–591.

Robinson, D.A., Gordon, J.L., and Gordon, S.E. (1986). A model of the smooth pursuit eye movement system. *Biol. Cybern.*, **55**, 43–57.

Schwartz, J.D. and Lisberger, S.G. (1994). Modulation of the level of smooth pursuit activation by initial tracking conditions in monkeys. *Visual Neuroscience*, **11**, 411–424.

Schwarz, U. and Ilg, U.J. (1999). Asymmetry in visual motion processing. *Neuroreport*, **10**(12), 2477–2480.

Schweigart, G., Mergner, T., and Barnes, G.R. (2003). Object motion perception is shaped by the motor control mechanism of ocular pursuit. *Experimental Brain Research*, **148**(3), 350–365.

Shagass, C., Roemer, R.A., and Amadeo, M. (1976). Eye-tracking performance and engagement of attention. *Archives of General Psychiatry*, **33**, 121–125.

Spering, M. and Gegenfurtner, K.R. (2007). Contrast and assimilation in motion perception and smooth pursuit eye movements. *Journal of Neurophysiology*, **98**(3), 1355–1363.

St-Cyr, G.J. and Fender, D.H. (1969). Nonlinearities of the human oculomotor system: gain. *Vision Research*, **9**, 1235–1246.

Steinbach, M.J. (1976). Pursuing the perceptual rather than the retinal stimulus. *Vision Research*, **16**, 1371–1376.

Stone, L.S. and Krauzlis, R.J. (2003). Shared motion signals for human perceptual decisions and oculomotor actions. *Journal of Vision*, **3**(11), 725–736.

Suehiro, K., Miura, K., Kodaka, Y., Inoue, Y., Takemura, A., and Kawano, K. (1999). Effects of smooth pursuit eye movement on ocular responses to sudden background motion in humans. *Neuroscience Research*, **30**(4), 329–338.

Sweeney, J.A., Haas, G.L., Li, S., and Weiden, P.J. (1994). Selective effects of antipsychotic medications on eye-tracking performance in schizophrenia. *Psychiatry Research*, **54**(2), 185–198.

van den Berg, A.V. (1988). Human smooth pursuit during transient perturbations of predictable and unpredictable target movement. *Experimental Brain Research*, **72**, 95–108.

van den Berg, A.V. and Collweijn, H. (1987). Voluntary smooth eye movements with foveally stabilized targets. *Experimental Brain Research*, **68**, 195–204.

van der Steen, J., Tamminga, E.P., and Collewijn, H. (1983). A comparison of oculomotor pursuit of a target in circular real, beta or sigma motion. *Vision Research*, **23**(12), 1655–1661.

Van Donkelaar, P. and Drew, A.S. (2002). The allocation of attention during smooth pursuit eye movements. *Progress in Brain Research*, **140**, 267–277.

Watamaniuk, S.N. and Heinen, S.J. (2003). Perceptual and oculomotor evidence of limitations on processing accelerating motion. *Journal of Vision*, **3**(11), 698–709.

Waterston, J.A., Barnes, G.R., and Grealy, M.A. (1992). A quantitative study of eye and head movements during smooth pursuit in patients with cerebellar disease. *Brain*, **115**, 1343–1358.

Whittaker, S.G. and Eaholtz, G. (1982). Learning patterns of eye motion for foveal pursuit. *Investigative Ophthalmology & Visual Science*, **23**, 393–397.

Worfolk, R. and Barnes, G.R. (1992). Interaction of active and passive slow eye movement systems. *Experimental Brain Research*, **90**, 589–598.

Wyatt, H.J. and Pola, J. (1983). Smooth pursuit eye movements under open-loop and closed-loop conditions. *Vision Research*, **23**, 1121–1131.

Wyatt, H.J. and Pola, J. (1987). Smooth eye movements with step-ramp stimuli: The influence of attention and stimulus extent. *Vision Research*, **27**, 1565–1580.

Yasui, S. and Young, L.R. (1975). Perceived visual motion as effective stimulus to pursuit eye movement system. *Science*, **190**, 906–908.

PART 2
Neural basis of eye movements

CHAPTER 8

The oculomotor plant and its role in three-dimensional eye orientation

Dora E. Angelaki

Abstract

Following years of controversy, a combined approach consisting of both single unit recordings from cyclovertical extraocular motoneurons and electrical microstimulation of the abducens nerve have shown that, for visually-guided eye movements, motoneuron commands balance out to appear two-dimensional (2D; i.e. horizontal/vertical). These studies have also shown that the mechanical properties of the eyeball (perhaps mediated by extraocular muscle pulleys) provide for an eye position-dependent muscle pulling direction, thus accounting for the 'half-angle rule', a property of three-dimensional (3D) eye rotations necessary to keep the eyes in Listing's plane during visually-guided eye movements. Yet, how eye movements that do not follow Listing's law (e.g. the rotational vestibulo-ocular reflex, VOR) use an eye plant that implements the half-angle rule remains a challenge for future studies.

Introduction: extraocular muscles and nuclei

The six extraocular muscles of each eye are organized in three agonist/antagonist muscle pairs. This arrangement allows rotations about any axis in three dimensions, turning the eye right or left, up or down, and clockwise or counterclockwise. Each muscle pair rotates the eye about one principal axis, which defines the plane of action for that muscle pair. For example, the medial and lateral recti rotate the eye in the horizontal plane. Contraction of the lateral rectus gives rise to abduction (temporal eye rotation, away from the nose). Contraction of the medial rectus results in adduction (nasally-directed movement). Elevation and depression of the eye are accomplished mainly by the superior and inferior recti, respectively. The superior and inferior oblique muscles are primarily responsible for intorsion and extorsion. The four vertical movers have secondary actions and are all associated with both elevation/depression and intorsion/extorsion of the eyes.

The pulling directions of the primary activated and inhibited muscles are closely aligned with the planes of the semicircular canals across species (see Ezure and Graf, 1984; Simpson and Graf, 1981). The six muscles are innervated by neurons in the nuclei of three cranial nerves: the III (oculomotor),

IV (trochlear), and IV (abducens). The abducens and trochlear nuclei each supply only one muscle, the ipsilateral lateral rectus and contralateral superior oblique, respectively. The oculomotor nuclei, which have four subdivisions, supply four muscles: the ipsilateral medial rectus, inferior rectus, inferior oblique, and the contralateral superior rectus. The abducens nuclei also contain internuclear neurons that cross the midline to excite medial rectus motoneurons. Although many studies have characterized the physiological properties of extraocular motoneurons, much still remains unknown about the diversity of neuronal fibre types, as well as their role in both the dynamic and kinematic control of the eyeball. Most of these studies have focused on describing the dynamics, recruitment thresholds and eye position sensitivities of cells in the abducens and oculomotor nuclei (de la Cruz et al., 1989; Delgado-Garcia et al., 1986; Fuchs and Luschei, 1970; Fuchs et al., 1988; Henn and Cohen, 1973; Henn et al., 1982; Hepp and Henn, 1985; Pastor et al., 1991; Robinson, 1970; Robinson and Keller, 1972; Schiller, 1970; Stahl and Simpson, 1995; Sylvestre and Cullen, 1999; Suzuki et al., 1999). A few studies have also characterized the firing rates of trochlear neurons (Fuchs and Luschei, 1971; Hepp and Henn, 1985; Mays et al., 1991; Precht et al., 1979; Suzuki et al., 1999). There is general agreement that the dynamics of most motoneurons are adequately described by a first- or second-order function, although differences in the dynamics between saccades, pursuit and the VOR have also been noted (Sylvestre and Cullen, 1999). This overview starts with a summary of a few basic properties of extraocular motoneurons and muscle fibres, followed by a most extensive coverage of the most prominent controversy in oculomotor research of the past decade: the role of the peripheral mechanical properties of the eyeball in the control of 3D eye movements.

Motor and sensory innervation of extraocular muscle fibres

For a long time it was thought that motoneurons form a relatively homogeneous group, which provides the final common path for muscle motor innervation. However, growing evidence suggests the opposite. Specifically, it has become increasingly clear that the structure of eye muscles is highly complex and not yet fully understood. It contains different types of muscle fibres in a global layer and an orbital layer (Shall et al., 1996; Spencer and Porter, 1988; Oh et al., 2001). The global layer inserts directly into the sclera, providing the primary force to rotate the eye. The orbital layer inserts on the sleeves of fibrous tissue around the recti (pulleys) that might modulate the pulling direction of the eye muscles (see below). Both twitch (singly-innervated fibres, which respond to electrical stimulation with a fast twitch propagated throughout the fibre) and non-twitch (multiply-innervated fibres, which respond to electrical stimulation with a slow and tonic nonpropagated contraction) muscle fibres exist for the global and orbital layers. Non-twitch muscle fibres are very resistant to fatigue and are suited to maintaining tension over long periods, suggesting a tonic function in eye muscle control.

The three extraocular nuclei contain two sets of motoneurons innervating twitch and non-twitch muscle types, each with different afferent inputs (Büttner-Ennever and Horn, 2002). Motoneurons innervating twitch muscle fibres are located within the classic boundaries of the oculomotor, trochlear and abducens nuclei. In contrast, motoneurons innervating non-twitch muscle fibres lie slightly separated around the periphery of the motor nuclei (Büttner-Ennever et al., 2001). Most recordings of motoneuron activities in alert animals have probably been from those innervating twitch muscle fibres. The few studies that have recorded from abducens motoneurons innervating non-twitch fibres support the hypothesis that non-twitch motoneurons have tonic properties (Dieringer and Precht, 1986; Goldberg et al., 1981). At present, no recordings have been made from identified non-twitch motoneurons in behaving mammals, thus it is unknown how they contribute to different types of eye movements.

In contrast to skeletal muscles that are typically innervated by proprioceptors, including spindles and Golgi tendon organs, these receptors are not typically found in extraocular muscles (Maier et al., 1974). Because there is also no evidence for a classic stretch reflex (Keller and Robinson, 1971), nor is proprioceptive information required to generate accurate eye movements (Guthrie et al., 1983), it had been often assumed that there is no proprioceptive input from eye muscles to the brain. However, several recent studies have provided abundant evidence that the brain utilizes information from eye muscle proprioceptors (Donaldson, 2000; Steinbach, 2000; Wang et al., 2007; Weir et al., 2000). In particular, the principal sensory afferent input from extraocular muscles probably arises from palisade endings. They form a cuff of nerve terminals around the tip of muscle fibres looking like 'inverted spindles' and are found exclusively on the multiply innervated, non-twitch fibres of the global layer (Donaldson, 2000; Spencer and Porter, 1988). Although not yet explicitly demonstrated for palisade endings, the eye muscle proprioceptive signals are thought to ascend to the brain via the trigeminal nerve, with at least some terminating in the spinal trigeminal nucleus, where proprioceptive activity has been recorded (Donaldson, 2000; Ruskell, 1999). Recently, eye muscle proprioception responses have been described in the macaque primary somatosensory cortex (Wang et al., 2007).

In summary, although the traditional thinking had been that all motoneurons participate in every type of eye movement regardless of whether it is saccadic, vestibular, or vergence in nature (Gamlin and Mays, 1992; Keller and Robinson, 1972), recent evidence raises doubt to this widespread assumption. In particular, although the function of non-twitch motoneurons is currently unknown, all available evidence points to the fact that it is different from that of twitch motoneurons. In support of a potentially differential role of twitch and non-twitch motoneurons, premotor neurons to the non-twitch motoneurons of the abducens nucleus have been shown to lie in areas that support gaze holding and vergence responses (e.g. the near response region, the adjacent central mesencephalic reticular formation and the neural integrator areas), rather than saccadic and VOR pathways that exclusively project to twitch motoneurons (Wasicky et al., 2004). Büttner-Ennever and Horn (2002) have put forward the hypothesis that twitch motoneurons are those important for the generation of eye rotations, whereas non-twitch motoneurons might participate in a proprioceptive system, important for setting and stabilizing the alignment of the eye ('dual motor control hypothesis'). A disruption of proprioceptive feedback might play a role in calibrating central oculomotor parameters over the long term in oculomotor disorders like strabismus and congential nystagmus (Steinbach, 2000; Weir et al., 2000).

Orbital mechanics: phasic and tonic innervation

The neural commands for all types of eye movements must take into account the mechanical constraints of the tissues supporting the eyeball. In particular, to move the eyes it is necessary to overcome viscous drag and elastic restoring forces imposed by the orbital supporting tissues (the inertia of the eyeball has been considered to be negligible). To overcome the viscous drag, motoneuron discharge must include a phasic component, which for saccades, consists of a burst in activity (*pulse of innervation*). Once in its new position, the eye must be held there against the elastic restoring forces that tend to return the eyeball to its central position. To overcome these elastic forces, motoneuron firing rates must include a tonic component (*step of innervation*). Indeed, motoneuron firing rates during saccades consist of both a burst and tonic component (Fig. 8.1A, top traces), as confirmed by studies of discharge characteristics of ocular motoneurons (Robinson, 1970; Robinson and Keller, 1972). Without the pulse, the eye movement could never sustain the high velocities of saccadic eye movements. Without the tonic component of motoneuron discharge, the eye could never be maintained at an eccentric orientation, since eye position would decay exponentially (Fig. 8.1A, bottom traces).

This tonic component in motoneuron activity is generated by neural populations that perform a function similar to time integration in calculus; this has been known as the velocity-to-position neural integrator (Cannon and Robinson, 1987; Robinson, 1981; Skavenski and Robinson, 1973), a basic component for the generation of all eye movements. Based on the discharge properties of extraocular motoneurons and quantitative modelling, the transfer function of the eye plant has been described to be a second- or third-order system, with a single dominant time constant of approximately 250 ms and a bandwidth of about 0.5–1 Hz (Fuchs et al., 1988; Robinson, 1970; Sylvestre and Cullen, 1999). In contrast to such a good understanding of the dynamics of the oculomotor plant

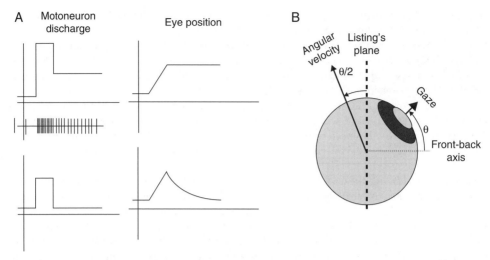

Fig. 8.1 A) Schematic illustrating the phasic-tonic motoneuron discharge required to overcome the viscous-elastic properties of the eye plant. Top traces: motoneurons must elicit a burst-tonic signal (left) to change and maintain eye position at a new steady-state level (right). The vertical lines indicate the occurrence of action potentials of a hypothetical ocular motoneuron. Bottom traces: schematic of eye position change (right) if motoneuron discharge only consisted of a burst but not tonic signal (left). Abscissa represents time. The phasic component is used to quickly rotate the eyes, whereas the tonic component ensures that the eye is held there against the elastic restoring forces. B) According to Listing's law, the axis of rotation of the eye (as defined by the angular velocity) is neither head-fixed nor eye-fixed, but rotates in the same direction as gaze through half the gaze angle ($\theta/2$; *half-angle rule*). Thus, during a horizontal saccade from eccentric eye positions, the axis of rotation of the eye is not purely horizontal (vertical dotted line) but also has a torsional component (horizontal dotted line). The orientation of this plane in a head-fixed coordinate system relative to straight ahead (i.e. the x-axis) is not always aligned with the animal's frontal plane. However, when eye positions are expressed relative to a unique eye position, referred to as primary position, then Listing's plane is aligned with the y–z plane and perpendicular to the x- (torsional) axis. For simplicity in the following discussion we consider *Listing's plane* to coincide with the *horizontal/vertical*, y–z plane. Reprinted from *Neuron*, **47**(2), 281–93, Ghasia and Angelaki, Do motoneurons encode the noncommutativity of ocular rotations?, © 2005, with permission from Elsevier.

and its contribution to eye movement generation along a single direction (typically horizontal, but sometimes vertical), until recently little was known about the kinematics and 3D properties of the eye plant. Next we describe attempts to quantify the properties of the eye plant in 3D. We start by first summarizing a controversy that has long faced the 3D oculomotor field.

The controversy about ocular torsion

How the brain controls ocular torsion has been a matter of considerable debate for many years. The controversy has been primarily centred on issues of neural versus mechanical contributions to the control of torsion during saccadic eye movements (Demer et al., 2000; Quaia and Optican, 1998; Raphan, 1998; Schnabolk and Raphan, 1994; Tweed et al., 1994). As summarized above, the eyeball has three degrees of freedom, and thus is capable of rotating in 3D. This is appropriate during head movements, as the head can rotate in roll, pitch, and yaw and compensatory eye movements are generated for all axes of head motion. However, unlike the VOR, the goal of saccades and pursuit is to re-direct the line of sight (referred to as 'gaze'); thus, only the horizontal and vertical degrees of freedom of the eye are functionally specified for visually-guided eye movements. What then happens to the third degree of freedom of the eyeball?

It is now well known that all saccades that originate from primary position are associated with rotation axes that are confined to a single horizontal/vertical plane, referred to as 'Listing's plane' (Ferman et al., 1987; Tweed and Vilis, 1987, 1990). When saccades are generated from non-primary eye positions, the angular velocity axis of the eye does not remain confined to Listing's plane but deviates towards the direction of gaze by approximately half as much ('half-angle rule'; Fig. 8.1B; see also Tweed and Vilis, 1987, 1990). Thus, when expressed in a head-fixed coordinate system, an eye position-dependent torsional component is 'added' to horizontal and vertical eye velocity during saccades that do not originate from primary position. In contrast, eye orientation and the derivative of eye orientation remain confined to the horizontal/vertical (Listing's) plane. This occurs because the mathematics of rotations do not follow simple (commutative) vector algebra, e.g. angular velocity is not equal to the derivative of eye orientation unless the eye is in primary position. Thus, eye positions in Listing's plane have zero torsion, but eye velocities must have a non-zero torsional component for the movement to stay in Listing's plane (for mathematical details, see Haslwanter, 1995, 2002; Tweed and Vilis, 1987, 1990; van Opstal, 1993).

How this torsional eye velocity component, necessary to keep eye position in Listing's plane during visually-guided eye movements, is generated was at the centre of the controversy for many years. This problem was first addressed in the late 1980s by Tweed and Vilis (1987, 1990). Specifically, because angular velocity is not the derivative of eye orientation in 3D, traditional oculomotor concepts that were well established for the horizontal system, like that of the velocity-to-position neural integrator (Cannon and Robinson, 1987; Robinson, 1981; Skavenski and Robinson, 1973), came under question. Tweed and Vilis proposed that an extension of the neural integration concept in 3D would require the incorporation of non-linear (multiplicative) mathematical operations (Tweed and Vilis, 1987, 1990; see also Angelaki and Hess, 2004). Perhaps not surprisingly, this proposal was soon challenged (Schnabolk and Raphan, 1994; Strauman and Zee, 1995). Moreover, Henn and colleagues failed to find evidence for a clear neural representation of 3D angular velocity in the premotor pathway for saccadic eye movements (Hepp et al., 1993, 1999; Scherberger et al., 2001; van Opstal et al., 1991, 1996). This led to the suggestion that these pathways could instead code the derivative of eye orientation, which does not include 'half angle' torsional tilts, and therefore can be integrated to provide the correct oculomotor position signal (Crawford 1994; Crawford and Guitton, 1997; Tweed, 1997). Thus, another explanation of the half angle rule was required. Simultaneously, 'pulleys' in the orbit were proposed to influence the pulling direction of the extraocular muscles (Demer et al., 2000; Kono et al., 2002).

Active pulley hypothesis

Since 1989, there has been steadily growing evidence that the peripheral ocular mechanics might be more complicated than once thought. Specifically, several studies have reported the existence of mobile, soft-tissue sheaths or 'pulleys' in the orbit that influence the pulling direction of the extraocular muscles (Demer et al., 1995, 2000; Miller, 1989; Miller et al., 1993). Based on theoretical arguments, it was then proposed that pulleys may simplify the brain's work in implementing Listing's law (Crawford and Guitton, 1997; Quaia and Optican, 1998; Raphan, 1997, 1998). In fact, a theoretical study by Quaia and Optican (1998) has shown that appropriately-placed pulleys in an otherwise idealized eye plant can generate both physiologically realistic saccades and implement the half-angle rule without a need to calculate a 'neural torsional signal' as originally proposed by Tweed and Vilis (1987, 1990). This is so because, as elegantly explained by Quaia and Optican (1998), with 'correctly' located pulleys the saccadic pulse is treated like the derivative of eye orientation. This allows for a simple approximation of the saccadic step from the pulse signal (Fig. 8.1A) and solves the problem of the 3D velocity-position transformation for saccades and pursuit (without directly dealing with the non-commutativity issue (Quaia and Optican, 1998)). Indeed, magnetic resonance imaging (MRI) of rectus muscle paths has shown that the arrangement of the pulleys is consistent with an oculomotor plant that could implement the eye position-dependence of Listing's law (Demer et al., 2000; Kono et al., 2002).

In summary, Demer's functional imaging results, combined with the modelling studies of Quaia and Optican (1998; also Raphan, 1998), whereby a commutative 2D (horizontal/vertical) neural pulse-step generator could be sufficient to generate accurate saccades and smooth pursuit eye movements in Listing's plane, created an alternative view to the original proposal of Tweed and Vilis (1987, 1990). This 'commutative controller' hypothesis was attractive because it simplified the premotor processing of eye movements such that the traditional 'Robinsonian' concepts of dynamic premotor processing, well-established for the horizontal system, could now be used to describe the pulse-step matching for saccades and pursuit in 3D. This was the theory, but what remained to be demonstrated was physiological proof for this scheme. However, as will be summarized next, recent neurophysiological experiments have provided further support for an implementation of the half angle-rule by the peripheral ocular mechanics.

Motoneuron discharge: is there any evidence for a neural implementation of the half-angle rule?

In the first of these studies, neural activities were recorded from cyclovertical motoneurons of the oculomotor and trochlear nerves. Cyclovertical motoneurons carry the appropriate motor drive to generate vertical and torsional eye velocities during pitch and roll VOR (referred to as 'sensory-driven torsion'). In contrast, during saccades and smooth pursuit, the stimulus constitutes a 2D retinal signal, where only the horizontal and vertical components of eye velocity are directly driven by the sensory stimulus. Thus, the torsional eye velocity necessary for the half-angle rule is not sensory-driven but a direct result of non-commutativity. Whether motoneurons carry the appropriate motor drive to generate this 'non-commutative-driven torsion' is fundamental to the differing predictions between the neural versus mechanical (active pulley hypothesis, APH) hypotheses. Specifically, if the non-commutative-driven torsion is neurally-generated (neural hypothesis), the firing rates of *all* cyclovertical (but not horizontal) motoneurons should change proportionally to both sensory-driven and non-commutative-driven torsion. In contrast, the APH hypothesis predicts no correlation between firing rates and non-commutative-driven torsion, because the latter is simply added on at the level of the oculomotor plant, due to eye position-dependent changes in the pulling direction of the rectus muscles.

The experiment illustrated in Fig. 8.2 examined these two alternative hypotheses in macaques during horizontal and vertical pursuit eye movements at different vertical and horizontal eccentricities, respectively. The small torsional velocity elicited during eccentric pursuit reflects the non-commutative-driven torsion. Unlike the sensory-driven torsion generated during roll head movements, the torsional eye velocity elicited during horizontal and vertical smooth pursuit (Angelaki et al., 2003; Tweed et al., 1992) is not in response to a sensory stimulus, but reflects the rather unintuitive consequences of the non-commutative mathematics of rotations. When eye velocity is plotted in head coordinates (see insets; A: side view; B: top view), eye velocity tilts in the same direction as gaze, by approximately half as much (accounting for the 'half-angle rule'; Fig. 8.1B). This torsional component of eye velocity is necessary to keep eye position in Listing's plane (Haslwanter et al., 1991; Tweed and Vilis, 1987, 1990; Tweed et al., 1992). According to the APH hypothesis, cyclovertical motoneurons should not change their activity to reflect the added torsional velocity during eccentric pursuit. In contrast, the neural hypothesis predicts that cyclovertical motoneurons would exhibit the same sensitivity to this non-commutative-driven torsion as they do for the roll head movement-driven torsion. As a result, their firing rates should systematically change as the ratio of torsional versus horizontal or vertical velocity changes at different ocular eccentricities.

By recording from oculomotor and trochlear nerve fibres, Ghasia and Angelaki (2005) showed that the small eye position-dependence of many cyclovertical motoneurons is not only much smaller in magnitude but also often in the wrong direction to be consistent with the predictions of the neural hypothesis (Ghasia and Angelaki, 2005). Thus, these results are inconsistent with motoneurons providing the motor drive for the non-commutative-driven torsion, a finding that would be consistent

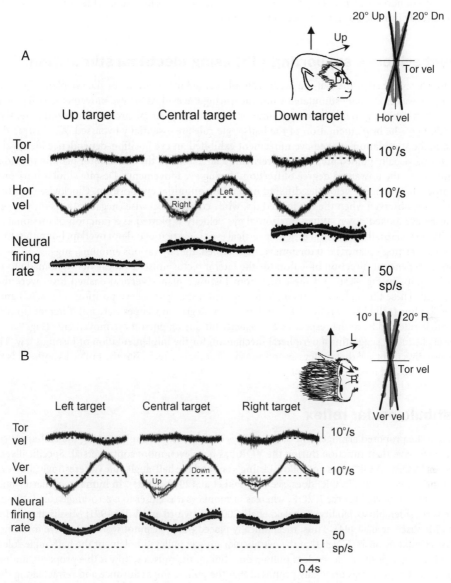

Fig. 8.2 Eye velocity and neural responses from a trochlear nerve fibre during (A) horizontal and (B) vertical pursuit of targets at different eccentricities. From left to right, data shown are for targets moving horizontally at vertical eccentricities of 20° Up, centre and 20° Down (A) and for targets moving vertically at horizontal eccentricities of 10° left (L), centre and 20° right (R) (B). From top to bottom, traces illustrate mean torsional eye velocity and mean horizontal (A) or mean vertical (B) eye velocity (±SD, grey lines). Bottom traces illustrate neural firing rate, with the superimposed sinusoidal fit (grey lines). Notice that, as typical of all motoneurons, mean firing rates increased when looking eccentrically in the cell's on-direction (down). However, it is the peak-to-trough firing rate modulation that is of interest in these comparisons. Insets on the top illustrate mean eye velocity plotted in head coordinates (see monkey's head drawing). Data are shown in grey, with superimposed black solid lines illustrating linear regression (for clarity only shown for eccentric targets). Notice that eye movements are expressed in space (not Listing's) coordinates. Reprinted from *Neuron*, **47**(2), 281–93, Ghasia and Angelaki, Do motoneurons encode the noncommutativity of ocular rotations?, © 2005, with permission from Elsevier.

with (but not necessarily proof of) the APH hypothesis. Next, positive support for the APH hypothesis is directly provided using electrical microstimulation.

Direct evidence supporting APH using electrical stimulation

To directly test whether the half-angle rule is implemented mechanically by the eye plant, the abducens nerve was electrically stimulated while measuring the evoked 3D eye movements (Klier et al., 2006). By stimulating so late in the oculomotor pathway, any neural circuits that could potentially contribute to the implementation of the half-angle rule are essentially bypassed. As illustrated in Fig. 8.3, the stimulation-evoked eye movement exhibited an eye position-dependence identical to that during visually-guided pursuit, thus verifying a large role for the oculomotor plant in providing a solution for the unwanted degree of freedom during eye movements. Despite similar horizontal responses, torsional eye velocities differed depending on initial eye position. Clockwise (positive) torsion was observed when the eye looked up, while counterclockwise (negative) torsion was seen when the eye looked down. When horizontal eye velocity is plotted as a function of torsional eye velocity (Fig. 8.3B), the data from different vertical eye eccentricities did not overlap, but rather tilted away from Listing's plane (i.e. 0 torsion, vertical dashed line) by various amounts, suggesting an eye position-dependent direction of action for the lateral rectus muscle. Linear fits were made to the velocity loops in Fig. 8.3B and their tilts from Listing's plane (vertical dashed line) were then compared. These tilt angles were then plotted against initial vertical eye position (Fig. 8.3C) and a regression line (solid black) is fitted through the data. Regression slopes were not different from the half-angle rule and from the respective eye velocity tilt during pursuit eye movements (Fig. 8.4A,B; Klier et al., 2006), suggesting a peripheral mechanism for the implementation of Listing's law. This does not directly prove that pulleys are responsible for these effects, but the pulley hypothesis is the best described and most testable explanation for these findings.

Vestibulo-ocular reflex

Whereas the proposed arrangement of the pulleys could work for implementing the half-angle rule of Listings' law, their function during the VOR has been even more controversial. Specifically, the rotational VOR (RVOR) does not follow Listing's law and the half-angle rule (interestingly, however, the translational VOR (TVOR) does; see Angelaki et al. (2000, 2003)). In humans, a quarter-angle rule has been reported for the RVOR, whereas in monkeys it is closer to a zero-angle rule (although there is considerable variability; Angelaki et al., 2003; Crawford and Vilis, 1991; Misslisch and Hess, 2000; Misslisch et al., 1994). Thus, mechanically placed pulleys cannot work for all eye movement systems simultaneously. Given that the extraocular muscle pulleys implement the half-angle rule by imposing an eye position-dependent pulling direction of the muscles, how is this property 'undone' during the RVOR? It was originally proposed that the pulleys might advance and retract along their muscle paths, adopting one arrangement for Listing's law and another for the RVOR (Demer et al., 2000; Thurtell et al., 1999, 2000). This theory, however, was later shown to be incorrect, as the required retraction to explain the RVOR would be so large as not to be physiologically plausible (Misslisch and Tweed, 2001). Furthermore, the proposed retraction, no matter how large, could not explain the full pattern of eye velocity tilts seen in the RVOR (Misslisch and Tweed, 2001). In particular, although during the pitch and yaw RVOR eye velocity tilts by only a quarter (or less) of the gaze angle in the same direction as gaze ('quarter-angle rule'), during the roll RVOR eye velocity tilts in the opposite direction as gaze and typically through an angle as large as the gaze angle (Misslisch and Hess, 2000; Misslisch and Tweed, 2001).

The exact amount of the eye position dependence for the RVOR depends systematically on the torsional RVOR gain: The higher the torsional RVOR gain, the weaker the eye position dependence of the RVOR; the lower the torsional RVOR gain, the stronger the eye position dependence of the RVOR. In the extreme (hypothetical) case that torsional RVOR gain is zero, pitch/yaw RVOR eye

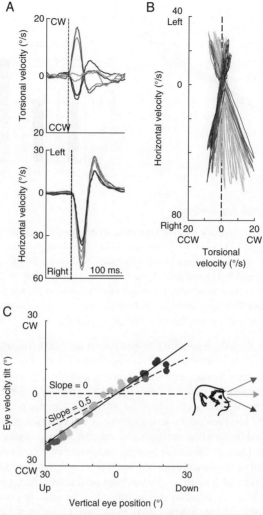

Fig. 8.3 (Also see Plate 4.) Characteristics of eye velocity during abducens nerve microstimulation. A) Temporal plots of eye velocity from different initial eye positions (green = straight ahead; red = 25° up; blue = 25° down) are similar in the horizontal domain (lower panel), but differ in the torsional domain (upper panel). B) Horizontal versus torsional velocity is plotted as the eye assumes different vertical positions. The eye's orientation when the stimulation was delivered is illustrated by a colour palette, ranging from 25° up (dark red) to 25° down (dark blue) in 5° intervals. The orientation of Listing's plane is indicated by the vertical dashed line at 0° torsion. C) Measures of eye velocity tilt angle are plotted against initial vertical eye position. A slope of 0 (indicating fixed axes of rotation and a zero-angle rule) and a slope of 0.5 (indicating eye position-dependent axes of rotation and proper implementation of the half-angle rule) are also shown (dashed lines). Replotted with permission from Klier et al. (2006).

velocity should tilt by half the gaze angle, whereas roll RVOR eye velocity should tilt in the opposite direction by 90° minus the gaze angle (Misslisch and Tweed, 2001). The fact that Demer's original proposal about pulleys during the RVOR is incorrect has been further supported by results during combined RVOR/TVOR (Angelaki, 2003). Specifically, during combined RVOR/TVOR (e.g. as experienced during eccentric rotation), eye velocity not only tilts in the opposite direction as gaze, but also exhibits slopes as large as ten times those expected from the half-angle rule (default position

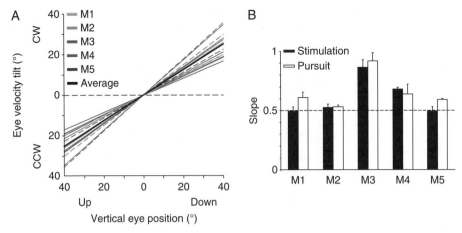

Fig. 8.4 (Also see Plate 5.) Stimulation-evoked eye movements have the same eye position-dependence as visually-guided pursuit. A) Slopes for all sites closely approximate the half-angle rule (slope = 0.5) and not a zero-angle rule (slope = 0) (black dashed lines). This finding is observed for both nerve (solid lines) and nucleus (dashed lines) stimulation. B) Comparison of median stimulation slopes (black bars) with half-angle rule slopes from pursuit (white bars), shown separately for each animal. Error bars illustrate 95% confidence intervals. Dashed line: half-angle rule slope of 0.5. Replotted with permission from Klier et al. (2006).

of the pulleys; Demer et al., 2000; Klier et al., 2006; Kono et al., 2002). These large, systematic deviations away from a Listing's law strategy would strongly argue for a neural component to 3D ocular kinematics for the VOR. How this occurs remains unclear and still represents a mystery.

Although we are currently no closer in understanding how the RVOR and associated neural commands are able to alter the half-angle rule of the default oculomotor plant, Demer (2002, see also Demer and Clark, 2005) has presented a new hypothesis: the violation of Listing's law during the RVOR might be mediated by the oblique extraocular muscles whose velocity axes are actively maintained orthogonal to the Listing's velocity axes of the rectus muscles. This new proposal is not based on any firm experimental or theoretical evidence, but it is the only remaining conjecture that has not yet been refuted. This proposal actually originated from MRI results during ocular convergence and static ocular counter-rolling, where rectus pulleys rotated in the orbit, but remained fixed relative to the pulling direction of the obliques (Demer and Clark, 2005; Demer et al., 2003). According to this hypothesis, appropriate neural signals during convergence and counter-rolling (and presumably also RVOR) would activate the oblique muscles, causing the eye not only to rotate torsionally but also to simultaneously rotate the rectus pulleys as well. As a result, the rectus muscle pulling directions would remain fixed relative to the obliques but change relative to the head. Thus, the rectus pulleys would function like a 'half-angle rule gimbal' that is under control by the obliques. This revised hypothesis could nicely explain the rotation or translation of Listing's plane during ocular convergence and static head tilts (Haslwanter et al., 1992; Minken and van Gisbergen, 1994; Mok et al., 1992; van Rijn and van den Berg, 1993). This hypothesis might also account for the shift in the preferred direction of burst neurons during saccades in static roll head positions (Scherberger et al., 2001). Although this evidence, particularly during ocular counter-rolling is sketchy (e.g. the observed pulley rotation is only half that of eyeball torsion), it provides a testable hypothesis that should be addressed in future studies.

Commutativity versus non-commutativity of rotations: is there a role for both the pulleys and the brain?

Throughout these years of controversy, there was often a confusion regarding the role of the brain (see also Crawford and Klier, Chapter 18, this volume). Now this controversy is also reaching a resolution: the brain still needs to deal with the issue of non-commutativity, despite the existence of appropriately placed pulleys (Smith and Crawford 1998; Tweed et al., 1999). At least three experimental findings argue for this: a) different eye movements exhibit different 3D kinematics. Specifically, as summarized above, Listing's law is relaxed or abandoned during the RVOR and optokinetic slow phases (Crawford and Vilis, 1991; Fetter et al., 1992; Misslisch et al., 1994). Furthermore, during eccentric rotations where both the RVOR and the TVOR are coactivated, a variable eye position dependent torsion is observed, with slopes that are as much as ten times larger than and often in the opposite direction from what would be expected based on extraocular muscle pulley location (Angelaki, 2003). These results are consistent with the hypothesis that the eye position dependent torsion is centrally computed separately for the RVOR and the TVOR (Angelaki, 2003). b) During head-free gaze shifts where slower head movements are routinely preceded by a saccade, the saccade normally drives the eyes out of Listing's plane in an anticipatory fashion, such that it ends up in Listing's plane after the whole movement is complete (Crawford and Guitton 1997; Crawford and Vilis 1991; Crawford et al., 1999; Tweed 1997). The fact that the saccade drives eye position out of Listing's plane in an anticipation of the whole gaze shift can not be explained without neural commands (Crawford et al., 1999). c) Other studies have also convincingly shown that the visuomotor transformations from retinal information into kinematically correct eye movements requires accurate neural control over horizontal, vertical and torsional eye position (Crawford and Guitton, 1997; Klier and Crawford, 1998). d) Finally, histological and imaging studies of the oculomotor plant continue to raise doubt about the exact mechanism that controls the 3D properties of eye rotations by the oculomotor plant (Dimitrova et al., 2003; Lee et al., 2007).

Conclusions and future directions

During the past decades, much has been learned about the oculomotor periphery and how it contributes in the generation of temporally and kinematically accurate eye movements. Many questions though remain. For example, what is the functional significance of the dual innervation, as well as the orbital and global layer motoneurons? What about twitch and non-twitch muscle fibres? Most of the neurophysiological recordings so far are most likely from twitch motoneurons innervating the global layer. Are the properties of the other motoneuron types similar? Furthermore, is there a differential role of orbital and global layer motoneurons in the control of the pulley arrangement during visually-guided eye movements versus the VOR? Finally, but equally importantly, only recently have studies started using more realistic plants consisting of 'biomechanically-correct' models that incorporate at least some of the known anatomical and physiological details of the oculomotor plant. For example, the torques exerted by a muscle, in addition to having a component proportional to innervation, are also characterized by a complicated, non-linear length–tension relationship (Simonsz, 1994). Because of their complexity, simulations of such models are usually restricted to static fixations (Porrill et al., 2000; Quaia and Optican, 2003). An extension of biomechanical models to include eye movement dynamics (thus, incorporating the complex properties of muscle force generation (Goldberg and Shall 1999; Goldberg et al., 1998; Miller and Robins, 1992)) would also be necessary. Research in future years must continue to address these complicated issues, as they are critical for a complete understanding of the generation of eye movements.

Acknowledgement

Supported by National Institutes of Health grant RO1-EY15271.

References

Angelaki, D.E. (2003). Three-dimensional ocular kinematics during eccentric rotations: evidence for functional rather than mechanical constraints. *Journal of Neurophysiology*, **89**, 2685–2696.

Angelaki, D.E. and Hess, B.J. (2004). Control of eye orientation: where does the brain's role end and the muscle's begin? *Europena Journal of Neuroscience*, **19**, 1–10.

Angelaki, D.E., McHenry, M.Q. and Hess, B.J. (2000). Primate translational vestibuloocular reflexes. I. High-frequency dynamics and three-dimensional properties during lateral motion. *Journal of Neurophysiology*, **83**, 1637–1647.

Angelaki, D.E., Zhou, H.H. and Wei, M. (2003). Foveal versus full-field visual stabilization strategies for translational and rotational head movements. *Journal of Neuroscience*, **23**, 1104–1108.

Büttner-Ennever, J.A. and Horn, A.K. (2002). Oculomotor system: a dual innervation of the eye muscles from the abducens, trochlear, and oculomotor nuclei. *Movement Disorders Supplement*, **2**, S2–3.

Büttner-Ennever, J.A., Horn, A.K., Scherberger, H. and D'Ascanio, P. (2001). Motoneurons of twitch and nontwitch extraocular muscle fibers in the abducens, trochlear, and oculomotor nuclei of monkeys. *Journal of Comparative Neurology*, **438**, 318–335.

Cannon, S.C. and Robinson, D.A. (1987). Loss of the neural integrator of the oculomotor system from brain stem lesions in monkey. *Journal of Neurophysiology*, **57**, 1383–1409.

Crawford, J.D. (1994). The oculomotor neural integrator uses a behavior-related coordinate system. *Journal of Neuroscience*, **14**(11 Pt 2), 6911–6923.

Crawford, J.D. and Guitton, D. (1997). Visual-motor transformations required for accurate and kinematically correct saccades. *Journal of Neurophysiology*, **78**, 1447–1467.

Crawford, J.D. and Vilis, T. (1991). Axes of eye rotation and Listing's law during rotations of the head. *Journal of Neurophysiology*, **65**, 407–423.

Crawford, J.D., Ceylan, M.Z., Klier, E.M. and Guitton, D. (1999). Three-dimensional eye-head coordination during gaze saccades in the primate. *Journal of Neuroscience*, **1**, 1760–1782.

De la Cruz, R.R., Escudero, M., and Delgado-Garcia, J.M. (1989). Behaviour of medial rectus motoneurons in the alert cat. *European Journal of Neuroscience*, **1**, 288–295.

Delgado-Garcia, J.M., Del Pozo, F., and Baker, R. (1986). Behavior of neurons in the abducens nucleus of the alert cat. I. Motoneurons. *Neuroscience*, **17**, 929–952.

Demer, J.L. (2002). The orbital pulley system: a revolution in concepts of orbital anatomy. *Annals of the New York Academy of Sciences*, **956**, 17–32.

Demer, J.L. and Clark, R.A. (2005). Magnetic resonance imaging of human extraocular muscles during static ocular counter-rolling. *Journal of Neurophysiology*, **94**, 3292–3302.

Demer, J.L., Kono, R., and Wright, W. (2003). Magnetic resonance imaging of human extraocular muscles in convergence. *Journal of Neurophysiology*, **89**, 2072–2085.

Demer, J.L., Miller, J.M., Poukens, V., Vinters, H.V., and Glasgow, B.J. (1995). Evidence for fibromuscular pulleys of the recti extraocular muscles. *Investigative Ophthalmology & Visual Science*, **36**, 1125–1136.

Demer, J.L., Oh, S.Y. and Poukens, V. (2000). Evidence for active control of rectus extraocular muscle pulleys. *Investigative Ophthalmology & Visual Science*, **41**, 1280–1290.

Dieringer, N. and Precht, W. (1986). Functional organization of eye velocity and eye position signals in abducens motoneurons of the frog. *Journal of Comparative Physiology*, **158**, 179–194.

Dimitrova, D.M., Shall, M.S., and Goldberg, S.J. (2003). Stimulation-evoked eye movements with and without the lateral rectus muscle pulley. *Journal of Neurophysiology*, **90**, 3809–3815.

Donaldson, I.M. (2000). The functions of the proprioceptors of the eye muscles. *Philosophical Transactions of the Royal Society B: Biological Science* **355**, 1685–1754.

Ezure, K. and Graf, W. (1984). A quantitative analysis of the spatial organization of the vestibule-ocular reflexes in lateral- and frontal-eyed animals–I. Orientation of semicircular canals and extraocular muscles. *Neuroscience*, **12**, 85–93.

Ferman, L., Collewijn, H., and Van den Berg, A.V. (1987). A direct test of Listing's law—I. Human ocular torsion measured in static tertiary positions. *Vision Research*, **27**, 929–938.

Fetter, M., Tweed, D., Misslisch, H., Fischer, D., and Koenig, E. (1992). Multidimensional descriptions of the optokinetic and vestibuloocular reflexes. *Annals of the New York Academy of Sciences*, **656**, 841–842.

Fuchs, A.F. and Luschei, E.S. (1970). Firing patterns of abducens neurons of alert monkeys in relationship to horizontal eye movement. *Journal of Neurophysiology*, **33**, 382–392.

Fuchs, A.F. and Luschei, E.S. (1971). The activity of single trochlear nerve fibers during eye movements in the alert monkey. *Experimental Brain Research*, **13**, 78–89.

Fuchs, A.F., Scudder, C.A., Kaneko, C.R. (1988). Discharge patterns and recruitment order of identified motoneurons and internuclear neurons in the monkey abducens nucleus. *Journal of Neurophysiology*, **60**, 1874–1895.

Gamlin, P.D. and Mays, L.E. (1992). Dynamic properties of medial rectus motoneurons during vergence eye movements. *Journal of Neurophysiology*, **67**, 64–74.

Ghasia, F.F. and Angelaki, D.E. (2005). Do motoneurons encode the noncommutativity of ocular rotations? *Neuron*, **47**, 281–293.

Goldberg, S.J., Clamann, H.P., and McClung, J.R. (1981). Relation between motoneuron position and lateral rectus motor unit contraction speed: an intracellular study in the cat abducens nucleus. *Neuroscience Letters*, **23**, 49–54.

Goldberg, S.J., Meredith, M.A., and Shall, M.S. (1998). Extraocular motor unit and whole-muscle responses in the lateral rectus muscle of the squirrel monkey. *Journal of Neuroscience*, **18**, 10629–10639.

Goldberg, S.J. and Shall, M.S. (1999). Motor units of extraocular muscles: Recent findings. *Progress in Brain Research*, **123**, 221–232.

Guthrie, B.L., Porter, J.D., and Sparks, D.L. (1983). Corollary discharge provides accurate eye position information to the oculomotor system. *Science*, **221**, 1193–1195.

Haslwanter, T. (1995). Mathematics of three-dimensional eye rotations. *Vision Research*, **35**, 1727–1739.

Haslwanter, T. (2002). Mechanics of eye movements: implications of the 'orbital revolution'. *Annals of the New York Academy of Sciences*, **956**, 33–41.

Haslwanter, T., Straumann, D., Hepp, K., Hess, B.J., and Henn, V. (1991). Smooth pursuit eye movements obey Listing's law in the monkey. *Experimental Brain Research*, **87**, 470–472.

Haslwanter, T., Straumann, D., Hess, B.J., and Henn, V. (1992). Static roll and pitch in the monkey: shift and rotation of Listing's plane. *Vision Research*, **32**, 1341–1348.

Henn, V., Büttner-Ennever, J.A., and Hepp, K. (1982). The primate oculomotr system. *Human Neurobiol* **1**, 77–85.

Henn, V. and Cohen, B. (1973). Quantitative analysis of activity in eye muscle motoneurons during saccadic eye movement and positions of fixation. *Journal of Neurophysiology*, **36**, 115–126.

Hepp, K., Cabungcal, J.H., Duersteler, M., Hess, B.J., Scherberger, H., Straumann, D., *et al.* (1999). 3D structure of the reticular saccade generator. *Society for Neuroscience Abstracts*, **25**, 661.6.

Hepp, K. and Henn, V. (1985). Iso-frequency curves of oculomotor neurons in the rhesus monkey. *Vision Research*, **25**, 493–499.

Hepp, K., Van Opstal, A.J., Straumann, D., Hess, B.J., and Henn, V. (1993). Monkey superior colliculus represents rapid eye movements in a two-dimensional motor map. *Journal of Neurophysiology*, **69**, 965–979.

Keller, E.L. and Robinson, D.A. (1971). Absence of a stretch reflex in extraocular muscles of the monkey. *Journal of Neurophysiology*, **34**, 908–919.

Keller, E.L. and Robinson, D.A. (1972). Abducens unit behavior in the monkey during vergence movements. *Vision Research*, **12**, 369–382.

Klier, E.M. and Crawford, J.D. (1998). Human oculomotor system accounts for 3-D eye orientation in the visual-motor transformation for saccades. *Journal of Neurophysiology*, **80**, 2274–2294.

Klier, E.M., Meng, H., and Angelaki, D.E. (2006). Three-dimensional kinematics at the level of the oculomotor plant. *Journal of Neuroscience*, **26**, 2732–2737.

Kono, R., Clark, R.A., and Demer, J.L. (2002). Active pulleys: magnetic resonance imaging of rectus muscle paths in tertiary gazes. *Investigative Ophthalmology & Visual Science*, **43**, 2179–2188.

Lee, K.M., Lai, A.P., Brodale, J., and Jampolsky, A. (2007). Sideslip of the medial rectus muscle during vertical eye rotation. *Investigative Ophthalmology & Visual Science*, **48**, 4527–4533.

Maier, A., DeSantis, M., and Eldred, E. (1974). The occurrence of muscle spindles in extraocular muscles of various vertebrates. *Journal of Morphology*, **143**, 397–408.

Mays, L.E., Zhang, Y., Thorstad, M.H., and Gamlin, P.D. (1991). Trochlear unit activity during ocular convergence. *Journal of Neurophysiology*, **65**, 1484–1491.

Miller, J.M. (1989). Functional anatomy of normal human rectus muscles. *Vision Research*, **29**, 223–240.

Miller, J.M. and Robins, D. (1992). Extraocular muscle forces in alert monkey. *Vision Research*, **32**, 1099–1113.

Miller, J.M., Demer, J.L., and Rosenbaum, A.L. (1993). Effect of transposition surgery on rectus muscle paths by magnetic resonance imaging. *Ophthalmology*, **100**, 475–487.

Minken, A.W. and Van Gisbergen, J.A. (1994). A three-dimensional analysis of vergence movements at various levels of elevation. *Experimental Brain Research*, **101**, 331–345.

Misslisch, H. and Hess, B.J. (2000). Three-dimensional vestibuloocular reflex of the monkey: optimal retinal image stabilization versus listing's law. *Journal of Neurophysiology*, **83**, 3264–3276.

Misslisch, H. and Tweed, D. (2001). Neural and mechanical factors in eye control. *Journal of Neurophysiology*, **86**, 1877–1883.

Misslisch, H., Tweed, D., Fetter, M., Sievering, D., and Koenig, E. (1994). Rotational kinematics of the human vestibuloocular reflex. III. Listing's law. *Journal of Neurophysiology*, **72**, 2490–2502.

Mok, D., Ro, A., Cadera, W., Crawford, J.D., and Vilis, T. (1992). Rotation of Listing's plane during vergence. *Vision Research*, **32**, 2055–2064.

Oh, S.Y., Poukens, V., Cohen, M.S., and Demer, J.L. (2001). Structure-function correlation of laminar vascularity in human rectus extraocular muscles. *Investigative Ophthalmology & Visual Science*, **42**, 17–22.

Pastor, A.M., Torres, B., Delgado-Garcia, J.M., and Baker, R. (1991). Discharge characteristics of medial rectus and abducens motoneurons in the goldfish. *Journal of Neurophysiology*, **66**, 2125–2140.

Porrill, J., Warren, P.A., and Dean, P. (2000). A simple control law generates Listing's positions in a detailed model of the extraocular muscle system. *Vision Research*, **40**, 3743–3758.

Precht, W., Anderson, J.H., and Blanks, R.H. (1979). Canal-otolith convergence on car ocular motoneurons. *Progress in Brain Research*, **50**, 459–468.

Quaia, C. and Optican, L.M. (1998). Commutative saccadic generator is sufficient to control a 3-D ocular plant with pulleys. *Journal of Neurophysiology*, **79**, 3197–3215.

Quaia, C. and Optican, L.M. (2003). Dynamic eye plant models and the control of eye movements. *Strabismus* **11**, 17–31.

Raphan, T. (1997). Modeling control of eye orientation in three dimensions. In M. Fetter, H. Haslwanter, H. Misslisch, and D. Tweed (eds.) *Three dimensional kinematics of eye, head, and limb movements* (pp. 359–374). Amsterdam: Harwood Academic Publishers.

Raphan, T. (1998). Modeling control of eye orientation in three dimensions. I. Role of muscle pulleys in determining saccadic trajectory. *Journal of Neurophysiology*, **79**, 2653–2667.

Robinson, D.A. (1970). Oculomotor unit behavior in the monkey. *Journal of Neurophysiology*, **33**, 393–403.

Robinson, D.A. (1981). The use of control systems analysis in the neurophysiology of eye movements. *Annual Review of Neuroscience*, **4**, 463–503.

Robinson, D.A. and Keller, E.L. (1972). The behavior of eye movement motoneurons in the alert monkey. *Bibliotheca Ophthalmologic*, **82**, 7–16.

Ruskell, G.L. (1999). Extraocular muscle proprioceptors and propioception. *Progress in Retinal and Eye Research*, **18**, 269–291.

Scherberger, H., Cabungcal, J.H., Hepp, K., Suzuki, Y., Straumann, D., and Henn, V. (2001). Ocular counterroll modulates the preferred direction of saccade-related pontine burst neurons in the monkey. *Journal of Neurophysiology*, **86**, 935–949.

Schiller, P.H. (1970). The discharge characteristics of single units in the oculomotor and abducens nuclei of the unanesthetized monkey. *Experimental Brain Research*, **10**, 347–362.

Schnabolk, C. and Raphan, T. (1994). Modeling three-dimensional velocity-to-position transformation in oculomotor control. *Journal of Neurophysiology*, **71**, 623–638.

Shall, M.S., Wilson, K.E., and Goldberg, S.J. (1996). Extraocular motoneuron stimulation frequency effects on motor unit tension in cats. *Acta Anatomica (Basel)*, **157**, 217–225.

Simonsz, H.J. (1994). Force-length recording of eye muscles during local-anesthesia surgery in 32 strabismus patients. *Strabismus*, **4**, 197–218.

Simpson, J.I. and Graf, W. (1981). Eye-muscle geometry and compensatory eye movements in lateral-eyed and frontal-eyed animals. *Annals of the New York Academy of Sciences*, **374**, 20–30.

Skavenski, A.A. and Robinson, D.A. (1973). Role of abducens neurons in vestibuloocular reflex. *Journal of Neurophysiology*, **36**, 724–738.

Smith, M.A. and Crawford, J.D. (1998). Neural control of rotational kinematics within realistic vestibuloocular coordinate systems. *Journal of Neurophysiology*, **80**, 2295–2315.

Spencer, R.F. and Porter, J.D. (1988). Structural organization of the extraocular muscles. *Reviews of Oculomotor Research*, **2**, 33–79.

Stahl, J.S. and Simpson, J.I. (1995). Dynamics of abducens nucleus neurons in the awake rabbit. *Journal of Neurophysiology*, **73**, 1383–1395.

Steinbach, M.J. (2000). The Palisade Ending: an afferent source for eye position information in humans. In G. Lennerstrand, J. Ygge, and T. Laurent (eds.) *Advances in Strabismus Research: Basic and Clinical Aspects* (pp. 33–42). London: Portland Press.

Straumann, D. and Zee, D.S. (1995). Three-dimensional aspects of eye movements. *Current Opinion in Neurology*, **8**(1), 69–71.

Suzuki, Y., Straumann, D., Simpson, J.I., Hepp, K., Hess, B.J., and Henn, V. (1999). Three-dimensional extraocular motoneuron innervation in the rhesus monkey. I: Muscle rotation axes and on-directions during fixation. *Experimental Brain Research*, **126**, 187–199.

Sylvestre, P.A. and Cullen, K.E. (1999). Quantitative analysis of abducens neuron discharge dynamics during saccadic and slow eye movements. *Journal of Neurophysiology*, **82**, 2612–2632.

Thurtell, M.J., Black, R.A., Halmagyi, G.M., Curthoys, I.S., and Aw, S.T (1999). Vertical eye position-dependence of the human vestibuloocular reflex during passive and active yaw head rotations. *Journal of Neurophysiology*, **81**, 2415–2428.

Thurtell, M.J., Kunin, M., and Raphan, T. (2000). Role of muscle pulleys in producing eye position-dependence in the angular vestibuloocular reflex: a model-based study. *Journal of Neurophysiology*, **84**, 639–650.

Tweed, D. (1997). Velocity-to-position transformation in the VOR and the saccadic system. In M. Fetter, H. Haslwanter, H. Misslisch, and D. Tweed (eds.) *Three-dimensional kinematics of eye, head, and limb movements* (pp. 375–386). The Netherlands: Harwood Academic.

Tweed, D. and Vilis, T. (1987). Implications of rotational kinematics for the oculomotor system in three dimensions. *Journal of Neurophysiology*, **58**, 832–849.

Tweed, D. and Vilis, T. (1990). Geometric relations of eye position and velocity vectors during saccades. *Vision Research*, **30**, 111–127.

Tweed, D., Fetter, M., Andreadaki, S., Koenig, E., and Dichgans, J. (1992). Three-dimensional properties of human pursuit eye movements. *Vision Research*, **32**, 1225–1238.

Tweed, D., Misslisch, H., Fetter M. (1994). Testing models of the oculomotor velocity-to-position transformation. *Journal of Neurophysiology*, **72**, 1425–1429.

Tweed, D.B., Haslwanter, T.P., Happe, V., and Fetter, M. (1999). Non-commutativity in the brain. *Nature*, **399**, 261–263.

Van Opstal, A.J. (1993). Representation of eye position in three dimensions. In A. Berthoz (ed.) *Multisensory Control of Movement* (pp. 27–41). Oxford: Oxford University Press.

Van Opstal, A.J., Hepp, K., Hess, B.J., Straumann, D., and Henn, V. (1991). Two- rather than three-dimensional representation of saccades in monkey superior colliculus. *Science*, **252**, 1313–1315.

Van Opstal, J., Hepp, K., Suzuki, Y., and Henn, V. (1996). Role of monkey nucleus reticularis tegmenti pontis in the stabilization of Listing's plane. *Journal of Neuroscience*, **16**, 7284–7296.

Van Rijn, L.J. and Van den Berg, A.V. (1993). Binocular eye orientation during fixations: Listing's law extended to include eye vergence. *Vision Research*, **33**, 691–708.

Wang, X., Zhang, M., Cohen, I.S., and Goldberg, M.E. (2007). The proprioceptive representation of eye position in monkey primary somatosensory cortex. *Nature Neuroscience*, **10**, 640–646.

Wasicky, R., Horn, A.K., and Büttner-Ennever, J.A. (2004). Twitch and nontwitch motoneuron subgroups in the oculomotor nucleus of monkeys receive different afferent projections. *Journal of Comparative Neurology*, **479**, 117–129.

Weir, C.R., Knox, P.C., and Dutton, G.N. (2000). Does extraocular muscle proprioception influence oculomotor control? *British Journal of Ophthalmology*, **84**, 1071–1074.

CHAPTER 9

Brainstem pathways and premotor control

Kathleen E. Cullen and Marion R. Van Horn

Abstract

The oculomotor system is one of the better understood motor systems. In contrast to locomotion—the control of posture or limb control—the structural features of the oculomotor system are mechanically simple. The oculomotor plant includes the eyeball, the extraocular muscles, and the surrounding orbital tissue. In particular, the eye has little inertia and rotates about a point that is relatively fixed such that there is only one 'joint' to consider. Moreover, there is no stretch reflex and activity in each of the three antagonistic muscles pairs is reciprocally related. As a result, a relatively simple relationship between motoneuron discharge and eye movements has facilitated our understanding of the central premotor circuitry that underlies the generation of oculomotor behaviours. In this chapter, the neural pathways that control eye movements are considered with a focus on the generation of appropriate motor commands at the level of the brainstem.

Overview and classification of eye movements

In the early 1900s Raymond Dodge described five distinct classes of eye movements used to redirect or stabilize a visual image on the fovea (Dodge, 1903). Three classes of eye movements, i) saccades, ii) smooth pursuit, and iii) vergence, are voluntarily initiated to redirect gaze to a particular object in the visual field. *Saccades*, the fastest and most common type of eye movement, are constantly used to redirect gaze between stationary objects and bring images onto the fovea (see Gilchrist, Chapter 5, this volume). *Smooth pursuit eye movements* are considerably slower movements (<100°/s) that are used to track targets moving across a stationary visual background (see Barnes, Chapter 7, this volume). *Vergence eye movements* rotate the two eyes in opposite directions to fixate on targets located at different depths.

The remaining two classes of eye movements, the iv) vestibulo-ocular reflex (VOR; see Hess, Chapter 3, this volume) and the v) optokinetic reflex (OKR; see Distler and Hoffman, Chapter 4, this volume), function to hold images stationary on the retina. The VOR and OKR function to move the eye in the direction opposite to ongoing head motion during our daily activities. The *VOR* keeps visual images stable on the retina when the head moves during everyday activities such as walking and running. In contrast to the VOR, the *OKR*, is a visually guided reflex and is used to stabilize vision when the head remains relatively stationary. The properties of these eye movements are summarized in Table 9.1.

Traditionally, these five classes of eye movements have been studied in isolation. This has led to an excellent understanding of the brainstem circuitry underlying each of these types of eye movements.

Table 9.1 Classes of eye movements

Eye movement classification		Function
Voluntary	Saccade	Fast redirection of gaze between stationary targets
	Pursuit	Slow eye movements used to track moving targets
	Vergence	Rotation of the eyes in opposite directions to fixation targets at different depths
Involuntary	Vestibulo-ocular	Uses vestibular inputs to hold images stationary on the retina as the head moves
	Optokinetic	Uses visual inputs to stabilize gaze in response to low frequency head movements

During most natural voluntary orienting and tracking behaviours, however, two or more subsystems work together to control gaze. In this chapter, the premotor pathways that control voluntary and reflex eye movements are considered with focus on the generation of appropriate motor commands at the level of the brainstem. To better appreciate the requirements inherent to the premotor control pathways, the anatomy and mechanical properties of the eye and orbit are first briefly reviewed. This is followed by a description of the premotor circuits that command each class of eye movement when preformed in isolation. Finally, we consider more recent work that has established how the brain coordinates the interactions between these eye movement subsystems to accurately control gaze in everyday life.

Ocular structure and functional implications

The extraocular eye muscles and their innervation

To provide a unified, clear view of the world the brain needs to precisely coordinate our eyes so that both foveas are aimed at the same point in visual space. The precise position of each eye in its orbit is controlled by six extraocular muscles. Extraocular muscles generate the forces necessary to overcome the elasticity and viscosity of the oculomotor plant (see Angelaki, Chapter 8, this volume). Horizontal eye movements are controlled by the medial and lateral rectus muscles, while vertical and torsional movements are controlled by the superior and inferior rectus muscles and superior and inferior oblique muscles. Together, these three pairs of muscles permit the eye to rotate with three degrees of freedom. While the VOR and OKR operate in three dimensions, orbital mechanics and possibly central mechanisms largely restrict saccades and smooth pursuit to two dimensions. The restriction of voluntary eye movements to two dimensions is referred to as Listing's law (Demer, 2006; Hess, 2008; Klier et al., 2006) (see also Crawford and Klier, Chapter 18, this volume).

The extraocular muscles are innervated by three groups of motoneurons located in the brainstem (Fig. 9.1A). The lateral rectus is innervated by the abducens nerve (cranial nerve VI), the medial, inferior and superior recti are innervated by the oculomotor nerve (cranial nerve III) and the inferior and superior obliques are innervated by the trochlear nerve (cranial nerve IV). Some neurons within the abducens and oculomotor nucleus are internuclear neurons, which project via the medial longitudinal fasciculus (MLF) to the contralateral oculomotor or abducens nucleus, respectively (Buttner-Ennever and Akert, 1981; Maciewicz et al., 1975).

Lesions of the extraocular muscles or nerves result in a serious limitation of the movement of the affected eye. A characteristic syndrome is associated with lesions of each muscle or nerve. For example, a lesion of the abducens nerve results in a loss of abduction beyond the midline. Accordingly, when the fovea of one eye is directed at an object of interest, the fovea of the paretic eye is deviated resulting in visual problems such as diplopia (i.e. double vision).

A novel feature of the oculomotor system is that each extraocular muscle is comprised of two distinct layers, a global layer and an orbital layer. These layers contain two types of muscle fibres: twitch and

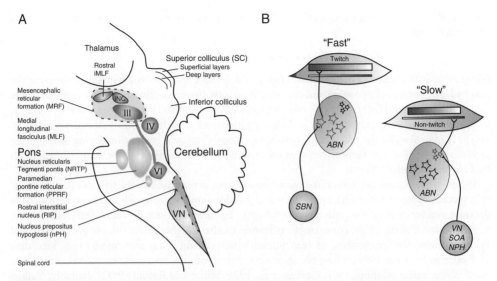

Fig. 9.1 A) Schematic diagram of the brainstem. Excitatory burst neurons (EBNs) for horizontal saccades lie in the paramedian pontine reticular formation (PPRF), and for vertical and torsional lie in the rostral interstitial nucleus of the medial longitudinal fasciculus (riMLF). Oculor motoneurons lie in the abducens nucleus (ABN; VI), the oculomotor nucleus (OMN; III) and the trochlear nucleus (IV). INC: interstitial nucleus of Cajal; NRTP: nucleus reticularis tegmentis pontis; nPH: nucleus prepositus hypoglossi. VN: vestibular nucleus. B) Schematic diagram of muscle fibre innervations. Twitch fibres receive innervations from large motoneurons whereas non-twitch fibres received innervations from small motoneurons, which tend to lie separately around the periphery of the nucleus (right). Large motoneurons receive premotor signals from the saccadic burst generator (SBN) whereas small motoneurons receive innervations from premotor sources involved in executing slow eye movements (e.g. VN, NPH and supraoculomotor nucleus (SOA)).

non-twitch fibres (Buttner-Ennever et al., 2001; Spencer and Porter, 1988). Recent retrograde studies have shown that twitch fibres receive innervations from large motoneurons, which lie within the oculomotor nuclei, whereas non-twitch fibres receive innervations from small motoneurons, which tend to lie separately around the periphery of the nucleus (Buttner-Ennever et al., 2001; Ugolini et al., 2006). In turn, larger motoneurons receive strong innervation from premotor sources involved in fast eye movements (e.g. the saccadic burst generator) while recent studies of the abducens nucleus suggest small motoneurons receive innervation from premotor sources involved in executing slow eye movements (e.g. vestibular nucleus (VN), nucleus prepositus hypoglossi (nPH) and supraoculomotor nucleus (SOA)) (Ugolini et al., 2006) (Fig. 9.1B).

Motoneuron discharges

Extracellular recordings have been made from single oculomotoneurons of alert monkeys during steady fixation, VOR, smooth pursuit, saccadic and vergence eye movements (Keller, 1973; Keller and Robinson, 1972; Mays and Porter, 1984; Robinson, 1970; Robinson and Keller, 1972; Skavenski and Robinson, 1973; Sylvestre and Cullen, 2002). Robinson and his collaborators showed that when the eye is centred in the orbit, motoneurons discharge at a constant firing rate (i.e. resting discharge). In addition, to drive saccades, motoneurons fire a burst of action potentials and once the eyes have reached an eccentric position motoneurons continue to generate a sustained tonic firing rate that is higher (or lower) than their resting discharge. Overall, it was concluded that, during saccades, the discharge activity of extraocular motoneurons is appropriate for overcoming the viscous-elastic properties of the oculomotor plant. Accordingly, the relationship between firing rate and eye motion can be well described using a simple, first-order model (Sylvestre and Cullen, 1999, 2002; Van Horn and Cullen, 2009):

$$FR(t) = b + k\,E(t - t_d) + r\,\dot{E}(t - t_d)$$

where $FR(t)$ is the neuron's instantaneous firing rate, b and k and r are constants that represent the bias and the neuron's eye position and eye velocity sensitivities, respectively. t_d refers to the dynamic lead time and $E(t)$ and $\dot{E}(t)$ refer to the instantaneous eye position and velocity, respectively. Notably, by expanding the model structure to include the movement of each eye, this first order model can also be used to describe the relationship between neuronal firing and eye motion during disconjugate saccades (see section 'Interactions between eye movement subsystems') (Sylvestre and Cullen, 2002; Van Horn and Cullen, 2009).

Although the general behaviour of a motoneuron is not determined by the type of eye movement (e.g. saccade or smooth pursuit), eye velocity and position sensitivities have been found to invariably decrease as a function of the generated eye velocity (Fuchs et al., 1988; Sylvestre and Cullen, 1999; Van Horn and Cullen, 2009). For example, motoneurons have higher sensitivities to eye position and velocity during slower movements (e.g. pursuit) than during faster movements (e.g. saccades) (Sylvestre and Cullen, 1999). These results are consistent with the proposal that the viscosity of the plant is non-linear (Collins, 1971; Collins et al., 1975; Miller and Robins, 1992). Notably, Collins (1971) showed that the viscosity of the extraocular muscle varies non-linearly as a function of the muscle's stretch velocity and that the viscosity of passive orbital tissues remains relatively constant as a function of eye velocity. Accordingly, faster movements encounter less viscous resistance and hence a smaller change in force (i.e. corresponding to smaller coefficients) is required to move the eye (see discussion, Sylvestre and Cullen, 1999). The premotor inputs to the motoneurons for each eye movement are further discussed below.

Premotor control of gaze redirection

Saccades

Accurate saccades can be made in less than 100 ms (Fig. 9.2A; top). To produce such rapid eye movements a motoneuron must generate a burst (or 'pulse') of action potentials to overcome the viscous drag on the eye as it moves in the orbit. Firing rate bursts can reach frequencies as high as 500 spikes/s. This is in striking contrast to other types of motoneurons, such as spinal motoneurons, which can reach maximal firing rates of only 10–30 spikes/s. Additionally, once the eye reaches its final position at the end of a saccade, it is then held steady by a sustained motoneuron firing that produces a fixed contraction of the extraocular muscle.

The difference between the neuron's sustained discharge rate at the initial and final eye positions is referred to as the 'step'. Thus, to a first approximation, the neural control of saccades requires the generation of a 'pulse-step' command signal (see also Fig. 8.1, Angelaki, Chapter 8, this volume). Evidence for the pulse-step command during saccades can be also found in recordings of muscle tension. Following initiation of the saccade, muscle tension rises to a peak whose amplitude and duration are proportional to the magnitude of the eye movement, at which point tension decays to a new steady state level within 350 ms (Robinson, 1964).

Generation of the neural pulse

The 'pulse' or burst signal required to drive horizontal and vertical saccades is generated by neurons in the paramedian pontine reticular formation (PPRF) and mesencephalic reticular formation (MRF), respectively. Physiological and anatomical tracing studies have demonstrated that excitatory burst neurons (EBNs), in the rostral portion of the PPRF are the source of the high frequency burst of discharges responsible for driving the lateral rectus muscle (Fig. 9.2A; bottom) (Sasaki and Shimazu, 1981; Strassman et al., 1986a) and vertical burst neurons, which lie in the rostral interstitial

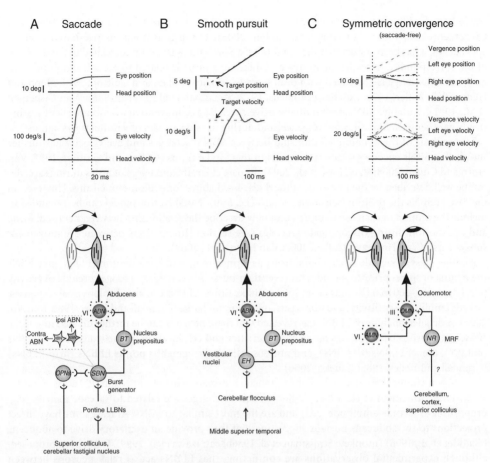

Fig. 9.2 Schematic of pathways that mediate the three different classes of voluntary eye movements. A) Saccadic eye movements can reach speeds of up to 900°/s (top).The bottom panel illustrates the premotor pathway for producing saccades. Command signals, issued in the deep layers of the superior colliculus, are delivered to burst neurons (BNs) in the PPRF. Not shown are cortical inputs received by superior colliculus. B) Pursuit eye movements are used to follow moving objects and lag target motion by ~90 ms (top). The bottom panel illustrates the brainstem circuit for the generation of smooth pursuit movements. C) Symmetric vergence eye movements, which are characteristically much slower than saccades, move the eyes in opposite directions to fixate objects lying at varying depths (top). The bottom panel illustrates how projections from near response neurons (NR) in the mesencephalic reticular formation (MRF) are thought to contribute to the generation of slow vergence eye movements. Cerebellum, cortex, and the superior colliculus are likely sources of vergence information.

nucleus of the medial longitudinal fasciculus (riMLF), are responsible for driving the inferior and superior recti (Moschovakis et al., 1991a, 1991b).

   To drive horizontal saccades, EBNs work together with a second group of inhibitory burst neurons (IBNs) in the caudal pontine reticular formation, which silence the antagonist motoneurons (i.e. contralateral abducens) (Hikosaka et al., 1978; Hikosaka and Kawakami, 1977; Strassman et al., 1986b; Yoshida et al., 1982; reviewed in Scudder et al. (2002) and Shinoda et al. (2008)) (Fig. 9.2A; bottom). Typically, EBNs and IBNs (collectively referred to as saccadic burst neurons; SBNs) burst most vigorously for ipsilaterally directed saccades, preceding the onset of a saccade by approximately 10–20 ms (Cullen and Guitton, 1997; Scudder et al., 1988). Far fewer spikes are observed during contralateral, oblique and vertical saccades (Cullen and Guitton, 1997; Scudder et al., 1988; Van Gisbergen et al., 1981; Van Horn and Cullen, 2008). Using traditional metric-based analysis approaches, it has been shown that the duration of a SBN's burst is tightly correlated to the duration of the corresponding saccade; the number of spikes in a burst is related to saccade amplitude and peak burst discharge is correlated with peak saccade velocity (Cullen and Guitton, 1997; Hepp and Henn, 1983; Keller, 1974; Luschei and Fuchs, 1972; Strassman et al., 1986a, 1986b; Van Gisbergen et al., 1981). Notably, SBNs preferentially drive saccadic eye movements—and are silent during steady gaze, smooth pursuit, slow vergence, and during the slow phases of vestibular nystagmus.

The analysis of the dynamic relationship between SBN discharges and eye velocity has further shown that SBNs encode saccade trajectories in their spike trains (Cullen and Guitton, 1997; Van Horn and Cullen, 2008; Van Horn et al., 2008). In particular, the discharge of SBNs during saccades can be well described by the first-order model discussed above for oculomotoneurons. However, in the case of SBNs the position sensitivity is zero (i.e. $k=0$). Notably, this model can be expanded to include the motion of each eye to more accurately describe the relationship between neuronal firing and eye motion during disconjugate saccades (see section 'Interactions between eye movement subsystems') (Van Horn and Cullen, 2008; Van Horn et al., 2008).

Another class of saccade related burst neurons termed long-lead burst neuron (LLBN)-like EBNs fire a burst of spikes prior to saccades however their burst is preceded by a longer prelude of activity (e.g. latency 16–200 ms) (Munoz et al., 2000). Unlike EBNs, LLBNs can also display visual responses, saccade amplitude sensitivity, and non-visual or motor discharge (Crandall and Keller, 1985; Kaneko, 2006). A detailed analysis of LLBNs has revealed that these neurons can be further divided into three classes of neurons based on discharge characteristics and cell location, namely: excitatory LLBNs (eLLBN), dorsal LLBNs (dLLBNs), and nucleus reticularis tegmentis pontis LLBNs (nrtp LLBNs) (Crandall and Keller, 1985; Kaneko, 2006).

eLLBNs are found throughout the pontine reticular formation in both EBN and IBN areas (Scudder et al., 1988; Strassman et al., 1986a, 1986b). Their discharges are related to saccade metrics (e.g. proportion to saccade amplitude, etc.) and are the most similar to EBNs. At least some have direct projections to the abducens nucleus suggesting that they provide an excitatory drive to abducens (Scudder et al., 1996) (monkey: Strassman et al. 1986b; cat: Izawa et al. 1999). It has been proposed, although experimental observations are conflicting, that LLBNs act as relay neurons between the superior colliculus and EBNs. Consistent with this proposal, Keller and colleagues (2000), in the monkey, were only able to activate LLBNs at monosynaptic latencies using a single electrical pulse applied to the deep layers of the superior colliculus (Fig. 9.1A). On the other hand, both EBNs and LLBNs could be activated at monosynaptic latencies in the cat (Chimoto et al. 1996).

In contrast, the burst of nrtp LLBNs are tuned for saccades of a particular direction and amplitude. Nrtp LLBNs project to the cerebellum (Crandall and Keller, 1985; Hepp and Henn, 1983) suggesting their role in saccade generation is less direct (see Scudder et al. 2002). Finally, dLLBNs, which are located dorsal to nrtp LLBNs and rostral to eLLBNs, are more similar to eLLBNs in that they are also ipsilaterally tuned. However they are preferentially tuned for smaller saccade amplitudes (<10°) and their discharge is not as well related to saccade metrics. Based on this, dLLBNs have been proposed to provide a trigger signal which could be used to initiate saccades (Kaneko, 2006; Raybourn and Keller, 1977).

Omnipause neurons

The generation of saccades relies on an additional class of brain stem neurons called omnipause neurons (OPNs). These neurons, which lie around the midline of the caudal pontine reticular formation in the nucleus raphe interpositus (RIP), are thought to act as an inhibitory gate for saccades. Using glycine as their primary neurotransmitter (Horn et al., 1994), OPNs tonically inhibit both horizontal and vertical and saccadic burst neurons (Buttner-Ennever et al., 1988; Furuya and Markham, 1982; Horn et al., 1994; Langer and Kaneko, 1990; Nakao et al., 1980; Ohgaki et al., 1989; Strassman et al., 1987). OPNs discharge at a constant rate when gaze is steady and pause their firing during saccades in all directions. Additionally, the duration of the pause is well correlated to saccade duration (Keller, 1974; Luschei and Fuchs, 1972). The role of OPNs in controlling fixation, and inhibiting saccadic eye movements is well supported by the results of studies, which have shown that microstimulation of the OPN region of the RIP cause complete cessation of eye movements (Keller, 1974).

Intracellular recordings have revealed tight relationships between the durations of OPN hyperpolarizations and saccades as well as the amplitudes of OPN hyperpolarizations and saccade velocities. Interestingly, the dynamic time course of OPN hyperpolarization also resembles the velocity profile of the corresponding eye movement (Yoshida et al., 1999). These findings suggest that OPN pauses are initiated by inputs carrying an eye velocity signal (Yoshida et al., 1999). Likely candidates are the saccade burst neurons in the PPRF and superior colliculus both of which have been show to have projections to OPNs (Buttner-Ennever et al., 1999; Scudder et al., 1996; Shinoda et al., 2008; Takahashi et al., 2005) (Fig. 9.2A; bottom).

Inputs to saccadic burst neurons

Excitatory projections originating from the superior colliculus and cerebellar caudal fastigial nucleus play an important role in the generation of saccades. Recent intracellular studies in cat have shown that caudal portion of the SC projects to contralateral EBNs and IBNs while the rostral SC projects more heavily to OPNs. The rostral SC, also sends bilateral disynaptic inhibition to IBNs through OPNs (Sugiuchi et al., 2005; Takahashi et al., 2005). These findings are in agreement with the proposal that the caudal SC is involved in driving saccades whereas the rostral SC is involving in maintaining fixation (Choi and Guitton, 2006; Hafed et al., 2009; Munoz and Wurtz, 1993, 1995). Notably, at the rostral tip of the SC, neurons have been found to encode multiple eye movements including very small saccades, microsaccades smooth pursuit, and fixation (Bergeron and Guitton, 2000; Choi and Guitton, 2006; Krauzlis et al., 1997; Munoz and Wurtz, 1992, 1993; Van Horn, 2009). Additionally, as noted above, eLLBNs, with somata in the PPRF, have projections to EBN and IBN regions supporting the proposal that LLBNs may act as interneurons between the caudal SC and EBNs (Scudder et al., 1996) (Fig. 9.2A; bottom).

Oculomotor integration

In order to hold the eyes steady at the end of a saccade the pulse command generated in the PPRF and MRF must be transformed into an appropriately scaled tonic discharge. The SBNs in the PPRF project to neurons in the nPH, which serves, in part, as a neural integrator for horizontal saccades (Fig. 9.2A; bottom) (Cannon and Robinson, 1987; reviewed in Fukushima et al. (1992) and McCrea (1988). Neurons in the nPH and interstitial nucleus of Cajal (INC) encode robust position signals and can also burst during saccades. These neurons are commonly referred to as burst-tonic neurons (BTs). Velocity integration is leaky or imperfect and as a result, in the dark, the eyes gradually drift back to centre from eccentric positions with a time constant of approximately 25 s. A lesion of either the nPH or INC will result in an inability to hold the eyes at a new position after a saccade. Taken together, the results of anatomical, lesion, and single-unit recordings in nPH or INC are consistent with their proposed role in integrating the pulse command (Cannon and Robinson, 1987). As discussed below, neurons in these two structures are also part of the velocity-position integrator required for the VOR.

Vertical saccades

As detailed above, the premotor control of horizontal saccades is well understood. A similar structured circuit has also been described for the control of vertical saccades. For example, both upwards and downwards vertical burst neurons are located in the riMLF (Moschovakis et al., 1991a, 1991b). These neurons project to neurons in the INC, which acts as a vertical neural integrator. Neurons in riMLF and INC send appropriate pulse and step commands, respectively, to motoneurons in the oculomotor and trochlear nuclei (Crawford et al., 1991). Similar to horizontal burst neurons excitatory projections originating from the superior colliculus are also considered to play an important role in the generation of vertical saccades.

Smooth pursuit

Smooth pursuit eye movements, which are considerably slower movements than saccades, are used to track targets moving targets (Fig. 9.2B; top). Pursuit signals access the brainstem circuitry via projections from descending pathways originating in cortical regions that process visual motion, including the middle temporal (MT) and medial superior temporal (MST) areas. Pursuit commands are conveyed to the premotor circuitry via a pathway originating in MST, which projects to the pontine nuclei (PONs) (Fig. 9.2B; bottom). The PONs, in turn, sends projections to the flocculus and ventral paraflocculus of the cerebellum (see also Thier, Chapter 10, this volume). A parallel pathway, which originates in the frontal eye field (FEF) and projects to the nrtp, is also thought to be involved in initiating and maintaining smooth pursuit eye movements.

During pursuit the simple spike activity of floccular Purkinje cells encodes eye position, eye velocity, and to a much smaller degree eye acceleration (Leung et al. 2000; Suh et al. 2000). Notably, lesions of the flocculus and paraflocculus cause large deficits in smooth pursuit eye movements (Zee et al., 1981). Floccular Purkinje cells have ipsilateral projections to the vestibular nuclei (VNs) which then convey the appropriate motor output signals to the extraocular motoneurons (Fig. 9.2B; bottom). The target neurons within the vestibular nuclei have similar discharge characteristics to floccular Purkinje cells. Specifically, eye-head (EH) neurons, also known as flocculus target neurons (FTNs), in the rostral MVN (medial vestibular nucleus) and LVN (lateral vestibular nucleus) receive direct inhibitory projections from the floccular lobe (Broussard and Lisberger, 1992; Lisberger and Pavelko, 1988; Lisberger et al., 1994a, 1994b). Within the vestibular nuclei there exists two classes of EH neurons, type I and type II neurons, which are characterized by ipsilateral and contralateral eye movement sensitivities, respectively.

The discharge of EH neurons during pursuit can be well described by a simple model that includes a resting discharge, eye position, and eye velocity terms (Roy and Cullen, 2003). While the eye movement information carried by EH neurons during pursuit (Cullen and McCrea, 1993; Roy and Cullen, 2003; Scudder and Fuchs, 1992) is considered to be the most significant input driving the motoneurons of the abducens nucleus during smooth pursuit eye movements (Cullen et al., 1993; Scudder and Fuchs, 1992), other premotor neurons also contribute. Notably, position vestibular pause neurons (PVPs) and BT neurons also show clear modulation during smooth pursuit eye movements (Cullen and McCrea, 1993; McCrea et al., 1987; Scudder and Fuchs, 1992). However, the pursuit-related discharges of PVP neurons are thought to be mediated indirectly via local projections from the BT (i.e. the neurons of the velocity-position integrators in the nPH). As discussed in more detail below, PVPs play a more prominent role in mediating the direct rotational VOR pathway.

Vergence

When redirecting gaze to objects along in the mid-sagittal plane the eyes rotate by the same angle, in opposite directions. This type of eye movement is known as symmetrical vergence (Fig. 9.2C; top). The dynamics of symmetrical vergence has been shown to be much more sluggish than saccades. For example, maximum vergence velocities are generally <60°/s. At the brainstem level, a group of neurons, called near response (NR) neurons, have been located in the MRF who discharge is proportional to vergence angle when tracking visual targets located along the midline (i.e. symmetric vergence) (Judge and Cumming, 1986; Mays, 1984; Zhang et al., 1992). Some neurons have been found to increase their activity during symmetric convergence (i.e. convergence neuron) while others decrease their activity during symmetric convergence (i.e. divergence neuron). Notably, these neurons do not respond during conjugate saccades. Moreover, neurons responsible for driving saccades (i.e. EBNs, IBNs, and OPNs) do not respond to slow changes in vergence angle (Busettini and Mays, 2003; Van Horn et al., 2008).

Anatomical studies have shown that NR neurons can be antidromically activated from the medial rectus subdivision of the oculomotor nucleus (Zhang et al., 1991, 1992) (Fig. 9.2C; bottom). To date, no vergence related neurons have been found to be antidromically activated from the abducens nucleus. A second class of neurons, which have activity related to vergence velocity, have also been identified in the MRF (Mays et al., 1986). Both convergence and divergence neurons have been described, although far fewer divergence neurons than convergence neurons have been reported. Vergence burst neurons have been identified in two regions of the MRF. One group is located in proximity to the neurons that encode vergence angle and a second group is located in a more ventral area, potentially in the rostral superior colliculus.

Under normal viewing conditions near and far objects are rarely perfectly aligned along the midline and hence symmetric vergence movements are uncommon. Usually saccadic and/or head movements will accompany vergence movements. The neural circuitry governing these interactions will be discussed in more detail later (see section 'Interactions between eye movement subsystems').

Premotor control of gaze stabilization

Vestibulo-ocular reflexes

The VOR uses information from both the semicircular canals and otolith organs to generate compensatory eye movements in response to head motion in three dimensional space (Fig. 9.3A; top). The rotational VOR (RVOR) is evoked by rotations of the head, which in turn activate hair cells in the semicircular canals. The three canals on each side are arranged at right angles to each other, sensing head rotation in three dimensions. The translational VOR (TVOR) is evoked by translations of the head through space, which in turn activate hair cells in the otolith organs (the saccule and utricle). The respective orientations of the hair cells in the saccule and utricle sense linear accelerations (i.e. the sum of gravitational and inertial accelerations).

Information encoded by the vestibular hair cells is sent to the brainstem via the vestibular nerve (i.e. VIIIth nerve). The vestibular nerve, in turn, projects to the ipsilateral vestibular complex in the dorsal part of the pons and medulla (Fig. 9.3A; bottom). The vestibular complex consists of four nuclei, the medial vestibular nucleus (MVN), the superior vestibular nucleus (SVN), the lateral vestibular nucleus (LVN), and the inferior (or descending) vestibular nucleus (IVN). Afferents from horizontal and vertical semicircular canals terminate mainly in the MVN and SVN, respectively. Utricular afferents terminate mainly in the LVN and SVN. Saccule fibres mainly innervate the LVN and IVN (Newlands et al., 2003).

Unlike other sensory systems, the information encoded by the vestibular system becomes strongly multisensory and multimodal at the first stage of central processing. This occurs because the VNs receive inputs from a wide range of cortical, cerebellar, and other brainstem structures in addition to direct inputs from the vestibular afferents. Somatosensory, proprioceptive, and visual sensory information, as well as premotor signals related to the generation of eye and head movements are relayed to the VNs. Recent studies have emphasized the importance of these extra-vestibular signals in shaping the sensory-motor transformations that mediate the VOR.

Neural substrates of the rotational VOR (RVOR)

To effectively stabilize gaze over a wide frequency range, signals from the semicircular canals must be sent as directly as possible to the eye muscles. The most direct connection involves only three neurons, and is called the 'three-neuron-arc'. This pathway, which was first described by Lorente de No' in 1933, consists of a series of projections: the primary afferent fibres in the vestibular nerve project to the secondary vestibular neurons in the vestibular nuclei, which in turn project to the motorneurons that innervate the extraocular muscles of the eyes. Consequently, the RVOR is one of

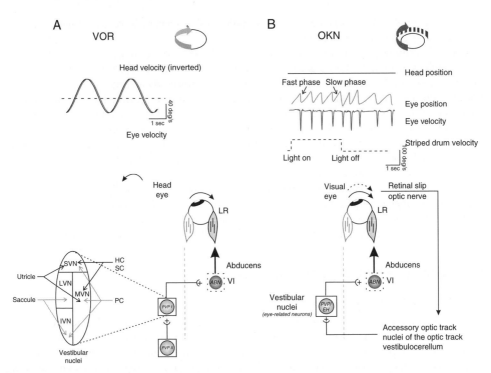

Fig. 9.3 Schematic of pathways that mediate reflexive eye movements. A) Example response to sinusoidal rotations. Eye and inverted head velocities are shown. Note that fast phases have been removed (top). During head rotations or translations information encoded by the vestibular hairs cells is sent to the brainstem via the vestibular nerve (i.e. VIIIth nerve) (bottom). The vestibular complex consists of four nuclei: the medial vestibular nucleus (MVN), the superior vestibular nucleus (SVN), the lateral vestibular nucleus (LVN), and the inferior (or descending) vestibular nucleus (IVN). Afferents from horizontal and vertical semicircular canals terminate mainly in the MVN and SVN, respectively. Utricular afferents terminate mainly in the MVN and SVN. Saccule fibres mainly innervate the LVN and IVN. Rotation of the head to the left excites neurons in the left vestibular nuclei (VN) (bottom). Position-vestibular-pause (PVP) neurons send excitatory projections to motoneurons in the right abducens (ABN) to generate rightwards eye movements of the eyes. B) The optokinetic reflex is activated by motion of large parts of the visual field, includes an initial rapid rise in eye velocity that begins within 100–200 ms of the start of visual motion and is followed 1–2 s later by a slower build up of eye velocity. During prolonged stimulation, the OKR is composed not only of compensatory movements, but also includes quick resetting eye movements in the opposite direction, which collectively give rise to optokinetic nystagmus (OKN) (top). Retinal information from pretectal and mesencephalic neurons in the nucleus of the optic tract and the accessory optic nuclei is sent to neurons in the VN and nPH, which in turn project directly to the extraocular motor nuclei. The quick resetting eye movements are produced by the same neurons in the brainstem that generate saccades (not shown).

the fastest reflexes, with the response latency of 5–6 ms in the primate (Huterer and Cullen, 2002; Minor et al., 1999).

PVP neurons, which make up most of the intermediate leg of the VOR pathway, derive their name from the signals they carry during passive head rotations and eye movements. The firing rates of type I PVP neurons increase with contralaterally directed eye *position;* they are sensitive to ipsilaterally directed head *velocity* and their discharge ceases (*pauses*) for ipsilaterally directed saccades and the quick phases of vestibular nystagmus. The majority of type I PVP neurons are located in the rostral MVN and send an excitatory projection to the motoneurons of the a) contralateral abducens nucleus or b) ipsilateral medial rectus subdivision of the oculomotor nucleus (Fig. 9.3A; bottom). A minority of type I PVP neurons also send inhibitory projections to the motoneurons of the ipsilateral abducens nucleus.

During sinusoidal passive whole-body rotation in the dark, the modulation of type I PVP neurons slightly lead ipsilateral head velocity, and neurons pause firing during ipsilaterally directed quick phases of vestibular nystagmus. Neglecting the small phase shift, neuronal responses during the compensatory slow phase VOR can be well described by the equation:

$$FR(t) = b + kE(t) + g\,\dot{H}(t)$$

where FR is the neuronal firing rate, b is the resting discharge, E is the eye position, k is the eye-position sensitivity during ocular fixation, $\dot{H}$ is head velocity, and g is the head-velocity sensitivity. In addition, these neurons also carry an eye velocity signal during smooth pursuit in the absence of head motion. Sensitivities to head velocity during rotation are typically more than 50% greater than those to eye velocity during pursuit.

In order to dissociate the vestibular-related modulation of PVP neurons from their eye-movement related responses, animals are typically trained to cancel their VOR by tracking a target that moves with the head. During cancellation of the VOR (i.e. in the absence of eye movement), type I PVP neurons respond robustly to ipsilaterally-directed head velocity, showing only a 30% decrease in modulation as compared to VOR in the dark (Cullen and McCrea, 1993; Scudder and Fuchs, 1992).

Within the vestibular nuclei also exists a second class of PVP neurons, type II neurons. These neurons are characterized by head and eye movement sensitivities that are opposite to those of type I PVP neurons, and their anatomical projections are less well known. It is thought that type II PVPs support inhibitory commissural pathways between vestibular nuclei (reviewed in Roy and Cullen, 2002) and that they contribute to the weaker three-neuron-arc that, in part, mediates the translational VOR (see section 'Neural substrates of the translational VOR (TVOR)'). It is also likely that the inhibitory inputs from type II PVP neurons contribute to the pause-behaviour of type I PVP neurons during ipsilaterally directed saccades, vestibular quick phases, and gaze shifts. This proposal is consistent with known interconnections between the brainstem saccade generator and the vestibular nuclei (Fig. 9.4A; reviewed in Roy and Cullen, 1998).

Neural substrates of the translational VOR (TVOR)

The latency of the TVOR is longer than that of the RVOR; compensatory eye movements generally lag head movements by greater than 10 ms in the primate (Angelaki and McHenry, 1999). Although a direct disynaptic pathway has been shown to exist between the utricular nerve and the abducens nucleus, the longer latency of the TVOR suggests that it is primarily mediated by more complex polysynaptic pathways. Accordingly, the TVOR is not as effective as the RVOR in stabilizing gaze (Paige and Seidman, 1999).

Since type I PVPs do not receive direct inputs from the otoliths, they do not contribute to the intermediate leg of the TVOR pathway. A typical type I PVP neuron shows negligible response modulation during translation when the subject fixates a head-fixed target (i.e. TVOR cancellation). However, when a subject fixates an earth-fixed target during translation (TVOR earth fixed), neurons modulate in a manner that is consistent with their oculomotor-related response during smooth pursuit (see earlier section on pursuit) (Meng et al., 2005). Neurons that do show modulation in response to TVOR suppression include eye-movement sensitive neurons in the vestibular nuclei with ipsilateral eye movement sensitivities. For example, type II PVP neurons and type I EH neurons show modest modulation during suppression of the TVOR.

The neural substrates mediating the optokinetic reflex

The optokinetic system has response dynamics complementary to those of the VOR, and thus functions to stabilize vision in response to low frequency and constant velocity head movements (Fig. 9.3B; top). In contrast to the VOR, the optokinetic system uses visual rather than vestibular

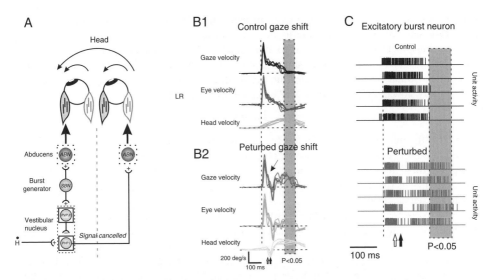

Fig. 9.4 A) Schematic of the interaction that occurs between the VOR and saccadic premotor pathways during gaze shifts. Type I PVPs receive monosynaptic projections from ipsilateral vestibular afferents and project to extraocular motoneurons. During saccades, vestibular quick phases and gaze shifts SBNs become active and provide inhibition of type I PVPs through type II PVPs (vestibular neurons that are active during contralateral head rotations. B1) Example of (control) active gaze shifts and (B2) perturbed gaze shifts. Vertical dashed line, gaze onset; shaded box, average increase in perturbed trials duration; open and filled arrows, average perturbation onset and time at which the resulting head perturbation reached maximum velocity, respectively. C) Example of neuronal activity of excitatory burst neuron (EBN) recorded during the control and perturbed trials. Traces were aligned on gaze shift onset. EBN saccade-related activity (before the perturbation) remained tightly coupled to gaze shift onset. If two completely independent premotor feedback circuits specified the eye and head movements, EBN should have been unaffected by the head perturbation. Instead, a substantial increase in the duration of the EBN burst was observed ($P < 0.05$). This finding that neurons are updated 'on-line' as a function of the artificially modified head-movement feedback signals is consistent with models that use a single integrated comparator to control gaze shifts.

inputs to stabilize gaze. This reflex is driven by the relative motion of the visual world across the retina (retinal slip) that occurs when the head moves. It produces as an optokinetic nystagmus that is similar to vestibular nystagmus in that it consists of alternating slow compensatory and quick resetting eye movements.

Physiological studies have shown that optokinetic eye movements are largely mediated by subcortical pathways. Retinal information from pretectal and mesencephalic neurons in the nucleus of the optic tract and the accessory optic nuclei is sent to neurons in the vestibular nuclei and nPH, which in turn project directly to the extraocular motor nuclei (Fig. 9.3B; bottom). Regions of the vestibulocerebellum are also thought to contribute to the production of optokinetic eye movements. Originally it was suggested that all classes of VN neurons are driven by optokinetic as well as vestibular stimulation (Boyle et al., 1985; Buettner and Buttner, 1979; Reisine and Raphan, 1992; Waespe and Henn, 1977). However, the results of more recent studies suggest that only eye-movement sensitive neurons are modulated during the optokinetic as well as VORs (Beraneck and Cullen, 2007).

During sustained motion in the light, the drive from the OKN system supplements the decaying velocity signal from the vestibular afferents to produce compensatory eye movements (see also Distler and Hoffman, Chapter 4, this volume). When the visual stimulus is extinguished, for example by turning out the lights, the stored velocity signal is manifested as a slowly decaying optokinetic after nystagmus (OKAN). Consistent with their role in OKR, the responses of eye-sensitive VN neurons decay with a time constant that mirrors the eye movement response. In real world situations, where vestibular and optokinetic stimulation occur simultaneously (as would be the case when moving through the room during the day), inputs from vestibular and visually driven reflex pathways are integrated within single VN neurons to produce a sustained responses, that in turn generate robust stabilizing eye movements.

Interactions between eye movement subsystems

The traditional method of studying, the VOR, optokinetic, and the oculomotor 'subsystems' that generate voluntary eye movements has led to an excellent understanding of the brainstem circuitry underlying each of these types of eye movements. However, it is important to keep in mind that during most natural voluntary orienting and tracking behaviours, two or more subsystems work together to control gaze. For example, when we shift our axis of gaze in space by making a combined eye-head gaze shift, the VOR and saccadic subsystems must work together to ensure that the axis of gaze is placed precisely on the target of interest. Similarly, anytime we rapidly reorient our eyes between targets located at different eccentricities and depths, the vergence and saccadic subsystem must work together to accurately control binocular positioning. In this section, recent work establishing how the brain coordinates interactions between different eye movement subsystems to accurately control gaze in everyday life is considered.

Voluntary gaze shifts: interactions between AVOR and saccadic pathways

Status of the VOR

As described in the earlier section 'Premotor control of gaze redirection', saccadic eye movements are used to rapidly redirect the axis of gaze to targets of interest. When the head is not restrained, combinations of rapid eye and head movements (gaze shifts; Fig. 9.4B1) are commonly used to redirect the gaze axis to a new target in space. During such movements, the VOR would be counterproductive since it would produce an eye movement in the direction opposite to that of the intended gaze shift. Nevertheless, it was initially proposed that the VOR remained functional during gaze shifts, such that it eliminated the head's contribution to the change in gaze. In this scheme, termed 'the linear summation hypothesis' (Lanman et al., 1978), the actual eye movement generated at the level of the extraocular motoneurons reflected the summation of two signals: an intact VOR from vestibular pathways (i.e. an oppositely directed eye movement signal), and a separate oculocentric saccadic eye movement signal from the brainstem 'saccade generator', which counters the VOR and redirects the axis of gaze.

Subsequent studies have shown that the linear summation hypothesis is incorrect (reviewed in Cullen and Roy 2004); the VOR is significantly suppressed during active gaze shifts. Notably, the VOR gain (defined as the change in eye velocity/change in head velocity resulting from a perturbation to the head movement) decreases as a function of increasing gaze shift amplitude. In particular, the VOR is partially suppressed during small gaze shifts (<50°) and almost completely suppressed during the early phase of larger gaze shifts. Moreover, the application of transient perturbations at precise times throughout the course of a gaze shift has established that VOR suppression is maximal early in the gaze shift and progressively recovers to reach normal values towards gaze shift end (Cullen, 2004).

An 'on-line' reduction in the activity of VOR pathways is directly responsible for reducing VOR gain during gaze shifts (Roy and Cullen, 1998, 2002). As discussed above, type I PVP neurons constitute most of the middle leg of the three-neuron RVOR pathway. The head-velocity related signals carried by type I PVP neurons are reduced during gaze shifts relative to passive whole-body rotation in the dark (i.e. during the VOR) (McCrea and Gdowski, 2003; Roy and Cullen, 1998, 2002). Notably, a model based on a neuron's response during passive rotation systematically over-predicts its discharge during gaze shifts. In contrast, the head velocity sensitivity of PVP neurons recovers immediately following the end of a gaze shift once gaze is stable, even when the head is still moving. Neuronal responses to head velocity are increasingly attenuated for larger amplitude gaze shifts (Roy and Cullen, 1998, 2002). Thus, consistent with the role of type I PVPs in driving the VOR, this neurophysiological trend mirrors the results of the behavioural studies that were discussed above.

The attenuation of the modulation of type I PVP neurons during gaze shifts can be accounted for by known brainstem mechanisms (Roy and Cullen, 1998), namely via projections from the brainstem saccade generator to the vestibular nuclei (Hikosaka and Kawakami, 1977; Hikosaka et al., 1978; Igusa et al., 1980; Sasaki and Shimazu, 1981) (Fig. 9.4A). During saccades, vestibular quick phases and gaze shifts, brainstem burst neurons (BNs) become active. As a result, BNs provide an inhibitory input related to eye velocity $\dot{E}$ and head velocity $\dot{H}$ to type I PVP neurons during gaze shifts via their projections to type II neurons in the vestibular nuclei. (Note: type II PVP neurons show comparable pauses (Roy and Cullen, 1998)).

Integrated feedback control of eye-head gaze shifts and implications for upstream control

Because the VOR is not fully operational during gaze shifts, it follows that the head, as well as the eyes, contribute to shifting the axis of gaze relative to space. Thus, a fundamental question is: how are the motor commands to the eye and head musculature coordinated to ensure accurate gaze shifts? Two general classes of models have emerged that can account for the control of gaze shifts (see also Corneil, Chapter 16, this volume). In the first model, a single controller is used to minimize gaze error rather than enforce a specific eye or head trajectory, making it conceptually analogous to optimal feedback control (Cullen et al., 2004; Guitton and Volle, 1987; Laurutis and Robinson, 1986). Alternatively, it has been proposed that a gaze displacement command is decomposed early on to control separate eye and head comparators. In this schema it is the individual displacements of the eye and head, rather than the overall accuracy of the movement per se, that are under feedback control (Freedman, 2001).

Firm evidence that gaze shift accuracy is ensured by a single comparator has been provided by single unit recording experiments. The responses of saccadic brainstem neurons are better correlated with gaze than eye motion during gaze shifts (Paré and Guitton, 1998; Phillips et al., 1999; Sylvestre and Cullen, 2006). Additionally, neural activity in the premotor circuit that controls saccadic eye movement is rapidly (~3 ms) updated following experimentally applied head perturbations (Fig. 9.4B; bottom) (Sylvestre and Cullen, 2006). The offset of all OPN and SBN responses during perturbed trials remains tightly synchronized to gaze shift onset, updating in parallel with the resultant increase in movement duration (e.g. EBN shown in Fig. 9.4C). This finding that neurons are updated 'on-line' as a function of the artificially modified head-movement feedback signals is consistent with models that use a single integrated comparator to control gaze shifts, but not models in which gaze shift accuracy is ensured by separate controllers.

The results of numerous studies have provided evidence that the movements of the eyes and head during gaze shifts are coordinated by a drive from the superior colliculus (see Corneil, Chapter 16, this volume). Electrical stimulation and single-unit recording experiments have provided firm evidence that neurons in the superior colliculus controls coordinated eye-head gaze saccades by controlling the direction and amplitude of the entire gaze shift (gaze = eye-in-head + head-in-space), rather than only of the saccadic component of the movement. In addition, the output neurons of the superior colliculus have direct access to both the saccadic and neck premotor circuitry, thereby providing a physiological substrate by which eye and head movements can be driven in a coordinated fashion during gaze shifts. Thus, the saccadic system is more than just an eye-movement system. It is a gaze-control system that plays an integral role in coordinating head and eye movements to make rapid, yet accurate gaze shifts.

Voluntary gaze pursuit: interactions between VOR and pursuit pathways

Head-restrained primates generate continuous, smooth-pursuit eye movements to follow a *moving* visual target of interest. When the head is <u>not</u> restrained, a combination of head and eye motion (i.e. gaze pursuit) is commonly used. Bizzi and colleagues proposed that the linear summation hypothesis (see previous section 'Voluntary gaze shifts: interactions between AVOR and saccadic pathways') could also be applied to eye-head pursuit (Lanman et al., 1978). Accordingly, in this schema the eye movement reflects the summation of two opposing command signals: a VOR, which cancels out the contribution of head motion to gaze, and an ocular pursuit signal of cerebellar origin.

For the same reason it is counterproductive during active gaze shifts, an intact VOR is also counterproductive during eye-head pursuit. In particular, the VOR would function to generate an eye movement command in the direction opposite to that of the ongoing tracking. Indeed, if transient head perturbations are applied while subjects cancel their VOR by tracking a head stationary target, the VOR is not cancelled by a smooth-pursuit signal. In this condition, the VOR is suppressed at latencies shorter (i.e. <30 ms) than could be produced by the smooth pursuit system (i.e. >90 ms; Cullen et al. (1991), Lisberger (1990)).

The idea that a non-visual (or parametric) adjustment of transmission in the VOR pathways contributes to VOR cancellation is consistent with the findings of many behavioural studies. First, humans can decrease the gain of their VOR in the absence of visual cues by simply imagining a target that moved with their heads (Barr et al., 1976). Moreover, humans are better at suppressing their VOR during passive, pseudorandom vestibular stimulation than they are at pursuing a visual target that is moved pseudo-randomly at similar velocities (McKinley and Peterson, 1985), and their ability to cancel torsional VOR is better than their ability to generate torsional smooth pursuit (Leigh et al., 1989). Finally, there is clinical evidence that the ability to generate smooth pursuit eye movements and to cancel the VOR is not always equally affected by CNS lesions (Chambers and Gresty, 1983).

What are the neurophysiological correlates of the non-visual gain adjustment of the VOR during gaze pursuit? The results of single-unit recording studies suggest that the attenuation of the head-velocity sensitivity of PVP neurons underlies parametric (i.e. non-visual) VOR suppression. The head velocity modulation of the direct VOR pathways (i.e. PVP neurons) is attenuated by 30% during cancellation of the VOR. Notably, this reduction in head-velocity sensitivity also occurs at latencies that are too short to be mediated by smooth pursuit pathways (Cullen et al., 1993). Comparable parametric adjustments of transmission in the direct VOR pathway are also observed during the active head movements made during coordinated eye-head pursuit (Roy and Cullen, 2002).

As described above, EH neurons play a major role in generating smooth pursuit eye movements. They receive a pursuit-related command from the cerebellar flocculus, and in turn project to the extraocular motoneurons. During VOR, VOR cancellation, and smooth pursuit, their responses can be well described by the linear summation of their gaze related activity (measured during smooth pursuit) and their vestibular related activity (measured during passive whole-body rotation in the dark). The findings of recent studies have further shown that this same description also well predicts the responses of EH neurons during eye-head gaze pursuit (Roy and Cullen, 2003). Thus the smooth pursuit inputs mediated via these neurons function in parallel with the attenuation in the gain of the direct VOR pathways (i.e. type I PVP neurons) to reduce VOR gain during VOR cancellation and eye-head pursuit.

Disconjugate saccades: interactions between vergence and saccadic pathways

In order to quickly and accurately redirect our gaze between near and far targets, we typically combine saccadic and vergence eye movements (Fig. 9.A). During such eye movements, termed disconjugate saccades, the eyes rotate by different angles and with different trajectories to precisely realign the two visual axes on the new target of interest. Traditionally, disconjugate saccades were thought to be controlled by linear summation of premotor commands from two distinct neural control pathways which separately encode the conjugate and vergence components of eye motion: i) a conjugate saccadic subsystem to quickly rotate the two eyes in a given direction, and ii) a separate vergence subsystem, to rotates the eyes in opposite directions (Hering, 1977; Mays, 1984, 1998). The premotor circuitry involved in generating horizontal saccades (e.g. SBNs of the PPRF) was generally assumed to provide the command to drive the horizontal conjugate component of such movements, whereas near response neurons in the MRF were thought to produce the required vergence command

(Busettini and Mays, 2005; Gamlin, 2002; Gamlin et al., 1989; Mays and Gamlin, 1995b; Mays et al., 1986; Zhang et al., 1992).

There is now considerable evidence that when we reorient our eyes between targets located at different eccentricities the speed of vergence eye movements is increased. In fact, vergence velocities reach values greater during disconjugate saccades than would be predicted by the linear summation of commands from separate saccadic and vergence premotor pathways (Busettini and Mays, 2005; Collewijn et al., 1997; Enright, 1984, 1992; Maxwell and King, 1992; Ono et al., 1978; Oohira, 1993; Van Horn and Cullen, 2008; van Leeuwen et al., 1998; Zee et al., 1992). These behavioural findings challenge the traditional view that there exists separate vergence and conjugate oculomotor subsystems and suggests that conjugate and vergence commands are integrated upstream of the level of the motoneurons.

Indeed, recent reports have now clearly shown that the neural structures previously assumed to form the conjugate saccadic system do not carry purely conjugate information during disconjugate saccades (McConville et al., 1994; Sylvestre and Cullen, 2002; Sylvestre et al., 2003; Van Horn and

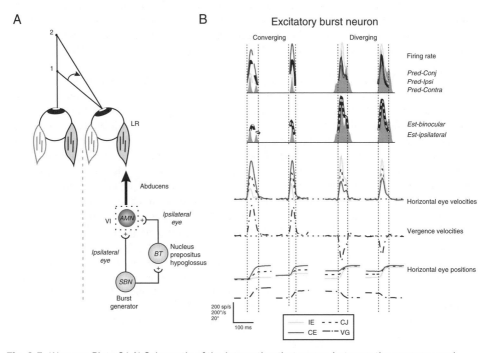

Fig. 9.5 (Also see Plate 6.) A) Schematic of the interaction that occurs between the vergence and saccadic premotor pathways during disconjugate saccades. When the lateral rectus is the agonist muscle the SBNs provide the abducens motoneurons with an integrated vergence/conjugate command (i.e. ipsilateral command) to drive the movement of the eye. B) Example discharges from an example EBN during (left) converging disconjugate saccades (contralateral eye moves more), and (right) diverging disconjugate saccades (ipsilateral eye moves more). The second row shows the same firing rate traces duplicated for clarity. Predicted model fits using conjugate, ipsilateral, and contralateral eye velocities as inputs to SBN model are shown in the top row in black, blue, and red respectively. Note the poor fits obtained when the conjugate and contralateral parameters are used to predict the firing rate of this neuron compared to the prediction using the ipsilateral eye (top row, red and black traces compared to blue trace). Estimated model fits using a binocular model (i.e. left eye and right eye as inputs) are shown in the second row (thick black curve). Estimated model fits using the reduced ipsilateral model are also shown (dashed grey curve). This finding is consistent with the hypothesis that burst neurons encode the movement of the ipsilateral eye rather than the conjugate component of the eye movements.

Cullen, 2008; Van Horn et al., 2008; Zhou and King, 1996, 1998). Individual SBNs in the PPRF (see earlier section 'Generation of the neural pulse') carry integrated conjugate and vergence-related signals. In particular, the majority of SBNs dynamically encode the movement of an individual eye (Van Horn and Cullen, 2008; Van Horn et al., 2008) (Fig. 9.5B). Accordingly, to model the firing rate of a neuron during disconjugate saccades a binocular expansion of the firing rate model is required. For example, for SBNs, terms proportional to the velocity of ipsilateral and contralateral eye should be included (Fig. 9.5B; second row; black trace superimposed on firing rate). In fact, for the majority SBNs this model can be further reduced to include only the movement of the ipsilateral eye (Van Horn et al., 2008; Van Horn and Cullen, 2008) (Fig. 9.5B; second row; grey dashed trace superimposed on firing rate).

Two likely sources of vergence information for SBNs are the MRF and SC (Fig. 9.1A). Both of these structures receive inputs from disparity sensitive cortical and subcortical regions (Ferraina et al., 2000; Genovesio and Ferraina, 2004; Gnadt and Beyer, 1998; Gnadt and Mays, 1995; Mimeault et al., 2004) and stimulation of both the MRF (goldfish: Luque et al. (2006); monkey: Waitzman et al. (2008)) and SC (monkey: Chaturvedi and Van Gisbergen (1999, 2000); cat: Suzuki et al. (2004)) have clear effects on vergence. Moreover, neurons in the SC (cat: Jiang et al. (1996); monkey: Walton and Mays (2003)) and the MRF (Gamlin et al., 1994; Judge and Cumming, 1986; Mays et al., 1986; Waitzman et al., 2008) are modulated during vergence eye movements.

Conclusion and future directions

In this chapter, the premotor pathways that control voluntary and reflex eye movements have been reviewed. Research over the last decade has provided a fundamental understanding of the premotor pathways that generate specific eye movements in isolation. More recently, experiments have begun to explore how the brain coordinates more complex movements when there is interaction between eye movement subsystems. We are now gaining a better understanding of how the brain coordinates movements to accurately control gaze in everyday life. For example, there is now considerable evidence that the saccadic system does not only control conjugate saccadic motion. Instead, recent studies have shown that the 'saccadic' premotor circuit plays an integral role in coordinating head and eye movements to make rapid, yet precise gaze shifts. Moreover when we reorient our two eyes between targets located at different depths and eccentricities, the saccadic system encodes integrated conjugate and vergence commands that ensure the accurate control of gaze in three dimensions. Future studies in higher level brain areas will be required to understand the sensorimotor computations and role of integrative feedback in coordinating multiple effectors (i.e. eye and head, or two eyes) to achieve precise multijoint movements during natural orienting behaviours.

References

Angelaki, D.E. and McHenry, M.Q. (1999). Short-latency primate vestibuloocular responses during translation. *Journal of Neurophysiology*, **871**, 136–147.

Barr, C., Schultheis, L., and Robinson, D. (1976). Voluntary, non-visual control of the human vestibulo-ocular reflex. *Acta Otolaryngology*, **181**(5–6), 365–375.

Beraneck, M. and Cullen, K.E. (2007). Activity of vestibular nuclei neurons during vestibular and optokinetic stimulation in the alert mouse. *Journal of Neurophysiology*, **98**(3), 1549–1565.

Bergeron, A. and Guitton, D. (2000). Fixation neurons in the superior colliculus encode distance between current and desired gaze positions. *Nature Neuroscience*, **3**, 932–939.

Boyle, R., Buttner, U., and Markert, G. (1985). Vestibular nuclei activity and eye movements in the alert monkey during sinusoidal optokinetic stimulation. *Experimental Brain Research*, **57**(2), 362–369.

Broussard, D. and Lisberger, S. (1992). Vestibular inputs to brain stem neurons that participate in motor learning in the primate vestibuloocular reflex. *Journal of Neurophysiology*, **68**(5), 1906–1909.

Buettner, U.W. and Buttner, U. (1979). Vestibular nuclei activity in the alert monkey during suppression of vestibular and optokinetic nystagmus. *Experimental Brain Research*, **37**(3), 581–593.

Busettini, C. and Mays, L.E. (2003). Pontine omnipause activity during conjugate and disconjugate eye movements in macaques. *Journal of Neurophysiology*, **90**(6), 3838–3853.

Busettini, C. and Mays, L.E. (2005). Saccade-vergence interactions in macaques. II. Vergence enhancement as the product of a local feedback vergence motor error and a weighted saccadic burst. *Journal of Neurophysiology*, **94**(4), 2312–2330.

Buttner-Ennever, J.A. and Akert, K. (1981). Medial rectus subgroups of the oculomotor nucleus ant their abducens internuclear input in the monkey. *Journal of Comparative Neurology*, **197**(1), 17–27.

Buttner-Ennever, J.A., Cohen, B., Pause, M., and Fries, W. (1988). Raphe nucleus of the pons containing omnipause neurons of the oculomotor system in the monkey, and its homologue in man. *Journal of Comparative Neurology*, **267**(3), 307–321.

Buttner-Ennever, J.A., Horn, A. K., Henn, V., and Cohen, B. (1999). Projections from the superior colliculus motor map to omnipause neurons in monkey. *Journal of Comparative Neurology*, **413**(1), 55–67.

Buttner-Ennever, J., Horn, A., Scherberger, H., and D' Ascanio, P. (2001). Motoneurons of twitch and nontwitch extraocular muscle fibers in the abducens, trochlear, and oculomotor nuclei of monkeys. *Journal of Comparative Neurology*, **438**, 318–335.

Cannon, S. and Robinson, D. (1987). Loss of the neural integrator of the oculomotor system from brain stem lesions in monkey. *Journal of Neurophysiology.*, **57**(5), 1383–1409.

Chambers, B.R. and Gresty, M.A. (1983). The relationship between disordered pursuit and vestibulo-ocular reflex suppression. *Journal of Neurology, Neurosurgery and Psychiatry*, **46**(1), 61–66.

Chaturvedi, V. and Van Gisbergen, J. (1999). Perturbation of combined saccade-vergence movements by microstimulation in monkey superior colliculus. *Journal of Neurophysiology*, **81**, 2279–2296.

Chaturvedi, V. and Van Gisbergen, J. (2000). Stimulation in the rostral pole of monkey superior colliculus: effects on vergence eye movements. *Experimental Brain Research*, **132**, 72–78.

Choi, W.Y. and Guitton, D. (2006). Responses of collicular fixation neurons to gaze shift perturbations in head-unrestrained monkey reveal gaze feedback control. *Neuron*, **50**(3), 491–505.

Collewijn, H., Erkelens, C.J., and Steinman, R.M. (1997). Trajectories of the human binocular fixation point during conjugate and non-conjugate gaze-shifts. *Vision Research*, **37**(8), 1049–1069.

Collins, C. (ed.) (1971). *The Control of Eye Movements*. New York: American Press.

Collins, C.C., O'Meara, D., and Scott, A.B. (1975). Muscle tension during unrestrained human eye movements. *J Physiol*, **245**(2), 351–369.

Crandall, W.F. and Keller, E.L. (1985). Visual and oculomotor signals in nucleus reticularis tegmenti pontis in alert monkey. *Journal of Neurophysiology*, **54**(5), 1326–1345.

Crawford, J.D., Cadera, W., and Vilis, T. (1991). Generation of torsional and vertical eye position signals by the interstitial nucleus of Cajal. *Science*, **252**(5012), 1551–1553.

Cullen, K.E. (2004). Sensory signals during active versus passive movement. *Current Opinion in Neurology*, **14**(6), 698–706.

Cullen, K. and McCrea, R. (1993). Firing behavior of brain stem neurons during voluntary cancellation of the horizontal vestibuloocular reflex. I. Secondary vestibular neurons. *Journal of Neurophysiology*, **70**(2), 828–843.

Cullen, K.E. and Guitton, D. (1997). Analysis of primate IBN spike trains using system identification techniques. I. Relationship To eye movement dynamics during head-fixed saccades. *Journal of Neurophysiology*, **78**(6), 3259–3282.

Cullen, K.E., Belton, T., and McCrea, R.A. (1991). A non-visual mechanism for voluntary cancellation of the vestibulo-ocular reflex. *Experimental Brain Research*, **83**, 237–252.

Cullen, K.E., Chen-Huang, C., and McCrea, R.A. (1993). Firing behavior of brain stem neurons during voluntary cancellation of the horizontal vestibuloocular reflex. II. Eye movement related neurons. *Journal of Neurophysiology*, **70**(2), 844–856.

Cullen, K.E., Huterer, M., Braidwood, D.A., and Sylvestre, P.A. (2004). Time course of vestibuloocular reflex suppression during gaze shifts. *Journal of Neurophysiology*, **92**(6), 3408–3422.

Demer, J.L. (2006). Current concepts of mechanical and neural factors in ocular motility. *Current Opinion in Neurology*, **19**(1), 4–13.

Dodge, R. (1903). Five types of eye movement in the horizontal meridian plane of the field of regard. *American Journal of Physiology*, **8**, 307–329.

Enright, J. (1984). Changes in vergence mediated by saccades. *Journal of Physiology*, **350**, 9–31.

Enright, J.T. (1992). The remarkable saccades of asymmetrical vergence. *Vision Research*, **32**(12), 2261–2276.

Everling, S., Paré, M., Dorris, M., and Munoz, D.P. (1998). Comparison of the discharge characteristics of brain stem omnipause neurons and superior colliculus fixation neurons in monkey: implications for control of fixation and saccade behavior. *Journal of Neurophysiology*, **79**, 511–528.

Ferraina, S., Paré, M., and Wurtz, R. (2000). Disparity sensitivity of frontal eye field neurons. *Journal of Neurophysiology*, **83**, 625–629.

Freedman, E. (2001). Interactions between eye and head control signals can account for movement kinematics. *Biological Cybernetics*, **84**, 453–462.

Fuchs, A.F., Scudder, C.A., and Kaneko, C. (1988). Discharge patterns and recruitment order of identified motoneurons and internuclear neurons in the monkey abducens nucleus. *Journal of Neurophysiology*, **60**, 1874–1895.

Fukushima, K., Kaneko, C., and Fuchs, A.F. (1992). The neuronal substrate of integration in the oculomotor system. *Progress in Neurobiology*, **39**, 609–639.

Furuya, N. and Markham, C.H. (1982). Direct inhibitory synaptic linkage of pause neurons with burst inhibitory neurons. *Brain Research*, **245**(1), 139–143.

Gamlin, P.D. (2002). Neural mechanisms for the control of vergence eye movements. *Annals of the New York Academy of Sciences*, **956**, 264–272.

Gamlin, P.D., Gnadt, J.W., and Mays, L.E. (1989). Abducens internuclear neurons carry an inappropriate signal for ocular convergence. *Journal of Neurophysiology*, **62**(1), 70–81.

Gamlin, P.D., Zhang, Y., Clendaniel, R.A., and Mays, L.E. (1994). Behavior of identified Edinger-Westphal neurons during ocular accommodation. *Journal of Neurophysiology*, **72**(5), 2368–2382.

Genovesio, A. and Ferraina, S. (2004). Integration of retinal disparity and fixation-distance related signals toward an egocentric coding of distance in the posterior parietal cortex of primates. *Journal of Neurophysiology*, **91**(6), 2670–2684.

Gnadt, J.W. and Beyer, J. (1998). Eye movements in depth: What does the monkey's parietal cortex tell the superior colliculus? *Neuroreport*, **9**, 233–238.

Gnadt, J.W. and Mays, L.E. (1995). Neurons in monkey parietal area LIP are tuned for eye-movement parameters in three-dimensional space. *Journal of Neurophysiology*, **73**(1), 280–297.

Guitton, D. and Volle, M. (1987). Gaze control in humans: eye-head coordination during orienting movements to targets within and beyond the oculomotor range. *Journal of Neurophysiology*, **58**(3), 427–459.

Hafed, Z.M., Goffart, L., and Krauzlis, R.J. (2009). A neural mechanism for microsaccade generation in the primate superior colliculus. *Science*, **323**(5916), 940–943.

Hepp, K. and Henn, V. (1983). Spatio-temporal recoding of rapid eye movement signals in the monkey paramedian pontine reticular formation (PPRF). *Experimental Brain Research*, **52**, 105–120.

Hering, E. (1977). *Lehre vom binokularen Sehen. (The theory of binocular vision) (1868)*. New York: Plenum Press.

Hess, B.J. (2008). Control of ocular torsion in the rotational vestibulo-ocular reflexes. *Progress in Brain Research*, **171**, 199–206.

Hikosaka, O., Igusa, Y., Nakao, S., and Shimazu, H. (1978). Direct inhibitory synaptic linkage of pontomedullary reticular burst neurons with abducens motoneurons in the cat. *Experimental Brain Research*, **33**, 337–352.

Hikosaka, O. and Kawakami, T. (1977). Inhibitory reticular neurons related to the quick phase of vestibular nystagmus—their location and projection. *Experimental Brain Research.*, **27**(3–4), 377–386.

Horn, A., Buttner-Ennever, J., Wahle, P., and Reichenberger, I. (1994). Neurotransmitter profile of saccadic omnipause neurons in nucleus raphe interpositus. *Journal of Neuroscience*, **14**, 2032–2046.

Huterer, M. and Cullen, K. (2002). Vestibuloocular reflex dynamics during high-frequency and high-acceleration rotations of the head on body in rhesus monkey. *Journal of Neurophysiology.*, **88**(1), 13–28.

Igusa, Y., Sasaki, S., and Shimazu, H. (1980). Excitatory premotor burst neurons in the cat pontine reticular formation related to the quick phase of vestibular nystagmus. *Brain Res*, **182**(2), 451–456.

Jiang, H., Guitton, D., and Cullen, K.E. (1996). Near-response-related neural activity in the rostral superior colliculus of the cat. *Soc Neurosci Abstr*, **22**(662).

Judge, S.J. and Cumming, B. (1986). Neurons in monkey midbrain with activity related to vergence eye movement and accomodation. *Journal of Neurophysiology*, **55**, 915–930.

Kaneko, C.R. (2006). Saccade-related, long-lead burst neurons in the monkey rostral pons. *Journal of Neurophysiology*, **95**(2), 979–994.

Keller, E.L. (1973). Accomodative vergence in the alert monkey. Motor unit analysis. *Vision Res*, **13**, 1565–1575.

Keller, E.L. (1974). Participation of medial pontine reticular formation in eye movement generation in monkey. *Journal of Neurophysiology*, **37**, 316–332.

Keller, E.L. and Robinson, D.A. (1972). Abducens unit behaviour in the monkey during vergence movements. *Vision Research*, **12**, 369–382.

Klier, E.M., Meng, H., and Angelaki, D.E. (2006). Three-dimensional kinematics at the level of the oculomotor plant. *Journal of Neuroscience*, **26**(10), 2732–2737.

Krauzlis, R.J., Basso, M.A., and Wurtz, R.H. (1997). Shared motor error for multiple eye movements. *Science*, **276**(5319), 1693–1695.

Langer, T.P. and Kaneko, C.R. (1990). Brainstem afferents to the oculomotor omnipause neurons in monkey. *Journal of Comparative Neurology*, **295**(3), 413–427.

Lanman, J., Bizzi, E., and Allum, J. (1978). The coordination of eye and head movement during smooth pursuit. *Brain Res*, **153**, 39–53.

Laurutis, V.P. and Robinson, D. A. (1986). The vestibulo-ocular reflex during human saccadic eye movements. *Journal of Physiology*, **373**, 209–233.

Leigh, R.J., Maas, E.F., Grossman, G.E., and Robinson, D.A. (1989). Visual cancellation of the torsional vestibulo-ocular reflex in humans. *Experimental Brain Research*, **75**(2), 221–226.

Leung, H.-C., Suh, M., and Kettner, R.E. (2000). Cerebellar flocculus and paraflocculus Purkinje cell activity during circular pursuit in monkey. *Journal of Neurophysiology*, **83**, 13–30.

Lisberger, S.G. (1990). Visual tracking in monkeys: evidence for short-latency suppression of the vestibuloocular reflex. *J. Neurophysiol*, **63**, 676–688.

Lisberger, S. and Pavelko, T. (1988). Brain stem neurons in modified pathways for motor learning in the primate vestibulo-ocular reflex. *Science*, **242**(4879), 771–773.

Lisberger, S.G., Pavelko, T.A., and Broussard, D.M. (1994a). Neural basis for motor learning in the vestibuloocular reflex of primates. I. Changes in the responses of brain stem neurons. *Journal of Neurophysiology*, **72**(2), 928–953.

Lisberger, S.G., Pavelko, T.A., and Broussard, D.M. (1994b). Responses during eye movements of brain stem neurons that receive monosynaptic inhibition from the flocculus and ventral paraflocculus in monkeys. *Journal of Neurophysiology*, **72**(2), 909–927.

Luque, M.A., Perez-Perez, M.P., Herrero, L., Waitzman, D.M., and Torres, B. (2006). Eye movements evoked by electrical microstimulation of the mesencephalic reticular formation in goldfish. *Neuroscience*, **137**(3), 1051–1073.

Luschei, E. and Fuchs, A.F. (1972). Activity of brain stem neurons during eye movements of alert monkeys. *Journal of Neurophysiology*, **35**, 445–461.

Maciewicz, R., Kaneko, C., Highstein, S.M., and Baker, R. (1975). Morphophysiological identification of interneurons in the oculomotor nucleus that project to the abducens nucleus in the cat. *Brain Res*, **96**, 60–65.

Maxwell, J.S. and King, W.M. (1992). Dynamics and efficacy of saccade-facilitated vergence eye movements in monkeys. *Journal of Neurophysiology*, **68**(4), 1248–1260.

Mays, L.E. (1984). Neural control of vergence eye movements: convergence and divergence neurons in midbrain. *Journal of Neurophysiology*, **51**(5), 1091–1108.

Mays, L.E. (1998). Has Hering been hooked? *Nature Med.*, **4**, 889–890.

Mays, L.E. and Gamlin, P.D. (1995b). A neural mechanism subserving saccade-vergence interactions. In W. R. Findlay J., Kentridge R.W. (eds.) *Eye movement research: mechanisms, processes and applications* (pp. 215–223). Amsterdam: Elsevier.

Mays, L.E. and Porter, J.D. (1984). Neural control of vergence eye movements: activity of abducens and oculomotor neurons. *Journal of Neurophysiology*, **52**(4), 743–761.

Mays, L.E., Porter, J.D., Gamlin, P.D., and Tello, C.A. (1986). Neural control of vergence eye movements: neurons encoding vergence velocity. *Journal of Neurophysiology*, **56**(4), 1007–1021.

McConville, K.M., Tomlinson, D., King, W.M., Paige, G.D., and Na, E.Q. (1994). Eye position signals in the vestibular nuclei: Consequences for models of integrator function. *J. Vest. Res.*, **4**, 391–400.

McCrea, R.A. (1988). Neuroanatomy of the oculomotor system. The nucleus prepositus. *Rev Oculomot Res*, **2**, 203–223.

McCrea, R.A. and Gdowski, G.T. (2003). Firing behaviour of squirrel monkey eye movement-related vestibular nucleus neurons during gaze saccades. *J Physiol.*, **546**(Pt 1), 207–224.

McCrea, R.A., Strassman, E.M., and Highstein, S.M. (1987). Anatomical and physiological characteristics of vestibular neurons mediating the horizontal vestibulo-ocular reflex of the squirrel monkey. *Journal of Comparative Neurology*, **264**, 547–570.

McKinley, P.A. and Peterson, B.W. (1985). Voluntary modulation of the vestibuloocular reflex in humans and its relation to smooth pursuit. *Experimental Brain Research*, **60**, 454–464.

Meng, H., Green, A.M., Dickman, J.D., and Angelaki, D.E. (2005). Pursuit—vestibular interactions in brain stem neurons during rotation and translation. *Journal of Neurophysiology*, **93**(6), 3418–3433.

Miller, J.M. and Robins, D. (1992). Extraocular muscle forces in alert monkey. *Vision Research*, **32**(6), 1099–1113.

Mimeault, D., Paquet, V., Molotchnikoff, S., Lepore, F., and Guillemot, J.P. (2004). Disparity sensitivity in the superior colliculus of the cat. *Brain Research*, **1010**(1–2), 87–94.

Minor, L.B., Lasker, D.M., Backous, D.D., and Hullar, T.E. (1999). Horizontal vestibuloocular reflex evoked by high-acceleration rotations in the squirrel monkey. I. Normal responses. *Journal of Neurophysiology*, **82**(3), 1254–1270.

Moschovakis, A.K., Scudder, C.A., and Highstein, S.M. (1991a). Structure of the primate oculomotor burst generator. I. Medium-lead burst neurons with upward on-directions. *Journal of Neurophysiology*, **65**(2), 203–217.

Moschovakis, A.K., Scudder, C.A., Highstein, S.M., and Warren, J.D. (1991b). Structure of the primate oculomotor burst generator. II. Medium-lead burst neurons with downward on-directions. *Journal of Neurophysiology*, **65**(2), 218–229.

Munoz, D.P. and Wurtz, R.H. (1992). Role of the rostral superior colliculus in active visual fixation and execution of express saccades. *Journal of Neurophysiology*, **67**(4), 1000–1002.

Munoz, D.P. and Wurtz, R.H. (1993). Fixation cells in monkey superior colliculus. I. Characteristics of cell discharge. *Journal of Neurophysiology*, **70**(2), 559–575.

Munoz, D.P. and Wurtz, R.H. (1995). Saccade-related activity in monkey superior colliculus. I. Characteristics of burst and buildup cells. *Journal of Neurophysiology*, **73**(6), 2313–2333.

Munoz, D.P., Dorris, M.C., Paré, M., and Everling, S. (2000). On your mark, get set: brainstem circuitry underlying saccadic initiation. *Can J Physiol Pharmacol*, **78**(11), 934–944.

Nakao, S., Curthoys, I.S., and Markham, C.H. (1980). Direct inhibitory projection of pause neurons to nystagmus-related pontomedullary reticular burst neurons in the cat. *Experimental Brain Research*, **40**(3), 283–293.

Newlands, S.D., Vrabec, J.T., Purcell, I.M., Stewart, C.M., Zimmerman, B.E., and Perachio, A.A. (2003). Central projections of the saccular and utricular nerves in macaques. *Journal of Comparative Neurology*, **466**(1), 31–47.

Ohgaki, T., Markham, C.H., Schneider, J.S., and Curthoys, I.S. (1989). Anatomical evidence of the projection of pontine omnipause neurons to midbrain regions controlling vertical eye movements. *Journal of Comparative Neurology*, **289**(4), 610–625.

Ono, H., Nakamizo, S., and Steinbach, M.J. (1978). Nonadditivity of vergence and saccadic eye movement. *Vision Res*, **18**(6), 735–739.

Oohira, A. (1993). Vergence eye movements facilitated by saccades. *Jpn J Ophthalmol*, **37**(4), 400–413.

Paige, G.D. and Seidman, S.H. (1999). Characteristics of the VOR in response to linear acceleration. *Annals of the New York Academy of Sciences*, **871**, 123–135.

Paré, M. and Guitton, D. (1998). Brain stem omnipause neurons and the control of combined eye-head gaze saccades in the alert cat. *Journal of Neurophysiology*, **79**(6), 3060–3076.

Phillips, J.O., Ling, L., and Fuchs, A.F. (1999). Action of the brain stem saccade generator during horizontal gaze shifts. I. Discharge patterns of omnidirectional pause neurons. *Journal of Neurophysiology*, **81**(3), 1284–1295.

Raybourn, M.S. and Keller, E.L. (1977). Colliculoreticular organization in primate oculomotor system. *Journal of Neurophysiology*, **40**(4), 861–878.

Reisine, H. and Raphan, T. (1992). Neural basis for eye velocity generation in the vestibular nuclei of alert monkeys during off-vertical axis rotation. *Experimental Brain Research*, **92**(2), 209–226.

Robinson, D.A. (1964). The mechanics of human saccadic eye movement. *J Physiol*, **174**, 245–264.

Robinson, D.A. (1970). Oculomotor unit behavior in the monkey. *Journal of Neurophysiology*, **33**(3), 393–403.

Robinson, D.A. and Keller, E.L. (1972). The behavior of eye movement motoneurons in the alert monkey. *Bibliotheca Ophthalmologic*, **82**, 7–16.

Roy, J.E. and Cullen, K.E. (1998). A neural correlate for vestibulo-ocular reflex suppression during voluntary eye-head gaze shifts. *Nature Neuroscience*, **1**, 404–410.

Roy, J.E. and Cullen, K.E. (2002). Vestibuloocular reflex signal modulation during voluntary and passive head movements. *Journal of Neurophysiology*, **87**, 2337–2357.

Roy, J.E. and Cullen, K.E. (2003). Brain stem pursuit pathways: dissociating visual, vestibular, and proprioceptive inputs during combined eye-head gaze tracking. *Journal of Neurophysiology*, **90**(1), 271–290.

Sasaki, S. and Shimazu, H. (1981). Reticulovestibular organization participating in generation of horizontal fast eye movement. *Annals of the New York Academy of Sciences*, **374**, 130–143.

Scudder, C.A. and Fuchs, A.F. (1992). Physiological and behavioural identification of vestibular nucleus neurons mediating the horizontal vestibuloocular reflex in trained rhesus monkeys. *Journal of Neurophysiology*, **68**, 244–264.

Scudder, C.A., Fuchs, A.F., and Langer, T.P. (1988). Characteristics and functional identification of saccadic inhibitory burst neurons in the alert monkey. *Journal of Neurophysiology*, **59**(5), 1430–1454.

Scudder, C.A., Kaneko, C.S., and Fuchs, A.F. (2002). The brainstem burst generator for saccadic eye movements: a modern synthesis. *Experimental Brain Research*, **142**(4), 439–462.

Scudder, C.A., Moschovakis, A.K., Karabelas, A.B., and Highstein, S.M. (1996). Anatomy and physiology of saccadic long-lead burst neurons recorded in the alert squirrel monkey. I. Descending projections from the mesencephalon. *Journal of Neurophysiology*, **76**(1), 332–352.

Shinoda, Y., Sugiuchi, Y., Izawa, Y., and Takahashi, M. (2008). Neural circuits for triggering saccades in the brainstem. *Progress in Brain Research*, **171**, 79–85.

Skavenski, A.A. and Robinson, D.A. (1973). Role of abducens neurons in vestibuloocular reflex. *Journal of Neurophysiology*, **36**(4), 724–738.

Spencer, R.F. and Porter, J.D. (1988). Structural organization of the extraocular muscles. *Rev Oculomot Res*, **2**, 33–79.

Strassman, A., Highstein, S.M., and McCrea, R.A. (1986a). Anatomy and physiology of saccadic burst neurons in the alert squirrel monkey. I. Excitatory burst neurons. *Journal of Comparative Neurology*, **249**(3), 337–357.

Strassman, A., Highstein, S.M., and McCrea, R.A. (1986b). Anatomy and physiology of saccadic burst neurons in the alert squirrel monkey. II. Inhibitory burst neurons. *Journal of Comparative Neurology*, **249**(3), 358–380.

Strassman, A., Evinger, C., McCrea, R.A., Baker, R.G., and Highstein, S.M. (1987). Anatomy and physiology of intracellularly labelled omnipause neurons in the cat and squirrel monkey. *Experimental Brain Research*, **67**(2), 436–440.

Sugiuchi, Y., Izawa, Y., Takahashi, M., Na, J., and Shinoda, Y. (2005). Physiological characterization of synaptic inputs to inhibitory burst neurons from the rostral and caudal superior colliculus. *Journal of Neurophysiology*, **93**(2), 697–712.

Suh, M., Leung, H.-C., and Kettner, R.E. (2000). Cerebellar flocculus and ventral paraflocculus Purkinje cellactivity during predictive and visually driven pursuit in monkey. *Journal of Neurophysiology*, **84**, 1835–1850.

Sylvestre, P.A. and Cullen, K.E. (1999). Quantitative analysis of abducens neuron discharge dynamics during saccadic and slow eye movements. *Journal of Neurophysiology*, **82**(5), 2612–2632.

Sylvestre, P.A. and Cullen, K.E. (2002). Dynamics of abducens nucleus neuron discharges during disjunctive saccades. *Journal of Neurophysiology*, **88**(6), 3452–3468.

Sylvestre, P.A. and Cullen, K.E. (2006). Premotor correlates of integrated feedback control for eye-head gaze shifts. *Journal of Neuroscience*, **26**(18), 4922–4929.

Sylvestre, P.A., Choi, J.T., and Cullen, K.E. (2003). Discharge dynamics of oculomotor neural integrator neurons during conjugate and disjunctive saccades and fixation. *Journal of Neurophysiology*, **90**(2), 739–754.

Takahashi, M., Sugiuchi, Y., Izawa, Y., and Shinoda, Y. (2005). Commissural excitation and inhibition by the superior colliculus in tectoreticular neurons projecting to omnipause neuron and inhibitory burst neuron regions. *Journal of Neurophysiology*, **94**(3), 1707–1726.

Ugolini, G., Klam, F., Doldan Dans, M., Dubayle, D., Brandi, A.M., Buttner-Ennever, J., *et al.* (2006). Horizontal eye movement networks in primates as revealed by retrograde transneuronal transfer of rabies virus: differences in monosynaptic input to 'slow' and 'fast' abducens motoneurons. *Journal of Comparative Neurology*, **498**(6), 762–785.

Van Horn, M.R. (2009). Tracking an invisible target reveals spatial tuning of neurons in the rostral superior colliculus is not dependent on visual stimuli. *Journal of Neuroscience*, **29**(3), 589–590.

Van Horn, M.R. and Cullen, K.E. (2008). Dynamic coding of vertical facilitated vergence by premotor saccadic burst neurons. *Journal of Neurophysiology*, **100**(4), 1967–1982.

Van Horn, M.R. and Cullen, K.E. (2009). Dynamic characterization of agonist and antagonist oculomotoneurons during conjugate and disconjugate eye movements. *Journal of Neurophysiology*, **102**, 28–40.

Van Gisbergen, J.A., Robinson, D.A., and Gielen, S. (1981). A quantitative analysis of generation of saccadic eye movements by burst neurons. *Journal of Neurophysiology*, **45**(3), 417–442.

Van Horn, M., Sylvestre, P.A., and Cullen, K.E. (2008). The brain stem saccadic burst generator encodes gaze in three-dimensional space. *Journal of Neurophysiology*, **99**(5), 2602–2616.

Van Leeuwen, A.F., Collewijn, H., and Erkelens, C.J. (1998). Dynamics of horizontal vergence movements: interaction with horizontal and vertical saccades and relation with monocular preferences. *Vision Res*, **38**(24), 3943–3954.

Waespe, W. and Henn, V. (1977). Vestibular nuclei activity during optokinetic after-nystagmus (OKAN) in the alert monkey. *Experimental Brain Research*, **30**(2–3), 323–330.

Waitzman, D.M., Van Horn, M.R., and Cullen, K.E. (2008). Neuronal evidence for individual eye control in the primate cMRF. *Progress in Brain Research*, **171**, 143–150.

Walton, M.M. and Mays, L.E. (2003). Discharge of saccade-related superior colliculus neurons during saccades accompanied by vergence. *Journal of Neurophysiology*, **90**(2), 1124–1139.

Yoshida, K., Iwamoto, Y., Chimoto, S., and Shimazu, H. (1999). Saccade-related inhibitory input to pontine omnipause neurons: an intracellular study in alert cats. *Journal of Neurophysiology*, **82**(3), 1198–1208.

Yoshida, K., McCrea, R., Berthoz, A., and Vidal, P.P. (1982). Morphological and physiological characteristics of inhibitory burst neurons controlling horizontal rapid eye movements in the alert cat. *Journal of Neurophysiology*, **48**(3), 761–784.

Zee, D.S., Fitzgibbon, E.J., and Optican, L.M. (1992). Saccade-vergence interactions in humans. *Journal of Neurophysiology*, **68**(5), 1624–1641.

Zee, D.S., Yamazaki, A., Butler, P.H., and Gucer, G. (1981). Effects of ablation of flocculus and paraflocculus of eye movements in primate. *Journal of Neurophysiology*, **46**(4), 878–899.

Zhang, Y., Gamlin, P.D., and Mays, L.E. (1991). Antidromic identification of midbrain near response cells projecting to the oculomotor nucleus. *Experimental Brain Research*, **84**(3), 525–528.

Zhang, Y., Mays, L.E., and Gamlin, P.D. (1992). Characteristics of near response cells projecting to the oculomotor nucleus. *Journal of Neurophysiology*, **67**(4), 944–960.

Zhou, W. and King, W.M. (1996). Ocular selectivity of units in oculomotor pathways. *Annals of the New York Academy of Sciences*, **781**, 724–728.

Zhou, W. and King, W.M. (1998). Premotor commands encode monocular eye movements. *Nature*, **393**(6686), 692–695.

CHAPTER 10

The oculomotor cerebellum

Peter Thier

Abstract

Several regions of the cerebellum contribute to eye movements. The one best known is the 'vestibular' cerebellum, modifying visual and vestibular reflexes. The second well-understood oculomotor region is the oculomotor vermis, the major substrate of short-term saccadic learning and the adjustment of the gain of the initial, open loop part of smooth pursuit eye movements. Several studies have provided evidence for yet a further oculomotor region in the hemispheric parts of the cerebellum, involving parts of Crus I, II, and the simple lobule. As the dorsal paraflocculus, adjoining the vestibular cerebellum, it seems to contribute to smooth-pursuit and to saccades. However, their specific contributions to these two forms of goal-directed eye movements have not yet been worked out.

The cerebellar cortex is a crystal-like structure consisting of highly stereotypic microcircuitry showing no relevant regional variability. Therefore, it may be firmly assumed that basically the same neuronal computations are performed throughout the cerebellar cortex. Moreover, as the horizontal extent of intracortical fibres is confined to a few millimetres only, these neuronal computations must necessarily remain local. Hence the type of motor—and possibly also non-motor—function a particular part of cerebellar cortex is committed to is fully determined by the specific pattern of afferent and efferent connections it maintains with functionally distinct extracerebellar structures. A discussion of the role of the cerebellum in eye movement control requires a brief recapitulation of the conspicuous anatomical organization of cerebellar cortex which constrains the possible function (for a more detailed account, see, for instance, Ito (1984) and Sultan (2000)).

The cerebellar cortex has three layers: the outermost molecular layer, the Purkinje cell (PC) layer, and the innermost granular layer, which borders on the white matter (Fig. 10.1A). PCs, whose cell bodies are located in the Purkinje cell layer, are the only output element of cerebellar cortex. Their long axons terminate in the deep cerebellar nuclei and in the vestibular nuclei, where they make GABAergic synapses. The planar dendritic tree of PCs, extended along the rostocaudal axis, is largely confined to the molecular layer. It collects input from a huge number of parallel fibres (PFs) (100,000–200,000 in rat: Napper and Harvey (1988)), which stem from granule cell (GC) axons. These axons ascend from the GC layer to the molecular layer, where they bifurcate into the PF. The PF run perpendicularly to the PC dendritic tree, which is densely covered by PF synapses. Whereas huge numbers of PF converge on individual PCs, the second PC input, the climbing fibre (CF), is much more selective. CF branches contact small groups of PCs and an individual PC typically receives input from just one CF making about 300–500 synaptic contacts (Hillman, 1969). The CF synapses are few but powerful: they are responsible for the generation of complex spikes (CSs) fired at conspicuously low frequencies by PCs. Their ional basis is the activation of calcium channels. The only source of the CF is the inferior olive. On the other hand, input to the GC layer originates from a number of precerebellar nuclei in the brainstem, among them many of the tegmental structures subserving eye movements such as the paramedian pontine reticular formation (PPRF) or the nucleus reticularis tegmenti pontis (NRTP) (see also Cullen and Horn, Chapter 9, this volume). In terms of numbers, the most important source of afferents are the pontine nuclei, linking large parts of cerebral cortex with the cerebellum. Activity in the GC layer/PF system is responsible for the second, more conventionally-shaped type of spike fired by PCs, the simple spike (SS), which is based on conventional sodium and potassium channels and may be fired at frequencies of several hundred spikes per second. SSs are typically observed even in the absence of any overt stimulus. A number of inhibitory interneurons modulate activity in the GC layer/PF system as well as activity of PCs. One of these inhibitory interneurons, the Golgi cell, receiving MF input and feeding back on GC cells, will be examined more closely when discussing the vermal control of saccades.

Several regions of the cerebellum have been implicated in the control of eye movements (Fig. 10.2). The one which has been investigated most intensively and whose specific role is probably best known is a complex comprising phylogenetically old parts of the cerebellum intimately involved in the control of vestibular (see also Hess, Chapter 3, this volume) and related optokinetic reflexes (see also Distler and Hoffmann, Chapter 4, this volume). This 'vestibular' cerebellum consists of the flocculus, the adjoining ventral paraflocculus, the uvula, and the nodulus. Also the dorsal paraflocculus, adjacent to the ventral paraflocculus, has oculomotor functions. Although as yet relatively little explored, its function seems to differ from that of the neighbouring vestibular cerebellum.

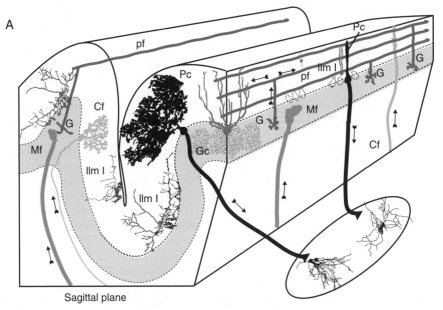

Fig. 10.1 A) Semidiagramatic three-dimensional representation of parts of two folia of cerebellar cortex showing the major neuronal elements. The granular layer is distinguished by grey shading. The planar build of Purkinje cells is revealed by showing them both in sagittal and transversal view. The two types of molecular interneurons, the stellate and basket cells, are shown as flat structures in the transversal view. Abbreviations: Cf, climbing fibre; IIml, interhibitory interneurons of the molecular layer; G, granule cell; Gc, golgi cell; Mf, mossy fibre; Pc, Purkinje cell; PF, parallel fibre. Based on Hamori and Szentagothai (1966) and Sultan (2000). With kind permission from Springer Science+Business Media: *Experimental Brain Research*, Identification under the electron microscope of climbing fibres and their synaptic contacts, **1**(1) 2003, J. Hamori.

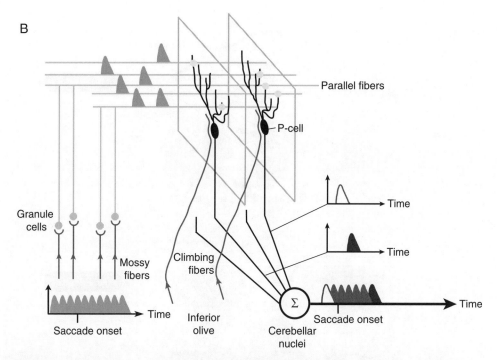

Fig. 10.1 *(continued)* B) Illustration of vermal population coding as basis of short-term saccadic adaptation. Purkinje cells fire saccade-related bursts (or saccade-related pauses, not shown) at different times. As their axons converge on individual target neurons in the deep cerebellar nuclei they act collectively as a population, depolarizing the target neurons as long as the population signal is up. In order to give the population signal the right shape, contributions from individual PCs have to be facilitated or, alternatively, to be suppressed. This is assumed to be due to the CF, modulating the impact of saccade-related parallel fibre input. The mossy fibre/parallel fibre input comprises saccade-related bursts occurring at very different times relative to saccade onset. Additional temporal dispersion of saccade-related bursts is added by different conduction delays arising from differences in the distances to individual PCs. For instance, in order to expand the duration of the PC population signal in time, the strength of those PC bursts would have to be increased that occur comparatively late (shown dark) relative to the ones already active (shown grey). This would require strengthening the impact of correspondingly late parallel fibre bursts. Expanding the population signal in time will delay the stop signal for saccades, thought to be provided by the post-inhibitory rebound fired by nuclear target neurons. The consequence will be larger amplitude saccades.

The second well-defined oculomotor region is the *oculomotor vermis*, comprising the caudal part of lobulus VI (VIc) and the rostral parts of lobulus VII (VIIA). As it receives input not only from the brainstem tegmentum but also substantial input from the pontine nuclei, it is much more dependent on cerebrocortical processing. Several studies have provided evidence for yet a further oculomotor region in the hemispheric parts of the cerebellum, probably adjoining the vermal oculomotor region. However, the extent and the boundaries of this third area, referred to as the *hemispheric oculomotor region* or HVII by Nagao and co-workers (Ohki et al., 2009; Xiong et al., 2002), as well as its functional role remain poorly defined. As excellent reviews of the 'vestibular' cerebellum and its role in the control of eye movements reflexes are available (Barmack, 2006; Highstein and Holstein, 2006; Ito, 1984; Voogd and Barmack, 2006), I will as far as possible restrict its discussion to its role in the control of goal-directed eye movements, namely smooth-pursuit eye movements (see also Barnes, Chapter 7, this volume) and saccades (see also Gilchrist, Chapter 5, this volume).

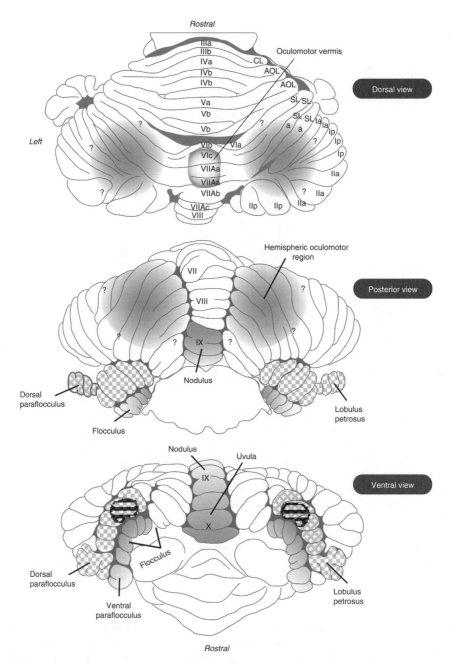

Fig. 10.2 Illustration of eye movement-related areas in the primate cerebellum. The boundaries of the *hemispheric oculomotor region* are ill-defined (?. . .?). The region in the dorsal paraflocculus distinguished by horizontal stripes represents the oculomotor 'hot spot' identified by Noda and Mikami (1986a). Views of the cerebellum modified from Madigan and Carpenter (1971).

The flocculus–paraflocculus complex

In the monkey, the paraflocculus consists of three parts, the dorsal paraflocculus, the ventral paraflocculus adjoining the flocculus, and the lobulus petrosus, a thin appendage of the dorsal para- flocculus, largely engulfed by petrosal bone (Fig. 10.2). In the older anatomical literature, the lobulus petrosus is usually seen as part of the ventral paraflocculus and the latter as being distinct from the flocculus (Madigan and Carpenter, 1971). However, recent studies of connectivity and function suggest that the lobulus petrosus is actually part of the dorsal paraflocculus (Glickstein et al., 1994; Xiong and Soichi, 2002), devoted to visual and oculomotor functions, probably distinct from the vestibulo-ocular functions, subserved by the second tandem, comprising the flocculus (lobuli I–V) and the ventral paraflocculus (lobuli VI–X), the two separated by the posterolateral fissure.

Flocculus and ventral paraflocculus

Although exhibiting clear phylogenetic, anatomical, and functional differences, unfortunately, in much of the relevant physiological literature on monkeys, the last two regions are often dealt with indiscriminatingly and referred to as the *floccular complex* or the *floccular region*. This makes it hard, if not impossible, to identify the specific roles of the two structures. For the sake of convenience, I will also resort to the term *floccular region* (FR), unless the work discussed clearly distinguishes the flocculus and the ventral paraflocculus. The FR helps stabilize visual images on the retina by moving the eyes in the direction of the expected image movement. The type of image motion the primate FR is concerned with is image motion arising from head and body rotation which is compensated by optokinetic and vestibular eye reflexes. In order to serve the goal of optimal ego-motion compensa- tion, the gains of these reflexes need continuous adjustment ('adaptation') in order to be useful under a wide range of behavioural conditions. A major need for modification is introduced by the availability of a fovea and the emergence of foveating eye and head tracking movements. For instance, if a distant target is foveated, the ideal gain of the vestibulo-ocular reflex (VOR) is −1, i.e. the angular velocity of the eye movement is equal and opposite to that of the head. However, for geometrical reasons the ideal gain for a target brought closer to the head needs to be larger than −1 (Viirre et al., 1986). In fact, an even more profound modification of the VOR is prompted by active head move- ments made in order to track slowly moving objects of interest. Any attempt to track a moving target with the head would fail, if the head movement evoked an unrestricted VOR, moving the eyes into the opposite direction. In other words, a VOR response evoked by an active head movement must be cancelled ('VOR-cancellation' or 'VOR-suppression'). The VOR must also be cancelled if the observer's head is moved passively while she or he at the same time tries to fixate a head-stationary target. By the same token, the optokinetic reflex (OKR), normally evoked by self-induced background motion, must be suppressed when the background motion is due to smooth-pursuit eye or head movements ('OKR-suppression'). Numerous studies have indeed established the ability of both reflexes to rapidly adapt to the requirements of the behavioural conditions (Faulstich et al., 2004; Ito et al., 1977; Lindner and Ilg, 2006; Miles and Fuller, 1974). Actually, the modifications of the two reflexes are not independent. This is a consequence of the fact that the two reflexes share a common 'velocity storage' mechanism, responsible for the persistence of eye velocity in the absence of stimulation (Cannon and Robinson, 1987). Adaptation of the VOR is accompanied by changes of the velocity storage, causing a modified decay of the optokinetic after-nystagus after the termination of the optokinetic stimulus (Blazquez et al., 2007). Experimental lesions clearly indicate that all these various types of VOR-adaptation and -cancellation depend on the FR (Ito et al., 1982; Lisberger et al., 1984; Rambold et al., 2002a; Zee et al., 1981). Lesions of the FR also impair the OKR and smooth-pursuit eye move- ments (Barmack and Pettorossi, 1985; Zee et al., 1981). In fact, the extent of the smooth-pursuit deficit seems to correlate with the extent of the VOR adaptation and cancellation deficits (Rambold et al., 2002b; Zee et al., 1981). The study by Rambold and co-workers, moreover, suggests that the critical part of the FR is the ventral paraflocculus rather than the flocculus proper. Large lesions of the FR basically annihilate VOR-adaptation, documenting the outstanding role of this part of the cerebellum in mediating this particular function. However, even large lesions of the FR that encroach on the neighbouring dorsal paraflocculus leave a substantial capacity for smooth pursuit eye movements. This finding is in line with increasing evidence for a role of a parallel non-floccular/non-parafloccular pathway for smooth-pursuit involving the *oculomotor vermis* and parts of the hemispheres, discussed later.

CFs to the flocculus arise from the dorsal cap region of the inferior olive and are thought to convey information on retinal image slip derived from the nucleus of the optic tract (Kato et al., 1995; Langer et al., 1985a). Mossy fibre input arises from floccular projection neurons in the vestibular nuclei (Langer et al., 1985a). In turn, PCs project to a subset of neurons in the central vestibular pathway, the flocculus target neurons (Langer et al., 1985c). Prevailing models of the oculomotor role of the flocculus usually stress additional input from parieto-occipital cortex including areas MT and MST as sources of visual information on target and background motion as well as non-visual smooth-pursuit related signals, implicating the dorsolateral pontine nuclei as intermediary. However, while there is compelling evidence for a role of MT/MST and the dorsolateral pontine nucleus (DLPN) in smooth-pursuit as well as the OKR (Ilg and Thier, 2008; Thier and Möck, 2006) and the availability of pursuit-related signals in the flocculus (Miles and Fuller, 1975; Stone and Lisberger, 1990a, 1990b), the concept of a significant parieto-occipital–ponto-floccular pathway remains disputable. This is a consequence of the fact that the main projections of the DLPN are to the dorsal paraflocculus and to the *oculomotor vermis* rather than to the FR. DLPN input to the FR is comparatively weak and, moreover, confined to the ventral paraflocculus (Brodal, 1979; Glickstein et al., 1994; Kralj-Hans et al., 2007; Langer et al., 1985b; Nagao et al., 1997a; Thielert and Thier, 1993). Hence, it seems worth considering the alternative speculation that pursuit-related information to the flocculus might actually arise from pursuit-related secondary vestibular neurons, most probably representing the final premotor element in the pathway for smooth pursuit (Roy and Cullen, 2003). Such signals could be conveyed by the strong projection from the vestibular nuclei to the FR (Brodal and Brodal, 1985; Langer et al., 1985a).

Studies in monkeys suggest that the role of the FR in smooth-pursuit may be confined to the smooth eye movement component of visual tracking, whereas active head tracking movements seem to be independent of the FR. This is indicated by experiments, in which the squirrel monkey FR was transiently inactivated by injections of muscimol. These injections led to a reduction of the ipsilateral OKR as well as to a yoked bilateral impairment of smooth eye movements and the suppression of the VOR, evoked by passive head movement. On the other hand, they had little effect on smooth head tracking and no effect on the VOR gain (Belton and McCrea, 2000a, 2000b).

A role of the FR in the control of smooth-pursuit eye movements is consistent with the existence of two major types of floccular PCs that are driven by smooth eye-velocity. A first class of floccular PCs implicated in smooth-pursuit are the so-called gaze-velocity PCs (Krauzlis and Lisberger, 1994; Miles and Fuller, 1975; Nagao et al., 1997b). Their responses seemed to be best explained by assuming that they sum eye velocity relative to head and head velocity in the world in order to represent gaze velocity in a world-centred frame of reference: this assumption can account for the fact that these neurons are activated by smooth-pursuit with the head immobile as well as by VOR-cancellation or visuo-vestibular conflict stimulation. During VOR-cancellation, a normal VOR response to passive head movement is suppressed by asking subjects to fixate a head stationary target (Miles and Fuller, 1975). During visuo-vestibular conflict stimulation, the VOR is suppressed by rotating the optokinetic drum with the vestibular turntable (Büttner and Waespe, 1984). On the other hand, these cells show no or little response to head movements that evoke a compensatory VOR stabilizing the eyes in space. Gaze-velocity PCs were first described in rhesus monkeys and reported to be, on average, equally sensitive to eye and to head velocity, which of course would be needed in order to veridically encode gaze velocity (Lisberger and Fuchs, 1978; Miles et al., 1980). They are assumed to contact floccular target neurons in the vestibular nuclei, supplying them with the signals needed to drive eye pursuit and to cancel VOR responses evoked by passive head movements. However, later work on squirrel and Japanese monkeys has suggested that floccular PCs with equal sensitivities to eye and to head velocity are actually more the exception than the rule (Belton and McCrea, 2000a;

Fukushima et al., 1999). Actually, at the population level, at least in squirrel monkeys, their sensitivity to head velocity is only half of the one to eye velocity (Belton and McCrea, 2000a). This does not mean, though, that gaze velocity PCs could not help to cancel vestibularly evoked eye velocity commands in VOR pathways during VOR cancellation or to contribute to the generation of eye pursuit. A further argument against the existence of floccular gaze-velocity PCs in the strict sense comes from studies in which typical gaze-velocity PCs were subjected to optokinetic and visuo-vestibular conflict stimulation (Büttner and Waespe, 1984). The cells studied were modulated by 30°/s peak velocity sinusoidal smooth pursuit eye movements. However, none of them responded when the same slow eye movement velocity was evoked by an optokinetic stimulus, except for transient responses to the onset and offset of the optokinetic stimulus.

A second class of floccular pursuit-related PCs that has been distinguished from gaze velocity PCs are the so-called eye velocity PCs that are modulated by smooth-pursuit eye movement as well as by the slow, reflex eye movements evoked by passive head movements. Eye velocity PCs ignore active head movements (Belton and McCrea, 2000a, 2000b, 2004). This holds for smooth head-tracking movements as well as for head movements, which are part of saccadic gaze shifts. Saccadic gaze shifts are based on initial targeting eye and head shifts, which are followed by a continuation of the head movement in the direction of the initial shifts, accompanied by a vestibularly mediated rollback of the eyes in the opposite direction. Eye velocity PCs of squirrel monkeys are only 1/20 as responsive to this gaze saccade associated VOR as they are to the VOR evoked by passive head movements (Belton and McCrea, 2004).

The overall conclusion suggested by the recording and lesion studies is that the primate FR uses information on eye pursuit as well as optokinetic and vestibular signals in order to adjust the gain of vestibulo-ocular and optokinetic reflexes evoked by passive head movements according to the needs of the behavioural framework. It has been suggested that this modulatory function of the FR might be confined to horizontal and vertical eye movements, while the neighbouring uvula and nodulus (see below) might be in charge of controlling the third degree of oculomotor freedom, namely torsion. This view tries to accommodate the fact that goal-directed eye movements, whose interaction with the eye movement reflexes is accommodated by the FR, obey Listing's law, i.e. they lack torsion and can be fully described in two-dimensional retinal coordinates (Straumann et al., 1991). Wäspe and Henn have suggested that the modulatory role the FR exerts on the vestibulo-ocular and the optokinetic reflexes is based on a direct action of floccular output on neurons in the vestibular nuclei (the 'flocculus/central-vestibular neuron complementarity' concept; Waespe and Henn (1985)). On the other hand, the control of active head pursuit and the modification of the VOR associated with active head movements seem to be largely independent of the FR and may rely on other cerebellar circuits.

The clinical signs of cerebellar disease involving the FR are deviant VOR gains in conjunction with deficient VOR adaptation and deficient VOR suppression, impaired smooth pursuit eye movements, and, last but not least, gaze-evoked nystagmus, the latter consisting of sequences of eye drifts back towards the centre and saccades bringing the eyes back to the excentric position (Leigh and Zee, 1991). Gaze-evoked nystagmus is also observed after experimental cerebellar lesions involving the FR (Zee et al., 1981). The usual explanation of this disturbance is the assumption of an inappropriate 'step' input to motoneurons due to the flocculus lesion. Motoneurons fire an initial burst (the 'pulse' input) in order to move the eyes at high speed towards the desired location. A subsequent tonic discharge (the 'step' input) is needed to maintain a sufficient amount of muscular contraction to ensure that elastic forces will not passively drive the eyes back towards the centre. According to prevailing models of saccades (Fuchs et al., 1985), the pulse is contributed by short-lead burst neurons and the step by tonic neurons, which on their part reflect the integrated pulse. The sizes of the pulse and the step need to be adjusted precisely in order to guarantee precise saccades. Non-optimal pulses will result in over- or undershoots of the eyes, dysmetria, with the need to generate corrective saccades. Non-optimal steps will jeopardize gaze holding and lead to gaze-evoked nystagmus. After total cerebellectomy, both the pulse and the step gains become inappropriate and vary depending on initial eye position (Optican and Robinson, 1980). As described elsewhere in this chapter, there is compelling evidence that the optimization of the pulse relies on the *oculomotor vermis*. On the other hand, the adjustment of the step requires the FR (Optican and Robinson, 1980), which is thought to be part of a generic circuit for gaze holding and drift suppression based on the conversion of residual image slip signals into appropriate corrective signals. The idea that gaze holding after saccades is based on the minimization of retinal image slip would be in line with the general role of the FR in the optimization of oculomotor reflexes subserving image stability. The features of saccade-related signals in the FR may suggest a speculative mechanism explaining how this conversion of retinal image slip into corrective signals may be put into action. Noda and co-workers collected a large sample of saccade-related PCs from the flocculus and neighbouring ventral paraflocculus that was dominated by units that paused during saccades and, moreover, showed pre- and postsaccadic activity whose size seemed to depend on eye position (Noda and Suzuki, 1979). Unfortunately, the eye position dependency was not assessed quantitatively and, moreover, the relationship of these pause neurons to other oculomotor behaviours subserved by the FR remains unclear. Nevertheless, it seems tempting to speculate that the discharge of these neurons might actually be interpreted as step-related. This speculation is nourished by the demonstration of the eye position dependency of the pre- and postsaccadic discharge and the fact that pause duration reflects saccade duration, which in turn parallels the duration of the pulse, determined by non-floccular circuitry. It is, moreover, supported by the availability of saccade- and position-related mossy fibre input that may introduce information on the default step size. Unfortunately, it is not known if the saccade-related FR PCs receive information on the adequacy of the step which would be needed in order to mediate adjustments. According to prevailing concepts, we would assume that this information would be contributed by CF input, reflected in the pattern of CS. Unfortunately, the CS discharge of saccade-related FR PCs has never been studied in any detail.

Dorsal paraflocculus

Probably the first indication of a possible role of the paraflocculus in eye movements came from attempts to reveal the roles of the flocculus/paraflocculus by lesions. As in many cases lesions involved the ventral paraflocculus as well as parts of the dorsal paraflocculus, it seemed possible that the smooth pursuit eye movement deficit and other oculomotor disturbances observed after the lesion actually reflected the loss of the ventral and dorsal paraflocculus, rather than the destruction of the flocculus proper (Zee et al., 1981). As discussed in the preceding paragraph, later lesion work has indeed confirmed the expected role of the ventral paraflocculus in smooth pursuit eye movements (Rambold et al., 2002a). It has also provided evidence for a role of at least some parts of the dorsal paraflocculus in pursuit (Hiramatsu et al., 2008).

In order to assess the oculomotor role of the dorsal paraflocculus (DPF), a recapitulation of its connectivity seems pertinent. The DPF is characterized by a pattern of connections, it shares with its appendage, the lobulus petrosus, that differ significantly from those of the flocculus and the adjoining ventral paraflocculus. The CF input originates from parts of the rostral medial accessory olive and the principal olive, known to receive input from multiple brain areas involved in the control of eye, head, or limb movements such as the rostral interstitial nucleus of the medial longitudinal fasciculus or the interstitial nucleus of Cajal (Buttner-Ennever et al., 1982; Jeneskog, 1987). The mossy fibre input comes predominantly from different subdivisions of the pontine nuclei (Kralj-Hans et al., 2007; Xiong and Nagao, 2002), including the dorsal subdivisions, which comprise distinct patches of neurons involved in saccades and smooth pursuit and hand movements (Dicke et al., 2004; Mustari et al., 1988; Suzuki and Keller, 1984; Thier et al., 1988; Tziridis et al., 2009). The projections from the dorsal paraflocculus are to the ventral part of the dentate nuclei and the ventrolateral region of the posterior interpositus nucleus, the latter known to contain neurons that are active in conjunction with saccades and vergence movements of the eyes (Robinson, 2000; van Kan et al., 1993; Zhang and Gamlin, 1998). In sum, the connectivity of the dorsal paraflocculus suggests a role of this part of the cerebellum in saccades rather than a selective role in smooth pursuit eye movements. The few electrophysiological studies available indeed come up with this expectation.

Noda and Mikami (1986b) demonstrated rich oculomotor activity in a circumscribed part of the DPF adjoining the flocculus. About two-thirds of the PCs studied showed SS responses to saccades with most of the PCs firing saccade-related bursts. Others displayed pauses or more complex burst-pause patterns. Other less frequently observed PCs exhibited interest in smooth pursuit eye movements or in eye position. By and large, a similar distribution of oculomotor response types was observed in the mossy fibre input, which, moreover, involved a substantial proportion of visual fibres. Qualitatively, similar response types of PCs and mossy fibres including saccade-related responses have been described by the same group in the FR (Noda and Suzuki, 1979). However, pause cells seem to be much more dominant in the FR (see above). Moreover, the temporal precision of saccade-related bursts and pauses as well as the degree of direction selectivity may be less in the DPF. Hence, the differences in the response properties of neurons in the oculomotor region of the dorsal paraflocculus explored (see Fig. 10.2) and the FR as well as the differences in the afferent as well as the efferent connections support the notion of independent oculomotor roles. Because of its difficult accessibility, the properties of neurons in the monkey lobulus petrosus of the DPF remain unknown. However, an oculomotor function of this area is clearly indicated by a recent lesion study. Injecting the neurotoxin ibotenic acid, Hiramatsu et al. demonstrated severe, albeit partly transient smooth pursuit eye movement deficits. Unfortunately, the analysis of the saccadic system was confined to catch-up saccades, which were reported to remain unaffected (Hiramatsu et al., 2008).

Nodulus/uvula

The nodulus (=lobulus IX) and uvula (X) represent the inferior aspect of the vermis located in the immediate vicinity of the flocculus/paraflocculus complex with which they share the intimate relationship with the brainstem vestibular system (see Voogd and Barmack, 2006 for a review of connections). Our understanding of the functional role of the primate nodulus and uvula, referred to here for the sake of convenience as *inferior vermis*, is largely based on studies of lesions. A common denominator of the lesion effects may be the assumption that the *inferior vermis* helps to represent sensory information in an inertial frame of reference for the control of eye movements and, eventually, also for the control of stance and gait. This suggestion accommodates the observations that an intact *inferior vermis* is required to generate adequate torsional vestibulo-ocular and optokinetic responses (Angelaki and Hess, 1994) and that it is needed to adjust the time constant (Waespe et al., 1985) and the orientation of angular velocity storage (Angelaki and Hess, 1995). Furthermore, it is required to tilt-suppress postrotatory nystagmus (Wiest et al., 1999) and to facilitate horizontal and vertical translational VOR responses (Walker et al., 2008b). Finally, lesions of the *inferior vermis* cause a rather selective and actually quite severe impairment of downward smooth-pursuit of foveal targets while sparing the ocular following of large field visual backgrounds (Walker et al., 2008a). A specific role of the *inferior vermis* in vertical pursuit may reflect a dominance of connections with pre-and postcerebellar structures on their part emphasizing vertical eye movements (see for discussion Walker et al. (2008a)). These authors also suggest that the downward pursuit deficit after inferior vermal lesions may be functionally related to the frequent occurrence of downward nystagmus in patients suffering from vestibulo-cerebellar lesions (Glasauer et al., 2005).

The hemispheric oculomotor region

Evidence for oculomotor contributions of regions in the hemispheres in the vicinity of the *oculomotor vermis* comes from clinical and functional magnetic resonance imaging (fMRI) observations on the human cerebellum as well as from experimental work on non-human primates. Patients with lesions of the hemispheres sparing the deep cerebellar nuclei may show impaired smooth pursuit (Robinson et al., 1997). Smooth pursuit as well as saccade deficits are observed after surgical lesions of cerebellocortical regions outside the *oculomotor vermis*, centring on the hemispheric parts of the simple lobule involving hemispheric folia VI and VII (HVI, HVII): lesions impair the velocity of initial pursuit responses as well as smooth pursuit adaptation. Moreover, visually guided saccades are delayed and show increased amplitude variability (Ohki et al., 2009). A role in saccadic adaptation is suggested by the fact that visual errors that drive saccadic adaptation evoke BOLD responses in regions neighbouring the human *oculomotor vermis*, including HVI and HVII (van Broekhoven et al., 2009) rather than activating the *oculomotor vermis*. On the other hand, Golla and co-workers observed an impairment of saccadic adaptation only in patients with vermal pathology, and not in patients, in which the pathology was confined to the lateral cerebellum (Golla et al., 2008). In any case, the precise location and boundaries of the *hemispheric oculomotor region* remain ill defined. This is for instance indicated by the fact that Mano et al. (1991) could not find saccade-related SS responses of PCs in the simple lobule. Rather in this study, hemispheric saccade-related PCs were confined to Crus I and IIa, a part of the cerebellum that adjoins the simple lobule anteriorly. On the other hand, Mano et al. (1991) recorded saccade-related PC SS responses from Crus I and II as well as from the simple lobule. A hemispheric eye movement representation involving Crus I, II, as well as the simple lobule seems more in line with the extent of the cerebellar region whose electric stimulation at currents up to 1000 μAmp gives rise to evoked saccades (Ron et al., 1972). Tracer studies show that this region receives mossy fibre input from the frontal eye field through the dorsal pontine nuclei and the NRTP. On the other hand, it projects back to the frontal lobe via the dentate nucleus (Xiong et al., 2002). This pattern of connections may suggest a role in the cognitive control of eye movements, rather than in elementary visuomotor transformations or the shaping of motor signals. On the other hand, Mano et al. (1991) reported larger SS responses of saccade-related PCs in Crus IIa for visually triggered saccades as compared to self-determined, spontaneous saccades. In a similar vein, hardly compatible with a primary role cognitive control, is the fact that a substantial part of the CF input to hemispheric folium VII originates from the dorsal cap region of the inferior olive, also projecting to the flocculus and ventral flocculus, known to receive visual motion input from the nucleus of the optic tract (Kitazawa et al., 2009). Obviously, much more work will be needed in order to replace the vague concepts on the role of the *hemispheric oculomotor region* currently available by more specific hypotheses. Future work will also have to clarify if this fairly large region actually does not comprise several distinct areas.

Oculomotor vermis

A contribution of the posterior vermis and neighbouring regions of the cerebellum to saccades was originally suggested by experiments in which surgical lesions of this part of the cerebellum were carried out. For instance, Aschoff and Cohen (1971) observed fewer ipsiversive saccades after unilateral lesions of the cerebellar vermis and Ritchie (1976) reported dysmetric visually-guided saccades following lesions of the posterior vermis. Dysmetric saccades have also been reported in the clinical literature as a consequence of cerebellar pathology involving the human vermis due to disease (Botzel et al., 1993). Ron and Robinson (1973) were the first to demonstrate that electric stimulation of the posterior vermis and neighbouring regions of the hemispheres is able to evoke saccadic eye movements. While this early work using electric stimulation with currents of up to 1 mA suggested a quite extended saccade representation in the posterior cerebellum, seemingly in accordance with the lessons learned from studies of lesions, Noda and co-workers, by resorting to electric microstimulation, could show that the saccade representation was actually much smaller than hitherto assumed (Fujikado and Noda, 1987; Noda and Fujikado, 1987b; Noda et al., 1990; Yamada and Noda, 1987). When stimulation currents were kept below 10 μA, saccades could only be evoked from lobuli VIc and VIIA of the posterior vermis, the *oculomotor vermis* (OV) proper, but not from the adjoining regions of the vermis and paravermis. Moreover, Noda and co-workers could demonstrate that the stimulation effects were actually a consequence of directly activating Purkinje cell axons. This was indicated by three observations: firstly, stimulation thresholds were lowest in the white matter. Secondly, blocking PC synapses by injecting the GABA blocker bicuculline into the target area in the caudal fastigial nucleus prevented stimulation-evoked saccades. Thirdly, stimulation-evoked saccades were eliminated by destroying PCs and other cerebellocortical neurons by injecting the neurotoxin kainic acid (Noda and Fujikado, 1987a). As vermal afferents were not affected by this manipulation, this experiment clearly ruled out that evoked saccades were a consequence of antidromically activating the brainstem centres for saccades by way of mossy fibres (Noda and Fujikado, 1987b). The horizontal component of saccades evoked from the OV is typically directed to the ipsilateral side. Unlike natural saccades, those evoked by microstimulating the OV are usually more or less curved. This is a consequence of asynchronous onset, offset, and peak velocity times of the horizontal and vertical components (Fujikado and Noda, 1987). Moreover, these authors observed that the two components could be varied independently by altering stimulus intensity. This is important as it may suggest separate vermal channels for the control of the horizontal and vertical components. On the other hand, recordings from PCs (see below) have not revealed any anatomical segregation of preferred saccade directions. Their velocity is influenced by the frequency of stimulation and also their amplitude and duration are increased by stimulation duration.

The OV projects to the saccade representation in the caudal fastigial nucleus (cFN), which in turn contacts the brainstem centres for saccades (Noda et al., 1990; Yamada et al., 1996). The cFN contains saccade-related as well as pursuit-related neurons. The timing of the bursts of saccade-related neurons depends on the direction as well as the amplitude of the saccade executed with most neurons firing earlier for contraversive compared to ipsiversive saccades (Fuchs et al., 1993; Kleine et al., 2003; Ohtsuka and Noda, 1991). Unilateral inactivation of the cFN leads to ipsiversive saccadic hypermetria (amplitudes too large) and controversive saccadic hypometria (amplitudes too small) (Robinson et al., 1993). This loss of endpoint precision is accompanied by abnormalities in saccade kinematics (Goffart et al., 2004).

Lesions of the OV in monkeys cause a transient hypometria of saccades and a permanent loss of short-term saccadic adaptation, accompanied by an increase in endpoint variability (Fig. 10.3A) (Barash et al., 1999; Takagi et al., 1998). Patients suffering from midline lesions of their cerebellum show very similar deficits (Golla et al., 2008). Moreover, their adaptation deficit is accompanied by an inability to compensate 'saccadic fatigue': when asked to make long sequences of saccades, healthy subjects show a drop in peak velocity, which is compensated by an upregulation of saccade duration. Patients lack this velocity duration trade-off. This observation strongly suggests an important role of the OV in optimizing the duration of a saccadic eye movement, a conclusion which is in full accordance with the discharge properties of saccade-related Purkinje cells discussed further below. Permanent saccadic hypometria, usually taken as the key clinical signs of cerebellar disease does not result from lesions of the OV. Moreover, covert shifts of attention remain affected by such lesions (Golla et al., 2005; Ignashchenkova et al., 2009). On the other hand, they lead to clear disturbances of smooth pursuit, emphasizing the open-loop period of smooth-pursuit eye movements elicited by ramp-like movements of the target (Takagi et al., 2000). This loss of pursuit gain was accompanied by an impairment of the ability of the lesioned monkeys to adapt the initial pursuit response to changes of target velocity (Fig. 10.3B). In general, the severity of the pursuit deficits was comparable to the saccade disturbances resulting from the lesion, suggesting a common functional contribution of the OV to saccades as well as to smooth pursuit. Actually, a common role of the OV in both types of goal-directed eye movements is in accordance with the fact that it houses not only saccade-related but also smooth-pursuit-related PCs. In many cases, these cells can be driven by both saccades and by smooth-pursuit eye movements (Suzuki and Keller, 1988). Collectively, as a population, these pursuit-related PCs can fully account for the changes in eye movement kinematics resulting from smooth-pursuit adaptation (Dash et al. 2009). As summarized before, the lesion work suggests that the OV ensures precise saccades by optimizing saccade duration. As discussed below we think that the control of duration may be based on a PC SS population response whose end determines the end of the saccade (Catz et al., 2008; Thier et al., 2000).

When tested in the memory-saccade paradigm, in which centre-out saccades are made in darkness towards the remembered location of a cue, turned off a couple of 100ms before the saccade is carried out, most saccade-related posterior vermal PCs exhibit pure saccade-related SS bursts, whereas others may exhibit saccade-related pauses of their spontaneous SS discharge (see Fig. 10.4A for an example). In any case, they only rarely display visual responses or activity in the period of time, in which the monkey is waiting for the go-signal to start the saccade. Saccade-related responses of OV

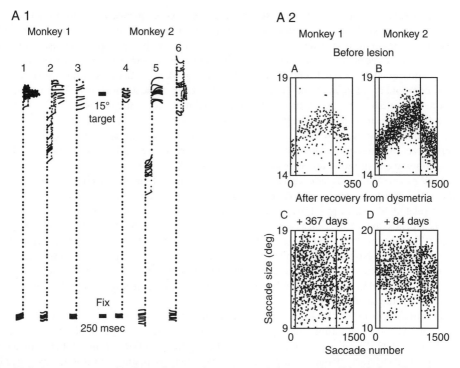

Fig. 10.3 Consequences of lesions of the *oculomotor vermis* for saccades (A1, A2; from Barash et al., 1999) and smooth pursuit eye movements (B; Takagi et al., 2000). A1) Exemplary visually guided saccades made before (1), early (2), and late (3) after an OV lesion. Note that the hypometria, obvious in the first days and weeks after the lesion (2), completely disappears after a few months (3). However, an increased variability of saccade end points remains. A2) Plots of saccade amplitude as function of trial number in a typical gain increase short-term saccadic adaptation experiment before and late after the lesion. Gain-increase adaptation was achieved by resorting to the classical McLaughlin paradigm (McLaughlin, 1967): the monkeys were presented a visual target at 15° excentricity which was shifted to 20° during the saccade. Initially the eyes land at 15° and a second, corrective saccade has to be added in order to bring the eyes to the final position of the target. However, in the course of the experiment, which involves many stereotypic repetitions of the target jump, the subjects learn to upregulate the amplitude of the first saccade, thereby bringing the eyes closer to the final position of the target and alleviating the need for a second saccade. Whereas the two monkeys showed the expected gain increase adaptation before the lesion, it was completely lost—probably permanently—after the lesion. Reproduced with permission of The Society for Neuroscience © 1999. B) Smooth-pursuit adaptation before and after OV lesions. In this particular experiment, initial pursuit velocity was adapted by doubling target velocity at the time the target reached the straight-ahead position. The dashed line describes the target position. Early after the activation of the velocity doubling the eyes are unable to keep up with the target as the visual delay prevents immediate reaction and the eye velocity is still determined by the lower target velocity seen 100 ms earlier. However, in the course of the adaptation experiment, pursuit gets better. This is a consequence of the fact that the gain of the conversion of the low target velocity before the velocity step is up-regulated. This adaptation is largely lost after the lesion and in general monkeys exhibit a significant decline in eye velocity post-lesion. Reproduced with permission of The American Physiological Society © 2000.

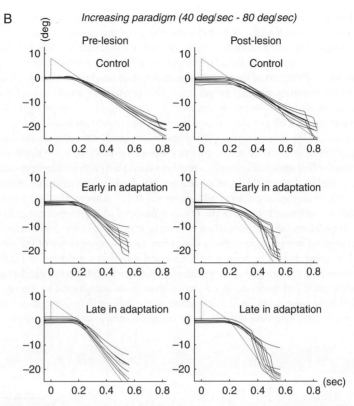

Fig. 10.3 (continued).

PCs are usually direction-selective. Saccade duration and amplitude are closely linked with saccade duration increasing linearly with amplitude for up to 40°. This tight linkage allows one to change saccade duration by simply asking monkeys to make saccades of different amplitude. When saccades of different amplitudes are carried out in the preferred direction of a given cell, the amplitude-dependency of the saccade-related bursts is highly idiosyncratic. Whereas some cells may show a monotonic increase in the number of spikes fired with increasing saccade amplitude, others show preferred amplitudes or no dependency on amplitude at all within a range of amplitudes up to 40°. In other words, one would most probably fail if one tried to determine the duration or amplitude of a saccade made by the monkey by monitoring the discharge pattern of individual OV PCs. Unlike individual cells, though, larger groups of these saccade-related Purkinje cells provide a precise signature of saccade duration and amplitude. This is suggested by the conspicuous relationship between saccade duration and the duration of the SS population burst, the instantaneous SS discharge rate of a larger group of saccade-related PCs, obtained by considering the timing of each spike fired by each cell in the sample. This population response (Fig. 10.4B) lasts longer, the longer the saccade lasts. Actually, the population signal ends exactly at the time the saccade ends, suggesting that there may be a causal relationship between the end of the population signal and the end of the saccade. The conclusion that individual PC's SS responses are not informative, whereas a SS population signal precisely determines the end of the saccade is fully supported by studies of gain-increase short-term saccadic adaptation. Recordings of SS of individual PCs during saccadic adaptation (Catz et al., 2008) typically reveal highly idiosyncratic changes, which in no case can be led back to changes in saccade kinematics accompanying the changes in saccade amplitude. In many cases these changes are dramatic as exemplified in Fig. 10.4A. This figure shows a SS unit, studied during gain increase adaptation, which started out as a saccade-related pause neuron. Towards the end of the adaptation period it had turned into a unit that fired a postsaccadic burst-tonic response only to gradually return to its pre-adaptation pause pattern in the course of the ensuing extinction period. Gain-increase adaptation increases saccade amplitude, largely because saccade duration increases. As shown in Fig. 10.4C, gain-increase adaptation shows the same precise relationship between the end of the saccade and the end of the population response as unadapted saccades. The difference is that the end of the population signal comes later. This is what one would expect if the end of the population signal determined the end of the saccade. This interpretation prompts three questions: 1) Is the assumption of a SS population signal encoding saccade duration biologically plausible? 2) If yes, how then can the time structure of the population signal be translated into the time structure of the saccade? 3) How does the time structure of the population signal adopt the shape needed?

The answer to the first question is that PCs must act collectively rather than in isolation as a simple consequence of the fact that several dozen up to a few hundred of them converge on individual target neurons in the deep cerebellar nuclei (Palkovits et al., 1977). This means that a cell in the caudal part of the fastigial nucleus, the target of the OV, is influenced by a compound signal, not too different from the population burst as described before. In other words, the population burst is not a mathematical artefact but most probably a direct functional consequence of the properties of the cerebellonuclear projection. The answer to the second question considers the GABAergic nature of this projection and the intriguing disposition of nuclear target neurons to fire postinhibitory bursts: the population burst will deliver a strong hyperpolarizing signal to the recipient nuclear neuron, probably turning it off while the saccade is carried out. *In vitro* studies have shown that nuclear neurons fire strong rebound bursts upon cessation of hyperpolarization as a consequence of

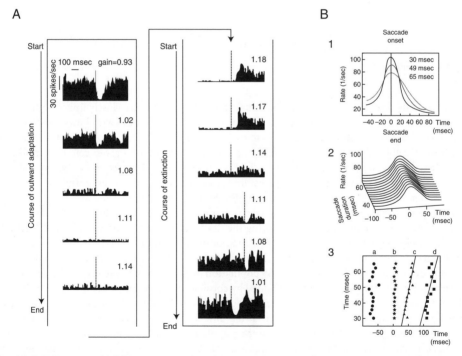

Fig. 10.4 A) Example of PC SS response studied during gain increase adaptation and subsequent recovery from adaptation (extinction). The individual histograms capture the response at different times during adaptation. The dashed line indicates saccade onset. The numbers on the right of each histogram give the saccadic gain (=saccade amplitude/target amplitude). Note the profound, but nevertheless fully reversible changes of the response pattern. From Catz et al., (2008). Copyright (2008) National Academy of Sciences, USA.

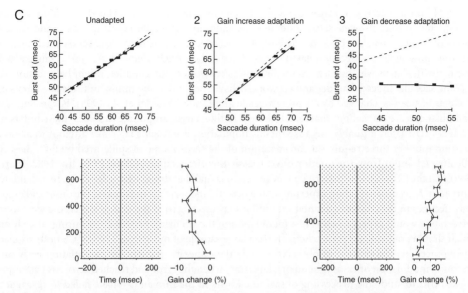

Fig. 10.4 (*continued*) B) 1) SS population burst profiles based on group of 94 saccade-related vermal PCs studied during normal, unadapted visually-guided saccades for three saccade durations of 30, 49, and 65 ms The population signal starts, independent of saccade duration, a couple of 10 ms before saccade onset, peaks right at saccade onset, again independent of saccade duration, and then declines. This decline takes the longer, the longer the saccade lasts (see also (3)). 2) The dependence of the duration of the population burst on saccade duration is not confined to the three durations shown in (1). (2) shows a pseudo three-dimensional plot of the population burst as function of saccade duration for a larger number of saccade durations. The x-axis plots the time relative to saccade onset at 0 ms, the y-axis saccade duration and the z-axis the mean instantaneous discharge rate of a population of 94 PCs. 3) Regression plots relating different parameters characterizing the population burst timing relative to the saccade. We measured the times of the onset (*a*), peak (*b*), and end (*c*) of the population burst relative to saccade onset for each saccade duration. (*d*) is the population burst duration given by *c–a*. We determined population onset and offset times as the times when the population burst reached four times the baseline firing rate when building up and when declining. The figure plots time t as a function of *a*, *b*, *c*, and *d*, respectively. In the case of *a*, *b* and *d*, t corresponds to saccade duration, in the case of *c* to the time of saccade termination. The plots are fitted by linear regressions. Both *c* and *d* increased significantly with the time of saccade termination and saccade duration, respectively, whereas neither *a* or *b* depended significantly on saccade duration. The end of the population burst (*c*) as predicted by the regression corresponds very closely to the end of the saccades. From Thier et al. (2002). Reproduced with permission of John Wiley and Sons © 2002. C) Effect of short-term saccadic adaptation on the end of the PC population burst. 1) Unadapted visually guided saccades: As shown in B3 (see parameter *c*) there is a tight correlation between saccade duration and the end of the population burst. 2) Gain increase adaptation: Saccade amplitudes are increased, but the same tight correlation is maintained. 3) Gain decrease adaptation: Saccade amplitude is decreased and the correlation between saccade duration and burst end is broken. The population burst now ends much earlier than the saccade, arguably too early to have a significant influence on the saccade. Saccades resulting from gain-decrease adaptation may actually be default saccades, not significantly influenced by a PC signal. From Catz et al. (2008). Copyright (2008) National Academy of Sciences, USA. D) The spiking activity of two exemplary saccade-related Golgi cells studied during gain-decrease (left) and gain-increase saccadic adaptation (right). Note that the discharge profiles do not change during adaptation. From Prsa et al. (2009). Reproduced with permission of The Society for Neuroscience © 2009.

hyperpolarization-activated mixed cation- and calcium-channels (Czubayko et al., 2001). If such rebound bursts were also generated under *in vivo* conditions, we would expect to see saccade-related bursts of nuclear neurons close to the end of a saccade. Actually, many saccade-related nuclear neurons show such late saccade-related bursts (Fuchs et al., 1993; Kleine et al., 2003; Ohtsuka and Noda, 1990), signals which if sent to the brainstem machinery for saccades, might help to stop an ongoing saccade. Indeed Scudder and co-workers have shown that the timing of these late bursts of cFN neurons can be changed by adapting saccade amplitude (Scudder et al., 1998). For instance, if manipulations are carried out that lead to longer lasting, larger amplitude saccades, these bursts in the cFN occur later, arguably, because the PC population input ends later. An attempt to answer question number three requires a consideration of the second type of spike fired by PCs, the CS, reflecting CF input from the inferior olive. Classic theories assume (Albus, 1971; Ito, 1982; Marr, 1969) that the CS discharge pattern conveys an error signal that drives motor learning. In a standard short-term saccadic adaptation experiment, the performance error is maximal at the onset and gradually declines in the course of adaptation until it may reach zero at the end. If the classic view were correct, one would expect to observe a modulation of the CS firing pattern early during adaptation which should gradually taper out. Actually, in a large sample of more than 170 OV CS units studied during saccadic adaptation, we observed exactly the opposite, namely, no modulation early but profound modulation of CS at the end of adaptation, when the error had reached zero. Also attempts to use fMRI to study the processing of saccadic errors in the human OV have failed to reveal any significant activity (van Broekhoven et al., 2009). On the other hand, CS are notoriously rare events, a fact that greatly diminishes the odds of detecting subtle, but nevertheless potentially informative changes in their firing statistics, let alone their reflections in the BOLD (blood oxygen-level dependent) response. Hence, it may be possible that the CS discharge of at least some PCs early during adaptation may hide information on the error and, actually, Soetedjo and Fuchs (2006) have reported an influence of a directional error in a small sample of 27 OV CS units studied. However, independent of the question if CS are influenced by saccadic errors or not, it is clear that OV CS exhibit a specific pattern of modulation that builds up in parallel with the development of saccadic adaptation, which is maximal at the end of adaptation that can be seen with the naked eye, without resorting to subtle statistical methods. Given the fact that the CS discharge is fully determined by the CF input, the conclusion is that adaptation-related information must be available at the level of group b of the medial inferior olivary nucleus (MAO), the source of CFs feeding the OV (Bowman and Sladek, 1973; Brodal and Brodal, 1981; Kitazawa, et al., 2009; Kralj-Hans, et al., 2007). This could be information that directly reflects the behavioural changes. Alternatively, it could be subliminal information on the performance error, amplified by an integration-like process accompanying the learning process. A potential source of information on saccadic errors impinging on the MAO are the deep layers of the superior colliculus, known to project to the MAO (Frankfurter et al., 1976; Harting, 1977). Amplification could be provided by feedback from PCs to the inferior olive by means of nucleo-olivary projections neurons in the cFN (Ikeda et al., 1989; see Sultan (2000), for general information on the internal architecture of the deep cerebellar nuclei). At any rate, in the case of gain-increase adaptation, the probability of observing CS decreases around the time of the saccade. Conversely, in the case of gain-decrease adaptation, leading to smaller amplitude saccade, the probability increases. The reciprocal changes of the CS responses during inward and outward adaptation may provide the key to understanding the specific role of the CS in saccadic learning. Maximal long-term depression (LTD) at parallel fibre synapses is observed when a CS occurs within 200 ms after simple spikes (Wang et al., 2000). Hence, the CS 'burst' during gain decrease adaptation that was found by Catz et al. (2005) to peak at −23 ms relative to saccade end might induce LTD if the saccade-related SS burst appeared between −220 and −20 ms relative to saccade offset. SS, which would normally have appeared in this period, would be suppressed. Consequently, the SS population signal would stop earlier. On the other hand, the suppression of CS during gain increase adaptation, maximal at −10 ms, might reduce LTD if the SS burst emerged between −210 and −10 ms, unleashing SS in this period and thereby extending the SS population signal. In other words, relative to non-adapted saccades, we would expect to see longer-lasting saccade-related SS activity in the case of gain increase adaptation, but shorter-lasting saccade-related SS activity for gain decrease adaptation. This is exactly what Catz et al. (2008) found in their study of SS activity during saccadic adaptation. Hence, specific changes of the CS discharge pattern may be responsible for behaviourally relevant changes in the SS population signal. In other words, we suggest that the PC SS population response develops the temporal structure needed based on CS facilitating the SS responses of individual PC whose timing is appropriate and, conversely, by suppressing those whose timing is inappropriate. Of course, for this mechanism to work, the spectrum of occurrences of individual SS responses is required to cover the full temporal range to be covered by the population signal. As SS responses depend on their parallel fibre input, which in turn reflects the mossy fibre input, the expectation is that the temporal dispersion of saccade-related mossy fibre activity is at least as wide as the temporal extent of the SS-PC signal. Actually, this expectation is surpassed as saccade-related mossy fibre signals cover a significantly wider range of times relative to the saccade. The same holds for the major interneuron, processing mossy fibre/parallel fibre input to PCs, the Golgi cell. Finally, saccade-related Golgi cell responses do not change as a consequence of saccadic adaptation (Prsa et al., 2009). This finding is important as it clearly indicates that learning-related changes do not take place before the level of the PC.

In a nutshell, these studies of the role of the OV in short-term saccadic adaptation suggest the hypothesis that the modification of the saccadic behaviour is based on sculpturing a PC SS population signal by selecting saccade-related mossy fibre/parallel fibre input from a wide spectrum of choices (Fig. 10.1B). The selection and the stabilization of selection are carried out by the CF system. The end of the population signal determines the size of the saccade by determining the end of the saccadic movement. The population signal may do more than that. Preliminary evidence suggests that the size of the population signal may influence saccade velocity. If this observation were confirmed, the population signal could rightly be regarded as a specific neuronal realization of an internal model fine-tuning saccade kinematics.

Conclusion

The cerebellum contributes to any type of eye movement mammals are able to perform. At first glance one might surmise a straightforward organization of the cerebellar cortex characterized by distinct regions devoted to specific types of eye movements. However, on closer scrutiny it becomes clear that distinct parts of the cerebellum actually accommodate specific *functional principles* involved in oculomotor control rather than types of eye movement. The need to prevent large field image slip on the retina is a case in point: this need has functional implications for types of eye movements as diverse as saccades, smooth pursuit, or the VOR. This is why the floccular region, the key cerebellar structure implicated in the prevention of large field image slip, contributes to all of them. By the same token, the oculomotor vermis is involved in saccades as well as in smooth pursuit initiation, most probably reflecting the common need to control an initial movement pulse. Given the highly stereotypic architecture of cerebellar cortex, it may be firmly assumed that one and the same *computational principle* underlies these cerebellar contributions to the distinct functional building blocks of eye movements. For the same reason, we may feel certain that insights on the computational principle accommodated by cerebellar cortex, provided by studies of eye movements, will be generally valid for any function supported by this most intriguing part of the mammalian brain.

References

Albus, J.S. (1971). A theory of cerebellar function. *Mathematical Biosciences*, 10, 25–61.

Angelaki, D.E. and Hess, B.J. (1994). The cerebellar nodulus and ventral uvula control the torsional vestibulo-ocular reflex. *Journal of Neurophysiology*, 72(3), 1443–1447.

Angelaki, D.E. and Hess, B.J. (1995). Lesion of the nodulus and ventral uvula abolish steady-state off-vertical axis otolith response. *Journal of Neurophysiology*, 73(4), 1716–1720.

Aschoff, J.C. and Cohen, B. (1971). Changes in saccadic eye movements produced by cerebellar cortical lesions. *Experimental Neurology*, 32(2), 123–133.

Barash, S., Melikyan, A., Sivakov, A., Zhang, M., Glickstein, M., and Thier, P. (1999). Saccadic dysmetria and adaptation after lesions of the cerebellar cortex. *Journal of Neuroscience*, **19**(24), 10931–10939.

Barmack, N.H. (2006). Inferior olive and oculomotor system. *Progress in Brain Research*, **151**, 269–291.

Barmack, N.H. and Pettorossi, V.E. (1985). Effects of unilateral lesions of the flocculus on optokinetic and vestibuloocular reflexes of the rabbit. *Journal of Neurophysiology*, **53**(2), 481–496.

Belton, T. and McCrea, R.A. (2000a). Role of the cerebellar flocculus region in cancellation of the VOR during passive whole body rotation. *Journal of Neurophysiology*, **84**(3), 1599–1613.

Belton, T. and McCrea, R.A. (2000b). Role of the cerebellar flocculus region in the coordination of eye and head movements during gaze pursuit. *Journal of Neurophysiology*, **84**(3), 1614–1626.

Belton, T. and McCrea, R.A. (2004). Context contingent signal processing in the cerebellar flocculus and ventral paraflocculus during gaze saccades. *Journal of Neurophysiology*, **92**(2), 797–807.

Blazquez, P.M., Davis-Lopez de Carrizosa, M.A., Heiney, S.A., and Highstein, S.M. (2007). Neuronal substrates of motor learning in the velocity storage generated during optokinetic stimulation in the squirrel monkey. *Journal of Neurophysiology*, **97**(2), 1114–1126.

Botzel, K., Rottach, K., and Buttner, U. (1993). Normal and pathological saccadic dysmetria. *Brain*, **116**(Pt 2), 337–353.

Bowman, J. and Sladek, J. J. (1973). Morphology of the inferior olivary complex of the rhesus monkey (macaca mulatta). *Journal of Computational Neurology*, **152**, 299–316.

Brodal, P. (1979). The pontocerebellar projection in the rhesus monkey: an experimental study with retrograde axonal transport of horseradish peroxidase. *Neuroscience*, **4**, 193–208.

Brodal, A. and Brodal, P. (1985). Observations on the secondary vestibulocerebellar projections in the macaque monkey. *Experimental Brain Research*, **58**(1), 62–74.

Brodal, P. and Brodal, A. (1981). The olivocerebellar projection in the monkey. Experimental studies with the method of retrograde tracing of horseradish peroxidase. *Progress in Brain Research*, **201**(3), 375–393.

Büttner, U. and Waespe, W. (1984). Purkinje cell activity in the primate flocculus during optokinetic stimulation, smooth pursuit eye movements and VOR-suppression. *Experimental Brain Research*, **55**, 97–104.

Buttner-Ennever, J.A., Buttner, U., Cohen, B., and Baumgartner, G. (1982). Vertical glaze paralysis and the rostral interstitial nucleus of the medial longitudinal fasciculus. *Brain*, **105**(Pt 1), 125–149.

Cannon, S.C. and Robinson, D.A. (1987). Loss of the neural integrator of the oculomotor system from brain stem lesions in monkey. *Journal of Neurophysiology*, **57**(5), 1383–1409.

Catz, N., Dicke, P., and Thier, H.-P. (2005). Cerebellar complex spike firing is suitable to induce as well as to stabilize motor learning. *Current Biology*, **15**, 2179–2189.

Catz, N., Dicke, P.W., and Thier, P. (2008). Cerebellar-dependent motor learning is based on pruning a Purkinje cell population response. *Proceedings of the National Academy of Sciences U S A*, **105**(20), 7309–7314.

Czubayko, U., Sultan, F., Thier, P., and Schwarz, C. (2001). Two types of neurons in the rat cerebellar nuclei as distinguished by membrane potentials and intracellular fillings. *Journal of Neurophysiology*, **85**(5), 2017–2029.

Dash, S.C., Nicolas, C., Dicke, P.W. (2009). A vermal Purkine cell simple spike population response encodes the changes in eye movements kinematics during smooth pursuit adaptation. *Society for Neuroscience*, **660**, 27.

Dicke, P.W., Barash, S., Ilg, U.J., and Thier, P. (2004). Single-neuron evidence for a contribution of the dorsal pontine nuclei to both types of target-directed eye movements, saccades and smooth-pursuit. *European Journal of Neuroscience*, **19**(3), 609–624.

Faulstich, B.M., Onori, K.A., and du Lac, S. (2004). Comparison of plasticity and development of mouse optokinetic and vestibulo-ocular reflexes suggests differential gain control mechanisms. *Vision Research*, **44**(28), 3419–3427.

Frankfurter, A., Weber, J.T., Royce, G.J., Strominger, N.L., and Harting, J.K. (1976). An autoradiographic analysis of the tecto-olivary projection in primates. *Brain Research*, **118**, 245–257.

Fuchs, A.F., Kaneko, C.R., and Scudder, C.A. (1985). Brainstem control of saccadic eye movements. *Annual Review of Neuroscience*, **8**, 307–337.

Fuchs, A.F., Robinson, F.R., and Straube, A. (1993). Role of the caudal fastigial nucleus in saccade generation. I. Neuronal discharge pattern. *Journal of Neurophysiology*, **70**(5), 1723–1740.

Fujikado, T., and Noda, H. (1987). Saccadic eye movements evoked by microstimulation of lobule VII of the cerebellar vermis of macaque monkeys. *Journal of Physiology*, **394**, 573–594.

Fukushima, K., Fukushima, J., Kaneko, C.R., and Fuchs, A.F. (1999). Vertical Purkinje cells of the monkey floccular lobe: simple-spike activity during pursuit and passive whole body rotation. *Journal of Neurophysiology*, **82**(2), 787–803.

Glasauer, S., Hoshi, M., and Buttner, U. (2005). Smooth pursuit in patients with downbeat nystagmus. *Annals of the New York Academy of Sciences*, **1039**, 532–535.

Glickstein, M., Gerrits, N., Kralj-Hans, I., Mercier, B., Stein, J., and Voogd, J. (1994). Visual pontocerebellar projections in the macaque. *Journal of Comparative Neurology*, **349**, 51–72.

Goffart, L., Chen, L.L., and Sparks, D.L. (2004). Deficits in saccades and fixation during muscimol inactivation of the caudal fastigial nucleus in the rhesus monkey. *Journal of Neurophysiology*, **92**(6), 3351–3367.

Golla, H., Thier, P., and Haarmeier, T. (2005). Disturbed overt but normal covert shifts of attention in adult cerebellar patients. *Brain*, **128**(Pt 7), 1525–1535.

Golla, H., Tziridis, K., Haarmeier, T., Catz, N., Barash, S., and Thier, P. (2008). Reduced saccadic resilience and impaired saccadic adaptation due to cerebellar disease. *European Journal of Neuroscience*, **27**(1), 132–144.

Hamori, J. and Szentagothai, J. (1966). Identification under the electron microscope of climbing fibers and their synaptic contacts. *Experimental Brain Research*, **1**(1), 65–81.

Harting, J.K. (1977). Descending pathways from the superior colliculus: an autoradiographic analysis in the rhesus monkey (Macaca mulatta). *Journal of Comparative Neurology*, **173**, 583–612.

Highstein, S.M. and Holstein, G.R. (2006). The anatomy of the vestibular nuclei. *Progress in Brain Research*, **151**, 157–203.

Hillman, D.E. (1969). Morphological organization of frog cerebellar cortex: a light and electron microscopic study. *Journal of Neurophysiology*, **32**(6), 818–846.

Hiramatsu, T., Ohki, M., Kitazawa, H., Xiong, G., Kitamura, T., Yamada, J., et al. (2008). Role of primate cerebellar lobulus petrosus of paraflocculus in smooth pursuit eye movement control revealed by chemical lesion. *Neuroscience Research*, **60**(3), 250–258.

Ignashchenkova, A.D., Dash, S., Dicke, P.W., Haarmeier, T., Glickstein, M., and Thier, P. (2009). Normal spatial attention but impaired saccades and visual motion perception after lesions of the monkey cerebellum. *Journal of Neurophysiology*, **102**, 3156–3168.

Ikeda, Y., Noda, H., and Sugita, S. (1989). Olivocerebellar and cerebellooivary connections of the oculomotor region of the fastigial nucleus in the macaque monkey. *Progress in Brain Research*, **284**(3), 463–488.

Ilg, U.J. and Thier, P. (2008). The neural basis of smooth pursuit eye movements in the rhesus monkey brain. *Brain and Cognition*, **68**(3), 229–240.

Ito, M. (1982). Cerebellar control of the vestibulo-ocular reflex—around the flocculus hypothesis. *Annual Review of Neurosciences*, **5**, 275–296.

Ito, M. (1984). *The cerebellum and neural control.* New York: Raven Press.

Ito, M., Nisimaru, N., and Yamamoto, M. (1977). Specific patterns of neuronal connexions involved in the control of the rabbit's vestibulo-ocular reflexes by the cerebellar flocculus. *Journal of Physiology*, **265**(3), 833–854.

Ito, M., Jastreboff, P. J., and Miyashita, Y. (1982). Specific effects of unilateral lesions in the flocculus upon eye movements in albino rabbits. *Experimental Brain Research*, **45**(1–2), 233–242.

Jeneskog, T. (1987). Termination in posterior and anterior cerebellum of a climbing fibre pathway activated from the nucleus of Darkschewitsch in the cat. *Brain Research*, **412**(1), 185–189.

Kato, I., Watanabe, S., Sato, S., and Norita, M. (1995). Pretectofugal fibers from the nucleus of the optic tract in monkeys. *Brain Research*, **705**(1–2), 109–117.

Kitazawa, H., Xiong, G., Hiramatsu, T., Ohki, M., and Nagao, S. (2009). Difference of climbing fiber input sources between the primate oculomotor-related cerebellar vermis and hemisphere revealed by a retrograde tracing study. *Neuroscience Letters*, **462**(1), 10–13.

Kleine, J. F., Guan, Y., and Buttner, U. (2003). Saccade-related neurons in the primate fastigial nucleus: what do they encode? *Journal of Neurophysiology*, **90**(5), 3137–3154.

Kralj-Hans, I., Baizer, J.S., Swales, C., and Glickstein, M. (2007). Independent roles for the dorsal paraflocculus and vermal lobule VII of the cerebellum in visuomotor coordination. *Experimental Brain Research*, **177**(2), 209–222.

Krauzlis, R.J., and Lisberger, S.G. (1994). Simple spike responses of gaze velocity Purkinje cells in the floccular lobe of the monkey during the onset and offset of pursuit eye movements. *Journal of Neurophysiology*, **72**(4), 2045–2050.

Langer, T., Fuchs, A.F., Scudder, C.A., and Chubb, M.C. (1985a). Afferents to the flocculus of the cerebellum in the rhesus macaque as revealed by retrograde transport of horseradish peroxidase. *Progress in Brain Research*, **235**(1), 1–25.

Langer, T., Fuchs, A.F., Scudder, C.A., and Chubb, M.C. (1985b). Afferents to the flocculus of the cerebellum in the rhesus macaque as revealed by retrograde transport of horseradish peroxidase. *Journal of Comparative Neurology*, **235**, 1–25.

Langer, T., Fuchs, A.F., Chubb, M.C., Scudder, C.A., and Lisberger, S.G. (1985c). Floccular efferents in the rhesus macaque as revealed by autoradiography and horseradish peroxidase. *Progress in Brain Research*, **235**(1), 26–37.

Leigh, R.J. and Zee, D.S. (1991). *The neurology of eye movements* (2nd edn.). Philadelphia, PA: F.A. Davis Company.

Lindner, A. and Ilg, U.J. (2006). Suppression of optokinesis during smooth pursuit eye movements revisited: the role of extra-retinal information. *Vision Research*, **46**(6–7), 761–767.

Lisberger, S.G. and Fuchs, A.F. (1978). Role of primate flocculus during rapid behavioral modification of vestibuloocular reflex. I. Purkinje cell activity during visually guided horizontal smooth-pursuit eye movements and passive head rotation. *Journal of Neurophysiology*, **41**(3), 733–763.

Lisberger, S.G., Miles, F.A., and Zee, D.S. (1984). Signals used to compute errors in monkey vestibuloocular reflex: possible role of flocculus. *Journal of Neurophysiology*, **52**(6), 1140–1153.

Madigan, J.C., and Carpenter, M.B. (1971). *Cerebellum of the rhesus monkey; atlas of lobules, laminae, and folia, in sections.* Baltimore, MA: University Park Press.

Mano, N., Ito, Y., and Shibutani, H. (1991). Saccade-related Purkinje cells in the cerebellar hemispheres of the monkey. *Experimental Brain Research*, **84**(3), 465–470.

Marr, D. (1969). A theory of cerebellar cortex. *Journal of Physiology*, **202**(2), 437–470.

McLaughlin, S. (1967). Parametric adjustment in saccadic eye movements. *Perception and Psychophysics*, **2**(8), 358–362.

Miles, F.A., and Fuller, J.H. (1974). Adaptive plasticity in the vestibulo-ocular responses of the rhesus monkey. *Brain Research*, **80**(3), 512–516.

Miles, F.A., and Fuller, J.H. (1975). Visual tracking and the primate flocculus. *Science*, **189**(4207), 1000–1002.

Miles, F.A., Fuller, J.H., Braitman, D.J., and Dow, B.M. (1980). Long-term adaptive changes in primate vestibuloocular reflex. III. Electrophysiological observations in flocculus of normal monkeys. *Journal of Neurophysiology*, **43**(5), 1437–1476.

Mustari, M. J., Fuchs, A. F., and Wallman, J. (1988). Response properties of dorsolateral pontine units during smooth pursuit in the rhesus monkey. *Journal of Neurophysiology*, **60**, No.2, 664–686.

Nagao, S., Kitamura, T., Nakamura, N., Hiramatsu, T., and Yamada, J. (1997a). Differences of the primate flocculus and ventral paraflocculus in the mossy and climbing fiber input organization. *Progress in Brain Research*, **382**(4), 480–498.

Nagao, S., Kitamura, T., Nakamura, N., Hiramatsu, T., and Yamada, J. (1997b). Differences of the primate flocculus and ventral paraflocculus in the mossy and climbing fiber input organization. *Journal of Comparative Neurology*, **382**, 480–498.

Napper, R.M., and Harvey, R.J. (1988). Number of parallel fiber synapses on an individual Purkinje cell in the cerebellum of the rat. *Progress in Brain Research*, **274**(2), 168–177.

Noda, H., and Fujikado, T. (1987a). Involvement of Purkinje cells in evoking saccadic eye movements by microstimulation of the posterior cerebellar vermis of monkeys. *Journal of Neurophysiology*, **57**(5), 1247–1261.

Noda, H. and Fujikado, T. (1987b). Topography of the oculomotor area of the cerebellar vermis in macaques as determined by microstimulation. *Journal of Neurophysiology*, **58**(2), 359–378.

Noda, H. and Mikami, A. (1986a). Discharges of neurons in the dorsal paraflocculus of monkeys during eye movements and visual stimulation. *Journal of Neurophysiology*, **56**(4), 1129–1146.

Noda, H. and Mikami, A. (1986b). Discharges of neurons in the dorsal paraflocculus of monkeys during eye movements and visual stimulation. *Journal of Neurophysiology*, **56**(4), 1129–1146.

Noda, H., and Suzuki, D.A. (1979). The role of the flocculus of the monkey in saccadic eye movements. *Journal of Physiology*, **294**, 317–334.

Noda, H., Sugita, S., and Ikeda, Y. (1990). Afferent and efferent connections of the oculomotor region of the fastigial nucleus in the macaque monkey. *Progress in Brain Research*, **302**(2), 330–348.

Ohki, M., Kitazawa, H., Hiramatsu, T., Kaga, K., Kitamura, T., Yamada, J., *et al.* (2009). Role of primate cerebellar hemisphere in voluntary eye movement control revealed by lesion effects. *Journal of Neurophysiology*, **101**(2), 934–947.

Ohtsuka, K. and Noda, H. (1990). Direction-selective saccadic-burst neurons in the fastigial oculomotor region of the macaque. *Experimental Brain Research*, **81**(3), 659–662.

Ohtsuka, K. and Noda, H. (1991). Saccadic burst neurons in the oculomotor region of the fastigial nucleus of macaque monkeys. *Journal of Neurophysiology*, **65**(6), 1422–1434.

Optican, L.M. and Robinson, D.A. (1980). Cerebellar-dependent adaptive control of primate saccadic system. *Journal of Neurophysiology*, **44**(6), 1058–1076.

Palkovits, M., Mezey, E., Hamori, J., and Szentagothai, J. (1977). Quantitative histological analysis of the cerebellar nuclei in the cat. I. Numerical data on cells and on synapses. *Experimental Brain Research*, **28**(1–2), 189–209.

Prsa, M., Dash, S., Catz, N., Dicke, P.W., and Thier, P. (2009). Characteristics of responses of Golgi cells and mossy fibers to eye saccades and saccadic adaptation recorded from the posterior vermis of the cerebellum. *Journal of Neuroscience*, **29**(1), 250–262.

Rambold, H., Churchland, A., Selig, Y., Jasmin, L., and Lisberger, S.G. (2002a). Partial ablations of the flocculus and ventral paraflocculus in monkeys cause linked deficits in smooth pursuit eye movements and adaptive modification of the VOR. *Journal of Neurophysiology*, **87**, 912–924.

Rambold, H., Churchland, A., Selig, Y., Jasmin, L., and Lisberger, S.G. (2002b). Partial ablations of the flocculus and ventral paraflocculus in monkeys cause linked deficits in smooth pursuit eye movements and adaptive modification of the VOR. *Journal of Neurophysiology*, **87**(2), 912–924.

Ritchie, L. (1976). Effects of cerebellar lesions on saccadic eye movements. *Journal of Neurophysiology*, **39**(6), 1246–1256.

Robinson, F.R. (2000). Role of the cerebellar posterior interpositus nucleus in saccades I. Effect of temporary lesions. *Journal of Neurophysiology*, **84**(3), 1289–1302.

Robinson, F.R., Straube, A., and Fuchs, A.F. (1993). Role of the caudal fastigial nucleus in saccade generation. II. Effects of muscimol inactivation. *Journal of Neurophysiology*, **70**(5), 1741–1758.

Robinson, F.R., Straube, A., and Fuchs, A.F. (1997). Participation of caudal fastigial nucleus in smooth pursuit eye movements. II. Effects of muscimol inactivation. *Journal of Neurophysiology*, **78**(2), 848–859.

Ron, S. and Robinson, D.A. (1973). Eye movements evoked by cerebellar stimulation in the alert monkey. *Journal of Neurophysiology*, **36**(6), 1004–1022.

Ron, S., Robinson, D.A., and Skavenski, A.A. (1972). Saccades and the quick phase of nystagmus. *Vision Research*, **12**(12), 2015–2022.

Roy, J.E. and Cullen, K.E. (2003). Brain stem pursuit pathways: dissociating visual, vestibular, and proprioceptive inputs during combined eye-head gaze tracking. *Journal of Neurophysiology*, **90**(1), 271–290.

Scudder, C.A., Batourina, E.Y., and Tunder, G.S. (1998). Comparison of two methods of producing adaptation of saccade size and implications for the site of plasticity. *Journal of Neurophysiology*, **79**(2), 704–715.

Soetedjo, R. and Fuchs, A.F. (2006). Complex spike activity of purkinje cells in the oculomotor vermis during behavioral adaptation of monkey saccades. *Journal of Neuroscience*, **26**(29), 7741–7755.

Stone, L.S. and Lisberger, S.G. (1990a). Visual responses of Purkinje cells in the cerebellar flocculus during smooth-pursuit eye movements in monkeys. I. Simple spikes. *Journal of Neurophysiology*, **63**(5), 1241–1261.

Stone, L.S. and Lisberger, S.G. (1990b). Visual responses of Purkinje cells in the cerebellar flocculus during smooth-pursuit eye movements in monkeys. II. Complex spikes. *Journal of Neurophysiology*, **63**(5), 1262–1275.

Straumann, D., Haslwanter, T., Hepp-Reymond, M.-C., and Hepp, K. (1991). Listing's law for eye, head and arm movements and their synergistic control. *Experimental Brain Research*, **86**, 209–215.

Sultan, F.M., Möck, M., and Thier, P. (2000). Functional architecture of the cerebellar system. In T. Klockgether (ed.) *Handbook of Ataxia Disorders* (Vol. 50, pp. 1–52). New York, Basel: Marcel Dekker, Inc.

Suzuki, D.A. and Keller, E.L. (1984). Visual signals in the dorsolateral pontine nucleus of the alert monkey: their relationship to smooth-pursuit eye movements. *Experimental Brain Research*, **53**, 473–478.

Suzuki, D.A. and Keller, E.L. (1988). The role of the posterior vermis of monkey cerebellum in smooth-pursuit eye movement control. I. Eye and head movement-related activity. *Journal of Neurophysiology*, **59**(1), 1–18.

Takagi, M., Zee, D.S., and Tamargo, R.J. (1998). Effects of lesions of the oculomotor vermis on eye movements in primate: saccades. *Journal of Neurophysiology*, **80**(4), 1911–1931.

Takagi, M., Zee, D.S., and Tamargo, R.J. (2000). Effects of lesions of the oculomotor cerebellar vermis on eye movements in primate: smooth pursuit. *Journal of Neurophysiology*, **83**(4), 2047–2062.

Thielert, C.-D. and Thier, P. (1993). Patterns of projections from the pontine nuclei and the nucleus reticularis tegmenti pontis to the posterior vermis in the rhesus monkey: a study using retrograde tracers. *Journal of Comparative Neurology*, **337**, 113–126.

Thier, P. and Möck, M. (2006). The oculomotor role of the pontine nuclei and the nucleus reticularis tegmenti pontis. *Progress in Brain Research*, **151**, 293–320.

Thier, P., Koehler, W., and Buettner, U.W. (1988). Neuronal activity in the dorsolateral pontine nucleus of the alert monkey modulatet by visual stimuli and eye movements. *Experimental Brain Research*, **70**, 496–512.

Thier, P., Dicke, P.W., Haas, R., and Barash, S. (2000). Encoding of movement time by populations of cerebellar Purkinje cells. *Nature*, **405**(6782), 72–76.

Thier, P., Dicke, P.W., Haas, R., Thielert, C.D., and Catz, N. (2002). The role of the oculomotor vermis in the control of saccadic eye movements. *Annals of the New York Academy of Sciences*, **978**, 50–62.

Tziridis, K., Dicke, P.W., and Thier, P. (2009). The role of the monkey dorsal pontine nuclei in goal-directed eye and hand movements. *Journal of Neuroscience*, **29**(19), 6154–6166.

van Broekhoven, P.C., Schraa-Tam, C.K., van der Lugt, A., Smits, M., Frens, M.A., and van der Geest, J.N. (2009). Cerebellar contributions to the processing of saccadic errors. *Cerebellum*, **8**(3), 403–415.

van Kan, P.L., Gibson, A.R., and Houk, J.C. (1993). Movement-related inputs to intermediate cerebellum of the monkey. *Journal of Neurophysiology*, **69**(1), 74–94.

Viirre, E., Tweed, D., Milner, K., and Vilis, T. (1986). A reexamination of the gain of the vestibuloocular reflex. *Journal of Neurophysiology*, **56**(2), 439–450.

Voogd, J. and Barmack, N.H. (2006). Oculomotor cerebellum. *Progress in Brain Research*, **151**, 231–268.

Waespe, W. and Henn, V. (1985). Cooperative functions of vestibular nuclei neurons and floccular Purkinje cells in the control of nystagmus slow phase velocity: single cell recordings and lesion studies in the monkey. *Reviews of Oculomotor Research*, **1**, 233–250.

Waespe, W., Cohen, B., and Raphan, T. (1985). Dynamic modification of the vestibulo-ocular reflex by the nodulus and uvula. *Science*, **228**, 199–202.

Walker, M.F., Tian, J., Shan, X., Tamargo, R.J., Ying, H., and Zee, D.S. (2008a). Lesions of the cerebellar nodulus and uvula impair downward pursuit. *Journal of Neurophysiology*, **100**(4), 1813–1823.

Walker, M.F., Tian, J., Shan, X., Tamargo, R.J., Ying, H., and Zee, D.S. (2008b). Lesions of the cerebellar nodulus and uvula in monkeys: effect on otolith-ocular reflexes. *Progress in Brain Research*, **171**, 167–172.

Wang, S.S., Denk, W., and Hausser, M. (2000). Coincidence detection in single dendritic spines mediated by calcium release. *Nat Neurosci*, **3**(12), 1266–1273.

Wiest, G., Deecke, L., Trattnig, S., and Mueller, C. (1999). Abolished tilt suppression of the vestibulo-ocular reflex caused by a selective uvulo-nodular lesion. *Neurology*, **52**(2), 417–419.

Xiong, G. and Soichi, N. (2002). The lobulus petrosus of the paraflocculus relays cortical visual inputs to the posterior interposed and lateral cerebellar nuclei:an anterograde and retrograde tracing study in the monkey. *Experimental Brain Research*, **147**, 252–263.

Xiong, G. and Nagao, S. (2002). The lobulus petrosus of the paraflocculus relays cortical visual inputs to the posterior interposed and lateral cerebellar nuclei: an anterograde and retrograde tracing study in the monkey. *Experimental Brain Research*, **147**(2), 252–263.

Xiong, G., Hiramatsu, T., and Nagao, S. (2002). Corticopontocerebellar pathway from the prearcuate region to hemispheric lobule VII of the cerebellum: an anterograde and retrograde tracing study in the monkey. *Neuroscience Letters*, **322**(3), 173–176.

Yamada, J. and Noda, H. (1987). Afferent and efferent connections of the oculomotor cerebellar vermis in the macaque monkey. *Progress in Brain Research*, **265**(2), 224–241.

Yamada, T., Suzuki, D. A., and Yee, R. D. (1996). Smooth pursuitlike eye movements evoked by microstimulation in macaque nucleus reticularis tegmenti pontis. *Journal of Neurophysiology*, **76**(5), 3313–3324.

Zee, D.S., Yamazaki, A., Butler, P.H., and Gucer, G. (1981). Effects of ablation of flocculus and paraflocculus of eye movements in primate. *Journal of Neurophysiology*, **46**(4), 878–899.

Zhang, H. and Gamlin, P.D. (1998). Neurons in the posterior interposed nucleus of the cerebellum related to vergence and accommodation. I. Steady-state characteristics. *Journal of Neurophysiology*, **79**(3), 1255–1269.

CHAPTER 11

The superior colliculus

Brian J. White and Douglas P. Munoz

Abstract

The mammalian superior colliculus (SC) serves the crucial function of guiding and coordinating the orienting response. Integrating multisensory, motor, and cognitive information, and sending motor commands directly to the brainstem circuitry, the SC initiates a rapid orienting response that can invoke much of the body. The phylogenetic preservation of this structure illustrates its ongoing significance for survival, but for higher mammals, evolutionary pressure for flexible control over orienting behaviour coincided with development of a much more complex set of corticotectal projections. As a result, orienting in higher mammals (e.g. primates) is controlled by a careful interplay between sensory-driven and goal-driven processes that converge in the SC. This review focuses on the SC as a critical locus for this interaction, whereby one compartment fits the role of a visual saliency map, and another a priority map that represents the integration of salience and behavioural relevance.

Introduction

Located on the dorsal surface of the midbrain, the mammalian SC is ideally situated to guide and coordinate orienting behaviour. By integrating multiple sources of sensory, motor, and cognitive signals, and in turn sending motor commands directly to the brainstem circuitry, the SC initiates a rapid orienting response that can invoke the eyes, neck, and shoulder muscles (Akert, 1949; Boehnke and Munoz, 2008; Corneil et al., 2008; Dean et al., 1989; Hess et al., 1946; Ingle, 1983; Pruszynski et al., 2010; Sokolov, 1963). For primates, the flexible control over orienting behaviour is essential, and resulted in the development of a more complex set of corticotectal projections compared with earlier mammals. In this review we highlight key findings that have emerged in predominantly primate research since earlier reviews of the SC have appeared (Krauzlis, 2005; Munoz et al., 2000; Robinson and McClurkin, 1989; Schiller, 1977; Sparks, 1986; Sparks and Hartwich-Young, 1989; Wurtz and Albano, 1980). We build off an idea first developed by Edwards and others (Casagrande et al., 1972; Edwards, 1980) that the mammalian SC represents two largely independent structures with functionally distinct roles. One compartment is consistent with the role of a *salience map*, where salience is defined as the sensory qualities that make a stimulus distinctive from its surroundings. The other compartment is consistent with the role of a *priority map* (Boehnke and Munoz, 2008; Fecteau and Munoz, 2006; Serences and Yantis, 2006), where priority is defined as the integration of visual salience and behavioural relevance, the relative importance of a stimulus for the goal of the observer.

We have two main aims: 1) we present an up-to-date summary of the intrinsic and extrinsic circuitry of the SC, primarily but not exclusively as it relates to the monkey, focusing on key aspects of laminar organization; 2) we outline the main functions of the SC, highlighting key findings that are changing and expanding our view of the SC for the flexible control of orienting behaviour.

Superior colliculus structure

SC layers

The mammalian SC is a laminated structure consisting of seven anatomically distinct layers that have been traditionally grouped into two functional regions (Edwards, 1980; Sprague, 1975), a *superficial* region concerned exclusively with visual processing (Goldberg and Wurtz, 1972a), and a *deeper* region concerned with multisensory (Meredith and Stein, 1983, 1985; Stein and Meredith, 1993), motor (Robinson, 1972; Sparks, 1978; Wurtz and Goldberg, 1971), and higher-level cognitive processes (Fig. 11.1A). The superficial layers consist of the three dorsal most laminae, residing within approximately the top 1 mm of the collicular surface: the *stratum zonale* (SZ), the *stratum griseum superficiale* (SGS), and the *stratum opticum* (SO). The deeper layers refer to the remaining four lower laminae: the *stratum griseum intermediale* (SGI), the *stratum album intermediale* (SAI), the *stratum griseum profundum* (SGP), and the *stratum album profundum* (SAP). The cytological and physiological characteristics of deeper layer SC cells are virtually indistinguishable from the underlying reticulum, and very different from superficial layer SC cells. So much so that the deeper layers have instead been considered to be part of the reticular core (Edwards, 1980), challenging the view of the SC as a unified structure. In this review we will highlight important functional differences between the superficial (SGS and SO) and intermediate (SGI and SAI) layers of the SC, which we henceforth refer to as the SCs and SCi, respectively.

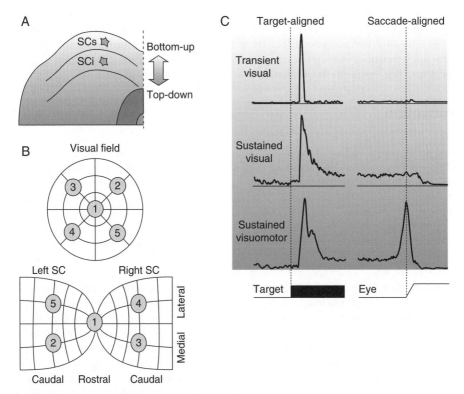

Fig. 11.1 The primate SC. A) Transverse view of the SC highlighting the superficial (SCs) and intermediate (SCi) layers. The progression from top to bottom represents a shift from mostly bottom-up towards increasing top-down processes. B) Topography of the correspondence between visual space (top) and SC space (bottom). C) Common response properties of SC neurons along the progression from the superficial to intermediate SC layers.

SC maps

Topographic maps are a central organizing principle of the brain, and play a crucial role in spatially-guided behaviour. It has long been known that neurons within the SC are organized into well-defined topographic maps, whereby each colliculus contains multisensory (Groh and Sparks, 1996; Jay and Sparks, 1987; Meredith and Stein, 1983, 1985; Stein and Meredith, 1993), and motor (Robinson, 1972; Sparks, 1978; Wurtz and Goldberg, 1971) representations of contralateral space (Fig. 11.1B). For example, the SCs contains a visual map such that a given neuron at a specific location on the map responds to stimuli presented in a restricted region of the contralateral visual field, which defines a receptive field (Cynader and Berman, 1972). The SCi on the other hand has both multisensory and motor representations, such that local stimulation of neurons at a given location on the map causes the eyes to move with a fixed vector of a specific direction and amplitude (Robinson, 1972). In terms of the visual and motor representations, the rostral, caudal, medial, and lateral SC represent the fovea, periphery, upper, and lower visual fields, respectively (Fig. 11.1B). As a general principle, the central region of vision defining the high acuity fovea has a much greater neural representation than the periphery (Van Essen et al., 1984). The same is true for the SC in which about one-third of its surface is devoted to the central 10° of visual angle (Cynader and Berman, 1972; Robinson, 1972; Schiller and Stryker, 1972). As such, the size of response fields in the SC increase as one moves from the rostral pole (representing the fovea) caudally (representing the periphery). The transformation of two-dimensional (2D) visual space into SC space is well understood (Cynader and Berman, 1972; Marino et al., 2008; Robinson, 1972; Schiller and Stryker, 1972), and can be best described by a logarithmic scaling factor (Ottes et al., 1986; Van Gisbergen et al., 1987). Furthermore, there is close spatial correspondence between the visual and motor representations in the SC (Marino et al., 2008).

SCs inputs and outputs

The SCs receives visual inputs from two primary sources (Fig. 11.2): 1) a direct projection from the retina (the retinotectal pathway) (Cowey and Perry, 1980; Hubel et al., 1975; Pollack and Hickey, 1979); and 2) direct projections from visual cortex, specifically primary visual cortex (V1), V2, V3, V4, and middle temporal area (MT) (Cusick, 1988; Fries, 1984; Graham, 1982; Lock et al., 2003; Tigges and Tigges, 1981; see Harting et al., 1992 for a detailed anatomical study of corticotectal projections in the cat). The retinotectal projection is most dense in the upper 200 μm (Hubel et al., 1975), and there is evidence that the progression from earlier to later cortical visual areas is represented by increasing depth in the SCs, with the V1 projection overlapping the retinotectal in the upper part of the SCs, and higher cortical visual areas projecting progressively deeper (Kawamura et al., 1974; Shipp, 2004; Sprague, 1975; Tigges and Tigges, 1981).

While visual activity in the primate SCs has been shown to persist after a temporary 'lesion' of visual cortex via cortical-cooling (Schiller et al., 1974), the retinotectal pathway has been somewhat superseded by a growing reliance on visual cortex in higher mammals. For example, the relative number of retinotectal fibres has systematically decreased with the increasing evolutionary elaboration of the geniculostriate system, with ratios of retinal fibres projecting to the SCs and LGN (lateral geniculate nucleus) that range from 3:1 in hamsters, to 2:1 in rats, and 1:8 in rhesus monkeys (Schiller, 1977). In short, for phylogenetically older mammals, the SC acted as the primary centre for visual analyses, a role that has been increasingly assigned to new areas of extrastriate visual cortex that have evolved in higher mammals, especially primates.

The primate SCs has three dominant outputs: the pulvinar complex (Berman and Wurtz, 2010; Casanova, 2004; Stepniewska et al., 2000), the LGN (Harting et al., 1978; Mathers, 1971), and intrinsic vertical connections with the SCi (Behan and Appell, 1992; Helms et al., 2004; Isa, 2002; Isa et al., 1998; Isa and Saito, 2001). The SCs projects to all layers of the pulvinar, and the magnocellular and interlaminar layers of the LGN, but the exact nature of these projections is not completely understood. Via such pathways, however, the SCs has substantial projections back into most of the extrastriate visual cortex, which places it in an ideal position to influence incoming visual signals as they enter the rest of the brain. The intrinsic vertical connection between the SCs and the premotor layers

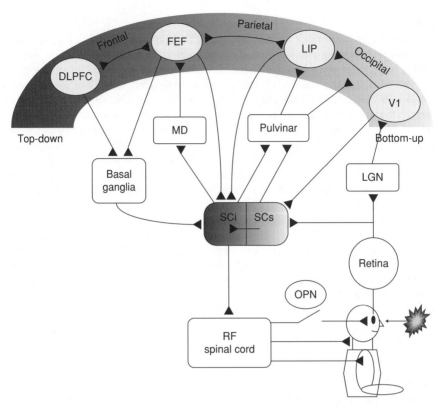

Fig. 11.2 Dominant extrinsic and intrinsic circuitry of the primate SC. Shading from light to dark represents the gradual shift from bottom-up to top-down processes respectively. DLPFC, dorsal lateral prefrontal cortex; FEF, frontal eye field; LIP, lateral intraparietal area; V1, primary visual cortex; MD, medial dorsal nucleus of the thalamus; LGN, lateral geniculate nucleus; RF, reticular formation; OPN, brainstem omnipause neuron region; SCs, superior colliculus superficial layers; SCi, superior colliculus intermediate layers.

of the SCi (Behan and Appell, 1992; Helms et al., 2004; Isa, 2002; Isa et al., 1998; Isa and Saito, 2001) has been proposed to mediate visually-guided orienting, and might act as an important locus for the interaction between sensory (bottom-up) and goal-related (top-down) processes (Dorris et al., 2007; Fecteau and Munoz, 2006; Olivier et al., 1999; Trappenberg et al., 2001).

SCi inputs and outputs

Compared to the SCs, the primate SCi receives a broader set of corticotectal projections (Fig. 11.2) from occipital, temporal, parietal, and frontal cortices (Cusick, 1988; Fries, 1984; Kunzle and Akert, 1977; Kunzle et al., 1976; Lock et al., 2003; see Harting et al., 1992 for corticotectal projections in the cat). These include lateral intraparietal area (LIP) (Lynch et al., 1985), the frontal eye fields (FEFs) (Kunzle and Akert, 1977; Kunzle et al., 1976; Stanton et al., 1995; Stanton et al., 1988), supplementary eye fields (SEFs) (Huerta and Kaas, 1990; Shook et al., 1990), dorsolateral prefrontal cortex (DLPFC) (Goldman and Nauta, 1976), and anterior cingulate cortex (ACC) (Leichnetz et al., 1981). The LIP-SCi projection carries both visual and motor-related information (Paré and Wurtz, 1997, 2001), and given LIP's role in covert spatial attention (Bisley and Goldberg, 2003, 2006; Goldberg et al., 2002, 2006; Ipata et al., 2006), it likely carries important signals in this regard as well. In terms of frontal projections, these may be thought of as representing the highest level top-down control to the SCi, and these inputs are critical for the flexible control of oculomotor behaviour (Everling and Munoz, 2000; Hanes and Wurtz, 2001; Johnston and Everling, 2006a, 2006b, 2008; Johnston et al., 2007; Segraves and Goldberg, 1987). A large proportion of SCi neurons have visual responses, but it is not absolutely clear whether these arise from direct projections from visual cortex, and/or the SCs, and/or through areas LIP or FEF. Nonetheless, corticotectal inputs appear to be crucial for visual activity in the SCi because visual responses are abolished when visual cortex is temporarily inactivated via cortical cooling (Schiller et al., 1974).

The SCi also receives important subcortical projections from the basal ganglia (Kunzle and Akert, 1977), cerebellum and brainstem (Edwards et al., 1979). The basal ganglia represent a group of substrates involved in the control of purposive motor behaviour, learning, and reward (Hikosaka et al., 2000, 2006). The primary means through which the basal ganglia influence the SCi is through direct inhibitory projections from the substantia nigra pars reticulata (SNr), an important output node of the basal ganglia (Jayaraman et al., 1977). The nigrotectal projection is believed to regulate saccadic burst initiation by imposing a blanket of tonic GABAergic inhibition over the SCi (Hikosaka, 1989; Hikosaka et al., 2000, 2006; Wurtz and Hikosaka, 1986), the release of which allows the SCi to trigger downstream premotor circuitry to drive the appropriate orienting response.

In terms of outputs, the SCi projects to the paramedian pontine reticular formation (PPRF) and rostral interstitial nucleus of the medial longitudinal fasciculus (riMLF) where the horizontal and vertical saccade premotor circuitry is located (Moschovakis et al., 1988; Rodgers et al., 2006; Sparks, 2002). The SCi also projects to the substantia nigra pars compacta (SNc) (Comoli et al., 2003; McHaffie et al., 2006). This projection carries transient visual activity to the basal ganglia dopaminergic system (Comoli et al., 2003), and is critical for reinforcing the context/actions that immediately precedes biologically relevant visual events (Dommett et al., 2005; Redgrave and Gurney, 2006). The SCi also projects to the FEF via the mediodorsal thalamus, MDN (Lynch et al., 1994; Sommer and Wurtz, 2004a). This projection serves to relay an internal copy (i.e. corollary discharge) of the saccadic motor command back to cortex immediately prior to movement onset to provide warning of an impending eye movement so that visual representations may be updated (Sommer and Wurtz, 2004b, 2006). This is thought to be responsible for maintaining our stable view of the world in the face of the rapid shifts of the visual axis caused by rapid eye movements (Sommer and Wurtz, 2006, 2008a, 2008b).

Finally, there is anatomical evidence of long-range connections within the SCi (Behan and Kime, 1996). There is also pharmacological (Meredith and Ramoa, 1998) and electrophysiological (Munoz and Istvan, 1998) evidence for a lateral inhibitory network across the SCi (see, however, Lee and Hall (2006)), whereby neurons with different spatial tuning functions are interconnected and compete in a push-pull relationship (Munoz and Istvan, 1998; Saito and Isa, 2004). Lateral inhibition is key to a winner-take-all mechanism that has been central to theories of visual attention and visual search (Itti and Koch, 2001; Treisman and Gelade, 1980; Wolfe et al., 1989; Wolfe and Horowitz, 2004), by controlling the allocation of overt/covert spatial attention via restricting all but one spatial location from reaching threshold. We elaborate on these important functions in the next section.

Superior colliculus function

SCs response properties

SCs neurons have been described as exclusively visual, with a characteristic transient visual response (Cynader and Berman, 1972; Goldberg and Wurtz, 1972a; Schiller and Koerner, 1971). That is, these neurons show a short, high-frequency, burst of action potentials as early as 40 ms following the appearance of a visual stimulus in their response field (a region of space in which the presence of a stimulus affects the firing of that neuron) (Fig. 11.1C). Other visual neurons typically found deeper in the SCs are the quasi-visual neurons described by Mays and Sparks (1980), and the tonic- or sustained-visual neurons described by McPeek and others (Li and Basso, 2008; McPeek and Keller, 2002;

White et al., 2009) (Fig. 11.1C). These neurons show an initial transient burst of action potentials followed by a lower frequency sustained firing pattern while a stimulus is present in the neuron's response field. They do not however show a burst of action potentials associated with a saccade that is characteristic of SCi neurons (Mays and Sparks, 1980; McPeek and Keller, 2002). It is not absolutely clear whether these neurons belong to the lower region of the SCs or the upper region of the SCi, but they are typically found above neurons with saccade-related activity (Li and Basso, 2008; Mays and Sparks, 1980; McPeek and Keller, 2002).

Like neurons throughout many areas of the visual system, SCs neurons are highly sensitive to stimulus intensity (Bell et al., 2006; Li and Basso, 2008). Despite large projections from visual cortex (Fries, 1984; Lock et al., 2003), SCs neurons show little preference for specific visual features, but there is evidence of some broad direction-of-motion tuning (Goldberg and Wurtz, 1972a), possibly arising from convergent projections from visual area MT (Fries, 1984; Lock et al., 2003), which is highly selective for visual motion (Born and Bradley, 2005). Similarly, SCs neurons show little preference for specific colours (Marrocco and Li, 1977; Schiller and Malpeli, 1977), and were thought to be driven exclusively from the broadband, achromatic visual pathway in early vision (the magnocellular path) (Schiller et al., 1979). However, recently we (White et al., 2009) found that the sustained-type of SC visual neurons are highly sensitive to luminant and isoluminant colour stimuli (i.e. isoluminant with the background). This suggests that they receive converging signals originating from both the broadband (magnocellular) and colour-opponent divisions of the geniculostrate pathway.

SCi response properties

SCi neurons have a much broader range of response properties than SCs neurons, owing to the fact that they integrate multisensory, motor, and cognitive signals from multiple cortical and subcortical brain areas (Fig. 11.2). Many SCi neurons (i.e. visuomotor neurons) discharge a burst of action potentials approximately 50 ms following the appearance of a visual stimulus in the neuron's response field, and a separate burst of action potentials associated with the occurrence of a saccade (Mohler and Wurtz, 1976) (Fig. 11.1C). The visual response of SCi neurons are also similar to SCs neurons in that they are highly sensitive to variations in stimulus luminance (Bell et al., 2006; Li and Basso, 2008), and often respond equally well to isoluminant colour stimuli (White et al., 2009). Saccade-related neurons in the SCi discharge action potentials for a range of saccade amplitudes and directions that define a movement field, the region of space to which a directed saccade affects the firing of that neuron (Munoz and Wurtz, 1995a; Sparks, 1978; Sparks and Mays, 1980; Wurtz and Goldberg, 1972a). Many neurons in the SCi have clearly defined closed movements fields. However, some saccade neurons discharge action potentials for all saccades equal to or greater in amplitude than their optimal, and these have been referred to as open-ended movement fields because they lack a distal border (Munoz et al., 1991a, 1991b; Munoz and Wurtz, 1995a, 1995b). A consequence of these open ended fields is that activity may move across the SC during the saccade as a hill or wave. This hypothesis generated vigorous debate and experimentation in the field and much follow-up work has failed to support the hypothesis (Anderson et al., 1998; Moschovakis et al., 2001; Soetedjo et al., 2002). However, experiments conducted on animals with head unrestrained have yielded the most convincing evidence to support this hypothesis (Choi and Guitton, 2006, 2009; Munoz et al., 1991a, 1991b; but see Freedman and Sparks, 1997).

There is also a close spatial correspondence between the visual and motor response fields of SCi neurons (Marino et al., 2008). This ensures that a visual response is mapped directly onto the appropriate SCi output neurons projecting to the brainstem premotor circuitry to trigger a saccade (Rodgers, Munoz, Scott, and Paré, 2006) and/or orienting head movement (Corneil et al., 2007; Corneil et al., 2002, 2004) to the visual stimulus.

Finally, a distinctive characteristic of many SCi neurons is 'prelude' or 'build-up' activity that precedes the saccade (Glimcher and Sparks, 1992; Munoz and Wurtz, 1995a). This low-frequency activity can begin well in advance of the movement itself and is associated with motor preparation

(Corneil et al., 2007; Dorris et al., 1997; Dorris and Munoz, 1998; Li and Basso, 2008; Munoz and Wurtz, 1995a), as well as various high-level processes such as a covert shift of attention (Ignashchenkova et al., 2004; Kustov and Robinson, 1996), expectation (Basso and Wurtz, 1997, 1998; Thevarajah et al., 2009), and target selection (Basso and Wurtz, 1997, 1998; Glimcher and Sparks, 1992; Horwitz and Newsome, 1999, 2001; McPeek and Keller, 2002).

Rostral SC responses

The rostrolateral pole of the SC contains the foveal and parafoveal representation of visual space (Fig. 11.1B) (Cynader and Berman, 1972; Robinson, 1972; Schiller and Stryker, 1972). Within the SCs, there are neurons with very small visual receptive fields that include the fovea. Within the SCi there is a continuation of the motor map (Hafed et al., 2009; Krauzlis et al., 1997), and at the rostral pole of the SCi there are neurons that discharge tonically during fixation and pause for most saccades, except very small contraversive saccades (Krauzlis, 2003; Munoz and Wurtz, 1993a, 1993b). These neurons have been labelled fixation neurons because of their tonic discharge recorded during periods of active fixation that persists without a visual stimulus (Dorris and Munoz, 1995; Munoz and Wurtz, 1993b). This tonic fixation-related activity is enhanced in an antisaccade task (Everling et al., 1999), when strong saccade suppression is necessary prior to target appearance. Most fixation neurons also increase their discharge for small contraversive saccades (Krauzlis, 2003; Munoz and Wurtz, 1993a) and neurons in the rostral SCi have now been shown to discharge for microsaccades (Hafed et al., 2009). Microstimulation of the extreme rostral SC has been shown to delay saccade initiation (Munoz and Wurtz, 1993b) and even interrupt ongoing saccades (Munoz et al., 1996). In addition, microinjection of the GABAA agonist muscimol into the rostral SC impairs the ability to delay saccades to suddenly appearing visual stimuli (Munoz and Wurtz, 1993b) (implying a critical role in saccade suppression), but it also impairs the ability to generate microsaccades (Hafed et al., 2009).

Recent findings suggest the rostral SC also plays a role in pursuit eye movements (Basso et al., 2000; Krauzlis and Dill, 2002; Krauzlis, 2001, 2003, 2004a, 2004b; Krauzlis et al., 2000), the smooth continuous movements of the eyes as they track a moving stimulus to keep it fixed on the fovea. Unlike saccades which can be guided by a range of visual and non-visual signals, pursuit eye movements are traditionally believed to be driven by visual motion signals mediated via substrates that are selective for motion (e.g. area MT and MST; Ilg (2008), Ilg and Thier (2003)), which then project to the motor nuclei via the cerebellum to initiate the movement (Krauzlis, 2004b). While the rostral SC lacks the motion tuning necessary to guide pursuit, recent findings suggest the pursuit system relies on much of the same circuitry as the saccade system (Krauzlis, 2004a), of which the rostral SC is an important component. One potential role of the rostral SC for pursuit is that the tonic activity associated with these neurons convey information about the position error between the tracked stimulus and the currently foveated position (Krauzlis et al., 2000), which is corroborated by microstimulation and inactivation experiments of the rostral SC during pursuit (Basso et al., 2000).

Finally, there is some evidence that the rostral SC is also involved in vergence eye movements (Chaturvedi and van Gisbergen, 1999, 2000; Suzuki et al., 2004; Van Horn et al., 2008), which serve to move the eyes in opposite directions in order to foveate stimuli at different depths.

SC and express saccades

Express saccades represent the fastest visually triggered eye movements with saccadic reaction times (SRT) that approach the minimal afferent (~50 ms) and efferent (~20 ms) limits (Fischer and Boch, 1983; Fischer and Ramsperger, 1984). They are believed to be produced when the incoming visual signal to the SCi is transformed directly into the saccade motor command (Dorris et al., 1997; Edelman and Keller, 1996). Express saccades are facilitated during a 'gap' paradigm (Saslow, 1967), in which a fixation spot is removed a few hundred milliseconds before the onset of a saccade target.

The early removal of the fixation spot is associated with a decrease in fixation-related activity at the rostral pole of the SC (Dorris and Munoz, 1995; Munoz and Wurtz, 1993b). Simultaneously, there is disinhibition of saccade-related neurons elsewhere in the SC, leading to an increase in low frequency build-up activity at loci that may drive the next saccade (Dorris and Munoz, 1998; Munoz and Wurtz, 1995a). This elevates the system closer to response threshold which when coupled with the target-evoked visual response can trigger express saccades.

SC lateral interactions

The saccade system is believed to be governed by a winner-take-all mechanism, which serves to restrict only one spatial location as the locus of visual attention/eye movements at any given moment. Such a mechanism has been central for theories of visual attention and visual search (Itti and Koch, 2001; Treisman and Gelade, 1980; Wolfe et al., 1989; Wolfe and Horowitz, 2004). A key component of a winner-take-all mechanism is a lateral inhibitory network that operates across the visual field (e.g. the maps in the SC, Fig. 11.1). At a given moment, two or more regions of distally represented activity on the SC map (generated by two or more discrete stimuli) are believed to compete in a winner-take-all manner, only one of which reaches the threshold necessary to evoke a saccade (Trappenberg et al., 2001). However, if the regions of activity are in close proximity on the SC map, their activity is mutually excitatory, pushing the saccade system closer to response threshold (Dorris et al., 2007; Trappenberg et al., 2001), and evoking even faster responses that are sometimes directed towards the centre-of-gravity of the two stimuli (Edelman and Keller, 1998; Findlay, 1982).

There is anatomical evidence for long-range connections within the SCi (Behan and Kime, 1996). There is also neurophysiological (Dorris et al., 2007; Munoz and Istvan, 1998) and pharmacological (Meredith and Ramoa, 1998) support for the existence of lateral inhibitory mechanisms in the SCi. However, a major criticism of these studies is that electrical stimulation can evoke inhibitory responses by activating axons of passage from GABAergic cell populations that project to the SC, e.g. nigrotectal projections, which are believed to impose a blanket of tonic GABAergic inhibition over the SCi (Hikosaka, 1989; Hikosaka et al., 2000, 2006; Wurtz and Hikosaka, 1986). A study using slice preparations failed to find support for the long-range inhibition hypothesized to exist across the SCi (Lee and Hall, 2006). However, slice preparations can damage long-range intracollicular fibres, and more recent slice work did find strong evidence for lateral inhibition across both the SCs (Phongphanphanee et al., 2009) and SCi (Isa et al., 2009).

An extrinsic source of inhibition that can support a winner-take-all mechanism is the nigrotectal projection. This projection is believed to regulate saccadic burst initiation by imposing a blanket of tonic GABAergic inhibition over the SCi (Hikosaka, 1989; Hikosaka et al., 2000, 2006; Wurtz and Hikosaka, 1986). The release of this inhibition allows the SCi to trigger the brainstem saccade generator. Recently, Jiang and colleagues (Jiang et al., 2003) described characteristics of the ipsilateral and contralateral nigrotectal pathway. Neurons comprising the ipsilateral projection may deliver spatially specific disinhibition to the SCi because they are tonically active (~100 Hz), and there is a discrete pause in their discharge for voluntary contraversive saccades to a restricted region of the visual field (Hikosaka and Wurtz, 1983). The function of the projection from the SNr to the contralateral SCi is less clear because it has only been studied in anesthetized animals (Jiang et al., 2003). Neurons that comprise the contralateral projection have tonic activity that increases following visual stimulation anywhere in the contralateral visual hemifield, and they have large termination fields in the contralateral SCi (Jiang et al., 2003). This suggests that these neurons may produce spatially global inhibition of the contralateral SCi. This type of global suppression signal is hypothesized to be required for successful suppression of the automatic prosaccade in the antisaccade task (Munoz and Everling, 2004).

SCs and salience

Salience refers to the sensory qualities that make a stimulus distinctive or conspicuous from its surroundings (e.g. a rapidly flickering bright red light against a dim stationary background). The concept of a visual salience map, a 2D representation of salience across the visual field, has been central to theories of visual attention and visual search (Itti and Koch, 2000, 2001; Treisman and Gelade, 1980; Wolfe et al., 1989). The salience map is believed to integrate the outputs of various visual feature maps, each representing a unique visual attribute such as intensity, motion, flicker, colour, orientation, etc. (Itti and Koch, 2001). The more salient the stimulus, the more likely it is to capture our attention (Theeuwes, 2004).

Several brain areas have been allocated the role of a visual salience map, for example visual area V1 (Koene and Zhaoping, 2007; Li, 2002; Zhaoping and May, 2007), V4 (Mazer and Gallant, 2003), LIP (Goldberg et al., 2006; Gottlieb, 2007; Gottlieb et al., 1998; Kusunoki et al., 2000), FEF (Thompson and Bichot, 2005; Thompson et al., 2005), and pulvinar (Robinson and Petersen, 1992). Several lines of evidence implicate the SCs as a particularly crucial component in this regard (Fecteau and Munoz, 2006). First, a visual salience map should be mostly concerned with the low-level visual attributes of a visual scene. Of course, top-down expectations can modulate early sensory responses of SCs neurons (Goldberg and Wurtz, 1972b; Li and Basso, 2008; Robinson and Kertzman, 1995; Wurtz and Goldberg, 1972b; Wurtz and Mohler, 1976), and even neurons as early as LGN (McAlonan et al., 2008), but not typically to the same degree as is observed in the SCi. Second, a visual salience map should have well defined spatial selectivity, but no significant feature selectivity, because it is thought to integrate inputs from feature maps tuned to various visual dimensions (Itti and Koch, 2000, 2001; Treisman and Gelade, 1980; Wolfe et al., 1989). In this way, visual cortical areas such as V1 (Koene and Zhaoping, 2007) or V4 (Mazer and Gallant, 2003) might better fit the role of feature maps because neurons in these areas show a high degree of tuning for specific visual properties (Gegenfurtner, 2003; Johnson et al., 2008; Sincich and Horton, 2005; Solomon and Lennie, 2007). Third, a salience map should have direct access to all feature selective areas. The SCs receives direct projections from visual cortical areas V1, V2, V3, and MT (Fries, 1984; Lock et al., 2003; Tigges and Tigges, 1981), and the progression from earlier to later areas is represented by increasing depth in the SCs (Kawamura et al., 1974; Sprague, 1975; Tigges and Tigges, 1981). Higher visual, motor and cognitive areas (e.g. V4, LIP, FEF) project to the SCi (Lock et al., 2003). This suggests a more gradual shift from mostly bottom-up to mostly top-down processes with increasing depth in the SC (which is emphasized by the shading in Figs. 11.1 and 11.2). Finally, a structure coding salience should have extensive feedback to higher levels of visual processing, and the SCs has substantial projections to pulvinar which then projects to multiple extrastriate visual areas.

SCi and priority

Earlier we referred to the idea of a winner-take-all mechanism that is important for the control of competing sources of information during the process of selection (see section 'SC lateral interactions'). For the flexible control of behaviour, such a mechanism ought to integrate sensory signals with the top-down signals related to the goals of the organism. Neurons in the SCi reflect both sensory *salience* and behavioural *relevance* (the relative importance of a stimulus for the goal of the observer) (Fecteau and Munoz, 2006), and the combined representation has been termed *priority* (Serences and Yantis, 2006, 2007). As such, the SCi has been functionally described as a *priority map* (Fecteau and Munoz, 2006). Below we describe some recent research that has implicated the SCi in this role.

SCi and target selection

In cluttered visual environments, the brain has the difficult task of selecting desired objects from undesired distractor information, the process of which has been termed target selection. Neurons throughout the network of visuosaccadic brain areas show neural activity reflecting this process (e.g. visual area V4 (Ogawa and Komatsu, 2004), LIP (Thomas and Paré, 2007), FEF (Schall, 1995, 2002), and the SC (Horwitz and Newsome, 1999, 2001; Kim and Basso, 2008; Krauzlis et al., 2004; Li and Basso, 2005; McPeek and Keller, 2002; Shen and Paré, 2007)).

Target selection processes provide a good example of the combined representation of bottom-up salience and top-down relevance. Target selection has been typically studied using simple visual search tasks in which the observer has to find a target amongst a set of distractors. In its most simple form, a target might differ from distractors along only one visual dimension (e.g. find the green target amongst the red distractors). Immediately following the onset of the visual search array, neurons that reflect target selection initially respond unselectively to the appearance of the target or distractor in the neuron's response field (reflecting the bottom-up component). Shortly thereafter the neuron begins to discriminate the two via a suppression of distractor-related activity, and an enhancement of target-related activity (reflecting the top-down goal-related component). This neural discrimination process typically begins before the eye is launched towards the target, demonstrating that the selection process is not simply motor-activity associated with launching a saccade into versus out of a neuron's movement field. Target selection processes have been observed in the activity of visuomotor neurons from the SCi (Horwitz and Newsome, 1999, 2001; Kim and Basso, 2008; Krauzlis et al., 2004; Li and Basso, 2005; McPeek and Keller, 2002; Shen and Paré, 2007). Furthermore, SCi inactivation (McPeek and Keller, 2004) impairs target selection, and SCi microstimulation (Carello and Krauzlis, 2004) can bias selection processes in favour of stimuli contralateral to the stimulation site. Visual neurons, which are located in the SCs, do not typically discriminate targets from distractors (McPeek and Keller, 2002). These results support the direct involvement of the SCi in target selection.

SCi and visuospatial attention

Because the brain cannot process all incoming sensory information at any given moment, it selects only certain objects/locations over others by a filtering mechanism that has been termed attention. In general, visuospatial attention is thought to follow eye movements, but a covert shift in visuospatial attention can be achieved without moving the eyes (Ignashchenkova et al., 2004; Posner, 1980; Robinson and Kertzman, 1995). Attention is also thought to be controlled either involuntarily by the salient properties of the stimulus itself (sometimes referred to as exogenous or 'stimulus-driven' attention), or voluntarily by prioritizing the selection of objects/locations relevant to the internal goals of the observer (sometimes referred to as endogenous or 'goal-driven' attention) (Klein, 1994; Theeuwes, 1994). There is now extensive literature showing that neurons within the SCi have discharges that correlate with both exogenous and endogenous shifts of visuospatial attention (Bell et al., 2004; Dorris et al., 2002, 2007; Fecteau and Munoz, 2005, 2006; Fecteau et al., 2004; Gattass and Desimone, 1996; Ignashchenkova et al., 2004; Kustov and Robinson, 1996; Lovejoy and Krauzlis, 2010; Lovejoy et al., 2009; Muller et al., 2005; Robinson and Kertzman, 1995). For example, visuomotor neurons in the SCi show enhanced activity during an endogenous shift of attention into their response fields, even in the absence of a visual stimulus (Ignashchenkova et al., 2004). Microstimulation of the SCi can facilitate visual discrimination performance at the spatially selective location represented by the stimulated site, which is indicative of a covert shift of visual attention (Muller et al., 2005). Also, inactivation of a selective region of the SC with muscimol caused monkeys to ignore critical spatial cues that appeared in the affected region of visual space, suggesting that the SC may act as a bottleneck for covert attention (Lovejoy and Krauzlis, 2010). Thus, the SCi can influence voluntary shifts of covert attention independent of eye movements.

Neural correlates of two conceptual mechanisms believed to be central to the control of reflexive visuospatial orienting, attentional capture (AC) and inhibition of return (IOR), are also found in the SC. Following an abrupt appearance of a visual stimulus, visuospatial attention is believed to be initially *captured* by the salient novel event (AC), but then subsequently *inhibited* from returning to that object/location (IOR). These concepts have been central to cognitive theories of attention, and are thought to facilitate visual search in complex scenes (Itti and Koch, 2001; Klein, 1988; Macinnes and Klein, 2003; Najemnik and Geisler, 2005; Posner, 1980).

AC and IOR are typically studied using the Posner cueing paradigm in which a cue stimulus precedes a target stimulus at the same spatial location (Posner, 1980). Saccadic reaction times (SRTs) to the target are shorter when the delay between the cue and target is short (~100 ms), but are prolonged when it is sufficiently long (~500 ms), reflecting AC and IOR respectively. When the delay is short, visual activity of SCi neurons in response to the cue and target combine to produce a greater response, which subsequently drives the faster SRTs reflected in AC (Fecteau and Munoz, 2005). Conversely, when the delay is long visually responsive neurons in the SCs and SCi display an attenuated target-related visual response that correlates with the slower SRTs reflected in IOR (Dorris et al., 2002). It is not entirely known whether these effects are driven directly from the intrinsic circuitry of the SC, but it is important to note that there is no evidence of actual inhibition of covert attention in the SCi during IOR (Dorris et al., 2002). Both these effects (AC and IOR) have neural correlates with *sensory* responses in the SC (Dorris et al., 2002; Fecteau and Munoz, 2005), and are therefore more closely related to modulations of bottom-up sensory processes (at least for these variants of AC and IOR as measured with saccades). In fact, some evidence suggests IOR may be explicable in terms of a simple low-level sensory adaptation/habituation mechanism, which might exist at various levels of visuomotor processing that include the SCs and SCi (Boehnke and Munoz, 2008).

SCi and reward expectancy

The expectation of reward has a significant effect on the top-down goals of the observer. This has been most clearly reflected in the responses of neurons in the SCi, most likely because the SCi receives direct inputs from brain areas that encode reward information including pre-frontal cortex and the basal ganglia (Ikeda and Hikosaka, 2007). When a visual stimulus signals an upcoming reward, both visual and preparatory activity of SCi neurons is enhanced (Ikeda and Hikosaka, 2003). The neurons encoding this enhanced signal tend to be the build-up or prelude-type neurons (Glimcher and Sparks, 1992; Munoz and Wurtz, 1995a). Similarly, the gain of SCi neurons is modulated by target spatial predictability, because predictable targets are associated with reward. That is, the activity of SCi neurons is modulated by the prior expectation that a target will appear in its response field: activity is enhanced if the probability is high, and suppressed if the probability is low (Basso and Wurtz, 1997, 1998; Dorris and Munoz, 1998; Glimcher and Sparks, 1992).

While reward-related gain modulation is observed in the SCi, it is not believed to be the cause (Ikeda and Hikosaka, 2003). There is, however, evidence that the SC itself plays an active role in encoding reward information during reinforcement learning via its projection to the SNc (Comoli et al., 2003). This projection carries transient visual activity to the basal ganglia dopaminergic system, which is critical for reinforcing the context/actions that immediately precede unpredicted, biologically relevant visual events (Dommett et al., 2005; Redgrave and Gurney, 2006). Also, subthreshold stimulation of the SCi can bias choice probability towards the stimulated site of two equally rewarded stimulus locations, implicating the SCi as an important part of the circuit that actively chooses strategic actions that produce positive rewards (Thevarajah et al., 2009).

Conclusion

The SC is arguably one of the most studied structures in the brain, yet there is still much to learn about its precise afferent and efferent circuitry to fully understand its role in the flexible control of the orienting response. Moreover, the SC contains many neurons with complex response properties that we know little about because they are either not modulated by the types of tasks used, or are modulated in ways that are difficult to interpret. In this review we highlighted recent research on the dominant functions of the SC that have led to insightful theoretical and computational models (e.g. Dean et al., 1989; Fecteau and Munoz, 2006; Hafed et al., 2009; Krauzlis, 2005; Krauzlis et al., 2004; Moschovakis et al., 1998; Trappenberg et al., 2001). We highlighted functional differences between the SC layers, emphasizing the SCs as a critical sensory node for bottom-up processes, and the SCi as a critical sensorimotor node for integrating bottom-up and top-down signals for the flexible control of orienting behaviour. With an expanding role of the SC in higher-level functioning (e.g. target selection, reward-expectation, covert visuospatial orienting, etc.), it continues to be a critical area of research in sensorimotor neuroscience.

References

Akert, K. (1949). Der visuelle Greifreflex. *Helvetica Physiologica et Pharmacolog*, **7**, 112–134.

Anderson, R.W., Keller, E.L., Gandhi, N.J., and Das, S. (1998). Two-dimensional saccade-related population activity in superior colliculus in monkey. *Journal of Neurophysiology*, **80**(2), 798–817.

Basso, M.A. and Wurtz, R.H. (1997). Modulation of neuronal activity by target uncertainty. *Nature*, **389**(6646), 66–69.

Basso, M.A. and Wurtz, R.H. (1998). Modulation of neuronal activity in superior colliculus by changes in target probability. *Journal of Neuroscience*, **18**(18), 7519–7534.

Basso, M.A., Krauzlis, R.J., and Wurtz, R.H. (2000). Activation and inactivation of rostral superior colliculus neurons during smooth-pursuit eye movements in monkeys. *Journal of Neurophysiology*, **84**(2), 892–908.

Behan, M. and Appell, P.P. (1992). Intrinsic circuitry in the cat superior colliculus: projections from the superficial layers. *Journal of Comparative Neurology*, **315**(2), 230–243.

Behan, M. and Kime, N.M. (1996). Intrinsic circuitry in the deep layers of the cat superior colliculus. *Visual Neuroscience*, **13**(6), 1031–1042.

Bell, A.H., Fecteau, J.H., and Munoz, D.P. (2004). Using auditory and visual stimuli to investigate the behavioral and neuronal consequences of reflexive covert orienting. *Journal of Neurophysiology*, **91**(5), 2172–2184.

Bell, A.H., Meredith, M.A., Van Opstal, A.J., and Munoz, D.P. (2006). Stimulus intensity modifies saccadic reaction time and visual response latency in the superior colliculus. *Experimental Brain Research*, **174**(1), 53–59.

Berman, R.A. and Wurtz, R.H. (2010). Functional identification of a pulvinar path from superior colliculus to cortical area MT. *Journal of Neuroscience*, **30**(18), 6342–6354.

Bisley, J.W. and Goldberg, M.E. (2003). Neuronal activity in the lateral intraparietal area and spatial attention. *Science*, **299**(5603), 81–86.

Bisley, J.W. and Goldberg, M.E. (2006). Neural correlates of attention and distractibility in the lateral intraparietal area. *Journal of Neurophysiology*, **95**(3), 1696–1717.

Boehnke, S.E. and Munoz, D.P. (2008). On the importance of the transient visual response in the superior colliculus. *Current Opinion in Neurobiology*, **18**(6), 544–551.

Born, R.T. and Bradley, D.C. (2005). Structure and function of visual area MT. *Annual Review of Neuroscience*, **28**, 157–189.

Carello, C.D. and Krauzlis, R.J. (2004). Manipulating intent: evidence for a causal role of the superior colliculus in target selection. *Neuron*, **43**(4), 575–583.

Casagrande, V.A., Harting, J.K., Hall, W.C., Diamond, I.T., and Martin, G.F. (1972). Superior colliculus of the tree shrew: a structural and functional subdivision into superficial and deep layers. *Science*, **177**(47), 444–447.

Casanova, C. (2004). The visual functions of the pulvinar. In L.M. Chalupa and J.S. Werner (eds.) *The Visual Neurosciences* (Vol. 1) (pp. 592–608). Cambridge, MA: MIT Press.

Chaturvedi, V. and van Gisbergen, J.A. (1999). Perturbation of combined saccade-vergence movements by microstimulation in monkey superior colliculus. *Journal of Neurophysiology*, **81**(5), 2279–2296.

Chaturvedi, V. and Van Gisbergen, J.A. (2000). Stimulation in the rostral pole of monkey superior colliculus: effects on vergence eye movements. *Experimental Brain Research*, **132**(1), 72–78.

Choi, W.Y. and Guitton, D. (2006). Responses of collicular fixation neurons to gaze shift perturbations in head-unrestrained monkey reveal gaze feedback control. *Neuron*, **50**(3), 491–505.

Choi, W.Y. and Guitton, D. (2009). Firing patterns in superior colliculus of head-unrestrained monkey during normal and perturbed gaze saccades reveal short-latency feedback and a sluggish rostral shift in activity. *Journal of Neuroscience*, **29**(22), 7166–7180.

Comoli, E., Coizet, V., Boyes, J., Bolam, J.P., Canteras, N.S., Quirk, R.H., *et al.* (2003). A direct projection from superior colliculus to substantia nigra for detecting salient visual events. *Nature Neuroscience*, **6**(9), 974–980.

Corneil, B.D., Olivier, E., and Munoz, D.P. (2002). Neck muscle responses to stimulation of monkey superior colliculus. II. Gaze shift initiation and volitional head movements. *Journal of Neurophysiology*, **88**(4), 2000–2018.

Corneil, B.D., Olivier, E., and Munoz, D.P. (2004). Visual responses on neck muscles reveal selective gating that prevents express saccades. *Neuron*, **42**(5), 831–841.

Corneil, B.D., Munoz, D.P., and Olivier, E. (2007). Priming of head premotor circuits during oculomotor preparation. *Journal of Neurophysiology*, **97**(1), 701–714.

Corneil, B.D., Munoz, D.P., Chapman, B.B., Admans, T., and Cushing, S.L. (2008). Neuromuscular consequences of reflexive covert orienting. *Nature Neuroscience*, **11**(1), 13–15.

Cowey, A. and Perry, V.H. (1980). The projection of the fovea to the superior colliculus in rhesus monkeys. *Neuroscience*, **5**(1), 53–61.

Cusick, C.G. (1988). Anatomical organization of the superior colliculus in monkeys: corticotectal pathways for visual and visuomotor functions. *Progress in Brain Research*, **75**, 1–15.

Cynader, M. and Berman, N. (1972). Receptive-field organization of monkey superior colliculus. *Journal of Neurophysiology*, **35**(2), 187–201.

Dean, P., Redgrave, P., and Westby, G.W. (1989). Event or emergency? Two response systems in the mammalian superior colliculus. *Trends in Neuroscience*, **12**(4), 137–147.

Dommett, E., Coizet, V., Blaha, C.D., Martindale, J., Lefebvre, V., Walton, N., *et al.* (2005). How visual stimuli activate dopaminergic neurons at short latency. *Science,* 307(5714), 1476–1479.

Dorris, M.C. and Munoz, D.P. (1995). A neural correlate for the gap effect on saccadic reaction times in monkey. *Journal of Neurophysiology,* 73(6), 2558–2562.

Dorris, M.C. and Munoz, D.P. (1998). Saccadic probability influences motor preparation signals and time to saccadic initiation. *Journal of Neuroscience,* 18(17), 7015–7026.

Dorris, M.C., Paré, M., and Munoz, D.P. (1997). Neuronal activity in monkey superior colliculus related to the initiation of saccadic eye movements. *Journal of Neuroscience,* 17(21), 8566–8579.

Dorris, M.C., Olivier, E., and Munoz, D.P. (2007). Competitive integration of visual and preparatory signals in the superior colliculus during saccadic programming. *Journal of Neuroscience,* 27(19), 5053–5062.

Dorris, M.C., Klein, R.M., Everling, S., and Munoz, D.P. (2002). Contribution of the primate superior colliculus to inhibition of return. *Journal of Cognitive Neuroscience,* 14(8), 1256–1263.

Edelman, J.A. and Keller, E.L. (1996). Activity of visuomotor burst neurons in the superior colliculus accompanying express saccades. *Journal of Neurophysiology,* 76(2), 908–926.

Edelman, J.A. and Keller, E.L. (1998). Dependence on target configuration of express saccade-related activity in the primate superior colliculus. *Journal of Neurophysiology,* 80(3), 1407–1426.

Edwards, S.B. (1980). The deep layers of the superior colliculus: their reticular characteristics and structural organization. In J.A. Hobson and M.A.B. Brazier (eds.) *The Reticular Formation Revisited* (pp. 193–209). New York: Raven Press.

Edwards, S.B., Ginsburgh, C.L., Henkel, C.K., and Stein, B.E. (1979). Sources of subcortical projections to the superior colliculus in the cat. *Journal of Comparative Neurology,* 184(2), 309–329.

Everling, S. and Munoz, D.P. (2000). Neuronal correlates for preparatory set associated with pro-saccades and anti-saccades in the primate frontal eye field. *Journal of Neuroscience,* 20(1), 387–400.

Everling, S., Dorris, M.C., Klein, R.M., and Munoz, D.P. (1999). Role of primate superior colliculus in preparation and execution of anti-saccades and pro-saccades. *Journal of Neuroscience,* 19(7), 2740–2754.

Fecteau, J.H. and Munoz, D.P. (2005). Correlates of capture of attention and inhibition of return across stages of visual processing. *Journal of Cognitive Neuroscience,* 17(11), 1714–1727.

Fecteau, J.H. and Munoz, D.P. (2006). Salience, relevance, and firing: a priority map for target selection. *Trends in Cognitive Science,* 10(8), 382–390.

Fecteau, J.H., Bell, A.H., and Munoz, D.P. (2004). Neural correlates of the automatic and goal-driven biases in orienting spatial attention. *Journal of Neurophysiology,* 92(3), 1728–1737.

Findlay, J.M. (1982). Global visual processing for saccadic eye movements. *Vision Research,* 22(8), 1033–1045.

Fischer, B. and Boch, R. (1983). Saccadic eye movements after extremely short reaction times in the monkey. *Brain Research,* 260(1), 21–26.

Fischer, B. and Ramsperger, E. (1984). Human express saccades: extremely short reaction times of goal directed eye movements. *Experimental Brain Research,* 57(1), 191–195.

Freedman, E.G. and Sparks, D.L. (1997). Eye-head coordination during head-unrestrained gaze shifts in rhesus monkeys. *Journal of Neurophysiology,* 77(5), 2328–2348.

Fries, W. (1984). Cortical projections to the superior colliculus in the macaque monkey: a retrograde study using horseradish peroxidase. *Journal of Comparative Neurology,* 230(1), 55–76.

Gattass, R. and Desimone, R. (1996). Responses of cells in the superior colliculus during performance of a spatial attention task in the macaque. *Revista Brasileira de Biologia,* 56(Supp 1 Pt 2), 257–279.

Gegenfurtner, K.R. (2003). Cortical mechanisms of colour vision. *Nature Reviews Neuroscience,* 4(7), 563–572.

Glimcher, P.W. and Sparks, D.L. (1992). Movement selection in advance of action in the superior colliculus. *Nature,* 355(6360), 542–545.

Goldberg, M.E. and Wurtz, R.H. (1972a). Activity of superior colliculus in behaving monkey. I. Visual receptive fields of single neurons. *Journal of Neurophysiology,* 35(4), 542–559.

Goldberg, M.E. and Wurtz, R.H. (1972b). Activity of superior colliculus in behaving monkey. II. Effect of attention on neuronal responses. *Journal of Neurophysiology,* 35(4), 560–574.

Goldberg, M.E., Bisley, J.W., Powell, K.D., and Gottlieb, J. (2006). Saccades, salience and attention: the role of the lateral intraparietal area in visual behavior. *Progress in Brain Research,* 155, 157–175.

Goldberg, M.E., Bisley, J., Powell, K.D., Gottlieb, J., and Kusunoki, M. (2002). The role of the lateral intraparietal area of the monkey in the generation of saccades and visuospatial attention. *Annals of the New York Academy of Sciences,* 956, 205–215.

Goldman, P.S. and Nauta, W.J. (1976). Autoradiographic demonstration of a projection from prefrontal association cortex to the superior colliculus in the rhesus monkey. *Brain Research,* 116(1), 145–149.

Gottlieb, J. (2007). From thought to action: the parietal cortex as a bridge between perception, action, and cognition. *Neuron,* 53(1), 9–16.

Gottlieb, J.P., Kusunoki, M., and Goldberg, M.E. (1998). The representation of visual salience in monkey parietal cortex. *Nature,* 391(6666), 481–484.

Graham, J. (1982). Some topographical connections of the striate cortex with subcortical structures in Macaca fascicularis. *Experimental Brain Research,* 47(1), 1–14.

Groh, J.M. and Sparks, D.L. (1996). Saccades to somatosensory targets. I. behavioral characteristics. *Journal of Neurophysiology*, **75**(1), 412–427.

Hafed, Z.M., Goffart, L., and Krauzlis, R.J. (2009). A neural mechanism for microsaccade generation in the primate superior colliculus. *Science*, **323**(5916), 940–943.

Hanes, D.P. and Wurtz, R.H. (2001). Interaction of the frontal eye field and superior colliculus for saccade generation. *Journal of Neurophysiology*, **85**(2), 804–815.

Harting, J.K., Casagrande, V.A., and Weber, J.T. (1978). The projection of the primate superior colliculus upon the dorsal lateral geniculate nucleus: autoradiographic demonstration of interlaminar distribution of tectogeniculate axons. *Brain Research*, **150**(3), 593–599.

Harting, J.K., Updyke, B.V., and Van Lieshout, D.P. (1992). Corticotectal projections in the cat: anterograde transport studies of twenty-five cortical areas. *Journal of Comparative Neurology*, **324**(3), 379–414, 1992.

Helms, M.C., Ozen, G., and Hall, W.C. (2004). Organization of the intermediate gray layer of the superior colliculus. I. Intrinsic vertical connections. *Journal of Neurophysiology*, **91**(4), 1706–1715.

Hess, W.R., Bürgi, S., and Bucher, V. (1946). Motorische funktion des tektal- und tegmentalgebietes. [Motor functions of tectal and tegmental areas.] *Monatsschrift für Psychiatrie und Neurologie*, **112**, 1–52.

Hikosaka, O. (1989). Role of basal ganglia in saccades. *Revue Neurologique (Paris)*, **145**(8–9), 580–586.

Hikosaka, O. and Wurtz, R.H. (1983). Visual and oculomotor functions of monkey substantia nigra pars reticulata. IV. Relation of substantia nigra to superior colliculus. *Journal of Neurophysiology*, **49**(5), 1285–1301.

Hikosaka, O., Takikawa, Y., and Kawagoe, R. (2000). Role of the basal ganglia in the control of purposive saccadic eye movements. *Physiological Review*, **80**(3), 953–978.

Hikosaka, O., Nakamura, K., and Nakahara, H. (2006). Basal ganglia orient eyes to reward. *Journal of Neurophysiology*, **95**(2), 567–584.

Horwitz, G.D. and Newsome, W.T. (1999). Separate signals for target selection and movement specification in the superior colliculus. *Science*, **284**(5417), 1158–1161.

Horwitz, G.D. and Newsome, W.T. (2001). Target selection for saccadic eye movements: prelude activity in the superior colliculus during a direction-discrimination task. *Journal of Neurophysiology*, **86**(5), 2543–2558.

Hubel, D.H., LeVay, S., and Wiesel, T.N. (1975). Mode of termination of retinotectal fibers in macaque monkey: an autoradiographic study. *Brain Research*, **96**(1), 25–40.

Huerta, M.F. and Kaas, J.H. (1990). Supplementary eye field as defined by intracortical microstimulation: connections in macaques. *Journal of Comparative Neurology*, **293**(2), 299–330.

Ignashchenkova, A., Dicke, P.W., Haarmeier, T., and Thier, P. (2004). Neuron-specific contribution of the superior colliculus to overt and covert shifts of attention. *Nature Neuroscience*, **7**(1), 56–64.

Ikeda, T. and Hikosaka, O. (2003). Reward-dependent gain and bias of visual responses in primate superior colliculus. *Neuron*, **39**(4), 693–700.

Ikeda, T. and Hikosaka, O. (2007). Positive and negative modulation of motor response in primate superior colliculus by reward expectation. *Journal of Neurophysiology*, **98**(6), 3163–3170.

Ilg, U.J. (2008). The role of areas MT and MST in coding of visual motion underlying the execution of smooth pursuit. *Vision Research*, **48**(20), 2062–2069.

Ilg, U.J. and Thier, P. (2003). Visual tracking neurons in primate area MST are activated by smooth-pursuit eye movements of an 'imaginary' target. *Journal of Neurophysiology*, **90**(3), 1489–1502.

Ingle, D.J. (1983). Brain mechanisms of visual localization by frogs and toads. In J.P. Ewert, R.R. Capranica, and D.J. Ingle (eds.) *Advances in Vertebrate Neuroethology* (pp. 177–226). New York: Plenum Press.

Ipata, A.E., Gee, A.L., Gottlieb, J., Bisley, J.W., and Goldberg, M.E. (2006). LIP responses to a popout stimulus are reduced if it is overtly ignored. *Nature Neuroscience*, **9**(8), 1071–1076.

Isa, T. (2002). Intrinsic processing in the mammalian superior colliculus. *Current Opinion in Neurobiology*, **12**(6), 668–677.

Isa, T. and Saito, Y. (2001). The direct visuo-motor pathway in mammalian superior colliculus; novel perspective on the interlaminar connection. *Neuroscience Research*, **41**(2), 107–113.

Isa, T. Endo, T., and Saito, Y. (1998). The visuo-motor pathway in the local circuit of the rat superior colliculus. *Journal of Neuroscience*, **18**(20), 8496–8504.

Isa, K., Phongphanphanee, P., Marino, R., Kaneda, K., Yanagawa, Y., Munoz, D.P., *et al.* (2009). The lateral interaction in the intermediate layers of the mouse superior colliculus slice. *Neuroscience Research*, **65**, S172.

Itti, L. and Koch, C. (2000). A saliency-based search mechanism for overt and covert shifts of visual attention. *Vision Research*, **40**(10–12), 1489–1506.

Itti, L. and Koch, C. (2001). Computational modelling of visual attention. *Nature Reviews Neuroscience*, **2**(3), 194–203.

Jay, M.F. and Sparks, D.L. (1987). Sensorimotor integration in the primate superior colliculus. II. Coordinates of auditory signals. *Journal of Neurophysiology*, **57**(1), 35–55.

Jayaraman, A., Batton, R.R., 3rd, and Carpenter, M.B. (1977). Nigrotectal projections in the monkey: an autoradiographic study. *Brain Research*, **135**(1), 147–152.

Jiang, H., Stein, B.E., and McHaffie, J.G. (2003). Opposing basal ganglia processes shape midbrain visuomotor activity bilaterally. *Nature*, **423**(6943), 982–986.

Johnson, E.N., Hawken, M.J., and Shapley, R. (2008). The orientation selectivity of color-responsive neurons in macaque V1. *Journal of Neuroscience*, **28**(32), 8096–8106.

Johnston, K. and Everling, S. (2006a). Monkey dorsolateral prefrontal cortex sends task-selective signals directly to the superior colliculus. *Journal of Neuroscience*, **26**(48), 12471–12478.

Johnston, K. and Everling, S. (2006b). Neural activity in monkey prefrontal cortex is modulated by task context and behavioral instruction during delayed-match-to-sample and conditional prosaccade-antisaccade tasks. *Journal of Cognitive Neuroscience*, **18**(5), 749–765.

Johnston, K. and Everling, S. (2008). Task-relevant output signals are sent from monkey dorsolateral prefrontal cortex to the superior colliculus during a visuospatial working memory task. *Journal of Cognitive Neuroscience*, **21**(5), 1023–1038.

Johnston, K., Levin, H.M., Koval, M.J., and Everling, S. (2007). Top-down control-signal dynamics in anterior cingulate and prefrontal cortex neurons following task switching. *Neuron*, **53**(3), 453–462.

Kawamura, S., Sprague, J.M., and Niimi, K. (1974). Corticofugal projections from the visual cortices to the thalamus, pretectum and superior colliculus in the cat. *Journal of Comparative Neurology*, **158**(3), 339–362.

Kim, B. and Basso, M.A. (2008). Saccade target selection in the superior colliculus: a signal detection theory approach. *Journal of Neuroscience*, **28**(12), 2991–3007.

Klein, R. (1988). Inhibitory tagging system facilitates visual search. *Nature*, **334**(6181), 430–431.

Klein, R.M. (1994). Perceptual-motor expectancies interact with covert visual orienting under conditions of endogenous but not exogenous control. *Canadian Journal of Experimental Psychology*, **48**(2), 167–181.

Koene, A.R. and Zhaoping, L. (2007). Feature-specific interactions in salience from combined feature contrasts: evidence for a bottom-up saliency map in V1. *Journal of Vision*, **7**(7), 6 1–14.

Krauzlis, R.J. (2001). Extraretinal inputs to neurons in the rostral superior colliculus of the monkey during smooth-pursuit eye movements. *Journal of Neurophysiology*, **86**(5), 2629–2633.

Krauzlis, R.J. (2003). Neuronal activity in the rostral superior colliculus related to the initiation of pursuit and saccadic eye movements. *Journal of Neuroscience*, **23**(10), 4333–4344.

Krauzlis, R.J. (2004a). Activity of rostral superior colliculus neurons during passive and active viewing of motion. *Journal of Neurophysiology*, **92**(2), 949–958.

Krauzlis, R.J. (2004b). Recasting the smooth pursuit eye movement system. *Journal of Neurophysiology*, **91**(2), 591–603.

Krauzlis, R.J. (2005). The control of voluntary eye movements: new perspectives. *Neuroscientist*, **11**(2), 124–137.

Krauzlis, R., and Dill, N. (2002). Neural correlates of target choice for pursuit and saccades in the primate superior colliculus. *Neuron*, **35**(2), 355–363.

Krauzlis, R.J., Basso, M.A., and Wurtz, R.H. (1997). Shared motor error for multiple eye movements. *Science*, **276**(5319), 1693–1695.

Krauzlis, R.J., Basso, M.A., and Wurtz, R.H. (2000). Discharge properties of neurons in the rostral superior colliculus of the monkey during smooth-pursuit eye movements. *Journal of Neurophysiology*, **84**(2), 876–891.

Krauzlis, R.J., Liston, D., and Carello, C.D. (2004). Target selection and the superior colliculus: goals, choices and hypotheses. *Vision Research*, **44**(12), 1445–1451.

Kunzle, H. and Akert, K. (1977). Efferent connections of cortical, area 8 (frontal eye field) in Macaca fascicularis. A reinvestigation using the autoradiographic technique. *Journal of Comparative Neurology*, **173**(1), 147–164.

Kunzle, H., Akert, K., and Wurtz, R.H. (1976). Projection of area 8 (frontal eye field) to superior colliculus in the monkey. An autoradiographic study. *Brain Research*, **117**(3), 487–492.

Kustov, A.A. and Robinson, D.L. (1996). Shared neural control of attentional shifts and eye movements. *Nature*, **384**(6604), 74–77.

Kusunoki, M., Gottlieb, J., and Goldberg, M.E. (2000). The lateral intraparietal area as a salience map: the representation of abrupt onset, stimulus motion, and task relevance. *Vision Research*, **40**(10–12), 1459–1468.

Lee, P. and Hall, W.C. (2006). An *in vitro* study of horizontal connections in the intermediate layer of the superior colliculus. *Journal of Neuroscience*, **26**(18), 4763–4768.

Leichnetz, G.R., Spencer, R.F., Hardy, S.G., and Astruc, J. (1981). The prefrontal corticotectal projection in the monkey; an anterograde and retrograde horseradish peroxidase study. *Neuroscience*, **6**(6), 1023–1041.

Li, Z. (2002). A saliency map in primary visual cortex. *Trends Cogn Sci*, **6**(1), 9–16.

Li, X. and Basso, M. A. (2005). Competitive stimulus interactions within single response fields of superior colliculus neurons. *Journal of Neuroscience*, **25**(49), 11357–11373.

Li, X. and Basso, M. A. (2008). Preparing to move increases the sensitivity of superior colliculus neurons. *Journal of Neuroscience*, **28**(17), 4561–4577.

Lock, T.M., Baizer, J.S., and Bender, D.B. (2003). Distribution of corticotectal cells in macaque. *Experimental Brain Research*, **151**(4), 455–470.

Lovejoy, L.P. and Krauzlis, R.J. (2010). Inactivation of primate superior colliculus impairs covert selection of signals for perceptual judgments. *Nature Neuroscience*, **13**(2), 261–266.

Lovejoy, L.P., Fowler, G.A., and Krauzlis, R.J. (2009). Spatial allocation of attention during smooth pursuit eye movements. *Vision Research*, **49**(10), 1275–1285.

Lynch, J.C., Graybiel, A.M., and Lobeck, L.J. (1985). The differential projection of two cytoarchitectonic subregions of the inferior parietal lobule of macaque upon the deep layers of the superior colliculus. *Journal of Comparative Neurology*, **235**(2), 241–254.

Lynch, J.C., Hoover, J.E., and Strick, P.L. (1994). Input to the primate frontal eye field from the substantia nigra, superior colliculus, and dentate nucleus demonstrated by transneuronal transport. *Experimental Brain Research*, **100**(1), 181–186.

Macinnes, J.W. and Klein, R.M. (2003). Inhibition of return biases orienting during the search of complex scenes. *Scientific World Journal*, **3**, 75–86.

Marino, R.A., Rodgers, C.K., Levy, R., and Munoz, D.P. (2008). Spatial relationships of visuomotor transformations in the superior colliculus map. *Journal of Neurophysiology*, **100**(5), 2564–2576.

Marrocco, R.T. and Li, R.H. (1977). Monkey superior colliculus: properties of single cells and their afferent inputs. *Journal of Neurophysiology*, **40**(4), 844–860.

Mathers, L.H. (1971). Tectal projection to the posterior thalamus of the squirrel monkey. *Brain Research*, **35**(1), 295–298.

Mays, L.E., and Sparks, D.L. (1980). Dissociation of visual and saccade-related responses in superior colliculus neurons. *Journal of Neurophysiology*, **43**(1), 207–232.

Mazer, J.A., and Gallant, J.L. (2003). Goal-related activity in V4 during free viewing visual search. Evidence for a ventral stream visual salience map. *Neuron*, **40**(6), 1241–1250.

McAlonan, K., Cavanaugh, J., and Wurtz, R.H. (2008). Guarding the gateway to cortex with attention in visual thalamus. *Nature*, **456**(7220), 391–394.

McHaffie, J.G., Jiang, H., May, P.J., Coizet, V., Overton, P.G., Stein, B.E., *et al.* (2006). A direct projection from superior colliculus to substantia nigra pars compacta in the cat. *Neuroscience*, **138**(1), 221–234.

McPeek, R.M. and Keller, E.L. (2002). Saccade target selection in the superior colliculus during a visual search task. *Journal of Neurophysiology*, **88**(4), 2019–2034.

McPeek, R.M. and Keller, E.L. (2004). Deficits in saccade target selection after inactivation of superior colliculus. *Nature Neuroscience*, **7**(7), 757–763.

Meredith, M.A. and Ramoa, A.S. (1998). Intrinsic circuitry of the superior colliculus: pharmacophysiological identification of horizontally oriented inhibitory interneurons. *Journal of Neurophysiology*, **79**(3), 1597–1602.

Meredith, M.A. and Stein, B.E. (1983). Interactions among converging sensory inputs in the superior colliculus. *Science*, **221**(4608), 389–391.

Meredith, M.A. and Stein, B.E. (1985). Descending efferents from the superior colliculus relay integrated multisensory information. *Science*, **227**(4687), 657–659.

Mohler, C.W. and Wurtz, R.H. (1976). Organization of monkey superior colliculus: intermediate layer cells discharging before eye movements. *Journal of Neurophysiology*, **39**(4), 722–744.

Moschovakis, A.K., Karabelas, A.B., and Highstein, S.M. (1988). Structure-function relationships in the primate superior colliculus. I. Morphological classification of efferent neurons. *Journal of Neurophysiology*, **60**(1), 232–262.

Moschovakis, A.K., Gregoriou, G.G., and Savaki, H.E. (2001). Functional imaging of the primate superior colliculus during saccades to visual targets. *Nature Neuroscience*, **4**(10), 1026–1031.

Moschovakis, A.K., Dalezios, Y., Petit, J., and Grantyn, A.A. (1998). New mechanism that accounts for position sensitivity of saccades evoked in response to stimulation of superior colliculus. *Journal of Neurophysiology*, **80**(6), 3373–3379.

Muller, J.R., Philiastides, M.G., and Newsome, W.T. (2005). Microstimulation of the superior colliculus focuses attention without moving the eyes. *Proceedings of the National Academy of Sciences U S A*, **102**(3), 524–529.

Munoz, D.P. and Everling, S. (2004). Look away: the anti-saccade task and the voluntary control of eye movement. *Nature Reviews Neuroscience*, **5**(3), 218–228.

Munoz, D.P., and Guitton, D. (1991). Control of orienting gaze shifts by the tectoreticulospinal system in the head-free cat. II. Sustained discharges during motor preparation and fixation. *Journal of Neurophysiology*, **66**(5), 1624–1641.

Munoz, D.P. and Istvan, P.J. (1998). Lateral inhibitory interactions in the intermediate layers of the monkey superior colliculus. *Journal of Neurophysiology*, **79**(3), 1193–1209.

Munoz, D.P. and Wurtz, R.H. (1993a). Fixation cells in monkey superior colliculus. I. Characteristics of cell discharge. *Journal of Neurophysiology*, **70**(2), 559–575.

Munoz, D.P. and Wurtz, R.H. (1993b). Fixation cells in monkey superior colliculus. II. Reversible activation and deactivation. *Journal of Neurophysiology*, **70**(2), 576–589.

Munoz, D.P. and Wurtz, R.H. (1995a). Saccade-related activity in monkey superior colliculus. I. Characteristics of burst and buildup cells. *Journal of Neurophysiology*, **73**(6), 2313–2333.

Munoz, D.P. and Wurtz, R.H. (1995b). Saccade-related activity in monkey superior colliculus. II. Spread of activity during saccades. *Journal of Neurophysiology*, **73**(6), 2334–2348.

Munoz, D.P., Guitton, D., and Pelisson, D. (1991a). Control of orienting gaze shifts by the tectoreticulospinal system in the head-free cat. III. Spatiotemporal characteristics of phasic motor discharges. *Journal of Neurophysiology*, **66**(5), 1642–1666.

Munoz, D.P., Pelisson, D., and Guitton, D. (1991b). Movement of neural activity on the superior colliculus motor map during gaze shifts. *Science*, **251**(4999), 1358–1360.

Munoz, D.P., Waitzman, D.M., and Wurtz, R.H. (1996). Activity of neurons in monkey superior colliculus during interrupted saccades. *Journal of Neurophysiology*, **75**(6), 2562–2580.

Munoz, D.P., Dorris, M.C., Paré, M., and Everling, S. (2000). On your mark, get set: brainstem circuitry underlying saccadic initiation. *Canadian Journal of Physiology and Pharmacology*, **78**(11), 934–944.

Najemnik, J. and Geisler, W.S. (2005). Optimal eye movement strategies in visual search. *Nature*, **434**(7031), 387–391.

Ogawa, T. and Komatsu, H. (2004). Target selection in area V4 during a multidimensional visual search task. *Journal of Neuroscience*, 24(28), 6371–6382.

Olivier, E., Dorris, M.C., and Munoz, D.P. (1999). Lateral interactions in the superior colliculus, not an extended fixation zone, can account for the remote distractor effect. Commentary on J.M. Findlay and R. Walker. *Behavioral and Brain Sciences*, 10, 35–38.

Ottes, F.P., Van Gisbergen, J.A., and Eggermont, J.J. (1986). Visuomotor fields of the superior colliculus: a quantitative model. *Vision Research*, 26(6), 857–873.

Paré, M. and Wurtz, R.H. (1997). Monkey posterior parietal cortex neurons antidromically activated from superior colliculus. *Journal of Neurophysiology*, 78(6), 3493–3497.

Paré, M. and Wurtz, R.H. (2001). Progression in neuronal processing for saccadic eye movements from parietal cortex area lip to superior colliculus. *Journal of Neurophysiology*, 85(6), 2545–2562.

Phongphanphanee, P., Marino, R., Kaneda, K., Yanagawa, Y., Munoz, D.P., and Isa, T. (2009). The lateral interaction in the superficial layers of the mouse superior colliculus slice. *Neuroscience Research*, 65, S172.

Pollack, J.G. and Hickey, T.L. (1979). The distribution of retino-collicular axon terminals in rhesus monkey. *Journal of Comparative Neurology*, 185(4), 587–602.

Posner, M.I. (1980). Orienting of attention. *Quarterly Journal of Experimental Psychology*, 32(1), 3–25.

Pruszynski, A.J., King, G.L., Boisse, L., Scott, S.H., Flanagan, R.J., and Munoz, D.P. (2010). Stimulus-locked responses on human arm muscles reveal a rapid neural pathway linking visual input to arm motor output. *European Journal of Neuroscience*, 32(6), 1049–1057.

Redgrave, P. and Gurney, K. (2006). The short-latency dopamine signal: a role in discovering novel actions? *Nature Reviews Neuroscience*, 7(12), 967–975.

Robinson, D.A. (1972). Eye movements evoked by collicular stimulation in the alert monkey. *Vision Research*, 12(11), 1795–1808.

Robinson, D.L. and Kertzman, C. (1995). Covert orienting of attention in macaques. III. Contributions of the superior colliculus. *Journal of Neurophysiology*, 74(2), 713–721.

Robinson, D.L. and McClurkin, J.W. (1989). The visual superior colliculus and pulvinar. *Reviews of Oculomotor Research*, 3, 337–360.

Robinson, D.L. and Petersen, S.E. (1992). The pulvinar and visual salience. *Trends in Neuroscience*, 15(4), 127–132.

Rodgers, C.K., Munoz, D.P., Scott, S.H., and Paré, M. (2006). Discharge properties of monkey tectoreticular neurons. *Journal of Neurophysiology*, 95(6), 3502–3511.

Saito, Y. and Isa, T. (2004). Laminar specific distribution of lateral excitatory connections in the rat superior colliculus. *Journal of Neurophysiology*, 92(6), 3500–3510.

Saslow, M.G. (1967). Effects of components of displacement-step stimuli upon latency for saccadic eye movement. *Journal of the American Optometric Association*, 57(8), 1024–1029.

Schall, J.D. (1995). Neural basis of saccade target selection. *Reviews in the Neurosciences*, 6(1), 63–85.

Schall, J.D. (2002). The neural selection and control of saccades by the frontal eye field. *Philosophical Transactions of the Royal Society B: Biological Science*, 357(1424), 1073–1082.

Schiller, P.H. (1977). The superior colliculus and visual function. In J.M. Brookhart, V.B. Mountcastle, and American Physiological Society (1887-) (eds.) *Handbook of physiology: a critical, comprehensive presentation of physiological knowledge and concepts* (Rev. and enl. ed., pp. v.). Bethesda, MA: American Physiological Society.

Schiller, P.H. and Koerner, F. (1971). Discharge characteristics of single units in superior colliculus of the alert rhesus monkey. *Journal of Neurophysiology*, 34(5), 920–936.

Schiller, P.H. and Malpeli, J.G. (1977). Properties and tectal projections of monkey retinal ganglion cells. *Journal of Neurophysiology*, 40(2), 428–445.

Schiller, P.H. and Stryker, M. (1972). Single-unit recording and stimulation in superior colliculus of the alert rhesus monkey. *Journal of Neurophysiology*, 35(6), 915–924.

Schiller, P.H., Malpeli, J.G., and Schein, S.J. (1979). Composition of geniculostriate input to superior colliculus of the rhesus monkey. *Journal of Neurophysiology*, 42(4), 1124–1133.

Schiller, P.H., Stryker, M., Cynader, M., and Berman, N. (1974). Response characteristics of single cells in the monkey superior colliculus following ablation or cooling of visual cortex. *Journal of Neurophysiology*, 37(1), 181–194.

Segraves, M.A. and Goldberg, M.E. (1987). Functional properties of corticotectal neurons in the monkey's frontal eye field. *Journal of Neurophysiology*, 58(6), 1387–1419.

Serences, J.T. and Yantis, S. (2006). Selective visual attention and perceptual coherence. *Trends in Cognitive Sciences*, 10(1), 38–45.

Serences, J.T. and Yantis, S. (2007). Spatially selective representations of voluntary and stimulus-driven attentional priority in human occipital, parietal, and frontal cortex. *Cerebral Cortex*, 17(2), 284–293.

Shen, K. and Paré, M. (2007). Neuronal activity in superior colliculus signals both stimulus identity and saccade goals during visual conjunction search. *Journal of Vision*, 7(5), 15 11–13.

Shipp, S. (2004). The brain circuitry of attention. *Trends in Cognitive Science*, 8(5), 223–230.

Shook, B.L., Schlag-Rey, M., and Schlag, J. (1990). Primate supplementary eye field: I. Comparative aspects of mesencephalic and pontine connections. *Journal of Comparative Neurology*, 301(4), 618–642.

Sincich, L.C., and Horton, J.C. (2005). The circuitry of V1 and V2: integration of color, form, and motion. *Annual Review of Neuroscience*, **28**, 303–326.

Soetedjo, R., Kaneko, C.R., and Fuchs, A.F. (2002). Evidence against a moving hill in the superior colliculus during saccadic eye movements in the monkey. *Journal of Neurophysiology*, **87**(6), 2778–2789.

Sokolov, E.N. (1963). Higher nervous functions; the orienting reflex. *Annual Review of Physiology*, **25**, 545–580.

Solomon, S.G. and Lennie, P. (2007). The machinery of colour vision. *Nature Reviews Neuroscience*, **8**(4), 276–286.

Sommer, M.A. and Wurtz, R.H. (2004a). What the brain stem tells the frontal cortex. I. Oculomotor signals sent from superior colliculus to frontal eye field via mediodorsal thalamus. *Journal of Neurophysiology*, **91**(3), 1381–1402.

Sommer, M.A. and Wurtz, R.H. (2004b). What the brain stem tells the frontal cortex. II. Role of the SC-MD-FEF pathway in corollary discharge. *Journal of Neurophysiology*, **91**(3), 1403–1423.

Sommer, M.A. and Wurtz, R.H. (2006). Influence of the thalamus on spatial visual processing in frontal cortex. *Nature*, **444**(7117), 374–377.

Sommer, M.A. and Wurtz, R.H. (2008a). Brain circuits for the internal monitoring of movements. *Annual Review of Neuroscience*, **31**, 317–338.

Sommer, M.A. and Wurtz, R.H. (2008b). Visual perception and corollary discharge. *Perception*, **37**(3), 408–418.

Sparks, D.L. (1978). Functional properties of neurons in the monkey superior colliculus: coupling of neuronal activity and saccade onset. *Brain Research*, **156**(1), 1–16.

Sparks, D.L. (1986). Translation of sensory signals into commands for control of saccadic eye movements: role of primate superior colliculus. *Physiological Reviews*, **66**(1), 118–171.

Sparks, D.L. (2002). The brainstem control of saccadic eye movements. *Nature Reviews Neuroscience*, **3**(12), 952–964.

Sparks, D.L. and Hartwich-Young, R. (1989). The deep layers of the superior colliculus. *Rev Oculomot Res*, **3**, 213–255.

Sparks, D.L., and Mays, L.E. (1980). Movement fields of saccade-related burst neurons in the monkey superior colliculus. *Brain Research*, **190**(1), 39–50.

Sprague, J.M. (1975). Mammalian tectum: intrinsic organization, afferent inputs, and integrative mechanisms. Anatomical substrate. *Neurosciences Research Program Bulletin*, **13**(2), 204–213.

Stanton, G.B., Bruce, C.J., and Goldberg, M.E. (1995). Topography of projections to posterior cortical areas from the macaque frontal eye fields. *Journal of Comparative Neurology*, **353**(2), 291–305.

Stanton, G.B., Goldberg, M.E., and Bruce, C.J. (1988). Frontal eye field efferents in the macaque monkey: II. Topography of terminal fields in midbrain and pons. *Journal of Comparative Neurology*, **271**(4), 493–506.

Stein, B.E. and Meredith, M.A. (1993). *The merging of the senses*. Cambridge, MA: MIT Press.

Stepniewska, I., Ql, H.X., and Kaas, J.H. (2000). Projections of the superior colliculus to subdivisions of the inferior pulvinar in New World and Old World monkeys. *Visual Neuroscience*, **17**(4), 529–549.

Suzuki, S., Suzuki, Y., and Ohtsuka, K. (2004). Convergence eye movements evoked by microstimulation of the rostral superior colliculus in the cat. *Neuroscience Research*, **49**(1), 39–45.

Theeuwes, J. (1994). Endogenous and exogenous control of visual selection. *Perception*, **23**(4), 429–440.

Theeuwes, J. (2004). Top-down search strategies cannot override attentional capture. *Psychonomic Bulletin and Review*, **11**(1), 65–70.

Thevarajah, D., Mikulic, A., and Dorris, M.C. (2009). Role of the superior colliculus in choosing mixed-strategy saccades. *Journal of Neuroscience*, **29**(7), 1998–2008.

Thomas, N.W., and Paré, M. (2007). Temporal processing of saccade targets in parietal cortex area LIP during visual search. *Journal of Neurophysiology*, **97**(1), 942–947.

Thompson, K.G. and Bichot, N.P. (2005). A visual salience map in the primate frontal eye field. *Progress in Brain Research*, **147**, 251–262.

Thompson, K.G., Bichot, N.P., and Sato, T.R. (2005). Frontal eye field activity before visual search errors reveals the integration of bottom-up and top-down salience. *Journal of Neurophysiology*, **93**(1), 337–351.

Tigges, J. and Tigges, M. (1981). Distribution of retinofugal and corticofugal axon terminals in the superior colliculus of squirrel monkey. *Investigative Ophthalmology and Visual Science*, **20**(2), 149–158.

Trappenberg, T.P., Dorris, M.C., Munoz, D.P., and Klein, R.M. (2001). A model of saccade initiation based on the competitive integration of exogenous and endogenous signals in the superior colliculus. *Journal of Cognitive Neuroscience*, **13**(2), 256–271.

Treisman, A.M. and Gelade, G. (1980). A feature-integration theory of attention. *Cognitive Psychology*, **12**(1), 97–136.

Van Essen, D.C., Newsome, W.T., and Maunsell, J.H. (1984). The visual field representation in striate cortex of the macaque monkey: asymmetries, anisotropies, and individual variability. *Vision Research*, **24**(5), 429–448.

Van Gisbergen, J.A., Van Opstal, A.J., and Tax, A.A. (1987). Collicular ensemble coding of saccades based on vector summation. *Neuroscience*, **21**(2), 541–555.

Van Horn, M.R., Cullen, K.E., and Waitzman, D.M. (2008). *The rostral superior colliculus encodes target location in three-dimensional space*. Paper presented at the Society for Neuroscience Abstracts, Washington, DC.

White, B.J., Boehnke, S.E., Marino, R.A., Itti, L., and Munoz, D.P. (2009). Color-related signals in the primate superior colliculus. *Journal of Neuroscience*, **29**(39), 12159–12166.

Wolfe, J.M., Cave, K.R., and Franzel, S.L. (1989). Guided search: an alternative to the feature integration model for visual search. *Journal of Experimental Psychology Human Perception and Performance*, **15**(3), 419–433.

Wolfe, J.M. and Horowitz, T.S. (2004). What attributes guide the deployment of visual attention and how do they do it? *Nature Reviews Neuroscience*, 5(6), 495–501.

Wurtz, R.H., and Albano, J.E. (1980). Visual-motor function of the primate superior colliculus. *Annual Review of Neuroscience*, 3, 189–226.

Wurtz, R.H. and Goldberg, M.E. (1971). Superior colliculus cell responses related to eye movements in awake monkeys. *Science,* 171(966), 82–84.

Wurtz, R.H. and Goldberg, M.E. (1972a). Activity of superior colliculus in behaving monkey. 3. Cells discharging before eye movements. *Journal of Neurophysiology*, 35(4), 575–586.

Wurtz, R.H. and Goldberg, M.E. (1972b). The primate superior colliculus and the shift of visual attention. *Investigative Ophthalmology*, 11(6), 441–450.

Wurtz, R.H. and Hikosaka, O. (1986). Role of the basal ganglia in the initiation of saccadic eye movements. *Progress in Brain Research*, 64, 175–190.

Wurtz, R.H., and Mohler, C.W. (1976). Organization of monkey superior colliculus: enhanced visual response of superficial layer cells. *Journal of Neurophysiology*, 39(4), 745–765.

Zhaoping, L. and May, K.A. (2007). Psychophysical tests of the hypothesis of a bottom-up saliency map in primary visual cortex. *PLoS Computational Biology*, 3(4), e62.

CHAPTER 12

Saccadic eye movements and the basal ganglia

Corinne R. Vokoun, Safraaz Mahamed, and Michele A. Basso

Abstract

Located deep within the telencephalon, the basal ganglia (BG) refer to an aggregate of subcortical structures that relay cortical signals through at least two pathways. The classical model of BG function suggests the existence of reciprocal pathways: a 'direct pathway' which releases movement and an 'indirect pathway' which prevents movement. However, more recent evidence suggests a more nuanced role of the BG in volitional movement, as well as more complex connectivity and pathways. Neuronal recordings and anatomical experiments within the BG and its output structures have provided a fairly comprehensive scheme for understanding the neuronal control of voluntary saccades. Thus, experiments using eye movements play a central role in revealing BG function and testing BG models.

Introduction

Many advances in our knowledge of BG circuitry have taken place since the classic work exploring the relationship of the BG and saccades occurred approximately 25 years ago. Currently, anatomically based models emphasizing the dichotomy between the direct and indirect striatonigral/pallidal pathways are being updated with models that emphasize the reciprocal and branching nature of the projections between BG structures. Similarly, physiological models based on increases and decreases in discharge rates are being replaced with models emphasizing the temporal structure of neuronal discharge properties (Israel and Bergman, 2008; Nini et al., 1995). Results from deep brain stimulation as a treatment for patients with movement disorders, such as Parkinson's disease and dystonia, have widened our view of the role of the BG to include cognition and even mood and emotion (Utter and Basso, 2008). In parallel with this, there has been a resurgence of interest in the role of BG dopaminergic circuits in mechanisms of reward and reinforcement learning. In this new context, experiments using eye movements play a central role in revealing BG function and testing BG models. There is certainly much left to do before we have a full picture of the role of the BG in general, or eye movement control in particular.

Voluntary saccadic eye movements are rapid movements of the eye serving to reorient the line of sight. Neuronal recordings and anatomical experiments over the last century provide a fairly comprehensive scheme for understanding the neuronal control of voluntary saccades. Cortical signals relaying eye movement information to the midbrain traverse at least two pathways. One pathway arises from frontal cortical neurons and targets the midbrain superior colliculus (SC) (Fries, 1984; Harting et al., 1992). These cortical projection neurons are excitatory, and they convey the results of their processing to the SC for the generation of voluntary saccades (Segraves and Goldberg, 1987; Sommer and Wurtz, 2000). A second pathway also arises from neurons of the frontal cerebral cortex and targets the SC, but this pathway traverses a series of synapses within the BG, before reaching the SC (Parthasarathy et al., 1992; Selemon and Goldman-Rakic, 1985, 1988; Stanton et al., 1988; Weyand and Gafka, 1998). The cortical projection neurons that make up this pathway are also excitatory, however most BG nuclei have high GABA content (Tepper and Bolam, 2004). Therefore, inhibition or disinhibition of SC neuronal activity can occur depending on which BG nuclei are firing (Chevalier and Deniau, 1990; Chevalier et al., 1981a, 1981b; Chevalier et al., 1984, 1985). For review of the SC see White and Munoz, Chapter 11, this volume. For review of the frontal cortex see Johnston and Everling, Chapter 15, this volume.

In what follows, we first provide a general overview of the structures that make up the BG. We then discuss the literature that shows a relationship between saccades and the neuronal activity in BG nuclei. Based on these data, we consider current models of BG function in saccade generation. Finally, we review more recent work in one output nucleus of the BG, the substantia nigra pars reticulata (SNr). This work, together with anatomical studies and physiological work *in vivo* and *in vitro*, suggest that the current model of BG function should be revisited. We conclude by high-lighting what we view as key future directions to advance our understanding of the BG and its role in eye movements.

Basal ganglia anatomy

Located deep within the telencephalon, the BG refer to an aggregate of subcortical structures. Most BG structures project exclusively to other parts of the BG. However, there are two output nuclei, the globus pallidus internal segment (GPi) and the SNr that target primarily the thalamus, the SC, and the pedunculopontine nucleus (PPN). Although BG output is mediated largely through these three structures, its influence is far reaching. Through thalamic targets such as the ventral lateral nucleus and the ventral anterior nucleus (Hoover and Strick, 1999), the BG influence cognitive, motor, and sensory cortical information processing (Middleton and Strick, 1996, 2000, 2002). Through the SC, the BG influence movements of the head and eyes (Hikosaka et al., 2000; see also Corneil, Chapter 16, this volume). Through the PPN, the BG influence spinal cord processing and other aspects of segmental movement control (Garcia-Rill et al., 1983; Lavoie and Parent, 1994; Shink et al., 1997).

The dorsal striatum (referred to as 'the striatum') is the main input nucleus of the BG and is made up of two nuclei: the caudate and putamen. Together, the caudate and putamen receive inputs from virtually the entire cerebral cortex. Of particular importance for saccadic eye movements are inputs to the striatum from regions of the prefrontal cortex: dorsolateral frontal cortex including the frontal eye fields (FEFs), dorsomedial frontal cortex including the supplementary eye fields (SEFs), and regions of the parietal cortex (Parthasarathy et al., 1992; Stanton et al., 1988) including lateral supra-sylvian cortex in cats (Niida et al., 1997). Striatal signalling is modulated by dopamine (DA) input from substantia nigra pars compacta (SNc) neurons. The ventral striatum, which contains the nucleus accumbens, also receives DA input largely from the ventral tegmental area (VTA) (Maeda and Mogenson, 1980). However, little work related to saccades has been performed in the nucleus accumbens and VTA, and therefore are beyond the scope of this review. The subthalamic nucleus (STN) can also be considered a BG input nucleus because, like the striatum, the STN receives direct input from the cerebral cortex (Nambu et al., 2000, 2002).

In the canonical model of the BG pathways (Albin et al., 1989, 1995), the direct pathway arises in the striatum and targets the GPi and SNr directly. An indirect pathway also arises in the striatum, but it targets the GPi and SNr indirectly, via relays in the globus pallidus external segment (GPe) and STN. Figure 12.1A illustrates schematically the different routes taken by the direct and indirect pathways. Subsequent anatomical work revealed that the connections within BG nuclei are more complicated than once thought. Current models include elaborated circuitry with both reciprocal projections and extensive branching (Lévesque and Parent, 2005; Lévesque et al., 2003) (Fig. 12.1B). For example, individual striatal axons branch to terminate in the GPe, GPi, and SNr (Lévesque and

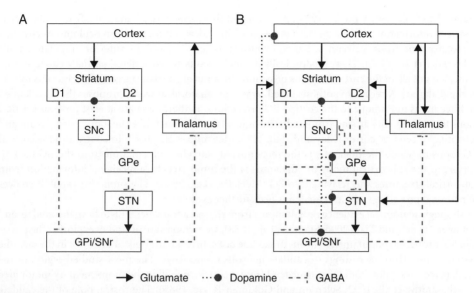

Fig. 12.1 Schematic diagrams of connections within BG nuclei and arising from cerebral cortex. A) The canonical anatomical model of the BG pathways (Albin et al., 1989, 1995). The direct pathway arises in the striatum and targets the GPi and SNr directly. The indirect pathway arises in the striatum and targets GPe which targets STN which targets GPi and SNr. B) Subsequent anatomical work reveals that the connections within BG nuclei are complicated and include reciprocal projections. This schematic reflects the results compiled from a number of sources (see text). In both panels, dashed lines show inhibitory connections mediated by GABA. Dotted lines show dopaminergic connections. Lines with arrows show excitatory connections mediated by glutamate. D1, D1 dopamine receptor; D2, D2 dopamine receptor; SNc, substantia nigra pars compacta; SNr, substantia nigra pars reticulata; STN, subthalamic nucleus; GPi, globus pallidus internal; GPe, globus pallidus external.

Parent, 2005; Lévesque et al., 2003; Parent et al., 2000). GPe neurons also project to the STN, often through branching collaterals of the GPi axons, as well as projecting back onto the striatum (Bevan et al., 1998; Smith et al., 1998). Again, the direct projection from the GPe to the GPi, excluding the STN projection, precludes a simple dichotomy between direct and indirect pathways. Also included in Fig. 12.1B is a third pathway from cortex to STN, referred to as the hyperdirect pathway (Nambu et al., 2000, 2002). This tangle of connections implicates the BG as the hub of a network of structures that can be modified by numerous influences. In what follows, we review each of the BG nuclei as they relate to the control of saccadic eye movements.

The striatum or caudate/putamen

The striatum, the major input structure of the BG, is comprised of two functionally similar nuclei, the caudate and putamen in mammals such as cats and monkeys. Rostrally, the caudate and putamen appear as one large structure, but they are separated by the internal capsule caudally. In rodents the striatum appears as one large structure throughout its rostrocaudal extent. Anatomical and physiological studies reveal that different cortical areas project to distinct regions of the caudate and putamen (Kemp and Powell, 1970; Parthasarathy et al., 1992; Selemon and Goldman-Rakic, 1985, 1988). For example, different regions of association cortex send projections to the anterior striatum that terminate in a complex, partially overlapping pattern (Calzavara et al., 2007; Haber et al., 2006; Selemon and Goldman-Rakic, 1985). On the other hand, sensory inputs largely arising from cortical visual areas, target posterior regions of the striatum, including the tail of the caudate and putamen

(Saint-Cyr et al., 1990; Updyke, 1993). As a result of this corticostriatal anatomy, five parallel corti-costriatal information processing circuits can be identified: a motor circuit, an oculomotor circuit, a dorsolateral prefrontal circuit, a lateral orbitofrontal circuit, and an anterior cingulate circuit (Alexander et al., 1986). These anatomically distinct circuits are considered partially closed in that some, but not all, of the cortical regions providing the input are also the targets of the outputs by way of the thalamus. A recent hypothesis based largely on anatomical work, proposes that this looped architecture is not unique to the cortico-BG projections. Rather, there are at least three subcortical loops through the BG arising from and returning to the SC, much like the loops arising from and returning to cerebral cortex (May and Hall, 1986; McHaffie et al., 2005). In contrast to the cortical BG loops in which the thalamus is the relay nucleus carrying information from the BG back to cortex, in the subcortical loops the thalamus is the input structure receiving information from subcortical structures and relaying it to BG (McHaffie et al., 2005). The similarities and differences of neuronal processing within these loops need further exploration.

Although anatomical evidence reveals inputs from the saccade-related FEF to both the caudate and putamen (Lynch and Tian, 2006; Stanton et al., 1988), we are unaware of studies exploring the physiological properties of putamen neurons in saccade tasks. Instead, the bulk of the work in the saccadic system comes from recordings of caudate neurons in monkeys. The most studied region of the caudate receives input from the dorsolateral frontal cortex, including the supplementary motor area (Parthasarathy et al., 1992; Selemon and Goldman-Rakic, 1985). The rostral pole of the caudate nucleus, where the parietal cortex projects, also remains relatively unexplored in saccade tasks (Calzavara et al., 2007; Haber et al., 2006; Selemon and Goldman-Rakic, 1985, 1988).

Striatal activity is modulated by dense innervation from dopaminergic neurons that are located primarily in the SNc, with lesser contributions from the VTA and lateral hypothalamus. The projections of the mesolimbic DA nuclei play an important role in mechanisms of reward and addiction (Kelley, 2004; Schultz, 1998, 1999). There is a large body of literature exploring reward modulation of BG neurons during saccade tasks. However, the control of the striatum by DA is beyond the scope of this review, so we refer the interested reader to a recent review (Hikosaka et al., 2006).

The initial studies in monkeys exploring the physiology of caudate neurons in saccade tasks identified two broad classes (Hikosaka et al., 1989a). One type of caudate neuron discharged with a low spontaneous rate, averaging 1.8 sp/s. The second type of caudate neuron discharged spontaneously, but irregularly, with an average rate of 5.6 sp/s. Striatal neurons are divided into two general classes that likely correspond to these types: phasically active neurons (PANs) and tonically active neurons (TANs). Based on combined physiological and anatomical experiments, PANs are considered to be the medium-sized spiny, GABAergic projection neurons, whereas the TANs are considered to be the large, aspiny, cholinergic interneurons (Bolam et al., 1984; Tepper and Bolam, 2004).

Caudate neurons discharge in relation to the appearance of visual stimuli, the generation of saccades, and events that intervene between vision and action, such as expectancy of reward. The discharges of caudate neurons are time-locked to the appearance of visual stimuli and the initiation of saccades. The sensory activity is highly dependent upon the context in which the saccade is produced. The amplitude of the saccade-related discharge is correlated with saccade velocity. Furthermore, individual caudate neurons exhibit different neuronal response profiles depending on the behavioural context. Therefore, it is more accurate to refer to 'neuronal response profiles' rather than 'neuronal types'. The most common neuronal response profile observed in the caudate nucleus is the memory-guided, saccade-related discharge. This pattern of activity is time-locked to the onset of saccades directed contralaterally, and appears when a saccade is made to a remembered target, in the absence of an actual visual stimulus to guide the saccade. The second most common type is the discharge associated with visually-guided saccades. This transient activity is time-locked to the onset of a saccade, when a visual target is used to guide the saccade. If a delay is imposed between the appearance of the target and the cue to make a saccade, neurons discharge action potentials at a lower rate for the duration of the delay. Importantly, this delay-period activity is contingent upon the presence of the visual stimulus. The third type of activity in caudate neurons is an increase in discharge rate occurring after the appearance of a saccade target and before the onset of a saccade. The fact that this activity is spatially selective and linked to the occurrence of a saccade indicates a role for this neuronal activity in saccade preparation.

In addition to saccade-related activity that is contingent upon behavioural context, many caudate neurons have transient sensory responses that correlate with the appearance of visual stimuli (Hikosaka et al., 1989b). These visual responses are also highly sensitive to the behavioural context in which the stimuli appear. The properties of caudate sensory responses differ from those of saccade-related discharges. First, when presented with the same saccade target repeatedly, visual discharges of caudate neurons habituate within a few trials, whereas saccade-related discharges do not. Second, some visual neurons respond only when the stimulus is associated with a subsequent reward. In contrast, caudate saccade-related discharges occur for both rewarded and unrewarded saccadic eye movements. A final important difference between visual and saccadic discharges of caudate neurons appears in memory-guided saccade tasks. The visual responses of caudate neurons are stronger when the target location is randomized. If the target location appears in blocks and is therefore predictable, the visual response does not occur. This suggests that caudate sensory activity is dependent on the relevance of the sensory information for an upcoming motor act. For example, if the activity signalled expectation, it would have been greater in the blocked target trials (Hikosaka et al., 1989b, 1989c). It would be interesting to explore these differences in sensorimotor activity of caudate neurons in light of more recent decision-making models (Beck et al., 2008; Gold and Shadlen, 2007; Ding and Gold, 2010).

Interestingly, TANs of the caudate, the presumed large, aspiny cholinergic interneurons (Bolam et al., 1984; Tepper and Bolam, 2004), also have visual responses. Since TANs have a low spontaneous discharge rate, the response to the appearance of a visual stimulus in these neurons is a decrease in discharge rate. One remarkable property of the visual responses of caudate neurons is that the directional selectivity of the visual responses can change depending upon the reward contingencies (Kawagoe et al., 1998). However, visual responses of TANs are not modulated by reward, but visual responses of PANs are (Aosaki et al., 1994, 1995; Shimo and Hikosaka, 2001). Based on these data, hypotheses regarding the role of TANs and PANs in reinforcement learning have flourished, but the relationship between these two neuronal classes with respect to control of saccadic eye movements is poorly understood.

Many of the visual responses of caudate neurons signal sensory information required to guide saccades in particular contexts. There are, however, signals expressed by caudate neurons that correlate with cognitive events such as expectancy of target appearance or reward (Hikosaka et al., 1989c). Activity also occurs at the end of a trial, when a monkey receives a reward. This post movement or reward-related activity of caudate neurons is thought to provide evaluative information needed to guide the learning of sensorimotor tasks (Lau and Glimcher, 2007; Nakamura and Hikosaka, 2006; Williams and Eskandar, 2006). These signals presumably modulate or enhance sensory processing for the guidance of future actions.

Although a role for thalamic inputs cannot be excluded (Harting and Updyke, 2006; Lin et al., 1984; May and Hall, 1986; McHaffie et al., 2005), the likely origin underlying some of the discharges in caudate neurons is the cerebral cortex (Niida et al., 1997; Parthasarathy et al., 1992; Selemon and Goldman-Rakic, 1985, 1988; Weyand and Gafka, 1998). There are clear similarities of the discharge profiles of cerebral cortical neurons and caudate neurons (Bruce and Goldberg, 1985; Bruce et al., 1985; Funahashi et al., 1989, 1991). Moreover, the transient discharge of caudate neurons correlating with sensory or cognitive events follows the pattern of inputs from the cortex. Sensory activity appears more commonly in the posterior region of the caudate and putamen, whereas memory and cognitive activity appear more commonly in the anterior regions of the caudate (Harting and Updyke, 2006; Hikosaka et al., 1989a, 1989b, 1989c). This distribution of activity correlates with the distribution of corticostriatal inputs from regions of cortex having similar features.

Future experiments in which striatal neuron activity during saccade tasks is recorded in combination with identification of cortical inputs will provide better insight into the specific role of corticostriatal pathways in the control of saccades. Furthermore, increasingly detailed assessments of intrastriatal organization, as it relates to saccades, are also needed. For example, is there a map of saccades or visual stimuli within the regions of caudate associated with the generation of saccades? Can the oculomotor circuit be subdivided further, such that there are segregated channels related to learning a sensorimotor relationship or related to producing movement? Do individual caudate neurons participate in multiple contexts, with different subpopulations being recruited at different times during the task, such as occurs in motor cortex (Riehle et al., 1997, 2000)? Recent advances in recording from multiple neurons and multiple sites will no doubt contribute to answers for these important, circuit-based questions.

Anatomical evidence supports both a segregated model and an overlapping model of cortical inputs to the striatum (Calzavara et al., 2007; Haber et al., 2006; Lynd-Balta and Haber, 1994; Parthasarathy et al., 1992; Selemon and Goldman-Rakic, 1985). Future work must also determine whether inputs from multiple, functionally related cortical areas, like SEF and FEF, converge on the same neurons. Furthermore, we need to know whether these striatal neurons in turn, are part of the direct or indirect pathway. Defining the functional connectivity of the striatum is crucial to understanding how the circuits underlie different aspects of behaviour.

The subthalamic nucleus

The subthalamic nucleus lies just ventral to the zona incerta. Early work emphasized the role of the STN within the indirect pathway, relaying caudate information to the output nuclei, the GPi and the SNr (Albin et al., 1989, 1995). However, STN has reciprocal connections with the GPe (Gillies et al., 2002; Plenz and Kital, 1999; Terman et al., 2002) indicating complexity beyond the direct/indirect model. The projections from STN are the only glutamatergic projections within the BG (Kitai and Deniau, 1981). Like the striatum, the STN can be considered an input nucleus since it receives input directly from the cerebral cortex. This pathway is often referred to as the hyperdirect pathway (Hartmann-von Monakow et al., 1978; Kunzle and Akert, 1977; Nambu et al., 2000, 2002). However, studies of the role of STN neurons in saccadic eye movements of monkeys are limited. In light of the anatomical relationship between dorsal medial frontal cortex and STN (Huerta and Kaas, 1990; Huerta et al., 1986), recent work focuses on the hyperdirect pathway.

Although STN activity has mostly been tied to skeletal motor behaviour (DeLong et al., 1985), there are neurons located in the ventral STN that discharge in relation to visual stimuli, cognitive events, and saccadic eye movements (Matsumura et al., 1992). The ventral location corresponds to the terminal regions of inputs arising from FEF and SEF (Huerta and Kaas, 1990; Huerta et al., 1986). *In vitro*, STN neurons show spontaneous discharges of action potentials with rates between 5 and 15 sp/s (Bevan et al., 2007). Importantly, these rates occur in the absence of synaptic input suggesting pacemaker-like biophysical properties of these neurons (Bevan et al., 2007). In monkeys, the discharge rates average between 5 and 48 sp/s and the response profiles of STN neurons include increases in discharge for the onset of visual stimuli and increases in discharge before the generation of saccades (Matsumura et al., 1992). Activity associated with attentive fixation and reward can also be found in STN. Typically, the saccade-related increases in discharge are greater for saccades guided by memory than for those guided by vision. Like the caudate, saccade-related activity in the STN is spatially restricted and shows maximal activity associated with saccades directed into the contralateral hemifield. The saccade-related activity of STN neurons precedes the onset of saccades and generally outlasts a saccadic eye movement by hundreds of milliseconds. This feature of STN neuronal activity is in contrast to caudate neuronal activity, which occurs primarily before saccades. Since neurons of the STN contain glutamate, its outputs depolarize their target neurons (Kitai and Deniau, 1981). This agrees with the classical model (Hikosaka et al., 2000) where increased activity in STN produces increases in the discharge rate of GABAergic output nuclei (SNr), thereby suppressing saccades. Furthermore, the timing of saccade-related activity in STN neurons is appropriate for a role in suppressing unwanted saccades (Matsumura et al., 1992). It is also likely that the STN suppresses saccades though its input to the GPi, but evidence is not yet available.

To assess the relationship of STN neurons to saccade suppression, in a recent study, trained monkeys made the same saccade on repeated trials or switched to a different saccade based on the appearance of a colour cue. Switching the saccade requirement from an automatic saccade to a volitional saccade requires suppression. Interestingly, STN neurons showed increased discharge rates on the switch trials, indicating a change in the required saccade (Isoda and Hikosaka, 2008). In the STN some neurons even increased in discharge after a 'no go' cue, indicating that the saccade should be suppressed. Indeed, similar increases in activity correlating with a change in saccade requirement appear in neurons of an area just adjacent to the SEF (pre-SMA) which provides input to the STN (Isoda and Hikosaka, 2007). Based on the similarities in neuronal discharge profiles between the STN and the SEF in these experiments, it is suggested that the hyperdirect pathway is at play (Isoda and Hikosaka, 2007, 2008). What remains unknown is whether the activation of the STN also arises via the indirect, striatal-pallidal pathway. Future work will also be needed to determine whether the suppression of saccades in this switching task is meditated through the SC, by virtue of the direct inputs from the BG output nuclei (either SNr or GPi) or whether the suppression of saccades is mediated by the BG-thalamocortical pathway.

Globus pallidus external/globus pallidus internal

The globus pallidus (GP) is separated into two nuclei by small fibres of passage and pallidal border cells. The more laterally positioned nucleus is the GPe, whereas the medially positioned nucleus is the GPi (entopeduncular nucleus in rodents). Both segments of GP receive GABAergic input from medium spiny striatal projection neurons, but these projections originate from different classes of medium spiny neurons. The direct pathway arises from GABA/substance P-containing medium spiny neurons, whereas the indirect pathway arises from the GABA/enkephalin containing medium spiny neurons (Albin et al., 1989, 1995; Gerfen et al., 1990; Surmeier et al., 1996), although, anatomical evidence shows that direct pathway neurons send collaterals to the GPe; therefore, these pathways are not mutually exclusive (Levesque and Parent, 2005).

In light of greater awareness of the complexity of the BG circuitry, the role of the GP in saccades has garnered more attention. In monkeys, GPe neurons discharge with an irregular tonic rate of approximately 50 sp/s (DeLong et al., 1985; Turner and Anderson, 2005), and are broadly tuned for saccade directions. This reflects a large convergence of inputs from the caudate. In one report, recordings of GPe neurons within the dorsal aspect of the nucleus, revealed that they display combinations of increases and decreases in activity, as well as combinations of phasic and tonic activity during performance of saccade tasks (Kato and Hikosaka, 1995). The types of signals recorded include increases in discharge with the appearance of visual stimuli and decreases in discharge associated with saccade generation. The decreases associated with saccade generation are generally transient whereas the increases associated with the appearance of visual stimuli can be transient or tonic. Increases in discharge of GPe neurons tend to occur earlier in the behavioural trials and the decreases tend to occur later. This general time-course of activity is consistent with the idea that increases in activity arise from cortico-STN input and decreases in activity arise from direct striatal input. It is worth noting that there is still no indication of whether GPe neuronal activity is preferential for memory-guided versus visually-guided saccades, as is the case for caudate neuronal activity. The role of GPi neurons in saccades is unclear. In one study, no GPi neurons were found that discharged in relation to visual-saccade behaviour (Kato and Hikosaka, 1995). This finding stands in contrast to recent work demonstrating that GPi neurons contain activity modulated in saccade tasks (Hong and Hikosaka, 2008; Shin and Sommer, 2010; Yoshida and Tanaka, 2009). Like other BG nuclei, the activity in the GP is highly context dependent. In GPe, neurons show increases for saccades made reflexively in a gap task, whereas neurons show decreases for saccades made voluntarily in a delay task (Shin and Sommer, 2010). Furthermore, the activity of GPi neurons appears more related to reward, whereas the activity of GPe neurons appears more tightly related to visually-guided saccades (Shin and Sommer, 2010).

Recent recordings from GP neurons suggest that the activity of GPe neurons also plays a role in suppressing unwanted or reflexive saccadic eye movements (Yoshida and Tanaka, 2009). This is a function similar to that proposed for STN. In an antisaccade task, neurons in the GPe showed both increasing and decreasing levels of activity around the time of a saccade. When monkeys were required to withhold a saccade to the visual stimulus and prepare one to the opposite hemifield (antisaccade) the increasing neurons increased activity further and the decreasing neurons similarly decreased activity further. Inactivation of GPe neurons resulted in increased errors in the antisaccade task. Based on this observation, the authors suggested that the activity of GPe neurons may be to suppress reflexive eye movements. However, it is difficult to understand how neurons with such broad tuning properties could suppress specific saccades (Hikosaka et al., 2000; Yoshida and Tanaka, 2009). Rather, the suppression may be more global. Clearly, further experiments in GP are needed to resolve these issues.

Substantia nigra pars reticulata

Like the GPi, the SNr is composed mainly of GABAergic projection neurons that inhibit target neuronal activity (Chevalier et al., 1981b; DiChiara et al., 1979; Yoshida and Omata, 1979). SNr neurons exhibit discharge properties distinct from the adjacent DA containing neurons of the SNc. SNr neurons display short-duration action potentials and spontaneous repetitive firing *in vivo* and *in vitro* with a mean rate of 12–100 sp/s (Atherton and Bevan, 2005; Deniau et al., 1978; Deniau et al., 2007; Nakanishi et al., 1987). The tonic discharge of action potentials by the SNr is thought to provide a sustained hyperpolarization of target neurons, such as those in the SC. Some SNr neurons decrease their discharge rate either transiently or in a sustained manner, with the appearance of visual stimuli (Basso and Wurtz, 2002; Boussaoud and Joseph, 1985; Handel and Glimcher, 1999). SNr neurons can also show transient decreases in discharge rate around the time of saccade generation in monkeys (Hikosaka and Sakamoto, 1986) or head movements in cats (Boussaoud and Joseph, 1985). Figure 12.2A shows examples of neuronal recordings from SNr in monkeys.

The SNr receives GABAergic afferents from the striatum and GPe, as well as glutamatergic afferents from the STN. The relationship between saccadic eye movements and SNr neuronal activity was first elucidated from recordings performed in cat and monkey (Boussaoud and Joseph, 1985; Hikosaka and Wurtz, 1983a, 1983b, 1983c). Studies of saccadic eye movements emphasize the SNr due to its direct projections to the SC (Basso and Liu, 2007; Basso and Wurtz, 2002; Bayer et al., 2002; Handel and Glimcher, 2000; Hikosaka and Wurtz, 1983a, 1983b,1983c, 1983d; Jayaraman et al., 1977; Liu and Basso, 2008; Sato and Hikosaka, 2002). Based on this and other work, the SNr is thought to act as a gate permitting SC burst neurons (predorsal bundle neurons) to signal the brainstem thereby generating saccadic eye movements (Moschovakis et al., 1996; Sparks and Hartwich-Young, 1989). Support for this model is derived from several lines of evidence. First, electrical stimulation of SC antidromically activates SNr neurons (Hikosaka and Wurtz, 1983d; Moschovakis and Karabelas, 1985). Second, stimulation of SNr neurons, which have GABA-positive terminals surrounding predorsal bundle neurons within the SC (Behan et al., 1987), evokes inhibitory postsynaptic potentials (IPSPs) in SC predorsal bundle neurons (Karabelas and Moschovakis, 1985). This is consistent with the notion that the SNr provides strong synaptic inhibition of SC predorsal bundle neurons (Bickford and Hall, 1992; May and Hall, 1984). Third, injection of a GABA antagonist, bicuculline, into the SC results in irrepressible saccadic eye movements in monkeys (Hikosaka and Wurtz, 1985a). Likewise, injection of a GABA agonist, muscimol, into the SNr also produces irrepressible saccades in monkeys (Hikosaka and Wurtz, 1985b), and orienting head and body movements in cats (Boussaoud and Joseph, 1985). Together these results are strong support for a direct inhibitory influence of SNr on SC saccade-related burst neurons.

The role of SNr in the classical model of saccadic eye movements

Based on the information presented thus far, the current model of saccade generation is as follows: the drive to make a voluntary saccade presumably originates from FEF neuronal activity. This FEF

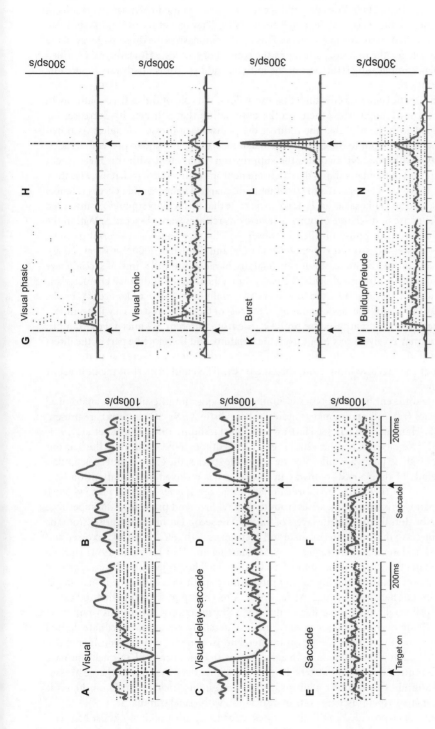

Fig. 12.2 Examples of response profiles of neurons in SNr and SC. Left) Three example neurons recorded from SC. Monkeys performed a visually-guided, delayed saccade task. Each tick represents the time of occurrence of an action potential. Each row of ticks indicates an individual trial. The gray lines show the spike density functions (σ = 12 ms for SNr and 10 ms for SC). The vertical dashed lines and upward arrows in each panel indicate the alignment times. Panels A, C, E, G, I, K, and M are aligned on the onset of the visual stimulus labelled 'Target on'. Panels B, D, F, H, J, L, and N are aligned on saccade onset, labelled 'Saccade'. Reprinted from *Current Opinion in Neurobiology*, **20**(6), Joel Shires, Siddhartha Joshi, and Michele A Basso, Shedding new light on the role of the basal ganglia-superior colliculus pathway in eye movements, pp. 717–752, Copyright (2010), with permission from Elsevier.

discharge activates the medium spiny GABAergic caudate neurons, which in turn inhibit tonic SNr activity (Hikosaka et al., 1993, 2000; Yoshida and Precht, 1971). The pause in SNr activity results in a transient disinhibition of the SC (Chevalier and Deniau, 1990; Chevalier et al., 1981a, 1981b, 1984; Hikosaka and Wurtz, 1983d) resulting in a saccade. This model emphasizes the direct pathway of the BG, yet provides no role for the indirect pathway in the control of saccades. However, as described above, there is evidence implicating structures of the indirect and hyperdirect pathways in saccadic eye movement generation.

Rather than releasing movement as the direct pathway does, the role of the indirect pathway in saccades is to prevent movement. How then can the observation that SNr activity decreases for saccades be reconciled with the idea that the indirect BG pathway suppresses saccades? As noted above, one possibility is that input to the GPi inhibits thalamocortical pathways to prevent saccades. A second possibility is that the SNr mediates the suppression. Consistent with this idea, recent evidence from recordings in monkeys shows that there are neurons within the SNr that increase their discharge rate after visual targets appear, and continue to discharge when a saccade occurs (Handel and Glimcher, 2000; Sato and Hikosaka, 2002). It is conceivable that this activity suppresses unwanted saccades whereas the pause in discharge of other SNr neurons releases wanted saccades. Within the SNr, a number of different response profiles are observed: discrete pausers, universal pausers, bursters, and pause-bursters (Basso and Wurtz, 2002; Handel and Glimcher, 2000; Sato et al., 2000). The last two are characterized by increases in neuronal discharge around the time of saccadic eye movements made into the contralateral field. The pause-bursters have the additional characteristic of decreasing their discharge rate around the time that ipsilaterally-directed saccades occur (Handel and Glimcher, 1999). For a complete understanding of the role of the BG in saccades it will be important to learn whether these different response profiles arise from different BG nuclei. For example, pausing SNr neurons may receive direct input from the striatum, and therefore be part of the direct pathway (Hikosaka et al., 1993). On the other hand, SNr neurons showing increases in discharge around saccade onset may receive input from the GPe or the STN, and be part of the indirect or hyperdirect pathways.

The target of these different neuronal types is another open question. Results from anatomical work in several species (rat, cat, and monkey) indicate three distinct SNr-SC pathways are present (Gerfen et al., 1982; Harting et al., 1988; Harting and Van Lieshout, 1991; Huerta et al., 1991; Jayaraman et al., 1977; Mana and Chevalier, 2001) (Fig. 12.3). Although the locations of the neurons of origin in the SNr for these pathways differ slightly across the species, the general pattern is similar. The anatomical details of the SNr-SC pathway in monkeys has received far less attention (e.g. Jayaraman et al., 1977) so there may be more similarities across species than current evidence suggests. The first pathway is uncrossed, arises from the lateral SNr, and projects to the superficial layers of the SC and the dorsal intermediate layers of the SC. The second is uncrossed, arises from the medial SNr, and projects to the lower intermediate and deep layers of the SC. The third is crossed and terminates in the contralateral SC (Gerfen et al., 1982; Harting and Van Lieshout, 1991; Harting et al., 1988; Jayaraman et al., 1977; Mana and Chevalier, 2001). The projection to the superficial layers may terminate on neurons making up the interlaminar pathways in SC, or it may target GABAergic interneurons (Behan et al., 2002; Mize, 1992). A recent report from anesthetized cats is consistent with the ipsilaterally and contralaterally directed SNr projections having a push-pull effect on their SC targets (Jiang et al., 2003). Specifically, the ipsilateral projection may facilitate desired saccades through focal disinhibition, while the contralateral projection may simultaneously suppress unwanted saccades through global inhibition. In agreement with this, uncrossed SNr neurons have small response fields centred on the contralateral hemifield and they decrease their discharge in association with visual stimuli. Crossed SNr neurons have large response fields centred on the same hemifield, and they increase their discharge rate in association with visual stimuli.

Work in the monkey has provided conflicting evidence for this push-pull hypothesis. As previously mentioned, muscimol inactivation of the SNr results in irrepressible saccades directed into the contralateral hemifield (Hikosaka and Wurtz, 1985b). A more profound, but lesser emphasized effect of the muscimol injections into the SNr is the lack of saccades into the ipsilateral hemifield.

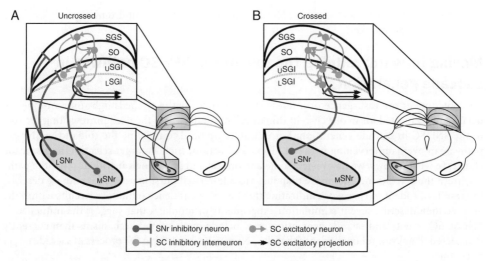

Fig. 12.3 (Also see Plate 7.) Schematic diagram of the connections between the SNr and the SC. A) A coronal section of the SC is shown with expanded views of the layers dorsally and the SNr ventrally indicated by the shaded portions in the inset. Uncrossed projections from the SNr to the SC arise from the lateral and medial SNr and target superficiale and intermediate layers of the SC. B) Crossed pathway from SNr to the SC. SGS, stratum griseum superficial; SO, stratum opticum; $_U$SGI, upper stratum griseum intermediale; $_L$SGI, lower stratum griseum intermediale; $_L$SNr, lateral substantia nigra pars reticulata; $_M$SNr, medial substantia nigra pars reticulata. Green arrows show excitatory SC connections; red lines show inhibitory SNr connections; blue lines show inhibitory SC connections; black arrows show excitatory projections.

Such antagonistic effects on saccades are consistent with the proposed push-pull organization. More recent experiments introducing electrical stimulation of the SNr also produced effects that differed for ipsilaterally and contralaterally directed saccades. Stimulation of the SNr reduces the likelihood of contralateral saccades, whereas the likelihood of ipsilateral saccades is unaffected (Basso and Liu, 2007).

However, some observations are difficult to reconcile with a simple push-pull scheme. First, the SNr neurons recorded in the anesthetized cat show transient increases in discharge time-locked to the presentation of moving visual stimuli. We are unaware of any reports in monkey showing that neurons in SNr respond to moving visual stimuli, although some neurons increase their activity when monkeys track moving stimuli with smooth pursuit eye movements (Basso et al., 2005). As described above, some SNr neurons show increases in activity to the presentation of visual stimuli, but whether these increases also correlate with orofacial movements or postural adjustments associated with saccade preparation remains unknown (Handel and Glimcher, 2000; Sato and Hikosaka, 2002). Second, the model proposed in the cat explains how visual information is conveyed from cortex through BG nuclei to influence the SC. Although some evidence suggests that SNr neurons do not distinguish between visually and non-visually-guided eye movements (Bayer et al., 2002), both the muscimol and stimulation experiments indicate that manipulating SNr neuronal activity preferentially alters saccades guided by memory with little effect on visually-guided saccades (Basso and Liu, 2007; Hikosaka and Wurtz, 1985b). The push–pull model applies particularly to visually-guided saccades. Finally, in the cat, the neurons with different response properties making up the crossed and uncrossed pathway appear to be segregated anatomically (Jiang et al., 2003), although contradictory evidence has been reported (Karabelas and Moschovakis, 1985). This segregation is less apparent in the monkey (Basso and Liu, 2007; Handel and Glimcher, 1999, 2000). Overall, whether these differences are species or methodologically driven will be an important direction for future investigation. For example, it would be important to test whether SNr burst neurons are driven antidromically only from the opposite side SC and whether SNr pause neurons are driven antidromically only from the same side SC in the monkey.

Moving forward: refining the role of the SNr-SC pathway in saccade generation

The outcome of the resurgence of interest in the SNr-SC pathway sheds light on a number of details not accounted for in our current thinking. This underscores the need for revisiting the role of the SNr-SC in saccade generation. For example, we need to redefine the role of the SNr-SC pathway in events intervening between vision and action, such as target selection and saccade choice. In what follows, we first review some anatomical and physiological evidence that the pathway from the SNr-SC includes more than just saccade-related burst neurons. Second, we describe the results of rodent *in vitro* work indicating that SNr may influence inhibitory circuits within the SC. We then describe recent stimulation experiments in monkeys that suggest the influence of SNr on SC activity and saccade generation may include more subtle mechanisms than currently considered. Finally, we show evidence that the SNr may be involved in the process of saccade target selection.

Anatomical experiments in rat, cat, and monkey suggest that the SNr-SC pathway is multifaceted, with different nigral source populations and different laminar targets within the SC (Beckstead and Frankfurter, 1983; Beckstead et al., 1981; Deniau and Thierry, 1997; Harting et al., 1988). Since the original experiments in cats and monkeys (Boussaoud and Joseph, 1985; Hikosaka and Wurtz, 1983a, 1983b, 1983c, 1983d; Joseph and Boussaoud, 1985) other types of SC neurons have been described (Glimcher and Sparks, 1992; Munoz and Wurtz, 1995). Furthermore, within the layers of the SC targeted by the nigra, at least two physiological populations of visuomotor neurons exist: one involved in target selection and one involved in saccade initiation (McPeek and Keller, 2002). Still other SC neurons are associated with perceptual decision-making (Horwitz and Newsome, 1999, 2001; Ratcliff et al., 2003, 2007) and saccade choice (Kim and Basso, 2008). Figure 12.2 illustrates some of the varied response profiles of SC neurons. For review of the SC see White and Munoz, Chapter 11, this volume. The focus of the original SNr-SC experiments was on saccade-related burst neurons. In the cat, the SNr to SC projection emphasized tectoreticulospinal neurons (Karabelas and Moschovakis, 1985) or neurons with visual responses (Jiang et al., 2003). It is likely that the tectoreticulospinal neurons in cat are homologous to the burst and build-up neurons in monkey (Glimcher and Sparks, 1992; Grantyn and Grantyn, 1982; Moschovakis et al., 1988a, 1988b; Munoz and Wurtz, 1995; Rodgers et al., 2006).

In recent work, the Isa group developed an *in vitro* preparation to study the SNr-SC pathway in mice genetically-modified to express green fluorescent protein in GABAergic SC interneurons (Kaneda et al., 2008). With this preparation, the investigators tested whether SNr influences different layers of the SC as predicted from anatomical experiments. They could also assess whether the SNr targets different neuron classes within the SC. Stimulation of the dorsolateral SNr caused monosynaptic IPSPs in both GABAergic and non-GABAergic neurons of the intermediate SC. Further analyses showed that the SNr-recipient GABAergic neurons were SC interneurons that project within or between layers of the SC, but generally do not leave the SC (Lee et al., 2007). Taken together, these findings reveal that the BG may also regulate the spatiotemporal properties of neuronal activity within the SC by regulating intrinsic inhibitory circuits. This example also shows how *in vitro* studies offer a number of advantages complementing *in vivo* recordings.

The role of the intrinsic inhibitory circuitry in the SC is poorly understood, particularly for monkeys (Behan et al., 2002; Mize, 1992). How intrinsic circuits are regulated by external inputs has received limited anatomical and physiological investigation (Kaneda et al., 2008). However, recent experiments in monkeys are consistent with a role for the SNr in modulating inhibitory circuits within the SC (Basso and Liu, 2007). Trained monkeys performed visually-guided and memory-guided saccades to locations throughout the visual field. On randomly interleaved trials, electrical stimulation of the SNr occurred. The current model of the SNr predicts that stimulation of the SNr should increase SNr neuronal discharge, further inhibiting the SC, therefore suppressing saccades. At the very least, the latency of saccades should increase. In contrast to the prediction, SNr stimulation resulted in only subtle effects on visually-guided saccades, and more profound effects on memory-guided saccades. Memory-guided saccades were rotated contralaterally and ipsilaterally. Increases and decreases in the latency of memory-guided saccades were observed. Moreover, the likelihood of memory-guided saccade occurrence was reduced by approximately 10%. Since a single stimulation site in the SNr could alter the amplitude and direction of many saccades, it seems likely that SNr influence on SC is widespread. The decreases in saccade latency produced by SNr stimulation for visually-guided saccades may result from effects on inhibitory interneurons like those shown by Kaneda and colleagues (2008).

The stimulation results reveal a conundrum. How can increased inhibition of the SC from the SNr produce a decrease in saccade latency? The context dependent nature of the effects of SNr stimulation makes it difficult to imagine how antidromic activation of SNr by stimulation of SC neurons could produce the changes in saccade latency (Comoli et al., 2003; May et al., 2009). There are two other pieces of evidence that argue against a mechanism involving direct excitation. First electrical stimulation of the SNr causes reliable reductions in the activity of SC buildup neurons, in spite of the decreases in saccade latency (Liu and Basso, 2008). Second, the variability of saccade latency also decreased with electrical stimulation of the SNr. In our view, inhibitory mechanisms more easily explain changes in variability than mechanisms based on direct excitation. In net, the evidence supports a scheme in which the SNr initially inhibits saccade-related activity in build-up and burst neurons through direct inputs, and then disinhibits the SC via inhibitory interneurons (Liu and Basso, 2008). Although they did not differ significantly, the longer latencies of IPSPs recorded in GABAergic compared to non-GABAergic neurons of the SC are consistent with this idea (Kaneda et al., 2008). Taken together, the results indicate that the effect of altering SNr output on saccades is not simply to gate the occurrence of saccades in an all or none fashion, but rather to sculpt the activity of populations of SC neurons, including inhibitory interneurons.

In addition to recent evidence supporting a more subtle role for SNr inhibition on SC, other recent work implicates the SNr in events that precede saccade generation, such as target selection. The relationship between SNr neurons showing pauses in discharge for saccades and SC neurons showing increases in discharge for saccades is shown in Fig. 12.2E,F and 12.2K,L, respectively. However, there are many other response profiles that can be found in SNr, as well as in SC (Glimcher and Sparks, 1992; Handel and Glimcher, 1999; Hikosaka and Wurtz, 1983a, 1983b, 1983c, 1983d; Li and Basso, 2005; Munoz and Wurtz, 1995). Examples of these different response profiles also appear in Fig. 12.2. A number of neurons in SNr show activity profiles that are modulated well in advance of saccadic eye movement generation. To test the hypothesis that SNr neuron activity is involved in mechanisms preceding saccade generation, we designed a simple task in which the probability of saccade targets varied. We measured SNr neuronal activity to determine whether the activity correlated with the probability of selecting a particular target, or whether it was obligately linked to the initiation of a saccade (Basso and Wurtz, 2002). Since we performed the same experiments in the SC previously, we could also compare directly the changes in SNr activity with the changes in SC activity (Basso and Wurtz, 1997, 1998). We found that SC neurons showed high levels of activity when only one target appeared. However, as the number of possible targets increased, this activity decreased, consistent with the reduced probability of any stimulus being the target. The SNr sensory responses exhibited a similar pattern, but of opposite sign. For example, when only one target appeared, SNr neurons showed a maximal pause in activity. When multiple possible targets appeared, the pause in activity was reduced. Thus, SNr neurons, like neurons in SC, reflect changes in the probability that a particular target will be identified for a saccadic eye movement. Therefore, these neurons signal events that precede saccadic eye movement generation.

The larger and longer pause in SNr neuronal activity that occurred with a single saccade target in the selection task would result in a larger disinhibition of SC when the probability of selecting a particular target is higher. Note that the visual responses of SNr are slightly longer than those of the SC (Basso and Wurtz, 2002; Hikosaka and Wurtz, 1983b). Thus, this decrease in activity could not contribute to the initial visual response changes in SC, but could influence the later visual or delay-period activity. However, during the delay period, before the saccade target was identified, SC neurons showed a dramatic modulation of activity, whereas the SNr activity was modulated very little. This indicates that the suppressive effect of the multiple stimuli seen in the SC during the delay period does not result from an increased inhibition from the SNr. Thus, this is an example of a condition in which the SNr and SC neuronal activity are not mirror images of one another (Basso and Wurtz, 2002). This finding pointedly conflicts with proposed mechanisms of saccade initiation in which SNr and SC activity are mirror-images and the inhibition from the SNr is thought to hold off the production of a saccadic eye movement.

We believe the apparent differences in SNr and SC occur because monkeys did not have to rely solely on internal information to make the saccade choice in this task. Rather, the change in luminance of the target provided a large visual drive that contained all the information required to make the choice. This interpretation is consistent with the idea that alterations in SNr activity preferentially influence movements occurring without visual stimuli to guide them (Basso and Liu, 2007; Hikosaka and Wurtz, 1985a, 1985b). Another finding consistent with this hypothesis is that when the probability of selecting a target changed from 12.5% (eight possible targets) to 100% (clearly identified target), SNr neurons paused well before the saccade was initiated. The pause in SNr activity during this time is important, because when monkeys made mistakes and chose the wrong target, the pause in SNr activity was not present (Basso and Wurtz, 2002). Thus, the SNr is involved in selection because the pause predicted the saccade choices independent of the visual cue, and well in advance of the movement. Exploring the role of the SNr in saccade choice is a promising direction for future research.

Conclusions and future outlook

It is still unclear whether the direct and indirect pathways operate in concert such that subtle imbalances alter BG output. It is possible that these pathways work in a competitive nature or synergistically. The classical model suggests that the direct pathway releases movement, whereas the indirect pathway prevents movements. Perhaps selective populations of neurons are recruited from both pathways, or from one or the other pathway, but only in specific behavioural contexts. With the recent improvements in methods for simultaneous neuronal recordings, we are well poised to begin addressing such questions. Experiments designed to record from multiple neurons across multiple nuclei within the BG during performance of saccade tasks employing different behavioural contingencies will reveal much about how the BG process cortical information to guide action. Recent anatomical evidence also reveals that cortical structures containing neurons involved in smooth pursuit eye movements target regions within the striatum distinct from those involved in saccades (Cui et al., 2003). Little is known about how the BG may be involved in other eye movements, such as pursuit (Basso et al., 2005; Yoshida and Tanaka 2009). As we learn more about the involvement of striatum in cognitive processing, a more general, but much overlooked question is: what happens downstream of the striatum? Are downstream structures such as GP and SNr also involved in the cognitive processes? Do structures downstream of the striatum in the direct and indirect pathways simply 'read out' these inputs as 'go' or 'no-go' signals for movements? Electrophysiological studies performed many years ago demonstrated branching collaterals from the SNr to the SC and thalamus (Anderson and Yoshida, 1980). The anatomical connections are reasonably well-known (Lynch et al., 1994; Sakai et al., 1996, 1998) but the role of the SNr-thalamic pathway in saccades is poorly if at all understood. Furthermore, the cerebellum targets regions of the thalamus that are distinct from the thalamic regions targeted by the SNr (Hoover and Strick, 1999; Middleton and Strick, 2000). For review of the cerebellum, see Thier, Chapter 10, this volume. How SNr and cerebellum interact at the level of the thalamus would be an important direction for further studies. These interactions between cerebellum and SNr are also evident at the level of the SC (Westby et al., 1994), making this an equally important direction for future studies in monkeys. There is no doubt that the results of studies of the role of BG in eye movements will continue to provide much insight into these important questions.

Acknowledgements

The work in our laboratory is supported by NIH EY13692 (MAB), NIH EY019663 (MAB), NCRR P51 RR000167 to the Wisconsin National Primate Research Center, and by a core grant for vision research (P30 EY0166665) from the National Institutes for Health. We are grateful to Dr Paul J. May, Dr Marc Sommer, and SooYoon Shin for providing helpful comments on our manuscript. Corinne R. Vokoun was also supported by the Alice R. McPherson Endowment for the Visual Sciences at the UW Eye Research Institute, and was supported in part by a Parkinson's Disease Foundation Summer Student Fellowship.

References

Albin, R.L., Young, A.B., and Penney, J.B. (1989). The functional anatomy of basal ganglia disorders. *Trends in Neurosciences*, **12**, 366–375.

Albin, R.L., Young, A.B., and Penney, J.B. (1995). The functional anatomy of disorders of the basal ganglia. *Trends in Neurosciences*, **18**, 63–63.

Alexander, G.E., DeLong, M.R., and Strick, P.L. (1986). Parallel organization of functionally segregated circuits linking basal ganglia and cortex. *Annual Review of Neuroscience*, **9**, 357–381.

Anderson, M.E. and Yoshida, M. (1980). Axonal branching patterns and location of nigrothalamic and nigrocollicular neurons in the cat. *Journal of Neurophysiology*, **43**, 883–895.

Aosaki, T., Kimura, M., and Graybiel, A.M. (1995). Temporal and spatial characteristics of tonically active neurons of the primate's striatum. *Journal of Neurophysiology*, **73**, 1234–1252.

Aosaki, T., Tsubokawa, H., Ishida, A., Watanabe, K., Graybiel, A.M., and Kimura, M. (1994). Responses of tonically active neurons in the primate's striatum undergo systematic changes during behavioral sensorimotor conditioning. *Journal of Neuroscience*, **14**, 3969–3984.

Atherton, J.F. and Bevan, M.D. (2005). Ionic mechanisms underlying autonomous action potential generation in the somata and dendrites of GABAergic substantia nigra pars reticulata neurons *in vitro*. *Journal of Neuroscience*, **25**, 8272–8281.

Basso, M.A. and Liu, P. (2007). Context-dependent effects of substantia nigra stimulation on eye movements. *Journal of Neurophysiology*, **97**, 4129–4142.

Basso, M.A. and Wurtz, R.H. (1998). Modulation of neuronal activity in superior colliculus by changes in target probability. *Journal of Neuroscience*, **18**, 7519–7534.

Basso, M.A. and Wurtz, R.H. (2002). Neuronal activity in substantia nigra pars reticulata during target selection. *Journal of Neuroscience*, **22**, 1883–1894.

Basso, M.A. and Wurtz, R.H. (1997). Modulation of neuronal activity by target uncertainty. *Nature*, **389**, 66–69.

Basso, M.A., Pokorny, J.J., and Liu, P. (2005). Activity of substantia nigra pars reticulata neurons during smooth pursuit eye movements in monkeys. *European Journal of Neuroscience*, **22**, 448–464.

Bayer, H.M., Handel, A., and Glimcher, P.W. (2002). Eye position and memory saccade related responses in substantia nigra pars reticulata. *Experimental Brain Research*, **154**, 428–441.

Beck, J.M., Ma, W.J., Kiani, R., Hanks, T., Churchland, A.K., Roitman, J., *et al.* (2008). Probabilistic population codes for bayesian decision making. *Neuron*, **60**, 1142–1152.

Beckstead, R.M. and Frankfurter, A. (1983). A direct projection from the retina to the intermediate gray layer of the superior colliculus demonstrated by anterograde transport of horseradish peroxidase in monkey, cat and rat. *Experimental Brain Research*, **52**, 261–268.

Beckstead, R.M., Edwards, S.B., and Frankfurter, A. (1981). A comparison of the intranigral distribution of nigrotectal neurons labeled with horseradish peroxidase in the monkey, cat, and rat. *Journal of Neuroscience*, **1**, 121–125.

Behan, M., Lin, C.S., and Hall, W.C. (1987). The nigrotectal projection in the cat: an electron microscope autoradiographic study. *Neuroscience*, **21**, 529–539.

Behan, M., Steinhacker, K., Jeffrey-Borger, S., and Meredith, M.A. (2002). Chemoarchitecture of GABAergic neurons in the ferret superior colliculus. *Journal of Comparative Neurology*, **452**, 334–359.

Bevan, M.D., Hallworth, N.E., and Baufreton, J. (2007). GABAergic control of the subthalamic nucleus. *Progress in Brain Research*, **160**, 173–188.

Bevan, M.D., Booth, P.A., Eaton, S.A., and Bolam, J.P. (1998). Selective innervation of neostriatal interneurons by a subclass of neuron in the globus pallidus of the rat. *Journal of Neuroscience*, **18**, 9438–9452.

Bickford, M.E. and Hall, W.C. (1992). The nigral projection to predorsal bundle cells in the superior colliculus of the rat. *Journal of Comparative Neurology*, **319**, 11–33.

Bolam, J.P., Wainer, B.H., and Smith, A.D. (1984). Characterization of cholinergic neurons in the rat neostriatum. A combination of choline acetyltransferase immuniocytochemistry, Golgi-impregnation and electron microscopy. *Neuroscience*, **12**, 711–718.

Boussaoud, D. and Joseph, J.P. (1985). Role of the cat substantia nigra pars reticulata in eye and head movements. II. Effects of local pharmacological injections. *Experimental Brain Research*, **57**, 297–304.

Bruce, C.J. and Goldberg, M.E. (1985). Primate frontal eye fields: I. Single neurons discharging before saccades. *Journal of Neurophysiology*, **53**, 603–635.

Bruce, C.J., Goldberg, M.E., Bushnell, M.C., and Stanton, G.B. (1985). Primate frontal eye fields. II. Physiological and anatomical correlates of electrically evoked eye movements. *Journal of Neurophysiology*, **54**, 714–734.

Calzavara, R., Mailly, P., and Haber, S.N. (2007). Relationship between the corticostriatal terminals from areas 9 and 46, and those from area 8A, dorsal and rostral premotor cortex and area 24c: an anatomical substrate for cognition to action. *European Journal of Neuroscience*, **26**, 2005–2024.

Chevalier, G.and Deniau, J.M. (1990). Disinhibition as a basic process in the expression of striatal functions. *Trends in Neurosciences*, **13**, 277–280.

Chevalier, G., Vacher, S., and Deniau, J.M. (1984). Inhibitory nigral influence on tectospinal neurons, a possible implication of basal ganglia in orienting behavior. *Experimental Brain Research*, **53**, 320–326.

Chevalier, G., Vacher, S., Deniau, J.M., and Desban, M. (1985). Disinhibition as a basic process in the expression of striatal functions. I. The striato-nigral influence on tecto-spinal/tecto-diencephalic neurons. *Brain Research*, **334**, 215–226.

Chevalier, G., Deniau, J.M., Thierry, A.M., and Feger, J. (1981a). The nigro-tectal pathway. An electrophysiological reinvestigation in the rat. *Brain Research*, **213**, 253–263.

Chevalier, G., Thierry, A.M., Shibazaki, T., and Feger, J. (1981b). Evidence for a GABAergic inhibitory nigrotectal pathway in the rat. *Neuroscience Letters*, **21**, 67–70.

Comoli, E., Coizet, V., Boyes, J., Bolam, J.P., Canteras, N.S., Quirk, R.H., *et al.* (2003). A direct projection from superior colliculus to substantia nigra for detecting salient visual events. *Nature Neuroscience*, **6**, 974–980.

Cui, D.-M., Yan, Y.-J., and Lynch, J.C. (2003). Pursuit subregion of the frontal eye field projects to the caudate nucleus in monkeys. *Journal of Neurophysiology*, **89**, 2678–2684.

DeLong, M.R., Crutcher, M.D., and Georgopoulos, A.P. (1985). Primate globus pallidus and subthalamic nucleus: Functional organization. *Journal of Neurophysiology*, **53**, 530–543.

Deniau, J.M. and Thierry, A.M. (1997). Anatomical segregation of information processing in the rat substantia nigra pars reticulata. *Advances in Neurology*, **74**, 83–96.

Deniau, J.M., Hammond, C., Riszk, A., and Feger, J. (1978). Electrophysiological properties of identified output neurons of the rat substantia nigra (pars compacta and pars reticulata): Evidences for the existence of branched neurons. *Experimental Brain Research*, **32**, 409–422.

Deniau, J.M., Mailly, P., Maurice, N., and Charpier, S. (2007). The pars reticulata of the substantia nigra: a window to basal ganglia output. *Progress in Brain Research*, **160**, 151–172.

DiChiara, G., Porceddu, M.L., Morelli, M.L., Mulas, M.L., and Gessa, G.L. (1979). Evidence for a GABAergic projection from the substantia nigra to the ventromedial thalamus and to the superior colliculus of the rat. *Brain Research*, **176**, 273–284.

Ding, L. and Gold, J.I. (2010). Caudate encodes multiple computations for perceptual decisions. *Journal of Neuroscience*, **30**, 15747–15759.

Fries, W. (1984). Cortical projections to the superior colliculus in the macaque monkey: A retrograde study using horseradish peroxidase. *Journal of Comparative Neurology*, **230**, 55–76.

Funahashi, S., Bruce, C.J., and Goldman-Rakic, P.S. (1989). Mnemonic coding of visual space in the monkey's dorsolateral prefrontal cortex. *Journal of Neurophysiology*, **61**, 331–349.

Funahashi, S., Bruce, C.J., and Goldman-Rakic, P.S. (1991). Neuronal activity related to saccadic eye movements in the monkey's dorsolateral prefrontal cortex. *Journal of Neurophysiology*, **65**, 1464–1483.

Garcia-Rill, E., Skinner, R.D., Jackson, M.B., and Smith, M.M. (1983). Connections of the mesencephalic locomotor region (MLR) I. Substantia nigra afferents. *Brain Research Bulletin*, **10**, 57–62.

Gerfen, C.R., Staines, W.A., Arbuthnott, G.W., and Fibiger, H.C. (1982). Crossed connections of the substantia nigra in the rat. *Journal of Comparative Neurology*, **207**, 283–303.

Gerfen, C.R., Engber, T.M., Mahan, L.C., Susel, Z., Chase, T.N., Monsma, F.J., Jr, *et al.* (1990). D1 and D2 dopamine receptor-regulated gene expression of striatonigral and striatopallidal neurons. *Science*, **250**, 1429–1432.

Gillies, A., Willshaw, D., and Li, Z. (2002). Subthalamic-pallidal interactions are critical in determining normal and abnormal functioning of the basal ganglia. *Proceedings of the Royal Society B: Biological Science*, **269**, 545–551.

Glimcher, P.W. and Sparks, D.L. (1992). Movement selection in advance of action in the superior colliculus. *Nature*, **355**, 542–545.

Gold, J.I. and Shadlen, M.N. (2007). The neural basis of decision making. *Annual Review of Neuroscience*, **30**, 535–574.

Grantyn, A. and Grantyn, R. (1982). Axonal patterns and sites of termination of cat superior colliculus neurons projecting in the tecto-bulbo-spinal tract. *Experimental Brain Research*, **46**, 243–256.

Haber, S.N., Kim, K.-S., Mailly, P., and Calzavara, R. (2006). Reward-related cortical inputs define a large striatal region in primates that interface with associative cortical connections, providing a substrate for incentive-based learning. *Journal of Neuroscience*, **26**, 8368–8376.

Handel, A. and Glimcher, P.W. (1999). Quantitative analysis of substantia nigra pars reticulata activity during a visually guided saccade task. *Journal of Neurophysiology*, **82**, 3458–3475.

Handel, A. and Glimcher, P.W. (2000). Contextual modulation of substantia nigra pars reticulata neurons. *Journal of Neurophysiology*, **83**, 3042–3048.

Harting, J.K. and Van Lieshout, D.P. (1991). Spatial relationships of axons arising from the substantia nigra, spinal trigeminal nucleus, and pedunculopontine tegmental nucleus within the intermediate gray of the cat superior colliculus. *Journal of Comparative Neurology*, **305**, 543–558.

Harting, J.K. and Updyke, B.V. (2006). Oculomotor-related pathways of the basal ganglia. *Progress in Brain Research*, **151**, 441–460.

Harting, J.K., Updyke, B.V., and Van Lieshout, D.P. (1992). Corticotectal projections in the cat: anterograde transport studies of twenty-five cortical areas. *Journal of Comparative Neurology*, **324**, 379–414.

Harting, J.K., Huerta, M.F., Hashikawa, T., Weber, J.T., and Van Lieshout, D.P. (1988). Neuroanatomical studies of the nigrotectal projection in the cat. *Journal of Comparative Neurology*, **278**, 615–631.

Hartmann-von Monakow, K., Akert, K., and Kunzle, H. (1978). Projections of the precentral motor cortex and other cortical areas of the frontal lobe to the subthalamic nucleus in the monkey. *Experimental Brain Research*, **33**, 395–403.

Hikosaka, O. and Sakamoto, M. (1986). Cell activity in monkey caudate nucleus preceding saccadic eye movements. *Experimental Brain Research*, **63**, 659–662.

Hikosaka, O. and Wurtz, R.H. (1983a). Visual and oculomotor functions of monkey substantia nigra pars reticulata. I. Relation of visual and auditory responses to saccades. *Journal of Neurophysiology*, **49**, 1230–1253.

Hikosaka, O. and Wurtz, R.H. (1983b). Visual and oculomotor functions of monkey substantia nigra pars reticulata. II. Visual responses related to fixation of gaze. *Journal of Neurophysiology*, **49**, 1254–1267.

Hikosaka, O. and Wurtz, R.H. (1983c). Visual and oculomotor functions of monkey substantia nigra pars reticulata. III. Memory-contingent visual and saccade responses. *Journal of Neurophysiology*, **49**, 1268–1284.

Hikosaka, O. and Wurtz, R.H. (1983d). Visual and oculomotor functions of monkey substantia nigra pars reticulata. IV. Relation of substantia nigra to superior colliculus. *Journal of Neurophysiology*, **49**, 1285–1301.

Hikosaka, O. and Wurtz, R.H. (1985a). Modification of saccadic eye movements by GABA-related substances. I. Effect of muscimol and bicuculline in monkey superior colliculus. *Journal of Neurophysiology*, **53**, 266–291.

Hikosaka, O. and Wurtz, R.H. (1985b). Modification of saccadic eye movements by GABA-related substances. II. Effects of muscimol in monkey substantia nigra pars reticulata. *Journal of Neurophysiology*, **53**, 292–308.

Hikosaka, O., Sakamoto, M., and Usui, S. (1989a). Functional properties of monkey caudate neurons. I. Activities related to saccadic eye movements. *Journal of Neurophysiology*, **61**, 780–798.

Hikosaka, O., Sakamoto, M., and Usui, S. (1989b). Functional properties of monkey caudate neurons. II. Visual and auditory responses. *Journal of Neurophysiology*, **61**, 799–813.

Hikosaka, O., Sakamoto, M., and Usui, S. (1989c). Functional properties of monkey caudate neurons. III. Activities related to expectation of target and reward. *Journal of Neurophysiology*, **61**, 814–832.

Hikosaka, O., Sakamoto, M., and Miyashita, N. (1993). Effects of caudate nucleus stimulation on substantia nigra cell activity in monkey. *Experimental Brain Research*, **95**, 457–472.

Hikosaka, O., Takikawa, Y., and Kawagoe, R. (2000). Role of the basal ganglia in the control of purposive saccadic eye movements. *Physiological Review*, **80**, 953–978.

Hikosaka, O., Nakamura, K., and Nakahara, H. (2006). Basal ganglia orient eyes to reward. *Journal of Neurophysiology*, **95**, 567–584.

Hong, S. and Hikosaka, O. (2008). The globus pallidus sends reward-related signals to the lateral habenula. *Neuron*, **60**, 720–729.

Hoover, J.E. and Strick, P.L. (1999). The organization of cerebellar and basal ganglia outputs to primary motor cortex as revealed by retrograde transneuronal transport of herpes simplex virus type 1. *Journal of Neuroscience*, **19**, 1446–1463.

Horwitz, G.D. and Newsome, W.T. (1999). Separate signals for target selection and movement specification in the superior colliculus. *Science*, **284**, 1158–1161.

Horwitz, G.D. and Newsome, W.T. (2001). Target selection for saccadic eye movements: direction-selective visual responses in the superior colliculus. *Journal of Neurophysiology*, **86**, 2527–2542.

Huerta, M.F. and Kaas, J.H. (1990). Supplementary eye field as defined by intracortical microstimulation: connections in macaques. *Journal of Comparative Neurology*, **293**, 299–330.

Huerta, M.F., Krubitzer, L.A., and Kaas, J.H. (1986). Frontal eye field as defined by intracortical microstimulation in squirrel monkeys, owl monkeys, and macaque monkeys: I. Subcortical connections. *Journal of Comparative Neurology*, **253**, 415–439.

Huerta, M.F., Van Lieshout, D.P., and Harting, J.K. (1991). Nigrotectal projections in the primate *Galago crassicaudatus*. *Experimental Brain Research*, **87**, 389–401.

Isoda, M. and Hikosaka, O. (2007). Switching from automatic to controlled action by monkey medial frontal cortex. *Nature Neuroscience*, **10**, 240–248.

Isoda, M. and Hikosaka, O. (2008). Role for subthalamic nucleus neurons in switching from automatic to controlled eye movement. *Journal of Neuroscience*, **28**, 7209–7218.

Israel, Z. and Bergman, H. (2008). Pathophysiology of the basal ganglia and movement disorders: from animal models to human clinical applications. *Neuroscience and Biobehavioral Reviews*, **32**, 367–377.

Jayaraman, A., Batton, R.R., 3rd, and Carpenter, M.B. (1977). Nigrotectal projections in the monkey: an autoradiographic study. *Brain Research*, **135**, 147–152.

Jiang, H., Stein, B.E., and McHaffie, J.G. (2003). Opposing basal ganglia processes shape midbrain visuomotor activity bilaterally. *Nature*, **423**, 982.

Joseph, J.P. and Boussaoud, D. (1985). Role of the cat substantia nigra pars reticulata in eye and head movements. I. Neural activity. *Experimental Brain Research*, **57**, 286–296.

Kaneda, K., Isa, K., Yanagawa, Y., and Isa, T. (2008). Nigral inhibition of GABAergic neurons in mouse superior colliculus. *Journal of Neuroscience*, **28**, 11071–11078.

Karabelas, A.B. and Moschovakis, A.K. (1985). Nigral inhibitory termination on efferent neurons of the superior colliculus: an intracellular horseradish peroxidase study in the cat. *Journal of Comparative Neurology*, **239**, 309–329.

Kato, M. and Hikosaka, O. (1995). Function of the indirect pathway in the basal ganglia oculomotor system: Visuo-oculomotor activities of external pallidum neurons. In M. Segawa and Y. Nomura (eds.) *Age-Related Dopamine-Deficient Disorders* (pp. 178–187). Basal: Karger.

Kawagoe, R., Takikawa, Y., and Hikosaka, O. (1998). Expectation of reward modulates cognitive signals in the basal ganglia. *Nature Neuroscience*, **1**, 411–416.

Kelley, A.E. (2004). Memory and addiction: shared neural circuitry and molecular mechanisms. *Neuron*, **44**, 161.

Kemp, J.M. and Powell, T.P.S. (1970). The cortico-striate projection in the monkey. *Brain*, **93**, 525–546.

Kim, B. and Basso, M.A. (2008). Saccade target selection in the superior colliculus: a signal detection theory approach. *Journal of Neuroscience*, **28**, 2991–3007.

Kitai, S.T. and Deniau, J.M. (1981). Cortical input to the subthalamus: intracellular analysis. *Brain Research*, **214**, 411–415.

Kunzle, H. and Akert, K. (1977). Efferent connections of cortical area 8 (frontal eye field) in *Macaca fascicularis*. A reinvestigation using the autoradiographic technique. *Journal of Comparative Neurology*, **173**, 147–164.

Lau, B. and Glimcher, P.W. (2007). Action and outcome encoding in the primate caudate nucleus. *Journal of Neuroscience*, **27**, 14502–14514.

Lavoie, B.and Parent, A. (1994). Pedunculopontine nucleus in the squirrel monkey: projections to the basal ganglia as revealed by anterograde tract-tracing methods. *Journal of Comparative Neurology*, **344**, 210–231.

Lee, P.H., Sooksawate, T., Yanagawa, Y., Isa, K., Isa, T., and Hall, W.C. (2007). Identity of a pathway for saccadic suppression. *Proceedings of the National Academy of Sciences USA*, **104**, 6824–6827.

Lévesque, M.and Parent, A. (2005). The striatofugal fiber system in primates: A reevaluation of its organization based on single-axon tracing studies. *Proceedings of the National Academy of Sciences USA*, **102**, 11888–11893.

Lévesque, M., Bédard, A., Cossette, M., and Parent, A. (2003). Novel aspects of the chemical anatomy of the striatum and its efferent projections. *Journal of Chemical Neuroanatomy*, **26**, 231–350.

Li, X. and Basso, M.A. (2005). Competitive stimulus interactions within single response fields of superior colliculus neurons. *Journal of Neuroscience*, **25**, 11357–11373.

Lin, C.-S., May, P.J., and Hall, W.C. (1984). Non-intralaminar thalamostriatal projections in the gray squirrel (Sciurus carolinensis) and tree shrew (Tupaia glis). *Journal of Comparative Neurology*, **230**, 33–46.

Liu, P. and Basso, M.A. (2008). Substantia nigra stimulation influences monkey superior colliculus neuronal activity bilaterally. *Journal of Neurophysiology*, **100**, 1098–1112.

Lynch, J.C. and Tian, J.R. (2006). Cortico-cortical networks and cortico-subcortical loops for the higher control of eye movements. *Progress in Brain Research*, **151**, 461–501.

Lynch, J.C., Hoover, J.E., and Strick, P.L. (1994). Input to the primate frontal eye field from the substantia nigra, superior colliculus, and dentate nucleus demonstrated by transneuronal transport. *Experimental Brain Research*, **100**, 181–186.

Lynd-Balta, E.and Haber, S.N. (1994). Primate striatonigral projections: A comparison of the sensorimotor-related striatum and the ventral striatum. *Journal of Comparative Neurology*, **345**, 562–578.

Maeda, H. and Mogenson, G.J. (1980). An electrophysiological study of inputs to neurons of the ventral tegmental area from the nucleus accumbens and medial preoptic-anterior hypothalamic areas. *Brain Research*, **197**, 365–377.

Mana, S. and Chevalier, G. (2001). The fine organization of nigro-collicular channels with additional observations of their relationships with acetylcholinesterase in the rat. *Neuroscience*, **106**, 357.

Matsumura, M., Kojima, J., Gardiner, T.W., and Hikosaka, O. (1992). Visual and oculomotor functions of monkey subthalamic nucleus. *Journal of Neurophysiology*, **67**, 1615–1632.

May, P.J. and Hall, W.C. (1984). Relationships between the nigrotectal pathway and the cells of origin of the predorsal bundle. *Journal of Comparative Neurology*, **226**, 357–376.

May, P.J. and Hall, W.C. (1986). The sources of the nigrotectal pathway. *Neuroscience*, **19**, 159–180.

May, P.J., McHaffie, J.G., Stanford, T.R., Jiang, H., Costello, M.G., Coizet, V., et al. (2009). Tectonigral projections in the primate: a pathway for pre-attentive sensory input to midbrain dopaminergic neurons. European Journal of Neuroscience, 29, 575–587.

McHaffie, J.G., Stanford, T.R., Stein, B.E., Coizet, V., and Redgrave, P. (2005). Subcortical loops through the basal ganglia. Trends in Neurosciences, 28, 401–407.

McPeek, R.M. and Keller, E.L. (2002). Saccade target selection in the superior colliculus during a visual search task. Journal of Neurophysiology, 88, 2019–2034.

Middleton, F.A. and Strick, P.L. (1996). The temporal lobe is a target of output from the basal ganglia. Proceedings of the National Academy of Sciences USA, 93(16), 8683–8687.

Middleton, F.A. and Strick, P.L. (2000). Basal ganglia and cerebellar loops: motor and cognitive circuits. Brain Research Reviews, 31, 236.

Middleton, F.A. and Strick, P.L. (2002). Basal-ganglia 'projections' to the prefrontal cortex of the primate. Cerebral Cortex, 12, 926–935.

Mize, R.R. (1992). The organization of GABAergic neurons in the mammalian superior colliculus. Progress in Brain Research, 90, 219–248.

Moschovakis, A.K. and Karabelas, A.B. (1985). Observations on the somatodendritic morphology and axonal trajectory of intracellularly HRP-labeled efferent neurons located in the deep layers of the superior colliculus of the cat. Journal of Comparative Neurology, 239, 276–308.

Moschovakis, A.K., Karabelas, A.B., and Highstein, S.M. (1988a). Structure-function relationships in the primate superior colliculus. I. Morphological classification of efferent neurons. Journal of Neurophysiology, 60, 232–262.

Moschovakis, A.K., Karabelas, A.B., and Highstein, S.M. (1988b). Structure-function relationships in the primate superior colliculus. II. Morphological identification of presaccadic neurons. Journal of Neurophysiology, 60, 263–302.

Moschovakis, A.K., Scudder, C.A., and Highstein, S.M. (1996). The microscopic anatomy and physiology of the mammalian saccadic system. Progress in Neurobiology, 50, 133–254.

Munoz, D.P. and Wurtz, R.H. (1995). Saccade-related activity in monkey superior colliculus. I. Characteristics of burst and buildup cells. Journal of Neurophysiology, 73, 2313–2333.

Nakamura, K. and Hikosaka, O. (2006). Role of dopamine in the primate caudate nucleus in reward modulation of saccades. Journal of Neuroscience, 26, 5360–5369.

Nakanishi, H., Kita, H., and Kitai, S.T. (1987). Intracellular study of rat substantia nigra pars reticulata neurons in an in vitro slice preparation: electrical membrane properties and response characteristics to subthalamic stimulation. Brain Research, 437, 45–55.

Nambu, A., Tokuno, H., and Takada, M. (2002). Functional significance of the cortico-subthalamo-pallidal 'hyperdirect' pathway. Neuroscience Research, 43, 111–117.

Nambu, A., Tokuno, H., Hamada, I., Kita, H., Imanishi, M., Akazawa, T., et al. (2000). Excitatory cortical inputs to pallidal neurons via the subthalamic nucleus in the monkey. Journal of Neurophysiology, 84, 289–1696.

Niida, T., Stein, B.E., and McHaffie, J.G. (1997). Response properties of corticotectal and corticostriatal neurons in the posterior lateral suprasylvian cortex of the cat. Journal of Neuroscience, 17, 8550–8565.

Nini, A., Feingold, A., Slovin, H., and Bergman, H. (1995). Neurons in the globus pallidus do not show correlated activity in the normal monkey, but phase-locked oscillations appear in the MPTP model of parkinsonism. Journal of Neurophysiology, 74, 1800–1805.

Parent, A., Sato, F., Wu, Y., Gauthier, J., Lévesque, M., and Parent, M. (2000). Organization of the basal ganglia: the importance of axonal collateralization. Trends in Neurosciences, 23, S20–27.

Parthasarathy, H.B., Schall, J.D., and Graybiel, A.M. (1992). Distributed but convergent ordering of corticostriatal projections: analysis of the frontal eye field and the supplementary eye field in the macaque monkey. Journal of Neuroscience, 12, 4468–4488.

Plenz, D. and Kital, S.T. (1999). A basal ganglia pacemaker formed by the subthalamic nucleus and external globus pallidus. Nature, 400, 677–682.

Ratcliff, R., Cherian, A., and Segraves, M. (2003). A comparison of macaque behavior and superior colliculus neuronal activity to predictions from models of two-choice decisions. Journal of Neurophysiology, 90, 1392.

Ratcliff, R., Hasegawa, Y. T., Hasegawa, R.P., Smith, P.L., and Segraves, M.A. (2007). Dual diffusion model for single-cell recording data from the superior colliculus in a brightness-discrimination task. Journal of Neurophysiology, 97, 1756–1774.

Riehle, A., Grun, S., Diesmann, M., and Aertsen, A. (1997). Spike synchronization and rate modulation differentially involved in motor cortical function. Science, 278, 1950–1953.

Riehle, A., Grammont, F., Diesmann, M., and Grun, S. (2000). Dynamical changes and temporal precision of synchronized spiking activity in monkey motor cortex during movement preparation. Journal of Physiology (Paris) 94, 569–582.

Rodgers, C.K., Munoz, D.P., Scott, S.H., and Paré, M. (2006). Discharge properties of monkey tectoreticular neurons. Journal of Neurophysiology, 95, 3502–3511.

Saint-Cyr, J.A., Ungerleider, L.G., and Desimone, R. (1990). Organization of visual cortical inputs to the striatum and subsequent outputs to the pallido-nigral complex in the monkey. Journal of Comparative Neurology, 298, 129–156.

Sakai, S.T., Inase, M., and Tanji, J. (1996). Comparison of cerebellothalamic and pallidothalamic projections in the monkey (Macaca fuscata): a double anterograde labeling study. Journal of Comparative Neurology, 368, 215–228.

Sakai, S.T., Grofova, I., and Bruce, K. (1998). Nigrothalamic projections and nigrothalamocortical pathway to the medial agranular cortex in the rat: single- and double-labeling light and electron microscopic studies. *Journal of Comparative Neurology*, **391**, 506–525.

Sato, M. and Hikosaka, O. (2002). Role of primate substantia nigra pars reticulata in reward-oriented saccadic eye movement. *Journal of Neuroscience*, **22**, 2363–2373.

Sato, F., Parent, M., Levesque, M., and Parent, A. (2000). Axonal branching pattern of neurons of the subthalamic nucleus in primates. *Journal of Comparative Neurology*, **424**, 142–152.

Schultz, W. (1998). Predictive reward signal of dopamine neurons. *Journal of Neurophysiology*, **80**, 1–27.

Schultz, W. (1999). The reward signal of midbrain dopamine neurons. *News in Physiological Sciences*, **14**, 249–255.

Segraves, M.A. and Goldberg, M.E. (1987). Functional properties of corticotectal neurons in the monkey's frontal eye field. *Journal of Neurophysiology*, **58**, 1387–1419.

Selemon, L.D. and Goldman-Rakic, P.S. (1985). Longitudinal topography and interdigitation of corticostriatal projections in the rhesus monkey. *Journal of Neuroscience*, **5**, 776–794.

Selemon, L.D. and Goldman-Rakic, P.S. (1988). Common cortical and subcortical targets of the dorsolateral prefrontal and posterior parietal cortices in the rhesus monkey: Evidence for a distributed neural network subserving spatially guided behavior. *Journal of Neuroscience*, **8**, 4049–4068.

Shimo, Y. and Hikosaka, O. (2001). Role of tonically active neurons in primate caudate in reward-oriented saccadic eye movements. *Journal of Neuroscience*, **21**, 7804–7814.

Shin, S. and Sommer, M.A. (2010). Activity of neurons in monkey globus pallidus during oculomotor behavior compared with that in substantia nigra pars reticulata. *Journal of Neurophysiology*, **103**, 1874–1887.

Shink, E., Sidibe, M., and Smith, Y. (1997). Efferent connections of the internal globus pallidus in the squirrel monkey: II. Topography and synaptic organization of pallidal efferents to the pedunculopontine nucleus. *Journal of Comparative Neurology*, **382**, 348–363.

Smith, Y., Bevan, M.D., Shink, E., and Bolam, J.P. (1998). Microcircuitry of the direct and indirect pathways of the basal ganglia. *Neuroscience*, **86**, 353–387.

Sommer, M.A. and Wurtz, R.H. (2000). Composition and topographic organization of signals sent from the frontal eye field to the superior colliculus. *Journal of Neurophysiology*, **83**, 1979–2001.

Sparks, D.L. and Hartwich-Young, R. (1989). The deep layers of the superior colliculus. *Reviews in Oculomotor Research*, **3**, 213–255.

Stanton, G.B., Goldberg, M.E., and Bruce, C.J. (1988). Frontal eye field efferents in the macaque monkey: I. Subcortical pathways and topography of striatal and thalamic terminal fields. *Journal of Comparative Neurology*, **271**, 473–492.

Surmeier, D.J., Song, W.J., and Yan, Z. (1996). Coordinated expression of dopamine receptors in neostriatal medium spiny neurons. *Journal of Neuroscience*, **16**, 6579–6591.

Tepper, J.M. and Bolam, J.P. (2004). Functional diversity and specificity of neostriatal interneurons. *Current Opinion in Neurobiology*, **14**, 685–692.

Terman, D., Rubin, J.E., Yew, A.C., and Wilson, C.J. (2002). Activity patterns in a model for the subthalamopallidal network of the basal ganglia. *Journal of Neuroscience*, **22**, 2963–2976.

Turner, R.S. and Anderson, M.E. (2005). Context-dependent modulation of movement-related discharge in the primate globus pallidus. *Journal of Neuroscience*, **25**, 2965–2976.

Updyke, B.V. (1993). Organization of visual corticostriatal projections in the cat, with observations on visual projections to claustrum and amygdala. *Journal of Comparative Neurology*, **327**, 159–193.

Utter, A.A. and Basso, M.A. (2008). The basal ganglia: an overview of circuits and function. *Neuroscience and Biobehavioral Reviews*, **32**, 333–342.

Westby, G.W., Collinson, C., Redgrave, P., and Dean, P. (1994). Opposing excitatory and inhibitory influences from the cerebellum and basal ganglia converge on the superior colliculus: an electrophysiological investigation in the rat. *European Journal of Neuroscience*, **6**, 1335–1342.

Weyand, T.G. and Gafka, A.C. (1998). Corticostriatal and corticotectal neurons in area 6 of the cat during fixation and eye movements. *Vision Neuroscience*, **15**, 141–151.

Williams, Z.M. and Eskandar, E.N. (2006). Selective enhancement of associative learning by microstimulation of the anterior caudate. *Nature Neuroscience*, **9**, 562–568.

Yoshida, A. and Tanaka, M. (2009). Enhanced modulation of neuronal activity during antisaccades in the primate globus pallidus. *Cerebral Cortex*, **19**, 206–217.

Yoshida, M. and Omata, S. (1979). Blocking by picrotoxin of nigra-evoked inhibition of neurons of ventromedial nucleus of the thalamus. *Experientia*, **35**, 794.

Yoshida, M. and Precht, W. (1971). Monosynaptic inhibition of neurons of the substantia nigra by caudato-nigral fibers. *Brain Research*, **32**, 225–228.

Yoshida, A and Tanaka, M. (2009). Neuronal activity in the primate globus pallidus during smooth pursuit eye movements. *Neuroreport*, **20**, 121–125.

CHAPTER 13

Thalamic roles in eye movements

Masaki Tanaka and Jun Kunimatsu

Abstract

The thalamus serves as the gateway to the cerebral cortex—all subcortical signals that ascend to the cortex are relayed by neurons in the thalamus. Different nuclei in the central thalamus receive inputs from the brainstem, the basal ganglia, and the cerebellum, and send outputs to the eye movement-related areas in the cortex, including the frontal eye field, the supplementary eye field, and the lateral prefrontal cortex. Consistent with the converging inputs, neurons in the central thalamus exhibit a variety of eye movement-related activities. Recent analyses of neural activity and eye movements in subjects with natural or experimentally-induced thalamic lesions suggest that signals in the central thalamus are essential for the online monitoring of self-motions and the generation of volitional saccades. In addition, the pathways through the central and the posterior thalamus appear to play a role in visuospatial attention that directly guides eye movements. We will describe recent findings and discuss the role for the thalamus in eye movements.

Introduction

Although the description of a role for the thalamus in eye movements appeared in the late 1930s, the first systematic studies were done by Schlag and Schlag-Rey in cats in the 1970s, and later in monkeys in the 1980s. By exploring the internal medullary lamina (IML) and adjacent paralaminar part of the mediodorsal (MD), ventrolateral (VL), ventroanterior (VA), and lateral dorsal (LD) nuclei with microelectrodes, they found a variety of neurons related to eye movements. These early studies suggest that this part of the thalamus—collectively called the 'IML complex' or 'oculomotor thalamus'—may transmit corollary discharge signals for eye movements and play roles in planning of self-paced saccades (for reviews, see Schlag and Schlag-Rey 1986, 1989). However, there have been little follow-up on these attractive hypotheses until recently, possibly because of the anatomical complexity of the thalamus and its apparent relay function (Sommer, 2003). Following the recent study by Sommer and Wurtz (2002), several laboratories have begun examining the physiology of the central thalamus in order to determine how the large-scale cortico-subcortical networks through the thalamus regulate eye movements. In this chapter, we first outline the early physiological studies and the anatomical connections with the central thalamus. Next, we consider the roles of the central thalamus in the monitoring of eye and other self-generated movements. Recent studies showing the thalamic involvement in saccade generation are then reviewed. Finally, the roles of the central and the posterior thalamus in spatial attention are discussed.

Overview of anatomy and early studies

Anatomy of the central thalamus

The IML is a fibre pathway segregating the medial and the ventral nuclei of the thalamus. Among the several nuclei located within the lamina, Schlag-Rey and Schlag (1984) found eye movement-related neurons in the central lateral (CL) and the paracentral nuclei. These nuclei belong to the anterior group of the intralaminar nuclei, and receive ascending inputs from a number of brainstem structures related to eye movements, including the deep layer of the superior colliculus (SC), the paramedian pontine reticular formation, the nucleus prepositus hypoglossi, the interstitial nucleus of Cajal, the vestibular nuclei, the substantia nigra pars reticulata (SNr), and the deep cerebellar nuclei (for reviews, see Schlag-Rey and Schlag (1989); Jones (2007, pp. 1160–1163) (Fig. 13.1A). In turn, those nuclei send diffuse, non-specific projections to the frontal and parietal cortices and dense projections to the anterior striatum (Smith et al., 2004; Jones (2007, pp. 1143–1157)).

Although Schlag-Rey and Schlag found some eye movement-related neurons in the paralaminar part of adjacent nuclei as well, they mostly considered the roles of the intralaminar nuclei. Recent studies in monkeys and humans showed that the paralaminar part of the MD, VL, and VA nuclei also participate in the control of eye movements. For example, neurons in the MD (Sommer and Wurtz, 2004a; Tanibuchi and Goldman-Rakic, 2003; Watanabe and Funahashi, 2004a) and the VA/VL nuclei (Tanaka, 2005b; Wyder et al., 2003) discharge during saccades. Furthermore, functional imaging studies have repeatedly detected activation in these thalamic nuclei during eye movements (Matsuda et al., 2004; Petit et al., 1993), and focal lesions in the MD and VL thalamus impair eye movements in a particular condition (Bellebaum et al., 2005). These observations are consistent with anatomical studies showing that different paralaminar nuclei receive signals from the basal ganglia, the cerebellum and the SC, and send projections to the frontal eye field (FEF), the supplementary eye field (SEF), and the prefrontal cortex (PFC) (for review, see Alexander et al., 1986; Middleton and Strick 2000). A summary of the recent studies by Lynch and his colleagues showing that different thalamocortical pathways regulate specific aspects of eye movements is shown in Fig. 13.1A (Tian and Lynch, 1997; for review, see Lynch and Tian, 2006). Thus, the oculomotor region in the central thalamus has access to virtually all stages of subcortical processing for eye movements and sends signals to cortical areas that regulate eye movements, suggesting that it may operate as a central controller (Schlag and Schlag-Rey, 1986). The anatomical connections with the thalamus and their roles in eye movements are also discussed in the chapters of the basal ganglia (by Vokoun et al., Chapter 12), the cerebellum (Thier, Chapter 10), the SC (White and Munoz, Chapter 11), and the frontal cortex (Johnston and Everling, Chapter 15) in this volume.

Effects of electrical stimulation

Electrical stimulation in the central thalamus evokes contraversive saccades in cats and monkeys. The stimulation current for evoking saccades can be lower than 20 µA, and the latency is typically 60–80 ms The elicited saccades are either fixed-vector or goal-directed depending on the site of stimulation (cats: Maldonado et al., 1980; monkeys: Schlag et al., 1990). Since there is no anatomical evidence for a direct projection that descends from the thalamus to the brainstem, Schlag and his colleagues considered several possible routes through which thalamic stimulation evokes saccades (for review, see Schlag-Rey and Schlag, 1989), as follows: 1) since neurons in the central thalamus send massive projections to the cortex, the stimulation may recruit cortical neurons that in turn send saccade commands to the brainstem, or 2) alternatively, stimulation in the central thalamus might excite passing fibres; Leichnetz et al. (1981) demonstrated in monkeys that some descending fibres from the FEF to the brainstem pass through the IML. To test these possibilities, Schlag and Schlag-Rey (1971) examined the effects of thalamic stimulation in cats following complete decortification plus destruction of the basal ganglia. However, saccades were still evoked from the central thalamus, even after a few weeks post surgery when any corticofugal fibre would die out. Because these results excluded both possibilities, they concluded that stimulation in the central thalamus antidromically excites

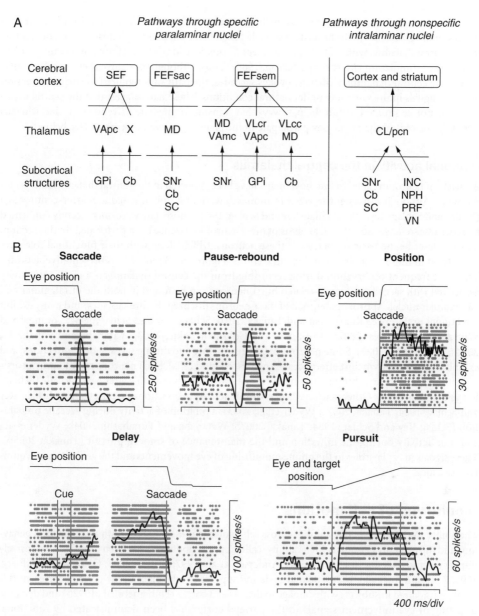

Fig. 13.1 A) Cortico-subcortical connections through the central thalamus. The different parts of the paralaminar nuclei collect signals from the cerebellum, the basal ganglia, and the brainstem, and send projections to specific cortical areas. The intralaminar nuclei receive inputs from many subcortical areas, and send diffuse, non-specific outputs to the cortex and the striatum. The diagram is modified from Tian and Lynch (1997) with permission. Cb, Cerebellar nuclei; CL, central lateral nucleus; FEFsac and FEFsem, saccadic and smooth eye movement subregions of frontal eye field, respectively; GPi, internal segment of the globus pallidus; INC, interstitial nucleus of Cajal; MD, mediodorsal nucleus; NPH, nucleus prepositus hypoglossi; pcn, paracentral nucleus; PRF, pontine reticular formation; SC, superior colliculus; SEF, supplementary eye field; SNr, substantia nigra pars reticulata; VAmc and VApc, ventroanterior nucleus pars magnocellularis and parvocellularis, respectively; VLcc and VLcr, caudal and rostral part of the ventrolateral nucleus pars caudalis, respectively; VN, vestibular nuclei; X, area X. B) Representative examples of neuronal activity in the central thalamus.

ascending collateral fibres of neurons in the brainstem, and the signal then orthodromically travels the descending branches to the brainstem saccade generator. Consistent with this, ablation of neurons in the central thalamus with a fibre-sparing agent (ibotenic acid) did not eliminate saccades evoked by electrical stimulation (Merker and Schlag, 1985). Thus, although low-current electrical stimulation in the central thalamus artificially evokes saccades, the pathways required to elicit saccades do not send signals in the same way under natural conditions. These data suggest that the central thalamus may not be situated within the pathways that transmit immediate drive for saccades, whereas signals in the central thalamus may participate in the planning of eye movements (see below).

Neuronal activity in the central thalamus

A variety of neurons related to eye movements have been reported in the central thalamus in cats and monkeys. Although most neuron types in monkeys were first documented a quarter-century ago (Schlag and Schlag-Rey, 1984; Schlag-Rey and Schlag, 1984), those data were only recently confirmed by other researchers, and detailed analysis of these neurons has since been performed. In this section, we only describe the basic properties of these neurons, which along with their functional roles, are considered in more detail in the following sections. Figure 13.1B plots five representative neurons. The most frequent observation during recording from the central thalamus is a transient activity associated with saccades. Saccade-related burst neurons can be found in both the intralaminar and paralaminar nuclei. Approximately half of these neurons discharge before saccades, and many exhibit directional preference (Kunimatsu and Tanaka, 2010; Schlag-Rey and Schlag, 1984; Sommer and Wurtz, 2004a; Tanaka, 2007a; Tanibuchi and Goldman-Rakic, 2003; Watanabe and Funahashi, 2004a; Wyder et al., 2003). Some neurons cease firing before and during saccade in all directions, and exhibit a burst of activity just after saccade (pause-rebound cells). Such neurons might inform cortical neurons as to the exact timing when new visual processing is available after each saccade (Schlag-Rey and Schlag, 1984). Other neurons display a tonic activity proportional to eye position (Schlag-Rey and Schlag, 1984; Tanaka, 2007a; Wyder et al., 2003), a buildup of activity during saccade preparation (Schlag-Rey and Schlag, 1984; Tanaka, 2007b; Watanabe and Funahashi, 2004b; Wyder et al., 2004) or activity during the initiation and the maintenance of smooth pursuit (Tanaka, 2005b). These signals may play roles in the online monitoring of eye movements and the generation of voluntary saccades.

Monitoring of self-motions

The ability to preserve spatial stability across self-motions is essential for both goal-directed behaviour and the perception of space. This ability, called 'spatial updating', has been examined extensively during eye movements (for reviews, see Andersen et al., 1997; Britten 2008; Colby and Goldberg, 1999; Klier and Angelaki, 2008). Spatial updating appears to take place in the parietal cortex, as this ability is impaired in subjects with damage to the parietal cortex (Duhamel et al., 1992b) and dynamic updating of eye movement signals in the parietal cortex has been demonstrated by functional magnetic resonance imaging (fMRI) (Medendorp et al., 2003). Since most neurons in the parietal cortex represent visual stimuli in eye-centred, rather than head-centred coordinate frames, information about eye movements must be combined with visual signals to establish space constancy (for reviews, see Andersen et al., 1993; Angelaki, 2005). These extraretinal signals may arise from either the proprioception of extraocular muscles or the internal feedback of eye movement commands in the oculomotor pathways ('efference copy' or 'corollary discharge' signals). Several lines of evidence suggest that the central thalamus transmits these eye movement signals for spatial updating.

Monitoring of saccade

Gaymard et al. (1994) asked subjects with focal lesions in the central thalamus, presumably involving the IML, to make a memory-guided saccade to the location of previously presented visual stimulus.

Compared with healthy controls, the memory saccades became less accurate in subjects with thalamic lesions only when the initial eye position was displaced by saccades during the delay period. Spatial updating has also been examined using the double-step saccade paradigm (Hallet and Lightstone, 1976) (Fig. 13.2A). In this paradigm, two targets are presented only briefly, and subjects make two successive saccades in the absence of the targets. The direction and amplitude of the first saccade can be easily computed from the retinotopic coordinate of the first target, while the second saccade in the sequence must be planned based on both the retinal coordinate of the second target and the direction

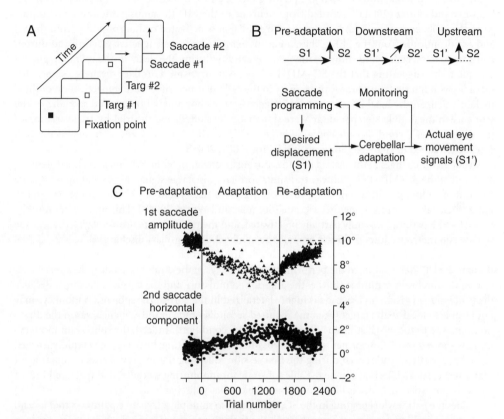

Fig. 13.2 The saccade system keeps track of adaptive changes in the first saccade in the double-step paradigm. A) Two targets are presented successively, and the subjects make a saccade to each. The first and the second targets are illuminated only briefly, say about 100 and 20 ms, respectively. Because both targets disappear before saccades, the subjects make saccades without any visual guidance. B) The upper panels represent the prediction of the results based on two alternative hypotheses. The lower diagram indicates the signal flow in the saccade system. If the brain monitors the first saccade using signals originating in the sites downstream from adaptation (S1'), the horizontal component of the second saccade in the sequence would compensate for the adaptive changes in the first saccade. Alternatively, if the brain monitors the first saccade using the signals upstream of cerebellar adaptation (S1), the direction and amplitude of the second saccade would not be altered during adaptation. C) Adaptation in the first saccade altered the horizontal component of the second saccade in the double-step paradigm in the monkey. Each symbol indicates horizontal component of saccades in the sequence. The double-step paradigm was presented at a lower probability (20%) during the course of saccade adaptation. Reprinted from *Journal of Neurophysiology*, **90**, Tanaka, M., Contribution of signals downstream from adaptation to saccade programming, pp. 2080–2086, figures 1 and 2 © 2003 The American Physiological Society, used with permission.

and amplitude of the first saccade. Using this paradigm, Bellebaum et al. (2005) showed that the subjects with lesions in either the MD or the VL nucleus of the thalamus failed to update the memorized location of visual stimulus during contraversive saccades. Further, the same authors demonstrated that the cortical potential recorded from the parietal cortex during spatial updating decreased for subjects with thalamic lesions (Bellebaum et al., 2006). Similar results were also reported for a subject with focal lesion in the MD thalamus, but the deficits were found during the monitoring of ipsiversive saccades (Ostendorf et al., 2010).

The role of the thalamus in spatial updating has been examined further in trained monkeys. Sommer and Wurtz (2004a) recorded from neurons in the MD thalamus, which received inputs from the ipsilateral SC and sends outputs to the FEF (those activated orthodromically from the SC and antidromically from the FEF). These neurons exhibited a transient activity before and during contraversive saccades, and showed only a weak activity during the delay in the memory-guided saccade tasks, suggesting that the SC–MD–FEF pathways transmit corollary discharge signals for saccades with filtering out of the tonic activity in the collicular neurons. During inactivation of these thalamic neurons by local injection of GABA agonist, the endpoints of the second saccades in the sequence in the double-step paradigm were systematically shifted, and the trial-by-trial variation of the direction of second saccades became larger, while both the latency and accuracy of the first saccade remained unchanged (Sommer and Wurtz, 2002, 2004b).

Although the changes in the second saccades during inactivation of the MD nucleus clearly demonstrated that the SC–MD–FEF pathway transmits corollary discharge signals for spatial updating, the amount of endpoint shift was only approximately 20% of that would be expected if the system did not entirely take account of the first saccade (Sommer and Wurtz, 2004b). This may be because the SC–MD–FEF pathway was only partially inactivated, and the remaining neurons relayed the saccade signals. Alternatively, other pathways may also be involved. The corollary discharge signals for spatial updating could come from other cortical areas via direct cortico-cortical projections. To test this, Berman et al. (2005) examined the performance of monkeys in the double-saccade tasks after dissection of the forebrain commissures (i.e. the anterior commissure and the corpus callosum). Because the processing of vision and saccade is highly lateralized in the cortex, the split-brain monkeys may not be able to localize the target when the required second saccade in the sequence was in the direction opposite to the visual stimulus ('across-hemifield' condition). Indeed, the split-brain monkeys initially showed severe impairments in the across-hemifield updating; however, they rapidly learned to make accurate saccades even during the first session following the surgery. These results suggest that direct cortical links may not be the sole substrate for monitoring saccades, and that a redundant cortical-subcortical network is likely to provide the corollary discharge signals.

Besides the pathway originating in the SC, there are also multiple alternative pathways that ascend from subcortical eye movement areas through the thalamus to the cortex, which may play a role in monitoring eye displacements to achieve space constancy (Fig. 13.1A). Using the double-step paradigm during the course of short-term saccadic adaptation, Tanaka (2003) examined the relative locations of the site of adaptation and the origin of eye movement signals for internal monitoring of saccades (Fig. 13.2B). When the target is relocated backward by 30–50% of the initial step during saccade to the target, the size of the targeting saccade gradually decreases (Deubel et al., 1986; Straube et al., 1997). This saccade adaptation is believed to occur in the cerebellum, downstream from the SC in the system, because a lesion in the vermal lobule of the cerebellum eliminates adaptation (Barash et al., 1999; Takagi et al., 1998), neuronal firing in the relevant cerebellar region alters during the course of adaptation (Inaba et al., 2003; Scudder et al., 2003), and adaptation also modifies saccades evoked by stimulation in the SC (Edelman and Goldberg, 2002; for review, see Robinson and Fuchs, 2001; see also Thier, Chapter 10, this volume). Because saccade adaptation takes place far downstream in the system, there are 'desired' and 'actual' eye movement signals in the brainstem during adaptation (Fig. 13.2B). Therefore, it is expected that if the second saccade in the double-step paradigm is computed based on the 'desired' eye movement signals for the first saccade (i.e. the signals upstream of adaptation), the direction and amplitude of the second saccade would not be altered during adaptation of the first saccade. Alternatively, if the signals arising from the sites downstream of saccade adaptation are used to monitor the first saccade, the second saccade would compensate for the adaptive changes in the first saccade. To distinguish these possibilities, the double-step paradigm was presented as a probe trial at a lower probability during the course of adaptation trials (Tanaka, 2003). They found that, as the horizontal displacement of the first saccade in the double-step paradigm decreased due to adaptation, the horizontal component of the second saccade in the sequence increased and the changes in the initial position of the second saccade was compensated (Fig. 13.2C). Thus, the saccade system takes account of the adaptive changes in the first saccade to update the location of the second target, suggesting that the pathways from the lower brainstem (sites downstream of adaptation) through the thalamus to the cortex may also transmit signals for internal monitoring of saccades. Similarly, Awater et al. (2004) examined the perisaccadic mislocalization of visual stimuli before and during adaptation: it was previously shown that a brief visual stimulus flashed around the time of saccade is mislocalized toward the endpoint of saccade under normal room lighting (Lappe et al., 2000; Morrone et al., 1997; Ross et al., 2001). During saccade adaptation, this perisaccadic compression of visual space was observed toward the actual saccade endpoints, rather than to the location of the target, indicating that signals after the cerebellar adaptation determine the perceived location of visual stimulus.

The neuronal correlates of spatial updating were first reported in the parietal cortex of monkeys. Duhamel et al. (1992a) demonstrated that neurons in the posterior parietal cortex responded to visual stimuli presented within the future receptive field immediately before saccade (for review, see Colby et al., 1995). This predictive remapping of visual receptive field has now been reported in several cortical and subcortical areas, including the FEF (Umeno and Goldberg, 1997), V3a (Nakamura and Colby, 2000), and SC (Edelman and Goldberg, 2002). Since the remapping occurs for saccades in multiple directions and amplitudes, the cortical neurons may have access to information on saccades in all directions, as well as visual stimuli in the entire visual field (Heiser and Colby, 2006). Recently, Sommer and Wurtz (2006) demonstrated that the SC–MD–FEF pathway described above is one of the sources of the extraretinal signals for the remapping in the FEF. They examined the predictive remapping of single FEF neurons during inactivation of the MD thalamus, and found that the predictive visual response decreased remarkably for contraversive saccades but not for ipsiversive saccades. Thus, the remapping in the FEF during contraversive saccades is controlled, at least in part, by the corollary discharge signals through the MD thalamus. The corollary discharge signals for ipsiversive saccades may come from the commissural fibres or from the other thalamocortical pathways.

Monitoring of smooth pursuit

Spatial updating has also been examined in smooth pursuit eye movements. In one paradigm, subjects are asked to track a slowly moving target with their eyes, and make an immediate saccade to a second, flashed target that appears in their peripheral visual field. If the saccade system takes account of the smooth changes in eye position during the reaction time of the saccades, their endpoints would be close to the actual location of the target, and the direction and amplitude of the saccades would be somewhat different from the retinal error of the target. In monkeys, McKenzie and Lisberger (1986) found that the endpoint of saccades was shifted systematically in the direction of pursuit, and that the retinal error and saccade amplitudes were closely correlated with each other. Similar results were also reported in humans (Gellman and Fletcher, 1992), suggesting that the saccade system may not take account of the smooth change in eye position. However, in a series of later studies in both humans and monkeys, when the subjects were asked to make a memory-guided saccade to the location of previously presented visual stimuli, they were able to compensate for the change in eye position resulting from intervening smooth pursuit during the delay period (Baker et al., 2003; Herter and Guitton, 1998; Ohtsuka, 1994; Schlag et al., 1990; Tanaka, 2005a; Zivotofsky et al., 1996). A potential explanation for these conflicting results was recently proposed by Blohm et al. (2005). They showed a strong correlation between the retinal error and the direction and amplitude of saccade with a short latency (<175 ms after the target flash), while saccades with longer latency were spatially accurate and compensated for the smooth change in eye position. Furthermore, it was suggested that saccades with short latency are processed through the direct striatal-SC pathway which uses only retinal information, while those with longer latency are processed through the striatal-parietal-SC pathway which may also take account of the extraretinal pursuit signals (Blohm et al., 2006).

Like saccades, the extraretinal signals for spatial updating during smooth pursuit may also come from the central thalamus. Previous studies have detected activation in the thalamus during pursuit (Berman et al., 1999; Tanabe et al., 2002). Subjects with a focal lesion in the central thalamus displayed difficulty in making accurate memory-guide saccades when the initial eye position was displaced by intervening pursuit (Gaymard et al., 1994). The similarities in the impairments of spatial updating for both saccade and pursuit in thalamic patients initially led to the hypothesis that the orbital eye position rather than eye movement signals might be used for spatial updating (Gaymard et al., 1994; for review, see Schlag-Rey and Schlag, 2002). However, Baker et al. (2003) found in monkeys that the memory-guided saccades following pursuit were more variable than those following saccades, suggesting that different extraretinal signals were used to monitor these eye movements. Further simulation experiments using a recurrent network model indicated that the velocity rather than the position signals play more important roles for spatial updating during pursuit (White and Snyder, 2004).

It was recently shown that a subset of neurons in the paralaminar part of the VL thalamus exhibit a sustained activity during pursuit (Tanaka, 2005b). Many neurons are directional and continue firing during the brief removal of tracking target, indicating that they carry extraretinal signals. The origin of these signals remains unknown, however, these neurons may transmit pursuit signals from the cerebellum (Stone and Lisberger, 1990; Suzuki and Keller, 1988) or the basal ganglia (Basso et al., 2005; Yoshida and Tanaka, 2009) for the monitoring of pursuit. The remapping of the visual receptive field of parietal neurons during pursuit was also reported (Powell and Goldberg, 1997).

Smooth pursuit operates as a negative feedback system (Fig. 13.3A). Because the motion of retinal images of the tracking target is greatly reduced during the maintenance of pursuit, the system itself must contain neural mechanisms for the internal monitoring of pursuit velocity in order to reconstruct target velocity in space (Robinson, 1986). The pursuit neurons in the central thalamus may lie within those pathways (for review, see Thier and Ilg, 2005). In addition, the transformation from visual motion to eye velocity is subject to a dynamic gain control (Schwartz and Lisberger, 1994), and this gain control mechanism is scaled by the signals related to eye velocity in the frontal cortex (Tanaka and Lisberger, 2001). A recent model of smooth pursuit suggests that the signals in the thalamocortical pathways may play a role in setting the gain higher during pursuit (Nuding et al., 2008). Consistent with these data, inactivation of the central thalamus reduces eye velocity both during the initiation and the maintenance of pursuit, without alteration of pursuit latency (Tanaka 2005b; Fig. 13.3B).

Monitoring of eye position

Information regarding orbital eye position is essential for the planning of eye movements to auditory or tactile stimuli from different initial eye positions, or for the computing of head-centred location of visual stimuli, which is necessary to plan, for example, reaching movements. The eye position signals in the cortex are likely to be transmitted from the brainstem via the thalamus. It was shown clinically that saccades to the auditory, but not visual, target presented contralateral to the side of lesion in the central thalamus become hypometric (Versino et al., 2000). Experimentally, a large lesion in the SC extending to the MD thalamus reduced the accuracy of fixation for the target presented contralateral to the lesion in monkeys (Albano and Wurtz, 1982).

A subset of neurons in the central thalamus of monkeys were shown to exhibit firing modulation proportional to orbital eye position (Schlag-Rey and Schlag, 1984; Tanaka, 2007a, Wyder et al., 2003). The preferred directions of these neurons are either along the horizontal or the vertical axis, indicating that the eye position signals in the central thalamus are decomposed into the cardinal axes,

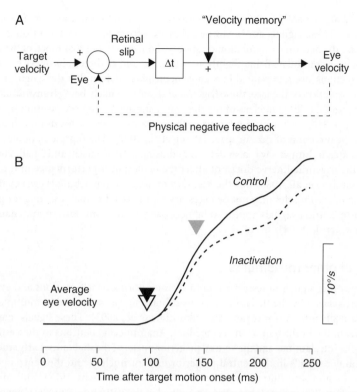

Fig. 13.3 Signals in the central thalamus monitor and regulate smooth pursuit eye movements. A) A diagram of the smooth pursuit system. This system converts target velocity into the command of eye velocity, and operates as a negative feedback system. The input of the brain is the motion of the retinal images ('retinal slip') that is defined as the difference between target velocity and eye velocity. During maintenance of smooth pursuit, the brain must keep track of pursuit velocity to reconstruct target velocity from motion of the retinal images. Many studies assume the internal positive feedback circuitry in the system for this purpose. B) Traces of eye velocity before and during inactivation of the central thalamus. Although inactivation of the central thalamus did not alter pursuit latency, eye velocity during the initiation and maintenance of pursuit was reduced, suggesting that the central thalamus lies within the internal feedback pathways. The first two triangles indicate the time of pursuit initiation before and during inactivation. The right, grey triangle indicates the time when the two traces become statistically different. See Tanaka (2005b) for details.

just as for eye position neurons in the brainstem. However, unlike neurons in the brainstem, activity of eye position-related neurons in the central thalamus exhibit a trace of preceding eye movements. For instance, for many neurons, the sustained activity during fixation was greater when the prior eye movement was in the preferred direction than in the opposite direction (Schlag-Rey and Schlag, 1984; Tanaka, 2007a), suggesting that the eye position signals are modified dynamically through the ascending pathways. The eye position neurons in the central thalamus appear to be composed of at least two different populations; neurons in the dorsal part of the thalamus (mostly in the LD nucleus) exhibit firing modulation slightly following the changes in eye position, while those in the deeper part (CL and paralaminar VL) discharge before saccades in the preferred direction (Schlag-Rey and Schlag, 1984; Tanaka 2007a). Furthermore, Schlag and his colleagues recorded from head-unrestrained cats (Maldonado and Schlag, 1984) and monkeys (Schlag and Schlag-Rey, 1986), and found that some eye position neurons in the central thalamus actually modulated their firing rate as a function of the direction of gaze (eye in space).

Wang et al. (2007) recently found the eye position representation in the primary somatosensory cortex (area 3a). These signals appear to be originated from the proprioception of extraocular muscles, because the neuronal modulation disappeared during retrobulbar block of the contralateral orbit. These neurons modulate firing slightly after saccade, and all directions of eye position, including oblique directions, are represented in a single hemisphere. Given that these neurons reside near the tactile representation of the face, these trigeminal signals are likely being transmitted through the ventral posteromedial (VPM) nucleus of the thalamus, although VPM eye position signals have not yet been recorded. The eye position neurons in the somatosensory cortex did not modulate firing depending on the direction of gaze in space (Wang et al., 2007). The representation of eye position in the relevant area in humans was also determined using fMRI (Balslev and Miall, 2008). Because dissection of the trigeminal nerve does not affect the oculomotor performance in the double-step saccade task (Guthrie et al., 1983) nor the accuracy of open-loop reaching (Lewis et al., 1998), the proprioception of eye muscles may not be necessary for the rapid spatial updating for goal-directed behaviour. Instead, these signals appear to be necessary for the long-term maintenance of ocular alignment (Lewis et al., 1994).

Monitoring of other movements

There are some other signals necessary for both the monitoring of self-motions and eye movement control that are relayed by the thalamus. First, vestibular signals are found in multiple areas in the frontal and parietal cortices (for review, see Fukushima et al., 2003). These signals may come from multiple nuclei in the brainstem or the cerebellum. Anatomically, neurons in the vestibular nuclei send axons to the intralaminar and the ventral posterior nuclei of the thalamus. Early studies reported thalamic vestibular signals in the ventral posterior inferior nucleus and the ventral posterolateral (VPL) nucleus in monkeys (Büttner and Henn, 1976; Magin and Fuchs, 1977), while more recently, the properties of vestibular signals have been examined in the VPL and VL nuclei (Meng et al., 2007). These studies showed that most neurons lack sensitivity to eye movements, indicating that the vestibular relay neurons are distinct from the eye movement related neurons reported in the central thalamus. Secondly, Fukushima et al. (2009) demonstrated that the pursuit-related neurons in the FEF receive proprioceptive inputs from the neck muscles. It was previously shown that neck proprioception can influence the cortical processing of visual spatial memory that guides saccades (Corneil et al., 2004). The VPL is likely the thalamic relay for neck proprioception (Marlinski and McCrea, 2008), although other pathway might exist for the monitoring of head movements.

Generation of voluntary saccades

For somatic motor control, it has been widely accepted that two subcortical structures—the basal ganglia and the cerebellum—contribute to the planning and generation of movements by sending signals through the thalamus to the cortex (for reviews, see Alexander and Crutcher, 1990; Middleton and Strick, 2000; Mink, 1996; Thach et al., 1992). In contrast, for ocular motor control, both the basal ganglia and the cerebellum are thought to form feedforward descending pathways that modulate signals from the cortex to the brainstem (for reviews, see Hikosaka et al., 2000; Optican, 2005; Robinson and Fuchs, 2001). As outlined above, the eye movement-related areas in the frontal cortex receive inputs from the basal ganglia and the cerebellum via multiple nuclei in the thalamus. These pathways may regulate the cortical processing for the planning and decisions of voluntary eye movements.

Planning of eye movements

As the MD thalamus reciprocally connects with the PFC, and also because it lies within the cortical–basal ganglia–thalamocortical pathways, Tanibuchi and Goldman-Rakic (2003) reasoned that neurons in the MD thalamus may contribute to executive processes such as working memory and decision making. Using the memory-guided saccade task, they found spatially selective neurons in the dorsolateral part of the MD nucleus where strong connection with the dorsolateral PFC was previously reported (Goldman-Rakic and Porrino, 1985; Siwek and Pandya, 1991). Further, they found neurons selective to object-features and selective to sounds in the ventrolateral and in posterior portions of the MD nucleus, respectively. Interestingly, most of these neurons exhibited no spatial selectivity, suggesting that the segregated spatial and non-spatial processing previously proposed in the PFC (Goldman-Rakic, 1988; O'Scalaidhe et al., 1997; Ungerleider et al., 1998; Wilson et al., 1993) might extend in the MD thalamus. However, it should also be noted that the idea of the segregated spatial and non-spatial processing in the PFC has been challenged by other studies (Rao et al., 1997; Rainer et al., 1998; for reviews, see Postle, 2006; Tanji and Hoshi, 2008).

The directionality of neurons recorded throughout the MD nucleus during memory-guided saccade tasks was quantified by Watanabe and Funahashi (2004a). A strong contralateral bias of the preferred direction was observed for the visual and presaccadic activities, whereas no such bias was found for the delay period activity. The authors further examined the roles of MD neurons in sensory-to-motor transformation during the delay period in the memory-guided saccade task, and compared the results with those obtained from the dorsolateral PFC (Watanabe and Funahashi, 2004b; Watanabe et al., 2009). In the rotatory oculomotor delayed response task, monkeys were required to make a memory-guided saccade in the direction 90° clockwise from the cue location. The population vector computed from directional neurons gradually altered its direction from the cue to saccade directions during the 3-s delay interval. Interestingly, the directional change in the population vector started earlier in the MD than in the PFC, suggesting that the MD thalamus may provide motor information about forthcoming saccades to the PFC (Watanabe et al., 2009).

Significant visual, motor, and delay period activity was recently demonstrated in neurons in the anterior intralaminar nuclei (CL and PCN) and in the paralaminar VA and VL nuclei during the delayed saccade task in monkeys (Wyder et al., 2003). Similarly to neurons in the MD thalamus, most visual neurons have contralateral receptive fields. However, the preferred directions of the presaccadic burst neurons in the paralaminar regions distribute all directions relative to the recording site without any bias toward a particular direction, while those in the MD nucleus exhibit a strong contralateral preference (Sommer and Wurtz, 2004a; Watanabe and Funahashi, 2004a). Many neurons in the paralaminar thalamus also elevate their firing rate during the delay period, suggesting their roles in the 'higher-order' visuomotor processing. One signature of cognitive control is the context-dependent firing modulation of saccade-related activity. Many neurons in the paralaminar VA and VL nuclei exhibit much greater activity for memory than for visually-guided saccades in the preferred direction (Tanaka, 2007b; Tanibuchi and Goldman-Rakic, 2005), as previously reported for neurons in the basal ganglia (Hikosaka and Wurtz, 1983; Hikosaka et al., 1989, but see Bayer et al., 2004).

The most compelling evidence for the involvement of the paralaminar thalamus in higher order visuomotor processing is the observation that neurons in the VA/VL thalamus exhibit context-dependent firing modulation during selection of the saccade target. In the visually guided choice task, monkeys were required to select from two targets for saccade depending on the color of the fixation point (Wyder et al., 2004). In addition to neurons that merely responded to visual stimuli in the receptive field, neurons in the VA/VL thalamus that signalled either the goal of the upcoming saccade or the location of the currently visible saccade goal during the imposed delay period were found. When taken together with their anatomical location within the cortico-subcortical network, the existence of neurons carrying combined information both on sensory stimuli and the behavioural context suggests the roles of the paralaminar VA/VL thalamus in flexible linkage of sensory signals and saccade commands.

Self-timed saccades

Current evidence suggests that subcortical signals play a role in the self-triggering of movements. For instance, besides the impairments of motor coordination, subjects with a cerebellar lesion also exhibit a delay of movement initiation (Holmes, 1939; Meyer-Lohmann et al., 1977). The slow cortical potential preceding the self-paced movements, known as readiness potential or Bereitschaftspotential, decreases following the lesion in the superior cerebellar peduncle (Ikeda et al., 1994). On the other hand, subjects with Parkinson's disease often have difficulty in self-initiation of movements, especially when external cues to move are unavailable (Kelly et al., 2002). Further, Parkinson's patients show decreased cortical potential during anticipation of an upcoming stimulus that triggers movements (contingent negative variation or CNV) (Ikeda et al., 1997). Experimentally, it has also been shown that inactivation of the thalamic nuclei receiving signals from the cerebellum or the basal ganglia impairs limb movements guided by external or internal cues (van Donkelaar et al., 2000).

The neural substrates for voluntary saccades were first explored with PET (positron emission tomography) by Petit et al. (1993). In addition to many cortical areas, a significant elevation of regional blood flow was found in the thalamus and the basal ganglia when subjects generated self-paced saccades, suggesting a role of the basal ganglia–thalamocortical pathways in saccade initiation. In monkeys, saccade-related neurons in the central thalamus were shown to elevate their firing rate long (>400 ms) before spontaneous saccade in the preferred direction (Schlag-Rey and Schlag, 1984). A similar prelude of activity before spontaneous saccade was also reported in the SEF (Schlag and Schlag-Rey, 1987). The reciprocal connection between the central thalamus and the SEF (Shook et al., 1990) suggests that these two areas are within the pathways that generate spontaneous saccades.

Recently, it was shown that signals in the paralaminar VA and VL thalamus play roles in the generation of self-timed saccades. In one study, monkeys were trained to make a memory-guided saccade to the location of a previously presented visual stimulus following the delay period (Tanaka, 2006). In one condition, the end of the delay period was instructed externally by the disappearance of the fixation point, and the monkeys were required to make an immediate saccade in response to the fixation point offset; this is the standard memory-guided saccade task developed originally by Hikosaka and Wurtz (1983). In the other condition, monkeys were required to make a self-timed saccade within the predetermined time widow (usually 0.8–1.6 s) following the cue, and the fixation point disappeared only after the saccade. When the paralaminar thalamus was inactivated with muscimol, the monkeys had difficulty in the generation of the self-timed saccade, and the timing of the self-initiated saccades was delayed markedly. The reaction time in the standard task was also prolonged, but the changes in latency were only less than 20% of those observed in the self-timed task.

Tanaka (2007) also described a subset of neurons in the paralaminar VA and VL thalamus that exhibited a gradual elevation of firing rate during saccade preparation. Although the time course of neuronal activity predicted the timing of the fixation point offset in the standard memory-guided saccade task, there was no correlation between the trial-by-trial variation in saccade latency and that in the time course (or the magnitude) of neuronal activity. Thus, neurons in the central thalamus appear to carry subjective time information, but these signals do not regulate the timing of externally-triggered saccades. On the other hand, the same neurons also exhibited a significant buildup of activity before the initiation of the self-timed saccade, and the variation in saccade timing was well-correlated with that in neuronal activity (Fig. 13.4A). Along with the results from the inactivation experiments, these data suggest a causal role of the paralaminar thalamus in regulating the timing of self-initiated saccades. The thalamocortical pathways provide subjective time information to the cortex, and the cortical network may use this information to determine the timing of self-timed, but not externally-triggered, saccades.

Antisaccades

The antisaccade paradigm has been used to investigate the voluntary control of eye movements. In this task, subjects suppress a reflexive saccade toward the sudden appearance of visual stimulus (prosaccade), and generate a saccade with the same amplitude as the target eccentricity but in the opposite direction (antisaccade) (Hallett, 1978). Since antisaccades are impaired in individuals with Parkinson's disease or Huntington's disease, the subcortical pathways through the basal ganglia and

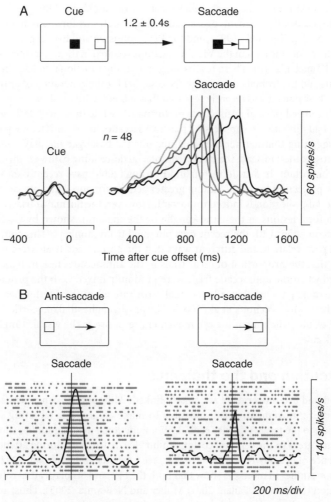

Fig. 13.4 Neuronal activity preceded the initiation of voluntary saccades. A) Time course of population activity before self-timed saccades. Monkeys were trained to make a saccade within a fixed time interval from the offset of visual cue. For each neuron, data were classified into five groups according to the time of saccades. The population activity was then computed for each group, and the trace was shifted in time so that the vertical line indicates the means of the saccade latency relative to the cue offset. Modified from Tanaka (2007b) with permission. B) An example of a VL neuron that showed greater firing modulation during antisaccades than prosaccades.

possibly the thalamus may be involved (for reviews, see Everling and Fischer, 1998; Munoz and Everling, 2004; see also Johnston and Everling, Chapter 15, and White and Munoz, Chapter 11, this volume). Consistent with this, many neurons in multiple nuclei of the basal ganglia exhibit enhanced firing modulation during antisaccades when compared with those during prosaccades (SNr: Gore et al., 2005, caudate nucleus: Ford and Everling 2009; Watanabe and Munoz 2009, globus pallidus: Yoshida and Tanaka 2009), and inactivation in the globus pallidus impairs antisaccades (Yoshida and Tanaka, 2009). In addition, many fMRI studies have revealed enhanced activity during antisaccades both in the basal ganglia and in the thalamus (Dyckman et al., 2007; Ettinger et al., 2008; Matsuda et al., 2004; O'Driscoll et al., 1995; Tu et al., 2006). Indeed, Kunimatsu and Tanaka (2010) recently found that neurons in the paralaminar thalamus of monkeys exhibit greater firing modulation during antisaccades than during prosaccades (Fig. 13.4B), as for many neurons in the basal ganglia, the SEF (Schlag-Rey et al., 1997), and the PFC (Johnston and Everling, 2006). Furthermore, inactivation of the recording sites in the VL/VA thalamus resulted in the impairments of antisaccades (Kunimatsu and Tanaka, 2010). These results suggest that the functional linkage between the basal ganglia, thalamus and the frontal cortex might be essential for the generation of antisaccades.

In contrast to these data, it was recently reported that subjects with focal lesions in the thalamus or the basal ganglia showed normal antisaccade performance, while those with lesions in the anterior internal capsule had difficulty in suppressing reflexive saccades in the antisaccade paradigm (Condy et al., 2004), suggesting that neither the thalamus nor the basal ganglia play a major role in the generation of antisaccades; instead, the direct frontotectal descending pathways through the internal capsule may be important. In fact, Johnston and Everling (2006) have recently shown that the PFC neurons directly projecting to the SC exhibit greater activity for anti- than prosaccades, suggesting that the frontotectal projection is indeed important. However, the normal antisaccade performance in subjects with focal lesions in the basal ganglia or the thalamus shown by Condy et al. (2004) appears to be inconsistent with the recent data obtained from monkeys. This contradictory result may, at least in part, relate to the different ways that the antisaccade trials were presented. It was recently shown that the proportion of error trials in the antisaccades task in Parkinson's patients greatly increased when the antisaccade trials were randomly mixed with the prosaccade trials in a block, while the same patients showed a normal error rate when they performed a block of only antisaccade trials (Rivaud-Péchoux et al., 2007). The basal ganglia–thalamocortical circuitry might be involved in flexible switching of the eye movement response to the visual stimuli depending on the imposed task rule.

Spatial attention and the thalamus

Spatial attention and eye movements are closely linked. Although we can orient spatial attention covertly without eye movement, it is impossible to make an accurate targeting saccade without directing attention to the target (Kowler et al., 1995). Functional imaging studies show that most eye movement-related areas in the cerebral cortex exhibit elevated activity during attentional orienting, even in the absence of eye movements (for review, see Corbetta and Shulman, 2002). Furthermore, recent stimulation studies in monkeys show that both the FEF and SC play causal roles in the shifting of spatial attention (Moore and Fallah, 2001; Müller and Newsome, 2005). Thus, attention and eye movements are controlled, at least partly, by a shared neural mechanism (see Part 3: Saccades and attention, this volume).

The intralaminar nuclei

Lesions of the central thalamus result in spatial neglect in cats, monkeys and humans (for review, see Schlag-Rey and Schlag, 1989). For instance, Orem et al. (1973) produced electrolytic lesions in the central thalamus of 19 cats and found deficits in 1) orienting to visual stimuli, 2) head and ocular following of a small moving object, 3) blinking in response to visual threat, and 4) optokinetic response to a rotating drum. These deficits were observed for stimuli presented in or moved toward the contralateral visual field, and when the lesion included the caudal part of the CL nucleus rather than only the adjacent MD, VL or centre median (CM) nuclei. Because lesions were produced electrolytically, these results could be attributed to the ablation of passing fibres. However, Merker and Schlag (1985) later showed that cats with ibotenic acid lesions in the central thalamus exhibited a remarkable lengthening of saccade latency (>1 s) when the visual target appeared in the contralateral visual field. Spatial neglect for visual, auditory, and somatosensory stimuli was also reported in monkeys (Watson et al., 1978) and humans (Watson and Heilman, 1979).

While those early studies mainly considered the effects of lesions in the CL and PCN, roles for the posterior group of the intralaminar thalamus have also been suggested. Watson et al. (1981) reported a hemineglect patient with a lesion in the right thalamus, and suggested a role of the CM and para-fascicular (Pf) nuclei in attention. A recent PET study demonstrated activation in the CM nucleus during an attention-demanding reaction time task in humans (Kinomura et al., 1996). Further, Minamimoto and Kimura (2002) demonstrated in monkeys that the visual responses of CM/Pf neurons were strongly enhanced by attention, and that inactivation of these neurons reduced the context-dependent modulation of manual response latency, suggesting a causal role. The CM/Pf nuclei may interact with the attentional (and possibly eye movement) networks through their incoming connections from the SC and other brainstem nuclei, and outgoing connections to the basal ganglia and the frontal cortex (for reviews, see Sadikot and Rymar, 2009; Smith et al., 2004).

The pulvinar nucleus

The pulvinar in the posterior thalamus is especially developed in primates and is known to play a role in visuospatial attention and eye movements. In both humans (Ogren et al., 1984; Zihl and von Cramon, 1979) and monkeys (Ungerleider and Christensen, 1977, 1979; but see Bender and Baizer, 1990), subjects with a lesion in the pulvinar exhibit decreased scanning eye movements during visual search and difficulty in directing both attention and eyes to visual stimuli presented in the contralateral visual field. A lesion in the right pulvinar can also cause hemispatial neglect (Karnath et al., 2002). In normal subjects, the latency of visually-guided saccades becomes shorter when the fixation point disappears at the time of target onset, as compared to when the fixation point remains on throughout the trial (overlap effect). However, subjects with a pulvinar lesion did not exhibit a change in latency between these conditions, suggesting a role in fixation disengagement (Rafal et al., 2004). Many fMRI studies also report elevated activity in the pulvinar during the tasks requiring attention (e.g. Kastner et al., 2004; Smith et al., 2009; Villeneuve et al., 2005; for review, see Kastner and Pinsk, 2004).

The pulvinar consists of several subnuclei, each of which has different cortical and subcortical connections (for reviews, see Kaas and Lyon, 2007; Shipp, 2003). The lateral pulvinar has reciprocal connections with most visual areas in the parietal, temporal, and occipital cortices. There exists a retinotopic map in this region (Petersen et al., 1985). Neurons respond strongly to moving visual stimuli, but the response is attenuated when the visual motion is induced by eye movements (Robinson et al., 1991), suggesting a gain modulation by the extraretinal signals. The dorsomedial portion of the lateral pulvinar has connections with the PFC and the posterior parietal cortex, and plays a role in spatial attention (for review, see Robinson and Petersen, 1992). The retinotopic organization in this region is unclear, and neurons often have a large, bilateral receptive field. Petersen et al. (1987) found that inactivation of this region with a GABA agonist inhibited attentional orienting to the contralateral visual field in monkeys, whereas excitation with a GABA antagonist causes the opposite effects. The medial part of the inferior pulvinar receives dense projections from the superficial layer of the SC. This region, in turn, sends outputs to the extrastriate visual cortices, especially those within the dorsal visual pathway, including the MT and MST. The retinal-SC-pulvinar-parietal pathway (the extrageniculate visual pathway) might be involved in visuomotor processing that guides eye movements, although its exact role remains unknown.

Summary and conclusions

Compared to the substantial knowledge of the anatomy of the thalamus, how signals in the thalamus control eye movements remains largely unknown. In particular, since the pioneering work by Schlag and Schlag-Rey in the mid-1980s, systematic analyses on signals in the central thalamus during eye movements have only recently been performed (Kunimatsu and Tanaka, 2010; Sommer and Wurtz, 2002, 2004a, 2004b, 2006; Tanaka 2005, 2006, 2007a, 2007b; Tanibuchi and Goldman-Rakic, 2003, 2005; Watanabe and Funahashi, 2004a, 2004b; Wyder et al., 2003, 2004). The anterior part of the intralaminar nuclei and adjacent paralaminar portion of the MD, VL, VA, and LD nuclei contain neurons related to eye movements. Anatomically, this part of the thalamus collects signals originated in virtually all stages of eye movement processing in the brainstem and the cerebellum, and send signals to many cortical areas including the FEF, SEF, and PFC. In addition, these paralaminar nuclei compose the 'oculomotor loop' with the basal ganglia and the frontal cortex (Alexander et al., 1986).

The thalamus plays at least three roles in the control of eye movements. First, it serves pathways for the monitoring of self-generating movements. Recent experiments on nonhuman primates showed that the corollary discharge signals through the SC–MD–FEF pathway are actually used for spatial updating in the double-step saccade paradigm and for the predictive remapping of visual receptive field before saccades (Sommer and Wurtz, 2002, 2006). Other studies also suggest a role of the central thalamus in the monitoring of smooth pursuit and eye position. Further, the central thalamus and nearby structures appear to transmit the vestibular and the proprioception signals from the neck and extraocular muscles during self-motions that directly control eye movements.

Secondly, the central thalamus is involved in the planning and generating of voluntary eye movements. Neurons in the central thalamus exhibit visual, movement, and delay period activity during the memory-guided saccade task suggesting their involvement in sensory-to-motor transformation. Many neurons in the VA/VL thalamus also show a buildup of activity that predicts both the timing of external event triggering saccades and the timing of self-initiated saccades. Inactivation of these neurons specifically delays the self-timed saccades, suggesting a role for the central thalamus in the generation of voluntary saccades. This hypothesis is supported by recent imaging studies during a variety of eye movement paradigms, including self-timed saccades, antisaccades, or sequential saccades.

Finally, accumulating evidence suggests that the central and the posterior thalami play roles in spatial attention and eye movements. Consistent with early observations in thalamic patients and animal experiments, recent imaging studies have detected activation in the intralaminar nuclei and the lateral pulvinar during attention-demanding tasks. Since spatial attention and eye movements are regulated by shared neural mechanisms, these thalamic areas may also participate in oculomotor control through the connections with the SC and the frontal and parietal cortices. However, their specific roles remain to be elucidated.

Acknowledgements

This research was supported by grants from the Japan Science and Technology Agency (JST) and the Ministry of Education, Culture, Sports, Science and Technology (MEXT) of Japan.

References

Albano, J.E. and Wurtz, R.H. (1982). Deficits in eye position following ablation of monkey superior colliculus, pretectum, and posterior-medial thalamus. *Journal of Neurophysiology*, **48**, 318–337.

Alexander, G.E. and Crutcher, M.D. (1990). Functional architecture of basal ganglia circuits: neural substrates of parallel processing. *Trends in Neurosciences*, **13**, 266–271.

Alexander, G.E., Delong, M.R., and Strick, P.L. (1986). Parallel organization of functionally segregated circuits linking basal ganglia and cortex. *Annual Review of Neuroscience*, **9**, 357–381.

Andersen, R.A., Snyder, L.H., Bradley, D.C., and Xing, J. (1997). Multimodal representation of space in the posterior parietal cortex and its use in planning movements. *Annual Review of Neuroscience*, **20**, 303–330.

Andersen, R.A., Snyder, L.H., Li, C.S., and Stricanne, B. (1993). Coordinate transformations in the representation of spatial information. *Current Opinion in Neurobiology*, **3**, 171–176.

Angelaki, D.E. and Hess, B.J. (2005). Self-motion-induced eye movements: effects on visual acuity and navigation. *Nature Reviews Neuroscience*, **6**, 966–976.

Awater, H. and Lappe, M. (2004). Perception of visual space at the time of pro- and anti-saccades. *Journal of Neurophysiology*, **91**, 2457–2464.

Baker, J.T., Harper, T.M., and Snyder, L.H. (2003). Spatial memory following shifts of gaze. I. Saccades to memorized world-fixed and gaze-fixed targets. *Journal of Neurophysiology*, **89**, 2564–2576.

Balslev, D. and Miall, R.C. (2008). Eye position representation in human anterior parietal cortex. *Journal of Neuroscience*, **28**, 8968–8972.

Barash, S., Melikyan, A., Sivakov, A., Zhang, M., Glickstein, M., and Their, P. (1999). Saccadic dysmetria and adaptation after lesions of the cerebellar cortex. *Journal of Neuroscience*, **19**, 10931–10939.

Basso, M.A., Pokorny, J.J., and Liu, P. (2005). Activity of substantia nigra pars reticulata neurons during smooth pursuit eye movements in monkeys. *Europeam Jornal of Neuroscience*, **22**, 448–464.

Bayer, H.M., Handel, A., and Glimcher, P. W. (2004). Eye position and memory saccade related responses in substantia nigra pars reticulata. *Experimental Brain Research*, **154**, 428–441.

Bellebaum, C., Daum, I., Koch, B., Schwarz, M., and Hoffmann, K.P. (2005) The role of the human thalamus in processing corollary discharge. *Brain*, **128**, 1139–1154.

Bellebaum, C., Hoffmann, K.P., Koch, B., Schwarz, M., and Daum, I. (2006). Altered processing of corollary discharge in thalamic lesion patients. *Europeam Jornal of Neuroscience*, **24**, 2375–2388.

Bender, D.B. and Baizer, J.S. (1990). Saccadic eye movements following kainic acid lesions of the pulvinar in monkeys. *Experimental Brain Research*, **79**, 467–478.

Berman, R.A., Heiser, L.M., Saunders, R.C., and Colby, C.L. (2005). Dynamic circuitry for updating spatial representations. I. Behavioral evidence for interhemispheric transfer in the split-brain macaque. *Journal of Neurophysiology*, **94**, 3228–3248.

Berman, R.A., Colby, C.L., Genovese, C.R., Voyvodic, J.T., Luna, B., Thulborn, K.R., and Sweeney, J.A. (1999). Cortical networks subserving pursuit and saccadic eye movements in humans: an fMRI study. *Human Brain Mapping*, **8**, 209–225.

Blohm, G., Missal, M., and Lefèvre, P. (2005). Processing of retinal and extraretinal signals for memory-guided saccades during smooth pursuit. *Journal of Neurophysiology*, **93**, 1510–1522.

Blohm. G., Optican, L.M., and Lefèvre, P. (2006). A model that integrates eye velocity commands to keep track of smooth eye displacements. *Journal of Computational Neuroscience*, **21**, 51–70.

Britten, K.H. (2008). Mechanisms of self-motion perception. *Annual Review of Neuroscience*, **31**, 389–410.

Büttner, U. and Henn, V. (1976). Thalamic unit activity in the alert monkey during natural vestibular stimulation. *Brain Research*, **103**, 127–132.

Colby, C.L. and Goldberg, M.E. (1999). Space and attention in parietal cortex. *Annual Review of Neuroscience*, **22**, 319–349.

Colby, C.L., Duhamel, J.R., and Goldberg, M.E. (1995). Oculocentric spatial representation in parietal cortex. *Cerebral Cortex*, **5**, 470–481.

Condy, C., Rivaud-Péchoux, S., Ostendorf, F., Ploner, C.J., and Gaymard, B. (2004). Neural substrate of antisaccades: role of subcortical structures. *Neurology*, **63**, 1571–1578.

Corbetta, M. and Shulman, G.L. (2002). Control of goal-directed and stimulus-driven attention in the brain. *Nature Reviews Neuroscience*, **3**, 201–215.

Corneil, B.D. and Andersen, R.A. (2004). Dorsal neck muscle vibration induces upward shifts in the endpoints of memory-guided saccades in monkeys. *Journal of Neurophysiology*, **92**, 553–566.

Deubel, H., Wolf, W., and Hauske, G. (1986). Adaptive gain control of saccadic eye movements. *Human Neurobiology*, **5**, 245–253.

Duhamel, J.R., Colby, C.L., and Goldberg, M.E. (1992a). The updating of the representation of visual space in parietal cortex by intended eye movements. *Science*, **255**, 90–92.

Duhamel, J.R., Goldberg, M.E., Fitzgibbon, E.J., Sirigu, A., and Grafman, J. (1992b). Saccadic dysmetria in a patient with a right frontoparietal lesion: the importance of corollary discharge for accurate spatial behaviour. *Brain*, **115**, 1387–1402.

Dyckman, K.A., Camchong, J., Clementz, B.A., and McDowell, J.E. (2007). An effect of context on saccade-related behavior and brain activity. *Neuroimage*, **36**, 774–784.

Edelman. J.A. and Goldberg. M.E. (2002). Effect of short-term saccadic adaptation on saccades evoked by electrical stimulation in the primate superior colliculus. *Journal of Neurophysiology*, **87**, 1915–1923.

Ettinger, U., Ffytche, D.H., Kumari, V., Kathmann, N., Reuter, B., Zelaya, F., and Williams, S.C.R. (2008). Decomposing the neural correlates of antisaccade eye movements using event-related fMRI. *Cerebral Cortex*, **18**, 1148–1159.

Everling, S. and Fischer, B. (1998). The antisaccade: a review of basic research and clinical studies. *Neuropsychologia*, **36**, 885–899.

Ford, K.A. and Everling, S. (2009). Neural activity in primate caudate nucleus associated with pro- and antisaccade. *Journal of Neurophysiology*, **102**, 2334–2341.

Fukushima, K. (2003). Frontal cortical control of smooth-pursuit. *Current Opinion in Neurobiology*, **13**, 647–654.

Fukushima, K., Kasahara, S., Akao, T., Kurkin, S., Fukushima, J., and Peterson, B.W. (2009). Eye-pursuit and reafferent head movement signals carried by pursuit neurons in the caudal part of the frontal eye fields during head-free pursuit. *Cerebral Cortex*, **19**, 263–275.

Gaymard, B., Rivaud, S., and Pierrot-Deseilligny, C. (1994). Impairment of extraretinal eye position signals after central thalamic lesions in humans. *Experimental Brain Research*, **102**, 1–9.

Gellman, R.S. and Fletcher, WA. (1992). Eye position signals in human saccadic processing. *Experimental Brain Research*, **89**, 425–434.

Goldman-Rakic, P.S. (1988). Topography of cognition: parallel distributed networks in primate association cortex. *Annual Review of Neuroscience*, **11**, 137–156.

Goldman-Rakic, P.S. and Porrino, L.J. (1985). The primate mediodorsal (MD) nucleus and its projection to the frontal lobe. *Journal of Comparative Neurology*, **242**, 535–560.

Gore, J.L., Marino, R.A., and Munoz, D.P. (2005). Neural correlates associated with pro- and anti-saccades in primate SNr. *Society for Neuroscience Abstract*, **35**, 167–6.

Guthrie, B.L., Porter, J.D., and Sparks, D.L. (1983). Corollary discharge provides accurate eye position information to the oculomotor system. *Science*, **221**, 1193–1195.

Hallett, P.E. (1978). Primary and secondary saccades to goals defined by instructions. *Vision Research*, **18**, 1279–1296.

Hallett, P.E. and Lightstone, A.D. (1976). Saccadic eye movements to flashed targets. *Vision Research*. **16**, 107–114.

Heiser, L.M. and Colby, C.L. (2006). Spatial updating in area LIP is independent of saccade direction. *Journal of Neurophysiology*, **95**, 2751–2767.

Herter, T.M. and Guitton, D. (1998). Human head-free gaze saccades to targets flashed before gaze-pursuit are spatially accurate. *Journal of Neurophysiology*, **80**, 2785–2789.

Hikosaka, O., Takikawa, Y., and Kawagoe, R. (2000). Role of the basal ganglia in the control of purposive saccadic eye movements. *Physiological Reviews*, **80**, 953–978.

Hikosaka, O. and Wurtz, R.H. (1983). Visual and oculomotor functions of monkey substantia nigra pars reticulata. III. Memory-contingent visual and saccade responses. *Journal of Neurophysiology*, **49**, 1268–1284.

Hikosaka, O., Sakamoto M., and Usui, S. (1989). Functional properties of monkey caudate neurons. I. Activities related to saccadic eye movements. *Journal of Neurophysiology*, **61**, 780–798.

Holmes, G. (1939). The cerebellum of man. *Brain*, **62**, 1–30.

Ikeda, A., Shibasaki, H., Nagamine, T., Terada, K., Kaji, R., Fukuyama, H., and Kimura, J. (1994). Dissociation between contingent negative variation and Bereitschaftspotential in a patient with cerebellar efferent lesion. *Electroencephalography and Clinical Neurophysiology*, **90**, 359–364.

Ikeda, A., Shibasaki, H., Kaji, R., Terada, K., Nagamine, T., Honda, M., and Kimura, J. (1997). Dissociation between contingent negative variation (CNV) and Bereitschaftspotential (BP) in patients with parkinsonism. *Electroencephalography and Clinical Neurophysiology*, **102**, 142–151.

Inaba, N., Iwamoto, Y., and Yoshida, K. (2003). Changes in cerebellar fastigial burst activity related to saccadic gain adaptation in the monkey. *Neuroscience Research*, **46**, 359–368.

Johnston, K. and Everling, S. (2006). Monkey dorsolateral prefrontal cortex sends task-selective signals directly to the superior colliculus. *Journal of Neuroscience*, **26**, 12471–12478.

Jones, E.G. (2007). *The thalamus*. New York: Cambridge University Press.

Kaas, J.H. and Lyon, D.C. (2007). Pulvinar contributions to the dorsal and ventral streams of visual processing in primates. *Brain Research Reviews*, **55**, 285–296.

Karnath, H.O., Himmelbach, M., and Rorden, C. (2002). The subcortical anatomy of human spatial neglect: putamen, caudate nucleus and pulvinar. *Brain*, **125**, 350–360.

Kastner, S. and Pinsk, M.A. (2004). Visual attention as a multilevel selection process. *Cognitive, Affective, and Behavioral Neuroscience*, **4**, 483–500.

Kastner, S., O'Connor, D.H., Fukui, M.M., Fehd, H.M., Herwig, U., and Pinsk, M.A. (2004). Functional imaging of the human lateral geniculate nucleus and pulvinar. *Journal of Neurophysiology*, **91**, 438–448.

Kelly, V.E., Hyngstrom, A.S., Rundle, M.M., and Bastian, A.J. (2002). Interaction of levodopa and cues on voluntary reaching in Parkinson's disease. *Movement Disorders*, **17**, 38–44.

Klier, E.M. and Angelaki, D.E. (2008). Spatial updating and the maintenance of visual constancy. *Neuroscience*, **156**, 801–818.

Kinomura, S., Larsson, J, Gulyás. B., and Roland, P.E. (1996). Activation by attention of the human reticular formation and thalamic intralaminar nuclei. *Science*, **271**, 512–515.

Kowler, E., Anderson, E., Dosher, B., and Blaser, E. (1995). The role of attention in the programming of saccades. *Vision Research*, **35**, 1897–1916.

Kunimatsu, J. and Tanaka, M. (2010). Roles of the primate motor thalamus in the generation of antisaccades. *Journal of Neuroscience*, **30**, 5108–5117.

Lappe, M., Awater, H., and Krekelberg, B., (2000). Postsaccadic visual references generate presaccadic compression of space. *Nature*, **403**, 892–895.

Leichnetz, G.R. (1981). The prefrontal cortico-oculomotor trajectories in the monkey. *Journal of the Neurological Sciences*, **49**, 387–396.

Lewis, R.F., Gaymard, B.M., and Tamargo, R.J. (1998). Efference copy provides the eye position information required for visually guided reaching. *Journal of Neurophysiology*, **80**, 1605–1608.

Lewis, R.F., Zee, D.S., Gaymard, B.M., and Guthrie, B.L. (1994). Extraocular muscle proprioception functions in the control of ocular alignment and eye movement conjugacy. *Journal of Neurophysiology*, **72**, 1028–1031.

Lynch, J.C. and Tian, J. -R. (2006). Cortico-cortical networks and cortico-subcortical loops for the higher control of eye movements. *Progress in Brain Research*, **151**, 461–501.

Magnin, M. and Fuchs, A.F. (1977). Discharge properties of neurons in the monkey thalamus tested with angular acceleration, eye movement and visual stimuli. *Experimental Brain Research*, **28**, 293–299.

Matsuda, T., Matsuura, M., Ohkubo, T., Ohkubo, H., Matsushima, E., Inoue, K., *et al.* (2004). Functional MRI mapping of brain activation during visually guided saccades and antisaccades: cortical and subcortical networks. *Psychiatry Research*, **131**, 147–155.

Maldonado, H. and Schlag, J. (1984), Unit activity related to head and eye movements in central thalamus of cats. *Experimental Neurology*, **86**, 359–378.

Maldonado, H., Joseph, J.P., and Schlag, J. (1980). Types of eye movements evoked by thalamic microstimulation in the alert cat. *Experimental Neurology*, **70**, 613–625.

Marlinski, V. and McCrea, R.A. (2008). Coding of self-motion signals in ventro-posterior thalamus neurons in the alert squirrel monkey. *Experimental Brain Research*, **189**, 463–472.

McKenzie, A. and Lisberger, S.G. (1986). Properties of signals that determine the amplitude and direction of saccadic eye movements in monkeys. *Journal of Neurophysiology*, **56**, 196–207.

Medendorp, W.P., Goltz. H.C., Vilis, T., and Crawford, J.D. (2003). Gaze-centered updating of visual space in human parietal cortex. *Journal of Neuroscience*, **23**, 6209–6214.

Meng, H., May, P.J., Dickman, J.D., and Angelaki, D.E. (2007). Vestibular signals in primate thalamus: properties and origins. *Journal of Neuroscience*, **27**, 13590–13602.

Merker, B. and Schlag, J. (1985). Role of intralaminar thalamus in gaze mechanisms: evidence from electrical stimulation and fiber-sparing lesions in cat. *Experimental Brain Research*, **59**, 388–394.

Meyer-Lohmann, J., Hore, J., and Brooks, V.B. (1977). Cerebellar participation in generation of prompt arm movements. *Journal of Neurophysiology*, **40**, 1038–1050.

Middleton, F.A. and Strick, P.L. (2000). Basal ganglia and cerebellar loops: motor and cognitive circuits. *Brain Research. Brain Research Reviews*, **31**, 236–250.

Minamimoto, T. and Kimura, M. (2002). Participation of the thalamic CM-Pf complex in attentional orienting. *Journal of Neurophysiology*, **87**, 3090–3101.

Mink, J.W. (1996). The basal ganglia: focused selection and inhibition of competing motor programs. *Progress in Neurobiology*, **50**, 381–425.

Moore, T. and Fallah, M. (2001). Control of eye movements and spatial attention. *Proceedings of the National Academy of Sciences of the U S A*, **98**, 1273–1276.

Morrone, M.C., Ross, J., and Burr, D.C. (1997). Apparent position of visual targets during real and simulated saccadic eye movements. *Journal of Neuroscience*, **17**, 7941–7953.

Müller, J.R., Philiastides, M.G., and Newsome, W.T. (2005). Microstimulation of the superior colliculus focuses attention without moving the eyes. *Proceedings of the National Academy of Sciences of the U S A*, **102**, 524–529.

Munoz, D.P. and Everling, S. (2004). Look away: the anti-saccade task and the voluntary control of eye movement. *Nature Reviews Neuroscience*, **5**, 218–228.

Nakamura, K. and Colby, C.L., (2000). Visual, saccade-related, and cognitive activation of single neurons in monkey extrastriate area V3A. *Journal of Neurophysiology*, **84**, 677–692.

Nuding, U., Ono, S., Mustari, M.J., Büttner, U., and Glasauer, S. (2008). A theory of the dual pathways for smooth pursuit based on dynamic gain control. *Journal of Neurophysiology*, **99**, 2798–2808.

O'Driscoll, G.A., Alpert, N.M., Matthysse, S.W., Levy, D.L., Rauch, S.L., and Holzman, P.S. (1995). Functional neuroanatomy of antisaccade eye movements investigated with positron emission tomography. *Proceedings of the National Academy of Sciences of the U S A*, **92**, 925–929.

Ogren, M.P., Mateer, C.A., and Wyler, A.R. (1984). Alterations in visually related eye movements following left pulvinar damage in man. *Neuropsychologia*, **22**, 187–196.

Ohtsuka, K. (1994). Properties of memory-guided saccades toward targets flashed during smooth pursuit in human subjects. *Investigative Ophthalmology and Visual Science*, **35**, 509–514.

Optican, L.M. (2005). Sensorimotor transformation for visually guided saccades. *Annals of the New York Academy of Sciences*, **1039**, 132–148.

Orem, J., Schlag-Rey, A., and Schlag, J. (1973). Unilateral visual neglect and thalamic intralaminar lesions in the cat. *Experimental Neurology*, **40**, 784–797.

O'Scalaidhe, S.P., Wilson, F.A., and Goldman-Rakic, P.S. (1997). Areal segregation of face-processing neurons in prefrontal cortex. *Science*, **278**, 1135–1138.

Ostendorf, F., Liebermann, D., and Ploner, C.J. (2010). Human thalamus contributes to perceptual stability across eye movements. *Proceedings of the National Academy of Sciences of the U S A*, **107**, 1229–1234.

Petersen, S.E., Robinson, D.L., and Morris, J.D. (1987). Contributions of the pulvinar to visual spatial attention. *Neuropsychologia*, **25**, 97–105.

Petersen, S.E., Robinson, D.L., and Keys, W. (1985). Pulvinar nuclei of the behaving rhesus monkey: visual responses and their modulation. *Journal of Neurophysiology*, **54**, 867–886.

Petit, L., Orssaud, C., Tzourio, N., Salamon, G., Mazoyer, B., and Berthoz, A. (1993). PET study of voluntary saccadic eye movements in humans: basal ganglia-thalamocortical system and cingulate cortex involvement. *Journal of Neurophysiology*, **69**, 1009–1017.

Postle, B.R. (2006). Working memory as an emergent property of the mind and brain. *Neurosciense*, **139**, 23–38.

Powell, K.D. and Goldberg, M.E. (1997). Remapping of visual response in primate parietal cortex during smooth changes in gaze. *Society for Neuroscience Abstract*, **23**, 14–11.

Rafal, R., McGrath, M., Machado, L., and Hindle, J. (2004). Effects of lesions of the human posterior thalamus on ocular fixation during voluntary and visually triggered saccades. *Journal of Neurology, Neurosurgery, and Psychiatry*, **75**, 1602–1606.

Rainer, G., Assad, W.F., and Miller, E.K. (1998). Memory fields of neurons in the primate prefrontal cortex. *Proceedings of the National Academy of Sciences of the U S A*, **95**, 15008–15013.

Rao S.C., Rainer, G., and Miller, E.K. (1997). Integration of what and where in the primate prefrontal cortex. *Science*, **276**, 821–824.

Rivaud-Péchoux, S., Vidailhet, M., Brandel, JP., and Gaymard, B. (2007). Mixing pro- and antisaccades in patients with parkinsonian syndromes. *Brain*, **130**, 256–264.

Robinson, D.A. (1986). The systems approach to the oculomotor system. *Vision Research*, **26**, 91–99.

Robinson, D.L. and Petersen, S.E. (1992). The pulvinar and visual salience. *Trends in Neurosciences*, **15**, 127–132.

Robinson, D.L., McClurkin, J.W., Kertzman, C., and Petersen, S.E. (1991). Visual responses of pulvinar and collicular neurons during eye movements of awake, trained macaques. *Journal of Neurophysiology*, **66**, 485–496.

Robinson, F.R. and Fuchs, A.F. (2001). The role of the cerebellum in voluntary eye movements. *Annual Review of Neuroscience*, **24**, 981–1004.

Ross, J., Morrone, M.C., Goldberg, M.E., and Burr, D.C. (2001). Changes in visual perception at the time of saccades. *Trends in Neurosciences*, **24**, 113–121.

Sadikot, A.F. and Rymar, V.V. (2009). The primate centromedian-parafascicular complex: anatomical organization with a note on neuromodulation. *Brain Research Bulletin*, **78**, 122–130.

Schlag, J. and Schlag-Rey, M. (1971). Induction of oculomotor responses from thalamic internal medullary lamina in the cat. *Experimental Neurology*, **33**, 498–508.

Schlag, J. and Schlag-Rey, M. (1984). Visuomotor functions of central thalamus in monkey. II. Unit activity related to visual events, targeting, and fixation. *Journal of Neurophysiology*, **51**, 1175–1195.

Schlag, J. and Schlag-Rey, M. (1986). Role of the central thalamus in gaze control. *Progress in Brain Research*, **64**, 191–201.

Schlag, J. and Schlag-Rey, M. (1987). Evidence for a supplementary eye field. *Journal of Neurophysiology*, **57**, 179–200.

Schlag, J., Schlag-Rey, M., and Dassonville, P. (1990). Saccades can be aimed at the spatial location of targets flashed during pursuit. *Journal of Neurophysiology*, **64**, 575–581.

Schlag-Rey, M. and Schlag, J. (1984). Visuomotor functions central thalamus in monkey. I. Unit activity related to spontaneous eye movements. *Journal of Neurophysiology*, **51**, 1149–1174.

Schlag-Rey, M. and Schlag, J. (1989). The central thalamus. *Reviews of Oculomotor Research*, **3**, 361–390.

Schlag-Rey, M. and Schlag, J. (2002). Through the eye, slowly: delays and localization errors in the visual system. *Nature Reviews Neuroscience*, **3**, 191–215.

Schlag-Rey, M., Amador, N., Sanchez, H., and Schlag, J. (1997). Antisaccade performance predicted by neuronal activity in the supplementary eye field. *Nature*, **390**, 398–401.

Schwartz, J.D. and Lisberger, S.G. (1994). Initial tracking conditions modulate the gain of visuo-motor transmission for smooth pursuit eye movements in monkeys. *Visual Neuroscience*, **11**, 411–424.

Scudder, C.A. and McGee, D.M. (2003). Adaptive modification of saccade size produces correlated changes in the discharges of fastigial nucleus neurons. *Journal of Neurophysiology*, **90**, 1011–1026.

Shipp, S. (2003). The functional logic of cortico-pulvinar connections. *Philosophical Transactions of the Royal Society Series B: Biological Sciences*, **358**, 1605–1624.

Shook, B.L., Schlag-Rey, M., and Schlag, J. (1990). Primate supplementary eye field: I. Comparative aspects of mesencephalic and pontine connections. *Journal of Comparative Neurology*, **301**, 618–642.

Siwek, D.F. and Pandya, D.N. (1991). Prefrontal projections to the mediodorsal nucleus of the thalamus in the rhesus monkey. *Journal of Comparative Neurology*, **312**, 509–524.

Smith, A.T., Cotton, P.L., Bruno, A., and Moutsiana, C. (2009). Dissociating vision and visual attention in the human pulvinar. *Journal of Neurophysiology*, **101**, 917–925.

Smith, Y., Raju, D.V., Pare, J.F., and Sidibe, M. (2004). The thalamostriatal system: a highly specific network of the basal ganglia circuitry. *Trends in Neurosciences*, **27**, 520–527.

Sommer, M.A. (2003). The role of the thalamus in motor control. *Current Opinion in Neurobiology*, **13**, 663–670.

Sommer, M.A. and Wurtz, R.H. (2002). A pathway in primate brain for internal monitoring of movements. *Science*, **296**, 1480–1482.

Sommer, M.A. and Wurtz, R.H. (2004a). What the brain stem tells the frontal cortex. I. Oculomotor signals sent from superior colliculus to frontal eye field via mediodorsal thalamus. *Journal of Neurophysiology*, **91**, 1381–1402.

Sommer, M.A. and Wurtz, R.H. (2004b). What the brain stem tells the frontal cortex. II. Role of the SC-MD-FEF pathway in corollary discharge. *Journal of Neurophysiology*, **91**, 1403–1423.

Sommer, M.A. and Wurtz, R.H. (2006). Influence of the thalamus on spatial visual processing in frontal cortex. *Nature*, **16**, 374–347.

Stone, L.S. and Lisberger, S.G. (1990). Visual responses of Purkinje cells in the cerebellar flocculus during smooth-pursuit eye movements in monkeys. I. Simple spikes. *Journal of Neurophysiology*, **63**, 1241–1261.

Straube, A., Fuchs, A.F., Usher, S., and Robinson, F.R. (1997). Characteristics of saccadic gain adaptation in rhesus macaques. *Journal of Neurophysiology*, **77**, 874–895.

Suzuki, D.A. and Keller, E.L. (1988). The role of the posterior vermis of monkey cerebellum in smooth-pursuit eye movement control. II. Target velocity-related Purkinje cell activity. *Journal of Neurophysiology*, **59**, 19–40.

Takagi, M., Zee, D.S., and Tamargo, R.J. (1998). Effects of lesions of the oculomotor vermis on eye movements in primate: saccades. *Journal of Neurophysiology*, **80**, 1911–1931.

Tanabe, J., Tregellas, J., Miller, D., Ross, R.G., and Freedman, R. (2002). Brain activation during smooth-pursuit eye movements. *Neuroimage,* **17,** 1315–1324.

Tanaka, M. (2003). Contribution of signals downstream from adaptation to saccade programming. *Journal of Neurophysiology,* **90,** 2080–2086.

Tanaka, M. (2005a). Effects of eye position on estimates of eye displacement for spatial updating. *Neuroreport,* **22,** 1261–1265.

Tanaka, M. (2005b). Involvement of the central thalamus in the control of smooth pursuit eye movements. *Journal of Neuroscience,* **25,** 5866–5876.

Tanaka, M. (2006). Inactivation of the central thalamus delays self-timed saccades. *Nature Neuroscience,* **9,** 20–22.

Tanaka, M. (2007a). Spatiotemporal properties of eye position signals in the primate central thalamus. *Cerebral Cortex,* **17,** 1504–1515.

Tanaka, M. (2007b). Cognitive signals in the primate motor thalamus predict saccade timing. *Journal of Neuroscience,* **27,** 12109–12118.

Tanaka, M. and Lisberger, S.G. (2001). Regulation of the gain of visually guided smooth-pursuit eye movements by frontal cortex. *Nature,* **409,** 191–194.

Tanibuchi, I. and Goldman-Rakic, P.S. (2003). Dissociation of spatial-, object-, and sound-coding neurons in the mediodorsal nucleus of the primate thalamus. *Journal of Neurophysiology,* **89,** 067–1077.

Tanibuchi, I. and Goldman-Rakic, P.S. (2005). Comparison of oculomotor neuronal activity in paralaminar and mediodorsal thalamus in rhesus monkey. *Journal of Neurophysiology,* **93,** 614–619.

Tanji, J. and Hoshi, E. (2008). Role of the lateral prefrontal cortex in executive behavioral control. *Physiological Reviews,* **88,** 37–57.

Thach, W.T., Goodkin, H.P., and Keating, J.G. (1992). The cerebellum and the adaptive coordination of movement. *Annual Review of Neuroscience,* **15,** 403–442.

Thier, P. and Ilg, U.J. (2005). The neural basis of smooth-pursuit eye movements. *Current Opinion in Neurobiology,* **15,** 645–652.

Tian, J.-R. and Lynch, J.C. (1997). Subcortical input to the smooth and saccadic eye movement subregions of the frontal eye field in Cebus monkey. *Journal of Neuroscience,* **17,** 9233–9247.

Tu, P.C., Yang, T.H., Kuo, W.J., Hsieh, J.C., and Su, T.P. (2006). Neural correlates of antisaccade deficits in schizophrenia, an fMRI study. *Journal of Psychiatric Research,* **40,** 606–612.

Umeno, M.M. and Goldberg, M.E. (1997). Spatial processing in the monkey frontal eye field. I. Predictive visual responses. *Journal of Neurophysiology,* **78,** 1373–1383.

Ungerleider, L.G. and Christensen, C.A. (1977). Pulvinar lesions in monkeys produce abnormal eye movements during visual discrimination training. *Brain Research,* **136,** 189–196.

Ungerleider, L.G. and Christensen, C.A. (1979). Pulvinar lesions in monkeys produce abnormal scanning of a complex visual array. *Neuropsychologia,* **17,** 493–501.

Ungerleider, L.G., Courtney, S.M., and Haxby, J.V. (1998). A neural system for human visual working memory. *Proceedings of the National Academy of Sciences of the U S A,* **95,** 883–890.

van Donkelaar, P., Stein, J.F., Passingham, R.E., and Miall, R.C. (2000). Temporary inactivation in the primate motor thalamus during visually triggered and internally generated limb movements. *Journal of Neurophysiology,* **83,** 2780–2790.

Versino, M., Beltrami, G., Uggetti, C., and Cosi, V. (2000). Auditory saccade impairment after central thalamus lesions. *Journal of Neurology, Neurosurgery, and Psychiatry,* **68,** 234–237.

Villeneuve, M.Y., Kupers, R., Gjedde, A., Ptito, M., and Casanova, C. (2005). Pattern-motion selectivity in the human pulvinar. *Neuroimage,* **28,** 474–480.

Wang, X., Zhang, M., Cohen, I.S., and Goldberg, M.E. (2007). The proprioceptive representation of eye position in monkey primary somatosensory cortex. *Nature Neuroscience,* **10,** 640–646.

Watanabe, M. and Munoz, D. (2009). Neural correlates of conflict resolution between automatic and volitional actions by basal ganglia. *European Journal of Neuroscience,* **30,** 2165–2176.

Watanabe, Y. and Funahashi, S. (2004a). Neuronal activity throughout the primate mediodorsal nucleus of the thalamus during oculomotor delayed-responses. I. Cue-, delay, and response-period activity. *Journal of Neurophysiology,* **92,** 1738–1755.

Watanabe, Y. and Funahashi, S. (2004b). Neuronal activity throughout the primate mediodorsal nucleus of the thalamus during oculomotor delayed-responses. II. Activity encoding visual versus motor signal. *Journal of Neurophysiology,* **92,** 1756–1769.

Watanabe, Y., Takeda, K., and Funahashi, S. (2009). Population vector analysis of primate mediodorsal thalamic activity during oculomotor delayed-response performance. *Cerebral Cortex,* **19,** 1313–1321.

Watson, R.T. and Heilman, K.M. (1979). Thalamic neglect. *Neurology,* **29,** 690–694.

Watson, R.T., Miller, B.D., and Heilman, K.M. (1978). Nonsensory neglect. *Annals of Neurology,* **3,** 505–508.

Watson, R.T., Valenstein, E., and Heilman, K.M. (1981). Thalamic neglect. Possible role of the medial thalamus and nucleus reticularis in behavior. *Archives of Neurology,* **38,** 501–506.

White, R.L. and Snyder, L.H. (2004). A neural network model of flexible spatial updating. *Journal of Neurophysiology,* **91,** 1608–1619.

Wilson, F.A.W., O'Scalaidhe. S.P., and Goldman-Rakic, P.S. (1993). Dissociation of object and spatial processing domains in primate prefrontal cortex. *Science*, **260**, 1955–1958.

Wyder, M.T., Massoglia, D.P., and Stanford, T.R. (2003). Quantitative assessment of the timing and tuning of visual-related, saccade-related, and delay period activity in primate central thalamus. *Journal of Neurophysiology*, **90**, 2029–2052.

Wyder, M.T., Massoglia, D.P., and Stanford, T.R. (2004). Contextual modulation of central thalamic delay-period activity: representation of visual and saccadic goals. *Journal of Neurophysiology*, **91**, 2628–2648.

Yoshida, A. and Tanaka, M. (2009). Enhanced modulation of neuronal activity during antisaccades in the primate globus pallidus. *Cerebral Cortex*, **19**, 206–217.

Zihl, J. and von Cramon, D. (1979). The contribution of the 'second' visual system to directed visual attention in man. *Brain*, **102**, 835–856.

Zivotofsky, A.Z., Rottach, K.G., Averbuch-Heller, L., Kori, A.A., Thomas, C.W., Dell'Osso, L.F., *et al.* (1996). Saccades to remembered targets: the effects of smooth pursuit and illusory stimulus motion. *Journal of Neurophysiology*, **76**, 3617–3632.

CHAPTER 14

The role of posterior parietal cortex in the regulation of saccadic eye movements

Martin Paré and Michael C. Dorris

Abstract

The posterior parietal cortex (PPC) is a node within the cerebral 'higher-order' network that has no clear homologue in non-primate mammals and is fully defined only in catarrhine primates, which include old world monkeys and hominoids. The late coming of the PPC in the eye movement circuit and the absence of an unequivocal role in saccade preparation and production suggests that the PPC should only be viewed as an innovation to enhance the sensory guidance and flexible control of visual behaviour. In line with this idea is the evidence that the lateral intraparietal area integrates sensory and goal-directed information into a map wherein representations of spatial locations can be maintained and selected as saccade targets through decision processes.

Evolutionary considerations

A wealth of data from neuroanatomical, neurophysiological, lesion, and imaging studies has yielded several hypotheses regarding the functions subserved and the operations performed by the several areas of the PPC. Advances on the role of PPC in space coding, coordinate transformation, visual attention, movement planning, and multisensory integration have been reviewed previously, and the reader is invited to consult this rather large literature. Together, many of these hypotheses form the outline of a PPC visuomotor theory (e.g. Goodale and Milner, 1992; Wise et al., 1997), but a full integration is wanting before we have a complete theoretical grounding. Towards that end, we think that there is one important area of investigation to integrate and develop further, namely, the evolutionary perspective.

Comparative studies, as reviewed by Kaas (2008), suggest that the neocortex of early mammals was composed of a limited number of distinct areas, mostly primary and secondary sensory fields. The growing predominance of vision in early primates was associated with an expansion of the occipital and temporal cortices. Concomitantly, the organization of the somatosensory areas in parietal cortex underwent a significant expansion of the forepaw representation, which may partially be related to the high manual dexterity demands of arboreal life (see for review Ross and Martin, 2007). The PPC came about from the concerted expansion of the somatosensory and visual cortices, linking the latter with motor fields of the frontal cortex (Fang et al., 2005). These evolutionary considerations provide supportive evidence for the basic role of the PPC in visually-guided behaviour, but they also indicate that it may be to confer primates with skilled visuomanual behaviour, including eye–hand coordination and grasping (see for review Disbrow et al., 2007; Preuss, 2007a; Ross and Martin, 2007). The more recent evolution of a fully opposable thumb in humans, clearly a prerequisite for tool use, certainly coincided with further expansion of the PPC in this species (Frey, 2007; Ramayya et al., 2010). This capability may have built upon phylogenetically older neural circuits controlling skilled forelimb movements, such as in food handling behaviour (see for review Iwaniuk and Whishaw, 2000; Whishaw, 2003), and perhaps also on existing visual processing circuits associated with navigation and locomotion-related obstacle avoidance, which are evident in rodents (Kolb and Walkey, 1987) and cats (see for review McVea and Pearson, 2009).

Consistent with the above hypothesis, sustained electrical stimulation of the anterior PPC in prosimian galagos evokes what look like 'primitives' of ethologically significant behaviours, such as reaching-and-grasping, hand-to-mouth movements, and coordinated defensive body movements (Stepniewska et al., 2005)—such defensive movements have also been observed following sustained electrical stimulation of the ventral intraparietal area of the macaque monkey PPC (Cooke et al., 2003). Although these coordinated movements certainly result from the activation of distributed neural circuits extending beyond the PPC, they seem to be topographically organized within the PPC: moving the stimulation electrode from the most ventral part of the PPC to its most dorsal part progressively evokes eye movements, facial expressions, grasping, reaching, and hind-limb movements. Overall, the specific PPC role in regulating eye movements, which is the topic of this chapter, may well be only understood in the context of this larger sensory-motor map with perhaps special consideration to complex behaviour, such as eye–hand coordination (Land, 2006; Johansson and Flanagan, 2009). The hypothesized role of the PPC in space coding and coordinate transformation is particularly relevant in this context (see for review Cohen and Andersen, 2002; Husain and Nachev, 2007).

The distinctive visual ability of primates is conferred, in part, by a fairly large ocular motility and a retina equipped with a well-defined fovea requires a sophisticated eye movement system to gather useful, detailed visual information. The large oculomotor range that primates possess appears to be evolutionarily recent. The human oculomotor range spans about ±50° of visual angle (Guitton and Volle, 1987; Stahl, 1999) and is comparable to that of the macaque monkey (Tomlinson and Bahra, 1986) and baboon (Marchetti et al., 1983). In contrast, the oculomotor range of early primates such as prosimians (Shepherd and Platt, 2006) as well as that of the new world squirrel monkey (McCrea and Gdowski, 2003) is limited to 20–25°. Limited ocular motility is commonly reported in frontal-eyed non-primates that lack a distinct fovea, such as the tree shrew (Remple et al., 2006) and the cat (Guitton et al., 1984). This augmented oculomotor facility may have paralleled an increasing involvement of the PPC in regulating eye movements. Anatomical studies have shown that the PPC is heavily interconnected with the prefrontal cortex (PFC) and the superior temporal sulcus cortex, as well as with the dorsal pulvinar and the superior colliculus (SC), and thus a node is what is best described as a 'higher-order' network (Preuss, 2007b). This network has no clear homologue in non-primate mammals and is fully defined only in catarrhine primates (Preuss, 2007a, 2007b), which include old world monkeys and hominoids. In comparison, the high-order saccade centre, the frontal eye field (FEF), is common to all primates (Kaas, 2008; Preuss, 2007a), as the optic tectum (the SC homologue) is to vertebrates. In addition, the projections to the SC that originate from the PPC have been shown to be negligible in platyrrhine primates (Collins et al., 2005), the new world monkeys that are extant members of the oldest branch of the anthropoid radiation. It is therefore reasonable to assume that the role of PPC in regulating orienting in general and eye movements in particular is also evolutionarily recent.

The link between PPC and behaviour is certainly much more indirect than that implied by the above electrical stimulation studies. The PPC is an ideal interface between the different sensory fields and the frontal cortex motor fields and it is an undeniably important player in the frontoparietal network that endows us with several of our cognitive abilities. Nevertheless, the PPC does not have direct access to the motor circuitry, per se. As evidenced in the rest of this chapter, oculomotor research suggests that PPC neuronal activity is not directly associated with the production of movements. A more accurate view is that PPC only provides signals that can regulate potential actions in the form of representations from which specific goals can be selected. With respect to eye movements, these regulatory signals could reflect several cognitive processes and their origins would be predominantly visual.

There is a vast literature on the role of PPC in regulating eye movements and related cognitive processes. Significant advances have been made in studying human patients and healthy subjects using many different approaches, such as psychophysics, functional brain imaging (see for review Curtis, Chapter 20, this volume), and transcranial magnetic stimulation (see for review Müri and Nyffeler, Chapter 21, this volume). A complete review of these findings is beyond the scope of this chapter, and we opted to focus this review on work conducted on the saccadic eye movement system in our best animal model, the macaque monkey. This chapter also emphasizes work, framed by work conducted in our laboratories, on saccade-related processes investigated with single-neuron recording in the lateral intraparietal (LIP) area, an area within the PPC vision-for-action processing stream with the strongest connections to the saccadic eye movement system. Along with evolutionary considerations, the advances in our understanding of the neuronal activity in this particular cortical area in the macaque monkey provide a framework to guide our general understanding of PPC and to interpret data from different approaches.

A vision-for-saccade interface

The primate PPC contains many subdivisions (Fig. 14.1) (Lewis and Van Essen, 2000a), several of which appear homologous in monkeys and humans (Grefkes and Fink, 2005; see also Shikata et al., 2008; Arcaro et al., 2011). The intraparietal sulcus divides this cortical region into superior and

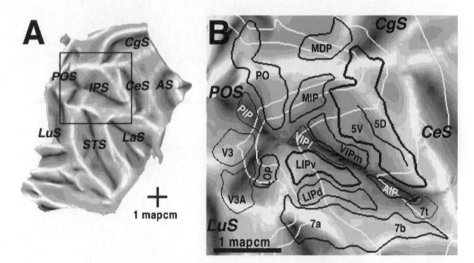

Fig. 14.1 Macaque posterior parietal cortex. **A.** Flat map of the macaque cerebral cortex showing the entire sulcal pattern and major subdivisions: arcuate sulcus (*AS*), central sulcus (*CeS*), cingulated sulcus (*CgS*), intra-parietal sulcus (*IPS*), the lateral sulcus (*LaS*), the lunate sulcus (*LuS*), the posterior-parietal sulcus (*POS*) and the superior temporal sulcus (*STS*). Anterior is to the right. **B.** Expanded view of the intra-parietal sulcus (*IPS*), showing the location of the dorsal (LIPd) and ventral (LIPv) portion of the lateral intraparietal area along with fifteen other architectonically identified subdivisions. White lines are layer IV contours. Adapted from Journal of Comparative Neurology, vol. 428, Lewis, J. W. & Van Essen, D. C., Mapping of architectonic subdivisions in the macaque monkey, with emphasis on parieto-occipital cortex. pp. 79-111, 2000, with permission from John Wiley and Sons.

inferior lobules, whose primary inputs are somatosensory and visual, respectively. One particular subdivision within the lateral bank of the intraparietal sulcus was found to contain neurons with both visually evoked responses and saccade-related activity (Andersen et al., 1987). Figure 14.2 illustrates the basic discharge properties of these neurons, including the sustained and persistent activity they often exhibit in delayed response tasks. All types of activity are spatially co-registered (Barash et al., 1991; Johnston et al., 2009) and give these neurons circumscribed, yet large response fields. Together, the neurons—located in what is now referred to as the LIP area—are organized into a coarse representation of the contralateral visual field (Ben Hamed et al., 2001; Blatt et al., 1990).

Anatomical studies have found that area LIP receives converging inputs from numerous visual areas and sends projections to the two brain regions necessary for saccade production, namely, the FEF within the anterior bank of the arcuate sulcus (see for review Johnston and Everling, Chapter 15, this volume) and the intermediate layers of the midbrain SC (see for review White and Munoz, Chapter 11, this volume) (Andersen et al., 1990; Baizer et al., 1991). Tracing of retrograde labels injected in FEF (Schall et al., 1995a) and SC (Lynch et al., 1985) confirmed this direct access to the saccadic eye movement system, and antidromic activation studies have identified that many of these projection neurons have saccade-related activity (Ferraina et al., 2002; Paré and Wurtz 1997, 2001). Lastly, there are also reciprocal connections from FEF (Ferraina et al., 2002; Lewis and Van Essen, 2000b; Schall et al., 1995a; Stanton et al., 1995) as well as from the SC (Clower et al., 2001), though the latter are via the inferior pulvinar and primarily from the more sensory superficial layers of the SC.

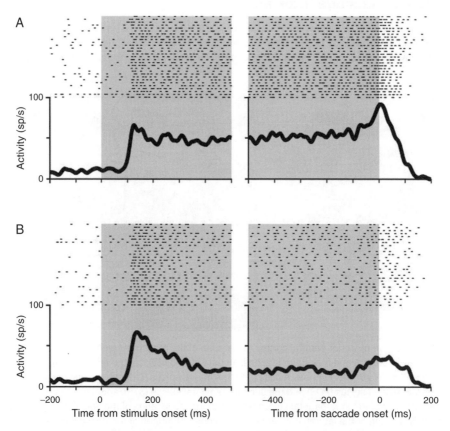

Fig. 14.2 LIP neuronal activity in delayed saccade tasks. Rasters and spike densities from one representative LIP neuron are shown for visual (**A**) and memory (**B**) delayed saccade tasks. [Paré M., & Wurtz, R. H., Journal of Neurophysiology, 1997, Am Physiol Soc, modified with permission.]

Area LIP itself may also be subdivided into an anterio-dorsal (LIVd) and posterio-ventral (LIPv) portion (Fig. 14.1), the latter being identified by its dense myelination (Blatt et al., 1990; Lewis and Van Essen, 2000a; Seltzer and Pandya, 1980). The stronger connections of LIPv with FEF and SC (Blatt et al., 1990; Lynch et al., 1985; Schall et al., 1995a) suggest that this portion of the lateral bank of the intraparietal sulcus is the main interface between the visual and saccadic eye movement systems. In contrast, the more exclusive connections of LIPd with visual areas of the temporal cortex (Blatt et al., 1990; Lewis and Van Essen, 2000b) suggest that this portion has a more sophisticated role in visual processing, perhaps at the expense of eye movement processing (but see Liu et al., 2010 for a different account). Consistent with this scheme, Bakola et al. (2006) have shown with C-deoxyglucose imaging that LIPv is recruited during both visually guided and memory-guided saccades, whereas LIPd is recruited primarily during visual fixation and visually-guided saccades. From this work, it is plausible that some of the different hypotheses regarding the functions of area LIP stemmed from results obtained from two distinct populations of neurons. For instance, the visual feature sensitivity identified in some LIP studies (Sereno and Amador 2006; Sereno and Maunsell, 1998; see also Janssen et al., 2008) could be limited to LIPd (Ogawa and Komatsu, 2009).

In summary, the role of PPC in regulating saccadic eye movements may be best investigated by examining the properties of area LIPv. In addition, given the general hypothesis that the PPC receives predominantly visual inputs, investigations should make particular considerations for visually guided eye movements.

Saccade production

The direct projections of area LIP to FEF and SC suggest that its neurons directly participate in the production of saccadic eye movements, but this is now proven not to be a tenable hypothesis. The first evidence for this original hypothesis is the original observation made by Mountcastle and colleagues of pre-saccade increase in activity in neurons of area 7—including portion of the lateral bank of the intraparietal sulcus, from which LIP neurons would likely have been sampled (Lynch et al., 1977; Yin and Mountcastle, 1977). This discharge patterns was subsequently attributed to neurons within area LIP (Andersen et al., 1987; Barash et al., 1991). More recent evidence suggests, however, that area LIP is not directly involved in saccade production. First, the magnitude of LIP pre-saccade activity shows visual dependence and is significantly reduced when saccades are made in the absence of a visual stimulus (Ferraina et al., 2002; Paré and Wurtz, 1997, 2001; see also Gottlieb and Goldberg, 1999) as well as when several stimuli are present (Thomas and Paré, 2007). In addition, large amount of electrical current is necessary to elicit saccadic eye movements when stimulating area LIP (Keating et al., 1983; Kurylo and Skavenski, 1991; Shibutani et al., 1984; Thier et al., 1998). Lastly, ablation of this cortical area does not impair saccade production (Lynch and McLaren, 1989). This body of evidence contrasts with the demonstration of the critical role of FEF and SC in the production of saccades. First, removal of both FEF and SC severely and irreversibly impairs the ability of monkey to produce saccades (Schiller et al., 1980). Second, low-current microstimulation of these brain regions produces saccades of predictable amplitudes and directions (Bruce et al., 1985; Robinson, 1972; Robinson and Fuchs, 1969). Third, SC and FEF contain neurons with pre-saccade increase in activity (Bruce and Goldberg, 1985; Wurtz and Goldberg, 1971) that is correlated with saccade occurrence (Hanes et al., 1998; Paré and Hanes, 2003; Sparks, 1978; see also Mohler and Wurtz, 1976). In light of these major differences, it appears premature to take the pre-saccadic increase in the activity of LIP neurons as evidence that this cortical area is directly involved in the production of saccades.

For any brain region hypothesized to be involved in saccade production, it is imperative to determine whether its neuronal activity is actually closely linked to saccade occurrence, i.e. sufficient to account for saccade production. One definitive test is provided by the countermanding paradigm, which has been adapted for monkeys making saccadic eye movements (Hanes and Schall, 1995, 1996). This paradigm tests one's ability to inhibit the initiation of a response when an infrequent stop signal follows the go signal, and modelling of task performance can estimate the length of time needed to cancel the commanded response (Logan and Cowan, 1984). In this context, for neurons to be involved in the process of saccade production, they must change their activity when a saccade is cancelled instead of executed, and they must do so before the saccade is cancelled. This has been found to be the case for nearly all SC movement neurons tested (Paré and Hanes, 2003) as well as for about half of such neurons in FEF (Hanes et al., 1998).

We recently conducted a study in which LIP neurons with saccade-related activity were submitted to the countermanding test (Brunamonti et al., 2008). Unlike what was observed in SC and FEF neurons, LIP neurons were found to change their activity when saccades were countermanded instead of executed only infrequently. In addition, this change in activity nearly always occurred later than when the saccade was cancelled, as estimated from the behaviour collected in the very same trials. This finding provides solid evidence that area LIP does not contain neurons with the signals necessary to control whether a saccade is to be produced. Similar result has been obtained in the supplementary eye field, despite the presence of pre-saccade activity observed in this PFC area since its discovery (Stuphorn et al., 2010). Figure 14.3 contrasts the results obtained from area LIP, FEF, and SC.

Altogether, the mere existence of a pre-saccadic increase in the activity of a neuron cannot be taken as evidence that this neuron is involved in saccade production. For example, some neurons in striate and extrastriate visual cortex have been shown to increase their activity just prior to a saccade made to a stimulus presented in their visual receptive fields (Moore, 1999; Nakamura and Colby, 2000; Supèr et al., 2004), but most would be cautious about describing this pre-saccade activity as playing a role in triggering saccades (see also Schiller and Tehovnik, 2001). Such activity can instead be interpreted as guiding saccades, and the strong dependence of LIP pre-saccade activity on visual stimulation is consistent with this interpretation. The evolutionary late emergence of PPC in the eye movement circuit may have limited its role in saccade regulation to processes that can only influence saccade production. This account agrees with the principle that the basic organization of neural

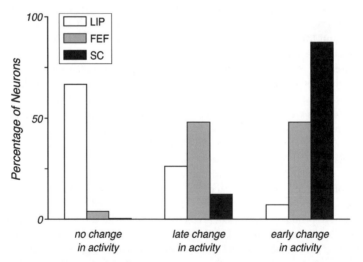

Fig. 14.3 Comparison of LIP, FEF, and SC neuronal responses associated with saccade countermanding. Graph shows the percentage of neurons with: 1) no significant change in activity around the time of saccade cancellation (no change in activity); 2) a significant change in activity, but occurring after saccade cancellation or after the efferent delay (late change in activity); and 3) a significant change in activity occurring early enough to account for saccade cancellation, i.e., within the efferent delay (early change in activity). Data are from samples of movement neurons: 42 in LIP (white), 51 in FEF (striped), and 32 in SC (dark). The shortest efferent delay is the minimal conduction time needed for signals from LIP, FEF, and SC to reach the eye muscles: 10 ms for both LIP and FEF, and 8 ms for SC (Paré & Hanes 2003). FEF data are from Hanes et al. (1998), SC data from Paré and Hanes (2003), and LIP data are from Brunamonti et al. (2008).

circuits is evolutionarily conservative, but that changes in behaviour can occur through adaptive changes in modulatory inputs to the control circuits (Katz and Harris-Warrick, 1999).

The evidence provided here argues against the idea that area LIP constitutes a parietal eye field (Andersen et al., 1992). The next sections consider the several hypotheses that LIP neuronal activity reflects more covert processes.

Saccade preparation and initiation

Response preparation refers to the neural processes by which response goals are specified and the execution of a specific response is facilitated (Riehle and Requin, 1989, 1993; Requin et al., 1990; see also Schall, 2004). For neurons to be involved in saccade preparation they must therefore: 1) change their activity in advance of an upcoming saccade, and the strength of their activity must predict both 2) the probability of occurrence, and 3) the timing of the saccade.

The involvement of area LIP in saccade preparation was first suggested by the observation that LIP neurons display a sustained activity during an imposed delay period between visual stimulation and saccade initiation. Andersen and colleagues (Andersen et al., 1987; Barash et al., 1991; Gnadt and Andersen, 1988) first showed that LIP neurons discharge long before specific saccadic vectors that correspond to their response fields. Specifically, the delay activity is maintained, albeit at a reduced level, when visual stimulation is interrupted or when the saccade is made within the response field without recent visual stimulation. These activity patterns meet the first operational criterion for response preparation, namely, that the activity must occur in advance of action.

Regarding the second criterion, some evidence suggests that LIP neuronal activity is predictive of an impending saccade in a neuron's response field. Several studies using various behavioural tasks have shown that LIP activity is sensitive to the information content of advanced instructions specifying whether or which saccade will be produced (Gottlieb et al., 1998; Paré and Wurtz, 2001; Platt and Glimcher, 1997; Shadlen and Newsome, 1996, 2001; Toth and Assad, 2002). Such activity has also been shown to be independent of the sensory modality and closely related to the occurrence of the next saccade (Mazzoni et al., 1996). Nevertheless, when compared with SC delay activity recorded in a Go/Nogo response task, the LIP activity is much less dependent on advanced instruction (Paré and Wurtz, 2001).

The third and highest-level operational criterion for response preparation refers to the predictive value of the neuronal activity for response initiation, i.e. the activity level should be related to the timing of the response. Neuronal activity can hardly be considered as preparatory if it does not affect the process for which it presumably prepares. This last criterion is been largely neglected in previous LIP studies. To date, studies have found relatively inconsistent and, at best, very weak evidence that the sustained activity of LIP neurons is predictive of saccade latency (e.g. Bendiksby and Platt, 2006; Dorris and Glimcher, 2004; Pesaran et al., 2002; Platt and Glimcher, 1999; Shadlen and Newsome, 2001; Roitman and Shadlen, 2002). These results contrast greatly with the preparatory nature of the activity of SC neurons recorded in a warned response task (Dorris and Munoz, 1998; Dorris et al., 1997; Paré and Munoz, 2001). In the gap saccade task, the early pre-target activity of SC neurons observed during the warming preparation period correlates with saccade latency. Our observations from the recording of LIP neurons in identical tasks are that these neurons generally lacked this early activity. Although some LIP neurons can display some activity in the absence of visual stimulation (Ben Hamed and Duhamel, 2002), they appear to reflect processes only once activated by sensory inputs.

In any given saccade task, response latency varies from trial to trial, and a useful framework to understand this variability is provided by accumulator models of response time performance (see for review Smith and Ratcliff, 2004). Studies in both FEF (Hanes and Schall, 1996) and SC (Dorris and Munoz, 1998; Dorris et al., 1997) have shown that saccades are initiated when the variable growth of pre-saccade activity reaches a fixed threshold (see for review Stuphorn and Schall, 2002). This saccade trigger threshold is reached very late in the response time interval, approximately 10–12 ms before saccade initiation (Paré and Hanes, 2003) and consistent with the anatomy and physiology of the premotor circuitry of the saccadic eye movement system (Hanes and Schall, 1996). Evidence for a similar rise-to-threshold pattern of activity in area LIP remains, however, limited. In the study conducted by Roitman and Shadlen (2002), a variable rate of growth in LIP neuronal activity was observed, but the timing of when it reaches threshold was estimated to be 70 ms before saccade initiation. This timing is at odds with the FEF and SC estimates of trigger activation threshold. It is, however, more in line with what is referred to as the saccade target selection threshold—when a visual stimulus is selected as the saccade goal—which has been estimated to have a comparable timing in both FEF (Thompson et al., 2005a) and SC (Shen and Paré, 2007).

These neurophysiological data provide only partial evidence regarding the existence of saccade preparation signals in area LIP. Data from human studies have provided converging evidence in showing that unilateral lesions of the parietal lobe do not result in enduring changes in saccade latency (Machado and Rafal, 2004; Pierrot-Deseilligny et al., 1991; Rafal, 2006). It has also been suggested the observed increases in latency of saccades made to visual, contralesional stimuli rather reflect a deficit in visual spatial attention (Rafal, 2006). The same interpretation may apply to data from monkeys with intraparietal lesions (Lynch and McLaren, 1989). Results from inactivation of area LIP with injections of the GABA$_A$ agonist muscimol have also been inconclusive. Some mild increases in saccade latency in the memory delayed response task were observed by Li et al. (1999), but subsequent single (Schiller and Tehovnik, 2003) and multiple injections (Wardak et al., 2002) failed to reproduce reliably these effects. In contrast, much more reliable increases in saccade latency following LIP inactivation are observed when monkeys perform alternative choice tasks (Wardak et al., 2002). Together with the decreases in saccade latency observed when LIP is microstimulated during choice tasks (Hank et al., 2006), these findings suggest that LIP neuronal activity reflects covert processes only indirectly related to saccade initiation.

Overall, the neuronal population in area LIP does not appear to carry the necessary neural signals to regulate when a saccade will be produced, i.e. it is most probably not involved in saccade preparation per se. The next sections examine whether area LIP participate in the covert processes that maintain saccade goal representations and select saccade goals.

Visual working memory

Saccadic eye movements can be directed not only to visual stimuli but also to their remembered location. Our ability to maintain information temporarily is critical for goal-driven behaviour, including eye movements. This cognitive process is referred to as working memory and significant experimental and theoretical advances have been made regarding its substrate. First, neural activity that persists in the absence of a sensory stimulus has been identified in a network of cortical areas, including the PPC (see for review Curtis, Chapter 20, this volume). Second, likely candidates for the underlying mechanism have been suggested to include the reverberatory process provided by the recurrent projections of cortical pyramidal neurons (Amit, 1995) and the slow dynamic of the NMDA glutamate receptor (Lisman et al., 1998), both of which playing predominant roles in our current models (see for review Durstewitz et al., 2000; Wang, 2001, 2010).

A large body of work on the neuronal persistent activity associated with working memory has been conducted within the PFC in delayed response tasks involving either skeletomotor (Fuster and Alexander, 1971; Kubota and Niki, 1971) or ocumolotor responses (Bruce and Goldberg, 1985; Funahashi et al., 1989). Persistent activity has also been observed in PPC (Fig. 14.1) (see for review Constantinidis and Procyk, 2004; Rawley and Constantinidis, 2009), and it is frequently used as a defining characteristic of neurons in area LIP, but not frequently studied as a mnemonic process (but see Mazzoni et al., 1996). As indicated in the section above, Andersen and colleagues were first to show that PPC neurons in area LIP and 7a discharge during the delay period (retention interval) intervening between the presentation of a stimulus in a neuron's receptive field and the ensuing eye movement made to that remembered location (Andersen et al., 1987; Gnadt and Andersen, 1988; Barash et al., 1991). This delay activity in area LIP has since most often been interpreted as being associated with saccade-related processes. Given the lack of strong evidence directly linking area LIP to movement processing, it is important to test the alternative hypothesis that its persistent activity reflects the process of retaining in memory the sensory stimulus presented in delayed response tasks.

There are extensive interconnections between PPC and PFC, including LIP and FEF, respectively (Andersen et al., 1990; Cavada and Goldman-Rakic, 1989; Petrides and Pandya, 1984; Schall et al., 1995a; Schwartz and Goldman-Rakic, 1984; Stanton et al., 1995). And the persistent activity of LIP neurons in the memory delayed saccade task is very similar to that found in PFC (Chafee and Goldman-Rakic, 1998). Furthermore, it has been shown that persistent activity in these areas is interdependent (Chafee and Goldman-Rakic, 2000), which suggests a cooperative role in working memory processes. The specific role of LIP persistent activity in working memory is, however, not as well established as for PFC (see for review Johnston and Everling, Chapter 15, this volume). For instance, correlational evidence that PFC persistent activity is mnemonic in nature has been provided by Funahashi et al. (1989), who showed that this activity is reduced, or absent, when monkeys incorrectly perform the delayed saccade task. Similar observations have yet to be made in area LIP. More causal evidence has also been provided in the demonstration that PFC deactivation impairs working memory performance (Funahashi et al., 1993). Again, such impairments have yet to be consistently observed following PPC deactivation (Chafee and Goldman-Rakic, 2000) or inactivation (Li et al., 1999; Wardak et al., 2002).

Nevertheless, some important observations have been made regarding the nature of LIP persistent activity in the memory delayed saccade task. First, LIP neurons have greater visually evoked responses than saccade-related activity in this task (Barash et al., 1991; Paré and Wurtz, 1997, 2001), and the directional tuning of their delay activity is better aligned with their visually evoked responses than their saccade activity (Barash et al., 1991). These data suggest that the LIP persistent activity reflects more retrospective than prospective representations. Second, the neural activity during the delay period possesses a temporal structure, which is not present during fixation and which include broadband oscillations within the gamma frequency range (Pesaran et al., 2002). These oscillations are comparable to those observed in human EEG during short-term memory (Tallon-Baudry et al., 1998; see for review Jensen et al., 2007; Wang, 2010) and consistent with the dynamics of slow reverberation networks capable of maintaining persistent activity (Wang, 1999; Compte et al., 2000; see for review Wang, 2010). Third, it was shown that the persistent activity of LIP pyramidal neurons that project to FEF does not differ from that of pyramidal neurons that project to SC (Ferraina et al., 2002). Because cortico-cortical and cortico-tectal neurons are nearly all confined to cortical layer III and V, respectively, this finding indicates that the persistent activity in both layers may rest on similar reverberatory processes. This may contrast with the emphasis on layer III microcircuitry within PFC as a substrate for working memory. Lastly, compared to the activity displayed by in response to prolonged visual stimulation, the rate of persistent activity of LIP neurons is both lower (Fig. 14.1) (Ferraina et al., 2002; Paré and Wurtz, 1997, 2001) and more irregular (Johnston et al., 2009), which suggest that LIP mnemonic representations are low-fidelity signals. It remains to be tested whether the limited information contained in LIP persistent activity accounts for the limited capacity of visuospatial working memory of macaque monkeys (Heyselaar et al., 2011).

The approach taken so far to study the neurophysiological basis of visual working memory has been almost exclusively limited to single-stimulus delayed response tasks, which obviously fail in manipulating working memory demands. It has therefore been difficult to establish a strong linking proposition between persistent activity and working memory content. Much stronger evidence that PPC plays an important role in visual working memory has been obtained in human studies using multiple-stimulus sequential comparison tasks while measuring brain activation with evoked related potentials (Vogel and Machizawa, 2004) and blood-oxygen-level dependent signals (Todd and Marois, 2004). These experiments have found that changes in activation localized to PPC to predict successful performance, to be modulated by the memory load imposed by the task (i.e. the number of objects being held in memory), and to saturate for memory arrays that meet or exceed the subject's memory capacity limit. Several pieces of evidence suggests that area LIP contain neurons carrying signals sufficient to maintain temporarily the goal of a saccade in the absence of visual stimulation, but new data and experimental approaches are needed to support unequivocally this hypothesis.

Visual attention

Visual attention relates to the neural processes by which visual information is filtered and selected, so that it can be more fully processed and possibly brought into perceptual awareness. In most natural situations, vision is active and visual processing involves the sequential sampling of details accomplished by overtly shifting perceptual resources, i.e. by reorienting the line of sight. Saccades are thus 'overt' shifts of visuospatial attention (see for review Kristjánsson, Chapter 25, this volume). Furthermore, experimental evidence suggests that saccade processing is closely related to 'covert' visuospatial attention. Shifting visual attention covertly to a spatial location facilitates the processing of saccades directed to that location, whereas planning a saccade to a spatial location facilitates perceptual processing of objects at that location (see for review Awh et al., 2006; Moore et al., 2003). Such a functional coupling between covert and overt shifts of visuospatial attention may result from the overlapping of their respective neural circuits (Corbetta et al., 1998; Nobre et al., 1997) and from the massive connections between brain areas with visual and oculomotor functions (e.g. Schall et al., 1995a). Consistent with this interconnectivity, voluntary shifts in visual attention are associated with enhanced activity not only in visual cortical areas (see for review Maunsell and Treue, 2006) but also in FEF and SC (see for review Awh et al., 2006; Moore et al., 2003).

Attention-related modulation in neuronal activity has also been observed in PPC (see for review Constantinidis, 2006; Goldberg et al., 2006). Early recording in area 7—including portion of the lateral bank of the intraparietal sulcus, from which LIP neurons would likely have been sampled—showed that the visually evoked responses of neurons are enhanced when a visual stimulus presented in their receptive fields specifies the goal of a saccade (Robinson et al., 1978; Yin and Mountcastle, 1977) or of a reaching arm movement (Bushnell et al., 1981). These findings paralleled those of Lynch et al. (1977), who recorded in the same PPC region neurons that showed enhanced activity during active fixation or tracking of a visual stimulus. Similar enhancements were observed when monkeys performed a peripheral attention task, which required detecting the dimming of a visual stimulus placed within the neuron's receptive field by releasing a lever, i.e. without making a saccade to that stimulus (Bushnell et al., 1981; see for review Colby and Goldberg, 1999). The independence of this enhancement from the animal's response is in line with the hypothesis that PPC provides guidance signals for actions in general as well as with the hypothesis that LIP neuronal activity reflects covert visuospatial attention, which is not necessarily associated with any action; see also Thompson et al. (2005b) for a similar account in the FEF. In summary, area LIP does appear to contain neural signals that are sufficient to regulate which stimulus is selected for further perceptual processing, which may then be used for guiding an action.

A significant body of work on visual attention has used the visual search paradigm, in which the ability of a subject to find a target within a multistimulus display can inform us about that subject's allocation of attentional resources (see for review Wolfe and Horowitz, 2004). This approach most often requires subjects to indicate the presence of the search target with a manual response without them being instructed to foveate that stimulus, but several studies have also monitored where subjects look while performing this task (e.g. Binello et al., 1995; Maioli et al., 2001; Scialfa and Joffe, 1998; Williams et al., 1997; Zelinsky and Sheinberg, 1995). As stressed above, the natural exploration of the visual world involves visuospatial attention being deployed by reorienting the line of gaze and the monitoring gaze fixations during visual search therefore provides almost a moment-by-moment measure of a subject's allocation of attention. The high rate of saccades in natural tasks such as visual search, text reading, and scene perception suggests that there are few attentional shifts besides those associated with the execution of saccades when the eyes are free to move (for a review see Findlay and Gilchrist, 2003). Covert shift of spatial attention may only assist overt shifts and the additional analysis of the visual periphery that it provides during each fixation contribute to the selection of the visual detail that will become the goal of the next saccade (see Henderson, 1992; Schall 2004; Schall and Thompson, 1999; Schneider, 1995).

The process of selecting a saccade target among the several alternatives available in a visual search display has been studied at the neural level (see for review Schall and Cohen, Chapter 19, this volume). For neurons to be involved in saccade target selection, they must discharge differently when a saccade target versus a distractor stimulus is presented in their receptive fields and they must do so in advance of saccade initiation. Such neurons have been recorded in both the FEF (Bichot and Schall, 1999; Sato and Schall, 2003; Schall and Hanes, 1993; Schall et al., 1995b; Thompson et al., 1996) and the SC (McPeek and Keller, 2002; Shen and Paré, 2007) as well as in visual cortical areas (area V4: Bichot et al., 2005; Chelazzi et al., 2001; Mazer and Gallant, 2003; Ogawa and Komatsu, 2004, 2006; area TEO: Chelazzi et al., 1993).

Several pieces of evidence indicate that the PPC in general and area LIP in particular participates in the process of selecting saccade targets during visual search. First, functional brain imaging studies have shown blood flow increases in human PPC during difficult visual search (Corbetta et al., 1993; Donner et al., 2000, 2002; Gitelman et al., 2002; Nobre et al., 2003). Interestingly, the location of this activation matches very closely a region previously associated with both covert and overt shifts of attention (Corbetta et al., 1993, 1998; Nobre et al., 1997). Second, transcranial magnetic stimulation of PPC selectively impairs performance in difficult visual search (Ashbridge et al., 1997; Hodsoll et al., 2009; Kalla et al., 2008; Muggleton et al., 2008). Third, human patients with PPC lesions show marked deficits in difficult visual search when targets fall in their contralesional visual field (Arguin et al., 1993; Eglin et al., 1989; Karatekin et al., 1999; Riddoch and Humphreys, 1987). In the monkey, the role of area LIP in the process of saccade target selection was first demonstrated by Wardak and colleagues (Wardak et al., 2002), who observed deficits in visual search following LIP inactivation; similar deficits in covert attention were also observed (Wardak et al., 2004).

Consistent with the visual search studies on saccade target selection cited above, LIP neurons were shown to discriminate a saccade target from distracter stimuli in advance of saccade initiation (Ipata et al., 2006; Mirpour et al., 2009; Ogawa and Komatsu, 2009; Thomas and Paré, 2007). The time at which LIP neuronal activity discriminates the saccade target was found to correlate with the latency of the search saccades (Ipata et al., 2006; Thomas and Paré, 2007). This finding is comparable to observations made in distinct neuronal populations within FEF (Sato and Schall, 2003; Thompson et al., 1996) and SC (McPeek and Keller, 2002), and it has been interpreted as evidence for the role of LIP in saccade generation (Bisley and Goldberg, 2010). This interpretation is, however, difficult to reconcile with previous findings that LIP neuronal activity does discriminate visual stimuli substantially in advance of saccade initiation in instructed, delayed saccade tasks (Paré and Wurtz, 2001; Platt and Glimcher, 1997; Toth and Assad, 2002). Furthermore, other studies have reported evidence for a similar visual selection in the complete absence of saccades (Balan and Gottlieb, 2006; Balan et al., 2008; Oristaglio et al., 2006). We have also argued elsewhere against such an interpretation, on the basis of the differences between the tasks performed by the monkeys in these studies (Paré et al., 2009). Visual and saccade selection processes may be more difficult to dissociate temporally in the LIP studies because the unconstrained nature of their search tasks emphasizes speed over accuracy. The correlation between the timing of LIP neuronal discrimination and saccade initiation may rather be evidence for a direct association between covert shift in visual attention and the selection of the next saccade in natural situations, when saccades are not associated directly with a reward or punishment (Findlay and Gilchrist, 2003). It remains to be tested whether this correlation is also manifest when FEF and SC neurons are recorded in unconstrained visual search tasks. Recent evidence suggests that it is the case in the SC (Shen et al., 2011).

Altogether, this collection of data implicates area LIP in selective visual processes guiding both covert and overt shifts in attention. The map of visual space within area LIP may thus instantiate the visual salience map postulated by models of visual search and selective attention (Cave and Wolfe, 1990; Findlay and Walker, 1999; Glimcher et al., 2005; Hamker, 2006; Itti and Koch, 2001; Logan, 1996; Treisman, 1988; Treisman and Gelade, 1980; Wolfe, 1994). According to these models, the stimulus-driven outputs from individual feature maps, which can be instantiated by extrastriate cortical areas, are integrated with goal-directed signals into a map of representations, whose magnitudes reflect the relative importance of each stimulus. Despite many similarities between the neuronal activity observed in FEF, area LIP, and SC (see for review Schall et al., 2007), it is unlikely that the visual salience map is simply replicated across these brain regions. With respect to saccade target selection, we posit that this process results from the progressive filtering of distracter representations and amplifying of target representations from area LIP to FEF onto SC. This is supported by our comparative analysis showing that the reliability of the target/distracter discrimination improves from cortex to SC (Thomas and Paré, 2007). Continuous flow of information between these brain regions could account for the discriminating activity observed simultaneously across these brain regions.

In summary, area LIP does appear to contain neurons carrying signals sufficient and perhaps necessary to regulate where a saccade will be directed.

Saccade decision

Saccade target selection in visual search implies a perceptual decision, which is the process by which a specific item is selected as the next target of an action. Anatomically, area LIP is ideally situated to integrate diverse sources of evidence that are involved in visual decision-making and to send guiding signals to saccade generating centres like the FEF and SC. Although some evidence suggests that LIP neuronal activity accumulates towards a bound (Churchland et al., 2008; Kiani et al., 2008), as we have outlined previously, it is unlikely that a saccade trigger threshold exists in LIP. Rather we argue that area LIP provides a map where evidence supporting the saliency of competing visual items accumulates. Decisional processes can then assist visual attention, visual working memory, saccade preparation and, if required, saccade execution (see for review Ludwig, Chapter 23, this volume).

Broadly speaking, evidence that favours one visual item over others can come in the form of immediate sensory cues or economic variables that are learned through experience. Researchers have developed tasks that employ instructive cues of varying quality or economic outcomes that are uncertain to examine how such forms of evidence are represented in LIP activity and related to one's choices. Recent evidence also suggests that decision processes in LIP are strongly modulated by the expected timing of environmental cues and required responses.

The motion discrimination task (Britten et al., 1992) has been particularly useful to study decision-making based on sensory evidence. In this task, monkeys view a random dot kinetogram, in which a minority of the dots is moving in a coherent direction amongst randomly moving dots. The monkey then indicates the overall perceived direction of motion by directing a saccade to one of two peripheral saccade targets. The location, size, speed, and direction of the random dot kinetogram are optimized to best activate the LIP neuron under study. Results from this work have demonstrated that LIP neuronal activity accumulates for preferred direction motion, the rate of which depends on the quality of the sensory evidence, i.e. motion coherence (Shadlen and Newsome, 1996, 2001). Moreover, the accumulation process continues with longer exposure, but like behavioural performance, tends to asymptote (Shadlen and Newsome, 2001). Together, these LIP properties are consistent with bounded accumulator models of simple decision-making, which provide a mechanism for integrating incoming sensory information over time.

LIP neuronal activity also encodes more economic variables that are not immediately sensory in nature but are learned through experience. Rather than base their decisions on sensory instructions, monkeys are required to choose based on the relative reward rates between options or through strategic competition. LIP neuronal activity is influenced by the probability of a saccade target yielding a reward, the magnitude of reward associated with that option and the degree of confidence in the decision (Fig. 14.4A) (Churchland et al., 2008; Dorris and Glimcher, 2004; Kiani and Shadlen, 2009; Platt and Glimcher, 1999; Rorie et al., 2010; Yang and Shadlen, 2007). Unlike the FEF and SC (Basso and Wurtz, 1998; Dorris and Munoz, 1998; Ikeda and Hikosaka, 2003; Roesch and Olson, 2003), economic information is not represented in baseline LIP activity but is only revealed immediately after target presentation (Fig. 14.4A). This finding strongly suggests that LIP is not where economic variables are stored; instead representations in area LIP are modulated by their potential economic impact from external sources.

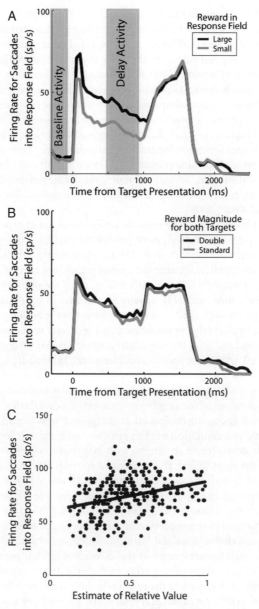

Fig. 14.4 LIP represents the relative value of potential visual targets. **A.** Population firing rate (n=30) when saccades were instructed to response field targets of differing reward. Note that there is no difference in firing rate during the baseline period preceding target presentation even though the location of the large and small rewarded targets are fixed throughout a block of trials. In addition, the difference in firing rate only occurs during the first 1000 ms after target presentation when the monkey is uncertain which target will be instructed. Once a cue indicates that the target in the response field is the target (approx. time 1000 ms) then uncertainty is removed and the neurons fire at the same rate regardless of reward magnitude. **B.** Trial by trial correlations between firing rate and an estimate of relative value during a strategic game. Activity was sampled for a single neuron during the delay period highlighted in **A. C.** Relative not absolute value is represented in LIP. Population firing rate (n=22) during a strategic game when standard reward magnitudes were used or the rewards for both targets were doubled. Adapted from Neuron, vol. 44, Dorris, M. C., & Glimcher, P. W., Activity in posterior parietal cortex is correlated with the relative subjective desirability of action, pp. 365-78, 2004, with permission from Elsevier.

More recently, a case has been made that LIP neuronal activity is not influenced by either probability or reward in isolation but something closer to their product, expected value. More specifically, activity is a function of relative expected value, i.e. the expected value of the neuron's preferred target divided by the sum of the expected values for the other potential visual targets (Fig. 14.4B) (Dorris and Glimcher, 2004; Platt and Glimcher, 1999; Rorie et al., 2010). This normalization of value across LIP is ideal from a decision-theoretic standpoint because it allows many multiple potential options to be represented simultaneously and compared across a wide range of values.

These decision processes do not evolve at a fixed rate but are strongly influenced by the expected timing of environmental events. For example, LIP neurons adjust their activity to reflect whether the duration of sensory events are shorter or longer than a standard time (Leon and Shadlen, 2003). LIP activity can also represent sophisticated probabilistic time distributions of when salient events are likely to occur (Janssen and Shadlen, 2005). Such timing signals are potentially important for initiating voluntarily actions especially those constrained by strict deadlines for choosing (Churchland et al., 2008; Maimon and Assad, 2006).

If area LIP is involved in the decision process, its activity must not only be influenced by sensory, economic, and timing evidence but also it must predict the choices that subjects ultimately make. Indeed, in the motion discrimination task, while LIP activity is clearly influenced by the coherence of the motion stimulus it also predicts whether the animal will choose correctly for a given coherence (Shadlen and Newsome, 1996, 2001). Particularly telling, when the monkey viewed motion stimuli below their psychophysical thresholds, LIP activity is predictive of upcoming choice. Lastly, artificially increasing LIP activity with electrical micro-stimulation manipulates perceptual decision formation as evidenced by decreases in the latency and increases in the proportion of choices in favour of the option associated with the site of stimulation (Hanks et al., 2006). Similarly, when saccadic choices are based on more economic considerations, LIP activity is influenced by the relative value of the options but also predicts the overall allocation of choices (Coe et al., 2002; Dorris and Glimcher, 2004; Seo et al., 2009; Sugrue et al., 2004). Similar to the ambiguous motion coherence, when the subjective values of the targets are, on average, equal during a strategic equilibrium, LIP activity is predictive of upcoming choices on a trial-by-trial basis (Fig.14.4C).

Together, the dynamic representation of both sensory and economic forms of evidence on the same maps can provide downstream structures with important information regarding which of the potential targets is the most salient at any moment in time. Decision theory posits that overt choice should be directed towards the most salient item, which would be the point of highest activity on the LIP map. Covert processes such as visual attention and saccade preparation, however, may be allocated in proportion to the salience representation of multiple options on this LIP map. Bounded integration models, influenced in large part by empirical findings, have been successful in reproducing patterns of behavioural choice (Huk and Shadlen, 2005; Kiani et al., 2008; Mazurek et al., 2003; Wong et al., 2007). Although further empirical and theoretical work is required to understand the rules by which sensory, economic and timing evidence are weighted and combined within this single map for the vast majority of decisions in the real world rely on all considerations (e.g. Feng et al., 2009; Gold and Shadlen, 2002). An initial examination of how sensory and reward information is integrated in LIP by Rorie et al. (2010) suggests that reward biases the starting position of the accumulation process but does not the affect the rate of accumulation which is determined by the quality of sensory information.

In summary, area LIP appears to contribute to saccade decision processes based on incoming sensory evidence, economic variables, and the expected timing of salient events.

Conclusion and future directions

We have reviewed the role of PPC in regulating saccadic eye movements. Our focus has been on area LIP, an evolutionarily recent outcropping of the PPC in primates presumably in response to their reliance on high acuity foveal vision and extended oculomotor range. Anatomically, area LIP is situated at the nexus between sensory and motor processing stages related to visual behaviour.

LIP neuronal activity is not as directly involved in the production of saccades as compared to the FEF and SC, but it forms representations about potential saccade targets. In sum, area LIP appears to be a recent innovation that supplements the saccadic eye movements system with guidance signals, thereby allowing primates more flexible behavioural control.

The guidance signal that LIP provides has been termed 'saliency', which is a subjective perceptual quality that causes some items to 'jump' out from their settings—the use of this term can be traced back to conditioning theory (see for review Rescorla, 1988; Rumbaugh, 2007). Saliency is a multifactorial quantity composed of diverse sensory and cognitive signals. We have reviewed how sensory evidence contributes to a saliency representation in area LIP during the discrimination of visual stimuli from alternatives. We have also reviewed cognitive evidence that are less immediate in nature but are gathered through experience. These include the relative value of potential targets, timing signals and a role for sensory working memory. In keeping with its evolutionary emergence, the salience map in area LIP should also be considered to regulate other behaviours, e.g. visual perception and visuomanual behaviour, including eye–hand coordination and grasping.

Future advances about the role of area LIP in saccade-related processes may be provided by new data from comparative studies that address the evolution of the PPC and of the 'high-order' network of which it is a constituent. This review highlighted the benefits of comparing results obtained in area LIP with those obtained in FEF and SC. This comparative approach is necessary to gain a comprehensive understanding of the neural circuit regulating saccadic eye movements. Further distinction between data collected from LIPd and LIPv will help resolve an already large and growing body of data. Substantially more data are needed to understand the role of LIP persistent activity in visual working memory, and new approaches are recommended to advance our understanding of the neural basis of this process within and beyond the PPC. Area LIP continues to be a model area to study decisional processes, but the study of selective visual attention in the context of visual search still deserves more attention.

Acknowledgements

We thank the support that we have benefited from Queen's University, the Canadian Institutes of Health Research, and the Natural Science and Engineering Research Council.

References

Amit, D.J. (1995). The Hebbian paradigm reintegrated: local reverberations as internal representations. *Behavioral and Brain Sciences*, **18**, 617–26.

Andersen, R.A., Essick, G.K., and Siegel, R.M. (1987). Neurons of area 7 activated by both visual stimuli and oculomotor behavior. *Experimental Brain Research*, **67**, 316–22.

Andersen, R.A., Brotchie, P.R., and Mazzoni, P. (1992). Evidence for the lateral intraparietal area as the parietal eye field. *Current Opinion in Neurobiology*, **2**, 840–6.

Andersen, R.A., Asanuma, C., Essick, G.K., and Siegel, R.M. (1990). Corticocortical connections of anatomically and physiologically defined subdivisions within the inferior parietal lobule. *Journal of Comparative Neurology*, **296**, 65–113.

Arcaro, M.J., Pinsk, M.A., Li, X., and Kastner, S. (2011). Visuotopic organization of macaque posterior parietal cortex: a functional magnetic resonance imaging study. *Journal of Neuroscience*, **31**, 2064–78.

Arguin, M., Joanette, Y., and Cavanagh, P. (1993). Visual search for feature and conjunction targets with an attention deficit. *Journal of Cognitive Neuroscience*, **5**, 436–52.

Ashbridge, E., Walsh, V., and Cowey, A. (1997). Temporal aspects of visual search studied by transcranial magnetic stimulation. *Neuropsychologia*, **35**, 1121–31.

Awh, E., Armstrong, K.M., and Moore, T. (2006). Visual and oculomotor selection: Links, causes and implications for spatial attention. *Trends in Cognitive Sciences*, **10**, 124–30.

Baizer, J.S., Ungerleider, L.G., and Desimone, R. (1991). Organization of visual inputs to the inferior temporal and posterior parietal cortex in macaques. *Journal of Neuroscience*, **11**, 168–90.

Bakola, S., Gregoriou, G.G., Moschovakis, A.K., and Savaki, H.E. (2006). Functional imaging of the intraparietal cortex during saccades to visual and memorized targets. *Neuroimage*, **31**, 1637–49.

Balan, P.F. and Gottlieb, J. (2006). Integration of exogenous input into a dynamic salience map revealed by perturbing attention. *Journal of Neuroscience*, **26**, 9239–49.

Balan, P.F., Oristaglio, J., Schneider, D.M., and Gottlieb, J. (2008). Neuronal correlates of the set-size effect in monkey lateral intraparietal area. *PLoS Biology*, **6**(7), e158.

Barash, S., Bracewell, R.M., Fogassi, L., Gnadt, J.W., and Andersen, R.A. (1991). Saccade-related activity in the lateral intraparietal area. I. Temporal properties; comparison with area 7a. *Journal of Neurophysiology*, **66**, 1095–108.

Basso, M.A. and Wurtz, R.H. (1998). Modulation of neuronal activity in superior colliculus by changes in target probability. *Journal of Neuroscience*, **18**, 7519–34.

Bendiksby, M.S. and Platt, M.L. (2006). Neural correlates of reward and attention in macaque area LIP. *Neuropsychologia*, **44**, 2411–20.

Ben Hamed, S. and Duhamel, J.R. (2002). Ocular fixation and visual activity in the monkey lateral intraparietal area. *Experimental Brain Research*, **142**, 512–28.

Ben Hamed, S., Duhamel, J.R., Bremmer, F., and Graf, W. (2001). Representation of the visual field in the lateral intraparietal area of macaque monkeys: a quantitative receptive field analysis. *Experimental Brain Research*, **140**, 127–44.

Bichot, N.P. and Schall, J.D. (1999). Effects of similarity and history on neural mechanisms of visual selection. *Nature Neuroscience*, **2**, 549–54.

Bichot, N.P., Rossi, A.F., and Desimone, R. (2005). Parallel and serial neural mechanisms for visual search in macaque area V4. *Science*, **308**, 529–34.

Binello, A., Mannan, S., and Ruddock, K.H. (1995). The characteristics of eye move- ments made during visual search with multi-element stimuli. *Spatial Vision*, **9**, 343–62.

Bisley, J.W. and Goldberg, M.E. (2010). Attention, intention, and priority in the parietal lobe. *Annual Review of Neuroscience*, **33**, 1–21.

Blatt, G.J., Andersen, R.A., and Stoner, G.R. (1990). Visual receptive field organization and cortico-cortical connections of the lateral intraparietal area (area LIP) in the macaque. *Journal of Comparative Neurology*, **299**, 421–45.

Britten, K.H., Shadlen, M.N., Newsome, W.T., and Movshon, J.A. (1992). The analysis of visual motion: a comparison of neuronal and psychophysical performance. *Journal of Neuroscience*, **12**, 4745–65.

Bruce, C.J. and Goldberg, M.E. (1985). Primate frontal eye fields. I. Single neurons discharging before saccades. *Journal of Neurophysiology*, **53**, 603–35.

Bruce, C.J., Goldberg, M.E., Bushnell, M.C., and Stanton, G.B. (1985). Primate frontal eye fields. II. Physiological and anatomical correlates of electrically evoked eye movements. *Journal of Neurophysiology*, **54**, 714–34.

Brunamonti, E., Thomas, N.W.D., and Paré, M. (2008). The activity patterns of lateral intraparietal area neurons is not sufficient to control visually guided saccadic eye movements. *Society for Neuroscience Abstracts*, **38**, 855–18.

Bushnell, M.C., Goldberg, M.E., and Robinson, D.L. (1981) Behavioral enhancement of visual responses in monkey cerebral cortex. I. Modulation in posterior parietal cortex related to selective visual attention. *Journal of Neurophysiology*, **46**, 755–72.

Cavada, C. and Goldman-Rakic, P.S. (1989). Posterior parietal cortex in rhesus monkey: II. Evidence for segregated cortico-cortical networks linking sensory and limbic areas with the frontal lobe. *Journal of Comparative Neurology*, **287**, 422–45.

Cave, K.R. and Wolfe, J.M. (1990). Modeling the role of parallel processing in visual search. *Cognitive Psychology*, **22**, 225–71.

Chafee, M.V. and Goldman-Rakic, P.S. (1998). Neuronal activity in macaque prefrontal area 8a and posterior parietal area 7ip related to memory guided saccades. *Journal of Neurophysiology*, **79**, 2919–40.

Chafee, M.V. and Goldman-Rakic, P.S. (2000). Inactivation of parietal and prefrontal cortex reveals interdependence of neural activity during memory-guided saccades. *Journal of Neurophysiology*, **83**, 1550–66.

Chelazzi, L., Miller, E.K., Duncan, J., and Desimone, R. (1993). A neural basis for visual search in inferior temporal cortex. *Nature*, **363**, 345–7.

Chelazzi, L., Miller, E.K., Duncan, J., and Desimone, R. (2001). Responses of neurons in macaque area V4 during memory-guided visual search. *Cerebral Cortex*, **11**, 761–72.

Churchland, A.K., Kiani, R., and Shadlen, M.N. (2008). Decision-making with multiple alternatives. *Nature Neuroscience*, **11**, 693–702.

Clower, D.M., West, R.A., Lynch, J.C., and Strick, P.L. (2001). The inferior parietal lobule is the target of output from the superior colliculus, hippocampus, and cerebellum. *Journal of Neuroscience*, **21**, 6283–91.

Coe, B., Tomihara, K., Matsuzawa, M., and Hikosaka, O. (2002). Visual and anticipatory bias in three cortical eye fields of the monkey during an adaptive decision-making task. *Journal of Neuroscience*, **22**, 5081–90.

Cohen, Y.E. and Andersen, R.A. (2002). A common reference frame for movement plans in the posterior parietal cortex. *Nature Reviews Neuroscience*, **3**, 553–62.

Colby, C.L. and Goldberg, M.E. (1999). Space and attention in parietal cortex. *Annual Review of Neuroscience*, **22**, 319–49.

Collins, C.E., Lyon, D.C., and Kaas, J.H. (2005). Distribution across cortical areas of neurons projecting to the superior colliculus in new world monkeys. *Anatomical Record, Part A, Discoveries in Molecular, Cellular, and Evolutionary Biology*, **285**, 619–27.

Compte, A., Brunel, N., Goldman-Rakic, P.S., and Wang, X.J. (2000). Synaptic mechanisms and network dynamics underlying spatial working memory in a cortical network model. *Cerebral Cortex*, **10**, 910–23.

Constantinidis, C. (2006). Posterior parietal mechanisms of visual attention. *Reviews in the Neurosciences*, **17**, 415–27.

Constantinidis, C. and Procyk, E. (2004). The primate working memory networks. *Cognitive, Affective, and Behavioral Neuroscience*, **4**, 444–65.

Cooke, D.F., Taylor, C.S., Moore, T., and Graziano, M.S. (2003). Complex movements evoked by microstimulation of the ventral intraparietal area. *Proceedings of the National Academy of Sciences USA*, **100**, 6163–68.

Corbetta, M., Miezin, F.M., Shulman, G.L., Petersen, S.E. (1993). A PET study of visuospatial attention. *Journal of Neuroscience*, **13**, 1202–26.

Corbetta, M., Akbudak, E., Conturo, T.E., Snyder, A.Z., Ollinger, J.M., Drury, H.A., et al. (1998). A common network of functional areas for attention and eye movements. *Neuron*, **21**, 761–73.

Disbrow, E., Hinkley, L., Padberg, J., and Krubitzer, L. (2007). Hand use and the evolution of posterior parietal cortex in primates. In J. H. Kaas, and T. M. Preuss (eds.) *Evolution of nervous systems (Vol. 4): the evolution of primate nervous systems* (pp. 407–15). Oxford: Elsevier.

Donner, T.H., Kettermann, A., Diesch E, Ostendorf, F., Villringer, A., and Brandt, S.A. (2000). Involvement of the human frontal eye field and multiple parietal areas in covert visual selection during conjunction search. *European Journal of Neuroscience*, **12**, 3407–14.

Donner, T.H., Kettermann, A., Diesch E, Ostendorf, F., Villringer, A., and Brandt, S.A. (2002). Visual feature and conjunction searches of equal difficulty engage only partially overlapping frontoparietal networks. *Neuroimage*, **15**, 16–25.

Dorris, M.C. and Glimcher, P.W. (2004). Activity in posterior parietal cortex is correlated with the relative subjective desirability of action. *Neuron*, **44**, 365–78.

Dorris, M.C. and Munoz, D.P. (1998). Saccadic probability influences motor preparation signals and time to saccadic initiation. *Journal of Neuroscience*, **18**, 7015–26.

Dorris, M.C., Paré, M., and Munoz, D.P. (1997). Neuronal activity in the monkey superior colliculus related to the initiation of saccadic eye movements. *Journal of Neuroscience*, **17**, 8566–79.

Durstewitz, D., Seamans, J.K., and Sejnowski, T.J. (2000). Neurocomputational models of working memory. *Nature Neuroscience*, **3(Suppl)**, 1184–91.

Eglin, M., Roberson, L., and Knight, R. (1989). Visual search performance in the neglect syndrome. *Journal of Cognitive Neuroscience*, **1**, 372–85.

Fang, P.C., Stepniewska, I., and Kaas, J.H. (2005). Ipsilateral cortical connections of motor, premotor, frontal eye, and posterior parietal fields in a prosimian primate, *Otolemur garnetti*. *Journal of Comparative Neurology*, **490**, 305–33.

Feng, S., Holmes, P., Rorie, A., and Newsome, W.T. (2009). Can monkeys choose optimally when faced with noisy stimuli and unequal rewards? *PLoS Computational Biology*, **5**(2), e1000284.

Ferraina, S., Paré, M., and Wurtz, R.H. (2002). Comparison of cortico-cortical and cortico-collicular signals for the generation of saccadic eye movements. *Journal of Neurophysiology*, **87**, 845–58.

Findlay, J.M. and Gilchrist, I.D. (2003). Active vision: the psychology of looking and seeing. New York: Oxford University Press.

Findlay, J.M. and Walker, R. (1999). A model of saccade generation based on parallel processing and competitive inhibition. *Behavioral and Brain Sciences*, **22**, 661–721.

Frey, S.H. (2007). Neurological specializations for manual gesture and tool use in humans. In J. H. Kaas, and T. M. Preuss (Eds.) *Evolution of nervous systems: the evolution of primate nervous systems*, **4**, 395–406). Oxford: Elsevier.

Funahashi, S., Bruce, C.J., and Goldman-Rakic, P.S. (1989). Mnemonic coding of visual space in the monkey's dorsolateral prefrontal cortex. *Journal of Neurophysiology*, **61**, 331–49.

Funahashi, S., Bruce, C.J., and Goldman-Rakic, P.S. (1993). Dorsolateral prefrontal lesions and oculomotor delayed-response performance: evidence for mnemonic 'scotomas'. *Journal of Neuroscience*, **13**, 1479–97.

Fuster, J.M. and Alexander, G.E. (1971). Neuron activity related to short-term memory. *Science*, **173**, 652–4.

Gitelman, D.R., Parrish, T.B., Friston, K.J., Mesulam, M.M. (2002). Functional anatomy of visual search: regional segregations within the frontal eye fields and effective connectivity of the superior colliculus. *Neuroimage*, **15**, 970–82.

Glimcher, P.W., Dorris, M.C, and Bayer, H.M. (2005). Physiological utility theory and the neuroeconomics of choice. *Games and Economic Behavior*, **52**, 213–56.

Gnadt, J.W. and Andersen, R.A. (1988). Memory related motor planning activity in posterior parietal cortex of macaque. *Experimental Brain Research*, **70**, 216–20.

Gold, J.I. and Shadlen, M.N. (2002). Banburismus and the brain: decoding the relationship between sensory stimuli, decisions and reward. *Neuron*, **36**, 299–308.

Goldberg, M.E., Bisley, J.W., Powell, K.D., and Gottlieb, J. (2006). Saccades, salience and attention: the role of the lateral intraparietal area in visual behavior. *Progress in Brain Research*, **155**, 157–75.

Goodale, M.A. and Milner, A.D. (1992). Separate visual pathways for perception and action. *Trends in Neurosciences*, **15**, 20–5.

Gottlieb, J.P. and Goldberg, M.E. (1999). Activity of neurons in the lateral intraparietal area of the monkey during an antisaccade task. *Nature Neuroscience*, **2**, 906–12.

Gottlieb, J.P., Kusunoki, M., and Goldberg, M.E. (1998). The representation of visual salience in monkey parietal cortex. *Nature*, **391**, 481–4.

Grefkes, C. and Fink, G.R. (2005). The functional organization of the intraparietal sulcus in humans and monkeys. *Journal of Anatomy*, **207**, 3–17.

Guitton, D. and Volle, M. (1987). Gaze control in humans: eye-head coordination during orienting movements to targets within and beyond the oculomotor range. *Journal of Neurophysiology*, **58**, 427–59.

Guitton, D., Douglas, R.M., and Volle, M. (1984). Eye-head coordination in cats. *Journal of Neurophysiology*, **52**, 1030–50.

Hamker, F.H. (2006). Modeling feature-based attention as an active top-down inference process. *Biosystems*, **86**, 91–9.

Hanes, D.P. and Schall, J.D. (1995). Countermanding saccades in macaque. *Visual Neuroscience*, **12**, 929–37.

Hanes, D.P. and Schall, J.D. (1996). Neural control of voluntary movement initiation. *Science*, **274**, 427–30.

Hanes, D.P., Patterson, W.F.III, and Schall, J.D. (1998). The role of frontal eye field in countermanding saccades: Visual, movement and fixation activity. *Journal of Neurophysiology*, **79**, 817–34.

Hanks, T.D., Ditterich, J., and Shadlen, M.N. (2006). Microstimulation of macaque area LIP affects decision-making in a motion discrimination task. *Nature Neuroscience*, **9**, 682–9.

Henderson, J. (1992). Visual attention and eye movement control during reading and picture viewing. In K. Rayner (ed.), *Eye movements and visual cognition* (pp. 261–283). Berlin: Springer.

Heyselaar, E., Johnston, K., and Paré, M. (2011). A change detection approach to study visual working memory of the macaque monkey. *Journal of Vision*, **11**(3), 1–10.

Hodsoll, J., Mevorach, C., and Humphreys, G.W. (2009). Driven to less distraction: rTMS of the right parietal cortex reduces attentional capture in visual search. *Cerebral Cortex*, **19**, 106–14.

Huk, A.C. and Shadlen, M.N. (2005). Neural activity in macaque parietal cortex reflects temporal integration of visual motion signals during perceptual decision making. *Journal of Neuroscience*, **25**, 10420–36.

Husain, M. and Nachev, P. (2007). Space and the parietal cortex. *Trends in Cognitive Sciences*, **11**, 30–6.

Ikeda, T. and Hikosaka, O. (2003). Reward-dependent gain and bias of visual responses in primate superior colliculus. *Neuron*, **39**, 693–700.

Ipata, A.E., Gee, A.L., Goldberg, M.E., and Bisley, J.W. (2006). Activity in the lateral intraparietal area predicts the goal and latency of saccades in a free-viewing visual search task. *Journal of Neuroscience*, **26**, 3656–61.

Itti, L. and Koch, C. (2001). Computational modelling of visual attention. *Nature Reviews Neuroscience*, **2**, 194–203.

Iwaniuk, A.N. and Whishaw, I.Q. (2000). On the origin of skilled forelimb movements. *Trends in Neurosciences* **23**, 372–76.

Janssen, P. and Shadlen, M.N. (2005). A representation of the hazard rate of elapsed time in macaque area LIP. *Nature Neuroscience*, **8**, 234–41.

Janssen, P., Srivastava, S., Ombelet, S., and Orban, G.A. (2008). Coding of shape and position in macaque lateral intraparietal area. *Journal of Neuroscience*, **28**, 6679–90.

Jensen, O., Kaiser, J., and Lachaux, J.P. (2007). Human gamma-frequency oscillations associated with attention and memory. *Trends in Neurosciences*, **30**(7), 317–24.

Johansson, R.S. and Flanagan, J.R. (2009). Coding and use of tactile signals from the fingertips in object manipulation tasks. *Nature Reviews Neuroscience*, **10**, 345–59.

Johnston, K., Brunamonti, E., Thomas, N.W.D., and Paré, M. (2009). Posterior parietal cortex persistent activity and visuo-spatial working memory. *Society for Neuroscience Abstracts*, **39**, 356–16.

Kaas, J.H. (2008). The evolution of the complex sensory and motor systems of the human brain. *Brain Research Bulletin*, **75**, 384–90.

Kalla, R., Muggleton, N.G., Juan, C.H., Cowey, A., and Walsh, V. (2008). The timing of the involvement of the frontal eye fields and posterior parietal cortex in visual search. *Neuroreport*, **19**, 1067–71.

Karatekin, C., Lazareff, J.A., and Asarnow, R.F. (1999). Parallel and serial search in two teenagers with lesions of the mesial parietal cortex. *Neuropsychologia*, **37**, 1461–8.

Katz, P.S. and Harris-Warrick, R.M. (1999). The evolution of neuronal circuits underlying species-specific behavior. *Current Opinion in Neurobiology*, **9**, 628–33.

Keating, E.G., Gooley, S.G., Pratt, S.E., and Kelsey, J.E. (1983). Removing the superior colliculus silences eye movements normally evoked from stimulation of the parietal and occipital eye fields. *Brain Research*, **269**, 145–8.

Kiani, R. and Shadlen, M.N. (2009). Representation of confidence associated with a decision by neurons in the parietal cortex. *Science*, **324**, 759–64.

Kiani, R., Hanks, T.D., and Shadlen, M.N. (2008). Bounded integration in parietal cortex underlies decisions even when viewing duration is dictated by the environment. *Journal of Neuroscience*, **28**, 3017–29.

Kolb, B. and Walkey, J. (1987). Behavioural and anatomical studies of the posterior parietal cortex in the rat. *Behavioural Brain Research*, **23**, 127–45.

Kubota, K. and Niki, H. (1971). Prefrontal cortical unit activity and delayed alternation performance in monkeys. *Journal of Neurophysiology*, **34**, 337–47.

Kurylo, D.D. and Skavenski, A.A. (1991). Eye movements elicited by electrical stimulation of area PG in the monkey. *Journal of Neurophysiology*, **65**, 1243–53.

Land, M.F. (2006). Eye movements and the control of actions in everyday life. *Progress in Retinal and Eye Research*, **25**, 296–324.

Leon, M.I. and Shadlen, M.N. (2003). Representation of time by neurons in the posterior parietal cortex of the macaque. *Neuron*, **38**, 317–27.

Lewis, J.W. and Van Essen, D.C. (2000a). Mapping of architectonic subdivisions in the macaque monkey, with emphasis on parieto-occipital cortex. *Journal of Comparative Neurology*, **428**, 79–111.

Lewis, J.W. and Van Essen, D.C. (2000b). Corticocortical connections of visual, sensorimotor, and multimodal processing areas in the parietal lobe of the macaque monkey. *Journal of Comparative Neurology*, **428**, 112–37.

Li, C.S., Mazzoni, P., and Andersen, R.A. (1999). Effect of reversible inactivation of macaque lateral intraparietal area on visual and memory saccades. *Journal of Neurophysiology* **81**, 1827–38.

Lisman, J.E., Fellous, J.M., and Wang, X.J. (1998). A role for NMDA-receptor channels in working memory. *Nature Neuroscience*, **1**, 273–5.

Liu, Y., Yttri, E.A., and Snyder, L.H. (2010). Intention and attention: different functional roles for LIPd and LIPv. *Nature Neuroscience*, **13**(4), 495–500.

Logan, G.D. (1996). The CODE theory of visual attention: an integration of space-based and object-based attention. *Psychological Review*, **103**, 603–49.

Logan, G.D. and Cowan, W.B. (1984). On the ability to inhibit thought and action: a theory of an act of control. *Psychological Review*, **91**, 295–327.

Lynch, J.C. and McLaren, J.W. (1989). Deficits of visual attention and saccadic eye movements after lesions of parietooccipital cortex in monkeys. *Journal of Neurophysiology*, **61**, 74–90.

Lynch, J.C., Graybiel, A.M., and Lobeck, L.J. (1985). The differential projection of two cytoarchitectural subregions of the inferior parietal lobule of macaques upon the deep layers of the superior colliculus. *Journal of Comparative Neurology*, **235**, 241–54.

Lynch, J.C., Mountcastle, V.B., Talbot, W.H., and Yin, T.C.T. (1977). Parietal lobe mechanisms for directed visual attention. *Journal of Neurophysiology*, **40**, 362–89.

Machado, L. and Rafal, R.D. (2004). Control of fixation and saccades in humans with chronic lesions of oculomotor cortex. *Neuropsychology*, **18**, 115–23.

Maimon, G. and Assad, J.A. (2006). A cognitive signal for the proactive timing of action in macaque LIP. *Nature Neuroscience*, **7**, 948–55.

Maioli, C., Benaglio, I., Siri, S., Sosta. K., and Cappa, S. (2001). The integration of parallel and serial processing mechanisms in visual search: Evidence from eye movement recording. *European Journal of Neuroscience*, **13**, 364–72.

Marchetti, E., Gauthier, G.M., and Pellet, J. (1983). Cerebellar control of eye movements studied with injection of harmaline in the trained baboon. *Archives Italiennes de Biologie*, **121**, 1–17.

Maunsell, J.H. and True, S. (2006). Feature-based attention in visual cortex. *Trends in Neurosciences*, **29**, 317–22.

Mazer, J.A. and Gallant, J.L. (2003). Goal-related activity in V4 during free viewing visual search: evidence for a ventral stream visual salience map. *Neuron*, **40**, 1241–50.

Mazurek, M.E., Roitman, J.D., Ditterich, J., and Shadlen, M.N. (2003). A role for neural integrators in perceptual decision making. *Cerebral Cortex*, **13**, 1257–69.

Mazzoni, P., Bracewell, R.M., Barash, S., and Andersen, R.A. (1996). Motor intention activity in the macaque's lateral intraparietal area. I. Dissociation of motor plan from sensory memory. *Journal of Neurophysiology*, **76**, 1439–56.

McCrea, R.A. and Gdowski, G.T. (2003). Firing behaviour of squirrel monkey eye movement-related vestibular nucleus neurons during gaze saccades. *Journal of Physiology*, **546**, 207–24.

McPeek, R.M. and Keller, E.L. (2002). Saccade target selection in the superior colliculus during a visual search task. *Journal of Neurophysiology*, **88**, 2019–34.

McVea, D.A. and Pearson, K.G. (2009). Object avoidance during locomotion. *Advances in Experimental Medicine and Biology*, **629**, 293–315.

Mirpour, K., Arcizet, F., Ong, W.G., and Bisley, J.W. (2009). Been there, seen that: a neural mechanism for performing efficient visual search. *Journal of Neurophysiology*, **102**, 3481–91.

Mohler, C.W. and Wurtz, R.H. (1976). Organization of monkey superior colliculus: intermediate layer cells discharging before eye movements. *Journal of Neurophysiology*, **39**, 722–44.

Moore, T. (1999). Shape representations and visual guidance of saccadic eye movements. *Science*, **285**, 1914–7.

Moore, T., Armstrong, K.M., and Fallah, M. (2003). Visuomotor origins of covert spatial attention. *Neuron*, **40**, 671–83.

Muggleton, N.G., Cowey, A., and Walsh, V. (2008). The role of the angular gyrus in visual conjunction search investigated using signal detection analysis and transcranial magnetic stimulation. *Neuropsychologia*, **46**, 2198–202.

Nakamura, K. and Colby, C.L. (2000). Visual, saccade-related, and cognitive activation of single neurons in monkey extrastriate area V3A. *Journal of Neurophysiology*, **84**, 677–92.

Nobre, A.C., Sebestyen, G.N., Gitelman, D.R., Mesulam, M.M., Frackowiak, R. S., and Frith, C. D. (1997). Functional localization of the system for visuospatial attention using positron emission tomography. *Brain*, **120**, 515–33.

Nobre, A.C., Coull, J.T., Walsh, V., and Frith, C.D. (2003). Brain activations during visual search: contributions of search efficiency versus feature binding. *Neuroimage*, **18**, 91–103.

Ogawa, T. and Komatsu, H. (2004). Target selection in area V4 during a multidimensional visual search task. *Journal of Neuroscience*, **24**, 6371–82.

Ogawa, T. and Komatsu, H. (2006). Neuronal dynamics of bottom-up and top-down processes in area V4 of macaque monkeys performing a visual search. *Experimental Brain Research*, **173**, 1–13.

Ogawa, T. and Komatsu, H. (2009). Condition-dependent and condition-independent target selection in the macaque posterior parietal cortex. *Journal of Neurophysiology*, **101**, 721–36.

Oristaglio, J., Schneider, D.M., Balan, P.F., and Gottlieb, J. (2006). Integration of visuospatial and effector information during symbolically cued limb movements in monkey lateral intraparietal area. *Journal of Neuroscience*, **26**, 8310–9.

Paré, M. and Hanes, D.P. (2003). Controlled movement processing: superior colliculus activity associated with countermanded saccades. *Journal of Neuroscience*, **23**, 6480–9.

Paré, M. and Munoz, D.P. (2001). Expression of a re-centering bias in saccade regulation by superior colliculus neurons. *Experimental Brain Research*, **137**, 354–68.

Paré, M. and Wurtz, R.H. (1997). Monkey posterior parietal cortex neurons antidromically activated from superior colliculus. *Journal of Neurophysiology*, **78**, 3493–7.

Paré, M. and Wurtz, R.H. (2001). Progression in neuronal processing for saccadic eye movements from parietal cortex area lip to superior colliculus. *Journal of Neurophysiology*, **85**, 2545–62.

Paré, M., Thomas, N.W.D., and Shen, K. (2009). Saccade target selection in unconstrained visual search. In L. Harris, and M. Jenkin (eds.) *Cortical mechanisms of vision* (pp. 299–320). Cambridge: Cambridge University Press.

Pesaran, B., Pezaris, J.S., Sahani, M., Mitra, P.P., and Andersen, R.A. (2002). Temporal structure in neuronal activity during working memory in macaque parietal cortex. *Nature Neuroscience*, **5**, 805–11.

Petrides, M. and Pandya, D.N. (1984). Projections to the frontal cortex from the posterior parietal region in the rhesus monkey. *Journal of Comparative Neurology*, **228**, 105–16.

Pierrot-Deseignilly, C., Rivaud, S., Gaymard, B., and Agid, Y. (1991). Cortical control of reflexive visually-guided saccades. *Brain*, **114**, 1473–85.

Platt, M.L. and Glimcher, P.W. (1997). Responses of intraparietal neurons to saccadic targets and visual distractors. *Journal of Neurophysiology*, **78**, 1574–89.

Platt, M.L. and Glimcher, P.W. (1999). Neural correlates of decision variables in parietal cortex. *Nature*, **400**, 233–8.

Preuss, T.M. (2007a). Primate brain evolution in phylogenetic context. In J. H. Kaas, and T. M. Preuss (eds.) *Evolution of nervous systems (Vol. 4): the evolution of primate nervous systems* (pp. 1–34). Oxford: Elsevier.

Preuss, T.M. (2007b). Evolutionary specializations of primate brain systems. In M. J. Ravosa, and M. Dagosto (eds.) *Primate origins: adaptations and evolution* (pp. 625–75). New York: Springer.

Rafal, R.D. (2006). Oculomotor functions of the parietal lobe: effects of chronic lesions in humans. *Cortex*, **42**, 730–9.

Ramayya, A.G., Glasser, M.F., and Rilling, J.K. (2010). A DTI investigation of neural substrates supporting tool use. *Cerebral Cortex*, **20**, 507–16.

Rawley, J.B., and Constantinidis, C. (2009). Neural correlates of learning and working memory in the primate posterior parietal cortex. *Neurobiology of Learning and Memory*, **91**, 129–38.

Remple, M.S., Reed, J.L., Stepniewska, I., and Kaas, J.H. (2006). Organization of frontoparietal cortex in the tree shrew (*Tupaia belangeri*). I. Architecture, microelectrode maps, and corticospinal connections. *Journal of Comparative Neurology*, **497**, 133–54.

Requin, J., Lecas, J.C., and Vitton, N. (1990). A comparison of preparation-related neuronal activity changes in the prefrontal, premotor, primary motor and posterior parietal areas of the monkey cortex: preliminary results. *Neuroscience Letters*, **111**, 151–6.

Rescorla, R.A. (1988). Behavioral studies of Pavlovian conditioning. *Annual Review of Neuroscience*, **11**, 329–52.

Riehle, A. and Requin, J. (1989). Monkey primary motor and premotor cortex: single-cell activity related to prior information about direction and extent of an intended movement. *Journal of Neurophysiology*, **61**, 534–49.

Riehle, A. and Requin, J. (1993). The predictive value for performance speed of preparatory changes in neuronal activity of the monkey motor and premotor cortex. *Behavioural Brain Research*, **53**, 35–49.

Riddoch, M.J. and Humphreys, G.W. (1987). A case of integrative visual agnosia. *Brain*, **110**, 1431–62.

Robinson, D.A. (1972). Eye movements evoked by collicular stimulation in the alert monkey. *Vision Research*, **12**, 1795–1808.

Robinson, D.A. and Fuchs, A.F. (1969). Eye movements evoked by stimulation of frontal eye fields. *Journal of Neurophysiology*, **32**, 637–48.

Robinson, D.L., Goldberg, M.E., and Stanton, G.B. (1978). Parietal association cortex in the primate: sensory mechanisms and behavioral modulations. *Journal of Neurophysiology*, **41**, 910–32.

Roesch, M.R. and Olson, C.R. (2003). Impact of expected reward on neuronal activity in prefrontal cortex, frontal and supplementary eye fields and premotor cortex. *Journal of Neurophysiology*, **90**, 1766–89.

Roitman, J.D. and Shadlen, M.N. (2002). Response of neurons in the lateral intraparietal area during a combined visual discrimination reaction time task. *Journal of Neuroscience*, **22**, 9475–89.

Rorie, A.E., Gao, J., McClelland, J.L., and Newsome W.T. (2010). Integration of sensory and reward information during perceptual decision-making in lateral intraparietal cortex (LIP) of the macaque monkey. *PLoS One*, **5**(2), e9308.

Ross, C.F., and Martin R.D. (2007). The role of vision in the origin and evolution of primates. In J. H. Kaas, and T. M. Preuss (eds.) *Evolution of nervous systems (Vol. 4): the evolution of primate nervous systems* (pp. 59–78). Oxford: Elsevier.

Rumbaugh, D.M., King, J.E., Beran, M.J., Washburn, D.A., and Gould K.L. (2007). A salience theory of learning and behavior: With perspectives on neurobiology and cognition. *International Journal of Primatology*, **28**, 973–96.

Sato, T.R. and Schall, J.D. (2003). Effects of stimulus-response compatibility on neural selection in frontal eye field. *Neuron*, **38**, 637–48.

Schall, J.D. (2004). On building a bridge between brain and behavior. *Annual Review of Psychology*, **55**, 23–50.

Schall, J.D. and Hanes, D.P. (1993). Neural basis of saccade target selection in frontal eye field during visual search. *Nature*, **366**, 467–9.

Schall, J.D. and Thompson, K.G. (1999). Neural selection and control of visually guided eye movements. *Annual Review of Neuroscience*, **22**, 241–59.

Schall, J.D., Paré, M., and Woodman, G.F. (2007). Comment on 'top-down versus bottom-up control of attention in the prefrontal and posterior parietal cortices.' *Science*, **318**, 44a–b.

Schall, J.D., Morel, A., King, D.J., and Bullier, J. (1995a). Topography of visual cortex connections with frontal eye field in macaque: convergence and segregation of processing streams. *Journal of Neuroscience*, **15**, 4464–87.

Schall, J.D., Hanes, D.P., Thompson, K.G., and King, D.J. (1995b). Saccade target selection in frontal eye field of macaque. I. Visual and premovement activation. *Journal of Neuroscience*, **15**, 6905–18.

Schiller, P.H. and Tehovnik, E.J. (2001). Look and see: how the brain moves your eyes about. *Progress in Brain Research*, **134**, 127–42.

Schiller, P.H. and Tehovnik, E.J. (2003). Cortical inhibitory circuits in eye-movement generation. *European Journal of Neuroscience*, **18**, 3127–33.

Schiller, P.H., True, S.D., and Conway, J.L. (1980). Deficits in eye movements following frontal eye-field and superior colliculus ablations. *Journal of Neurophysiology*, **44**, 1175–89.

Schneider, W. (1995). VAM: a neuro-cognitive model for visual attention control of segmentation, object recognition and space-based motor action. *Visual Cognition*, **2**, 331–76.

Schwartz, M.L. and Goldman-Rakic, P.S. (1984). Callosal and intrahemispheric connectivity of the prefrontal association cortex in rhesus monkey: relation between intraparietal and principal sulcal cortex. *Journal of Comparative Neurology*, **226**, 403–20.

Scialfa, C.T. and Joffe, K.M. (1998). Response times and eye movements in feature and conjunction search as a function of target eccentricity. *Perception and Psychophysics*, **60**, 1067–82.

Seltzer, B. and Pandya, D.N. (1980). Converging visual and somatic sensory cortical input to the intraparietal sulcus of the rhesus monkey. *Brain Research*, **192**, 339–51.

Seo, H., Barraclough, D.J., and Lee, D. (2009). Lateral intraparietal cortex and reinforcement learning during a mixed-strategy game. *Journal of Neuroscience*, **29**, 7278–89.

Sereno, A.B. and Maunsell, J.H. (1998). Shape selectivity in primate lateral intraparietal cortex. *Nature*, **395**, 500–3.

Sereno, A.B. and Amador, S.C. (2006). Attention and memory-related responses of neurons in the lateral intraparietal area during spatial and shape-delayed match-to-sample tasks. *Journal of Neurophysiology*, **95**, 1078–98.

Shadlen, M.N. and Newsome, W.T. (1996). Motion perception: seeing and deciding. *Proceedings of the National Academy of Sciences U S A*, **93**, 628–33.

Shadlen, M.N. and Newsome, W.T. (2001). Neural basis of a perceptual decision in the parietal cortex (area LIP) of the rhesus monkey. *Journal of Neurophysiology*, **86**, 1916–36.

Shen, K. and Paré, M. (2007). Neuronal activity in superior colliculus signals both stimulus identity and saccade goals during visual conjunction search. *Journal of Vision*, **7**(5), 15.1–13.

Shen, K., Valero, J., Day, G.S., and Paré M. (2011). Investigating the role of the superior colliculus in active vision with the visual search paradigm. *European Journal of Neuroscience*, **33**(11), 2003–16.

Shepherd, S.V. and Platt, M.L. (2006). Noninvasive telemetric gaze tracking in freely moving socially housed prosimian primates. *Methods*, **38**, 185–94.

Shibutani, H., Sakata, H., and Hyvarinen, J. (1984). Saccades and blinking evoked by microstimulation of the posterior parietal association cortex of the monkey. *Experimental Brain Research*, **55**, 1–8.

Shikata, E., McNamara, A., Sprenger, A., Hamzei, F., Glauche, V., Büchel, C., *et al.* (2008). Localization of human intraparietal areas AIP, CIP, and LIP using surface orientation and saccadic eye movement tasks. *Human Brain Mapping*, **29**, 411–21.

Smith, P.L. and Ratcliff, R. (2004). Psychology and neurobiology of simple decisions. *Trends in Neurosciences*, **27**, 161–8.

Sparks, D.L. (1978). Functional properties of neurons in the monkey superior colliculus: Coupling of neuronal activity and saccade onset. *Brain Research*, **156**, 1–16.

Stahl, J.S. (1999). Amplitude of human head movements associated with horizontal saccades. *Experimental Brain Research*, **126**, 41–54.

Stanton, G.B., Bruce, C.J., and Goldberg, M.E. (1995). Topography of projections to posterior cortical areas from the macaque frontal eye fields. *Journal of Comparative Neurology*, **353**, 291–305.

Stepniewska, I., Fang, P.C., and Kaas, J.H. (2005). Microstimulation reveals specialized subregions for different complex movements in posterior parietal cortex of prosimian galagos. *Proceedings of the National Academy of Sciences USA*, **102**, 4878–83.

Stuphorn, V. and Schall, J.D. (2002). Neuronal control and monitoring of initiation of movements. *Muscle and Nerve*, **26**, 326–9.

Stuphorn, V., Brown, J.W., and Schall, J.D. (2010). Role of supplementary eye field in saccade initiation: executive, not direct, control. *Journal of Neurophysiology*, **103**, 801–16.

Sugrue, L.P., Corrado, G.S., and Newsome, W.T. (2004). Matching behavior and the representation of value in the parietal cortex. *Science*, **304**, 1782–7.

Supèr, H., van der Togt, C., Spekreijse, H., and Lamme, V.A. (2004). Correspondence of presaccadic activity in the monkey primary visual cortex with saccadic eye movements. *Proceedings of the National Academy of Sciences U S A*, **101**, 3230–5.

Tallon-Baudry, C., Bertrand, O., Peronnet, F., and Pernier, J. (1998). Induced gamma-band activity during the delay of a visual short-term memory task in humans. *Journal of Neuroscience*, **18**, 4244–54.

Their, P. and Andersen, R.A. (1998). Electrical microstimulation distinguishes distinct saccade-related areas in the posterior parietal cortex. *Journal of Neurophysiology*, **80**, 1713–35.

Thomas, N.W.D. and Paré, M. (2007). Temporal processing of saccade targets in parietal cortex area LIP during visual search. *Journal of Neurophysiology*, **97**, 942–7.

Thompson, K.G., Bichot, N.P., and Sato, T.R. (2005a). Frontal eye field activity before visual search errors reveals the integration of bottom-up and top-down salience. *Journal of Neurophysiology*, **93**, 337–51.

Thompson, K.G., Biscoe, K.L., and Sato, T.R. (2005b). Neuronal basis of covert spatial attention in the frontal eye field. *Journal of Neuroscience*, **25**, 9479–87.

Thompson, K.G., Hanes, D.P., Bichot, N.P., and Schall, J.D. (1996). Perceptual and motor processing stages identified in the activity of macaque frontal eye field neurons during visual search. *Journal of Neurophysiology*, **76**, 4040–55.

Todd, J.J. and Marois, R. (2004). Capacity limit of visual short-term memory in human posterior parietal cortex. *Nature*, **428**, 751–4.

Tomlinson, R.D. and Bahra, P.S. (1986). Combined eye-head gaze shifts in the primate. I. Metrics. *Journal of Neurophysiology*, **56**, 1542–57.

Toth, L.J. and Assad, J.A. (2002). Dynamic coding of behaviourally relevant stimuli in parietal cortex. *Nature*, **415**, 165–8.

Treisman, A. (1988). Features and objects: The fourteenth Bartlett memorial lecture. *Quarterly Journal of Experimental Psychology, Section A*, **40**, 201–37.

Treisman, A.M. and Gelade, G. (1980). A feature-integration theory of attention. *Cognitive Psychology*, **12**, 97–136.

Vogel, E.K. and Machizawa, M.G. (2004). Neural activity predicts individual differences in visual working memory capacity. *Nature*, **428**, 748–51.

Wang, X.J. (1999). Synaptic basis of cortical persistent activity: the importance of NMDA receptors to working memory. *Journal of Neuroscience*, **19**, 9587–603.

Wang, X.J. (2001). Synaptic reverberation underlying mnemonic persistent activity. *Trends in Neurosciences*, **24**, 455–63.

Wang, X.J. (2010). Neurophysiological and computational principles of cortical rhythms in cognition. *Physiological Review*, **90**, 1195–268.

Wardak, C., Olivier, E., and Duhamel, J.R. (2002). Saccadic target selection deficits after lateral intraparietal area inactivation in monkeys. *Journal of Neuroscience*, **22**, 9877–84.

Wardak, C., Olivier, E., and Duhamel, J.R. (2004). A deficit in covert attention after parietal cortex inactivation in the monkey. *Neuron*, **42**, 501–8.

Whishaw, I.Q. (2003). Did a change in sensory control of skilled movements stimulate the evolution of the primate frontal cortex? *Behavioral Brain Research*, **146**, 31–41.

Williams, D.E., Reingold, E.M., Moscovitch, M., and Behrmann, M. (1997). Patterns of eye movements during parallel and serial visual search tasks. *Canadian Journal of Experimental Psychology*, **51**, 151–64.

Wise, S.P., Boussaoud, D., Johnson, P.B., and Caminiti, R. (1997). Premotor and parietal cortex: corticocortical connectivity and combinatorial computations. *Annual Review of Neuroscience*, **20**, 25–42.

Wolfe, J.M. (1994). Guided search 2.0: a revised model of visual search. *Psychonomic Bulletin and Review*, **1**, 202–38.

Wolfe, J.M. and Horowitz, T.S. (2004). What attributes guide the deployment of visual attention and how do they do it? *Nature Reviews Neuroscience*, **5**, 1–7.

Wong, K.F., Huk, A.C., Shadlen, M.N., and Wang, X.J. (2007). Neural circuit dynamics underlying accumulation of time-varying evidence during perceptual decision making. *Frontiers in Computational Neuroscience*, **1**(6), 1–11.

Wurtz, R.H. and Goldberg, M.E. (1971). Superior colliculus cell responses related to eye movements in awake monkeys. *Science*, **171**, 82–4.

Yang, T. and Shadlen, M.N. (2007). Probabilistic reasoning by neurons. *Nature*, **447**, 1075–80.

Yin, T.C. and Mountcastle, V.B. (1977). Visual input to the visuomotor mechanisms of the monkey's parietal lobe. *Science*, **197**, 1381–3.

Zelinsky, G. and Sheinberg, D. (1995). Why some search tasks take longer than others: using eye movements to redefine reaction times. In J.M. Findlay, R. Walker, and R.W. Kentridge (eds.) *Eye movement research: mechanisms, processes and applications* (pp. 325–36). New York: Elsevier.

CHAPTER 15

Frontal cortex and flexible control of saccades

Kevin Johnston and Stefan Everling

Abstract

The frontal cortex has been associated with the control of eye movements since the 19th century. More recently, detailed anatomical studies and physiological investigations in awake non-human primates performing sophisticated oculomotor tasks have revealed the existence of a set of distinct interconnected areas within frontal cortex with roles ranging from direct control of saccade initiation, to indirect control driven by cognitive processes and instantiated by modulation of oculomotor structures. Here we review studies of the frontal and supplementary eye fields, prefrontal and anterior cingulate cortices, and the pre-supplementary motor area in the awake behaving primate which highlight their functional contribution to the control of saccadic eye movements.

Historical overview

It has been known for well over a century that the primate frontal cortex is involved in the control of eye movements. In the early 1870, the Scottish physiologist David Ferrier conducted a series of careful experiments in which he applied electrical stimulation to exposed cortical and subcortical areas in anaesthetized monkeys (Ferrier, 1876). He observed contralateral eye and head movements following stimulation of the parietal cortex and a region in frontal cortex, which in primates comprised the area dorsal and medial to the upper arm of the arcuate suclus. Ferrier noted that:

> Among the reactions excited by electrisation of the anterior of motor part of the hemispheres, is one of a special character, viz., that which results from stimulation of (12) in the monkey. . . . The head and eyes are directed to the opposite side and at the same time pupils dilate widely . . . the attitude is also one of excited attention or surprise.
>
> (Ferrier, 1876, p. 229).

Subsequent stimulation experiments by Horlsey and Schaefer (1888) confirmed Ferrier's observations but these authors also found that stimulation of almost the entire cortex within the principal sulcus and dorsal to the midline evoked contralateral eye and head movements. The authors found no deficits following extirpation of this area, however, even if performed bilaterally. Further electrical stimulation experiments by Mott and Schaefer (1890) found directional tuning for eye movements from upward movements following ventral stimulation to downward movements following dorsal stimulation. Levinsohn (1909) suggested that the frontal cortical area was the primary motor area for eye movements in monkeys since the threshold for evoking movements was lower in the frontal cortex than in partietal and occipital cortex (Levinsohn, 1909). Levinsohn also narrowed down the frontal eye movement area by showing that contralateral eye movements were most frequently evoked by stimulation of the cortical surface between the posterior tip of the principal suclus and the arcuate sulcus. Only rarely did stimulation of the area dorsal or ventral of the principal sulcus evoke eye movements. Levinsohn found that stimulation of the upper arm of the arcuate sulcus evoked combined eye and head movements whereas stimulation of the area dorsal to the upper arm of the arcuate mainly evoked head movements. Like Horlsey and Schaefer (1888), Levinsohn observed no effects on eye or head movements following unilateral or bilateral frontal cortex lesions. Many studies have confirmed the existence of a frontal eye movement-related area in other Old World monkeys, great apes (Leyton and Sherrington, 1917), and humans (Penfield and Boldrey, 1937). More recently, combined evidence from human functional magnetic resonance imaging (fMRI) and cytoarchitectural studies have identified a region at the junction of the precentral sulcus and superior frontal sulcus that appears to be homologous to frontal eye field (FEF) in monkeys (Amiez et al., 2006a; Paus, 1996; Rosano, et al., 2002, 2003).

In 1969, Robinson and Fuchs performed the first systematic study of the FEF in monkeys by using modern methods of intracortical microstimulation with much smaller currents combined with precise eye movement recordings in alert monkeys. They demonstrated that the eye movements evoked by microstimulation were indeed saccades that were indistinguishable from naturally occurring saccades. Robinson and Fuchs (1969) also discovered that the amplitude of the evoked saccade varied systematically with the stimulation site. Dorsomedial sites evoked large amplitude saccades, whereas the amplitude decreased gradually when the stimulation electrode was moved towards ventrolateral sites. Bruce and Goldberg (1985) employed stimulation currents of less than 50 μA and localized FEF in the rostral bank and fundus of the arcuate suclus (Fig. 15.1). They also confirmed and refined the map of saccade amplitude in FEF. This is now the generally accepted anatomical location of the FEF in monkeys.

Although these studies narrowed down the initially large eye movement-related frontal area to this small area in the rostral bank of the arcuate suclus, several studies suggested that another eye field may exist in the dorsomedial region of the frontal lobe. In humans, Penfield showed in his pioneering electrical stimulation studies that gaze shifts could be evoked by stimulation of the rostral part of the supplementary motor area (SMA) (Penfield and Boldrey, 1937).

In monkeys, Brinkman and Porter (1979) found neurons in the rostral SMA that responded during gaze shifts and Gould et al. (1986) reported that microstimulation of the rostral SMA evoked gaze shifts in owl monkeys. Analogous to the definition of the FEF, Schlag and Schlag Rey (1985, 1987) eventually defined the supplementary eye field (SEF) as an area in the rostral part of the SMA in which low currents (<50 μA) evoked saccades and in which saccade-related single unit activity was found (Fig. 15.1).

Anatomical, lesion, and physiological studies suggest that many frontal cortical areas beyond these two traditional eye fields may also play a role in the control of eye movements. These include the prefrontal cortex (PFC), anterior cingulate cortex (ACC), and pre-supplementary motor area (pre-SMA). Although microstimulation of these areas does not elicit saccades at physiologically relevant current levels, they have been associated with a multitude of cognitive functions, including attention, target selection, spatial working memory, arbitrary stimulus-response mapping, response suppression, and reward. In addition to task-related activity in eye movement tasks, tract-tracing studies have shown that these areas, like FEF and SEF, contain neurons that project directly to the intermediate and deep layers of the superior colliculus (SC) (Fries, 1984; Goldman and Nauta, 1976; Leichnetz et al., 1981), an area strongly involved in saccade generation (Munoz et al., 2000; Sparks, 2002) (see White and Munoz, Chapter 11, this volume). Recently, a retrograde transneuronal viral tracer study has shown that all these frontal areas are oligosynaptically connected with extraocular motoneurons (Moschovakis, et al., 2004).

In this chapter we will review tract tracing, lesion, and electrophysiological studies regarding the oculomotor function and connectivity of the FEF, SEF, PFC, ACC, and the pre-SMA. We will focus

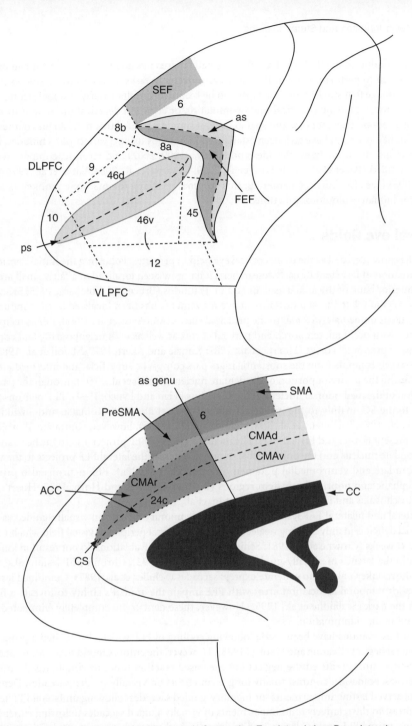

Fig. 15.1 Frontal cortical areas involved in control of saccades. Top, lateral view. Dorsolateral prefrontal cortex (DLPFC) corresponds to regions lying dorsal to the principal suclus (ps), and anterior to the frontal eye fields (FEF). Ventrolateral prefrontal cortex (VLPFC), to areas lying ventral to ps, and anterior to FEF. Bottom, medial view. Pre-supplementary motor area (Pre-SMA) corresponds to shaded area anterior to line denoting the genu of the arcuate sulcus (as genu), supplementary motor area (SMA), shaded area posterior to as genu. Anterior cingulate cortex (ACC) encompasses both dorsal and ventral banks of the rostral cingulate motor area, (CMAr), which corresponds to cytoarchitectonic area 24c. a, arcuate sulcus; CC, corpus callosum; CMAd, dorsal cingulate motor area; CMAv, ventral cingulate motor area; CS, cingulate sulcus; SEF, supplementary eye fields. See text for full description.

on studies conducted in Old World monkeys, usually rhesus macaques. These non-human primates can be trained to perform many of the same eye movement tasks used in human studies with the added advantage that single neuron activity can be recorded simultaneously and that neural activity can be manipulated using electrical microstimulation or chemical deactivation or activation techniques at a very precise temporal and spatial scale. It should be noted that homologues of these areas in non-human primates have also been established in humans using a variety of techniques, including cytoarchitectonic analyses (Petrides and Pandya, 1999, 2002) and recently, comparative high-resolution fMRI (Baker et al., 2005; Ford et al., 2009; Koyama, et al., 2004; Luna, et al., 1998; Orban, et al., 2006) (see also Curtis, Chapter 20, this volume) verifying the macaque monkey as a useful model for human oculomotor functions.

Frontal eye fields

The FEF is now regarded as the main cortical eye field in primates. Following the initial considerable overestimation of its extent by early researchers, it has now been localized to a fairly small area deep in the anterior bank of the arcuate sulcus and in its fundus (Bruce and Goldberg, 1985; Bruce et al., 1985). A region related to smooth pursuit eye movements has been localized at the fundus of the arcuate sulcus immediately caudal to the principal sulcus (MacAvoy et al., 1991). FEF is reciprocally connected with occipital, temporal, and parietal cortex as well as with neighbouring and contralateral areas of prefrontal cortex (Huerta et al., 1987; Kunzle and Akert, 1977; Maioli et al., 1983). The FEF also receives inputs from the substantia nigra pars compacta, superficial and intermediate layers of the SC, and the posterior portion of the dentate nucleus (Lynch et al., 1994) through the paralaminar region of the mediodorsal nucleus of the thalamus (Tian and Lynch, 1997). FEF neurons project heavily to the SC, mainly to the ipsilateral side (Huerta et al., 1986; Komatsu and Suzuki, 1985; Kunzle et al., 1976; Leichnetz, et al., 1981; Stanton et al., 1988b), however, contralateral projections are also present (Distel and Fries, 1982). The medial aspects of FEF project also to the head and body of the caudate nucleus and the dorsomedial putamen whereas the lateral FEF projects to the ventrolateral caudate and ventromedial putamen (Stanton et al., 1988a). FEF neurons also project to mesencephalic and pontine brainstem regions (Buttner-Ennever and Horn, 1997; Huerta, et al., 1986; Moschovakis and Highstein, 1994; Stanton, et al., 1988b).

Unilateral and bilateral FEF lesions produce only temporary deficits on visually-guided saccades. The initial deficit is mainly a strong neglect of the contralateral peripheral visual field which recovers within 2–4 weeks (Crowne et al., 1981; Schiller et al., 1980). FEF ablations do not result in long-term changes in the latency of visually-guided saccades (Lynch, 1992). Chronic FEF lesions also do not impair the monkey's ability to generate express saccades (Schiller et al., 1987). Combined lesions of the superior temporal association areas with FEF impair the animal's ability to foveate a fixation point in the dark (Scalaidhe et al., 1995). However, these deficits are completely eliminated under conditions of dim illumination.

Similar observations have been made following cooling of FEF which also elicited a pronounced contralateral neglect (Keating and Gooley, 1988). However, the authors found that cooling at slightly higher temperatures reduced the neglect but increased reaction times to visual targets and led to hypometric saccades. In contrast to any long-term effects on visually-guided saccades, Deng et al. (1986) observed lasting impairments for memory-guided saccades following unilateral FEF lesions.

In contrast to the relatively mild impairments of visually-guided saccades following either FEF or SC lesions, paired FEF and SC lesion lead to dramatic and relatively permanent deficits in saccadic eye movements with a severe impairment in the range of saccades (Schiller et al., 1979, 1980). Schiller and colleagues suggested that FEF and SC form parallel pathways in eye movement control because although they observed significant permanent decrements in several saccade parameters (velocity, frequency, size) following SC lesions, the animals were still able to generate saccades (Schiller, et al., 1980). Moreover, Schiller was still able to evoke saccades by intracortical FEF stimulation in animals with ablated superior colliculi (Schiller, 1977). A more recent study has questioned this hypothesis. Hanes and Wurtz chemically deactivated the SC using lidocaine or muscimol injections (Hanes and

Wurtz, 2001). They then applied electrical microstimulation to corresponding saccade sites in FEF and found that precisely aligned small injections or large injections in the SC abolished electrically evoked saccades. This finding suggests that in the non-ablated animal, the pathway from FEF to the brainstem is not functionally sufficient to evoke saccades in the absence of the signal from FEF to SC. Hanes and Schall suggested that the mild deficits seen in ablation studies are the result of recovery which might occur through a strengthening of projections from FEF to the brainstem. Although it had been initially proposed that FEF neurons project directly to premotor and oculomotor neurons in the brainstem (Leichnetz, 1981), no projection from FEF to premotor burst neurons has yet been identified. FEF neurons have a projection to omnipause neurons in the brainstem (Buttner-Ennever and Horn, 1997; Moschovakis and Highstein, 1994; Segraves, 1992). However, this pathway cannot carry any directional information because omnipause neurons pause for saccades in all directions (Cohen and Henn, 1972; Everling et al., 1998a; Keller, 1974; Luschei and Fuchs, 1972). Potentially other multisynapse pathways, for example through the reticularis tegmenti pontis nucleus or the nucleus of Darkschewitsch (Huerta, et al., 1986; Stanton, et al., 1988b), might be strengthened following SC lesions.

It has also been demonstrated that acute inactivations of FEF are associated with much stronger behavioural effects than previously observed following ablations. Dias et al. (1995) used muscimol injections to inactivate sites in FEF while monkeys performed visually-guided and memory-guided saccades. They found that muscimol injections impaired both visually-guided and memory-guided saccades to targets at the centre of the area represented by the injection site. In addition, monkeys generated many early errors in a memory-guided saccade task towards the stimulus on the side ipsilateral to the injection.

Electrical stimulation of the FEF has been shown to evoke fixed vector saccades with a clear amplitude coding. Stimulation of the ventrolateral FEF in head-restrained monkeys evokes small amplitude saccades and the amplitude increases when the electrode is moved to the dorsomedial portion (Bruce, et al., 1985; Robinson and Fuchs, 1969). The threshold and amplitude of electrically elicited saccades varies with the monkey's behavioural state when stimulation is applied. Smaller amplitude saccades with lower velocities are evoked during attentive visual fixation (Goldberg et al., 1986).

It has been known since Ferrier's pioneering experiments that FEF stimulation in anaesthetized monkeys also evokes contralateral head movements (Ferrier, 1876). This early observation has recently been confirmed in awake head unrestrained monkeys (Elsley et al., 2007; Knight and Fuchs, 2007). These findings suggest that FEF is not just an eye movement area, but more likely involved in more general orienting responses. This idea is also consistent with many recent studies that have indicated a role for FEF in the control of visual attention (Armstrong and Moore, 2007; Armstrong et al., 2006; Moore and Armstrong, 2003; Schafer and Moore, 2007).

Early single-unit recording studies in FEF raised doubts about a role of FEF in saccade generation, as the activity of FEF neurons followed rather than preceded spontaneous saccades (Bizzi, 1968; Bizzi and Schiller, 1970). Wurtz and Mohler (1976) provided new insights into the activity pattern of FEF neurons by demonstrating that about half the neurons had visual responses. They further showed that many neurons selectively enhanced their responses when the monkeys made a saccade toward the stimulus. Goldberg and Bushnell (1981) demonstrated that this enhancement was spatially selective and that it was presaccadic. They hypothesized that this activity represented the neural correlate for the initiation of visually-guided eye movements. Strong support for saccade-related activity in FEF was then provided by Bruce and Goldberg (1985) who recorded single-unit activity in FEF of monkeys while they performed several oculomotor tasks (Fig. 15.2). They observed presaccadic activity in about 50% of FEF neurons. They further classified this activity as visual, movement, and anticipatory. About 40% of presaccadic neurons had visual activity but no movement-related activity. Twenty per cent had movement-related activity, i.e. they discharged before purposive saccades with or without a visual target. These neurons were much less active or not active at all when the monkey made spontaneous saccades in the dark. The remaining 40% had both visual and movement activity and were classified as visuomovement cells. These neurons responded to visual stimuli but also discharged for saccades made with or without a visual target. An interesting feature of predominately movement and visuomovement neurons was anticipatory activity that preceded the cue to initiate a saccade when the monkey could predict the future saccade. The independence of presaccade activity from visual stimulation was demonstrated by Russo and Bruce (1994) who demonstrated that all FEF neurons with movement activity preceding visually-guided saccades were also active for saccades to auditory targets. The activity of movement neurons was similar for visually-guided and aurally-guided saccades, whereas visuomotor neurons were less active for aurally guided saccades. More recently, it has also been shown that FEF neurons display vergence-related activity (Ferraina et al., 2000).

A few studies have demonstrated that FEF neurons send a variety of task-related signals directly to the SC (Everling and Munoz, 2000; Segraves and Goldberg, 1987; Sommer and Wurtz, 2000). The original report by Segraves and Goldberg (1987) indicated that the majority of corticotectal FEF neurons were movement neurons and to a smaller extent foveal visual neurons. Subsequent studies by Sommer and Wurtz (2000), and Everling and Munoz (2000), suggested that FEF neurons also send visual and cognitive signals to the SC. Sommer and Wurtz (2000) recorded from corticotectal FEF neurons while monkeys performed delayed and gap saccade tasks. In addition to visual and saccade-related activity, they found that many corticotectal FEF neurons exhibited tonic delay activity and increases in activity during the gap period. They therefore concluded that FEF continuously influences the SC during oculomotor tasks. Everling and Munoz (2000) recorded from corticotectal FEF neurons while monkeys performed a task with randomly interleaved pro- and antisaccade trials. The colour of the central fixation point instructed the animal to either look towards a flashed peripheral stimulus on prosaccade trials or to look away from the stimulus on antisaccade trials (for review see Munoz and Everling, 2004). Everling and Munoz (2000) found that FEF neurons discharged for both prosaccades and antisaccades into their response field. The level of presaccadic activity and the motor burst, however, were lower on antisaccade trials. They also found that many FEF neurons had higher levels of activity before the peripheral stimulus was presented on prosaccade than on antisaccade trials. They suggested that these differences in preparatory activity reflected the different preparatory sets (Evarts et al., 1984) necessary to perform pro- and antisaccades. The authors proposed that the lower preparatory activity of saccade-related neurons and the reduced stimulus-related responses on antisaccade trials reduced the excitation of saccade-related neurons in the SC (Everling et al., 1998b, 1999) and therefore reduced the risk of generating a task-inappropriate saccade towards the stimulus.

Supplementary eye fields

In addition to the FEF, a second frontal cortical eye field has been identified. The SEF lies dorsomedial to the FEF within area 6 (Schlag and Schlag Rey, 1985, 1987) (Fig. 15.2). The region corresponding to the SEF can be separated from the pre-SMA medially, and the SMA caudally, based on functional and anatomical grounds (Tanji, 1994). The SEF was originally characterized by Schlag and Schlag-Rey (1985, 1987), who observed that electrical microstimulation of this region at currents as low as 20 µA evoked saccadic eye movements, and that single neurons within this area exhibited changes in activity time-locked to visual stimuli and saccadic eye movements. Several lines of evidence suggest functional differences between the FEF and SEF. First, there are clear differences between microstimulation evoked saccades in these two areas. Microstimulation of SEF evokes saccades at longer latencies than FEF stimulation, suggesting that the FEF may be more strongly connected to downstream circuitry involved in generation of saccades (Bruce, et al., 1985; Mann et al., 1988; Schlag and Schlag-Rey, 1985, 1987). In addition, saccades evoked by microstimulation of the FEF are fixed vector, and long trains of stimulation result in multiple saccades (Bruce, et al., 1985; Schall, 1991a). In comparison, microstimulation of the SEF can evoke fixed vector saccades, or saccades which drive the eye to a specific location of visual space (Bon and Lucchetti, 1992; Bruce, et al., 1985; Mann, et al., 1988; Mitz and Godschalk, 1989; Schall, 1991a; Schlag and Schlag-Rey, 1985, 1987; Tehovnik and Lee, 1993; but see Russo and Bruce, 1993, 1996). In the SEF, long trains of stimulation drive the eye to a specific location in space, and maintain it at that position (Schall, 1991a).

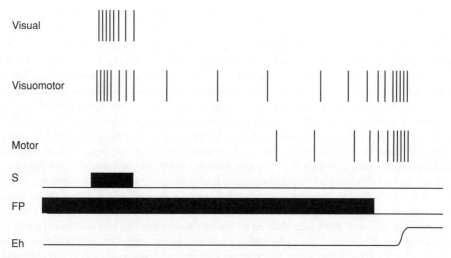

Fig. 15.2 Activity patterns of different neurons in the frontal eye fields. Visual neurons respond to the presentation of the stimulus in their response field. Visuomotor neurons respond to the presentation of the stimulus, discharge during the delay period and exhibit a burst of action potentials for the saccade in their response field. Motor neuron discharge for the saccade. S, stimulus, FP, fixation point, Eh, horizontal eye position. Each tickmark represents the time of an action potential.

Such findings suggest that the SEF may encode visual space in 'head centred' coordinates (Tehovnik et al., 2000). Second, lesions of the FEF and SEF have differential effects on saccades. FEF lesions produce pronounced changes in the accuracy, velocity, and reaction times of saccades made to visual targets, while those produced by lesions of the SEF are more mild (Schiller and Chou, 1998), again suggesting that the SEF is less directly involved in saccade control than the FEF. Third, the response properties of FEF and SEF neurons show subtle differences. The response latencies of FEF neurons to visual stimuli are typically shorter than neurons in SEF (Pouget et al., 2005), and the timing of presaccadic activity is generally more variable with respect to saccade onset in the SEF than FEF (Hanes et al., 1995). In addition, the response fields of presaccadic FEF neurons may be slightly smaller than those of SEF neurons (Schall, 1991a).

In addition to the physiological properties noted above, the anatomical connectivity of the SEF supports a critical role in oculomotor function. The SEF sends direct projections to virtually all subcortical and cortical regions involved in oculomotor control, including the SC and structures of the brainstem saccade generator (Huerta and Kaas, 1990) the nucleus raphe interpositius, which contains omnipause neurons (Shook et al., 1988), the oculomotor region of the caudate nucleus (Parthasarathy et al., 1992), and the FEF (Huerta and Kaas, 1990). In addition to its connections to oculomotor structures, it is also extensively interconnected with other frontal areas including the prefrontal and anterior cingulate cortices (Huerta and Kaas, 1990).

Although the physiological properties of the SEF and its intimate connections with oculomotor circuitry suggest a role in initiation of saccades, investigation of the detailed response properties of SEF neurons suggest that it does not carry signals sufficient for saccade initiation. Stuphorn et al (2000) recorded the activity of SEF neurons while monkeys performed a saccade countermanding task, in which they were required to either generate or withhold a saccade toward a visual stimulus depending upon the presence of a suddenly presented stop signal. Performance in this task can be modelled as a race between two processes, a *go* process, invoked by the appearance of a visual target, representing the command to generate saccade toward the target, and a *stop* process, invoked by the reappearance of the fixation point, representing the command to maintain fixation (Logan et al., 1984). Behaviour on a given trial is dictated by which of these processes is first to reach a threshold.

In the context of the saccade system, these processes are embodied by the activity of neurons sending saccade-related signals, underlying gaze-shifting, and those carrying fixation signals, underlying gaze-holding. In the countermanding paradigm, it is possible to compute the amount of time required to successfully withhold a planned movement on stop signal trials. This is referred to as the stop signal reaction time (SSRT). By comparing the activity of single neurons on trials in which animals successfully cancel saccades with those on which no stop signal is presented, and noting the correspondence between the timing of neuronal modulation and the SSRT, it is possible to determine whether such signals are sufficient for the cancellation of saccades. Specifically, neuronal differences in activity between cancelled and no stop signal trials must occur before the SSRT in order to be related to cancellation of saccades. This has been found to be the case in the FEF (Brown et al., 2008; Hanes and Schall, 1996). In contrast, although modulation of SEF neurons was found to be greater on successfully cancelled than no stop signal trials, the timing of this modulation was after the SSRT, too late to be directly involved in withholding saccades. Interestingly however, the magnitude of the activity of some SEF neurons on cancelled trials increased as the probability of failing to cancel saccades increased. Since both gaze-shifting and gaze-holding mechanisms are concurrently activated on stop signal trials, and since gaze holding mechanisms are more strongly activated on trials in which saccades are not cancelled, the authors interpreted this signal as a neural correlate of response conflict, a result of the coactivation these two mechanisms. In addition, they found neural signals related to performance errors and reinforcement. Taken together, these signals suggest that the SEF is not directly involved in the control of saccades, but rather is engaged when executive control of eye movements is required. This contention is further supported by the fact that microstimulation improves performance in this task in a context-dependent fashion. Stimulation delivered on stop signal trials during this task improves performance by slowing reaction times, while stimulation delivered on no stop signal trials produces the opposite effect (Stuphorn and Schall, 2006). Such context-dependent stimulation effects have been observed in other oculomotor paradigms as well (Fujii et al., 1995; Mann, et al., 1988).

SEF neurons have been shown to carry signals related to saccadic eye movements in a number of other cognitive tasks including those requiring learning of sequences of saccades (Isoda and Tanji, 2002), conditional oculomotor associations (Chen and Wise, 1995, 1996), eye–hand coordination (Mushiake et al., 1996), object-centred representations (Olson and Gettner, 1995), and oculomotor rules (Kim et al., 2005). In general, such paradigms require the linking of an abstract representation with a specific eye movement, for example, a saccade directed to the left side of a particular object (Olson and Gettner, 1995). The antisaccade paradigm is another example of an eye movement task requiring an arbitrary association between a behavioural instruction and an eye movement (Munoz and Everling, 2004). In this task, SEF neurons consistently discharge at higher rates in relation to behavioural instructions, visual stimuli, and saccades on antisaccade trials than prosaccade trials. Moreover, activity on incorrect antisaccade trials, in which monkeys generate erroneous prosaccades, is substantially lower than that on correct antisaccade trials, suggesting that the enhancement in activity observed on such trials is critical for successful performance of antisaccades (Amador et al., 2003; Schlag-Rey et al., 1997). This enhanced activity has been linked to various cognitive processes including encoding of the arbitrary stimulus-response association, suppression of reflexive prosaccades, and generation of the voluntary saccade away from the visual stimulus (Amador, et al., 2003). In any case, this finding, in combination with those described above, highlights the role of the SEF in control of eye movements based on cognitive variables.

Prefrontal cortex

Perhaps no other cortical area has been associated with a greater assortment of cognitive functions than the PFC. Human patients suffering from PFC lesions display a bewildering array of cognitive deficits, including hyperactivity, hypoactivity, impulsiveness, and perseveration (Fuster, 2008; Nauta, 1971). Similarly varied behavioural effects have been observed following lesions in experimental animals, including deficits in working memory (Jacobsen, 1935), response suppression (Weiskrantz and Mishkin, 1958), and perseveration (Mishkin, 1964). This complexity of function is matched by the complexity of organization of this area. The region generally referred to as PFC is a set of highly interconnected areas, receiving diverse inputs from essentially all sensory systems, and in return, sending outputs to essentially all motor and sensory systems (Barbas, 2000; Petrides and Pandya, 1999). The PFC can be loosely divided into two sets of areas lying on the lateral surface of the frontal lobe: regions dorsal to the principal sulcus including the dorsal portions of areas 8 and 46, and area 9, collectively referred to as dorsolateral prefrontal cortex (DLPFC), and areas ventral to the principal sulcus, including the ventral portion of area 46, area 45 and area 12, referred to as the ventrolateral prefrontal cortex (VLPFC) (see Fig. 15.1). These regions share reciprocal projections with higher order visual, auditory, somatosensory, and polysensory areas, including the superior temporal sulcus (Barbas and Mesulam, 1985; Barbas, et al., 2005; Petrides and Pandya, 1999). With respect to oculomotor function, areas 8 and 46 have been by far the most extensively investigated. This has undoubtedly been motivated by the results of the aforementioned studies which revealed that eye movements could be evoked by electrical stimulation of these areas in the macaque monkey (Robinson and Fuchs, 1969), and the subsequent identification of the FEFs, in the anterior bank of the arcuate sulcus within area 8. This area can be differentiated from the remainder of the PFC by the fact that microstimulation evokes saccades at low currents (<50 μA) (Bruce, et al., 1985), and the greater density of large layer V output neurons in this region in comparison to the more rostral portions of areas 8 and 46 (Stanton et al., 1989).

Anatomically, the DLPFC is ideally situated to play a role in oculomotor control. It is reciprocally connected to higher order cortical visual areas including the lateral intraparietal area (LIP) (Petrides and Pandya, 1984; Selemon and Goldman-Rakic, 1988), and FEF (Stanton et al., 1993). In addition, it sends direct projections to midbrain and brainstem oculomotor structures including the SC (Fries, 1984; Goldman and Nauta, 1976; Leichnetz, et al., 1981), and pontine nuclei (Leichnetz et al., 1984). Consistent with this pattern of connectivity, early investigations of the response properties of DLPFC neurons in oculomotor tasks revealed changes in activity in response to visual stimuli and saccadic eye movements (Boch and Goldberg, 1989; Joseph and Barone, 1987; Kojima, 1980). Three pieces of evidence suggest, however, that it is unlikely that these perisaccadic signals represent motor commands for saccadic eye movements. First, as mentioned above, saccades cannot be evoked from the DLPFC at low currents. Second, the onset of activity with respect to saccade onset is highly variable, occurring in some cases only *after* the saccade has started (Boch and Goldberg, 1989). Third, the activity level of DLPFC neurons does not correlate with saccadic reaction time on a trial-by-trial basis, even for those neurons sending direct projections to oculomotor structures (Johnston and Everling, 2009). Taken together, the anatomical and physiological evidence suggest that the DLPFC acts to *modulate* oculomotor function, rather than playing a direct role in saccade *initiation*.

Neurophysiological investigations in awake behaving monkeys have revealed that single PFC neurons carry diverse sets of signals representing neural correlates of a vast array of cognitive constructs, including task set (Asaad et al., 2000; Wallis et al., 2001; White and Wise, 1999), learning (Asaad et al., 1998), working memory (Fuster, 1973; Fuster and Alexander, 1971; Goldman-Rakic, 1995; Miller et al., 1996; Rainer et al., 1998a), numerosity (Nieder and Miller, 2003), attention (Everling et al., 2002; Lebedev et al., 2004; Rainer et al., 1998b), decision-making (Kim and Shadlen, 1999), abstract categories (Freedman et al., 2001; Nieder et al., 2002), response strategies (Genovesio et al., 2005), reward (Tsujimoto and Sawaguchi, 2004; Watanabe, 1996), and response suppression (Hasegawa et al., 2004). These signals have been observed in many tasks, using different effectors. A common theme underlying all of these signals and their associated functions is that they fall within the realm of what is typically considered 'executive' or cognitive control. More specifically, they are thought to represent flexible mappings between sensory inputs, goals, and the behavioural means by which such goals can be achieved (Miller and Cohen, 2001). It has been suggested that the PFC carries out such flexible control via active maintenance of patterns of activity representing task rules and goals, which in turn bias the activity of connected brain areas. The aim of this section is to illustrate the role of the PFC in the cognitive control of eye movements by focusing specifically on research using oculomotor paradigms to investigate three cardinal functions of the PFC: working memory, response suppression, and flexible control. We direct the reader interested in further details regarding PFC functions to the many excellent reviews available in the extant literature (Miller and Cohen, 2001; Sakai, 2008; Tanji and Hoshi, 2008).

No cognitive process has been more strongly linked to the DLPFC than working memory. Historically, PFC lesions have been shown to result in severe performance deficits in delayed response tasks in both humans (Fuster, 1997) and animals (Passingham, 1985). The response properties of prefrontal neurons in monkeys are also consistent with such a function. Early investigations revealed that prefrontal neurons showed sustained activity during the delay period intervening between stimulus presentation and behavioural responses in delayed-response tasks (Fuster, 1973; Fuster and Alexander, 1971). This property has been generally considered a neural correlate of working memory, since it persists after the offset of a sensory stimulus, and bridges the temporal gap between stimulus and response.

Studies of the response properties of prefrontal neurons in working memory tasks such as those carried out by Fuster and colleagues required animals to perform a manual response based on working memory. In the oculomotor domain, the memory-guided saccade task has been used extensively to investigate activity of DLPFC neurons in relation to visuospatial working memory. This task is essentially an oculomotor version of the classical delayed-response task used to assess working memory in human and animal subjects. In this task, a visual stimulus is briefly flashed, and the subject is required to make a saccade to the remembered location of the stimulus following a delay period. In a seminal series of studies, Funahashi and colleagues (Funahashi et al., 1989, 1990, 1991) demonstrated that DLPFC neurons showed phasic modulations in activity time-locked to visual stimulus onset and saccades, and sustained activity during the delay period. In many neurons, these responses were directional: they were tuned such that the firing rate of a given neuron was highest when a visual stimulus is presented at a particular spatial location, and lower at others. The spatial tuning exhibited by these neurons is contralaterally biased, with a high percentage of neurons preferring stimuli presented in the hemifield contralateral to the recording site, and of highly variable size, ranging from a few degrees to almost an entire hemifield (Funahashi, et al., 1989). They also observed a rough correspondence in tuning across trial epochs; a neuron responding most strongly to a visual stimulus appearing in the upper contralateral quadrant of the visual field tended to exhibit the highest delay and saccade related activity for those directions (Funahashi, et al., 1989, 1990, 1991). The area of the visual field to which a neuron responds best in this task has correspondingly been referred to as the 'memory field' of that neuron (Funahashi, et al., 1989). It has been shown that all of these signals are sent directly to the SC, a finding supporting a role of such PFC signals in top-down modulation of memory-based responses (Johnston and Everling, 2009) (Fig. 15.3).

In general, memory fields of neurons in the monkey prefrontal cortex do not appear to be organized in an orderly topographic fashion across the cortical surface, as are receptive fields in visual areas, but may be represented in local circuits on a smaller scale (Wang et al., 2004). It has been suggested that memory fields are constructed from the complex interaction between inhibitory interneurons and pyramidal neurons at the local level (Rao et al., 2000; Wilson et al., 1994), and that horizontal projections connect local and distant areas with similar tuning to form a cortical network (Constantinidis and Wang, 2004; Constantinidis et al., 2001a; Goldman-Rakic, 1996). Evidence for such a punctate representation is supported by lesion (Funahashi et al., 1993) and inactivation (Sawaguchi and Iba, 2001) studies, in which it has been shown that inactivation or destruction of localized areas of prefrontal cortex result in spatially restricted performance deficits in memory-guided saccades, referred to as 'mnemonic scotomas'. Interestingly, these deficits are also dependent on delay duration; deficits tend to be most pronounced at longer delay intervals, a finding supporting a direct and critical involvement of the prefrontal cortex in visuospatial working memory.

Spatial working memory is only one of many cognitive functions for which neural correlates can be found in the PFC, and it is as yet not clear exactly what is represented by the neural responses observed in DLPFC neurons during memory-guided saccades. For example, sustained delay period activity could potentially reflect the location of the visual stimulus, (a retrospective code), or the direction of the forthcoming saccade (a prospective code). Evidence in support of both of these

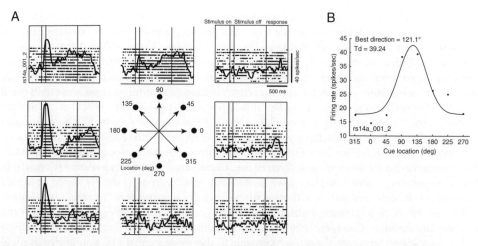

Fig. 15.3 Activity of a corticotectal dorsolateral prefrontal cortex neuron in a memory-guided saccade task. A) Each panel depicts activity of the neuron for trials on which the cue stimulus was presented in the location depicted in the schematic at centre. Rasters and spike density functions aligned on fixation offset (response). This neuron showed directionally-selective activity during the delay epoch, with best responses for stimuli presented in the upper quadrant of the visual field contralateral to the recorded. B) Gaussian tuning function for cue epoch activity for the neuron shown in (A). Function was fit to the mean delay epoch activity for each direction (see methods).

possibilities has been found (Constantinidis et al., 2001b; Funahashi, et al., 1993; Hasegawa et al., 1998). Another alternative is that delay activity represents neither of these alternatives, but is instead linked to a different process supporting performance in the task, such as attention (Lebedev et al., 2004). The extent to which attentional and memory processes have been truly dissociated to date remains open to debate. It is clear, however, that our current understanding regarding the role of sustained PFC delay activity in cognitive processes is less than complete.

An inability to inhibit inappropriate responses, including saccades, has been one of the most commonly observed consequences of PFC dysfunction in both human patients (Milner, 1963; Ploner et al., 2005) and monkeys (Dias et al., 1996; Iversen and Mishkin, 1970). This has been supported by the results of neurophysiological studies. Hasegawa et al. (2004) recorded the activity of PFC neurons while monkeys performed a delayed spatial matching/non-matching task, which required them to either make or withhold saccades. They identified a subset of neurons that were most active when monkeys were required to withhold a saccade to a specific spatial location, and thus concluded that the responses of these 'don't look' neurons encoded suppression of saccades. Thus, behavioural inhibition mediated by the PFC is not necessarily global in nature, but rather can reflect specific responses, in this case, a saccade of a particular direction and amplitude.

The antisaccade task has been used extensively to investigate inhibition of reflexive saccades (Everling and Fischer, 1998; Nigg, 2000). In this task, subjects are required to make a saccade in the direction opposite to that of a suddenly appearing visual stimulus. Correct performance in this task requires suppression of an automatic saccade toward the visual stimulus, or prosaccade, and programming of an antisaccade to the mirror location. As such, this task embodies several cognitive functions linked to the PFC, including inhibition of automatic in favour of voluntary goal-directed responses, and arbitrary stimulus response association (Asaad, et al., 2000; Miller and Cohen, 2001). Single neuron recordings and fMRI studies in monkeys have revealed differences in preparatory activity preceding onset of the visual stimulus between prosaccade and antisaccade trials in PFC (Everling and Desouza, 2005; Ford, et al., 2009), suggesting that it is involved in the active maintenance of activity selective for the pro and antisaccade task-sets. Johnston and Everling (2006) employed antidromic activation to determine whether such task-selective signals were sent directly to the SC. It has been shown that SC saccade neurons show lower levels of activity in response to visual stimuli and saccades on antisaccade trials than prosaccade trials, while SC fixation neurons, responsible for gaze-holding (see White and Munoz, Chapter 11, this volume) have enhanced responses on antisaccade relative to prosaccade trials (Everling, et al., 1999). This finding suggests that a top-down signal inhibiting saccade neurons, and thus generation of reflexive, stimulus driven saccades, or an excitatory signal enhancing the activity of fixation neurons on antisaccade trials could be critical for performance in this task. The authors found that the activity of PFC-SC projection neurons carried an enhanced signal around the time of visual stimulus presentation on antisaccade trials, and that the level of this activity was negatively correlated with saccadic reaction times on antisaccade trials. This finding demonstrates that PFC output signals are associated with a facilitation of performance in the antisaccade task. Since all cortical outputs are excitatory in nature (Creutzfeldt, 1993), the authors proposed that top-down modulation of SC neurons by the PFC could be carried out either via fixation neurons, or activation of the extensive network of SC interneurons (Munoz and Istvan, 1998). In combination with the results of microstimulation (Wegener et al., 2008) and muscimol inactivation (Condy et al., 2007) studies demonstrating a causal link between PFC activity and antisaccade performance, these results provide further evidence that PFC output signals could act to modulate the activity of target structures in the service of behavioural goals, and thus support guided-activation accounts of PFC function. Recent findings suggest that PFC output signals, carried by layer V pyramidal neurons, could be gated by inhibitory interneurons (Johnston et al., 2009). Thus both local PFC circuitry and outputs may be critical to antisaccade performance.

Anterior cingulate cortex

The cingulate cortex lies in the medial wall of the cerebral hemispheres, surrounding the corpus callosum from its rostral to caudal extent. It can be roughly subdivided into dorsal and ventral zones, separated by the cingulate sulcus (Fig. 15.1). This large cortical region has been subdivided based on cytoarchitectural (Dum and Strick, 1991; Vogt et al., 1987, 2005), anatomical (Dum and Strick, 1992; Vogt, et al., 1987), and neurophysiological (Luppino et al., 1991) criteria. Cingulate cortex can be separated into three broad regions, two caudal, and one rostral, divided roughly by the genu of the arcuate sulcus (Picard and Strick, 1996). This anatomical division has been related to functional differences between rostral and caudal cingulate areas (Isomura et al., 2003). Caudal regions include the dorsal and ventral cingulate motor areas (CMAd and CMAv) lying in the dorsal and ventral banks of the cingulate sulcus, respectively. These areas are thought to play a role in motor function based on their connectivity to the spinal cord (Dum and Strick, 1991), the fact that application of electrical microstimulation evokes body movements that are organized in a somatotopic fashion (Luppino, et al., 1991), and the observation that neurons in these regions display activity related to limb movements (Shima, et al., 1991). Neurons in the CMAv have also been show to exhibit saccade-related activity (Olson et al., 1996). The rostral cingulate motor area (CMAr), corresponding to area 24c, encompasses both the dorsal and ventral banks, and has been implicated in higher cognitive functions. It is this region that is typically referred to as anterior cingulate cortex (ACC), and it is to this area that we refer when using this term henceforth.

Several lines of evidence support a role of the ACC in cognitive as opposed to strictly motor function. Anatomically, the ACC shares dense reciprocal connections with the PFC (Bates and Goldman-Rakic, 1993; Vogt and Pandya, 1987). ACC neurons also display cytoarchitectural features linked to involvement in cognitive processes (Elston et al., 2005). In monkeys, microstimulation of the ACC only rarely evokes body movements, and movements which are evoked are not somatotopically organized (Luppino, et al., 1991), suggesting a weak influence on the spinal cord, and a less direct role in motor control (Picard and Strick, 1996). Single neuron recordings have revealed that single ACC neurons carry signals related to cognitive variables including expected reward (Amiez et al., 2006b; Shidara and Richmond, 2002), use of reward history to guide selection of upcoming motor movements (Shima and Tanji, 1998), and monitoring of movement sequences (Hoshi et al., 2005). Lesions or inactivation of the ACC impair these functions (Kennerley et al., 2006; Shima and Tanji, 1998), suggesting a direct and causal role. These findings have been corroborated by numerous fMRI studies in humans demonstrating activation of the ACC in a range of cognitive tasks (Dosenbach, et al., 2006; Paus, 2001).

Similarly convergent lines of evidence support a role of the ACC in the control of eye movements. Human fMRI studies have provided support for the existence of a cingulate eye field (CEF) within this area (Paus et al., 1993; Petit, et al., 1993), and human patients with lesions corresponding to the CEF exhibit deficiencies in oculomotor control (Gaymard, et al., 1998). In non-human primates, the ACC has been shown to have oligosynaptic connections to the eye muscles (Moschovakis, et al., 2004), and it is directly connected to a number of cortical and subcortical areas known to be involved in oculomotor function, including the FEF (Wang et al., 2004), SEF (Huerta and Kaas, 1990; Luppino et al., 2003), and pontine nuclei (Leichnetz, et al., 1984; Vilensky and van Hoesen, 1981). Conflicting evidence exists regarding direct connections from ACC to SC (Fries, 1985; Leichnetz, et al., 1981).

Saccades can be evoked by ACC microstimulation (Mitz and Godschalk, 1989). It should be noted however, that such stimulation is effective at only a small number of sites. Moreover, the response latency of ACC neurons to visual inputs is substantially longer than that of other cortical oculomotor areas (Pouget, et al., 2005), and neither the responses of single ACC neurons (Ito et al., 2003), nor intracranially recorded LFPs (Emeric, et al., 2008) are sufficient to control initiation of saccades. These findings, combined with the extensive evidence for a cognitive function of the ACC, suggest that it is involved more in modulation of oculomotor function based on behavioural context than the issuing of saccade commands. In this sense, its role in oculomotor function can be seen as similar and perhaps complementary to that of the DLPFC.

Theories regarding the specific role of the ACC in cognitive function have been based almost entirely upon the results of studies carried out with human subjects. Studies of event-related potentials (ERPs) have revealed large negative deflections following performance errors in several tasks (Falkenstein et al., 1991b; Gehring et al., 1995). This error-related negativity has been localized to the ACC, and has been variously linked to error (Gehring, et al., 1995), reinforcement (Holroyd and Coles, 2002), and conflict-monitoring (van Veen and Carter, 2002) functions. Error monitoring theories suggest that the ERN reflects the mismatch between representations of correct and incorrect responses (Falkenstein et al., 1991a; Gehring, et al., 1995), while reinforcement monitoring accounts suggest that this response is a result of dopaminergic inputs from the midbrain signalling errors, reinforcement, or punishment (Holroyd and Coles, 2002). The conflict-monitoring hypothesis (Botvinick et al., 2001) suggests that the ACC acts as a monitor of response conflict, defined as coactivation of incompatible stimulus-response processes, and that this conflict signal is used to recruit cognitive control to reduce conflict and improve performance on subsequent trials. Evidence in support of the conflict-monitoring hypothesis has been provided by numerous fMRI and ERP investigations using tasks thought to engender conflict, such as the Stroop colour-naming task (see Carter and van Veen, 2007; van Veen and Carter, 2002 for review). In these studies, signals consistent with response conflict are observed around the time of behavioural responses, when conflict between incompatible processes would be expected to be greatest, as well as following performance errors (Botvinick, et al., 2001; Carter, et al., 2000; Kerns, et al., 2004; MacDonald et al., 2000; van Veen and Carter, 2002). ACC activation is commonly observed in oculomotor tasks that encompass incompatibility between stimulus and required saccades (Merriam, et al., 2001; Sweeney, et al., 1996). Thus, a potential role of the ACC in oculomotor control may be to signal the mismatch between intended and actual eye movements, or to monitor for conflict between incompatible oculomotor commands and resolve this conflict by activating other cortical areas.

Neurophysiological studies in behaving primates have examined the various theories concerning ACC function. Ito and colleagues (2003) recorded the activity of single ACC neurons while monkeys performed a saccade countermanding task. This task is ideal for investigating conflict-related signals in the oculomotor system since stop signal trials explicitly set two competing and incompatible stimulus-response processes against one another. If conflict-related signals are present in single ACC neurons, a difference in activity should be observed between successful stop signal trials, in which gaze-shifting and gaze-holding mechanisms are coactivated, and no stop signal trials, in which no response conflict is present due to the activation of gaze shifting mechanisms alone. Contrary to conflict-monitoring accounts, Ito and colleagues found no such differences. Interestingly, they found that many neurons showed activity related to performance errors, as well as reinforcement related activity. Such activity was found in relation to rewards earned on correct trials, omission of earned rewards, or unexpected rewards delivered during the interval between trials. Altogether, these data are consistent with the notion that the ACC signals the mismatch between expected and actual consequences, rather than conflict. This result has been corroborated by other studies using other oculomotor tasks (Nakamura et al., 2005).

One possible explanation for the discrepancy between the results of single neuron recording and fMRI and ERP studies is the manner in which neural responses are measured. fMRI and ERPs represent the activity of large populations of neurons, and may represent neural events occurring at synapses which are not sufficient to evoke the action potentials measured in single neuron recordings. To address this, Emeric and colleagues (2008) measured intracranial local field potentials (LFPs) while monkeys performed the saccade countermanding task. LFPs are thought to reflect potential changes occurring in dendrites, similar to ERPs, and have been shown to be more highly correlated with the fMRI signal than the action potentials of single neurons (Logothetis et al., 2001). Similar to the study by Ito et al. (2003) the authors found no evidence for conflict related signals in LFPs. As in previous studies, signals related to errors and reinforcement were observed (Ito et al., 2003, Shidara and Richmond, 2002). Thus, the failure to find neural signals consistent with conflict in primate ACC are not likely the result of differences in the types of such signals measured by different techniques.

A core tenet of the conflict-monitoring hypothesis is that the conflict related signal generated by the ACC is used to recruit the other brain areas related to executive function, most notably the PFC, which in turn engage control. Thus, the ACC is ascribed a strictly 'evaluative' role, and does not engage control mechanisms itself (Botvinick et al., 2004). A prediction of this model is that the ACC should be active during the response period since this is the time at which conflict would be present, while the PFC should be most active during preparatory periods prior to behavioural responses since this would reflect the invocation of control to deal with upcoming conflict. Indeed such results have been observed in fMRI studies comparing the relative roles of the PFC and ACC in cognitive control using the Stroop task (MacDonald et al., 2000). To investigate the relative roles of the PFC and ACC in control processes at the single neuron level, Johnston et al. (2007) recorded the activity of PFC and ACC neurons while monkeys performed a task-switching version of a pro/antisaccade task. In this task, the animals performed alternating blocks of pro or antisaccade trials. Following a fixed number of correct trials, the task rule changed, and the animals were required to switch to the previously unrewarded response. Task switching is a common example of a behaviour requiring cognitive control, and has been extensively investigated in human subjects in a variety of paradigms (Allport et al., 1994). The authors found clear differences in both the magnitude and onset times of the task selective preparatory responses of ACC and PFC neurons following a task switch. ACC neurons were most selective immediately following a task switch, and this selectivity declined as the number of post-switch trials increased. This pattern contrasted with that observed in the PFC. The magnitude of task selectivity observed was comparable immediately following a task switch and later in the task block. Thus, the magnitude of ACC selectivity varied with the increase in task demands and thus control requirements imposed by the task switch, while such changes were absent in PFC neurons. These findings are inconsistent with a strict conflict monitoring interpretation on two counts. First, differences in ACC selectivity were observed during the response preparation period in response to changes in control requirements. Such differences would not be expected in a structure carrying out a purely evaluative role. Second, conflict monitoring would predict that changes in ACC activity should result in concomitant changes in PFC activity. The very different patterns of activity observed suggest that this is not the case. To further investigate this, and the behavioural relevance of such task-selective signals, the authors compared the activity of PFC and ACC neurons on correct trials, trials on which the monkeys made performance errors, and correct trials following errors. In both PFC and ACC, task selectivity was significantly lower on error than correct trials, consistent with a role of such activity in task performance. On trials immediately following a performance error, a different pattern of results emerged. Selectivity of ACC neurons was enhanced on the first trial following a performance error, while selectivity of PFC neurons was not. According to the conflict-monitoring hypothesis, performance errors should be signalled by the ACC and lead to an enhancement of PFC activity on the following trial. This was not the case. Instead, a neural correlate of a change in control following performance errors was observed in the ACC itself. Taken together, these findings suggest that the ACC is strongly recruited to deal with increases in task demands, and that it could act to engage control itself, rather than performing a strictly evaluative function. Although it is clear that ACC signals are not sufficient to initiate saccades, there are extensive connections to other cortical and subcortical areas within the oculomotor system by which it could modulate the activity of the saccade network. Further studies will be necessary to determine whether ACC control signals are sent directly to subcortical structures such as the SC.

Supplementary motor area and pre-supplementary motor area

The SMA is another frontal cortical area located in the medial wall of the cerebral hemispheres that has been associated with high-level control of motor function. The SMA is located in the medial portion of Brodmann's area 6, immediately adjacent to cingulate cortex (Fig. 15.1). The division between these two areas has been placed in the middle portion of the dorsal bank of the cingulate sulcus (Dum and Strick, 1991; Luppino, et al., 2003). This area was originally defined by electrical stimulation studies that revealed that movements of the limbs and body could be evoked in a topographically organized fashion (Luppino, et al., 2003; Picard and Strick, 1996; Tanji, 1994). Similar to cingulate cortex, this area has been subdivided into a rostral zone with a more strongly cognitive function, the pre-SMA, and a caudal zone more closely related to motor execution, the SMA proper (Picard and Strick, 1996; Tanji, 1994, 1996). As in cingulate cortex, the genu of the arcuate sulcus provides a rough landmark for this division (Picard and Strick, 1996). Evidence in support of this division has been provided by differences in cyotoarchitecture (Matelli et al., 1991; Zilles, et al., 1995), connectivity (Dum and Strick, 1991), and neurophysiological properties (Matsuzaka et al., 1992). For example, the SMA proper has direct connections to primary motor cortex, and the spinal cord (Dum and Strick, 1991; Hummelsheim et al., 1986), pattern of connectivity typical of motor areas. In contrast, the pre-SMA is not directly connected to motor areas, but sends and receives direct projections from the anterior cingulate and prefrontal cortices (Luppino et al., 1993; Wang et al., 2005), consistent with a more modulatory, cognitive role. In addition, single neuron recordings in pre-SMA and SMA have demonstrated that SMA neurons display changes in activity closely related to movement onset (Alexander and Crutcher, 1990), while the activity of pre-SMA neurons is more closely linked to cognitive aspects of motor tasks including preparatory set (Hoshi and Tanji, 2004), changing ongoing behaviour (Shima et al., 1996), and movement sequencing (Shima and Tanji, 2000).

In contrast to other frontal cortical areas such as the FEF, SEF, and PFC, conflicting evidence exists regarding the presence of direct projections from the pre-SMA to the SC and brainstem oculomotor structures (Fries, 1985; Leichnetz, 1981). Microstimulation of the pre-SMA does not evoke eye movements (Luppino, et al., 1991; Matsuzaka, et al., 1992), suggesting that this area is only indirectly related to the control of saccades. In spite of the distant role of the pre-SMA in oculomotor control, both imaging studies in humans (Curtis and D'Esposito, 2003; Merriam, et al., 2001), and single neuron recordings in monkeys (Isoda and Tanji, 2004; Schall, 1991b) have demonstrated activity changes in relation to saccadic eye movements in this region. Further, Isoda (2005) demonstrated that microstimulation of the preSMA, applied at different times during a delayed saccade task, resulted in changes in saccadic reaction times. Thus, although saccades cannot be directly evoked by stimulation of this area, it does appear to play a causal role in modulation of saccade plans already in progress. Based on these findings, the large body of evidence supporting a role of the pre-SMA in cognitive aspects of limb motor control (Tanji, 1994), and the fact that pre-SMA neurons have been shown to exhibit activity changes in relation to movements of the eyes, arm, or both effectors (Fuji et al., 2002), it has been suggested that the pre-SMA plays a general purpose, effector non-selective, role in the control of behaviour (Isoda and Tanji, 2004; Picard and Strick, 2001).

One high level form of control that has been linked to the pre-SMA is the ability to change ongoing movements. Several studies have demonstrated modulations of activity in single pre-SMA neurons in relation to changing the direction of forthcoming arm movements (Matsuzaka and Tanji, 1996), or changing a sequence of movements (Shima, et al., 1996). Based on the hypothesis of 'effector non-selectivity' it would be predicted that the pre-SMA plays a similar role in oculomotor control. Isoda and Hikosaka, (2007) investigated this possibility. They recorded single pre-SMA neurons while monkeys performed a saccade overriding task in which they were instructed to saccade to one of two stimuli depending upon the colour of a centrally presented instruction cue. Trials on which the instruction colour was the same as the previous trial were classified as 'non-switch' while those on which the instruction colour changed were classified as 'switch' trials. The monkeys' behaviour in this task showed a behavioural cost of the instruction change; their saccadic reaction times were slower on 'switch' than 'non-switch trials'. A substantial number of pre-SMA neurons reflected this behavioural difference. Many showed robust differences in activity between switch and non-switch trials. Moreover, the timing of this 'switch' signal was critical to correct performance in the task. The 'switch' signal preceded saccade onset on correct trials, but occurred after saccade onset on trials in which the animals made performance errors. Finally, switching was facilitated when microstimulation was delivered concurrently with presentation of the instruction cue, providing support for a causal role of pre-SMA activity in behavioural switching. These data demonstrate that the pre-SMA plays a distinct role in switching saccades, and together with single neuron recordings during tasks involving limb movements provide support for the notion that the pre-SMA is involved in the ongoing control of behaviour in an effector non-selective manner. Although this area does not have strong or direct projections to oculomotor structures, it does have substantial projections to the basal ganglia (Parent and Hazrati, 1995). It has been hypothesized that the pre-SMA could act to modulate saccades by the so called 'hyperdirect' pathway, through which it is polysynaptically linked to the SC via the substantia nigra pars reticulata (SNr) and subthalamic nucleus (STN) (Nambu et al., 2002). This conceptualization has been supported by the finding that STN neurons exhibit similar 'switch' related activity to that observed in pre-SMA neurons in the same oculomotor overriding task (Isoda and Hikosaka, 2008).

Summary

Since Ferrier's pioneering investigation of the functions of frontal cortical areas in motor control, our understanding of the role of frontal cortex in saccade control has expanded immensely. In Ferrier's hands, only a relatively small portion of the frontal cortex seemed to be devoted to direct oculomotor control with the remainder lying dormant and speculatively described as 'inhibitory motor'. In the last 25 years, sophisticated behavioural paradigms combined with advanced neurophysiological techniques have been brought to bear on the problem of identifying the role of frontal cortex in the control of behaviour and saccadic control in particular. In relation to eye movements, there appears to be a continuum from FEF, which plays a direct role in saccadic initiation to areas like SEF, PFC, ACC, and pre-SMA that enables flexible control of eye movements by modulating activity in the oculomotor system on the basis of cognitive processes. Ultimately, a more complete understanding of the function of these frontal cortical areas in eye movement control hinges on determining the way in which activity in these areas influences processing in downstream oculomotor areas such as the superior colliculus.

References

Alexander, G.E. and Crutcher, M.D. (1990). Preparation for movement: neural representations of intended direction in three motor areas of the monkey. *Journal of Neurophysiology*, **64**(1), 133–150.

Allport, A., Styles, E.A., Hsieh, S., Umilta, C., and Moscovitch, M. (1994). Shifting intentional set: exploring the dynamic control of tasks *Attention and Performance XV* (p. 421). Cambridge, MA: MIT Press.

Amador, N., Schlag-Rey, M., and Schlag, J. (2003). Primate antisaccade ii. supplementary eye field neuronal activity predicts correct performance. *Journal of Neurophysiology*, **91**, 1672–1689.

Amiez, C., Kostopoulos, P., Champod, A.S., and Petrides, M. (2006a). Local morphology predicts functional organization of the dorsal premotor region in the human brain. *Journal of Neuroscience*, **26**(10), 2724–2731.

Amiez, C., Joseph, J.P., and Procyk, E. (2006b). Reward encoding in the monkey anterior cingulate cortex. *Cerebral Cortex*, **16**(7), 1040–1055.

Armstrong, K.M. and Moore, T. (2007). Rapid enhancement of visual cortical response discriminability by microstimulation of the frontal eye field. *Proceedings of the National Academy of Sciences U S A*, **104**(22), 9499–9504.

Armstrong, K.M., Fitzgerald, J.K., and Moore, T. (2006). Changes in visual receptive fields with microstimulation of frontal cortex. *Neuron*, **50**(5), 791–798.

Asaad, W.F., Rainer, G., and Miller, E.K. (1998). Neural activity in the primate prefrontal cortex during associative learning. *Neuron*, **21**(6), 1399.

Asaad, W.F., Rainer, G., and Miller, E.K. (2000). Task-specific neural activity in the primate prefrontal cortex. *Journal of Neurophysiology*, **84**(1), 451.

Baker, J.T., Patel, G.H., Corbetta, M., and Snyder, L.H. (2005). Distribution of activity across the monkey cerebral cortical surface, thalamus and midbrain during rapid, visually guided saccades. *Cerebral Cortex*, **16**, 447–459.

Barbas, H. (2000). Complementary roles of prefrontal cortical regions in cognition, memory, and emotion in primates. *Advances in Neurology*, **84**, 87–110.

Barbas, H. and Mesulam, M.M. (1985). Cortical afferent input to the principalis region of the rhesus monkey. *Neuroscience*, **15**(3), 619–637.

Barbas, H., Medalla, M., Alade, O., Suski, J., Zikopoulos, B., and Lera, P. (2005). Relationship of prefrontal connections to inhibitory systems in superior temporal areas in the rhesus monkey. *Cerebral Cortex*, **15**(9), 1356–1370.

Bates, J.F. and Goldman-Rakic, P.S. (1993). Prefrontal connections of medial motor areas in the rhesus monkey. *Journal of Comparative Neurology*, **336**(2), 211.

Bizzi, E. (1968). Discharge of frontal eye field neurons during saccadic and following eye movements in unanesthetized monkeys. *Experimental Brain Research*, **6**(1), 69–80.

Bizzi, E. and Schiller, P.H. (1970). Single unit activity in the frontal eye fields of unanesthetized monkeys during eye and head movement. *Experimental Brain Research*, **10**(2), 150–158.

Boch, R.A. and Goldberg, M.E. (1989). Participation of prefrontal neurons in the preparation of visually guided eye movements in the rhesus monkey. *Journal of Neurophysiology*, **61**(5), 1064.

Bon, L. and Lucchetti, C. (1992). The dorsomedial frontal cortex of the macaca monkey: fixation and saccade-related activity. *Experimental Brain Research*, **89**(3), 571.

Botvinick, M.M. Braver, T.S., Barch, D.M., Carter, C.S., and Cohen, J.D. (2001). Conflict monitoring and cognitive control. *Psychology Review*, **108**(3), 624.

Botvinick, M.M, Cohen, J.D., Carter, C.S. (2004). Conflict monitoring and anterior cingulate cortex: an update. *Trends in Cognitive Sciences*, **8**(12), 539–546.

Brinkman, C. and Porter, R. (1979). Supplementary motor area in the monkey: activity of neurons during performance of a learned motor task. *Journal of Neurophysiology*, **42**, 681–709.

Brown, J.W., Hanes, D.P., Schall, J.D., and Stuphorn, V. (2008). Relation of frontal eye field activity to saccade initiation during a countermanding task. *Experimental Brain Research*, **190**(2), 135–151.

Bruce, C.J. and Goldberg, M.E. (1985). Primate frontal eye fields. I. Single neurons discharging before saccades. *Journal of Neurophysiology*, **53**(3), 603.

Bruce, C.J., Goldberg, M.E., Bushnell, M.C., and Stanton, G.B. (1985). Primate frontal eye fields. II. Physiological and anatomical correlates of electrically evoked eye movements. *Journal of Neurophysiology*, **54**(3), 714–734.

Buttner-Ennever, J.A. and Horn, A.K. (1997). Anatomical substrates of oculomotor control. *Current Opinion in Neurobiology*, **7**(6), 872–879.

Carter, C.S. and van Veen, V. (2007). Anterior cingulate cortex and conflict detection: an update of theory and data. *Cognitive, Affective, and Behavioral Neuroscience*, **7**(4), 367–379.

Carter, C.S., Macdonald, A.M., Botvinick, M., Ross, L.L., Stenger, V.A., Noll, D., *et al.* (2000). Parsing executive processes: strategic vs. evaluative functions of the anterior cingulate cortex. *Proceedings of the National Academy of Sciences U S A*, **97**(4), 1944–1948.

Chen, L.L. and Wise, S.P. (1995). Neuronal activity in the supplementary eye field during acquisition of conditional oculomotor associations. *Journal of Neurophysiology*, **73**(3), 1101–1121.

Chen, L.L. and Wise, S.P. (1996). Evolution of directional preferences in the supplementary eye field during acquisition of conditional oculomotor associations. *Journal of Neuroscience*, **16**(9), 3067.

Cohen, B. and Henn, V. (1972). Unit activity in the pontine reticular formation associated with eye movements. *Brain Research*, **46**, 403–410.

Condy, C., Wattiez, N., Rivaud-Pechoux, S., Tremblay, L., and Gaymard, B. (2007). Antisaccade deficit after inactivation of the principal sulcus in monkeys. *Cerebral Cortex*, **17**, 221–229.

Constantinidis, C. and Wang, X.J. (2004). A neural circuit basis for spatial working memory. *Neuroscientist*, **10**(6), 553–565.

Constantinidis, C., Franowicz, M.N., and Goldman-Rakic, P.S. (2001a). Coding specificity in cortical microcircuits: a multiple-electrode analysis of primate prefrontal cortex. *Journal of Neuroscience*, **21**(10), 3646.

Constantinidis, C., Franowicz, M.N., and Goldman-Rakic, P.S. (2001b). The sensory nature of mnemonic representation in the primate prefrontal cortex. *Nature Neuroscience*, **4**(3), 311.

Creutzfeldt, O.D. (1993). *Cortex Cerebri*. Goettingen: Springer.

Crowne, D.P., Yeo, C.H., and Russell, I.S. (1981). The effects of unilateral frontal eye field lesions in the monkey: visual-motor guidance and avoidance behaviour. *Behavioural Brain Research*, **2**(2), 165–187.

Curtis, C.E. and D'Esposito, M. (2003). Success and failure suppressing reflexive behavior. *Journal of Cognitive Neuroscience*, **15**(3), 409–418.

Deng, S., Goldberg, M.E., Segraves, M.A., Ungerleider, L.G., and Mishkin, M. (Eds). (1986). *Removal of frontal eye field impairs ability to make saccades to remembered targets*. New York: Pergamon.

Dias, E.C., Kiesau, M., and Segraves, M.A. (1995). Acute activation and inactivation of macaque frontal eye field with GABA-related drugs. *Journal of Neurophysiology*, **74**(6), 2744.

Dias, R., Robbins, T.W., and Roberts, A.C. (1996). Primate analogue of the Wisconsin Card Sorting Test: effects of excitotoxic lesions of the prefrontal cortex in the marmoset. *Behavioural Neuroscience*, **110**(5), 872.

Distel, H. and Fries, W. (1982). Contralateral cortical projections to the superior colliculus in the macaque monkey. *Experimental Brain Research*, **48**(2), 157–162.

Dosenbach, N.U., Visscher, K.M., Palmer, E.D., Miezin, F.M., Wenger, K.K., Kang, H.C., *et al.* (2006). A core system for the implementation of task sets. *Neuron*, **50**(5), 799–812.

Dum, R.P. and Strick, P.L. (1991). The origin of corticospinal projections from the premotor areas in the frontal lobe. *Journal of Neuroscience*, **11**(3), 667–689.

Dum, R.P. and Strick, P.L. (1992). Medial wall motor areas and skeletomotor control. *Current Opinion in Neurobiology*, **2**(6), 836–839.

Elsley, J.K., Nagy, B., Cushing, S.L., and Corneil, B.D. (2007). Widespread presaccadic recruitment of neck muscles by stimulation of the primate frontal eye fields. *Journal of Neurophysiology*, **98**(3), 1333–1354.

Elston, G.N., Benavides-Piccione, R., and Defelipe, J. (2005). A study of pyramidal cell structure in the cingulate cortex of the macaque monkey with comparative notes on inferotemporal and primary visual cortex. *Cerebral Cortex*, **15**(1), 64–73.

Emeric, E.E., Brown, J.W., Leslie, M., Pouget, P., Stuphorn, V., and Schall, J.D. (2008). Performance monitoring local field potentials in the medial frontal cortex of primates: anterior cingulate cortex. *Journal of Neurophysiology*, **99**(2), 759–772.

Evarts, E.V., Shinoda, Y., and Wise, S.P. (1984). *Neurophysiological approaches to higher brain function*. New York: Wiley.

Everling, S. and Fischer, B. (1998). The antisaccade: a review of basic research and clinical studies. *Neuropsychologia*, **36**(9), 885–899.

Everling, S. and Munoz, D.P. (2000). Neuronal correlates for preparatory set associated with pro-saccades and anti-saccades in the primate frontal eye field. *Journal of Neuroscience*, **20**(1), 387–400.

Everling, S. and Desouza, J.F. (2005). Rule-dependent activity for prosaccades and antisaccades in the primate prefrontal cortex. *Journal of Cognitive Neuroscience*, **17**, 1483–1496.

Everling, S., Dorris, M.C., and Munoz, D.P. (1998b). Reflex suppression in the anti-saccade task is dependent on prestimulus neural processes. *Journal of Neurophysiology*, **80**(3), 1584–1589.

Everling, S., Paré, M., Dorris, M.C., and Munoz, D.P. (1998a). Comparison of the discharge characteristics of brain stem omnipause neurons and superior colliculus fixation neurons in monkey: implications for control of fixation and saccade behavior. *Journal of Neurophysiology*, **79**(2), 511.

Everling, S., Dorris, M.C., Klein, R.M., and Munoz, D.P. (1999). Role of primate superior colliculus in preparation and execution of anti-saccades and pro-saccades. *Journal of Neuroscience*, **19**(7), 2740–2754.

Everling, S., Tinsley, C.J., Gaffan, D., and Duncan, J. (2002). Filtering of neural signals by focused attention in the monkey prefrontal cortex. *Nature Neuroscience*, **5**(7), 671.

Falkenstein, M., Hohnsbein, J., Hoormann, J., and Blanke, L. (1991a). Effects of crossmodal divided attention on late ERP components. II. Error processing in choice reaction tasks. *Electroencephalography and Clinical Neurophysiology*, **78**(6), 447–455.

Falkenstein, M., Hohnsbein, J., Hoormann, J., and Blanke, L. (1991b). Effects of crossmodal divided attention on late ERP components. II. Error processing in choice reaction tasks. *Electroencephalography and Clinical Neurophysiology*, **78**(6), 447.

Ferraina, S., Paré, M., and Wurtz, R.H. (2000). Disparity sensitivity of frontal eye field neurons. *Journal of Neurophysiology*, **83**(1), 625–629.

Ferrier, D. (1876). *The functions of the brain*. London: Smith, Elder and Co.

Ford, K.A., Gati, J.S., Menon, R.S., and Everling, S. (2009). BOLD fMRI activation for anti-saccades in nonhuman primates. *Neuroimage*, **45**(2), 470–476.

Freedman, D.J., Riesenhuber, M., Poggio, T., and Miller, E.K. (2001). Categorical representation of visual stimuli in the primate prefrontal cortex. *Science*, **291**(5502), 312.

Fries, W. (1984). Cortical projections to the superior colliculus in the macaque monkey: a retrograde study using horseradish peroxidase. *Journal of Comparative Neurology*, **230**(1), 55.

Fries, W. (1985). Inputs from motor and premotor cortex to the superior colliculus of the macaque monkey. *Behavioural Brain Research*, **18**(2), 95–105.

Fujii, N., Mushiake, H., Tamai, M., and Tanji, J. (1995). Microstimulation of the supplementary eye field during saccade preparation. *Neuroreport*, **6**(18), 2565.

Fujii, N., Mushiake, H., and Tanji, J. (2002). Distribution of eye- and arm-movement-related neuronal activity in the SEF and in the SMA and pre-SMA of monkeys. *Journal of Neurophysiology*, **87**(4), 2158–2166.

Funahashi, S., Bruce, C.J., and Goldman-Rakic, P.S. (1989). Mnemonic coding of visual space in the monkey's dorsolateral prefrontal cortex. *Journal of Neurophysiology*, **61**(2), 331.

Funahashi, S., Bruce, C.J., and Goldman-Rakic, P.S. (1990). Visuospatial coding in primate prefrontal neurons revealed by oculomotor paradigms. *Journal of Neurophysiology*, **63**(4), 814.

Funahashi, S., Bruce, C.J., and Goldman-Rakic, P.S. (1991). Neuronal activity related to saccadic eye movements in the monkey's dorsolateral prefrontal cortex. *Journal of Neurophysiology*, **65**(6), 1464.

Funahashi, S., Bruce, C.J., and Goldman-Rakic, P.S. (1993). Dorsolateral prefrontal lesions and oculomotor delayed-response performance: evidence for mnemonic 'scotomas'. *Journal of Neuroscience*, **13**(4), 1479.

Fuster, J.M. (1973). Unit activity in prefrontal cortex during delayed-response performance: neuronal correlates of transient memory. *Journal of Neurophysiology*, **36**(1), 61–78.

Fuster, J.M. (2008). *The prefrontal cortex*. London: Elsevier.

Fuster, J.M. and Alexander, G.E. (1971). Neuron activity related to short-term memory. *Science*, **173**(997), 652.

Gaymard, B., Rivaud, S., Cassarini, J.F., Dubard, T., Rancurel, G., Agid, Y., et al. (1998). Effects of anterior cingulate cortex lesions on ocular saccades in humans. *Experimental Brain Research*, **120**(2), 173–183.

Gehring, W.J., Coles, M.G., Meyer, D.E., and Donchin, E. (1995). A brain potential manifestation of error-related processing. *Electroencephalography and Clinical Neurophysiology Supplement*, **44**, 261.

Genovesio, A., Brasted, P.J., Mitz, A.R., and Wise, S.P. (2005). Prefrontal cortex activity related to abstract response strategies. *Neuron*, **47**(2), 307–320.

Goldberg, M.E. and Bushnell, M.C. (1981). Behavioral enhancement of visual responses in monkey cerebral cortex. II. Modulation in frontal eye fields specifically related to saccades. *Journal of Neurophysiology*, **46**(4), 773–787.

Goldberg, M.E., Bushnell, M.C., and Bruce, C.J. (1986). The effect of attentive fixation on eye movements evoked by electrical stimulation of the frontal eye fields. *Experimental Brain Research*, **61**(3), 579.

Goldman-Rakic, P.S. (1995). Cellular basis of working memory. *Neuron*, **14**(3), 477.

Goldman-Rakic, P.S. (1996). Regional and cellular fractionation of working memory. *Proceedings of the National Academy of Sciences U S A*, **93**(24), 13473.

Goldman, P.S. and Nauta, W.J. (1976). Autoradiographic demonstration of a projection from prefrontal association cortex to the superior colliculus in the rhesus monkey. *Brain Research*, **116**(1), 145.

Gould, H.J., 3rd, Cusick, C.G., Pons, T.P., and Kaas, J.H. (1986). The relationship of corpus callosum connections to electrical stimulation maps of motor, supplementary motor, and the frontal eye fields in owl monkeys. *Journal of Comparative Neurology*, **247**(3), 297–325.

Hanes, D.P. and Schall, J.D. (1996). Neural control of voluntary movement initiation. *Science*, **274**(5286), 427.

Hanes, D.P. and Wurtz, R.H. (2001). Interaction of the frontal eye field and superior colliculus for saccade generation. *Journal of Neurophysiology*, **85**(2), 804–815.

Hanes, D.P., Thompson, K.G., and Schall, J.D. (1995). Relationship of presaccadic activity in frontal eye field and supplementary eye field to saccade initiation in macaque: Poisson spike train analysis. *Experimental Brain Research*, **103**(1), 85.

Hasegawa, R., Sawaguchi, T., and Kubota, K. (1998). Monkey prefrontal neuronal activity coding the forthcoming saccade in an oculomotor delayed matching-to-sample task. *Journal of Neurophysiology*, **79**(1), 322.

Hasegawa, R.P., Peterson, B.W., and Goldberg, M.E. (2004). Prefrontal neurons coding suppression of specific saccades. *Neuron*, **43**(3), 415–425.

Holroyd, C.B. and Coles, M.G. (2002). The neural basis of human error processing: reinforcement learning, dopamine, and the error-related negativity. *Psychology Review*, **109**(4), 679–709.

Horlsey, V.A. and Schaefer, E.A. (1888). Experimental Researches in Cerebral Physiology. II. On the Muscular Contractions Which Are Evoked by Excitation of the Motor Tract. *Philosophical Transactions of the Royal Society B: Biological Science*, **39**, 404–409.

Hoshi, E. and Tanji, J. (2004). Differential roles of neuronal activity in the supplementary and presupplementary motor areas: from information retrieval to motor planning and execution. *Journal of Neurophysiology*, **92**(6), 3482–3499.

Hoshi, E., Sawamura, H., and Tanji, J. (2005). Neurons in the rostral cingulate motor area monitor multiple phases of visuomotor behavior with modest parametric selectivity. *Journal of Neurophysiology*, **94**(1), 640–656.

Huerta, M.F. and Kaas, J.H. (1990). Supplementary eye field as defined by intracortical microstimulation: connections in macaques. *Journal of Comparative Neurology*, **293**(2), 299–330.

Huerta, M.F., Krubitzer, L.A., and Kaas, J.H. (1986). Frontal eye field as defined by intracortical microstimulation in squirrel monkeys, owl monkeys, and macaque monkeys: I. Subcortical connections. *Journal of Comparative Neurology*, **253**(4), 415–439.

Huerta, M.F., Krubitzer, L.A., and Kaas, J.H. (1987). Frontal eye field as defined by intracortical microstimulation in squirrel monkeys, owl monkeys, and macaque monkeys. II. Cortical connections. *Journal of Comparative Neurology*, **265**(3), 332–361.

Hummelsheim, H., Wiesendanger, M., Bianchetti, M., Wiesendanger, R., and Macpherson, J. (1986). Further investigations of the efferent linkage of the supplementary motor area (SMA) with the spinal cord in the monkey. *Experimental Brain Research*, **65**(1), 75–82.

Isoda, M. (2005). Context-dependent stimulation effects on saccade initiation in the presupplementary motor area of the monkey. *Journal of Neurophysiology*, **93**(5), 3016–3022.

Isoda, M. and Hikosaka, O. (2007). Switching from automatic to controlled action by monkey medial frontal cortex. *Nature Neuroscience*, **10**(2), 240–248.

Isoda, M. and Hikosaka, O. (2008). Role for subthalamic nucleus neurons in switching from automatic to controlled eye movement. *Journal of Neuroscience*, **28**(28), 7209–7218.

Isoda, M. and Tanji, J. (2002). Cellular activity in the supplementary eye field during sequential performance of multiple saccades. *Journal of Neurophysiology*, **88**(6), 3541–3545.

Isoda, M. and Tanji, J. (2004). Participation of the primate presupplementary motor area in sequencing multiple saccades. *Journal of Neurophysiology*, **92**(1), 653–659.

Isomura, Y., Ito, Y., Akazawa, T., Nambu, A., and Takada, M. (2003). Neural coding of 'attention for action' and 'response selection' in primate anterior cingulate cortex. *Journal of Neuroscience*, **23**(22), 8002–8012.

Ito, S., Stuphorn, V., Brown, J.W., and Schall, J.D. (2003). Performance monitoring by the anterior cingulate cortex during saccade countermanding. *Science*, **302**(5642), 120–122.

Iversen, S.D. and Mishkin, M. (1970). Perseverative interference in monkeys following selective lesions of the inferior prefrontal convexity. *Experimental Brain Research*, **11**(4), 376–386.

Jacobsen, C.F. (1935). Functions of the frontal association area in primates. *Archives of Neurology and Psychiatry*, **33**, 558–569.

Johnston, K. and Everling, S. (2006). Monkey dorsolateral prefrontal cortex sends task-selective signals directly to the superior colliculus. *Journal of Neuroscience*, **26**(48), 12471–12478.

Johnston, K. and Everling, S. (2009). Task-relevant output signals are sent from monkey dorsolateral prefrontal cortex to the superior colliculus during a visuospatial working memory task. *Journal of Cognitive Neuroscience*, **21**(5), 1023–1038.

Johnston, K., Levin, H.M., Koval, M.J., and Everling, S. (2007). Top-down control-signal dynamics in anterior cingulate and prefrontal cortex neurons following task switching. *Neuron*, **53**(3), 453–462.

Johnston, K., De Souza, J.F.X., and Everling, S. (2009). Monkey prefrontal cortical pyramidal and putative interneurons exhibit differential patterns of activity between pro- and antisaccade tasks. *Journal of Neuroscience*, 29(17), 5516–5524.

Joseph, J.P. and Barone, P. (1987). Prefrontal unit activity during a delayed oculomotor task in the monkey. *Experimental Brain Research*, **67**(3), 460.

Keating, E.G. and Gooley, S.G. (1988). Saccadic disorders caused by cooling the superior colliculus or the frontal eye field, or from combined lesions of both structures. *Brain Research*, **438**(1–2), 247.

Keller, E.L. (1974). Participation of medial pontine reticular formation in eye movement generation in monkey. *Journal of Neurophysiology*, **37**(2), 316.

Kennerley, S.W., Walton, M.E., Behrens, T.E., Buckley, M.J., and Rushworth, M.F. (2006). Optimal decision making and the anterior cingulate cortex. *Nature Neuroscience*, **9**(7), 940–947.

Kerns, J.G., Cohen, J.D., MacDonald, A.W., 3rd, Cho, R.Y., Stenger, V.A., and Carter, C.S. (2004). Anterior cingulate conflict monitoring and adjustments in control. *Science*, **303**(5660), 1023–1026.

Kim, J.N. and Shadlen, M.N. (1999). Neural correlates of a decision in the dorsolateral prefrontal cortex of the macaque. *Nature Neuroscience*, **2**(2), 176.

Kim, Y.G., Badler, J.B., and Heinen, S.J. (2005). Trajectory interpretation by supplementary eye field neurons during ocular baseball. *Journal of Neurophysiology*, **94**(2), 1385–1391.

Knight, T.A. and Fuchs, A.F. (2007). Contribution of the frontal eye field to gaze shifts in the head-unrestrained monkey: effects of microstimulation. *Journal of Neurophysiology*, **97**(1), 618–634.

Kojima, S. (1980). Prefrontal unit activity in the monkey: relation to visual stimuli and movements. *Experimental Neurology*, **69**(1), 110–123.

Komatsu, H. and Suzuki, H. (1985). Projections from the functional subdivisions of the frontal eye field to the superior colliculus in the monkey. *Brain Research*, **327**(1–2), 324–327.

Koyama, M., Hasegawa, I., Osada, T., Adachi, Y., Nakahara, K., and Miyashita, Y. (2004). Functional magnetic resonance imaging of macaque monkeys performing visually guided saccade tasks: comparison of cortical eye fields with humans. *Neuron*, **41**(5), 795.

Kunzle, H. and Akert, K. (1977). Efferent connections of cortical, area 8 (frontal eye field) in Macaca fascicularis. A reinvestigation using the autoradiographic technique. *Journal of Comparative Neurology*, **173**(1), 147–164.

Kunzle, H., Akert, K., and Wurtz, R.H. (1976). Projection of area 8 (frontal eye field) to superior colliculus in the monkey. An autoradiographic study. *Brain Research*, **117**(3), 487–492.

Lebedev, M.A., Messinger, A., Kralik, J.D., and Wise, S.P. (2004). Representation of attended versus remembered locations in prefrontal cortex. *PLoS Biology*, **2**(11), e365.

Leichnetz, G.R. (1981). The prefrontal cortico-oculomotor trajectories in the monkey. *Journal of the Neurological Sciences*, **49**(3), 387–396.

Leichnetz, G.R., Spencer, R.F., and Smith, D.J. (1984). Cortical projections to nuclei adjacent to the oculomotor complex in the medial dien-mesencephalic tegmentum in the monkey. *Journal of Comparative Neurology*, **228**(3), 359–387.

Leichnetz, G.R., Spencer, R.F., Hardy, S.G., and Astruc, J. (1981). The prefrontal corticotectal projection in the monkey; an anterograde and retrograde horseradish peroxidase study. *Neuroscience*, **6**(6), 1023.

Levinsohn, G. (1909). Über die Beziehungen der Grosshirnrinde beim Affebn zu den Bewegungen des Auges. *Archiv für Opthalmologie*, **71**, 313–378.

Leyton, A.S.F. and Sherrington, C.S. (1917). Observations on the excitable cortex of the chimpanzee, orang-utan, and gorilla. *Quarterly Journal of Experimental Physiology*, **11**, 135–222.

Logan, G.D., Cowan, W.B., and Davis, K.A. (1984). On the ability to inhibit simple and choice reaction time responses: a model and a method. *Journal of Experimental Psychology Human Perception and Performance*, **10**(2), 276.

Logothetis, N.K., Pauls, J., Augath, M., Trinath, T., and Oeltermann, A. (2001). Neurophysiological investigation of the basis of the fMRI signal. *Nature*, **412**(6843), 150–157.

Luna, B., Thulborn, K.R., Strojwas, M.H., McCurtain, B.J., Berman, R.A., Genovese, C.R., *et al.* (1998). Dorsal cortical regions subserving visually guided saccades in humans: an fMRI study. *Cerebral Cortex*, **8**(1), 40.

Luppino, G., Matelli, M., Camarda, R., and Rizzolatti, G. (1993). Corticocortical connections of area F3 (SMA-proper) and area F6 (pre-SMA) in the macaque monkey. *Journal of Comparative Neurology*, **338**(1), 114–140.

Luppino, G., Rozzi, S., Calzavara, R., and Matelli, M. (2003). Prefrontal and agranular cingulate projections to the dorsal premotor areas F2 and F7 in the macaque monkey. *European Journal of Neuroscience*, **17**(3), 559–578.

Luppino, G., Matelli, M., Camarda, R.M., Gallese, V., and Rizzolatti, G. (1991). Multiple representations of body movements in mesial area 6 and the adjacent cingulate cortex: an intracortical microstimulation study in the macaque monkey. *Journal of Comparative Neurology*, **311**(4), 463–482.

Luschei, E.S. and Fuchs, A.F. (1972). Activity of brain stem neurons during eye movements of alert monkeys. *Journal of Neurophysiology*, **35**(4), 445.

Lynch, J.C. (1992). Saccade initiation and latency deficits after combined lesions of the frontal and posterior eye fields in monkeys. *Journal of Neurophysiology*, **68**(5), 1913.

Lynch, J.C., Hoover, J.E., and Strick, P.L. (1994). Input to the primate frontal eye field from the substantia nigra, superior colliculus, and dentate nucleus demonstrated by transneuronal transport. *Experimental Brain Research*, **100**(1), 181.

MacAvoy, M.G., Gottlieb, J.P., and Bruce, C.J. (1991). Smooth-pursuit eye movement representation in the primate frontal eye field. *Cerebral Cortex*, **1**(1), 95.

MacDonald, A.W., III, Cohen, J.D., Stenger, V.A., and Carter, C.S. (2000). Dissociating the role of the dorsolateral prefrontal and anterior cingulate cortex in cognitive control. *Science*, **288**(5472), 1835.

Maioli, M.G., Squatrito, S., Galletti, C., Battaglini, P.P., and Sanseverino, E. R. (1983). Cortico-cortical connections from the visual region of the superior temporal sulcus to frontal eye field in the macaque. *Brain Research*, **265**(2), 294–299.

Mann, S.E., Thau, R., and Schiller, P.H. (1988). Conditional task-related responses in monkey dorsomedial frontal cortex. *Experimental Brain Research*, **69**(3), 460–468.

Matelli, M., Luppino, G., and Rizzolatti, G. (1991). Architecture of superior and mesial area 6 and the adjacent cingulate cortex in the macaque monkey. *Journal of Comparative Neurology*, **311**(4), 445–462.

Matsuzaka, Y. and Tanji, J. (1996). Changing directions of forthcoming arm movements: neuronal activity in the presupplementary and supplementary motor area of monkey cerebral cortex. *Journal of Neurophysiology*, **76**(4), 2327–2342.

Matsuzaka, Y., Aizawa, H., and Tanji, J. (1992). A motor area rostral to the supplementary motor area (presupplementary motor area) in the monkey: neuronal activity during a learned motor task. *Journal of Neurophysiology*, **68**(3), 653–662.

Merriam, E.P., Colby, C.L., Thulborn, K.R., Luna, B., Olson, C.R., and Sweeney, J.A. (2001). Stimulus-response incompatibility activates cortex proximate to three eye fields. *Neuroimage*, **13**(5), 794–800.

Miller, E.K. and Cohen, J.D. (2001). An integrative theory of prefrontal cortex function. *Annual Review of Neuroscience*, **24**, 167.

Miller, E.K., Erickson, C.A., and Desimone, R. (1996). Neural mechanisms of visual working memory in prefrontal cortex of the macaque. *Journal of Neuroscience*, **16**(16), 5154.

Milner, B. (1963). Effects of different brain lesions on card sorting. *Archives of Neurology*, **9**, 90.

Mishkin, M. (1964). Perseveration of central sets after frontal lesions in monkeys. In J.M. Warren and K. Akert (eds.) *The frontal granular cortex and behavior* (pp. 219–241). New York: MacGraw Hill.

Mitz, A.R. and Godschalk, M. (1989). Eye-movement representation in the frontal lobe of rhesus monkeys. *Neuroscience Letters*, **106**(1–2), 157–162.

Moore, T. and Armstrong, K.M. (2003). Selective gating of visual signals by microstimulation of frontal cortex. *Nature*, **421**(6921), 370–373.

Moschovakis, A.K., Gregoriou, G.G., Ugolini, G., Doldan, M., Graf, W., Guldin, W., *et al.* (2004). Oculomotor areas of the primate frontal lobes: a transneuronal transfer of rabies virus and [14C]-2-deoxyglucose functional imaging study. *Journal of Neuroscience*, **24**(25), 5726–5740.

Moschovakis, A.K., and Highstein, S.M. (1994). The anatomy and physiology of primate neurons that control rapid eye movements. *Annual Review of Neuroscience*, **17**, 465–488.

Mott, F.W. and Schaefer, E.A. (1890). On associated eye-movements produced by cortical faradization of the monkey's brain. *Brain*, **13**, 165–173.

Munoz, D.P. and Istvan, P.J. (1998). Lateral inhibitory interactions in the intermediate layers of the monkey superior colliculus. *Journal of Neurophysiology*, **79**(3), 1193.

Munoz, D.P. and Everling, S. (2004). Look away: the anti-saccade task and the voluntary control of eye movement. *Nature Reviews Neuroscience*, **5**(3), 218–228.

Munoz, D.P., Dorris, M.C., Paré, M., and Everling, S. (2000). On your mark, get set: brainstem circuitry underlying saccadic initiation. *Canadian Journal of Physiology and Pharmacology*, **78**(11), 934.

Mushiake, H., Fujii, N., and Tanji, J. (1996). Visually guided saccade versus eye-hand reach: contrasting neuronal activity in the cortical supplementary and frontal eye fields. *Journal of Neurophysiology*, **75**(5), 2187.

Nakamura, K., Roesch, M.R., and Olson, C.R. (2005). Neuronal activity in macaque SEF and ACC during performance of tasks involving conflict. *Journal of Neurophysiology*, **93**(2), 884–908.

Nambu, A., Tokuno, H., and Takada, M. (2002). Functional significance of the cortico-subthalamo-pallidal 'hyperdirect' pathway. *Neuroscience Research*, **43**(2), 111–117.

Nauta, W.J. (1971). The problem of the frontal lobe: a reinterpretation. *Journal of Psychiatric Research*, **8**(3), 167–187.

Nieder, A., Freedman, D.J., and Miller, E.K. (2002). Representation of the quantity of visual items in the primate prefrontal cortex. *Science*, **297**(5587), 1708–1711.

Nieder, A. and Miller, E.K. (2003). Coding of cognitive magnitude: compressed scaling of numerical information in the primate prefrontal cortex. *Neuron*, **37**(1), 149–157.

Nigg, J.T. (2000). On inhibition/disinhibition in developmental psychopathology: views from cognitive and personality psychology and a working inhibition taxonomy. *Psychological Bulletin*, **126**(2), 220–246.

Olson, C.R. and Gettner, S.N. (1995). Object-centered direction selectivity in the macaque supplementary eye field. *Science*, **269**(5226), 985–988.

Olson, C.R., Musil, S.Y., and Goldberg, M.E. (1996). Single neurons in posterior cingulate cortex of behaving macaque: eye movement signals. *Journal of Neurophysiology*, **76**(5), 3285.

Orban, G.A., Claeys, K., Nelissen, K., Smans, R., Sunaert, S., Todd, J.T., *et al.* (2006). Mapping the parietal cortex of human and non-human primates. *Neuropsychologia*, **44**(13), 2647–2667.

Parent, A. and Hazrati, L.N. (1995). Functional anatomy of the basal ganglia. I. The cortico-basal ganglia-thalamo-cortical loop. *Brain Research. Brain Research Reviews*, **20**(1), 91–127.

Parthasarathy, H.B., Schall, J.D., and Graybiel, A.M. (1992). Distributed but convergent ordering of corticostriatal projections: analysis of the frontal eye field and the supplementary eye field in the macaque monkey. *Journal of Neuroscience*, **12**(11), 4468.

Passingham, R.E. (1985). Memory of monkeys (Macaca mulatta) with lesions in prefrontal cortex. *Behavioural Neuroscience*, **99**(1), 3–21.

Paus, T. (1996). Location and function of the human frontal eye-field: a selective review. *Neuropsychologia*, **34**(6), 475–483.

Paus, T. (2001). Primate anterior cingulate cortex: where motor control, drive and cognition interface. *Nature Reviews Neuroscience*, **2**(6), 417–424.

Paus, T., Petrides, M., Evans, A.C., and Meyer, E. (1993). Role of the human anterior cingulate cortex in the control of oculomotor, manual, and speech responses: a positron emission tomography study. *Journal of Neurophysiology*, **70**(2), 453.

Penfield, W. and Boldrey, E. (1937). Somatic motor and sensory representation in the cerebral cortex of man as studied by electrical stimulation. *Brain*, **60**, 389–443.

Petit, L., Orssaud, C., Tzourio, N., Salamon, G., Mazoyer, B., and Berthoz, A. (1993). PET study of voluntary saccadic eye movements in humans: basal ganglia-thalamocortical system and cingulate cortex involvement. *Journal of Neurophysiology*, **69**(4), 1009–1017.

Petrides, M. and Pandya, D.N. (1984). Projections to the frontal cortex from the posterior parietal region in the rhesus monkey. *Journal of Comparative Neurology*, **228**(1), 105–116.

Petrides, M. and Pandya, D.N. (1999). Dorsolateral prefrontal cortex: comparative cytoarchitectonic analysis in the human and the macaque brain and corticocortical connection patterns. *European Journal of Neuroscience*, **11**(3), 1011–1036.

Petrides, M. and Pandya, D.N. (2002). Comparative cytoarchitectonic analysis of the human and the macaque ventrolateral prefrontal cortex and corticocortical connection patterns in the monkey. *Eur.Journal of Neuroscience*, **16**(2), 291–310.

Picard, N. and Strick, P.L. (1996). Motor areas of the medial wall: a review of their location and functional activation. *Cerebral Cortex*, **6**(3), 342–353.

Picard, N. and Strick, P.L. (2001). Imaging the premotor areas. *Current Opinion in Neurobiology*, **11**(6), 663–672.

Ploner, C.J., Gaymard, B.M., Rivaud-Pechoux, S., and Pierrot-Deseilligny, C. (2005). The prefrontal substrate of reflexive saccade inhibition in humans. *Biological Psychiatry*, **57**(10), 1159–1165.

Pouget, P., Emeric, E.E., Stuphorn, V., Reis, K., and Schall, J.D. (2005). Chronometry of visual responses in frontal eye field, supplementary eye field, and anterior cingulate cortex. *Journal of Neurophysiology*, **94**(3), 2086–2092.

Rainer, G., Asaad, W.F., and Miller, E.K. (1998a). Memory fields of neurons in the primate prefrontal cortex. *Proceedings of the National Academy of Sciences U S A*, **95**(25), 15008.

Rainer, G., Asaad, W.F., and Miller, E.K. (1998b). Selective representation of relevant information by neurons in the primate prefrontal cortex. *Nature*, **393**(6685), 577.

Rao, S.G., Williams, G.V., and Goldman-Rakic, P.S. (2000). Destruction and creation of spatial tuning by disinhibition: GABA(A) blockade of prefrontal cortical neurons engaged by working memory. *Journal of Neuroscience*, **20**(1), 485.

Robinson, D.A. and Fuchs, A.F. (1969). Eye movements evoked by stimulation of frontal eye fields. *Journal of Neurophysiology*, **32**(5), 637.

Rosano, C., Sweeney, J.A., Melchitzky, D.S., and Lewis, D.A. (2003). The human precentral sulcus: chemoarchitecture of a region corresponding to the frontal eye fields. *Brain Research*, **972**(1–2), 16–30.

Rosano, C., Krisky, C.M., Welling, J.S., Eddy, W.F., Luna, B., Thulborn, K.R., *et al.* (2002). Pursuit and saccadic eye movement subregions in human frontal eye field: a high-resolution fMRI investigation. *Cerebral Cortex*, **12**(2), 107–115.

Russo, G.S. and Bruce, C.J. (1993). Effect of eye position within the orbit on electrically elicited saccadic eye movements: a comparison of the macaque monkey's frontal and supplementary eye fields. *Journal of Neurophysiology*, **69**(3), 800.

Russo, G.S. and Bruce, C.J. (1994). Frontal eye field activity preceding aurally guided saccades. *Journal of Neurophysiology*, **71**(3), 1250.

Russo, G.S. and Bruce, C.J. (1996). Neurons in the supplementary eye field of rhesus monkeys code visual targets and saccadic eye movements in an oculocentric coordinate system. *Journal of Neurophysiology*, **76**(2), 825.

Sakai, K. (2008). Task set and prefrontal cortex. *Annual Review Neuroscience*, **31**, 219–245.

Sawaguchi, T. and Iba, M. (2001). Prefrontal cortical representation of visuospatial working memory in monkeys examined by local inactivation with muscimol. *Journal of Neurophysiology*, **86**(4), 2041–2053.

Scalaidhe, S.P., Albright, T.D., Rodman, H.R., and Gross, C.G. (1995). Effects of superior temporal polysensory area lesions on eye movements in the macaque monkey. *Journal of Neurophysiology*, **73**(1), 1.

Schafer, R.J. and Moore, T. (2007). Attention governs action in the primate frontal eye field. *Neuron*, **56**, 541–551.

Schall, J.D. (1991a). Neuronal activity related to visually guided saccades in the frontal eye fields of rhesus monkeys: comparison with supplementary eye fields. *Journal of Neurophysiology*, **66**(2), 559.

Schall, J.D. (1991b). Neuronal activity related to visually guided saccadic eye movements in the supplementary motor area of rhesus monkeys. *Journal of Neurophysiology*, **66**(2), 530.

Schiller, P.H. (1977). The effect of superior colliculus ablation on saccades elicted by cortical stimulation. *Brain Research*, **122**(1), 154–156.

Schiller, P.H. and Chou, I.H. (1998). The effects of frontal eye field and dorsomedial frontal cortex lesions on visually guided eye movements. *Nature Neuroscience*, **1**(3), 248–253.

Schiller, P.H., True, S.D., and Conway, J.L. (1979). Effects of frontal eye field and superior colliculus ablations on eye movements. *Science*, **206**(4418), 590–592.

Schiller, P.H., True, S.D., and Conway, J.L. (1980). Deficits in eye movements following frontal eye-field and superior colliculus ablations. *Journal of Neurophysiology*, **44**(6), 1175.

Schiller, P.H., Sandell, J.H., and Maunsell, J.H. (1987). The effect of frontal eye field and superior colliculus lesions on saccadic latencies in the rhesus monkey. *Journal of Neurophysiology*, **57**(4), 1033.

Schlag, J. and Schlag-Rey, M. (1985). Unit activity related to spontaneous saccades in frontal dorsomedial cortex of monkey. *Experimental Brain Research*, **58**(1), 208.

Schlag, J. and Schlag-Rey, M. (1987). Evidence for a supplementary eye field. *Journal of Neurophysiology*, **57**(1), 179.

Schlag-Rey, M., Amador, N., Sanchez, H., and Schlag, J. (1997). Antisaccade performance predicted by neuronal activity in the supplementary eye field. *Nature*, **390**(6658), 398–401.

Segraves, M.A. (1992). Activity of monkey frontal eye field neurons projecting to oculomotor regions of the pons. *Journal of Neurophysiology*, **68**(6), 1967.

Segraves, M.A. and Goldberg, M.E. (1987). Functional properties of corticotectal neurons in the monkey's frontal eye field. *Journal of Neurophysiology*, **58**(6), 1387.

Selemon, L.D. and Goldman-Rakic, P.S. (1988). Common cortical and subcortical targets of the dorsolateral prefrontal and posterior parietal cortices in the rhesus monkey: evidence for a distributed neural network subserving spatially guided behavior. *Journal of Neuroscience*, **8**(11), 4049.

Shidara, M. and Richmond, B.J. (2002). Anterior cingulate: single neuronal signals related to degree of reward expectancy. *Science*, **296**(5573), 1709–1711.

Shima, K. and Tanji, J. (1998). Role for cingulate motor area cells in voluntary movement selection based on reward. *Science*, **282**(5392), 1335–1338.

Shima, K. and Tanji, J. (2000). Neuronal activity in the supplementary and presupplementary motor areas for temporal organization of multiple movements. *Journal of Neurophysiology*, **84**(4), 2148–2160.

Shima, K., Mushiake, H., Saito, N., and Tanji, J. (1996). Role for cells in the presupplementary motor area in updating motor plans. *Proceedings of the National Academy of Sciences U S A*, **93**(16), 8694–8698.

Shima, K., Aya, K., Mushiake, H., Inase, M., Aizawa, H., and Tanji, J. (1991). Two movement-related foci in the primate cingulate cortex observed in signal-triggered and self-paced forelimb movements. *Journal of Neurophysiology*, **65**(2), 188–202.

Shook, B.L., Schlag-Rey, M., and Schlag, J. (1988). Direct projection from the supplementary eye field to the nucleus raphe interpositus. *Experimental Brain Research*, **73**(1), 215–218.

Sommer, M.A. and Wurtz, R.H. (2000). Composition and topographic organization of signals sent from the frontal eye field to the superior colliculus. *Journal of Neurophysiology*, **83**(4), 1979.

Sparks, D.L. (2002). The brainstem control of saccadic eye movements. *Nature Reviews Neuroscience*, **3**(12), 952.

Stanton, G.B., Goldberg, M.E., and Bruce, C.J. (1988a). Frontal eye field efferents in the macaque monkey: I. Subcortical pathways and topography of striatal and thalamic terminal fields. *Journal of Comparative Neurology*, 271(4), 473–492.

Stanton, G.B., Goldberg, M.E., and Bruce, C.J. (1988b). Frontal eye field efferents in the macaque monkey: II. Topography of terminal fields in midbrain and pons. *J.Comp Neurol*, 271(4), 493.

Stanton, G.B., Bruce, C.J., and Goldberg, M.E. (1993). Topography of projections to the frontal lobe from the macaque frontal eye fields. *Journal of Comparative Neurology*, 330(2), 286–301.

Stanton, G.B., Deng, S.Y., Goldberg, M.E., and McMullen, N.T. (1989). Cytoarchitectural characteristic of the frontal eye fields in macaque monkeys. *Journal of Comparative Neurology*, 282(3), 415.

Stuphorn, V. and Schall, J.D. (2006). Executive control of countermanding saccades by the supplementary eye field. *Nature Neuroscience*, 9(7), 925–931.

Stuphorn, V., Taylor, T.L., and Schall, J.D. (2000). Performance monitoring by the supplementary eye field. *Nature*, 408(6814), 857.

Sweeney, J.A., Mintun, M.A., Kwee, S., Wiseman, M.B., Brown, D.L., Rosenberg, D.R., *et al.* (1996). Positron emission tomography study of voluntary saccadic eye movements and spatial working memory. *Journal of Neurophysiology*, 75(1), 454.

Tanji, J. (1994). The supplementary motor area in the cerebral cortex. *Neuroscience Research*, 19(3), 251–268.

Tanji, J. (1996). New concepts of the supplementary motor area. *Current Opinion in Neurobiology*, 6(6), 782–787.

Tanji, J., and Hoshi, E. (2008). Role of the lateral prefrontal cortex in executive behavioral control. *Physiological Review*, 88(1), 37–57.

Tehovnik, E.J. and Lee, K. (1993). The dorsomedial frontal cortex of the rhesus monkey: topographic representation of saccades evoked by electrical stimulation. *Experimental Brain Research*, 96(3), 430.

Tehovnik, E.J., Sommer, M.A., Chou, I.H., Slocum, W.M., and Schiller, P.H. (2000). Eye fields in the frontal lobes of primates. *Brain Research. Brain Research Reviews*, 32(2–3), 413–448.

Tian, J. and Lynch, J.C. (1997). Subcortical input to the smooth and saccadic eye movement subregions of the frontal eye field in Cebus monkey. *Journal of Neuroscience*, 17(23), 9233–9247.

Tsujimoto, S. and Sawaguchi, T. (2004). Neuronal representation of response-outcome in the primate prefrontal cortex. *Cerebral Cortex*, 14(1), 47–55.

van Veen, V. and Carter, C.S. (2002). The anterior cingulate as a conflict monitor: fMRI and ERP studies. *Physiology and Behavior*, 77(4–5), 477–482.

Vilensky, J.A. and van Hoesen, G.W. (1981). Corticopontine projections from the cingulate cortex in the rhesus monkey. *Brain Research*, 205(2), 391–395.

Vogt, B. A. and Pandya, D. N. (1987). Cingulate cortex of the rhesus monkey: II. Cortical afferents. *Journal of Comparative Neurology*, 262(2), 271–289.

Vogt, B.A., Pandya, D.N., and Rosene, D.L. (1987). Cingulate cortex of the rhesus monkey: I. Cytoarchitecture and thalamic afferents. *Journal of Comparative Neurology*, 262(2), 256–270.

Vogt, B.A., Vogt, L., Farber, N.B., and Bush, G. (2005). Architecture and neurocytology of monkey cingulate gyrus. *Journal of Comparative Neurology*, 485(3), 218–239.

Wallis, J.D., Anderson, K.C., and Miller, E.K. (2001). Single neurons in prefrontal cortex encode abstract rules. *Nature*, 411(6840), 953.

Wang, X.J., Tegner, J., Constantinidis, C., and Goldman-Rakic, P.S. (2004). Division of labor among distinct subtypes of inhibitory neurons in a cortical microcircuit of working memory. *Proceedings of the National Academy of Sciences U S A*, 101(5), 1368.

Wang, Y., Matsuzaka, Y., Shima, K., and Tanji, J. (2004). Cingulate cortical cells projecting to monkey frontal eye field and primary motor cortex. *Neuroreport*, 15(10), 1559–1563.

Wang, Y., Isoda, M., Matsuzaka, Y., Shima, K., and Tanji, J. (2005). Prefrontal cortical cells projecting to the supplementary eye field and presupplementary motor area in the monkey. *Neuroscience Research*, 53(1), 1–7.

Watanabe, M. (1996). Reward expectancy in primate prefrontal neurons. *Nature*, 382(6592), 629.

Wegener, S.P., Johnston, K., and Everling, S. (2008). Microstimulation of monkey dorsolateral prefrontal cortex impairs antisaccade performance. *Experimental Brain Research*, 190(4), 463–473.

Weiskrantz, L. and Mishkin, M. (1958). Effects of temporal and frontal cortical lesions on auditory discrimination in monkeys. *Brain*, 81(3), 406–414.

White, I.M. and Wise, S.P. (1999). Rule-dependent neuronal activity in the prefrontal cortex. *Experimental Brain Research*, 126(3), 315.

Wilson, F.A., O'Scalaidhe, S.P., and Goldman-Rakic, P.S. (1994). Functional synergism between putative gamma-aminobutyrate-containing neurons and pyramidal neurons in prefrontal cortex. *Proceedings of the National Academy of Sciences U S A*, 91(9), 4009.

Wurtz, R.H. and Mohler, C.W. (1976). Enhancement of visual responses in monkey striate cortex and frontal eye fields. *Journal of Neurophysiology*, 39(4), 766–772.

Zilles, K., Schlaug, G., Matelli, M., Luppino, G., Schleicher, A., Qu, M., *et al.* (1995). Mapping of human and macaque sensorimotor areas by integrating architectonic, transmitter receptor, MRI and PET data. *Journal of Anatomy*, 187(Pt 3), 515–537.

CHAPTER 16

Eye-head gaze shifts

Brian D. Corneil

Abstract

Large gaze shifts bring about rapid and accurate realignment of the line of sight via coordinated movements of the eyes and head. In this chapter, I review first the kinematic characteristics of eye-head gaze shifts, and then the biomechanical differences inherent to eye and head motion. A recognition of these differences provides a framework for the interpretation of recent neuroanatomical and neurophysiological results. A central theme is that investigations of eye-head gaze shifts provide an opportunity to more fully address the natural capabilities of the oculomotor system. Such capabilities include solutions to challenges faced by many motor control systems, such as the contextual control of reflexes and the selection of particular coordination patterns from an unlimited set of solutions that could achieve a given goal.

Humans and other primates are predominantly visual animals. This dependency on vision necessitates a refined oculomotor system to change the line of sight (gaze). Although many *gaze shifts* can be brought about via saccadic movements of the eyes within the head, large gaze shifts require movements of both the eyes and head. As with eye-only saccades, gaze shifts realign the fovea as quickly and as accurately as possible; unlike saccades, gaze shifts require coordination between multiple motor systems. The study of gaze shifts therefore provides an opportunity to investigate how the brain carries out such coordination. Many of the challenges faced by the brain in coordinating eye-head gaze shifts mirror those present in other motor systems, such as the limb. Indeed, one of the hallmarks of this system is that no one pattern of eye-head motion is adopted for a given gaze shift. How can the gaze shifting system, which at the level of the brainstem is renowned for its automaticity and consistency (see also Cullen and Van Horn, Chapter 9, this volume), produce such flexible patterns of coordination?

This chapter outlines what is known about eye-head gaze shifts. The first part of the chapter provides a basic kinematic description of eye-head gaze shifts, focusing predominantly on horizontal movements since they have been more thoroughly studied compared to vertical, oblique, or torsional gaze shifts. The second section of the chapter considers the biomechanical and musculoskeletal differences inherent to eye and head motion, emphasizing how recordings of neck muscle activity can aid in the identification of underlying neural control strategies. The third part of the chapter outlines neurophysiological findings from the oculomotor brainstem and cortex, with a particular emphasis on the neural substrates that enable the gaze shifting system with its hallmark flexibility.

Kinematics of eye-head gaze shifts

Terminology for describing eye-head gaze shifts

Figure 16.1 shows a gaze shift made by a human in response to the presentation of a visual target 60° to the right. This movement sequence displays a number of features common to large gaze shifts, and serves to introduce conventions used to describe such movements. Because the target lies beyond the customary oculomotor range (the limits of excursion of the eyes within the head, usually ~45° in humans (Stahl, 1999)), movements of the eye-in-head (termed 'eye') and head-in-space (termed 'head') must be coordinated to land gaze (eye-in-space) on target (gaze = eye-in-space = eye-in-head + head-in-space). In this case, the gaze shift is launched by a high-velocity eye movement with head motion beginning somewhat later. During the latter portion of the gaze shift, both the eye and head are moving in the same direction at the same time, hence the gaze shift during this portion results from the combined motion of two body segments, since the eyes are nested within the head. Head motion typically persists after the end of the gaze shift, with gaze stability being ensured by a compensatory vestibulo-ocular reflex (VOR; see also Cullen and Van Horn, Chapter 9, this volume).

While this sequence of events appears simple, the underlying neural processing is surprisingly complex. The comparative timing and amplitude of the component movements of the eyes and head are highly variable in that no single pattern dictates the coordination for a given gaze shift. Despite such variability, the rapidity and accuracy of the gaze shift means that the brain relies on internal feedback to land gaze on target. Finally, the trajectory of eye motion within the head, which changes

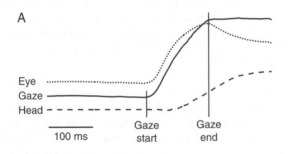

A

Eye ···········
Gaze ——
Head – – – –

———— 100 ms

Gaze start

Gaze end

B

_____

Comparison of eye and head motor systems

_____

Eye

    Visco-elastic plant
    6 extraocular muscles
    3 rotational axes about single point
    Simple musculoskeletal organization

Head

    Visco-inertial plant
    > 20 muscles
    3 rotational and 3 translational axes, multiple vertebra
    Complex musculoskeletal organization

Fig. 16.1 A) Depiction of a 60° rightward eye-head gaze shift. Gaze, the position of the eye-in-space (solid line), is the sum of the position of the eye within the head (dotted line) and the head in space (dashed line; gaze = eye-in-space = eye-in-head + head-in-space). B) Comparison of biomechanical and musculoskeletal properties underlying eye and head motion.

from a gaze shifting to a compensatory mode at the end of the gaze shift, implies intimate interplay between the oculomotor and vestibular systems.

Variability in eye and head motion during gaze shifts

A basic description of eye-head gaze shifts was first provided by Mowrer in 1932, who used successive images taken by a 16-Hz camera to illustrate the comparative timing of eye and head motion during large gaze shifts, and the importance of the vestibular system in compensating for head motion following the end of the gaze shift (Mowrer, 1932). Subsequent studies by Bartz (1966) and Fleming and colleagues (1969) provided more thorough descriptions of the timing of comparative motion of the eyes and head, as well as the first formal description of *head contribution*, or how much of the gaze shift was due to head motion (Bartz, 1966; Fleming et al., 1969). The advent of equipment enabling more resolved measures of motor performance allowed experiments to begin to study the coordination of eye-head gaze shifts in different experimental contexts. In this regard, studies by Bizzi and colleagues in monkeys (Bizzi et al., 1971, 1972), Guitton in cats (Guitton et al., 1984), and Zangemeister and Stark in humans (Zangemeister and Stark, 1981, 1982) are particularly relevant, as they were amongst the first to formally address eye-head variability during gaze shifts. These investigations differentiated between 'triggered' modes of orienting, wherein orienting commands to the eyes and head were issued almost simultaneously in response to presentation of an unpredictable target, and 'predictive' modes, wherein the head moved well in advance of the gaze shift (the VOR maintained gaze stability during such early head movements).

The past decades have witnessed a proliferation of studies of eye-head coordination in multiple species. Although each species, and every subject within a given species, displays idiosyncratic eye-head coordination preferences that are stable within a given context (Fuller, 1992; Fuller et al., 1992; Stahl, 1999), it is now widely recognized that a host of variables influence eye-head coordination within a given subject. In addition to the influence of target predictability, the comparative timing and contribution of the eyes and head are also modified readily by target amplitude and direction (Freedman and Sparks, 1997b; Gretsy, 1974; Guitton and Volle, 1987; Tomlinson and Bahra, 1986), target modality (Fuller, 1996a; Goossens and Van Opstal, 1997; Populin, 2006), the initial position of the eyes and head (Becker et al., 1992; Freedman and Sparks, 1997b; Fuller, 1996b; Goossens and Van Opstal, 1997; McCluskey and Cullen, 2007; Pélisson et al., 1988; Phillips et al., 1995; Tomlinson, 1990; Volle and Guitton, 1993), subject instruction and alertness (Fuller, 1992), foreknowledge of future orienting locations (Oommen et al., 2004), expectation of reward (Rezvani and Corneil, 2008), and a host of other task-related demands or conditions (Gandhi and Sparks, 2001; Herst et al., 2001; Kowler et al., 1992; Oommen and Stahl, 2005b; Smeets et al., 1996; Stahl, 2001). What is lacking is a mechanistic understanding of how such variability is instantiated by the oculomotor system.

Gaze shifts in complex environments

Additional insights into the capabilities of the oculomotor system have been gained by examining eye-head coordination during more complex environments involving multiple stimuli, or situations in which the behavioural goal is rapidly changed. In such environments, the head can orient independently of the gaze axis, suggesting that the orienting drive to the head is not simply a replica of that issued to the oculomotor system (Corneil and Munoz, 1999; Ron and Berthoz, 1991; Ron et al., 1993). Eye-head coordination during a *countermanding* task, wherein subjects are instructed to try to abruptly cancel an upcoming gaze shift, can also be quite informative. Success on such countermanding trials depends on the timing of the cancellation instruction, and as observed for head-restrained saccades (Hanes and Carpenter, 1999), subjects can either successfully withhold a gaze shift or not. Importantly, a lack of head restraint enabled observation of a third movement sequence, wherein the head oriented toward the target while gaze remained stable due to a compensatory VOR movement gaze shift (Corneil and Elsley, 2005). This sequence demonstrates that a commitment to orient the head is made first, allowing more time for the oculomotor system to cancel a gaze shift.

Van Opstal and colleagues (Vliegen et al., 2004, 2005) have recently examined eye-head gaze shifts in a dynamic double-step task, in which a secondary auditory or visual stimulus is presented during an ongoing gaze shift. Gaze shifts to secondary stimuli are perfectly accurate, demonstrating that the oculomotor system is capable of dynamically integrating visual stimuli (encoded relative to the retina) or auditory stimuli (encoded relative to the head) during ongoing gaze shifts to accurately reconstruct the absolute position of the stimuli in the world (Vliegen et al., 2004, 2005). These observations complement studies showing that the oculomotor system can generate accurate movements even when the desired goal of a gaze shift is changed in mid-flight (Corneil et al., 1999), necessitating continuous feedback about ongoing eye-head gaze shifts.

Bottom-up control for eye-head gaze shifts

Detailed examinations of the trajectories of the eyes and head during gaze shifts have provided other important insights into the operating principles of the gaze control system. For example, during large gaze shifts to targets well beyond the oculomotor range, the excursion of the eye within the orbit is halted well before it reaches its mechanical limit, suggesting neurally-imposed constraints to eye-in-head position (Guitton and Volle, 1987). A separate series of experiments involving 'pin-hole' goggles, which constrain the range of eye-in-head positions in which a target can be seen, provided additional evidence for how closely the brain controls eye-in-head trajectories during gaze shifts (Ceylan et al., 2000; Crawford and Guitton, 1997). In response to these goggles, monkeys relied on a reduced amount of eye motion and a greater amount of head motion during gaze shifts. More importantly, the position of the eye at the end of the saccadic portion of the gaze shift anticipated the upcoming intended head movement, so that the eye-in-head position following the compensatory eye movement aligned with the aperture of the pin-hole goggles. More extreme examples of a similar phenomenon are seen in large gaze shifts incorporating torsional components. During such movements, the amount the eye-in-head departs from Listing's plane anticipates the compensatory eye movement that will accompany head motion after the end of the gaze shift (Crawford and Vilis, 1991; Tweed et al., 1998; see also Angelaki, Chapter 8, this volume for a definition of Listing's plane). These findings emphasize a *bottom-up* nature to the neural control of eye-head gaze shifts that arises because of the nested nature of the eye within the head. Regardless of whether eye movement leads head movement or not, optimal control of the gaze axis requires that eye-in-head motion is informed about the upcoming movement of the head in space.

In summary, kinematic investigations of eye-head gaze shift have revealed a number of principles. First, although a given subject adopts a seemingly 'lawful' pattern of eye-head coordination in a given behavioural context, such coordination can be readily modified by a host of factors and processes. Second, although the initial portion of a gaze shift is usually generated by an eye-in-head movement, there is compelling evidence that the brain issues an orienting command to the head first, and controls the eye-in-head trajectory in anticipation of what the head is going to do. Third, continuous feedback about ongoing eye and head motion is available to the oculomotor system, permitting the production of accurate gaze shifts to stimuli presented dynamically, or following mid-flight changes in the desired goal. Clarification of these principles helps refine models of oculomotor function, and guide neurophysiological investigations.

Biomechanical and musculoskeletal factors influencing head motion

Comparison of eye and head movement control

Despite the preference for head-restraint in the laboratory, the oculomotor system evolved to operate with the head unrestrained. The researcher studying gaze shifts with the head unrestrained has the advantage of studying a system in its more natural setting. However, in addition to challenges associated with working with head-unrestrained preparations (particularly when uncooperative animals are involved), freeing the head forces the experimenter to confront two very different motor effectors. Comparatively, the eye is the far simpler structure (Fig. 16.1B), and the basic mechanics of saccadic eye movements were described over 40 years ago (Robinson, 1964). Briefly, the main forces resisting eye motion are viscous and elastic in nature, arising from the orbital tissues supporting the eyeball; the rotational inertia of the eyeball due to its mass is negligible. The anatomical arrangement of the six extraocular muscles that move the eye within the orbit is also relatively straightforward. Finally, extraocular muscle fibres are amongst the fastest contracting fibres in the body (Goldberg et al., 1998). These biomechanical and musculoskeletal properties, combined with the machine-like nature of saccadic control, means that eye movements can serve as a proxy for underlying neuromuscular control (see also Cullen and Van Horn, Chapter 9, this volume). For example, given a 10° rightward head-restrained saccade, one can infer with a high degree of certainty which extraocular muscles generated the movements, and the timing of the immediate premotor events.

A similar degree of inference is simply not possible with the head. Biomechanically, the head is characterized by a considerable rotational inertia (Winters et al., 1988; Zangemeister and Stark, 1981) that introduces a substantial lag between muscle contraction and the onset of head movement (effectively, the head acts as a low-pass filter). The musculoskeletal organization of the neck is also extremely complicated: upwards of two dozen neck muscles interconnecting the skull, cervical vertebrae, and/or shoulder girdle can induce head movement (Kamibayashi and Richmond, 1998; Richmond et al., 1988, 2001). Many of these muscles also appear to have redundant functions based on their anatomical pulling directions. Accordingly, one simply cannot infer the immediate motor and premotor events based on measurements of head movement kinematics with any degree of spatial (i.e. which muscles generated a movement) or temporal (i.e. when those muscles were activated) certainty. These realities constrain the development of realistic models of head movement control, and the integration of such models with well-studied elements within the oculomotor system.

Some of the complexities inherent to head motion can be circumvented by measuring the electromyographic (EMG) activity on neck muscles. Although the cascade from EMG activity through to force development is itself highly complicated and non-linear (influenced, in part, by muscle fibre type, length, and velocity), EMG measurements can at least inform about the neural command issued to the head plant. For example, one can ascertain whether a specific muscle is recruited for a given task, and when such recruitment took place. From a temporal perspective, the resolution provided by measuring neck EMG is at a millisecond timescale, comparable to the inferences that can be made by measuring eye movements. In humans, the seminal work by Zangemeister and colleagues in the early 1980s (Zangemeister and Stark, 1981, 1982; Zangemeister et al., 1982) investigated neck muscle recruitment via surface recordings of large, superficial muscles that turn the head, in part describing the comparative timing of neck muscle recruitment during eye-head gaze shifts. Various groups have also used intramuscular recordings of neck muscles of some of the deeper muscles to isolate single muscle fibres and circumvent concerns about cross-talk from overlying muscles (André-Deshays et al., 1988, 1991; Benhamou et al., 1995; Mayoux-Benhamou et al., 1997). More recently, ultrasound-guided insertion of intramuscular electrodes into the deepest layers of neck muscles has been achieved (Bexander et al., 2005; Blouin et al., 2007), and while these techniques are extremely promising, they are only just beginning to be paired with more complex behavioural paradigms.

Animal models for head movement control

Much of what we know about the control of head movements in humans has come from animal models (Richmond et al., 1999). The use of animal models offers the opportunity for a more extensive (albeit still incomplete) sampling of neck muscles, and the chance to pair these recordings with neurophysiological, neuroanatomical, and behavioural techniques. Cats traditionally served as the model of choice for such studies (e.g. Isa and Sasaki, 2002; Peterson and Richmond, 1988; Richmond et al., 1992; Thomson et al., 1994), but the use of non-human primates has more recently come into favour (e.g. Corneil et al., 2001; Lestienne et al., 1995) given their closer resemblance to humans, and their amenability to performing complex oculomotor tasks. As with all animal models, however, the interpretation of results obtained from animals as they pertain to humans must be done in light of obvious species differences in preferred modes of locomotion (quadrupeds vs. bipeds) and musculoskeletal organization.

Figure 16.2 shows the comparative anatomy of a number of small muscles that invest the deepest layer of the dorsal neck, spanning the upper cervical vertebra and skull. These suboccipital muscles form the core of the muscle synergies used to turn the head horizontally (Corneil et al., 2001;

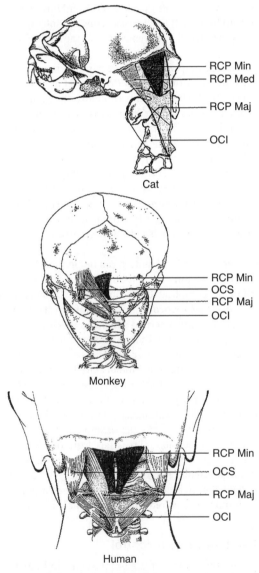

Fig. 16.2 Anatomical sketches of the suboccipital muscles in the dorsal neck of cats, monkeys, and humans. The suboccipital muscles invest the deepest layer of dorsal musculature, spanning the upper cervical vertebrae and skull, and form the core of many movement synergies. OCI, obliquus capitis inferior; OCS, obliquus capitis superior; RCP maj, rectus capitis posterior major; RCP min, rectus capitis posterior minor; RCP med, rectus capitis posterior medius.

Richmond et al., 1992). From a comparative standpoint, the organization of this muscle layer appears more similar between the monkey and human compared to the cat, further supporting use of the primate as an animal model for horizontal head turns. Concerns about comparative modes of locomotion must also be informed by radiographic studies which have demonstrated that many quadrupeds, cats and monkeys included, adopt a resting posture wherein the cervical vertebral column is oriented vertically, due to a marked dorsal inflection at the C7/T1 junction (Graf et al., 1995; Vidal et al., 1986). Thus, differences relating to habitual modes of locomotion may be targeted at the cervicothoracic junction, whereas common organizational principles applicable to cats, monkeys, and humans may be at work in the upper cervical areas that are primarily involved in horizontal head turns.

Neck muscle recruitment during horizontal gaze shifts

Neck muscle recruitment during horizontal head movements has been well studied in both cats and monkeys (Corneil et al., 2001; Richmond et al., 1992). These studies have involved the chronic implantation of indwelling EMG electrodes into both superficial and deep neck muscles, permitting the simultaneous characterization of recruitment of more than ten neck muscles in a variety of dynamic tasks and stable postures. Such studies have revealed a number of consistent principles. One principle is that the small and deep suboccipital muscles (Fig. 16.2) are recruited for all head movements and postures, suggesting that such muscles form the core of various coordination synergies. Additional recruitment of larger more superficial neck muscles is added to this core synergy for more eccentric postures or larger and faster head movements. These characterizations are important because they reflect a 'hardwired' neuromuscular solution to the apparent muscular redundancy that arises from the complex musculoskeletal organization of the head plant. Although the brain could theoretically achieve a given head movement task with an infinite number of recruitment solutions, the targeting of descending neural systems onto specific neck muscle motoneurons constrains the available solutions. An excellent example of such hardwiring is seen in the vestibulospinal system, where signals from each semicircular canal innervate a unique set of neck muscles appropriate to produce compensatory head movements (Sugiuchi et al., 2004). It appears likely that similar hardwired synergies are accessed by the descending tectoreticulospinal system that controls head orienting (Shinoda et al., 2006), presumably aiding the contextual control and integration of voluntary and reflexive head movements.

A second principle from these studies is the influence of initial posture on neck muscle recruitment. Systematic variations in initial head position in cats and monkeys revealed that the brain recruits ancillary muscles for horizontal head turns when the cervical column is held horizontally (Thomson et al., 1994), and elegantly exploits elastic recoil for centrifugal head movements that cross midline (Corneil et al., 2001). Each of these posturally-dependent strategies act in concert with the posturally-invariant core turning synergy, presumably simplifying the computations required for different behavioural tasks.

A third principle that has emerged concerns the timing of neck muscle recruitment, particularly compared to the initiation of saccadic gaze shifts. Figure 16.3 shows neck muscle recruitment from a head-restrained monkey of some of the small suboccipital muscles that turn the head in the ipsilateral direction (i.e. left OCI turns the head to the left). These representations of muscle activity are aligned to target onset, and segregated for leftward and rightward target presentation. Despite head-restraint, two features of recruitment stand out. First, all muscles increased activity following ipsilateral target presentation, and decreased activity following contralateral target presentation. Such lateralized recruitment forms the core of the head turning synergy, despite head restraint. Second, such recruitment began approximately 90 ms after ipsilateral target presentation (asterisks in Fig. 16.3), regardless of the ensuing saccadic reaction time. This demonstrates that a neural circuit permits an orienting command to access the head while the decision to commit to a gaze shift is ongoing (Corneil et al., 2004). Put another way, differences exist in the constraints dictating the initiation of an orienting drive at the head or the gaze axis.

In summary, the eyes and head are very different motor effectors. The eye is comparatively the far simpler structure, and measurements of eye movement permit accurate estimations of the immediate

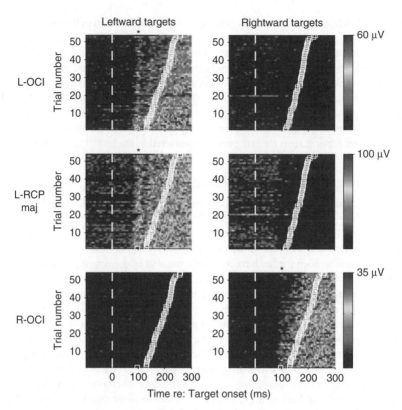

Fig. 16.3 (Also see Plate 8.) Representation of recruitment of bilateral OCI and left RCP maj muscles in a head-restrained monkey, aligned to the presentation of a visual target 27° to the left or right. Data segregated by side of target presentation (vertical dashed line), and sorted by saccadic reaction time (white square). Each row represents a different trial, with the grey scale colour conveying the magnitude of recruitment. Note the time-locked nature of recruitment following ipsilateral target presentation (asterisks), regardless of the time of initiation of the ensuing saccade. A prominent band of time-locked inhibition is also seen on left RCP maj following rightward target presentation. Such lateralized recruitment forms the core of the head turning synergy, despite head restraint.

motor and premotor events. The biomechanical and musculoskeletal complexities inherent to head motion prevent a similar degree of inference, but such complexities can be circumvented in part by measuring neck muscle recruitment to directly assess the motor command issued to the head. Techniques for recording the activity of a large sample of neck muscles have been developed in both cats and monkeys, and these recordings have revealed a number of recruitment solutions that simplify the control of a highly complex motor effector. As discussed in the next section, recordings of neck muscle activity can be paired with neurophysiological approaches to begin to address the neurobiological architectures that instantiate such solutions.

Brainstem control of eye-head gaze shifts

Superior colliculus

A key brainstem structure in the control of orienting is the superior colliculus, a layered structure within the midbrain (see also White and Munoz, Chapter 11, this volume). The intermediate and deep layers of the superior colliculus (dSC) subserve a motor function, emitting high-frequency bursts of neural activity slightly (~20 ms) before movement onset. These layers receive strong afferent projections from frontal oculomotor areas (see also Johnston and Everling, Chapter 15, this volume), which presumably play an important role in relaying behavioural context (see below). In turn, dSC neurons project to reticular premotor centres for eye and head movements located throughout the brainstem (see Isa and Sasaki (2002) and Scudder et al. (2002) for recent reviews). Thus, the dSC receives converging information from many cortical areas and distributes the primary signal to the premotor centres that generate the commands for the impending gaze shift.

Physiological evidence for the involvement of the dSC in eye-head gaze shifts comes from both stimulation and recording studies. Stimulation of the dSC in head-unrestrained animals elicits eye-head gaze shifts that resemble natural movements (Freedman et al., 1996; Klier et al., 2003; Roucoux et al., 1980). The amount the head contributes during evoked gaze shifts, and the magnitude of neck EMG activity associated with such head movements, increases progressively for more caudal stimulation locations (Corneil et al., 2002a; Roucoux et al., 1980). Recording studies have also shown that dSC neurons are involved in the execution of eye-head gaze shifts. In the cat, identified tectoreticulospinal neurons emit high-frequency bursts of activity prior to eye-head gaze shifts, and transient increases in the activity of tectoreticulospinal neurons during such bursts induce short-latency re-accelerations of both the eyes and head (Grantyn and Berthoz, 1985; Munoz et al., 1991). In the monkey, by varying the amount the eyes and head contribute to an isometric gaze shift, (Freedman and Sparks, 1997a) demonstrated that the high-frequency burst of dSC activity best related to the gaze shift, rather than the component movement of the eyes or head. Such physiological results are consistent with the extensive branching and termination of efferent collicular projections into both eye and head premotor areas (Grantyn, 1989; Scudder et al., 1996).

Omnipause neurons and the brainstem burst generator

The decomposition of a gaze-related command into the component commands to move the eyes and head occurs downstream of the SC. Head-restrained studies have demonstrated that collicular inputs to the brainstem burst generator trigger a saccade. Within the brainstem burst generator, mesencephalic and pontine saccadic excitatory and inhibitory burst neurons (collectively referred to as SBNs) discharge high-frequency bursts of action potentials that produce the 'pulse' of activity in extraocular motoneuron pools that drive high-velocity saccades (see also Cullen and Van Horn, Chapter 9, this volume for further details). Briefly, SBN activity is thought to be governed in part by the combined actions of long-lead burst neurons, which gradually increase activity prior to saccade onset, and omnipause neurons (OPNs), which are tonically-active during fixation and not active during saccades. OPNs potently inhibit SBNs, and thus must be silenced prior to saccade onset. Levels of dSC activity that exceed saccade threshold, either introduced artificially via electrical stimulation or acquired during behavioural tasks, initiate a cascade of events that culminate in a pause of OPN activity and a burst of SBN activity to drive a saccade.

While the sequence of immediate premotor events leading up to head-restrained saccades is fairly well understood, a number of neurophysiological observations bolster the behavioural evidence that the initiation of orienting head movements is not governed in a similar manner. First, although high-levels of stimulation current in the dSC initiate eye-head gaze shifts, lower levels of stimulation current below saccadic threshold evoke neck EMG responses and 'head-only' movements either without or well in advance of a gaze shift—a compensatory eye-movement maintains gaze stability during such head-only movements (Corneil et al., 2002a,b; Pélisson et al., 2001). These evoked head-only movements resemble those that can be elicited by a variety of behavioural tasks (Corneil and Elsley, 2005; Corneil and Munoz, 1999; Pélisson et al., 2001; Zangemeister and Stark, 1982). Second, dSC activity can be grossly subdivided into high-frequency levels of activity aligned to either the onset of a visual target or the initiation of a saccadic gaze shift, and low-frequency 'buildup' or 'prelude' levels of activity that are not necessarily associated with saccade (Glimcher and Sparks, 1992; Munoz and Wurtz, 1995). Previous head-restrained studies have emphasized that increases in low-frequency dSC activity are divorced from motor output, since the eyes remain stable, yet associated with a diversity of high-level processes such as target selection, attentional allocation, motor preparation, decision-making, and representation of reward variables (Basso and Wurtz, 1997; Dorris and Munoz, 1998; Fecteau et al., 2004; Horwitz and Newsome, 1999; Ignashchenkova et al., 2004; Ikeda and Hikosaka, 2003; McPeek and Keller, 2002). By employing a reward-related paradigm, we recently demonstrated that increasing levels of low-frequency dSC activity are associated with the recruitment of a contralateral head turning synergy (Rezvani and Corneil, 2008).

The observations above suggest that dSC activity need not be relayed through the brainstem burst generator to initiate a motor response at the head. The neural architecture shown in Fig. 16.4A suggests that the inhibitory influence of OPNs acts selectively on the eye premotor circuits, but not the head premotor circuits. This concept was first proposed in the early 1990s (Galiana and Guitton, 1992; Guitton et al., 1990), and recently received direct support in a study which stimulated the OPN region either before or during an eye-head gaze shift (Gandhi and Sparks, 2007). OPN stimulation selectively delayed gaze shifts or arrested them in mid-flight, but did not influence the timing or kinematics of head motion. Thus, in spite of OPN activation, the head continued to receive an orienting command. Such *selective gating* of descending dSC activity provides a plausible neurophysiological solution for the host of behavioural and neurophysiological observations that demonstrate that head orienting can be initiated before, or at lower levels of activity than, orienting of the gaze axis.

There appear to be important species differences in the downstream processing of dSC information in cats and monkeys. A direct tectospinal projection exists in cats (Alstermark et al., 1992; Anderson et al., 1971), but is either absent or very weak in monkeys (Nudo et al., 1993; Robinson et al., 1994). In both species however, the interstitial nucleus of Cajal within the mesencephalon and

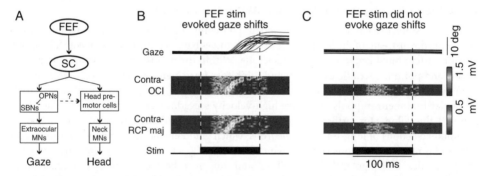

Fig. 16.4 (Also see Plate 9.) A) Conceptual schematic outlining role of various brainstem centres in eye-head gaze shifts. Descending commands from the dSC (superior colliculus), which receives converging information from a number of cortical areas including the FEF (frontal eye fields), is distributed to premotor centres governing gaze shifts and head movements. Gaze shifts are generated by saccadic burst neurons (SBNs), which are potently inhibited by omnipause neurons (OPNs). OPNs selectively inhibit the SBNs without exerting a similar influence on head premotor neurons. At the current time, it is unknown whether SBNs distribute a drive to the head when engaged ('?' in figure). Regardless, this schematic provides a plausible explanation for how head orienting can begin before, or in advance of, gaze orienting. B) Gaze shifts and neck muscle activity evoked by stimulation of the left FEF in a head-restrained monkey. Here, 100 ms of 50 μA of stimulation current evoked a 7° rightward gaze shift (upper traces), and recruitment of the contralateral (rightward) OCI and RCP maj muscles (same format as Fig. 16.3). Note how evoked neck muscle activity lead the evoked gaze shift. C) From the same FEF location, stimulation occasionally failed to evoke a gaze shift (top traces). However, evoked neck muscle activity persisted on such 'no gaze' trials. These results are consistent with the schematic in (A), whereby activity that was unable to engage the brainstem burst generator engaged an orienting drive on the head.

the nucleus reticularis gigantocellularis serve as key nodes pathway leading to the development of a vertical or horizontal orienting command at the head, respectively (Cowie and Robinson, 1994; Farshadmanesh et al., 2008; Isa and Naito, 1995; Isa and Sasaki, 2002; Quessy and Freedman, 2004). There is also some question regarding the role of SBNs in eye-head coordination. In cats, reticulospinal neurons project to the abducens nucleus (Grantyn and Berthoz, 1987; Grantyn et al., 1987) and SBNs are thought to distribute their signals to both the eyes and head (Cullen et al., 1993), potentially providing the neuroanatomical substrate for the strong coupling between eye and head trajectories during gaze shifts. There is less agreement as to whether a similar coupling exists in monkeys (see Fig. 16.4A). Bursts of neck EMG activity are seen at gaze onset in monkeys (Corneil et al., 2002b), but this could result from gaze-related discharges on dSC neurons that bypass the OPNs. The coupling between eye and head trajectories is also generally not as strong in the monkey versus the cat, even though the discharge patterns of SBNs correlate in part with head velocity as in the cat (Cullen and Guitton, 1997).

It is important to emphasize that this concept of selective gating of descending dSC activity applies only to those movement-related dSC neurons studied in head-restrained preparations. Other functional classes of dSC neurons can be observed if one departs from the traditional head-restrained preparation. For example, by training monkeys via head-mounted lasers to make head movements without moving the line of sight, Gandhi and colleagues observed a class of putative 'head cells' that were specifically modulated during head movements, regardless of whether such movements were associated with a gaze shift or not (Walton et al., 2007). Such head cells were intermingled with classical movement-related dSC neurons, but did not display their characteristic topographic relationship. While the functional contribution of head-only neurons to movement requires further investigation (simultaneous recordings with neck EMG activity could be particularly informative), these results revealed a hetereogeneity of functional cell types within the dSC. Similar lessons have been learned by studying the contribution of the dSC to reaching, which have revealed a class of reach-related neurons correlated with the activity of shoulder muscles and hand conformation (Nagy et al., 2006; Stuphorn et al., 1999). These results may reflect monkeys' use of quadrupedal locomotion and the requirements for limb responses to whole-body orienting, or fulfil a more direct role in eye-hand coordination.

Cortical control of eye-head gaze shifts

Although the concept of selective gating of descending dSC commands provides a plausible solution for how the oculomotor system could orient the head before a gaze shift, its relevance requires that cortical inputs access this circuit to appropriately modify the amount the head moves in different behavioural contexts. Currently, a mechanistic understanding for how the brain contextually modulates eye-head coordination during a given gaze shift is lacking. From a circumstantial aspect, many of the high-level processes known to increase the amounts of low-frequency dSC activity (e.g. motor preparation, target predictability, or representation of reward variables) are associated with increasing amounts of head contribution during eye-head gaze shifts (Corneil et al., 2007; Moschner and Zangemeister, 1993; Rezvani and Corneil, 2008). The frontal cortex has long been recognized as a source for such high-level processes, implementing the contextually-based rules necessary for goal-driven behaviours (see also Johnston and Everling, Chapter 15, this volume).

Within the frontal cortex, the contribution of both the frontal eye fields (FEFs) and supplementary eye field (SEF) to eye-head coordination has been investigated, primarily via electrical stimulation. Like the dSC, electrical stimulation of the FEFs and the SEF in monkeys or the FEF analogue in cats elicits coordinated eye-head gaze shifts, with most studies reporting predictable variations in the coordination of the eyes and head with initial eye position (Chen and Walton, 2005; Guitton and Mandl, 1978b; Knight and Fuchs, 2007; Martinez-Trujillo et al., 2003; Tu and Keating, 2000; but see Chen (2006) for an alternative interpretation of the FEFs' contribution to eye-head gaze shifts). FEF stimulation also elicits short-latency neck muscle responses in both species (Fig. 16.4B) (Elsley et al., 2007; Guitton and Mandl, 1978b). Importantly, neck muscle responses evoked by FEF stimulation persists even on those trials in which stimulation failed to evoke an accompanying gaze shift (Fig. 16.4c) (Elsley et al., 2007), and stimulation in the SEF can evoke head movements without gaze shifts (Chen and Walton, 2005).

These results are generally consistent with the notion that the frontal influences on eye-head coordination are relayed through the dSC, providing a plausible means by which high-level signals conveying behavioural context could access brainstem centres that ultimately implement flexible eye-head coordination. However, it should be noted that permanent ablation or reversible inactivation of the dSC or FEF leaves orienting head movements unimpaired (van der Steen et al., 1986; Walton et al., 2008). These effects are all the more surprising given the stimulation results noted above, and may attest to alternative or additional pathways for head orienting that have yet to be thoroughly studied. Furthermore, while the few recordings studies performed in the oculomotor cortex with the head-unrestrained have described units that relate to either gaze shifts or head-only movements as in the dSC (Bizzi and Schiller, 1970; Guitton and Mandl, 1978a), such studies were not designed to specifically address the functional role of such units in contextual eye-head coordination. Recent studies have described a host of behavioural paradigms which will facilitate the study of contextual eye-head coordination in monkeys (Rezvani and Corneil, 2008; Sparks et al., 2001; Stahl, 2002), and the pairing of such paradigms with neurophysiological approaches should yield a more comprehensive understanding of the role of the frontal cortex, and its interactions with the oculomotor brainstem, in eye-head gaze shifts.

Using neck EMG recordings as a tool for cognitive neuroscience

The oculomotor system has served as an excellent model system for studying many aspects of cognitive neuroscience. There exists a close association between the oculomotor system and the covert allocation of visuospatial attention (see also Kristjánsson, Chapter 25, this volume), and the discrete nature of head-restrained saccades aids in the discrimination of neural activity related to the eye movement from that related to preparation and planning. However, the oculomotor system evolved to control the line of sight without head-restraint, and the core idea behind the concept of selective gating is that the mechanisms governing the initiation of eye movements (via OPNs) are different from those governing the initiation of head movements. In particular, this implies that neural processes within the oculomotor system that percolate below the threshold for initiating saccades, such as those linked to visuospatial attention, may nevertheless culminate in motor commands at the head plant.

We have recently investigated this issue by recording neck EMG signals while monkeys performed a cueing task (Corneil et al., 2008). In this task, a visual cue is flashed briefly before target onset, which reflexively draws covert attention to the cue. The response of a subject to subsequent target presentation depends on cue timing and location relative to the target. Despite head-restraint, target presentation induced neck muscle activation (i.e. as shown in Fig. 16.3), but this response was highly modulated by the allocation of visuospatial attention in response to cue presentation (Corneil et al., 2008). Importantly, the profiles of neck muscle activity paralleled activity recorded from the dSC in the same task (Fecteau et al., 2004), demonstrating that a process that appears 'covert' from the perspective of one effector (since the visual axis remains stable) need not be divorced from motor output.

In monkeys, therefore, recordings of neck EMG activity can reflect subsaccadic levels of activity within the oculomotor system. Although the correlation between dSC and neck EMG activity is stronger for more eccentric targets (Rezvani and Corneil, 2008), small head movements and low levels of neck muscle activity are also observed for small-amplitude gaze shifts approximately 10° in amplitude in both humans and monkeys (Corneil et al., 2008, 2002a; Oommen and Stahl, 2005a). Perhaps the most exciting implication of the selective gating concept is that it is readily transferable to humans. Attentional tasks in humans influence eye-head coordination (Khan et al., 2009), and simply turning the head without shifting gaze influences manual response latencies in a manner similar to those observed for saccades (Cicchini et al., 2008). In theory, recordings of neck muscle activity should provide insights into the human oculomotor system at a millisecond-by-millisecond, perhaps paralleling the insights that have been gained by examining the linkage between microsaccades and covert orienting (Engbert and Kliegl, 2003; Hafed and Clark, 2002; see also Martinez-Conde and Macknik, Chapter 6, this volume).

Summary and future directions

Eye-head gaze shifts provide an excellent model for addressing multiple questions within systems neuroscience. Many of the brain areas involved in the control of saccadic eye movements contribute to eye-head gaze shifts, thus the knowledge base gained from saccadic eye movements can be leveraged to address eye-head gaze shifts. The head plant is a particularly complicated structure from both biomechanical and anatomical perspectives, yet converging findings from neurophysiological studies recording neck muscle recruitment and anatomical studies of the patterns of projections onto neck muscle motoneurons have begun to identify some of the core recruitment synergies that help simplify motor control. The accuracy of eye-head gaze shifts, even in spite of a variety of perturbations or changes in desired goal, attests to a system capable of virtually instantaneous integration of dynamic sensory stimuli with signals from vestibular sources and the ongoing movement. Finally, the flexibility with which component movements of the eyes and head can be combined within a given gaze shifts parallels that found within many motor actions involving multiple effectors, such as eye-hand coordination. Perhaps most importantly, the neural substrates of this system are present within the cortex and brainstem, and hence accessible to conventional neurophysiology.

One control principle that has emerged consistently from studies of eye-head gaze shifts is that the orienting command issued to the head usually precedes that issued to the eye. Thus, the kinematic sequence of eye and head initiation (due to its biomechanics, the eye movement is usually launched first) does not specify the sequence of neuromuscular events at the eye and head plants. This 'bottom-up' neuromuscular sequencing likely arises because of the nested nature of the eye within the head; optimal control of the gaze (eye-in-space) axis requires that the eye-in-head trajectory is programmed in light of the impending head-in-space movement. OPNs selectively inhibit the eye premotor circuits, thus a higher threshold of activity is required to generate saccadic eye movements compared to head movements. Such selective gating also imparts a behavioural benefit given the nature of foveal vision, ensuring a stable visual axis while the decision to commit to a gaze shift is ongoing, even if the head begins to move. The control of the visual axis therefore has a binary nature unique amongst voluntary motor control systems, in that the visual axis is either stable (and compensated for by vestibular reflexes), or moving as quickly as possible. In other inertial-laden systems, like the head or the arm, the separation between planning and execution is not so discrete. Within the oculomotor system, processes which appear 'premotor' (since the eyes remain stable) recruit neck muscles, implying that neck muscle recordings can assay the oculomotor system during various stages of sensorimotor transformations.

This review has focused on the role of the tectoreticulospinal system, and cortical inputs into this circuit, in implementing flexible eye-head coordination. It is important to stress that this represents only one of many descending systems that ultimately converge on neck muscle motoneurons. Other brainstem areas, such as the cerebellum (e.g. Goffart et al., 1998; Quinet and Goffart, 2007) or central mesencephalic reticular formation (Pathmanathan et al., 2006) have the requisite cortical and premotor connections to implement flexible eye-head coordination, and likely play a very important role. The surprisingly small influence of FEF or dSC lesions on orienting head movement (van der Steen et al., 1986; Walton et al., 2008) may attest to the importance of these non-tectal pathways. However, as with cortical oculomotor areas, future studies that incorporate more nuanced behavioural paradigms are required for a more comprehensive understanding of the functional role of such brainstem areas in eye-head coordination. Furthermore, while modulation of activity within the tectoreticulospinal system provides a plausible explanation of how the head leads the eye, perhaps representing the default mode of the oculomotor system, it does not explain how the brain can generate large gaze shifts with little or no head component. Indeed, the neuromuscular strategies preventing head motion may be just as interesting as those that generate motion, as head and gaze direction convey important societal cues in many species (Kaminski et al., 2004; Tomasello et al., 1998, 2007). At this point, it is not known precisely how head motion is prevented during gaze shifts. Plausible neuromuscular strategies include neck muscle co-contraction to stiffen the head plant, neck muscle activation at a level insufficient to overcome the head's inertia, or the absence of neck muscle activation altogether; although each strategy would prevent head motion, the underlying neural substrates are likely to be quite different.

The past decade has seen substantial advances in our understanding of how the brain controls eye-head gaze shifts. Work in both cats and monkeys have revealed similarities as well as species-specific differences, and these advances have begun to be leveraged to lead to a better understanding of the human brain. Key questions, however, remain. For example, it is still unclear precisely how the gaze-related command represented by the dSC is decomposed into the component commands to drive the eyes and head. This issue is surprisingly complicated given the correlation between eye and head trajectories during gaze shifts, and the extensive neuronal branching of the network ultimately carrying out this transformation. Debates about whether a given neural element encodes 'eye', 'head', or 'gaze' commands have not produced consensus. One need only consider the firing patterns of neck muscle motoneurons, which signal motor output, to illustrate the difficulties inherent to strict semantic classifications. Neck muscle motoneurons display time-locked bursts of activity following visual target onset that would be termed 'sensory' anywhere else (Corneil et al., 2004). Low-frequency activity within the dSC can also play a motor role by virtue of projections to the neck (Rezvani and Corneil, 2008), a premotor role by virtue of projections to the brainstem burst generator (Dorris and Munoz, 1998), and various high-level roles (e.g. associated with attention) by virtue of ascending projections through the thalamus (Sommer and Wurtz, 2004). The functional role of a neuron depends in large part on where the signal is sent, and hence future advances in understanding the head-unrestrained oculomotor system will be found at the intersection of anatomical and neuro-physiological studies.

References

Alstermark, B., Pinter, M.J., and Sasaki, S. (1992). Tectal and tegmental excitation in dorsal neck motoneurones of the cat. *Journal of Physiology*, **454**, 517–532.

Anderson, M.E., Yoshida, M., and Wilson, V.J. (1971). Influence of superior colliculus on cat neck motoneurons. *Journal of Neurophysiology*, **34**(5), 898–907.

André-Deshays, C., Berthoz, A., and Revel, M. (1988). Eye-head coupling in humans. I. Simultaneous recording of isolated motor units in dorsal neck muscles and horizontal eye movements. *Experimental Brain Research*, **69**(2), 399–406.

André-Deshays, C., Revel, M., and Berthoz, A. (1991). Eye-head coupling in humans. II. Phasic components. *Experimental Brain Research*, **84**(2), 359–366.

Bartz, A.E. (1966). Eye and head movements in peripheral vision: Nature of compensatory eye movements. *Science*, **152**, 1644–1645.

Basso, M.A. and Wurtz, R.H. (1997). Modulation of neuronal activity by target uncertainty. *Nature*, **389**(6646), 66–69.

Becker, W., Jurgens, R., Berthoz, A., Graf, W., and Vidal, P.P. (1992). Gaze saccades to visual targets: Does head movement change the metrics? In A. Berthoz, W. Graf, and P.P. Vidal (eds.) *The Head-Neck Sensory Motor System* (pp. 427–433). New York: Oxford University Press.

Benhamou, M.A., Revel, M., and Vallee, C. (1995). Surface electrodes are not appropriate to record selective myoelectric activity of splenius capitis muscle in humans. *Experimental Brain Research*, **105**(3), 432–438.

Bexander, C.S., Mellor, R., and Hodges, P.W. (2005). Effect of gaze direction on neck muscle activity during cervical rotation. *Experimental Brain Research*, **167**(3), 422–432.

Bizzi, E. and Schiller, P.H. (1970). Single unit activity in the frontal eye fields of unanesthetized monkeys during eye and head movement. *Experimental Brain Research*, **10**(2), 150–158.

Bizzi, E., Kalil, R.E., and Tagliasco, V. (1971). Eye-head coordination in monkeys: evidence for centrally patterned organization. *Science*, **173**, 452–454.

Bizzi, E., Kalil, R.E., and Morasso, P. (1972). Two modes of active eye-head coordination in monkeys. *Brain Research*, **40**(1), 45–48.

Blouin, J.S., Siegmund, G.P., Carpenter, M.G., and Inglis, J.T. (2007). Neural control of superficial and deep neck muscles in humans. *Journal of Neurophysiology*, **98**(2), 920–928.

Ceylan, M., Henriques, D.Y., Tweed, D.B., and Crawford, J.D. (2000). Task-dependent constraints in motor control: pinhole goggles make the head move like an eye. *Journal of Neuroscience*, **20**(7), 2719–2730.

Chen, L.L. (2006). Head movements evoked by electrical stimulation in the frontal eye field of the monkey: evidence for independent eye and head control. *Journal of Neurophysiology*, **95**(6), 3528–3542.

Chen, L.L. and Walton, M.M. (2005). Head movement evoked by electrical stimulation in the supplementary eye field of the rhesus monkey. *Journal of Neurophysiology*, **94**(6), 4502–4519.

Cicchini, G.M., Valsecchi, M., and de'Sperati, C. (2008). Head movements modulate visual responsiveness in the absence of gaze shifts. *Neuroreport*, **19**(8), 831–834.

Corneil, B.D. and Elsley, J.K. (2005). Countermanding eye-head gaze shifts in humans: marching orders are delivered to the head first. *Journal of Neurophysiology*, **94**(1), 883–895.

Corneil, B.D. and Munoz, D.P. (1999). Human eye-head gaze shifts in a distractor task. II. Reduced threshold for initiation of early head movements. *Journal of Neurophysiology*, **82**(3), 1406–1421.

Corneil, B.D., Olivier, E., and Munoz, D.P. (2002a). Neck muscle responses to stimulation of monkey superior colliculus. I. Topography and manipulation of stimulation parameters. *Journal of Neurophysiology*, **88**(4), 1980–1999.

Corneil, B.D., Olivier, E., and Munoz, D.P. (2002b). Neck muscle responses to stimulation of monkey superior colliculus. II. Gaze shift initiation and volitional head movements. *Journal of Neurophysiology*, **88**(4), 2000–2018.

Corneil, B.D., Olivier, E., and Munoz, D.P. (2004). Visual responses on neck muscles reveal selective gating that prevents express saccades. *Neuron*, **42**(5), 831–841.

Corneil, B.D., Munoz, D.P., and Olivier, E. (2007). Priming of head premotor circuits during oculomotor preparation. *Journal of Neurophysiology*, **97**(1), 701–714.

Corneil, B.D., Hing, C.A., Bautista, D.V., and Munoz, D.P. (1999). Human eye-head gaze shifts in a distractor task. I. Truncated gaze shifts. *Journal of Neurophysiology*, **82**(3), 1390–1405.

Corneil, B.D., Olivier, E., Richmond, F.J., Loeb, G.E., and Munoz, D.P. (2001). Neck muscles in the rhesus monkey. II. Electromyographic patterns of activation underlying postures and movements. *Journal of Neurophysiology*, **86**(4), 1729–1749.

Corneil, B.D., Munoz, D.P., Chapman, B.B., Admans, T., and Cushing, S.L. (2008). Neuromuscular consequences of reflexive covert orienting. *Nature Neuroscience*, **11**(1), 13–15.

Cowie, R.J. and Robinson, D.L. (1994). Subcortical contributions to head movements in macaques. I. Contrasting effects of electrical stimulation of a medial pontomedullary region and the superior colliculus. *Journal of Neurophysiology*, **72**(6), 2648–2664.

Crawford, J.D. and Guitton, D. (1997). Primate head-free saccade generator implements a desired (post-VOR) eye position command by anticipating intended head motion. *Journal of Neurophysiology*, **78**(5), 2811–2816.

Crawford, J.D. and Vilis, T. (1991). Axes of eye rotation and Listing's law during rotations of the head. *Journal of Neurophysiology*, **65**(3), 407–423.

Cullen, K.E. and Guitton, D. (1997). Analysis of primate IBN spike trains using system identification techniques. II. Relationship to gaze, eye, and head movement dynamics during head-free gaze shifts. *Journal of Neurophysiology*, **78**(6), 3283–3306.

Cullen, K.E., Guitton, D., Rey, C.G., and Jiang, W. (1993). Gaze-related activity of putative inhibitory burst neurons in the head-free cat. *Journal of Neurophysiology*, **70**(6), 2678–2683.

Dorris, M.C. and Munoz, D.P. (1998). Saccadic probability influences motor preparation signals and time to saccadic initiation. *Journal of Neuroscience*, **18**(17), 7015–7026.

Elsley, J.K., Nagy, B., Cushing, S. L., and Corneil, B.D. (2007). Widespread presaccadic recruitment of neck muscles by stimulation of the primate frontal eye fields. *Journal of Neurophysiology*, **98**(3), 1333–1354.

Engbert, R. and Kliegl, R. (2003). Microsaccades uncover the orientation of covert attention. *Vision Research*, **43**(9), 1035–1045.

Farshadmanesh, F., Chang, P., Wang, H., Yan, X., Corneil, B.D., and Crawford, J.D. (2008). Neck muscle synergies during stimulation and inactivation of the interstitial nucleus of Cajal (INC). *Journal of Neurophysiology*, **100**, 1677–1685.

Fecteau, J.H., Bell, A.H., and Munoz, D.P. (2004). Neural correlates of the automatic and goal-driven biases in orienting spatial attention. *Journal of Neurophysiology*, **92**(3), 1728–1737.

Fleming, D.G., Vossius, G.W., Bowman, G., and Johnson, E.L. (1969). Adaptive properties of the eye-tracking system as revealed by moving-head and open-loop studies. *Annals of the New York Academy of Sciences*, **156**, 825–850.

Freedman, E.G. and Sparks, D.L. (1997a). Activity of cells in the deeper layers of the superior colliculus of the rhesus monkey: evidence for a gaze displacement command. *Journal of Neurophysiology*, **78**(3), 1669–1690.

Freedman, E.G. and Sparks, D.L. (1997b). Eye-head coordination during head-unrestrained gaze shifts in rhesus monkeys. *Journal of Neurophysiology*, **77**(5), 2328–2348.

Freedman, E.G., Stanford, T.R., and Sparks, D.L. (1996). Combined eye-head gaze shifts produced by electrical stimulation of the superior colliculus in rhesus monkeys. *Journal of Neurophysiology*, **76**(2), 927–952.

Fuller, J.H. (1992). Head movement propensity. *Experimental Brain Research*, **92**(1), 152–164.

Fuller, J.H. (1996a). Comparison of horizontal head movements evoked by auditory and visual targets. *Journal of Vestibular Research,* **6**(1), 1–13.

Fuller, J.H. (1996b). Eye position and target amplitude effects on human visual saccadic latencies. *Experimental Brain Research,* **109**(3), 457–466.

Fuller, J.H., Berthoz, A., Graf, W., and Vidal, P.P. (1992). Comparison of Head Movement Strategies among Mammals *Head-neck sensory-motor system* (pp. 101–112). Oxford: Oxford University Press.

Galiana, H.L., and Guitton, D. (1992). Central organization and modeling of eye-head coordination during orienting gaze shifts. *Annals of the New York Academy of Sciences,* **656**, 452–471.

Gandhi, N.J. and Sparks, D.L. (2001). Experimental control of eye and head positions prior to head-unrestrained gaze shifts in monkey. *Vision Research,* **41**(25–26), 3243–3254.

Gandhi, N.J. and Sparks, D.L. (2007). Dissociation of eye and head components of gaze shifts by stimulation of the omnipause neuron region. *Journal of Neurophysiology,* **98**(1), 360–373.

Glimcher, P.W. and Sparks, D.L. (1992). Movement selection in advance of action in the superior colliculus. *Nature,* **355**(6360), 542–545.

Goffart, L., Pélisson, D., and Guillaume, A. (1998). Orienting gaze shifts during muscimol inactivation of caudal fastigial nucleus in the cat. II. Dynamics and eye-head coupling. *Journal of Neurophysiology,* **79**(4), 1959–1976.

Goldberg, S.J., Meredith, M.A., and Shall, M.S. (1998). Extraocular motor unit and whole-muscle responses in the lateral rectus muscle of the squirrel monkey. *Journal of Neuroscience,* **18**(24), 10629–10639.

Goossens, H.H. and Van Opstal, A.J. (1997). Human eye-head coordination in two dimensions under different sensorimotor conditions. *Experimental Brain Research,* **114**(3), 542–560.

Graf, W., De, W.C., and Vidal, P.P. (1995). Functional anatomy of the head-neck movement system of quadrupedal and bipedal mammals. *Journal of Anatomy,* **186** *(Pt 1),* 55–74.

Grantyn, A. (1989). How visual inputs to the ponto-bulbar reticular formation are used in the synthesis of premotor signals during orienting. *Progress in Brain Research,* **80**, 159–170.

Grantyn, A. and Berthoz, A. (1985). Burst activity of identified tecto-reticulo-spinal neurons in the alert cat. *Experimental Brain Research,* **57**(2), 417–421.

Grantyn, A. and Berthoz, A. (1987). Reticulo-spinal neurons participating in the control of synergic eye and head movements during orienting in the cat. I. Behavioral properties. *Experimental Brain Research,* **66**(2), 339–354.

Grantyn, A., Ong-Meang, J.V., and Berthoz, A. (1987). Reticulo-spinal neurons participating in the control of synergic eye and head movements during orienting in the cat. II. Morphological properties as revealed by intra-axonal injections of horseradish peroxidase. *Experimental Brain Research,* **66**(2), 355–377.

Gretsy, M.A. (1974). Coordination of head and eye movements to fixate continuous and intermittent targets. *Vision Research,* **14**, 395–403.

Guitton, D., Douglas, R.M., and Volle, M. (1984). Eye-head coordination in cats. *Journal of Neurophysiology,* **52**(6), 1030–1050.

Guitton, D. and Mandl, G. (1978a). Frontal 'oculomotor' area in alert cat. II. Unit discharges associated with eye movements and neck muscle activity. *Brain Research,* **149**(2), 313–327.

Guitton, D. and Mandl, G. (1978b). Frontal 'oculomotor' area in alert cat. I. Eye movements and neck activity evoked by stimulation. *Brain Research,* **149**(2), 295–312.

Guitton, D. and Volle, M. (1987). Gaze control in humans: eye-head coordination during orienting movements to targets within and beyond the oculomotor range. *Journal of Neurophysiology,* **58**(3), 427–459.

Guitton, D., Munoz, D.P., and Galiana, H.L. (1990). Gaze control in the cat: studies and modeling of the coupling between orienting eye and head movements in different behavioral tasks. *Journal of Neurophysiology,* **64**(2), 509–531.

Hafed, Z.M. and Clark, J.J. (2002). Microsaccades as an overt measure of covert attention shifts. *Vision Research,* **42**(22), 2533–2545.

Hanes, D.P. and Carpenter, R.H. (1999). Countermanding saccades in humans. *Vision Research,* **39**(16), 2777–2791.

Herst, A.N., Epelboim, J., and Steinman, R.M. (2001). Temporal coordination of the human head and eye during a natural sequential tapping task. *Vision Research,* **41**(25–26), 3307–3319.

Horwitz, G.D. and Newsome, W.T. (1999). Separate signals for target selection and movement specification in the superior colliculus. *Science,* **284**(5417), 1158–1161.

Ignashchenkova, A., Dicke, P.W., Haarmeier, T., and Thier, P. (2004). Neuron-specific contribution of the superior colliculus to overt and covert shifts of attention. *Nature Neuroscience,* **7**(1), 56–64.

Ikeda, T. and Hikosaka, O. (2003). Reward-dependent gain and bias of visual responses in primate superior colliculus. *Neuron,* **39**(4), 693–700.

Isa, T. and Naito, K. (1995). Activity of neurons in the medial pontomedullary reticular formation during orienting movements in alert head-free cats. *Journal of Neurophysiology,* **74**(1), 73–95.

Isa, T. and Sasaki, S. (2002). Brainstem control of head movements during orienting; organization of the premotor circuits. *Progress in Neurobiology,* **66**(4), 205–241.

Kamibayashi, L.K. and Richmond, F.J. (1998). Morphometry of human neck muscles. *Spine,* **23**(12), 1314–1323.

Kaminski, J., Call, J., and Tomasello, M. (2004). Body orientation and face orientation: two factors controlling apes' behavior from humans. *Animal Cognition,* **7**(4), 216–223.

Khan, A.Z., Blohm, G., McPeek, R.M., and Lefevre, P. (2009). Differential influence of attention on gaze and head movements. *Journal of Neurophysiology,* **101**(1), 198–206.

Klier, E.M., Wang, H., and Crawford, J.D. (2003). Three-dimensional eye-head coordination is implemented downstream from the superior colliculus. *Journal of Neurophysiology*, **89**(5), 2839–2853.

Knight, T.A. and Fuchs, A.F. (2007). Contribution of the frontal eye field to gaze shifts in the head-unrestrained monkey: effects of microstimulation. *Journal of Neurophysiology*, **97**(1), 618–634.

Kowler, E., Pizlo, Z., Guo-Liang, Z., Erkelens, C.J., Steinman, R.M., Collewijn, H., *et al.* (1992). Coordination of head and eyes during the performance of natural (and unnatural) visual tasks. In A. Berthoz, W. Graf, and P.P. Vidal (eds.) *The Head-Neck Sensory Motor System* (pp. 101–104). New York: Oxford University Press.

Lestienne, F.G., Le, G.B., and Liverneaux, P.A. (1995). Head movement trajectory in three-dimensional space during orienting behavior toward visual targets in rhesus monkeys. *Experimental Brain Research*, **102**(3), 393–406.

Martinez-Trujillo, J.C., Wang, H., and Crawford, J.D. (2003). Electrical stimulation of the supplementary eye fields in the head-free macaque evokes kinematically normal gaze shifts. *Journal of Neurophysiology*, **89**(6), 2961–2974.

Mayoux-Benhamou, M.A., Revel, M., and Vallee, C. (1997). Selective electromyography of dorsal neck muscles in humans. *Experimental Brain Research*, **113**(2), 353–360.

McCluskey, M.K. and Cullen, K.E. (2007). Eye, head, and body coordination during large gaze shifts in rhesus monkeys: movement kinematics and the influence of posture. *Journal of Neurophysiology*, **97**(4), 2976–2991.

McPeek, R.M. and Keller, E.L. (2002). Saccade target selection in the superior colliculus during a visual search task. *Journal of Neurophysiology*, **88**(4), 2019–2034.

Moschner, C. and Zangemeister, W.H. (1993). Preview control of gaze saccades: efficacy of prediction modulates eye-head interaction during human gaze saccades. *Neurological Research*, **15**(6), 417–432.

Mowrer, O.H. (1932). Concerning the normal function of the vestibular apparatus. *Annals of Otology, Rhinology and Laryngology*, **41**, 412–421.

Munoz, D.P. and Wurtz, R.H. (1995). Saccade-related activity in monkey superior colliculus. I. Characteristics of burst and buildup cells. *Journal of Neurophysiology*, **73**(6), 2313–2333.

Munoz, D.P., Guitton, D., and Pélisson, D. (1991). Control of orienting gaze shifts by the tectoreticulospinal system in the head-free cat. III. Spatiotemporal characteristics of phasic motor discharges. *Journal of Neurophysiology*, **66**(5), 1642–1666.

Nagy, A., Kruse, W., Rottmann, S., Dannenberg, S., and Hoffmann, K.P. (2006). Somatosensory-motor neuronal activity in the superior colliculus of the primate. *Neuron*, **52**(3), 525–534.

Nudo, R.J., Sutherland, D.P., and Masterton, R.B. (1993). Inter- and intra-laminar distribution of tectospinal neurons in 23 mammals. *Brain Behavior and Evolution*, **42**(1), 1–23.

Oommen, B.S. and Stahl, J.S. (2005a). Amplitudes of head movements during putative eye-only saccades. *Brain Research*, **1065**(1–2), 68–78.

Oommen, B.S. and Stahl, J.S. (2005b). Inhibited head movements: a risk of combining phoning with other activities? *Neurology*, **65**(5), 754–756.

Oommen, B.S., Smith, R.M., and Stahl, J.S. (2004). The influence of future gaze orientation upon eye-head coupling during saccades. *Experimental Brain Research*, **155**(1), 9–18.

Pathmanathan, J.S., Presnell, R., Cromer, J.A., Cullen, K.E., and Waitzman, D.M. (2006). Spatial characteristics of neurons in the central mesencephalic reticular formation (cMRF) of head-unrestrained monkeys. *Experimental Brain Research*, **168**(4), 455–470.

Pélisson, D., Prablanc, C., and Urquizar, C. (1988). Vestibuloocular reflex inhibition and gaze saccade control characteristics during eye-head orientation in humans. *Journal of Neurophysiology*, **59**(3), 997–1013.

Pélisson, D., Goffart, L., Guillaume, A., Catz, N., and Raboyeau, G. (2001). Early head movements elicited by visual stimuli or collicular electrical stimulation in the cat. *Vision Research*, **41**(25–26), 3283–3294.

Peterson, B.W. and Richmond, F.J. (1988). *Control of Head Movement*. New York: Oxford University Press.

Phillips, J.O., Ling, L., Fuchs, A.F., Siebold, C., and Plorde, J.J. (1995). Rapid horizontal gaze movement in the monkey. *Journal of Neurophysiology*, **73**(4), 1632–1652.

Populin, L.C. (2006). Monkey sound localization: head-restrained versus head-unrestrained orienting. *Journal of Neuroscience*, **26**(38), 9820–9832.

Quessy, S. and Freedman, E.G. (2004). Electrical stimulation of rhesus monkey nucleus reticularis gigantocellularis. I. Characteristics of evoked head movements. *Experimental Brain Research*, **156**(3), 342–356.

Quinet, J. and Goffart, L. (2007). Head-unrestrained gaze shifts after muscimol injection in the caudal fastigial nucleus of the monkey. *Journal of Neurophysiology*, **98**(6), 3269–3283.

Rezvani, S. and Corneil, B.D. (2008). Recruitment of a head-turning synergy by low-frequency activity in the primate superior colliculus. *Journal of Neurophysiology*, **100**(1), 397–411.

Richmond, F.J., Corneil, B.D., and Singh, K. (1999). Animal models of motor systems: cautionary tales from studies of head movement. *Progress in Brain Research*, **123**, 411–416.

Richmond, F.J., Vidal, P.P., and Peterson, B.W. (1988). The motor system: joints and muscles of the neck *Control of Head Movement* (pp. 1–21). New York: Oxford University Press.

Richmond, F.J., Thomson, D.B., and Loeb, G.E. (1992). Electromyographic studies of neck muscles in the intact cat. I. Patterns of recruitment underlying posture and movement during natural behaviors. *Experimental Brain Research*, **88**(1), 41–58.

Richmond, F.J., Singh, K., and Corneil, B.D. (2001). Neck muscles in the rhesus monkey. I. Muscle morphometry and histochemistry. *Journal of Neurophysiology*, **86**(4), 1717–1728.

Robinson, D.A. (1964). The mechanics of human saccadic eye movement. *Journal of Physiology, 174*, 245–264.

Robinson, F.R., Phillips, J.O., and Fuchs, A.F. (1994). Coordination of gaze shifts in primates: brainstem inputs to neck and extraocular motoneuron pools. *Journal of Comparative Neurology, 346*(1), 43–62.

Ron, S. and Berthoz, A. (1991). Eye and head coupled and dissociated movements during orientation to a double step visual target displacement. *Experimental Brain Research, 85*(1), 196–207.

Ron, S., Berthoz, A., and Gur, S. (1993). Saccade-vestibulo-ocular reflex co-operation and eye-head uncoupling during orientation to flashed target. *Journal of Physiology, 464*, 595–611.

Roucoux, A., Guitton, D., and Crommelinck, M. (1980). Stimulation of the superior colliculus in the alert cat. II. Eye and head movements evoked when the head is unrestrained. *Experimental Brain Research, 39*(1), 75–85.

Scudder, C.A., Kaneko, C.S., and Fuchs, A.F. (2002). The brainstem burst generator for saccadic eye movements: a modern synthesis. *Experimental Brain Research, 142*(4), 439–462.

Scudder, C.A., Moschovakis, A.K., Karabelas, A.B., and Highstein, S.M. (1996). Anatomy and physiology of saccadic long-lead burst neurons recorded in the alert squirrel monkey. II. Pontine neurons. *Journal of Neurophysiology, 76*(1), 353–370.

Shinoda, Y., Sugiuchi, Y., Izawa, Y., and Hata, Y. (2006). Long descending motor tract axons and their control of neck and axial muscles. *Progress in Brain Research, 151*, 527–563.

Smeets, J.B., Hayhoe, M.M., and Ballard, D.H. (1996). Goal-directed arm movements change eye-head coordination. *Experimental Brain Research, 109*(3), 434–440.

Sommer, M.A. and Wurtz, R.H. (2004). What the brain stem tells the frontal cortex. I. Oculomotor signals sent from superior colliculus to frontal eye field via mediodorsal thalamus. *Journal of Neurophysiology, 91*(3), 1381–1402.

Sparks, D.L., Freedman, E.G., Chen, L.L., and Gandhi, N.J. (2001). Cortical and subcortical contributions to coordinated eye and head movements. *Vision Research, 41*(25–26), 3295–3305.

Stahl, J.S. (1999). Amplitude of human head movements associated with horizontal saccades. *Experimental Brain Research, 126*(1), 41–54.

Stahl, J.S. (2001). Adaptive plasticity of head movement propensity. *Experimental Brain Research, 139*(2), 201–208.

Stahl, J.S. (2002). Knowledge of future target position influences saccade-associated head movements. *Annals of the New York Academy of Sciences, 956*, 418–420.

Stuphorn, V., Hoffmann, K.P., and Miller, L.E. (1999). Correlation of primate superior colliculus and reticular formation discharge with proximal limb muscle activity. *Journal of Neurophysiology, 81*(4), 1978–1982.

Sugiuchi, Y., Kakei, S., Izawa, Y., and Shinoda, Y. (2004). Functional synergies among neck muscles revealed by branching patterns of single long descending motor-tract axons. *Progress in Brain Research, 143*, 411–421.

Thomson, D.B., Loeb, G.E., and Richmond, F.J. (1994). Effect of neck posture on the activation of feline neck muscles during voluntary head turns. *Journal of Neurophysiology, 72*(4), 2004–2014.

Tomasello, M., Call, J., and Hare, B. (1998). Five primate species follow the visual gaze of conspecifics. *Animal Behavior, 55*(4), 1063–1069.

Tomasello, M., Hare, B., Lehmann, H., and Call, J. (2007). Reliance on head versus eyes in the gaze following of great apes and human infants: the cooperative eye hypothesis. *Journal of Human Evolution, 52*(3), 314–320.

Tomlinson, R.D. (1990). Combined eye-head gaze shifts in the primate. III. Contributions to the accuracy of gaze saccades. *Journal of Neurophysiology, 64*(6), 1873–1891.

Tomlinson, R.D. and Bahra, P.S. (1986). Combined eye-head gaze shifts in the primate. I. Metrics. *Journal of Neurophysiology, 56*(6), 1542–1557.

Tu, T.A. and Keating, E.G. (2000). Electrical stimulation of the frontal eye field in a monkey produces combined eye and head movements. *Journal of Neurophysiology, 84*(2), 1103–1106.

Tweed, D., Haslwanter, T., and Fetter, M. (1998). Optimizing gaze control in three dimensions. *Science, 281*(5381), 1363–1366.

van der Steen, J., Russell, I.S., and James, G.O. (1986). Effects of unilateral frontal eye-field lesions on eye-head coordination in monkey. *Journal of Neurophysiology, 55*(4), 696–714.

Vidal, P.P., Graf, W., and Berthoz, A. (1986). The orientation of the cervical vertebral column in unrestrained awake animals. I. Resting position. *Experimental Brain Research, 61*(3), 549–559.

Vliegen, J., Van Grootel, T.J., and Van Opstal, A.J. (2004). Dynamic sound localization during rapid eye-head gaze shifts. *Journal of Neuroscience, 24*(42), 9291–9302.

Vliegen, J., Van Grootel, T.J., and Van Opstal, A.J. (2005). Gaze orienting in dynamic visual double steps. *Journal of Neurophysiology, 94*(6), 4300–4313.

Volle, M. and Guitton, D. (1993). Human gaze shifts in which head and eyes are not initially aligned. *Experimental Brain Research, 94*(3), 463–470.

Walton, M.M., Bechara, B., and Gandhi, N.J. (2007). Role of the primate superior colliculus in the control of head movements. *Journal of Neurophysiology, 98*(4), 2022–2037.

Walton, M.M., Bechara, B., and Gandhi, N.J. (2008). Effect of reversible inactivation of superior colliculus on head movements. *Journal of Neurophysiology, 99*(5), 2479–2495.

Winters, J., Peterson, B.W., and Richmond, F.J. (1988). Biomechanical modeling of the human head and neck. In B.W. Peterson and F.J.R. Richmond (eds) *Control of Head Movement* (pp. 22–36). New York: Oxford University Press.

Zangemeister, W.H. and Stark, L. (1981). Active head rotations and eye-head coordination. *Annals of the New York Academy of Sciences*, **374**, 540–559.

Zangemeister, W.H. and Stark, L. (1982). Types of gaze movement: variable interactions of eye and head movements. *Experimental Neurology*, **77**(3), 563–577.

Zangemeister, W.H., Stark, L., Meienberg, O., and Waite, T. (1982). Neural control of head rotation: electromyographic evidence. *Journal of the Neurological Sciences*, **55**(1), 1–14.

CHAPTER 17

Interactions of eye and eyelid movements

Neeraj J. Gandhi and Husam A. Katnani

Abstract

Eyelid movements introduce a profound and transient modification in the positions of the eyes. This chapter describes the types of eye position perturbations and highlights the neural signatures within the oculomotor neuraxis that may mediate them. Such results imply that neural commands considered to encode a coordinated movement of the eyes and the head may, in fact, also integrate movements of the eyelid musculature as well as other skeletomotor effectors. This review also considers the use of blinks as a tool to evaluate the time-course of motor preparation of saccades and to probe whether a premotor signal is present during cognitive processes requiring executive control.

Neural commands for the generation of eye movements are routinely relayed to non-extraocular effectors. For example, electromyography (EMG) activity in neck muscles precedes the generation of a saccadic eye movement (see also Corneil, Chapter 16, this volume), even when a head movement is not required or generated. Likewise, activity observed in numerous cortical and subcortical regions encodes integrated movements of the eyes and hand (e.g. Buneo and Andersen, 2006; Lünenburger et al., 2001). Similarly, eyelid musculature is innervated in association with eye movements (Evinger et al., 1994; Fuchs et al., 1992; Gandhi, 2007; Williamson et al., 2005). The objective of this chapter is to review the integration of eyelid and eye movements. The first section of this chapter will briefly characterize eyelid movements. The second will discuss the neural pathways that produce eyelid movements and emphasizes the loci of overlapping control for blinks and eye movements, particularly saccades. The third section will review the effects of blinks on characteristics of eye movements, and the neural signatures that correlate with the observed behaviour will be highlighted. The final section will consider the use of blinks as a tool to evaluate the time-course of motor preparation and to probe whether a motor signal is present during cognitive processes requiring executive control. Another important topic on disorders associated with eyelid musculature is not considered here but is covered in a recent review by Helmchen and Rambold (2007).

Characteristics of eyelid movements

Two types of lid movements are prevalent. The first is a lid saccade, for which the movement of the upper eyelid is yoked primarily to the vertical component of the eye movement. During upward vertical movements (Fig. 17.1A) the levator palpebrae (LP) muscle contracts and raises the upper eyelid to prevent obstruction of vision. The speed of the lid movement matches that of the eye movement, generating lid saccades with rapid eye movements or more gradual changes during smooth pursuit (Becker and Fuchs, 1988). Downward eye movements (Fig. 17.1B) are accompanied by a depression of the eyelid, which is mediated by a reduction in LP muscle activity. During downward saccades, in particular, LP EMG ceases and the lid 'falls'. Such downward lid movements are considered passive since they are controlled entirely by the viscoelastic properties of the ligaments and connective tissue surrounding the lid (Becker and Fuchs, 1988; Evinger et al., 1984; Guitton et al., 1991).

The second type of lid movement occurs when the eyelid musculature produces a blink. It can be a reflexive movement, triggered by mechanical stimulation of the cornea or the periorbital skin including the eyelashes. It can also be evoked by electrical stimulation of the supraorbital branch of the trigeminal nerve and by exposure to strong visual and acoustic stimuli. It can be produced as a conditioned response as well. Nevertheless, a blink is most prevalent as a spontaneous movement, likely serving to wet and protect the cornea. In addition, it can be voluntary and accompany facial movements such as winking or grimacing. It can also occur as a gaze-evoked blink that accompanies a head-restrained and head-unrestrained gaze shift (Evinger et al., 1994; Gandhi, 2007) (Fig. 17.1C). This chapter will only consider gaze-evoked blinks and reflexive blinks triggered through trigeminal activation.

Blinks are initiated as a rapid depression of the upper eyelid. This response is due to a cessation of activity in the LP muscle plus a burst of activity in the orbicularis oculi (OO) muscle. In contrast to lid saccades, however, the eyelid gradually returns to an elevated position as a result of a decrease in OO discharge and an increase in LP activity (Björk and Kugelberg, 1953; Evinger et al., 1984). The amplitude of a lid movement during a blink can span a large range, depending on the strength of the mechanical or electrical stimulation. Regardless of the triggering mechanism, all blinks exhibit similar characteristics (Evinger et al., 1991; Gruart et al., 1995). The peak speeds of both downward and ensuing upward phases of the blink are linearly related to blink amplitude. However, the duration of the downward component is relatively constant, approximately 30 ms for reflexive blinks and approximately 75 ms for spontaneous blinks; while the return or upward component is slower and

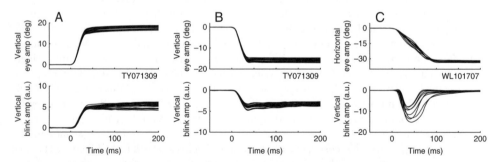

Fig. 17.1 Coordination of eye and eyelid movements. Temporal traces of eye and corresponding eyelid movements during upward (A) and downward (B) head-restrained saccades. Each trace corresponds to one trial, and movements are aligned on saccade onset. The magnetic search coil technique was used to record the position signals. For the eyelid, a small coil was taped to the upper lid (Gandhi and Bonadonna, 2005). Note that these lid saccades are fast movements executed in the same direction as the vertical saccades they accompany. The lid saccade data were collected on the same day from one animal. Thus, although the blink signals are shown in arbitrary units, their calibration is identical for the two panels. C) Temporal traces of horizontal, head-restrained saccades (top) accompanied by gaze-evoked blinks (bottom). Data obtained from another animal. The initial, downward phase of the blink is rapid, while the returning upward phase has a slower time course.

lasts 100–200 ms, with a modest increase in duration with blink amplitude. Thus, the main sequence trends for blinks are different from those observed for saccades, for which duration increases linearly with amplitude and peak velocity obeys a saturating function (Bahill et al., 1975).

Integration of neural pathways for eye and eyelid movements

The tight coordination of saccade–blink interaction can be attributed to the neural circuits which integrate the generation of saccades with the musculature of the eyelid. The OO muscle resembles a skeletal muscle and is controlled by motoneurons in the facial nucleus (Fig. 17.2). Most of the neural projections are from the dorsolateral and intermediate divisions of the ipsilateral nucleus (Porter et al., 1989). The firing rates of the motoneurons are correlated with lid velocity (Trigo et al., 1999a). With respect to oculomotor structures, evidence for contralateral tectofacial and tectoreticulofacial projections exists in the rat and cat (Dauvergne et al., 2004; May et al., 1990; Morcuende et al., 2002; Vidal et al., 1988), although it can be argued that these collicular signals may encode movement commands for the vibrissae and pinnae (Cowie and Robinson, 1994; Hemelt and Keller, 2008; Miyashita and Mori, 1995; Vidal et al., 1988). The superior colliculus also relays information to the facial nucleus via the regions of sensory trigeminal nucleus complex that receives dense afferents from the eyelids (Dauvergne et al., 2004; May and Porter, 1998). Even neural signals in cortical structures like the frontal eye fields are polysynaptically relayed to OO muscles (Gong et al., 2005). Thus, neural commands from numerous oculomotor structures have multiple avenues to innervate the OO muscle for coordinating blinks with saccadic eye movements. In addition, anatomical studies have also identified trigeminotectal pathways (Huerta et al., 1981, 1983; Ndiaye et al., 2002) through which blinks can contribute to the activity in superior colliculus and other oculomotor regions. This sensory information does not appear to encode lid position but is most likely limited to information arising from cutaneous receptors (Trigo et al., 1999b).

The LP is considered an extraocular muscle because it shares its embryogenesis with the superior rectus and is innervated by a branch of the superior division of the oculomotor nerve (Fig. 17.2). The cell bodies of these motoneurons reside bilaterally within the central caudal division of the

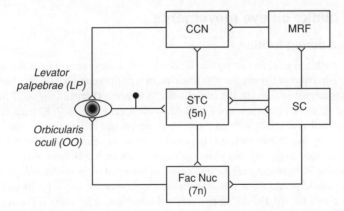

Fig. 17.2 A simplified representation of the neural circuit involved in the control of coordinated eye and eyelid movements. Sensory afferents are relayed by the trigeminal nerve to various subnuclei in the sensory trigeminal complex (STC). Direct inhibition of the levator palpebrae (LP) motoneurons in the central caudal nucleus (CCN) results in rapid depression of the LP muscle. Direct projections from the STC to the facial nucleus (Fac Nuc) terminate on motoneurons that innervate the orbicularis oculi (OO) muscle. These two pathways produce the blink reflex associated with the trigeminal reflex. Interactions of neural elements involved in controlling eyelid musculature and eye movements are known to occur at the level of the superior colliculus (SC) and the mesencephalic reticular formation (MRF). See text for details.

oculomotor nucleus complex (Porter et al., 1989). Like extraocular motoneurons, the LP moto-neurons are recruited at a threshold lid position and exhibit a tonic firing rate that increases linearly with upward positions. Burst-tonic profiles are observed for upward lid saccades, and a pause in activity precedes fast downward deflections (Fuchs et al., 1992). It has been proposed that premotor inputs for upward lid movements originate from the ipsilateral M-group neurons (Horn et al., 2000), which reside in the rostral mesencephalon and in the vicinity of the rostral interstitial nucleus of the medial longitudinal fasciculus (riMLF). Neurons in the M-group, in turn, receive inputs from oculo-motor structures like the riMLF and the superior colliculus (Horn and Büttner-Ennever, 2008). Passive downward deflection of the lid during a downward saccade requires inhibition of activity in LP motoneurons. This could be implemented as direct inhibition by GABA-ergic neurons that encode downward saccades (Horn and Büttner-Ennever, 2008). Such cells are found in the intersti-tial nucleus of Cajal (INC) (Horn et al., 2003). They could also inhibit the M-group neurons, thereby reducing or removing their excitatory drive to the LP motoneurons. Additional inhibition of LP motoneurons is postulated to stem from projections from the sensory trigeminal complex, either directly or via an interneuron (May et al., 2002; van Ham and Yeo, 1996).

The omnipause neurons (OPNs) in the paramedian pontine reticular formation are normally associated with saccadic eye movements (see also Cullen and Van Horn, Chapter 9, this volume). They serve to 'gate' saccades (Keller, 1974) by inhibiting the burst generator neurons. In addition, they also become quiescent during blinks (Fuchs et al., 1991; Mays and Morrisse, 1994), although the cessation of activity appears linked to the transient eye movement associated with the blink instead of the blink itself (Schultz et al., 2010). While this result downplays the potential association between OPNs and blinks, they cannot explain why stimulation of the OPNs prevents reflexive blinks (Mays and Morrisse, 1995). More recently, Horn and Büttner-Ennerver (2008) reported that a subgroup of OPNs inhibit LP motoneurons in the central caudal nucleus. This observation is counterintuitive because inhibition of OPNs would disinhibit the LP motoneurons, which would prevent the rapid depression of the upper lid. We speculate that the source of suppression on the OPNs also imposes a potent inhibition of the LP motoneurons such that the resulting disinhibition from OPNs is negligi-ble. The source of this inhibition is not known and needs to be addressed by future investigations.

Effects of blinks on eye movements

Blinks evoked during fixation

The eyes rotate within the orbits during blinks. Blink-induced eye movements during fixation are caused by co-contraction of the extraocular muscles, except the superior oblique. For blinks gener-ated when fixation is maintained in the straight-ahead location (Bergamin et al., 2002; Bour et al., 2000; Evinger et al., 1984; Helmchen and Rambold, 2007; Riggs et al., 1987; Rottach et al., 1998), the eyes move downward and nasally with an extorsional component during the downward phase. They then return in a loop-like fashion towards the original position before the end of the upward phase of the blink. It has been suggested that these eye movements are too slow to be considered saccades (Collewijn et al., 1985). Furthermore, the movement of the eye during a blink is dependent on initial eye position. For blinks produced or evoked with the eyes in more eccentric positions, the horizontal component increases for the abducting eye, while the vertical component increases with increas-ingly upward gaze. In contrast, the two components decrease with adduction and downward gaze, respectively. These results conform to the notion that the blink induced eye movement brings the eyes toward a primary position during the downward phase, and the eyes return towards the initial position as the eyes reopen.

Mechanical interactions of the eyelid and the globe do not fully account for the observed eye move-ment patterns. Neural activity recordings from oculomotor and abducens motoneurons reflect changes associated with the movement (Delgado-Garcia et al., 1990; Evinger and Manning, 1993; Trigo et al., 1999a). The blink-related signal most likely originates from the ophthalmic region of the trigeminal nucleus which projects to the supraoculomotor area that has connections with oculomotor motoneurons (Evinger et al., 1987). Trigeminal inputs have also been identified in the abducens motoneurons (Baker et al., 1980; Cegavske et al., 1979).

Saccade–blink interactions

A reflexive blink, timed to occur during a saccade, grossly perturbs the spatiotemporal properties of the eye movement. Such eye movements have been useful in probing neural mechanisms that trigger and control the accuracy of saccades. For a normal saccade, the spatial trajectory is a relatively straight line between the initial and final positions, and the temporal velocity waveform exhibits a bell-shaped profile. For a saccade accompanied by a blink, in contrast, the trajectory is highly curved, typically upwards (Goossens and Van Opstal, 2000a); the peak velocity is substantially reduced; and the duration of the movement increases. The endpoint accuracy is preserved even in the absence of visual feedback (Gandhi and Bonadonna, 2005; Goossens and Van Opstal, 2000a; Rambold et al., 2002; Rottach et al., 1998). These eye movement patterns observed during blink-perturbed saccades cannot be accounted for by a linear superposition of a normal saccade and a blink-associated eye movement observed during fixation (Goossens and Van Opstal, 2000a). Blinks also influence the latency of saccades. In particular, a blink triggered around a typical saccade reaction time reduces the latency (Evinger et al., 1994; Gandhi and Bonadonna, 2005; Goossens and Van Opstal, 2000a; Rambold et al., 2002). A comprehensive examination of latency effects is considered later in this chapter, in the section on motor preparation.

The effect of *reflexive blinks* on saccades is represented in the neural activity patterns of saccade related neurons in various oculomotor structures. The initial effect of the air puff, which evokes the reflexive blink, is an immediate attenuation of activity in superior colliculus neurons (Goossens and Van Opstal, 2000b). The weakened discharge is prolonged in duration such that the total number of action potentials fired by the neuron remains comparable in the control and blink perturbations conditions. The fast response time of approximately 10 ms suggests that the trigeminotectal pathway most likely produces the suppressive effect, either directly or through interneurons. Nigrotectal input, which imposes global inhibition on the superior colliculus, may also participate in blink induced modulation (Basso et al., 1996; Evinger et al., 1993).

To the best of our knowledge, published accounts of neural recordings performed during saccades accompanied by *gaze-evoked blinks* are limited. One reason is that the probability of generating a blink during small saccades is negligible, although the likelihood does increase with saccade amplitude (Williamson et al., 2005). Furthermore, the tendency of blink generation is also modulated by extraretinal factors, such as the cognitive set of performing an oculomotor task, because blinks are routinely generated during the 'return saccades' in the intertrial interval (Williamson et al., 2005). The limited published data indicate that the high-frequency, premotor burst of superior colliculus neurons does not appear to be compromised during saccades accompanied by gaze-evoked blinks (Goossens and Van Opstal, 2000b).

Effects of blinks on head-unrestrained gaze shifts

Like head-restrained saccades, head-unrestrained gaze shifts generate a rapid change in the line of sight, except that the action is produced as a coordinated movement of the eyes and the head. The velocity profile of the saccadic eye component of large amplitude head-unrestrained gaze shifts is generally not the bell-shaped curve typically seen with head-restrained saccades. The waveform will often exhibit two pronounced peaks with a significant attenuation in-between. The observation has led to the hypothesis that the head command attenuates the gain of the eye pathway: the saccade proceeds more slowly and takes longer to complete (Freedman, 2001; Freedman and Sparks, 2000).

As described above, blinks grossly attenuate the spatiotemporal profile of saccades. Furthermore, the probability of gaze-evoked blinks, assessed by the EMG of OO muscle, increases with both gaze and head amplitude (Evinger et al., 1994). This enhanced EMG is observed even during large head movements generated with the eyes closed. Hence, Evinger et al. (1994) concluded that one component of the command for large amplitude gaze shifts is used to generate a gaze-evoked blink. Therefore, the attenuation in the eye velocity could also be accounted for by gaze-evoked blinks (see Gandhi (2007) for a preliminary study). Gaze, head, eye, and eyelid signals were measured as monkeys oriented to visual targets. For matched eye, head, and target positions, the gaze shifts were separated into movements with and without gaze-evoked blinks. Figure 17.3A shows temporal plots of head and eye-in-head velocities, and blink amplitude of individual trials aligned on gaze onset.

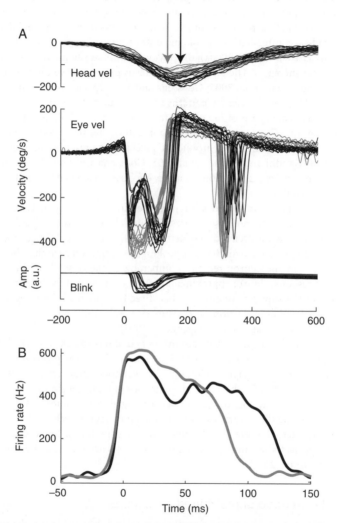

Fig. 17.3 Effects of gaze-evoked blinks on coordinated eye-head movements. A) Temporal traces of head velocity (top), eye-in-head velocity (middle) and eyelid amplitude (bottom) for large amplitude gaze shifts matched for initial eye and head position. Each trace represents one movement, and all traces are aligned on gaze onset. Black traces represent trials with gaze-evoked blinks, denoted by the deflection in the blink signal. Grey traces are trials without an accompanying blink. The vertical arrows denote the average times of peak head velocity in the two conditions. For gaze-evoked blink trials the head velocity reaches its peak later, and its average magnitude is greater also. B) Mean discharge profile of an excitatory burst neuron recorded during gaze shifts with (black trace) and without (grey trace) gaze-evoked blinks. Time zero corresponds to gaze onset. The neural activity does *not* correspond to the data shown in panel (A). The purpose of the panel is only to demonstrate blink related modulation in the neural activity. Also note that the time scale is different from panel (A). Adapted from Gandhi (2007).

The initial head and fixation target was 30° to the right, thus the eyes were centred in the orbits. Gaze shifts were directed to a target presented 36° to the left. For these movements, the average head amplitude was 55°. Blinks overlapped with gaze shifts on trials in which the eye velocity profiles showed distinct multiple peaks (two peaks in black traces). The eye velocity profiles on trials without blinks did not exhibit pronounced multiple peaks (grey traces). Neural activity of excitatory burst neurons in the oculomotor pons also reflect the multiple peaks observed in the eye and gaze velocity profiles of gaze shifts accompanied by gaze-evoked blinks, and the multiple peaks are absent in non-blink trials (Fig. 17.3B). Our unpublished data also indicate that the temporal pattern of multiple peaks in eye velocity depends on the relative timing of the blink and gaze shift, which can vary between animals. These results collectively provide another, perhaps additional, explanation for the multiple peaks observed in the eye velocity waveform. We do not view these observations as either test or rejection of the eye-head coupling hypothesis (Freedman, 2001; Freedman and Sparks, 2000). We instead prefer the interpretation that the brain issues a command for an integrated movement of the eyes, eyelids, and the head, and the altered eye velocity profiles during such movements could be due to both eye-head coupling and eye-eyelid interactions.

Head-unrestrained gaze shifts associated with blinks show other interesting characteristics also. When a reflexive blink is triggered just prior to the onset of a gaze shift, the latency of both gaze and head components are reduced (Evinger et al., 1994). The blink induced perturbation in the eye velocity increases the duration of the gaze shift. We have observed that both the magnitude and time of peak head velocity also increase (see black and grey arrows in Fig. 17.2A) (Gandhi, 2007), such that the peak aligns with the end of the gaze shift (Chen, 2006).

Effects of blinks on slow eye movements

The effects observed for saccade-blink interactions also extend to slow eye movements. For example, blinks attenuate the speed of ongoing smooth pursuit regardless of direction of pursuit (Rambold et al., 2005), and evoking a reflexive blink just before the typical onset of smooth pursuit reduces the latency by approximately 10 ms (Rambold et al., 2004). For vergence eye movements accompanied by a blink, the initial response is a transient convergence followed by a divergence independent of the direction of the eye movement. This pattern is followed by an attenuation in the velocity and increase in duration (Rambold et al., 2002), comparable to the effects seen for head-restrained and head-unrestrained gaze shifts and smooth pursuit.

Behavioural evaluation of motor preparation

A typical saccadic eye movement is initiated approximately 200 ms after a stimulus is presented in the visual periphery. Approximately 60–80 ms are required for afferent processes, such as the relay of sensory signals from the retina to various cortical and subcortical regions. Another 20 ms are accounted for by efferent pathways to send motor commands from the superior colliculus, for example, to the extraocular muscles. Thus the transduction time for a neural signal to travel from the retina to the extraocular muscles is substantially shorter than the typical reaction time of a saccade (Carpenter, 1981). A subset of saccade related burst neurons in the frontal eye fields (Hanes and Schall, 1996; see also Johnston and Everling, Chapter 15, this volume) and superior colliculus (Paré and Hanes, 2003; see also White and Munoz, Chapter 11, this volume) exhibits a low frequency discharge that increases its firing rate gradually during the intervening (approximately 100 ms) sensory-to-motor transformation period. When the firing rate reaches a threshold activation level, which can vary from neuron to neuron, the cell emits a high frequency burst, which leads to the inhibition of OPNs and initiation of the planned saccade. Furthermore, the firing rate level of the low-frequency response is negatively correlated with the saccade reaction time (Dorris et al., 1997). It has been hypothesized that the low frequency discharge represents a motor preparation signal that encodes both timing and metrics of the desired saccade (Glimcher and Sparks, 1992).

Gandhi and Bonadonna (2005) asked whether it was possible to obtain a behavioural readout of the planned movement. They reasoned that if prematurely inhibiting the OPNs before they ordinarily become quiescent is equivalent to reducing or eliminating the activation threshold, then an eye move-ment should be triggered at a reduced latency if the low frequency activity in neurons of the oculomo-tor neuraxis indeed encodes a motor component. Testing this hypothesis requires transient inhibition of the OPNs, which was accomplished by invoking the trigeminal blink reflex. Monkeys were required to make visually-guided saccades from a central fixation point to another stimulus that was illumi-nated briefly at one of two locations. On randomly selected trials and at unpredictable times during these trials, a puff of air was delivered to evoke a blink. The latency, accuracy, and kinematics of the saccade were measured. This approach allowed experimental control of evoking the blink at various times relative to stimulus onset, thereby permitting the characterization of the time-course of blink effects on saccade latency.

Figure 17.4 plots saccade latency as a function of blink time for three different oculomotor tasks performed on separate days. In the step paradigm (Fig. 17.4A), the offset of fixation point coincided with the presentation of the peripheral stimulus, and this event served as the cue to initiate the saccade (time=0). For blinks evoked more than 150 ms before the target presentation, saccade latency remained constant (~225 ms in panel A), and this value was comparable to the latency observed in non-blink trials. For blinks evoked between 150 before to 100 ms after target onset, saccade latency increased linearly (Gandhi and Bonadonna, 2005; Rambold et al., 2002). The most logical explana-tion for the increase is that the eyes are closed or closing when the target is illuminated. The visual target is sufficiently processed only after the eyes reopen. Thus the later the blink occurs within this period, the later the eyes re-open, and the longer the saccade latency. If the blink is evoked some time after the peripheral target is turned on, then there exists the possibility that the sensory neural channels in the brain may have processed the stimulus before the eyes closed. In such cases, the blink triggers the eye movement at a reduced latency. Indeed blinks triggered more than 60 ms after

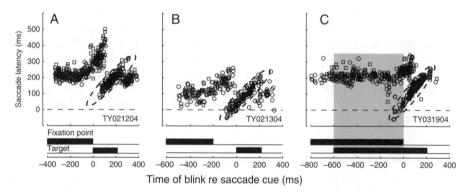

Fig. 17.4 Saccade onset is plotted as a function of the time of the trigeminal blink reflex during performance in the step (A), gap (B), and delayed (C) saccade tasks. Both parameters are measured with respect to the cue to initiate the saccade, which is defined as the later of fixation point offset or target onset. Note the lawful relationship between blink time and saccade latency across the three tasks. Blinks evoked well before (< 200 ms) the cue epoch typically did not influence saccade time; the values are similar for non-puff trials. This is followed by a period for which blinks increase saccade latencies. Then, there is an abrupt decrease in latencies, to values lower than control. We refer to these as *blink-triggered saccades* because the blink and saccade onset temporally overlap (enclosed within the dashed ellipses). In the delayed saccade task, the shaded area denotes the overlap period for which both fixation point and the eccentric saccade target remain illuminated. Both rightward (circles) and leftward (squares) target presentation trials are shown. Horizontal dashed lines are drawn to mark a latency of zero (equal to cue to initiate saccade). The bottom portion of each panel shows the time course of the behavioural task.

Reprinted from *Journal of Neurophysiology*, **93**(3), Gandhi and Bonadonna, Temporal interactions of air-puff evoked blinks and saccadic eye movements: Insights into motor preparation pp. 1718–1729 © 2005 The American Physiological Society, used with permission.

stimulus onset are often accompanied by a saccade towards the stimulus (Gandhi and Bonadonna, 2005; Rambold et al., 2004). Additionally delaying the blink also prolongs the onset of the saccade, and saccade latency increases linearly with blink time until the typical reaction time of saccades is reached (points enclosed within dashed ellipse). An air puff, timed to evoke a blink even later, typically results in an average latency saccade that precedes the blink.

Figure 17.4A also highlights a window of time around stimulus onset during which blinks can either reduce or prolong saccade latency. It has been suggested that the rate of increase in activity in saccade related burst neurons in the oculomotor system is a stochastic property (Carpenter and Williams, 1995; Hanes and Schall, 1996). If the low frequency discharge at blink onset is high enough to exceed the blink-reduced threshold, then a combined saccade-blink movement will occur. On the other hand, if the instantaneous firing rate is too low at the time of blink onset, the visual target would need to be reprocessed after the eyes reopen, which will result in an increase in saccade reaction time.

In the gap task (Fig. 17.4B), a fixed 200-ms interval elapses between the offset of the fixation point and the onset of the peripheral stimulus. This permits fixation to become disengaged prior to saccade preparation. The overall effects of blinks on saccade latency were comparable to those observed with the step task. Interestingly, blinks generated towards the end of the gap period often triggered saccades to one of the two possible target locations. Thus, saccade latency can lead stimulus onset, and the endpoint of the eye movement can land at the future target location on approximately 50% of the trials. This result is consistent with the observation that disengaged fixation introduced by the gap period allows preparatory activity encoding the two possible goals to begin accumulating in superior colliculus neurons (Dorris et al., 1997). When the blink occurs towards the end of the gap period, the saccade that gets generated is the one encoded by the winner of the competing low frequency activity at the separate sites in two colliculi.

In the delayed saccade task (Fig. 17.4C), the fixation point remains illuminated for few hundred milliseconds after the saccade target is presented. In this paradigm, the animal must implement top-down control to inhibit the tendency to reflexively orient to the stimulus. The animal is rewarded for looking at the peripheral stimulus only after the fixation point is extinguished. Neural recordings from various oculomotor regions show sustained low-frequency discharge during the 'overlap period' during which both the fixation point and saccade target are illuminated (e.g. Wurtz et al., 2001). The effect of a blink evoked *after* the animal receives the cue to initiate (fixation offset) the saccade is very similar to that observed for the step and gap tasks. Of chief interest in this task, however, is the overlap period (shaded region in Fig. 17.4C). In general, blinks evoked during much of the overlap period are not effective in triggering saccades (Gandhi and Bonadonna, 2005).

Multiple, non-exclusive interpretations can be extracted from the data and additional experiments are required to test them. On one hand, it is possible that the premotor signal isn't formulated unless the animal is operating in a reflexive mode or until the animal receives permission to trigger the saccade. On the other hand, the blink-induced attenuation in the low frequency activity in saccade related neurons (Goossens and Van Opstal, 2000b) might not exceed the activation threshold during the overlap period, even though the OPNs presumably cease to fire during the eye closure. Note that the blink-induced suppression in activity must be greater during the overlap period of the delayed saccade task compared to that seen during visually-guided step saccades because, in the latter condition, the blink does trigger a saccade. Another potential explanation is that OPNs are not the only source of inhibition that must be overcome to trigger a saccade, and that these inputs are not suppressed during blinks produced across periods requiring top-down control (such as during the overlap period). Both the basal ganglia (substantia nigra pars reticulata and caudate nucleus) and the so-called fixation neurons in the rostral superior colliculus are viable candidates since each is postulated to prevent saccade generation (Hikosaka and Wurtz, 1983; Munoz and Wurtz, 1993a, 1993b; Watanabe and Munoz, 2010). However, the activity patterns of these structures during blinks, both with and without saccades, remain to be investigated.

The results of blink-triggered saccades conform to the hypothesis that the low-frequency discharge observed during sensorimotor integration encodes motor preparation, although it does not discount the possibility that other cognitive processes, such as target selection (e.g. Basso and Wurtz, 1997) and reward expectation (e.g. Ikeda and Hikosaka, 2003), may be represented also. If so, what aspect(s) of motor preparation are signalled by the low frequency activity? For the blink-triggered saccades in all three oculomotor tasks, the endpoint accuracy of the saccade was preserved even though the eye movements were highly curved, attenuated in peak velocity, lengthened in duration, and directed to a remembered location. Thus, the metrics of the saccade are not reflected in the firing rate; the saccade vector is encoded by the locus of population activity in the superior colliculus and cortical eye fields. The temporally evolving low frequency discharge likely indicates the speed of the desired movement. For saccades triggered soon after stimulus onset, when the low frequency activity is minimal, the initial speed of the eye movement is very slow. As the time of the evoked blink is delayed, the low frequency activity has the opportunity to accumulate, and the initial speed of the accompanying saccade is higher (Gandhi and Bonadonna, 2005). The notion that the location of active population encodes the saccade metrics while the firing rate determines the speed of the movement has been termed dual-coding hypothesis, at least for the superior colliculus (Sparks and Mays, 1990).

Executive control

Existing data indicates that air-puff perturbation is most effective at producing a blink-triggered saccade once the animal has permission to produce the eye movement, in other words, when the animal is performing reflexive oculomotor tasks (Gandhi and Bonadonna, 2005). It is possible to implement conditions that employ executive or top-down control even within the context of such reflexive tasks. We consider the use of blinks to gain insights into executive control for two such tasks.

Movement cancellation

Voluntary control of action has been studied through behavioural, theoretical, and neurophysiological frameworks associated with the cancellation of an intended movement, also called the countermanding task (e.g. Hanes and Schall, 1995, 1996; Lappin and Eriksen, 1966; Logan and Cowan, 1984; Mirabella et al., 2006; Paré and Hanes, 2003). The standard procedure employed in the laboratory is to perform visually-guided saccades, as in the step task discussed above. On a subset of trials, a second cue is illuminated, instructing the subject to cancel the intended movement. The time elapsed between the onset of the saccade target and the presentation of the stop cue generally dictates the likelihood of successfully cancelling the movement. Analyses of the behavioural data have been used to *estimate* the minimum time required to cancel a planned movement, also known as the stop signal reaction time (SSRT). Note that the SSRT is unobservable because if the movement is successfully withheld, there is no way to know exactly when the movement was cancelled. Thus, the SSRT has been estimated using statistical techniques. Walton and Gandhi (2006) attempted to provide a behavioural readout of the SSRT estimate and thereby test its validity. They argued that evoking a blink ceases activity in the OPNs (Fuchs et al., 1991; Mays and Morrisse, 1994; Schultz et al., 2010), which in turn would 'unmask' the existing motor preparation signal as long as it is not successfully inhibited after presentation of the stop cue. As observed for visually guided saccades, blinks evoked approximately 50 ms after presentation of the saccade target generally resulted in a prematurely triggered eye movement. On countermanding trials, blink-triggered saccades were rarely observed approximately 70 ms after the stop cue. This value closely matches the estimated value of SSRT and therefore grants validity to the statistical approach as well as neurophysiological studies that rely on this assumption.

Antisaccades

In general, the default action plan is to orient to a stimulus presented in the periphery. For a stimulus-response mapping that requires the generation of an eye movement to the mirror location of the stimulus (antisaccade), a reflexive motor plan to the stimulus must be inhibited and the antisaccade movement plan must be formulated (Munoz and Everling, 2004). Katnani and Gandhi (2008) explored whether the trigeminal blink reflex can be used as a behavioural readout of the motor planning that takes place during an antisaccade task. They employed a modified version of the visual search task used by Schall and colleagues (Juan et al., 2004; Sato and Schall, 2003). Each trial began with several hundred milliseconds of fixation on a central visual target. The stimulus was then extinguished and fixation was maintained at the central location for another 200 ms. Following this gap period, a visual search array consisting of four stimuli spaced apart by 90° was presented. Randomly, on each trial, one of the four stimuli could be either red or green in colour indicating the singleton stimulus in the array, while the other three targets were purple. The monkeys were trained to make a saccade to the singleton if it was green and to the opposite distractor, 180° from the singleton, if red. Working on the premise that 1) blinks can provide a readout of the motor plan (Gandhi and Bonadonna, 2005) and 2) an underlying motor preparation signal is present during this task, the transition in the motor command from the singleton to the opposite distractor should be revealed by a blink reflex at some short time after the search array is presented. For the prosaccade condition, in contrast, all blink-triggered saccades should be directed to the singleton across the entire range of blink times.

Figure 17.5, panels A and B, show saccade latency as a function of blink time for prosaccade and antisaccade trials, respectively. Note that the distribution of data observed with the visual search task is very similar to that observed for the single target condition (Fig. 17.4), suggesting that the blink-induced effects are also present during performance in the visual search paradigm. For prosaccade trials the majority of the blink-triggered saccades, the subset shown within the dashed ellipse, are to the singleton. This is better visualized when the direction of the saccade is plotted as a function of saccade latency for only the blink-triggered movements (Fig. 17.5C). A moving average through the points (black curve) shows that most of the movements are directed toward the singleton. There are a small percentage of trials directed to the opposite distractor, but this fraction is not significantly different from the likelihood of errors the animal made during control trials. For antisaccade trials the correct response should be directed 180° away from the singleton; however, many reduced latency movements are directed to the oddball stimulus. A plot of saccade direction against its latency for blink-triggered saccades (Fig. 17.5D) reveals that nearly all movements with latency less than 120 ms are directed to the singleton. As saccade latency increases, the blink-triggered movement is more likely to be directed to the correct location, indicating that the initial motor plan to the singleton was inhibited and the corrected mirror movement was programmed.

The premotor theory of attention (Rizzolatti et al., 1987) posits that the neural elements that allocate spatial attention to the singleton also encode a motor command. A competing hypothesis states that spatial allocation and motor preparation can be dissociated, and both electrophysiological and anatomical studies of frontal eye field neurons have been used to support this view (Juan et al., 2004; Pouget et al., 2009; Sato and Schall, 2003). While the blink triggered saccade results (Katnani and Gandhi, 2008) conform to the principles of the premotor theory of attention, at least within the context of the reflexive saccade task, they do not distinguish whether the neural signals in individual responsive neurons encode spatial attention, motor preparation or both. Interestingly, however, recordings in the frontal eye fields and the superior colliculus during comparable visual search paradigms have revealed neural correlates for target discrimination (allocation of attention) around 100–150 ms after stimulus onset (McPeek and Keller, 2002; Murthy et al., 2001; Sato and Schall, 2003). Note that in Fig. 17.5A and B, blink-triggered saccades occurred within a similar time window after stimulus onset, suggesting that motor preparation can exist at the same time scale as allocation of attention.

Conclusions and future directions

The purpose of this chapter was to convey two important features of the interactions between eye movements and blinks. First, the eyelid musculature serves a purpose far greater than physically protecting the eye. Coordinated contraction of the LP and OO muscles induces a transient change in

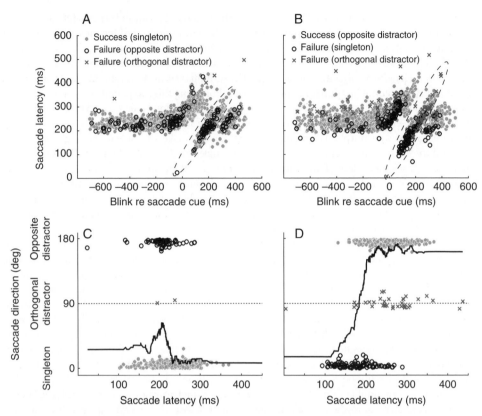

Fig. 17.5 Behavioural test of motor preparation during a behavioural task requiring executive control. (A, B) Saccade latency is plotted as a function of blink time for an animal performing the visual search array within the context of a gap task. Blink-triggered saccades are the subsets enclosed within the dashed ellipses. A) Performance in the prosaccade condition, in which the required saccade was to the 'green' singleton embedded within three purple distractors. Solid grey circles indicate saccades correctly directed to the oddball stimulus. Open black circles denote saccades incorrectly directed to the distractor located 180° away. Grey crosses mark movements directed to an orthogonal distractor. B) Performance in the antisaccade condition, in which a 'red' singleton indicated that the correct response was a saccade to the opposite distractor. Solid grey circles represent a correct response to the opposite location. Open black circles mark error trials with eye movements directed to the singleton. Grey crosses also denote error trials but the saccade ended near an orthogonal distractor. C) and D) Saccade direction is plotted as a function of its reaction time for only blink-triggered saccades for prosaccade and antisaccade trials, respectively. Saccades toward the singleton are represented near a direction of 0°, while saccades directed to the opposite distractor cluster near 180°. The continuous, black trace represents a computed moving average of data specified in 30-ms time epochs through the distribution. Note the transition from near 0° to close to 180° in the antisaccade condition. Data obtained from a conference proceeding (Katnani and Gandhi, 2008).

eye position. If the eyes are fixating at the onset of a blink, the perturbation is observed as a small, slow and 'loopy' eye movement. If the blink overlaps temporally with a saccade, its trajectory is altered, and its speed is often grossly reduced. Nevertheless, a reacceleration allows the saccade to land near the desired location. This interaction cannot solely be accounted for by biomechanical factors. Modulation of the high-frequency bursts of neurons in the superior colliculus (Goossens and Van Opstal, 2000b) and paramedian pontine reticular formation (Fig. 17.3B) correlates with the attenuation in eye velocity associated with such blink-perturbed saccades. The presence of a neuro-physiological contribution raises many questions that future studies must address. Some examples include the following: 1) it remains to be determined how activity in other higher-order oculomotor structures such as the frontal eye fields, which project to the OO muscles (Gong et al., 2005), is modified during blink-perturbed saccades. 2) Another avenue of research needs to consider whether trigeminally-induced and gaze-evoked blinks have similar neural signatures. A comparative approach may help to clarify whether the activity reflects (trigeminal) feedback signals or a feedforward command that already accounts for the dynamics associated with the combined blink-saccade movement. 3) Stimulation of the superior colliculus can introduce mono- and disynaptic potentials in parts of the facial nucleus that contains motoneurons innervating the OO muscle (Vidal et al., 1988). Furthermore, anatomy studies have identified tectofugal pathways that can mediate this response (Dauvergne et al., 2004). Such results permit the possibility that the oculomotor output of the colliculus is not limited to gaze shifts produced as coordinated eye-head movements, but that the neural command may in fact also integrate activation of eyelid musculature (Evinger et al., 1994) as well as other skeletomotor systems (Lünenburger et al., 2001). Additional studies are necessary to understand the coordination of movements across many effectors. 4) The OPNs have long been considered to gate both saccades and blinks. Support for this view comes from an anatomy study that reported connectivity between the regions that house the OPNs and LP motoneurons (Horn and Büttner-Ennever, 2008). A similar study is needed to check for connections between the OPNs and facial nucleus motoneurons innervating the OO muscle. In contrast, a neurophysiological study (Schultz et al., 2010) reported that the cessation of the tonic OPN activity is better synchronized with the transient eye movement than with the blink itself. These seemingly conflicting conclusions of the anatomical and electrophysiological studies need to be resolved.

The second major point of this chapter is to demonstrate the use of reflexive blinks as a tool to probe the time-course of motor preparation of saccades. Gandhi and Bonadonna (2005) reasoned that cessation of OPN activity during a blink would also remove its inhibition of the saccadic system. If true, then the neural activity associated with the developing motor programme could be expressed as a saccade accompanied with a blink, effectively offering an instantaneous behavioural readout of the motor preparation process. As detailed earlier in the chapter, this was indeed the case, as long as the animal was operating in a paradigm that required reflexive behaviour. Success with this approach has also led to a characterization of the time-course of motor preparation during behaviours requiring greater cognitive or top-down control; some examples include the countermanding task (Walton and Gandhi, 2006) and generation of antisaccades within the context of a visual search paradigm (Katnani and Gandhi, 2008). Future research questions can be extended in several directions: 1) one conspicuous finding is that a blink can only trigger saccades after the animal has the permission to initiate it. In the delayed saccade task, for example, a blink evoked during the overlap period, before the animal received the permission to initiate the eye movement, was not accompanied with a saccade. One interpretation of this outcome is that the OPNs serve as a low-level gate. Investigations that systematically manipulate higher-order gates (e.g. fixation-like neurons in the superior colliculus and frontal eye fields, and global inhibition from the substantia nigra) may reveal a motor preparation process in tasks that require voluntary control. 2) Neural recordings in the frontal eye fields during the visual search paradigm with pro- and antisaccades (Sato and Schall, 2003) have generated exciting data on spatial attention and motor preparation. Incorporating the blink perturbation approach with neurophysiological recordings during the visual search array can be a potentially powerful test. The results should provide a temporal reference frame of the neural activity that correlates with the blink perturbations behavioural readout. This information can provide crucial insight to how and where attention and motor preparation unfold.

Acknowledgments

This work was supported by NIH grants R01-EY015485 (N.J.G), P30-DC0025205, and T32-GM081760.

References

Bahill, A.T., Clark, M.R., and Stark, L. (1975). The main sequence, a tool for studying human eye movements. *Mathematical Biosciences*, **24**, 191–204.

Baker, R., McCrea, R.A., and Spencer, R.F. (1980). Synaptic organization of cat accessory abducens nucleus. *Journal of Neurophysiology*, **43**(3), 771–791.

Basso, M.A. and Wurtz, R.H. (1997). Modulation of neuronal activity by target uncertainty. *Nature*, **389**(6646), 66–69.

Basso, M.A., Powers, A.S., and Evinger, C. (1996). An explanation for reflex blink hyperexcitability in Parkinson's disease. I. Superior colliculus. *Journal of Neuroscience*, **16**(22), 7308–7317.

Becker, W. and Fuchs, A.F. (1988). Lid-eye coordination during vertical gaze changes in man and monkey. *Journal of Neurophysiology*, **60**(4), 1227–1252.

Bergamin, O., Bizzarri, S., and Straumann, D. (2002). Ocular torsion during voluntary blinks in humans. *Investigative Ophthalmology & Visual Science*, **43**(11), 3438–3443.

Björk, A. and Kugelberg, E. (1953). The electrical activity of the muscles of the eye and eyelids in various positions and during movement. *Electroencephalography and Clinical Neurophysiology*, **5**(4), 595–602.

Bour, L.J., Aramideh, M., and de Visser, B.W. (2000). Neurophysiological aspects of eye and eyelid movements during blinking in humans. *Journal of Neurophysiology*, **83**(1), 166–176.

Buneo, C.A. and Andersen, R.A. (2006). The posterior parietal cortex: sensorimotor interface for the planning and online control of visually guided movements. *Neuropsychologia*, **44**(13), 2594–2606.

Carpenter, R.H.S. (1981). Oculomotor procrastination. In D.F. Fischer and R.A. Monty (eds.) *Eye movements: cognition and visual perception* (pp. 237–246). Hillsdale, NJ: Erlbaum.

Carpenter, R.H. and Williams, M.L. (1995). Neural computation of log likelihood in control of saccadic eye movements [see comments]. *Nature*, **377**(6544), 59–62.

Cegavske, C.F., Patterson, M.M., and Thompson, R.F. (1979). Neuronal unit activity in the abducens nucleus during classical conditioning of the nictitating membrane response in the rabbit (Oryctolagus cuniculus). *Journal of Comparative & Physiological Psychology*, **93**(4), 595–609.

Chen, L.L. (2006). Head movements evoked by electrical stimulation in the frontal eye field of the monkey: evidence for independent eye and head control. *Journal of Neurophysiology*, **95**(6), 3528–3542.

Collewijn, H., van der Steen, J., and Steinman, R.M. (1985). Human eye movements associated with blinks and prolonged eyelid closure. *Journal of Neurophysiology*, **54**(1), 11–27.

Cowie, R.J. and Robinson, D.L. (1994). Subcortical contributions to head movements in macaques. I. Contrasting effects of electrical stimulation of a medial pontomedullary region and the superior colliculus. *Journal of Neurophysiology*, **72**(6), 2648–2664.

Dauvergne, C., Ndiaye, A., Buisseret-Delmas, C., Buisseret, P., Vanderwerf, F., and Pinganaud, G. (2004). Projections from the superior colliculus to the trigeminal system and facial nucleus in the rat. *Journal of Comparative Neurology*, **478**(3), 233–247.

Delgado-Garcia, J.M., Evinger, C., Escudero, M., and Baker, R. (1990). Behavior of accessory abducens and abducens motoneurons during eye retraction and rotation in the alert cat. *Journal of Neurophysiology*, **64**(2), 413–422.

Dorris, M.C., Paré, M., and Munoz, D.P. (1997). Neuronal activity in monkey superior colliculus related to the initiation of saccadic eye movements. *Journal of Neuroscience*, **17**(21), 8566–8579.

Evinger, C. and Manning, K.A. (1993). Pattern of extraocular muscle activation during reflex blinking. *Experimental Brain Research*, **92**(3), 502–506.

Evinger, C., Graf, W.M., and Baker, R. (1987). Extra- and intracellular HRP analysis of the organization of extraocular motoneurons and internuclear neurons in the guinea pig and rabbit. *Journal of Comparative Neurology*, **262**(3), 429–445.

Evinger, C., Manning, K.A., and Sibony, P.A. (1991). Eyelid movements. Mechanisms and normal data. *Investigative Ophthalmology & Visual Science*, **32**(2), 387–400.

Evinger, C., Shaw, M.D., Peck, C.K., Manning, K.A., and Baker, R. (1984). Blinking and associated eye movements in humans, guinea pigs, and rabbits. *Journal of Neurophysiology*, **52**(2), 323–339.

Evinger, C., Basso, M.A., Manning, K.A., Sibony, P.A., Pellegrini, J.J., and Horn, A.K. (1993). A role for the basal ganglia in nicotinic modulation of the blink reflex. *Experimental Brain Research*, **92**(3), 507–515.

Evinger, C., Manning, K.A., Pellegrini, J.J., Basso, M.A., Powers, A.S., and Sibony, P.A. (1994). Not looking while leaping: the linkage of blinking and saccadic gaze shifts. *Experimental Brain Research*, **100**(2), 337–344.

Freedman, E.G. (2001). Interactions between eye and head control signals can account for movement kinematics. *Biological Cybernetics*, **84**, 453–462.

Freedman, E.G. and Sparks, D.L. (2000). Coordination of the eyes and head: movement kinematics. *Experimental Brain Research*, **131**(1), 22–32.

Fuchs, A.F., Ling, L., Kaneko, C.R.S., King, W.M., and Usher, S.D. (1991). The timing of the response of brainstem omni-pause neurons relative to saccadic eye movements in rhesus monkeys. *Society for Neurosciences Abstract*, **17**, 462.

Fuchs, A.F., Becker, W., Ling, L., Langer, T.P., and Kaneko, C.R. (1992). Discharge patterns of levator palpebrae superioris motoneurons during vertical lid and eye movements in the monkey. *Journal of Neurophysiology*, **68**(1), 233–243.

Gandhi, N.J. (2007). Consequence of blinks on interactions between the eye and head components of gaze shifts. *Society for Neurosciences Abstract,* Program No. 178.2.

Gandhi, N.J. and Bonadonna, D.K. (2005). Temporal interactions of air-puff evoked blinks and saccadic eye movements: Insights into motor preparation. *Journal of Neurophysiology,* **93**(3), 1718–1729.

Glimcher, P.W. and Sparks, D.L. (1992). Movement selection in advance of action in the superior colliculus. *Nature,* **355**(6360), 542–545.

Gong, S., DeCuypere, M., Zhao, Y., and LeDoux, M.S. (2005). Cerebral cortical control of orbicularis oculi motoneurons. *Brain Research,* **1047**(2), 177–193.

Goossens, H.H. and Van Opstal, A.J. (2000a). Blink-perturbed saccades in monkey. I. Behavioral analysis. *Journal of Neurophysiology,* **83**(6), 3411–3429.

Goossens, H.H. and Van Opstal, A.J. (2000b). Blink-perturbed saccades in monkey. II. Superior colliculus activity. *Journal of Neurophysiology,* **83**(6), 3430–3452.

Gruart, A., Blazquez, P., and Delgado-Garcia, J.M. (1995). Kinematics of spontaneous, reflex, and conditioned eyelid movements in the alert cat. *Journal of Neurophysiology,* **74**(1), 226–248.

Guitton, D., Simard, R., and Codere, F. (1991). Upper eyelid movements measured with a search coil during blinks and vertical saccades. *Investigative Ophthalmology & Visual Science,* **32**(13), 3298–3305.

Hanes, D.P., and Schall, J.D. (1995). Countermanding saccades in macaque. *Visual Neuroscience,* **12**(5), 929–937.

Hanes, D.P. and Schall, J.D. (1996). Neural control of voluntary movement initiation. *Science,* **274**(5286), 427–430.

Helmchen, C. and Rambold, H. (2007). The eyelid and its contribution to eye movements. *Developments in Ophthalmology,* **40**, 110–131.

Hemelt, M.E. and Keller, A. (2008). Superior colliculus control of vibrissa movements. *Journal of Neurophysiology,* **100**(3), 1245–1254.

Hikosaka, O. and Wurtz, R.H. (1983). Visual and oculomotor functions of monkey substantia nigra pars reticulata. IV. Relation of substantia nigra to superior colliculus. *Journal of Neurophysiology,* **49**(5), 1285–1301.

Horn, A.K. and Büttner-Ennever, J.A. (2008). Brainstem circuits controlling lid-eye coordination in monkey. *Progress in Brain Research,* **171**, 87–95.

Horn, A.K., Buttner-Ennever, J.A., Gayde, M., and Messoudi, A. (2000). Neuroanatomical identification of mesencephalic premotor neurons coordinating eyelid with upgaze in the monkey and man. *Journal of Comparative Neurology,* **420**(1), 19–34.

Horn, A.K., Helmchen, C., and Wahle, P. (2003). GABAergic neurons in the rostral mesencephalon of the macaque monkey that control vertical eye movements. *Annals of the New York Academy of Sciences,* **1004**, 19–28.

Huerta, M.F., Frankfurter, A.J., and Harting, J.K. (1981). The trigeminocollicular projection in the cat: patch-like endings within the intermediate gray. *Brain Research,* **211**(1), 1–13.

Huerta, M.F., Frankfurter, A., and Harting, J.K. (1983). Studies of the principal sensory and spinal trigeminal nuclei of the rat: projections to the superior colliculus, inferior olive, and cerebellum. *Journal of Comparative Neurology,* **220**(2), 147–167.

Ikeda, T. and Hikosaka, O. (2003). Reward-dependent gain and bias of visual responses in primate superior colliculus. *Neuron,* **39**(4), 693–700.

Juan, C.H., Shorter-Jacobi, S.M., and Schall, J.D. (2004). Dissociation of spatial attention and saccade preparation. *Proceedings of the National Academy of Sciences U S A,* **101**(43), 15541–15544.

Katnani, H.A. and Gandhi, N.J. (2008). Evaluation of the premotor theory of attention using blink-triggered saccades *Society for Neurosciences Abstract,* Program No. 165.2.

Keller, E.L. (1974). Participation of medial pontine reticular formation in eye movement generation in monkey. *Journal of Neurophysiology,* **37**(2), 316–332.

Lappin, J.S. and Eriksen, C.W. (1966). Use of a delayed signal to stop a visual reaction-time response. *Journal of Experimental Psychology,* **72**, 805–811.

Logan, G.D. and Cowan, W.B. (1984). On the ability to inhibit thought and action: a theory of an act of control. *Psychological Review,* **91**, 295–327.

Lünenburger, L., Kleiser, R., Stuphorn, V., Miller, L.E., and Hoffmann, K.P. (2001). A possible role of the superior colliculus in eye-hand coordination. *Progress in Brain Research,* **134**, 109–125.

May, P.J. and Porter, J.D. (1998). The distribution of primary afferent terminals from the eyelids of macaque monkeys. *Experimental Brain Research,* **123**(4), 368.

May, P.J., Vidal, P.P., and Baker, R. (1990). Synaptic organization of tectal-facial pathways in cat. II. Synaptic potentials following midbrain tegmentum stimulation. *Journal of Neurophysiology,* **64**(2), 381–402.

May, P.J., Baker, R.G., and Chen, B. (2002). The eyelid levator muscle: servant of two masters. *Movement Disorders,* **17**(Suppl 2), S4–7.

Mays, L.E. and Morrisse, D.W. (1994). Activity of pontine omnipause neurons during eye blinks. *Society for Neurosciences Abstract,* **20**, 1404.

Mays, L.E. and Morrisse, D.W. (1995). Electrical stimulation of the pontine omnipause area inhibits eye blink. *Journal of the American Optometric Association,* **66**(7), 419–422.

McPeek, R.M. and Keller, E.L. (2002). Saccade target selection in the superior colliculus during a visual search task. *Journal of Neurophysiology,* **88**(4), 2019–2034.

Mirabella, G., Pani, P., Paré, M., and Ferraina, S. (2006). Inhibitory control of reaching movements in humans. *Experimental Brain Research*, **174**(2), 240–255.

Miyashita, E. and Mori, S. (1995). The superior colliculus relays signals descending from the vibrissal motor cortex to the facial nerve nucleus in the rat. *Neuroscience Letters*, **195**(1), 69–71.

Morcuende, S., Delgado-Garcia, J.-M., and Ugolini, G. (2002). Neuronal premotor networks involved in eyelid responses: retrograde transneuronal tracing with rabies virus from the orbicularis oculi muscle in the rat. *Journal of Neuroscience*, **22**(20), 8808–8818.

Munoz, D.P. and Everling, S. (2004). Look away: the anti-saccade task and the voluntary control of eye movement. *Nat Rev Neurosci*, **5**(3), 218–228.

Munoz, D.P. and Wurtz, R.H. (1993a). Fixation cells in monkey superior colliculus. I. Characteristics of cell discharge. *Journal of Neurophysiology*, **70**(2), 559–575.

Munoz, D.P. and Wurtz, R.H. (1993b). Fixation cells in monkey superior colliculus. II. Reversible activation and deactivation. *Journal of Neurophysiology*, **70**(2), 576–589.

Murthy, A., Thompson, K.G., and Schall, J.D. (2001). Dynamic dissociation of visual selection from saccade programming in frontal eye field. *Journal of Neurophysiology*, **86**(5), 2634–2637.

Ndiaye, A., Pinganaud, G., Buisseret-Delmas, C., Buisseret, P., and Vanderwerf, F. (2002). Organization of trigeminocollicular connections and their relations to the sensory innervation of the eyelids in the rat. *Journal of Comparative Neurology*, **448**(4), 373–387.

Paré, M. and Hanes, D.P. (2003). Controlled movement processing: superior colliculus activity associated with countermanded saccades. *Journal of Neuroscience*, **23**(16), 6480–6489.

Porter, J.D., Burns, L.A., and May, P.J. (1989). Morphological substrate for eyelid movements: innervation and structure of primate levator palpebrae superioris and orbicularis oculi muscles. *Journal of Comparative Neurology*, **287**(1), 64–81.

Pouget, P., Stepniewska, I., Crowder, E.A., Leslie, M.W., Emeric, E.E., Nelson, M.J., *et al.* (2009). Visual and motor connectivity and the distribution of calcium-binding proteins in macaque frontal eye field: implications for saccade target selection. *Frontiers in Neuroanatomy*, **3**, 2.

Rambold, H., El Baz, I., and Helmchen, C. (2004). Differential effects of blinks on horizontal saccade and smooth pursuit initiation in humans. *Experimental Brain Research*, **156**(3), 314–324.

Rambold, H., El Baz, I., and Helmchen, C. (2005). Blink effects on ongoing smooth pursuit eye movements in humans. *Experimental Brain Research*, **161**(1), 11–26.

Rambold, H., Sprenger, A., and Helmchen, C. (2002). Effects of voluntary blinks on saccades, vergence eye movements, and saccade-vergence interactions in humans. *Journal of Neurophysiology*, **88**(3), 1220–1233.

Riggs, L., Kelly, J., Manning, K., and Moore, R. (1987). Blink-related eye movements. *Investigative Ophthalmology & Visual Science*, **28**(2), 334–342.

Rizzolatti, G., Riggio, L., Dascola, I., and Umilta, C. (1987). Reorienting attention across the horizontal and vertical meridians: evidence in favor of a premotor theory of attention. *Neuropsychologia*, **25**(1A), 31–40.

Rottach, K.G., Das, V.E., Wohlgemuth, W., Zivotofsky, A.Z., and Leigh, R.J. (1998). Properties of horizontal saccades accompanied by blinks. *Journal of Neurophysiology*, **79**(6), 2895–2902.

Sato, T.R. and Schall, J.D. (2003). Effects of stimulus-response compatibility on neural selection in frontal eye field. *Neuron*, **38**(4), 637–648.

Schultz, K.P., Williams, C.R., and Busettini, C. (2010). Macaque pontine omnipause neurons play no direct role in the generation of eye blinks. *Journal of Neurophysiology*, **103**(4), 2255–2274.

Sparks, D.L. and Mays, L.E. (1990). Signal transformations required for the generation of saccadic eye movements. *Annual Review of Neuroscience*, **13**, 309–336.

Trigo, J.A., Gruart, A., and Delgado-Garcia, J.M. (1999a). Discharge profiles of abducens, accessory abducens, and orbicularis oculi motoneurons during reflex and conditioned blinks in alert cats. *Journal of Neurophysiology*, **81**(4), 1666–1684.

Trigo, J.A., Gruart, A., and Delgado-Garcia, J.M. (1999b). Role of proprioception in the control of lid position during reflex and conditioned blink responses in the alert behaving cat. *Neuroscience*, **90**(4), 1515–1528.

van Ham, J.J., and Yeo, C.H. (1996). Trigeminal inputs to eyeblink motoneurons in the rabbit. *Experimental Neurology*, **142**(2), 244–257.

Vidal, P.P., May, P.J., and Baker, R. (1988). Synaptic organization of the tectal-facial pathways in the cat. I. Synaptic potentials following collicular stimulation. *Journal of Neurophysiology*, **60**(2), 769–797.

Walton, M.M.G. and Gandhi, N.J. (2006). Behavioral evaluation of movement cancellation. *Journal of Neurophysiology*, **96**(4), 2011–2024.

Watanabe, M. and Munoz, D.P. (2010). Saccade suppression by electrical microstimulation in monkey caudate nucleus. *Journal of Neuroscience*, **30**(7), 2700–2709.

Williamson, S.S., Zivotofsky, A.Z., and Basso, M.A. (2005). Modulation of gaze-evoked blinks depends primarily on extraretinal factors. *Journal of Neurophysiology*, **93**(1), 627–632.

Wurtz, R.H., Sommer, M.A., Paré, M., and Ferraina, S. (2001). Signal transformations from cerebral cortex to superior colliculus for the generation of saccades. *Vision Research*, **41**(25–26), 3399–3412.

CHAPTER 18

Neural control of three-dimensional gaze shifts

J. Douglas Crawford and Eliana M. Klier

Abstract

In laboratory conditions, with the head restrained and held upright, eye-in-head orientation vectors are constrained to a tilted two-dimensional (2D) range called Listing's plane. However, in most real-world conditions gaze control utilizes a three-dimensional (3D) range. For example, when the head is allowed to move naturally, the accompanying saccades and vestibulo-ocular reflex movements include coordinated torsional components, out of, and then back into Listing's plane. The head itself rotates more like a set of Fick gimbals, resulting in a non-planar range of orientation vectors. To control this complex behaviour, the brainstem reticular formation appears to have struck upon an elegant solution: it encodes the 3D components of posture and movement in coordinates that align with the Listing and Fick behavioural constraints, such that its control signals collapse to 2D (zero torsion) when these constraints are upheld, but it retains the capacity for torsional control whenever required. In contrast, the superior colliculus and cortex appear to only encode 2D gaze direction. Surprisingly, after many years of research on this topic, we still know very little—other than a few clues—about the neural mechanisms that transform high-level 2D gaze direction commands into the 3D control signals for eye and head orientation.

Listing's and Donders' laws

Most oculomotor studies are primarily concerned with the control of 2D gaze direction, i.e. how the brain points the visual axis towards objects of interest. However, there are two important areas where one needs to consider the 3D orientation of the eye. The first involves any kind of visual stimulus that activates the retina beyond the fovea, because here the spatial pattern of retinal stimulation depends both on the configuration of the stimulus in space and the *torsional* orientation of the eyes around the visual axis. The second (which will be the focus of this review) relates to gaze *control*: the eye is equipped with the musculature to rotate in 3D. As we shall see, the eyes can and do rotate about nearly any combination of components about the vertical (left/right), horizontal (up/down) and torsional (clockwise/counterclockwise) axes (note that directions are defined here from the subject's perspective). As we shall see, torsion is not allowed to vary randomly: the brain usually sets a certain amount of torsion for a given 2D gaze direction, and sometimes it actively generates a muscular contraction to rapidly change the direction and amount of ocular torsion.

In the 19th century Donders proposed that for any one gaze direction, the eye assumes a unique orientation (one torsional value), no matter how it got there (Donders, 1848). The precise value of this torsion was then described in Listing's law. The origins of Listing's law are somewhat obscure. Listing was a German mathematician who somehow intuited that the eye assumes only those orientations that can be reached from some central reference position by rotations about axes within a single plane. For one special reference position, the line of gaze is orthogonal to the associate plane of axes; this is called primary position, and the associated plane is called Listing's plane. The best coordinate system to describe Listing's law (Listing's coordinates) can be defined by expressing eye orientations in terms of vectors aligned with the axes of rotation from primary position, scaling these vectors to the angle of rotation, and defining torsion as rotation about the head-fixed axis aligned with the primary gaze direction. Once this coordinate system is defined, Listing's law is simple: it just says that torsion equals zero (Westheimer, 1957). Examples of such data, in Listing's coordinates, are provided by Angelaki in Chapter 8 in this volume, and are also shown later in this chapter in Figs. 18.3C and 18.6B.

The description of Listing's law in terms of axes of rotation is more complicated. Intuitively, one would think that the eye would rotate about an axis in Listing's plane, but this is not what happens. In fact, if this is done, it causes a violation of Listing's law (Crawford and Vilis, 1991). As illustrated in Chapter 8 by Angelaki, in order to keep eye position in Listing's plane, the axis of eye rotation must tilt out of Listing's plane in a position-dependent manner. This is a requirement of the laws of rotational kinematics (Tweed and Vilis, 1987). (Many people find that this makes intuitive sense only after a couple of years of intense study; otherwise it is best left for mathematicians.)

Listing's law was first described, and confirmed, by Helmholtz, with the clever use of visual after-images (Helmholtz, 1867). Modern recording techniques are more direct, and usually involve the placement of two search coils in the eye within a set of orthogonal magnetic fields. So far these experiments have not revealed any behavioural differences between the human and monkey, so we will cite literature from both species together. These experiments have shown that Listing's law is obeyed when the head is held upright and stationary during saccades and fixations (Crawford and Vilis, 1991; Ferman et al., 1987a, 1987b; Straumann et al., 1991; Tweed and Vilis, 1990). In monkeys Listing's plane generally tilts back in the head whereas in humans its orientation seems to vary highly from subject to subject. Listing's law is also obeyed during smooth pursuit eye movements (Haslwanter et al., 1991; Tweed et al. 1992) and gaze fixation during purely translational head movements (Angelaki, 2003; Angelaki et al., 2003). It is obeyed in modified form during vergence movements (where the Listing's planes of the two eyes tilt outward (Mok et al., 1992; Van Rijn et al., 1993)) and when the head is stationary but not upright (resulting in either shifts or tilts (Crawford and Vilis, 1991; Haslwanter et al., 1992)). However, when the head rotates, vestibular and/or visual inputs can stabilize the retinal image of distant targets by rotating the eye about the same axis, but opposite direction, as the head, thus violating Listing's law (Crawford and Vilis, 1991; Fetter et al., 1992; Misslisch and Hess, 2000). The common theme of these rules is that whenever there is a degrees of freedom problem (gaze direction is specified but not torsion) Listing's law or some variant is used, but when specific torsional movements are required Listing's law is violated (Crawford et al., 2003).

There has been a surprisingly long-lived, and often obscure controversy about whether Listing's law is implemented mechanically or neurally (Angelaki, 2003; Angelaki and Hess, 2004; Crawford and Guitton, 1997; Crawford and Vilis, 1991; Misslisch and Tweed, 2001; Quaia and Optican, 1998; Raphan, 1998; Schnabolk and Raphan, 1994; Tweed and Vilis, 1987, 1990). Rather than review this entire controversy we will simply state our own view, which is that in retrospect this argument was largely based on the conflation of two different computational issues. In order to produce Listing's law, the oculomotor system must do two things: it must specify the desired 3D orientation of the eye, and it then choses the correct axis of eye rotation for a given initial position. In the first kinematically correct model of the 3D saccade generator, these two computations were done 'neurally' within one 'Listing's law box'. However, as described by Angelaki (Chapter 8, this volume), there is good evidence to suggest that the position-dependent axis tilts required to maintain eye position in Listing's plane are implemented mechanically by the tissues surrounding the eye (Demer et al., 1995;

Ghasia and Angelaki, 2005; Klier et al., 2006; Kono et al., 2002). This simplifies some of the control issues associated with generating eye movements that stay within Listing's plane. However, these mechanical position-dependencies cannot *constrain* the eye to Listing's plane (if they did, the system would not be able to violate Listing's law, which it often does).

More recent models of the 3D saccade generator have separated the neural process of selecting the desired orientation of the eye (and then choosing the movement vector that will get it there) from the mechanical process that determines the required axis tilts (Crawford and Guitton, 1997; Glasauer et al., 2001a, 2001b; Tweed, 1997). These models demonstrate that an eye 'plant' optimized for Listing's law will still only produce Listing's law if it is given the right neural signals, and will violate Listing's law if given different signals (Smith and Crawford, 1998). Thus, Listing's law is both neural and mechanical: it is the sequential product of neuromechanical control system.

Perhaps a second factor that has skewed our view of Listing's law is that 90% of the studies done on 3D ocular kinematics are done with the head artificially restrained. When the head is allowed to move naturally, a different picture emerges.

What happens to these rules when the head is not restrained?

Listing's law is only upheld continuously when the head is restrained. When the head is allowed to move naturally the gaze control system shows quite different properties (again, the story is quite similar for both the human and the monkey, so we will refer to both literatures equally). Despite the additional complexity of eye-head coordination, the system still appears to follow certain 'lawful' kinematic relationships (see Corneil, Chapter 16, this volume), and 3D control is no exception. If one understands the oculomotor rules described in the previous section, then one can understand the rules for eye-head coordination: 1) by understanding how these rules interact, and 2) by understanding the analogous rules that apply to head movement.

Rule 1: as long as the subject holds the eye and head stationary in space, the eye-in-head range (Fig. 18.1C) is statistically indistinguishable from Listing's plane (Crawford et al., 1999; Glenn and Vilis, 1992; Radeau et al., 1994; Straumann et al., 1991). However, *during* gaze shifts torsional control becomes more complicated. It is well known that during large rapid gaze shifts, typically a visually-guided saccade occurs while the head is just starting to build up momentum in the same general direction. Once the eye reaches its target, the vestibular-ocular reflex (VOR) turns on, causing the eye to roll back in the head so that gaze stays on target while the head completes its trajectory (Guitton, 1992; see also Hess (Chapter 3) and Corneil (Chapter 16) this volume). The conundrum here for 3D control is that, as stated above, saccades obey Listing's law and the VOR does not. Left unchecked, the VOR would generally drive the eye quite far out of Listing's plane. Apparently to avoid this, during head-free gaze shifts saccades take on anticipatory torsional components that are opposite and approximately equal to the oncoming torsional component of the VOR (Crawford et al., 1999; Crawford and Vilis, 1991; Tweed, 1997). This results in the eye ending up back in Listing's plane when the whole sequence is done (Fig. 18.1D). Tweed and colleagues exploited this property to induced the 'world record' for eye torsion in healthy subjects, inducing people to generate saccades with torsional components up to 17°. Thus, continuous adherence to Listing's law is an artefact of immobilizing the head.

In terms of the head movement itself, during gaze shifts the head follows its own version of Donders' law, albeit less precisely than the eye and in a different form (Crawford et al., 1999; Glenn and Vilis, 1992; Radeau et al., 1994). Instead of following Listing's law, the head acts as if it rotates horizontally about a body-fixed vertical axis but vertically about a head-fixed horizontal axis, like a set of Fick gimbals (Fig. 18.2). Torsion in this new coordinate system is again kept at a minimum in Fick coordinates, but when these data are plotted in Listing's coordinates, this results in a non-planar range of orientation vectors that is consistently twisted at the oblique corners (Fig. 18.1B).

Like eye movements, head torsion is not always held at zero, even in Fick coordinates: during oblique gaze shifts the head takes the shortest path from one corner of the range to the other in position space rather than curving along its Donders' range (Crawford et al., 1999). Moreover, the

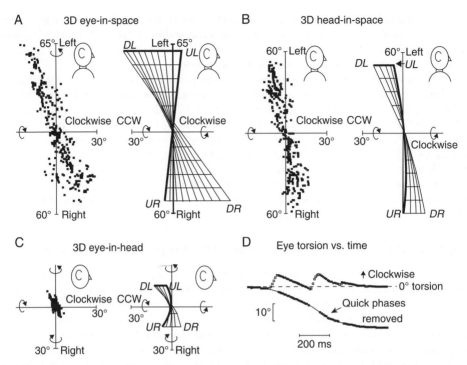

Fig. 18.1 Donders' laws for eye, head, and eye-in-space during head-free gaze fixations in the monkey (human data look the same). In each case torsional orientation is restricted compared to vertical and horizontal orientation. Panels (A–C) (left sides) plot tips of 3D eye position vectors (horizontal component as a function of torsional component) in an orthogonal right-hand coordinate system. The right sides show 2D surfaces fit to these ranges. In the 3D gaze literature this is known as a 'side view', because it views axes of rotation (relative to the zero vector reference position) are viewed from the side. *DL*, *UL*, *UR*, and *DR* represent Down-Left, Up-Left, Up-Right, and Down-Right orientations. A) The range of eye orientation in space consistently follows a twisted 'Fick' range. B) The range of head orientation in space also follows a Fick range. C) The range of eye orientation relative to the head shows variable twists that are not significantly different from the (Listing's) planar range seen in head-fixed saccades. D) Torsional eye-in-head position plotted during one multistep gaze shift including a large horizontal head movement (not shown). Without the anticipatory torsional components in saccades (quick phases) the eye would be driven far from Listing's plane. Reprinted from *Journal of Neurophysiology*, **97**, Klier, E.M., Wang, H., and Crawford, J.D., Interstitial nucleus of cajal encodes three-dimensional head orientations in Fick-like coordinates, p. 604, figure 3 © 2007 The American Physiological Society, used with permission.

Fick range is modified by gravity (shifting and tilting for body roll and pitch, respectively) in a fashion similar to Listing's law (Misslisch et al., 1994), can be modified to Listing's plane when the head alone is used to point gaze or to a shortest path strategy (resulting in a break down of Donders' law) when head pointing is dissociated from gaze (Ceylan et al., 2000). Thus, much like Donders' law for the eye, Donders' law for the head is associated with its own intrinsic coordinate system, where zero torsion can be selected, or not, depending on task requirements.

The final range to consider is that of eye orientation in space, which one can think of as a 3D version of gaze. Since Listing's plane is fixed in the head, and since eye position contributes relatively little to head-free gaze fixations over a wide range, the eye and head constraints interact to produce a range of eye-in-space (gaze) orientations that also resemble the range produced by Fick gimbals (Fig. 18.1A). Moreover, since the control of head torsion is much sloppier than control of eye torsion (in the order of ±5° compared to ±°1), the resulting torsional range of the eye-in-space is even sloppier (Crawford et al., 1999; Glenn and Vilis, 1992).

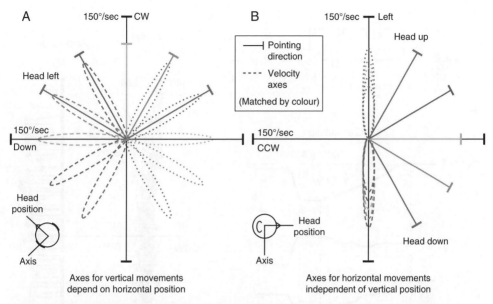

Fig. 18.2 (Also see Plate 10.) Schematic axes of rotation, and their dependence on orientation, in a Fick system, plotted in orthogonal Cartesian coordinates. Angular velocity (broken lines) is a vector parallel to the axis of rotation, scaled by the speed of rotation. The angular velocity of the eye and head generally follows the loops, starting at zero velocity, growing to maximum velocity, and then returning to zero. In each panel, five head pointing directions are shown (solid lines), each colour coded to two velocity loops in opposite directions (dashed vs. dotted lines). A) Velocity loops for vertical rotations at five horizontal positions, viewed from above. B) Velocity loops for horizontal rotations at five vertical positions, viewed from the side. Real head data follow the same pattern, but are never as symmetric. Reprinted from *Journal of Neurophysiology*, **97**, Klier, E.M., Wang, H., and Crawford, J.D., Interstitial nucleus of Cajal encodes three-dimensional head orientations in Fick-like coordinates, p. 604, figure 3 © 2007 The American Physiological Society, used with permission.

Premotor control of 3D eye velocity and orientation

Figure 18.3A shows the classic Robinsonian model for oculomotor control (Robinson, 1981). In this highly influential model, eye movements are encoded by a velocity signal, that is then integrated to provide a position signal, and the two are then summed at the level of motoneurons to rotate the eye against resistive viscous forces and hold it against elastic forces in the surrounding tissues. It turns out that this model does not translate well into 3D if the movement signal encodes angular velocity (i.e. degrees/second about the physical axis of rotation) because 3D orientation is not the derivative of 3D velocity (Tweed and Vilis, 1987). For example, during saccades angular velocity has torsional components (for the position-dependent axis tilts described above) that would be integrated to produce inappropriate torsional position signals. However, if the movement signal encodes derivatives—small changes in eye orientation divided by time (Crawford, 1994; Crawford and Guitton, 1997; Quaia and Optican, 1998)—and feeds this to motoneurons for a plant that mechanically implements the torsional axis tilts (Demer et al., 1995; Kono et al., 2002), then this scheme works just fine for saccades. Angelaki and colleagues have verified this scheme by correlating motoneuron firing rate against the torsional components of eye velocity (Ghasia and Angelaki, 2005), and analysing the changes in eye position produced by motoneuron stimulation (Klier et al., 2006). This works nicely for saccades, but complicates the VOR, which does not receive eye orientation derivatives from the semicircular canals and does not like position-dependent axis tilts (these would destabilize vision). However, it is a fairly simple matter for the VOR to undo these tilts with the right interaction between

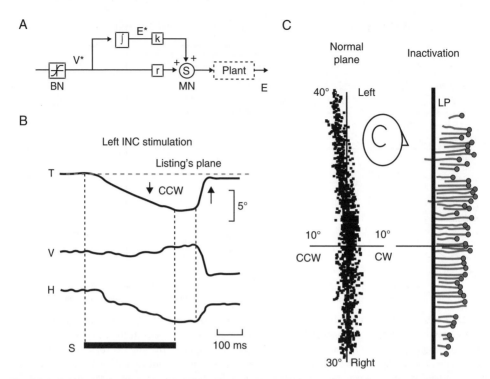

Fig. 18.3 Evidence of a 3D neural integrator for eye orientation, organized in Listing's coordinates, in the interstitial nucleus of Cajal (INC). A) David A. Robinson's seminal 1D model of the saccade generator. Reticular formation burst neurons (*BN*) have a saturating estimate of desired eye velocity (V*) which is sent to the neural integrator (∫), which converts this into a desired eye position signal (E*). V* and E* are then scaled and summed at the motoneurons (*MN*) to provide the required signal to control the *PLANT* (eye and muscles). B) Torsional (T), vertical (V), and horizontal (H) components of eye position plotted against time during INC stimulation (S). The eye rotates primarily counterclockwise (CCW) or clockwise (CW) out of Listing's plane during left and right INC stimulation respectively. Final eye position is held until the next saccade, which returns it to Listing's plane. Similar data published in Crawford et al. (1991). C) Left side: eye orientation vectors during head-fixed fixations, plotted in Listing's coordinates and viewed from the side. Right panel: following injection of muscimol into the the left INC, the eye drifts (grey traces) clockwise, orthogonal to Listing's plane (LP) until the start of the next saccade (○). Right INC injection produces the opposite pattern. Similar data plotted in Crawford (1994).

eye position and velocity signals before integration (Smith and Crawford, 1998; see also Cullen and Horn, Chapter 9, this volume).

So where then do the premotor signals arise for 3D saccades and eye position? At this time, human brain imaging techniques have too many spatiotemporal limitations to address this question, so nearly everything we know about this system comes from physiological studies with awake, behaving animals. The horizontal velocity components of saccades are encoded by burst neurons in the paramedian pontine reticular formation (PPRF) (e.g. Luschei and Fuchs, 1972) and the corresponding neural integrator for horizontal eye position is located in the nucleus prepositus hypoglossi (NPH) (e.g. Cannon and Robinson, 1987). The corresponding circuits for vertical and torsional saccades are located in the midbrain. The rostral interstitial nucleus of the medial longitudinal fasciculus (riMLF) possess burst neurons whose activity correlates to the vertical/torsional components of rapid eye movements (Buttner et al., 1977; Crawford and Vilis, 1992; Hepp et al., 1988; King et al., 1979).

The interstitial nucleus of Cajal (INC) appears to be the neural integration for vertical and torsional components (Crawford et al., 1991; Fukushima, 1987; Helmchen et al., 1998). It has the right anatomy: the riMLF projects to the INC, and both project to the motoneurons for eye muscles that control vertical/torsional rotation. Moreover, we know of this arrangement because: 1) the INC has activity related to vertical/torsional eye position, 2) pharmacological inactivation obliterates the ability to hold vertical/torsional eye positions (Fig. 18.3C), and 3) electrical stimulation of the INC produces vertical/torsional eye movements that hold their final position, as if one had 'charged up' a neural integrator (Fig. 18.3B).

The riMLF and INC appear to be similarly organized into pools of neurons with specific directional control very similar to those of the eye muscles and semicircular canals (see also Hess, Chapter 3, this volume). Units on both sides of the midline can be divided into randomly intermingled populations with upward or downward velocity or position tuning. However these same units are also tuned for clockwise components on the left side of midline and counterclockwise components on the right side (Crawford et al., 1991; Crawford and Vilis, 1992). Taken together with the horizontal populations in the PPRF/NPH, this creates a set of neuron pools like those illustrated in Fig. 18.4. This configuration is fully 3D but easily collapses to 2D: whenever the oculomotor system requires a torsional component (as in the saccades that occur with head-free gaze shifts) it need only create an imbalance between activity in the left and right riMLF (and thus INC) so that clockwise and counterclockwise components do not balance to zero. But as long as these two sides are balanced (as in saccades with the head fixed) torsion will cancel and the residual horizontal and vertical components of activation will determine saccade direction (Crawford et al., 1991; Crawford and Vilis, 1992).

This is all very well, but there is one hitch that is all too easy to take for granted. It depends on the non-trivial assumption that the neuron pools in Fig. 18.4 are organized in a coordinate system that aligns with Listing's plane. It has been shown many times that the orientation of Listing's plane in the head varies considerably from one subject to the next. If, for example, the PPRF encoded rotations about an earth-vertical axis with the head upright, in most subjects PPRF activation would drive eye position out of Listing's plane. However, there is evidence that these coordinates do in fact align. First, inactivation of the riMLF leaves axes of rotation for horizontal saccades (presumably generated by the PPRF) that align with Listing's plane, and unilateral coactivation of the up and down neuron populations of the riMLF produce rotations about an axis orthogonal to Listing's plane (Crawford and Vilis, 1992). Third, torsional drift during unilateral INC is perfectly orthogonal to Listing's plane (Fig. 18.3C) and settles to a range of positions parallel to Listing's plane (Crawford, 1994). Each of these observations is only possible with the coordinate system we want: Listing's coordinates.

To sum up, a series of observations simplify the control of 3D saccades: 1) eye muscles encode derivatives, not angular velocity, 2) torsional control is arranged symmetrically across the brainstem, 3) the brainstem coordinates for saccades align with Listing's plane. With this, and only this arrangement, saccades in Listing's plane will result from the planar coding of 2D movement vectors. But this still requires a very delicate balance of neural activation—no accident or trivial default—and torsional saccade components must be programmed very precisely when the head moves.

Premotor control of head orientation

As with the eye, there may be mechanical advantages for using a Fick-like coordinate system for head control. For gaze shifts to distant targets, one is mainly concerned with head orientation, but the head does not rotate in-place like the eye. Instead it rotates (and translates) much like an inverted pendulum, except that base is a flexible multijointed column (the cervical spine). The lower cervical vertebrae act somewhat like the vertical axis (for horizontal rotation), whereas vertical rotation (about the horizontal axis) occurs mainly about the higher cervical vertebrae (Graf et al., 1995a, 1995b; Vidal et al. 1986), as in a nested set of Fick axes. Nevertheless, it is once again clear that these mechanical factors do not constrain the head to a zero-torsion range. To convince oneself of this, one need only voluntarily roll the head torsionally from side to side. This means that, as in the

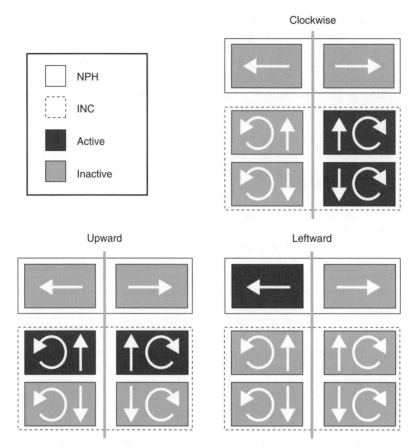

Fig. 18.4 Schema of populations of neurons for eye and head orientation control in the nucleus preopositus hypoglossi (NPH) and interstitial nucleus of Cajal (INC). Six neural populations are shown, divided across the brainstem midline (vertical bar) with arrows indicating their directional control in a fashion very similar to the semicircular canals and eye muscles (where vertical and torsional components are combined). The filled colour blocks show how these populations would be activated during clockwise (upper right panel), upward (lower left panel), and leftward (lower right panel) orientations. This schema only works if these populations coordinates align with the intrinsic coordinates of behaviour, i.e. Listing's plane for the eye and Fick coordinates for the head. A similar organization is seen in the burst neurons that provide the velocity signal for the eye. Reprinted from *Journal of Neurophysiology*, **68**, Crawford, J.D. and Vilis, T., Symmetry of, oculomotor burst neuron coordinates about Listing's plane, p. 432 figure 15 © 1992 The American Physiological Society, used with permission.

oculomotor system, the neural control system for the head must be optimally matched to the mechanical stages of the control system.

Little is known about the neural control of 3D head orientation (head movement studies are essentially impossible with current brain imaging techniques). However, there are a few clues from animal models that, at least so far as gaze control is concerned, the oculomotor and head motor systems share both circuitry and control principles. First of all, electrical stimulation of higher-level gaze structures in the cortex, superior colliculus (SC), and cerebellum evokes gaze shifts that involve movements of both the eyes and head (this topic will be taken up further in the next section). Moreover, this circuitry is shared down to the level of the brainstem. For example, in animals with unilateral stimulation of most PPRF sites produces ramp-like ipsilateral rotations of both the eyes and head (Gandhi et al., 2008). This implicates the PPRF in the control of both eye and head motion.

Similar observations have been made for the INC. The INC projects to spinal cord neurons involved in neck control via the interstitiospinal tract (Fukushima, 1987; Fukushima et al., 1980; 1994). Unilateral stimulation of the INC (Fig. 18.5B) produces vertical/torsional head rotations following very similar directions and patterns similar to those seen in the eye (clockwise for left INC stimulation, counterclockwise for right INC stimulation, and final positions that are held until corrected) (Klier et al., 2002, 2007). As with the eye, unilateral inactivation of the INC produces a transient nystagmus-like pattern of torsional head drift (Fig. 18.5A) with corrective 'quick phases' that eventually dissipate, leaving the head tilted in a torticollis-like posture (Farshadmanesh et al., 2007; Klier et al., 2002). These observations have led us to suggest that the INC is the 3D integrator not only for the eye, but also for head posture. However, head control is much more complex than eye control—with vastly greater inertia, an inverted pendulum structure, over-redundant musculature, multiple joints, and a nest of vestibular and proprioceptive reflex pathways (Fukushima et al., 1994; Graf et al., 1995a; 1995b; Perlmutter et al., 1999)—one might better think of this 'head integrator' as determining a set-point for reflex control pathways.

We do not know enough about these head premotor circuits to say if they are organized into the same neuron pools as their corresponding oculomotor pools (or to what degree these eye and head pools share member units) but what we know so far is consistent with this notion. Moreover, there is also evidence that the head controller utilizes a coordinate system aligned with the head's Donders constraint. Following INC inactivation, horizontal head positions continue to hold along the vertical axis of the Fick coordinate (Farshadmanesh et al., 2007; Klier et al., 2002), and during unilateral INC

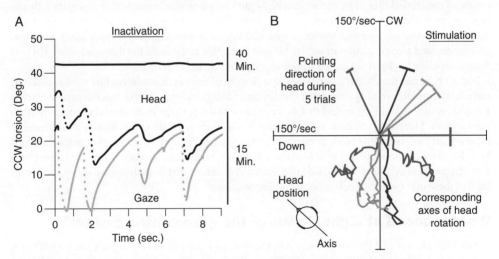

Fig. 18.5 (Also see Plate 11.) Evidence of a neural integrator for head orientation in the INC, organized in Fick coordinates. A) Head (dark line) and gaze/eye-in-space (grey line) torsion plotted against time following muscimol injection. Shortly after injection (15 min here) both drift away from the regular upright position, while rapid movements attempt to correct this. Later (40 min here) the head settles in a torsionally shifted position, i.e. corrective movements cease. From Klier et al., *Science* **295**, 1314 © 2002. Reprinted with permission from AAAS. B) During unilateral INC stimulation with the head free, the head rotates around vertical-torsional axes (clockwise for left INC; counterclockwise for right INC) that stay fixed relative to horizontal head orientation, as in a Fick gimbal. Conventions similar to Fig. 18.2A, but here real data are shown. Reprinted from *Journal of Neurophysiology*, **97**, Klier, E.M., Wang, H., and Crawford, J.D., Interstitial nucleus of Cajal encodes three-dimensional head orientations in Fick-like coordinates, p 604, figure 5 © 2007 The American Physiological Society, used with permission.

stimulation the head rotates about head-fixed horizontal axes—like the vertical axis for head rotation in Fick coordinates (Fig. 18.5B) (Klier et al. 2007). Thus, it appears likely that: 1) both the eye and head are controlled by neural populations organized into coordinates like those shown in Fig. 18.4, and that 2) there is a continuous synergy between the neural, mechanical, and behavioural coordinates for head control, which would have the same advantages as described above for the eye.

Clinical significance

One of the many things that healthy people take for granted is that (other than some random scatter) Donders' laws of the eye and head are normally obeyed during gaze fixations. However, this is not true in many clinical populations, for example those that experience ocular tilt (a tonic torsional offset of the eyes (Brandt and Strupp, 1992; Halmagyi et al., 1991; Ohashi et al., 1998; Westheimer and Blair, 1975)), torsional nystagmus (torsional drift with intermittent corrective eye movements (Glasauer et al., 2001; Halmagyi and Hoyt, 1991; Straumann et al., 2000)), and spasmodic torticollis (Agrawal et al., 2009; Medendorp et al., 1999; Patterson and Little, 1943). The last of these (also known as cervical dystonia) is the most common type of dystonia, and involves abnormal offset in head posture that very often have a significant torsional component. Disorders of the motoneurons and eye muscles, including strabismus, are also generally associated with abnormal torsional positions (Sharpe et al., 2008). Each of these symptoms can be debilitating; physically, functionally, emotionally, and socially.

Damage or inappropriate activation of the reticular formation can explain some of these symptoms, at least some of the time. This basic science review does not have space for a comprehensive review of the clinical literature, but we can highlight one particular example that ties in directly the previous physiology. Acute unilateral damage to the INC produces an array of clinical symptoms including vertical gaze-paretic nystamus (an inability to hold eccentric eye positions), torsional nystagmus, and a combination of ocular tilt and torticollis away from the damaged side). Each of these symptoms has been associated with midbrain damage in the human.

It must be noted that, when comparing physiology to pathology, most laboratory studies measure early, acute, rapidly evolving affects that the clinician would rarely see. By the time the patient reaches a specialist they have likely settled to a more chronic state, perhaps even involving compensatory mechanisms. Moreover, nature is unlikely to be as pin-point accurate in her neurological insults as experimentalists are, so one needs to interpret patients in light of the overall function of the damaged area. Finally, behaviours that resemble ocular tilt and torticollis can also occur from unilateral INC stimulation (here on the ipsilateral side to the tilt). This means that in pathological states, structures such as these may be involved, but not the ultimate cause.

What is coded at higher levels of the gaze control system?

In the 1990s it was not known at what point in the gaze control system signals became 3D (i.e. included a specified torsional command). Clearly this is the case in structures such as the INC and riMLF, but how far upstream does this go? As mentioned above, the first kinematically correct model of the 3D saccade generator proposed that points on the SC encode specific 3D saccade axes (Tweed and Vilis, 1990), including the torsional axis components required to keep eye position in Listing's plane. However, Van Opstal and colleagues showed, with a combination of unit recording and microstimulation, that the SC does not encode 3D axes (Hepp et al., 1993; Van Opstal et al., 1991). Figure 18.6B replicates their result that stimulation of the SC (in the head-fixed monkey) evokes saccades with zero torsional components (and thus variable axes) independent of initial eye position. The latter results seems less surprising two decades later, now that we know that the position-dependent torsional axis tilts are still not implemented at the level of motoneurons (Klier et al., 2006). However, we also know now that in natural head-free conditions saccades are often accompanied by variable torsional components. At what point in the system are these added on? Does the SC produce

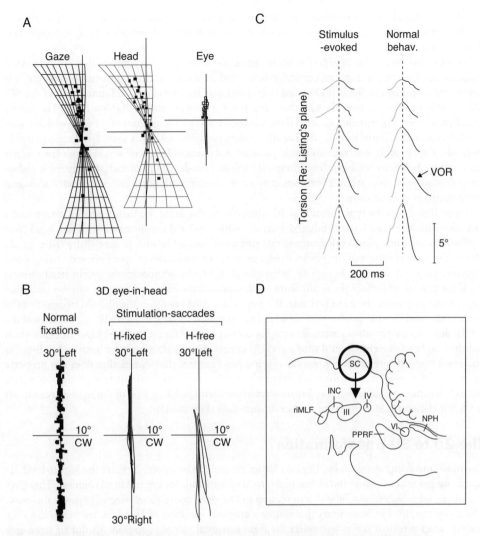

Fig. 18.6 Stimulation of the superior colliculus (SC) produces gaze shifts with normal 3-D kinematics. A) At the end of stimulation-evoked movements, Gaze (eye-in space), Head, and Eye orientation vectors fall within the normal Donders' ranges (compare to Fig. 18.1A–C). B) When the head is immobilized, stimulation-evoked saccades (center plot) stay within the normal Listing's plane range (left plot), viewed here from the side. When the head is freed, stimulation of the same site produces saccades (right plot) that flare out of Listing's plane. Why? C) Plotting torsion against time, one can see that both head-free stimulation evoked saccades (left plots) and normal saccades (right plots) show the same pattern of anticipatory torsion (grey traces): negating the torsion in the following VOR (black traces). A–C adapted from Klier et al. 2003. D) Schematic sagittal slice of monkey brainstem. The previous data suggest that the SC (black circle) encodes desired 2D gaze, and this is somehow elaborated into 3D commands at the level of the rostral intersititial nucleus of medial longitudinal fasciculus (riMLF), interstitial nucleus of Cajal (INC), paramedian pontine reticular formation (PPRF) and nucleus prepositus hypoglossi (NPH). III, IV, VI: 3rd, 4th, 6th cranial nuclei contain motoneurons for eye muscles. Adapted from Henn et al. 1982 with kind permission from Springer Science+Business Media B.V.

a vector command with zero torsion, parallel to some other variable torsional controller, or does the SC simply code a 2D gaze target, which is then converted somehow into a 3D command downstream?

We tested this in a series of experiments in the head-free monkey, in combination with electrical stimulation of the SC, and several cortical gaze control structures, including the supplementary eye fields (SEFs) frontal eye fields (FEFs) and lateral intraparietal cortex (LIP). Stimulation of the SC, SEFs, and FEFs is known to evoke gaze shifts that involve both eye and head movements. The simple logic behind these experiments was that if the site encodes a specific amount of torsion (whether zero or non-zero) stimulation should consistently evoke gaze shifts with that same fixed torsional eye-in-head component. In general, this would produce violations of Donders' and Listing's law (even if the saccades had zero torsion). In contrast, if the site encodes 2D gaze and 3D control is elaborated downstream, then stimulation should evoke gaze shifts with normally coordinated torsional components in their saccades.

Figure 18.6 shows the typical result of SC stimulation. The same site that produced zero-torsion saccades with the head fixed produced saccades with torsional components with the head free, opposed to the oncoming VOR components just as in normal head-free gaze shifts (Klier et al., 2003). The final positions of the eye-in-head, eye-in-space, and head-in-space obeyed Listing's and Donders' laws just as well as in normal behaviour (Fig. 18.6A). Moreover, the eye-in-head showed the same pattern of torsional coordination, with saccades showing anticipatory torsion (interestingly, these stop when the head is fixed). We found the same results in the SEF (Martinez-Trujillo et al., 2003) and FEF (Monteon et al., 2005). The exception so far has been LIP (Constantin et al., 2009): this structure produces saccades with the correct torsion for an expected head-free gaze shift, but then no head movement (and thus no VOR) occurs. This might simply be because LIP is so far upstream from the premotor centres for eye and head control that stimulation does not properly access the full motor circuitry for a natural gaze shift. But, in general, stimulation of high-level gaze control structures suggests that they are only concerned with pointing gaze in the right direction: 3D control is elaborated at some point further downstream (Fig. 18.6D).

The 2D to 3D transformation

The most interesting question in 3D gaze control remains to be solved: how are the higher-level 2D signals for gaze decomposed and elaborated into 3D commands for eye and head rotation? This gives rise to several subquestions: how is zero torsion in Donders' coordinates selected? How is this position range modified in behaviours that follow a different variation of Donders' law? How does the brain correct torsional errors and select the right torsional saccade components during head-free gaze shifts?

To repeat, we are not looking for the mechanism that causes saccade axes to tilt as a function of position: as explained above, there is now good agreement that this is done by orbital mechanics (Crawford and Guitton, 1997; Demer et al., 1995; Ghasia and Angelaki, 2005; Klier et al., 2006; Kono et al., 2002; Quaia and Optican, 1998; Raphan, 1998; Smith and Crawford, 1998; Tweed, 1997). Similarly, the neck may be mechanically suited for the axes used in the Fick strategy (Graf et al., 1995a, 1995b; Vidal et al., 1986).

What we are looking for is the mechanism that actively chooses which Donders' surface to use, when to modify it, when to correct deviations from this range. One cannot dismiss the theoretical possibility that eye muscle position-dependencies might be neurally modified in ways that could modify Listing's plane (Demer et al., 2000), but this would require more, not less, neural complexity, and does not explain active torsional control. We first need to understand the main mechanism that sets torsional signals in the brainstem. It's unlikely that this exists in a single, separate 'Listing's law box'. For example, in neural networks trained to perform these transformations the solution is distributed as torsional modulations in units that are also involved in other functions (Keith et al., 2007; Smith and Crawford, 2005). Therefore, this may not be any easy process to pin down. However, there are several clues.

One way to examine this is to start at both ends of the system and see where 2D meets 3D. Searching from the highest level downward: if the cortex and superior colliculus normally just encode 2D gaze direction (Klier et al., 2003; Van Opstal et al., 1991), then the 2D to 3D transformation for both the eyes and head must occur downstream (closer to the muscles). Searching from the lowest level up: since eye and head muscles, motoneurons, the neural integrator (INC and NHP), and premotor burst neurons (riMLF and PPRF) can rotate the eye about any axis and then hold it there (Crawford and Vilis, 1992; Hepp et al., 1988), then the 2D to 3D transformation must occur at a functional level between the superior colliculus and premotor burst neurons (Fig. 18.6C). Finally, since premotor burst neuron (and neural integrator) coordinates align with Donders' coordinates, with clockwise and counterclockwise control symmetric across midline (Crawford, 1994; Crawford and Vilis, 1992), the 2D to 3D transformation simplifies to balancing torsion to zero during head-fixed saccades and smooth pursuit.

These factors suggest that there may be a default mapping from 2D SC outputs onto the correct balance of burst neuron activity to encode zero torsion displacements in Listing's plane (and the Fick strategy for the head). However, this does not explain how these strategies are modified, and how the system maintains these ranges in the face of fairly common but brief violations. To do this, the system requires a modifiable set-point (technically, a set-*surface*) with a comparator (Ceylan et al., 2000; Crawford and Guitton, 1997; Glasauer et al., 2001a, 2001b). In support of this, when the torsional neural integrator is inactivated and the head is tilted, saccades keep aiming the eye toward the torsionally shifted Listing's plane even though the integrator deficit will not allow it to hold there (Crawford et al., 2003). This demonstrates that: 1) the saccade generator actively maintains the desired set point for torsion, and 2) this set point is modulated by vestibular inputs. Furthermore, small errors in torsion (whether naturally or experimentally induced) are usually corrected by forth-coming saccades (Lee et al., 2000; Van Opstal et al., 1996) and these corrective components corre-lated to neural activity in the nucleus reticularis tegmenti pontis (NRTP) (Van Opstal et al., 1996). Since this is a cerebellar input nucleus, this implicates the cerebellum in the active control of torsion through saccades. Consistent with this, patients with cerebellar damage show offsets and widening of Listing's planes (Baier and Dieterich, 2009; Straumann et al., 2000). In addition, the cerebellar floc-culus and paraflocculus may output inhibitory torsional eye velocity components to the vestibular nuclei (Ghasia et al., 2008). Finally, another potential contributor is the central mesencephalic retic-ular formation (cMRF) nucleus located just lateral to the INC, which has functions related to saccades and eye-head coordination (Graf and Ugolini, 2006; Pathmanathan et al., 2006), and has also been implicated in torticollis (Waitzman et al., 2000), but its role in 3D eye control is not known. We will not understand the complete role of these structures until they are studied in 3D/head free prepara-tions—where torsional control of the eye is most obvious and most complex.

Finally, although this review has focused on the control of 3D gaze, as stated above, the 3D orienta-tions of the eyes and head have extensive implications for higher-level vision and early aspects of gaze control. Because of the high variability of eye torsion in space, and its effects on visual receptive fields (Keith et al., 2009), the visual system must account both for systematic and variable torsion. For example, the brain must monitor 3D eye and head orientation to solve the binocular correspondence problem (Blohm et al., 2008), and to convert eye-centred visual information into useful commands for motor effectors (such as the eyes, head, and limb) organized in head or body coordinates (Klier et al., 2001). Such reference frame transformations can be done trivially—without comparisons with position—in purely translational systems, but the eyes and head primarily rotate. Thus, even when cortical mechanisms are primarily concerned with aiming 2D gaze direction (or depth), they cannot operate independently from internal knowledge of 3D eye and head orientation.

Conclusions

3D gaze control is complex because it is not just the control of torsion: it is the control of horizontal, vertical, and torsional components of rotation and all their interactions. Both theory and physiology show that torsion cannot be neatly separated from the other components. This 3D view forces us to give up comfortable intuitions grounded in translational mathematics and leap into the odd, counterintuitive world of rotational kinematics. In this review, we have tried to illustrate that some aspects of 3D control are mechanical and some are neural, but overall it must be understood as a neuromechanical system. Moreover, 3D gaze control is inseparable from the topics of eye-head coordination, and visual-vestibular integration. These factors combine to dictate that one cannot understand 3D gaze control without understanding the complete neurophysiology of gaze control, and conversely, one cannot understand any component of this system without understanding how it fits within the 3D entirety.

Acknowledgments

Supported by the Canadian Institutes of Health Research and the Canada Research Chair Program.

References

Agrawal, A., Cincu, R., Joharapurkar, S.R., Bhake, A., and Hiwale, K.M. (2009). Hemorrhage in brain stem cavernoma presenting with torticollis. *Pediatric Neurosurgery*, **45**, 49–52.

Angelaki, D.E. (2003). Three-dimensional ocular kinematics during eccentric rotations: evidence for functional rather than mechanical constraints. *Journal of Neurophysiology*, **89**, 2685–2696.

Angelaki, D.E. and Hess, B.J. (2004). Control of eye orientation: where does the brain's role end and the muscle's begin? *European Journal of Neuroscience*, **19**, 1–10.

Angelaki, D.E., Zhou, H.H., and Wei, M. (2003). Foveal versus full-field visual stabilization strategies for translational and rotational head movements. *Journal of Neuroscience*, **23**, 1104–1108.

Baier, B. and Dieterich, M. 2009. Ocular tilt reaction: a clinical sign of cerebellar infarctions? *Neurology*, **72**, 572–573.

Blohm, G., Khan, A.Z., Ren, L., Schreiber, K.M., and Crawford, J.D. (2008). Depth estimation from retinal disparity requires eye and head orientation signals. *Journal of Vision*, **8**, 1–23.

Buttner, U., Buttner-Ennever, J.A., and Henn, V. (1977). Vertical eye unit related activity in the rostral mesencephalic reticular formation of the alert monkey. *Brain Research*, **130**, 239–252.

Brandt, T. and Strupp, M. (1992). Otoneurology. *Current Opinion in Neurology and Neurosurgery*, **5**, 727–732.

Cannon, S.C. and Robinson, D.A. (1987). Loss of the neural integrator of the oculomotor system from brain stem lesions in monkey. *Journal of Neurophysiology*, **57**, 1383–1409.

Ceylan, M., Henriques, D.Y., Tweed, D.B., and Crawford, J.D. (2000). Task-dependent constraints in motor control: pinhole goggles make the head move like an eye. *Journal of Neuroscience*, **20**, 2719–2730.

Constantin, A.G., Wang, H., Monteon, J.A., Martinez-Trujillo, J.C., and Crawford, J.D. (2009). 3-D eye-head coordination in gaze shifts evoked during stimulation of the lateral intraparietal cortex (LIP). *Neuroscience*, **164**, 1284–1302.

Crawford, J.D. (1994). The oculomotor neural integrator uses a behavior-related coordinate system. *Journal of Neuroscience*, **14**, 6911–6923.

Crawford, J.D. and Guitton, D. (1997). Visual-motor transformations required for accurate and kinematically correct saccades. *Journal of Neurophysiology*, **78**, 1447–1467.

Crawford, J.D. and Vilis, T. (1991). Axes of eye rotation and Listing's law during rotations of the head. *Journal of Neurophysiology*, **65**, 407–423.

Crawford, J.D. and Vilis, T. (1992). Symmetry of oculomotor burst neuron coordinates about Listing's plane. *Journal of Neurophysiology*, **68**, 432–448.

Crawford, J.D., Cadera, W., and Vilis, T. (1991). Generation of torsional and vertical eye position signals by the interstitial nucleus of Cajal. *Science*, **252**, 1551–1553.

Crawford, J.D., Ceylan, M.Z., Klier, E.M., and Guitton, D. (1999). Three-dimensional eye-head coordination during gaze saccades in the primate. *Journal of Neurophysiology*, **81**, 1760–1782.

Crawford, J.D., Tweed, and D.B., Vilis, T. (2003). Static ocular counterroll is implemented through the 3-D neural integrator. *Journal of Neurophysiology*, **90**, 2777–2784.

Demer, J.L. (2002). The orbital pulley system: a revolution in concepts of orbital anatomy. *Annals of the New York Academy of Sciences*, **956**, 17–32.

Demer, J.L., Oh, S.Y., and Poukens, V. (2000). Evidence for active control of rectus extraocular muscle pulleys. *Investigative Ophthalmology & Visual Science*, **41**, 1280–1290.

Demer, J.L., Miller, J.M., Poukens, V., Vinters, H.V., and Glasgow, B.J. (1995). Evidence for fibromuscular pulleys of the recti extraocular muscles. *Investigative Ophthalmology & Visual Science*, **36**, 1125–1136.

Donders, F.C. (1848). Beitrag zur lehre von den bewegungen des menschlichen auges. [translation: The movements of the human eye] *Holländ Beitr Anat Physiol Wiss*, **1**, 104–145.

Farshadmanesh, F., Klier, E.M., Chang, P., Wang, H., and Crawford, J.D. (2007). Three-dimensional eye-head coordination after injection of muscimol into the interstitial nucleus of Cajal (INC). *Journal of Neurophysiology*, **97**, 2322–2338.

Ferman, L., Collewijn, H., and Van den Berg, A.V. (1987). A direct test of Listing's law—I. Human ocular torsion measured in static tertiary positions. *Vision Research*, **27**, 929–938.

Ferman, L., Collewijn, H., and Van den Berg, A.V. (1987). A direct test of Listing's law—II. Human ocular torsion measured under dynamic conditions. *Vision Research*, **27**, 939–951.

Fetter, M., Tweed, D., Misslisch, H., Fischer, D., and Koenig, E. (1992). Multidimensional descriptions of the optokinetic and vestibuloocular reflexes. *Annals of the New York Academy of Sciences*, **656**, 841–842.

Fukushima, K. (1987). The interstitial nucleus of Cajal and its role in the control of movements of head and eyes. *Progress in Neurobiology*, **29**, 107–192.

Fukushima, K., Ohashi, T., and Fukushima, J. (1994). Effects of chemical deactivation of the interstitial nucleus of Cajal on the vertical vestibulo-collic reflex induced by pitch rotation in alert cats. *Neuroscience Research*, **20**, 281–286.

Fukushima, K., Murakami, S., Matsushima, J., and Kato, M. (1980). Vestibular responses and branching of interstitiospinal neurons. *Experimental Brain Research*, **40**, 131–145.

Gandhi, N.J., Barton, E.J., and Sparks, D.L. (2008). Coordination of eye and head components of movements evoked by stimulation of the paramedian pontine reticular formation. *Experimental Brain Research*, **189**, 35–47.

Ghasia, F.F. and Angelaki, D.E. (2005). Do motoneurons encode the noncommutativity of ocular rotations? *Neuron*, **47**, 281–293.

Ghasia, F. F., Meng, H., and Angelaki, D.E. (2008). Neural correlates of forward and inverse models for eye movements: evidence from three-dimensional kinematics. *Journal of Neuroscience*, **28**, 5082–5087.

Glasauer, S., Dieterich, M., and Brandt, T. (2001a). Modeling the role of the interstitial nucleus of Cajal in otolithic control of static eye position. *Acta Otolaryngologica Supplumentum*, **545**, 105–107.

Glasauer, S., Dieterich, M., and Brandt, T. (2001b). Central positional nystagmus simulated by a mathematical ocular motor model of otolith-dependent modification of Listing's plane. *Journal of Neurophysiology*, **86**, 1546–1554.

Glenn, B. and Vilis, T. (1992). Violations of Listing's law after large eye and head gaze shifts. *Journal of Neurophysiology*, **68**, 309–318.

Graf, W.M., and Ugolini, G. (2006). The central mesencephalic reticular formation: its role in space-time coordinated saccadic eye movements. *Journal of Physiology*, **570**, 433–434.

Graf, W., de Waele, C., and Vidal, P.P. (1995a). Functional anatomy of the head-neck movement system of quadrupedal and bipedal mammals. *Journal of Anatomy*, **186**, 55–74.

Graf, W., de Waele, C., Vidal, P.P., Wang, D.H., and Evinger, C. (1995b). The orientation of the cervical vertebral column in unrestrained awake animals. II. Movement strategies. *Brain, Behavior and Evolution*, **45**, 209–231.

Guitton, D. (1992). Control of eye-head coordination during orienting gaze shifts. *Trends in Neurosciences*, **15**, 174–179.

Halmagyi, G.M. and Hoyt, W.F. (1991). See-saw nystagmus due to unilateral mesodiencephalic lesion. *Journal of Clinical Neuroophthalmology*, **11**, 79–84.

Halmagyi, G.M., Curthoys, I.S., Brandt, T., and Dieterich, M. (1991). Ocular tilt reaction: clinical sign of vestibular lesion. *Acta Otolaryngologica Supplumentum*, **481**, 47–50.

Haslwanter, T., Straumann, D., Hess, B.J., and Henn, V. (1992). Static roll and pitch in the monkey: shift and rotation of Listing's plane. *Vision Research*, **32**, 1341–1348.

Haslwanter, T., Straumann, D., Hepp, K., Hess, B.J., and Henn, V. (1991). Smooth pursuit eye movements obey Listing's law in the monkey. *Experimental Brain Research*, **87**, 470–472.

Helmchen, C., Rambold, H., Fuhry, L., and Büttner, U. (1998). Deficits in vertical and torsional eye movements after uni- and bilateral muscimol inactivation of the interstitial nucleus of Cajal of the alert monkey. *Experimental Brain Research*, **119**, 436–452.

Helmholtz, H. (1867). Handbuch der Physiologischen Optik [Treatise of optical physiology] *Treatise on Physiological Optics* 3(1). Hamburg: Voss. [English translation, vol 3 (trans. J.P.C. Southall). Rochester: Optical Society of America (1925) pp. 44–51.]

Henn, V., Büttner-Ennever, J.A., and Hepp, K. (1982). The primate oculomotor system. I. Motoneurons. A synthesis of anatomical, physiological, and clinical data. *Human Neurobiology*, **1**, 77–85.

Hepp, K., Vilis, T., and Henn, V. (1988). On the generation of rapid eye movements in three dimensions. *Annals of the New York Academy of Sciences*, **545**, 140–153.

Hepp, K., Van Opstal, A.J., Straumann, D., Hess, B.J., and Henn, V. (1993). Monkey superior colliculus represents rapid eye movements in a two-dimensional motor map. *Journal of Neurophysiology*, **69**, 965–979.

Keith, G.P., Smith, M.A., and Crawford, J.D. (2007). Functional organization within a neural network trained to update target representations across 3-D saccades. *Journal of Computational Neuroscience*, **22**, 191–209.

Keith, G.P., Desouza, J.F., Yan, X., Wang, H., and Crawford, J.D. (2009). A method for mapping response fields and determining intrinsic reference frames of single-unit activity: applied to 3D head-unrestrained gaze shifts. *Journal of Neuroscience Methods*, **180**, 171–184.

King, W.M. and Fuchs, A.F. (1979). Reticular control of vertical saccadic eye movements by mesencephalic burst neurons. *Journal of Neurophysiology*, **42**, 861–876.

Klier, E.M., Wang, H., and Crawford, J.D. (2001). The superior colliculus encodes gaze commands in retinal coordinates. *Nature Neuroscience*, **4**, 627–632.

Klier, E.M., Wang, H., and Crawford, J.D. (2003). Three-dimensional eye-head coordination is implemented downstream from the superior colliculus. *Journal of Neurophysiology*, **89**, 2839–2853.

Klier, E.M., Meng, H., and Angelaki, D.E. (2006). Three-dimensional kinematics at the level of the oculomotor plant. *Journal of Neuroscience*, **26**, 2732–2737.

Klier, E.M., Wang, H., and Crawford, J.D. (2007). Interstitial nucleus of Cajal encodes three-dimensional head orientations in Fick-like coordinates. *Journal of Neurophysiology*, **97**, 604–617.

Klier, E.M., Wang, H., Constantin, A.G., and Crawford, J.D. (2002). Midbrain control of three-dimensional head orientation. *Science*, **295**, 1314–1316.

Kono, R., Clark, R.A., and Demer, J.L. (2002). Active pulleys: magnetic resonance imaging of rectus muscle paths in tertiary gazes. *Investigative Ophthalmology & Visual Science*, **43**, 2179–2188.

Lee, C., Zee, D.S., and Straumann, D. (2000). Saccades from torsional offset positions back to listing's plane. *Journal of Neurophysiology*, **83**, 3241–3253.

Luschei, E.S. and Fuchs, A.F. (1972). Activity of brain stem neurons during eye movements of alert monkeys. *Journal of Neurophysiology*, **35**, 445–461.

Martinez-Trujillo, J.C., Wang, H., and Crawford, J.D. (2003). Electrical stimulation of the supplementary eye fields in the head-free macaque evokes kinematically normal gaze shifts. *Journal of Neurophysiology*, **89**, 2961–2974.

Medendorp, W.P., Van Gisbergen, J.A., Horstink, M.W., and Gielen, C.C. (1999). Donders' law in torticollis. *Journal of Neurophysiology*, **82**, 2833–2838.

Misslisch, H. and Hess, B.J. (2000). Three-dimensional vestibuloocular reflex of the monkey: optimal retinal image stabilization versus listing's law. *Journal of Neurophysiology*, **83**, 3264–3276.

Misslisch, H. and Tweed, D. (2001). Neural and mechanical factors in eye control. *Journal of Neurophysiology*, **86**, 1877–1883.

Misslisch, H., Tweed, D., Fetter, M., and Vilis, T. (1994). The influence of gravity on Donders' law for head movements. *Vision Research*, **34**, 3017–3025.

Mok, D., Ro, A., Cadera, W., Crawford, J.D., and Vilis, T. (1992). Rotation of Listing's plane during vergence. *Vision Research*, **32**, 2055–2064.

Monteon, J.A., Wang, H., Martinez-Trujillo, J.C., and Crawford, J.D. (2005). Gaze shifts evoked by electrical stimulation of the frontal eye field in the head-free macaque. Society for Neuroscience International Meeting, Washington, DC, USA.

Ohashi, T., Fukushima, K., Chin, S., Harada, T., Yoshida, K., Akino, M., and Matsuda, H. (1998). Ocular tilt reaction with vertical eye movement palsy caused by localized unilateral midbrain lesion. *Journal of Neuroophthalmology*, **18**, 40–42.

Pathmanathan, J.S., Presnell, R., Cromer, J.A., Cullen, K.E., and Waitzman, D.M. (2006). Spatial characteristics of neurons in the central mesencephalic reticular formation (cMRF) of head-unrestrained monkeys. *Experimental Brain Research*, **168**, 455–470.

Patterson, R.M. and Little, S.C. (1943). Spasmodic torticollis. *Journal of Nervous and Mental Disease*, **98**, 571–599.

Perlmutter, S.I., Iwamoto, Y., Baker, J.F., and Peterson, B.W. (1999). Spatial alignment of rotational and static tilt responses of vestibulospinal neurons in the cat. *Journal of Neurophysiology*, **82**, 855–862.

Quaia, C. and Optican, L.M. (1998). Commutative saccadic generator is sufficient to control a 3-D ocular plant with pulleys. *Journal of Neurophysiology*, **79**, 3197–3215.

Radau, P., Tweed, D., and Vilis, T. (1994). Three-dimensional eye, head, and chest orientations after large gaze shifts and the underlying neural strategies. *Journal of Neurophysiology*, **72**, 2840–2852.

Raphan, T. (1998). Modeling control of eye orientation in three dimensions. I. Role of muscle pulleys in determining saccadic trajectory. *Journal of Neurophysiology*, **79**, 2653–2667.

Robinson, D.A. (1981). The use of control systems analysis in the neurophysiology of eye movements. *Annual Review of Neuroscience*, **4**, 463–503.

Smith, M.A. and Crawford, J.D. (1998). Neural control of rotational kinematics within realistic vestibuloocular coordinate systems. *Journal of Neurophysiology*, **80**, 2295–2315.

Smith, M.A. and Crawford, J.D. (2005). Distributed population mechanism for the 3-D oculomotor reference frame transformation. *Journal of Neurophysiology*, **93**, 1742–1761.

Schnabolk, C. and Raphan, T. (1994). Modeling three-dimensional velocity-to-position transformation in oculomotor control. *Journal of Neurophysiology*, **71**, 623–638.

Sharpe, J.A., Wong, A.M., and Fouladvand, M. (2008). Ocular motor nerve palsies: implications for diagnosis and mechanisms of repair. *Progress in Brain Research*, **171**, 59–66.

Straumann, D., Zee, and D.S., Solomon, D. (2000). Three-dimensional kinematics of ocular drift in humans with cerebellar atrophy. *Journal of Neurophysiology*, **83**, 1125–1140.

Straumann, D., Haslwanter, Th., Hepp-Reymond, M.C., and Hepp, K. (1991). Listing's law for the eye, head and arm movements and their synergistic control. *Experimental Brain Research*, **86**, 209–215.

Tweed, D. (1997). Three-dimensional model of the human eye-head saccadic system. *Journal of Neurophysiology*, **77**, 654–666.

Tweed, D. and Vilis, T. (1987). Implications of rotational kinematics for the oculomotor system in three dimensions. *Journal of Neurophysiology*, **58**, 832–849.

Tweed, D. and Vilis, T. (1990). Geometric relations of eye position and velocity vectors during saccades. *Vision Research*, **30**, 111–127.

Tweed, D., Fetter, M., Andreadaki, S., Koenig, E., and Dichgans, J. (1992). Three-dimensional properties of human pursuit eye movements. *Vision Research*, **32**, 1225–1238.

Van Opstal, A.J., Hepp, K., Hess, B.J., Straumann, D., and Henn, V. (1991). Two- rather than three-dimensional representation of saccades in monkey superior colliculus. *Science*, **252**, 1313–1315.

Van Opstal, J., Hepp, K., Suzuki, Y., and Henn, V. (1996). Role of monkey nucleus reticularis tegmenti pontis in the stabilization of Listing's plane. *Journal of Neuroscience*, **16**, 7284–7296.

Van Rijn, L.J. and Van den Berg, A.V. (1993). Binocular eye orientation during fixations: Listing's law extended to include eye vergence. *Vision Research*, **33**, 691–708.

Vidal, P.P., Graf, W., and Berthoz, A. (1986). The orientation of the cervical vertebral column in unrestrained awake animals. I. Resting position. *Experimental Brain Research*, **61**, 549–559.

Waitzman, D.M., Silakov, V.L., DePalma-Bowles, S., and Ayers, A.S. (2000). Effects of reversible inactivation of the primate mesencephalic reticular formation. I. Hypermetric goal-directed saccades. *Journal of Neurophysiology*, **83**, 2260–2284.

Westheimer, G. and Blair, S.M. (1975). The ocular tilt reaction—a brainstem oculomotor routine. *Investigative Ophthalmology*, **14**, 833–839.

Westtheimer, G. (1957). Kinematics of the eye. *Journal of the Optical Society of America*, **47**, 967–974.

CHAPTER 19

The neural basis of saccade target selection

Jeffrey D. Schall and Jeremiah Y. Cohen

It would be an important subject of pedagogical methodology to provide firm and necessary rules for the perceptual activity of the eye.

(Purkinje 1819, in Wade and Brožek 2001).

Abstract

The neural basis of saccade target selection reviews how the visual system locates objects that are salient through their visual features relative to surrounding objects or through their importance based on task goals and then produces an appropriate overt response like a gaze shift. The neural processes responsible for locating salient or important locations and producing saccades occur in a large number of visual and visuomotor structures and cortical areas. We will describe findings from primary visual cortex and extrastriate visual areas that represent object features and findings from the parietal lobe, the superior colliculus and the frontal eye field that represent target salience and generate motor commands.

Introduction

Primate visual behaviour is organized around a fovea which provides high acuity vision over a limited range of the central visual field. Consequently, to identify an object in a scene, gaze must shift so that the image of that object projects onto the fovea. Because gaze can be directed to only one place at a time, some process must distinguish among possible locations to select the target for a saccade. Consequently, some items may be overlooked. The outcome of the selection process is purposeful in the context of visually guided behaviour (see Hayhoe and Ballard, Chapter 34, this volume). As reviewed elsewhere in this volume, patterns of eye movements express regularities such as concentrating on conspicuous and informative features of an image under diverse conditions (see Reingold and Sheridan, Chapter 29, and Geisler and Cormack, Chapter 24, this volume).

This chapter will review our current understanding of the neural basis of saccade target selection. The process of selecting the target for pursuit eye movements is similar (see Barnes, Chapter 7, this volume). This topic has been reviewed by ourselves and others recently (Bichot and Desimone, 2006; Fecteau and Munoz, 2006; Schall, 2003, 2004a; Schall et al., 2003; Schiller and Tehovnik, 2005; Thompson and Bichot, 2005), so this chapter will frame the major issues and highlight more recent developments.

Visual search, selection, attention, and action

To investigate how the brain selects the target for an eye movement, multiple stimuli that can be distinguished in some way must be presented. This experimental design is referred to as visual search. The visual search paradigm has been used extensively to investigate visual selection and attention (e.g. Wolfe and Horowitz, 2004). In a visual search task, multiple stimuli are presented among which a target is discriminated and located. Search is efficient (with fewer errors and faster response times) if stimuli differ along basic visual feature dimensions, such as colour, form or direction of motion. Search becomes less efficient (more errors, longer response times) if the distractors resemble the target or no single feature clearly distinguishes the stimuli. Recently, another approach to investigating the visual and other factors guiding saccade target selection has required participants to locate a more or less vague target embedded in an image of random or structured noise or texture (e.g. Eckstein et al., 2001; Najemnik and Geisler, 2009). A general conclusion drawn from these studies is that humans can direct gaze under these circumstances in a statistically optimal manner. By introducing rapid variation over time in the structure of the image, it is possible to measure the interval of visual input that most effectively guides saccades (e.g. Caspi et al., 2004; Ludwig et al., 2005). These experiments have found that in the 100 ms before a saccade is initiated, changes of visual input have little or no influence except on subsequent saccades (see also Camalier et al., 2007).

Saccade target selection cannot be discussed without consideration of the allocation of visual attention. In fact, several lines of evidence indicate that visual target selection and the allocation of visual attention may be synonymous. For example, perceptual sensitivity is reduced and saccade latency is elevated if attention is directed away from the target for a saccade (e.g. Deubel and Schneider, 1996; Kowler et al., 1995), but this relationship varies with task demands (Deubel, 2008). Also, the visual conspicuousness of an oddball stimulus can drive covert (e.g. Theeuwes, 1991) and overt (Theeuwes et al., 1998) selection, and non-target elements that resemble a designated target can be inadvertently selected covertly (e.g. Kim and Cave, 1995) and overtly (e.g. Bichot and Schall, 1999b; Motter and Belky, 1998; Zelinsky and Sheinberg, 1997). Finally, target selection is influenced by implicit memory representations arising through short-term priming of location or stimulus features for covert (e.g. Maljkovic and Nakayama, 1994, 1996) and overt (Bichot and Schall, 1999b; McPeek et al., 1999) orienting. These observations are explained most commonly by postulating the existence of a map of salience derived from converging bottom-up and top-down influences (e.g. Itti and Koch, 2001; Rodriguez-Sanchez et al., 2007; Wolfe, 2007). One major input to the salience map is the maps of the features (colour, shape, motion, depth) of elements of the image. Another major input is top-down modulation based on goals and expectations. Peaks of activation in the salience map that develop as a result of competitive interactions represent locations to which attention has become allocated for enhanced visual processing.

Some researchers have suggested that shifts of attention and eye movements are tightly linked (Deubel and Schneider, 1996; Henderson, 1991; Hoffman and Subramaniam, 1995; Hunt and Kingstone, 2003; Kowler et al., 1995; Sheliga et al., 1994, 1995; Shepherd et al., 1986). This view is known as the oculomotor readiness hypothesis (Klein, 1980; Klein and Pontefract, 1994) or the premotor theory of attention (Rizzolatti, 1983; Sheliga et al., 1994, 1995). However, the link between directing attention and shifting gaze is not obligatory (Crawford and Muller, 1992; Eriksen and Hoffman, 1972; Jonides, 1980; Klein et al., 1992; Posner, 1980; Remington, 1980; Reuter-Lorenz and Fendrich, 1992; Shepherd et al., 1986). Certainly, when observers scan an image, the timing of saccade production is not under immediate visual control (e.g. Hooge and Erkelens, 1996, 1998, 1999; Van Loon et al., 2002). These observations highlight the problem of explaining the timing of saccade production.

We propose that the allocation of attention refers to the manifestation of a particular process or state of the brain during a behaviour in the context of alternative stimuli. Accordingly, the allocation of attention across the image need be no more or less than the selective differential activation of neurons in the appropriate network of brain structures. In other words, attention is allocated when and to the extent that the activity of particular neurons represent one as opposed to another location.

This measure of the allocation of attention can be distinguished in time and neural process from when, whether and where gaze shifts.

A key measurement in describing stages of processing during eye-movement decisions has been response time, the time taken from visual stimulus onset to saccade. Separating a task into stages of processing allows for experimental manipulation of one stage (e.g. target selection) while holding constant another (e.g. saccade preparation) (Donders, 1868; Miller, 1988; Schall, 2004a; Sternberg, 1969). The decision to make a saccade to a target has been described using the principle of accumulation of evidence to a threshold (e.g. Carpenter and Williams, 1995; Reddi and Carpenter 2000; Reddi et al., 2003; Smith and Ratcliff, 2004). As we shall see later in this chapter, the activity of distinct populations of neurons have been associated with different stages of processing during saccade decisions.

The neural processes described as saccade target selection occur throughout the visual pathway and ocular motor system. Pedagogically, it is easiest to review the experimental evidence for each part of the brain in turn, but the reader should not gain the mistaken impression that the various areas and structures operate in isolation or sequence. In fact, the neural processes responsible for selecting a target and shifting gaze transpire concurrently in an interconnected network woven through the brain from front to back, top to bottom (Fig. 19.1).

Primary visual cortex and the ventral stream

Selecting a particular element in an image requires that the element be distinguished from others in the image. Such a distinction can be derived from differences in colour, shape, motion or depth. Therefore, selection of a target for a visually guided saccade must begin with neural signals that distinguish the features of elements in the image. A cornerstone of visual neuroscience is the fact that neurons in the visual cortex respond selectively according to the colour, shape, motion and depth of stimuli. A signal sufficient to distinguish the features of visual objects is available in the first few spikes produced by neurons in primary and extrastriate visual cortex (reviewed by Orban, 2008). Selectivity of neural responses for visual features forms the necessary substrate for visual target selection; however, it is not sufficient because targets are distinguished only through a comparison to the features of other stimuli in the image. When more than one stimulus is presented, interactions occur between neurons responding to stimuli in neighbouring parts of the scene. Different forms of response modulation by surrounding stimuli has been observed in some neurons primary visual cortex (e.g. Knierim and Van Essen, 1992; Rossi et al., 2001; Zipser et al., 1996), areas MT and MST (e.g. Saito et al., 1986) and area V4 (Desimone and Schein, 1987). Modulation of the response of neurons to a stimulus in the receptive field by stimuli present in the surrounding region provides the substrate for identifying the location of features that are conspicuously different from surrounding features.

Having larger receptive fields, the responses of neurons in area V4 appear to relate more directly to the guidance of saccades. Neurons in V4 exhibit modulated discharge rates before saccade initiation (Fischer and Boch, 1981) that seems to signal enhanced selectivity for the features of the stimulus at the location of the saccade (Moore, 1999; Moore and Chang, 2009). Also, the receptive fields of V4 neurons have been characterized as reducing in size to effectively focus around the target of the saccade (Tolias et al., 2001), resembling a shift of sensitivity within the receptive field in a spatial attention task (Connor et al., 1997). More direct information about how extrastriate cortex select targets has been obtained in studies that present multiple stimuli. This line of research has been framed by the seminal observation that when two stimuli are presented in the receptive field of many neurons in area V4, the response to the preferred stimulus is modulated according to which of the two stimuli is selected for guiding a behavioural response (reviewed by Reynolds and Chelazzi, 2004). For example, several studies have shown that neurons in V4 respond initially indiscriminately to target and distractor stimuli in their receptive fields but then the activity is modulated to signal through maximal activation the location of the target stimulus, whether it is defined by similarity to a cue stimulus or distinctiveness relative to non-target distractors (Chelazzi et al., 2001;

Mirabella et al., 2007; Motter, 1994a, 1994b; Ogawa and Komatsu, 2004; 2006). The selective activation took some time, on the order of 150 ms, to arise (Fig. 19.1). The time needed to distinguish and locate a target depends on the similarity of the target to non-target objects in the image (e.g. Hayden and Gallant, 2005). Nevertheless, this selective activation occurs as well when targets are selected during natural scanning eye movements (Bichot et al., 2005; David et al., 2008; Gallant et al., 1998; Mazer and Gallant, 2003).

Measurements of event-related potentials over extrastriate visual cortex of human participants performing tasks that require target selection and attention allocation have identified a signature of the locus and time of attention allocation (e.g. Luck and Hillyard, 1994; Woodman and Luck, 1999). Referred to as N2pc, it is a slightly more negative polarization arising approximately 200 ms after stimulus presentation in electrodes contralateral as compared to ipsilateral to the attended hemifield. Source localization procedures indicate that the N2pc arises from an early parietal source and a later occipitotemporal source (Hopf et al., 2000). A recent study demonstrated that a homologue of the N2pc can be recorded from electrodes in the surface of the skull in macaque monkeys (Woodman et al., 2007).

The modulation of neural activity that has been observed in, for example, area V4 has also been found in areas in inferior temporal cortex where neural representations of conjunctions of features and of objects arise. The stimulus selectivity of neurons in inferior temporal lobe seems the same during active scanning in a cluttered image as compared to passive presentation (DiCarlo and Maunsell, 2000). Studies have described modulation of neurons to attended versus non-attended stimuli (e.g. Richmond and Sato, 1987; Sato, 1988) and during natural scene viewing and search (Sheinberg and Logothetis, 2001; Rolls et al., 2003). The process of selection by modulation of neural activity for target and non-target stimuli that was described for V4 has also been observed in inferior temporal cortex (Chelazzi et al., 1998).

A general conclusion of these studies is that multiple stimuli compete for an explicit neural representation, and the competition among stimuli can be biased by other neural signals that reflect experience or instruction (e.g. Desimone and Duncan, 1995). Ultimately, though, enhanced activity in visual cortex represents the features characterizing the target and not that it is a target per se. A more general representation of the location of a target regardless of its features is necessary to guide saccadic eye movements. Such a representation has been referred to as a salience map. We will now describe results indicating that neurons instantiating this salience map are present in the superior colliculus as well as areas in the parietal and frontal lobes.

Superior colliculus

This chapter focuses on cortical areas, but it should be appreciated that subcortical structures contribute to saccade target selection equally. The most thorough descriptions have been provided for the superior colliculus. These data will lead to the view that certain neurons in the superior colliculus embody a representation of the image that can be identified with a salience map (reviewed by Findlay and Walker, 1999; see also Krauzlis et al., 2004) while other neurons contribute to the production of gaze shifts (see White and Munoz, Chapter 11, this volume).

To learn how the superior colliculus contributes to visual selection processes, many investigators have trained monkeys to identify a target location based on implicit cuing (Goldberg and Wurtz, 1972; Wurtz and Mohler, 1976) or by the timing of stimuli or other visual cues (Basso and Wurtz, 1998; Glimcher and Sparks, 1992; Horwitz and Newsome, 2001; Ignashchenkova et al., 2004; Kustov and Robinson, 1996; Li and Basso, 2005; Port and Wurtz, 2009; Ratcliff et al., 2003). Of more relevance for our consideration are studies in which multiple stimuli were presented simultaneously, and the target was distinguished from non-target stimuli by properties such as colour (Kim and Basso, 2008; McPeek and Keller, 2002a; Ottes et al., 1987; Shen and Paré, 2007). While details about the design and the nature or quality of the results for each study vary, the results can be summarized briefly. Initially, when multiple stimuli are presented, activation increases at all locations in the superior colliculus map corresponding to the potential saccade targets. This happens because neurons in the macaque superior colliculus are not naturally selective for visual features like colour; however, the neurons can respond to isoluminant chromatic stimuli (White et al., 2009). Following the initial volley, activation becomes relatively lower at locations that would produce saccades to non-target objects and is sustained or grows at locations corresponding to more conspicuous or important potential targets. When the target is easily distinguished from distractors (e.g. a red spot among green spots), then the difference in activity that signals target location arises 100–150 ms after the array appears (Fig. 19.1) and ~50 ms before saccade initiation. Obviously, to contribute to guiding gaze, saccade target selection must occur before saccade initiation, although curiously some authors describe a selection process that follows the saccade (Buschmann and Miller, 2007). As we will see, this pattern of activity of neurons in the superior colliculus closely resembles what has been observed in parietal and frontal areas from which these signals may arise through direct cortical afferents or to which these signals may contribute through thalamic relay nuclei.

The visual selection of the target is accomplished by different types of neurons in SC, both those with tonic visual responses and those described as build-up or visuomovement neuons. As will be emphasized in the section describing the frontal eye field below, the selection of the target as a visual location to which to orient attention does inevitably and immediately lead to re-orienting of the eyes.

Recent studies using microstimulation and inactivation have demonstrated a causal role of superior colliculus in target selection (Carello and Krauzlis, 2004; McPeek, 2008; McPeek and Keller, 2004). In one study, reversible inactivation of superior colliculus with lidocaine or muscimol caused deficits in target selection (McPeek and Keller, 2004). In this study, monkeys searched for a pop-out target among three distractors. Before superior colliculus inactivation, monkeys performed with 100% accuracy. After injections, monkeys made saccades to distractors on many trials when the target appeared in the location corresponding to the injection site. This deficit in target selection occurred without deficits in saccade production and occurs when overt orienting is not required among competing stimuli (Lovejoy and Krauzlis, 2010), providing further evidence for the dissociation of these processes.

Posterior parietal cortex

A great deal is known about parietal cortex contributions to attention and gaze (e.g. Andersen and Buneo, 2002; Behrmann et al., 2004; Constantinidis, 2006; Gottlieb, 2007), and we will only point to studies testing saccade target selection because a more comprehensive account can be found in Paré and Dorris, Chapter 14, this volume. Posterior parietal cortex consists of multiple areas; we will focus on results from area 7A and the lateral intraparietal area (LIP).

The importance of LIP in performing visual search is demonstrated by the deficits observed consequent to inactivation of LIP (Wardak et al., 2002, 2004). Recent studies have investigated the responses of neurons in posterior parietal cortex in monkeys confronted with displays consisting of a target and one or more distractors (Balan et al., 2008; Buschman and Miller, 2007; Constantinidis and Steinmetz, 2001a, 2001b; Gottlieb et al., 1998; Ipata et al., 2006; Ogawa and Komatsu, 2009; Platt and Glimcher, 1997; Thomas and Paré, 2007). Neurons in area 7a signal the location of a stimulus of one colour among distractors of another colour (Constantinidis and Steinmetz, 2001a). Other studies have examined how neural activity in area LIP participates in target selection (Balan et al., 2008; Buschman and Miller, 2007; Gottlieb et al., 1998; Ipata et al., 2006; Thomas and Paré, 2007). As observed in the superior colliculus and, as we shall see, the frontal eye field, the initial response to the array did not distinguish the location of the oddball, but when the target was easily distinguished from visual search distractors, then within 100–150 ms the activation increased if the oddball was in the receptive field and decayed if only distractors were in the receptive field (Fig. 19.1). This neural activity is sufficient to represent the location of a conspicuous target. A similar pattern of modulation has been observed in experiments in which monkeys shift gaze to the object in an array of eight distinct objects that matches a sample stimulus. If the object in the receptive field was designated the target, neurons exhibited a significant elevation of activity. When the sample was presented during fixation in the centre of the array, the augmented activity for the target arose more than 200 ms after the target was specified. This time is longer than that observed in simple pop-out search because

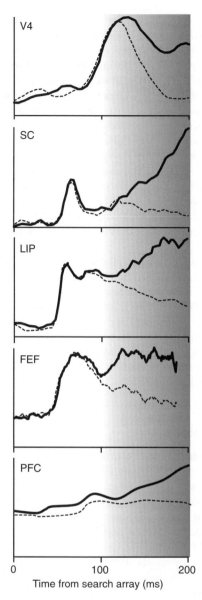

Fig. 19.1 Illustration of visual and saccade target selection of representative single neurons in area V4 (adapted from Ogawa and Komatsu, 2004), superior colliculus (SC) (adapted from McPeek and Keller, 2002a), area LIP (adapted from Thomas and Paré, 2007), FEF (adapted from Thompson et al. 1996), and area 46 of prefrontal cortex (adapted from Hasegawa et al. 2000). The average discharge rate on trials when the target appeared in the response field (thick line) is plotted with the average discharge rate on trials when distractors appeared in the response field, and the target was elsewhere (thin dashed line). Although the data were collected in different areas and under different stimulus and task conditions, it is clear that a concurrent process of target selection occurs throughout the network. Reprinted from *Journal of Neurophysiology*, **97**, Thomas, N.W.D., M. Paré, Temporal processing of saccade targets in parietal cortex area LIP during visual search, p 942, figure 1 © 2007 The American Physiological Society, used with permission.

more time was needed to encode the properties of the sample and locate the matching element. The modulation of activity is probably related to the enhancement of responses if it is to be the target for a saccade (e.g. Bushnell et al., 1981; Mountcastle et al., 1981; Robinson et al., 1978) or the attenuation of responses to a stimulus appearing at a location where attention is already allocated (Robinson et al., 1995; Powell and Goldberg 2000; Steinmetz and Constantinidis 1995; Steinmetz et al., 1994).

Overall, current results indicate that the visual representation in posterior parietal cortex represents the location of conspicuous and relevant stimuli, i.e. likely targets for orienting either covertly or overtly. Thus, neurons in posterior parietal cortex embody the properties of units in a salience map (reviewed by Gottlieb, 2007; Kusunoki et al., 2000).

Frontal eye field

FEF is an area in prefrontal cortex that contributes to transforming visual signals into saccade commands (reviewed by Schall 1997, 2003, 2004b; Schall and Thompson 1999; see also Johnston and Everling, Chapter 15, this volume). It is well known that microstimulation of FEF elicits saccades to the visual field contralateral to the stimulated hemisphere (e.g. Bruce et al., 1985), mediated by a population of neurons that controls whether and when saccades are initiated (e.g. Bruce and Goldberg, 1985; Hanes and Schall, 1996; Hanes et al., 1998). These neurons project to superior colliculus (Segraves and Goldberg, 1987; Sommer and Wurtz, 2000, 2001) and the brainstem (Segraves, 1992), which in turn generate saccades via outputs to the oculomotor nuclei (see Cullen and Van Horn Chapter 9, this volume). Although traditionally regarded as a motor area, the FEF is equally part of the visual system, being strongly interconnected with numerous visual areas, cortically (e.g. Barone et al., 2000; Jouve et al., 1998; Schall et al., 1995b) and subcortically (e.g. Huerta et al., 1986; Stanton et al., 1988). Most FEF neurons have transient or sustained responses to visual stimuli (Bruce and Goldberg, 1985; Mohler et al., 1973; Schall, 1991) with relatively fast latencies on the order of 50 ms after the appearance of the stimulus (Schmolesky et al., 1998).

Thus, the clear engagement of FEF in visual and motor processing make it a prime locus in which to investigate the signals involved in visual search and attentional target selection. This approach is validated by the observation that ablation or inactivation of FEF causes specific deficits in producing saccades when distractors are present as in visual search (e.g. Schiller and Chou, 2000; Wardak et al., 2006). In addition, a number of studies in human participants have demonstrated that trans-cranial magnetic stimulation over FEF in a limited timeframe relative to array presentation influences visual search performance, especially when the target is more difficult to locate (Muggleton et al., 2003; O'Shea et al., 2004).

A series of investigations has described specific neural correlates of target selection for visually guided saccades by recording the activity of neurons in the FEF of monkeys trained to shift gaze directly to a target in visual search arrays (Bichot and Schall, 1999a; Bichot et al., 2001a,b; Cohen et al., 2009b; Murthy et al., 2009; Sato et al., 2001; Sato and Schall, 2003; Schall, 2004b; Schall and Hanes, 1993; Schall et al., 1995a, 2004; Thompson et al., 1996; see also Ogawa and Komatsu, 2006). The extensive evidence for the involvement of FEF in saccade target selection has led to the suggestion that it, like the superior colliculus and parietal cortex, can be understood in terms of a saliency map (reviewed by Thompson and Bichot 2005; Thompson et al., 2001).

Following presentation of an array with a single target among uniform distractors, visually responsive neurons in FEF respond initially indiscriminately to the target or the distractors of the search array in their receptive field. However, before a saccade to the target was generated, a selection process proceeded by which visually responsive neurons in FEF ultimately signalled the location of the oddball target stimulus. If the target of the saccade was in the response field, FEF activity was greatest. If non-target distractors were in the response field, the activity was suppressed. This selection process requires more time when that target is less distinct from the distractors (Bichot et al., 2001; Cohen et al., 2009b; Sato et al., 2001) and occurs if no overt response is made (Thompson et al., 1997) or if target location or property is signalled by through a manual response (Thompson et al., 2005). Furthermore, in monkeys producing sequences of saccades to search for a target embedded in natural scenes FEF neurons signal not only the endpoint of the next saccade but also up to two subsequent saccades (Phillips and Segraves, 2010). Clearly, then, the target selection process can be preplanned through a sequence of saccades during natural scanning.

In FEF the target selection process includes spike timing cooperation and competition between pairs of neurons (Cohen et al., 2010). When pairs of neurons with overlapping receptive fields select the target, they cooperate more than when one or neither neuron in the pair selected the target. The amount of cooperation varies with target location, being highest when the target is within both neurons' receptive fields than when it was inside one but not the other, or outside both. This elevation of spike timing coincidences occurred at the time of target selection derived from the modulation of discharge rates. However, correlation in discharge rates of FEF neurons over longer time scales has been reported even before stimulus presentation (Ogawa and Komatsu, 2010). Neurons with non-overlapping receptive fields exhibited competition through negative spike timing correlations. Thus, perhaps not surprisingly, the neural process of saccade target selection involves dynamic and task-dependent cooperation and competition among neurons.

Further evidence for the network character of the selection process has been obtained in recordings of local field potentials. The target selection process has also been described in local field potentials recorded from FEF (Cohen et al., 2009a; Monosov et al., 2008); in fact the spatially selective activity identifying the location of the target in the visual search array appeared in the spikes ~30 ms before it appeared in the local field potentials. If local field potentials reflect dendritic input and spikes measure neuronal output from a brain region, then this temporal relationship suggests that spatial selection necessary for attention and eye movements is computed locally in FEF from spatially non-selective inputs. When gaze shift errors occur during these visual search tasks, the selection process erroneously guides gaze to a distractor (Thompson et al., 2005), and the errant selection process is evident in the N2pc as well (Heitz et al., 2010). However, when manual response errors occur, the selection process locates the singleton in the search array correctly (Trageser et al., 2008).

Clearly, the visual selection observed in FEF depends on the afferents from the various visual areas conveying feature selectivity. However, FEF also provides extensive feedback connections to extrastriate visual cortex (Barone et al., 2000; Schall et al., 1995b), so the state of neural activity in FEF can influence neural processing in visual cortex. In fact, this connection from FEF to visual cortex is a central feature of models of visual attention (e.g. Hamker and Zirnsak, 2006). Several recent studies have described the relationship between activity in FEF and extrastriate cortex. Microstimulation of FEF biases V4 activity in a manner similar to what is observed when attention is allocated (Armstrong and Moore, 2007; Armstrong et al., 2006; Moore and Armstrong, 2003).

In monkeys trained to maintain fixation and report with a forelimb movement the identity of a visual search target consisting of complex objects, a recent study demonstrated convincingly the contribution of FEF activity to covert spatial attention necessary for target detection and identification (Monosov and Thompson, 2009). The location of the target object was cued by the location of a colour singleton in an array of rings at each object location. The cues could be valid, invalid or neutral. The magnitude of spatially selective activity signalling the location of the cue prior to the presentation of the search object array was correlated with trends in behavioural performance across valid, invalid, and neutral cue trial conditions. However, the speed and accuracy of target identification on individual trials were predicted by the magnitude of spatially selective activity for the target object and not the spatial cue. Inactivation of FEF produced spatially selective perceptual deficits in the covert search task that were strongest on invalid cue trials that require an endogenous attention shift. Another study performed simultaneous single-unit recordings from FEF and from the region of inferotemporal cortex in which neurons contributed to the object recognition (Monosov et al., 2010). Neural signals specifying target location arose in FEF before neural activity specifying target identity arose in temporal cortex. This sequence is consistent with other evidence that spatial selection precedes and guides formation of complex object representations.

The relationship between FEF and processes in extrastriate visual cortex has also been investigated by comparing the timing of target selection signals in FEF with the N2pc, the signal of target selection measured in an event-related potential over extrastriate cortex (Cohen et al., 2009a). In this study, three signals measuring target selection time were recorded simultaneously while monkeys searched for a target defined by form among distractors: FEF single neurons, FEF local field potentials and ERPs over extrastriate cortex. Single FEF neurons selected the target among distractors first, followed by FEF local field potentials, followed by ERPs (Fig. 19.2). Recent anatomical work suggests that target-selecting neurons in the upper layers of FEF project to V4 (Pouget et al., 2009), providing the major anatomical substrate for the functional signals flowing from FEF to V4.

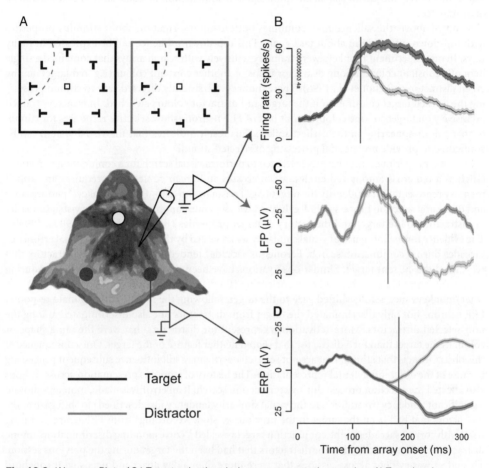

Fig. 19.2 (Also see Plate 12.) Target selection during a representative session. A) Top: visual search display (shown here with a set size of 8) with the target (L) inside the neuron's receptive field (indicated by the dashed arc) (left) and opposite the receptive field (right). Monkeys searched for a T or L target among 1, 3 or 7 L or T distractors. Bottom: schematic of recording sites and signals. Single unit discharges (blue) and local field potentials (green) were recorded intracranially from the frontal eye field. Event-related potentials were recorded from electrodes over extrastriate visual cortex (red). B) Average activity of one neuron when the search target was inside (dark) and opposite (light) its receptive field. Bands around average firing rates show time-varying standard error of the mean. Vertical line indicates target selection time when the two curves became statistically significantly different. C) FEF LFP with the target inside (dark) and opposite (light) the simultaneously recorded neuron's receptive field. D) ERP over extrastriate visual cortex from trials with the target inside (dark) and opposite (light) the receptive field of the concomitantly recorded FEF neuron. This component is the macaque homologue of the human N2pc (m-N2pc). Reprinted from *Journal of Neurophysiology*, **102**, Cohen, J.Y., R.P. Heitz, J.D. Schall, G.F. Woodman, On the origin of event-related potentials indexing covert attentional selection during visual search, pp. 2375–2386, figure 2 © 2009 The American Physiological Society, used with permission.

Evidence that FEF neurons can convey signals related to endogenous spatial attention has been presented recently (Zhou and Thompson, 2009). Neurons in FEF exhibit elevated activity when a cue informs monkeys that one of two choice stimuli would appear in their response field. This spatially selective anticipatory activity occurred without any visual stimulus appearing in the neuron's response field and was not related to motor preparation. These results provide evidence that FEF is a source of a purely top-down spatial attention signal in anticipation of visual stimuli that need to be discriminated.

As noted above, the salience map combines bottom-up information about stimulus properties with top-down information about task goals. This top-down influence can be expressed in many ways. In one experiment monkeys were trained exclusively with search arrays that contained a single item of a constant colour among distractor items of another constant colour (e.g. red target among green distractors) (Bichot et al., 1996). These monkeys persistently directed gaze to stimuli possessing the learned target colour even if the target and distractor colours switched. In monkeys trained exclusively on targets of one colour, about half of FEF neurons show selective responses for stimuli of that colour appearing in the earliest spikes. This result indicates that the visual system can be configured to provide preferential processing of selected stimuli.

In another experiment monkeys were trained to perform visual search for a conjunction of features (such as a red cross among red circles, green crosses and green circles); this requires an explicit memory representation to identify the target (e.g. Treisman and Sato, 1990). Monkeys' performance and the neural selection process in FEF exhibited two, separate contextual influences: visual similarity of distractors to the target and the history of target properties (Bichot and Schall, 1999a, 1999b). The evidence for the influence of visual similarity was revealed by the pattern of occasional erroneous saccades during conjunction search. Erroneous saccades tended to direct gaze to distractors that resembled the current target. Similar observations have been made with human observers during covert (Kim and Cave, 1995) and overt orienting (Findlay, 1997; Motter and Belky, 1998). Now, when monkeys successfully shifted gaze to the target, following the initial indiscriminate response, FEF neurons not only discriminated the target from distractors but also discriminated among the non-selected distractors. More activation was present for distractors that were the same shape or colour as the target than for a distractor that shared neither feature of the target. One consequence of this observation is that stimuli that are not selected overtly may still influence subsequent processing because of the differential neural representation. The history of stimulus presentation across sessions also affected the selection process during conjunction search. If an error was made, monkeys showed a significant tendency (in addition to the visual similarity tendency just described) to shift gaze to the distractors that had been the target in the previous session. Recordings from FEF neurons during trials with correct saccades to the conjunction target revealed a corresponding discrimination among distractors with more activation for distractors that had been the target during the previous session. This effect was evident across sessions that were more than a day apart and persisted throughout experimental sessions.

Another expression of cognitive control of visual search is expressed on a shorter time scale. Humans and monkeys are affected by trial-to-trial changes in stimulus features and target location during pop-out visual search. For example, repetition of stimulus features improves performance. This feature-based facilitation of return was manifested in the target discrimination process in FEF; neurons discriminated the target from distractors earlier and better with repetition of stimulus features, corresponding to improvements in saccade latency and accuracy, respectively. In contrast to the repetition of features, repetition of target position increased saccade latency. This location-based inhibition of return was reflected in the neuronal discrimination process but not in the base-line activity in FEF. These results show adjustments of the target selection process in FEF contributing to changes in performance across trials due to sequential regularities in display properties.

A major question in this line of research concerns the relationship of the visual target selection process to saccade preparation and production. This question touches on multiple major questions. First, what is the origin of the variability of fixation duration between saccades made during scanning a scene or reading? Multiple studies have found that the time spent fixating elements of an image cannot be explained just by the properties of the image (e.g. Jacobs, 1987; Hooge and Erkelens, 1996); however, more recent work has provided evidence for immediate control of some fixation periods (Henderson and Graham, 2008). In general, fixation duration seems to be adjusted according to the difficulty of finding the desired target, but moment-by-moment control of fixation duration based on the properties of the image does not seem to occur. This observation indicates that a form of executive control can be exerted on saccade production. Second, the relation of target selection and associated attention allocation with saccade production has been the focus of the oculomotor readiness or premotor theory of attention. Neurophysiological and anatomical data have been obtained that address specific claims of this theory. Finally, understanding how target selection leads to adaptive saccade production is an instance of the more general problem of understanding the mechanisms responsible for response times. A marriage of neurophysiological measurements and mental chronometry has provided new insights supporting the theory that response times are the outcome of successive, stochastic stages of processing.

The neural process of target selection occupies a certain amount of time that can be measured with reasonable accuracy. This provides an opportunity to determine how the time of visual target selection relates to the time of saccade initiation. This work is motivated by the general hypothesis that behavioural response times are occupied by more or less distinct stages of processing (Donders, 1868; Miller, 1988; Sternberg, 1969; Schall, 2004a). Recent studies have investigated how the time taken to select a target relates to the time taken to initiate the saccade.

One approach to this is the well-known method of selective influence. Different stages of processing should be influenced by different manipulations. The time of target selection by FEF neurons depends on the quality of the stimuli and, as described above, the cognitive context. When the discrimination of the target is easy because the target is visually distinct from the distractors, then the time taken by neurons in FEF to locate the target is relatively short (~140 ms for pop-out displays) and on average does not account for the variability and duration of saccade latency (Fig. 19.3A).[1] When the discrimination of the target is more difficult because the target more closely resembles the distractors, then the time taken by neurons in FEF to locate the target increases and accounts for a larger fraction but not all of the variability and duration of saccade latency (Bichot et al., 2001a; Cohen et al., 2009b; Sato et al., 2001). For example, in monkeys performing a search for a T (or L) among randomly oriented L's (or T's) with arrays of 2, 4, or 8 elements, the time taken for FEF neurons to locate the target increases with the number of objects in the array. However, even in the most difficult search in the 8-object array, saccades were initiated well after the target was selected.

If the time of visual target selection during search does not account for the full duration and variability of saccade initiation times, then some other process must occur to prepare and produce the saccade. As described above, a population of neurons in FEF and superior colliculus linked through the basal ganglia and thalamus provides the input to the brainstem network that produces the saccade. The activation of these neurons in FEF corresponds to the process of saccade preparation with the activation of these presaccadic movement neurons (also referred to as build-up, prelude or long-lead burst neurons). Saccades are initiated when the level of activation in this network reaches a certain level that may vary across task conditions but appears to be constant within a condition (Dorris et al., 1997; Fecteau and Munoz, 2007; Hanes and Schall, 1996; Woodman et al., 2008) (Fig. 19.3B). Most of the variability of the latencies of saccades to a visual target can be accounted for by randomness in the rate of growth of activity to the threshold (Hanes and Schall, 1996), although

---

[1] Studies of LIP (Ipata et al. 2006; Thomas and Paré, 2007) have not found this relationship. These investigators found that the time of target selection by LIP neurons was more correlated with response time. One possible account for this difference is the behavioural requirements in the respective experiments. In all of the experiments in our laboratory monkeys are required to produce a single saccade to the target; this emphasizes accuracy. In the experiments on LIP monkeys were permitted to produce multiple saccades to locate the target; this allows a strategy of speed over accuracy of the saccade. Experimental verification of this possibility has not been obtained to date.

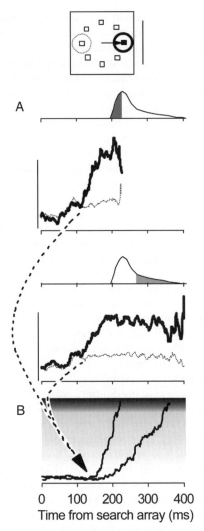

Fig. 19.3 Relation of time of neural target selection to time of saccade initiation during efficient search for a green target among red distractors. The activity of an FEF neuron representing the target (thick) or distractors (thin) is shown during trials with saccades of the shortest (top) or longest (bottom) latencies. The upper plots in each panel indicate the distribution of saccade latencies with the range selected for the analysis of activity shaded. The time at which the activity distinguished whether a target or distractor was in the receptive field is marked by the dashed vertical line. The neuron discriminated the target from distractors following a relatively constant interval after presentation of the search array. Reprinted from *Neuron*, **38**(4) Takashi R. Sato, Jeffrey D. Schall, Effects of Stimulus-Response Compatibility on Neural Selection in Frontal Eye Field pp. 637-648, Copyright (2003), with permission from Elsevier.

other studies in other task conditions find variability of the baseline activity as well (Dorris et al., 1997; Fecteau and Munoz, 2007). When saccade latencies are delayed because the target selection process takes longer, this is accomplished by a delay in the time when the activity begins to accumulate (Woodman et al., 2008).

A recent model was developed to investigate how the signals from the visual selection neurons can be transformed into a saccade command (Purcell et al., 2010). The model consists of a network of deterministic units that integrate through time the actual physiological signals recorded from ensembles of tonic visual neurons in FEF that select the target during visual search. Response times were specified by the time at which the integrated signal reached a threshold. The model explored the role of leak in the integration process and of feedforward and lateral inhibition by determining model parameters that provided the best fit to the actual distributions of response times and produced activation profiles that quantitatively corresponded to the form of actual movement neuron activity. To account for both behavioural and neural data, it was found that the model must include another form of inhibition that gates the flow of perceptual evidence to the accumulator.

Thus, the picture that emerges is that the process of visual selection occupies a certain amount of time that can be shorter and less variable if the target is conspicuous, or it can be longer and more variable if the target is less conspicuous. If subjects wish to prevent a saccade to a non-target stimulus, then the preparation of the saccade can be delayed until the visual selection process has proceeded to a high degree of resolution. Neural activity mediating saccade preparation begins to grow as the selection process is completed and (for reasons that are not clear) the rate of growth of activity leading to the movement varies apparently randomly such that sometimes gaze shifts sooner and sometimes gaze shifts later. Systematic adjustments of saccade latency, though, appear to arise through changes in the time that the accumulation of activity begins. In fact, further evidence for the distinction between target selection and saccade preparation is the observation that the movement neurons in FEF do not discharge at all above baseline when monkeys maintain fixation when monkeys report target location through a manual response (Thompson et al., 2005).

On the other hand, occasionally it is possible for the saccade preparation process to become activated before identification of the currently fixated element and selection of the next target are completed. For example, during visual search neurons in FEF with no visual response and only presaccadic movement activity can exhibit partial activation for non-target stimuli that resemble the target (Bichot et al., 2001b). Such activation of movement neurons can, if excessive, result in premature, erroneous saccades. Independence of visual selection and response preparation is also necessary to explain the production of saccades that are not directed to the location of the selected target.

The dynamics of visual selection and saccade preparation by the frontal eye field has been investigated in macaque monkeys performing a search-step task that combines the classic double-step saccade task with visual search (Camalier et al., 2007). In most trials the target appeared in an array of distractors and reward was earned for producing a saccade to the target. On random trials before the saccade was initiated, the target and one distractor swapped locations, and monkeys were rewarded for shifting gaze to the new target location. Performance of this task is unpredictable, but on average, the longer the delay of the target step, the less likely will monkeys (or humans) correctly shift gaze to the new target location. If target selection and saccade preparation are too far advanced before the target step, then they will shift gaze to the old target location. These errors are commonly followed by corrective saccades to the new target location. Now, some investigators use double-step target presentation as an explicit means of dissociating retinal error from motor error, but performance of this task under the instruction to follow the target steps is different from performance under the instruction to redirect gaze to the final target location (Ray et al., 2004).

Performance of this task can be accounted for as the outcome of a race between processes producing the two saccades and a process that inhibits production of the first saccades (Camalier et al., 2007). The race model provides a powerful framework in which to interpret and understand the activity of the different types of neurons. Central to this model is the duration of the process that interrupts preparation of the first saccade on trials when the target steps. This interval is referred to as *target step reaction time*. The physiological properties of neurons in FEF of monkeys performing this task have been described in several papers (Murthy et al., 2007, 2009). When the target stepped out of a movement field, non-compensated saccades to the original target location were produced when movement-related activity grew rapidly to a threshold. Compensated saccades to the final target location were produced when the growth of the original movement-related activity was interrupted within target step reaction time and was replaced by activation of other neurons producing the compensated saccade. When the target stepped into a receptive field, visual neurons selected the new target location regardless of the monkeys' response. In other words, even when gaze shifted away from the pop-out oddball of a search array, visual neurons in FEF represented the current location of the target. A modulation of this form has also been described in the superior colliculus (McPeek and Keller, 2002b). When the target stepped out of a receptive field most visual neurons maintained the representation of the original target location, but a minority of visual neurons showed reduced activity. These findings indicate that visual activity in the frontal eye field signals the location of targets for orienting while movement-related activity instantiates saccade preparation.

During natural scanning eye movements one observes occasional instances of saccades initiated after fixation intervals that are too short to permit visual analysis of the image sufficient to guide gaze. In the double-step or search-step task corrective saccades are observed following similarly short fixation of the original target location (Becker and Jürgens, 1979; Camalier et al., 2007; Sharika et al., 2008). In fact, the race model provides an explanation for the incidence and timing of these corrective saccades that includes an account of why midflight corrections are rare. The latency of these corrective saccades is predicted by the timing of movement-related activity in the FEF. Preceding rapid corrective saccades, the movement-related activity of many neurons began before visual feedback of the error was registered and that of a few neurons began before the error saccade was completed (Murthy et al., 2007; see also Phillips and Segraves, 2010). Corrective saccade can be produced, though, only if other neurons in the brain have located the new target location and maintain that representation through the production of the error. As noted above, this is just what the visual neurons in FEF do. However, this selection process is itself a variable process that may be more or less complete at the time of saccade initiation. Thus, incomplete suppression of distractor-related activity results in curvature of saccades toward the distractor (McPeek, 2006; see also McPeek et al., 2003).

The double-step or search-step condition dissociates visual target location from saccade endpoint incidentally. The dissociation can also be accomplished explicitly through instruction. For example, it is possible to shift gaze in the direction opposite a visual target, referred to as antisaccade. In monkeys producing antisaccades visually responsive neurons in the superior colliculus and FEF respond if the target falls in the receptive field, and movement neurons are active for saccades into the movement field whether it is a prosaccade or an antisaccade (Everling and Munoz, 2000; Everling et al., 1999). To investigate the relationship of visual target selection to saccade preparation explicitly, monkeys were trained to make a prosaccade to a colour singleton or an antisaccade to the distractor located opposite the singleton; the shape of the singleton cued the direction of the saccade (Sato and Schall, 2003; Schall, 2004). As observed in previous studies, the response time for antisaccades was greater than that for prosaccades. A goal of this experiment was to account for this difference in terms of the neural processes that locate the singleton, encode its shape, map the stimulus onto the response, select the endpoint of the saccade and finally initiate the saccade. Two types of visually-responsive neurons could be distinguished in FEF. The first, called Type I, exhibited the typical pattern of initially indiscriminate activity followed by selection of the singleton in the response field through elevated discharge rate regardless of whether the singleton's features cue a prosaccade or an anti saccade. Some of these Type I neurons maintained the representation of singleton location in antisaccade trials until the saccade was produced. However, the majority of the Type I neurons exhibited a remarkable and dramatic modulation of discharge rate before the antisaccade was initiated (Fig. 19.4A). After showing higher discharge rates for the singleton as compared to a distractor in the receptive field, the firing rates changed such that higher discharge rates were observed for the endpoint of the antisaccade relative to the singleton location. This modulation could be described as the focus of attention shifting from one location to the other before the saccade. The second type of neuron, called Type II, resembled qualitatively the form of modulation of Type I neurons in prosaccade trials, but in antisaccade trials, these neurons did not select the location of the singleton and only selected the endpoint of the saccade (Fig. 19.4B). This endpoint selection was distinct from movement neuron activation, but the selection times of Type II, but not Type I, neurons accounted from some of the variability of saccade response time on prosaccade or antisaccade trials.

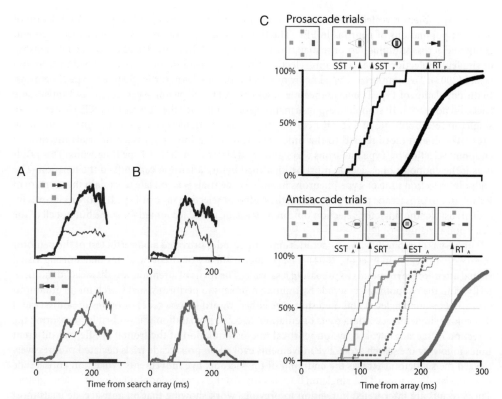

Fig. 19.4 (Also see Plate 13.) Pattern and timing of neural activity in FEF when mapping between location of visual target and endpoint of saccade is varied. A) Activity of FEF neuron with activity that can be identified with the allocation of attention (Type I). Average spike density function when the singleton fell in the neuron's receptive field (thick line) and when the singleton was located opposite the receptive field (thin line) in prosaccade (top) and antisaccade (bottom) trials. Bracket on abscissa marks range of RT. Scale bar represents 100 spikes/s. B) Activity of FEF neuron with activity that can be identified with selection of the saccade endpoint (Type II). C) Cumulative distributions of modulation times in prosaccade (top) and antisaccade (bottom) trials for Type I (thin) and Type II (thicker) neurons with corresponding RT (thickest). The inset arrays indicate hypothesized functional correlates. After presentation of the array, selection of the singleton location occurs at the SST of Type I neurons (indicated by the spotlight on the singleton); this occurs at the same time in prosaccade and antisaccade trials and does not relate to whether or when gaze shifts. In prosaccade but not antisaccade trials Type II neurons select the singleton at a later time which accounts for some of the variability of RT. A comparison of activation in prosaccade and antisaccade trials reveals the time at which the shape of the singleton is encoded to specify the correct saccade direction; this follows singleton selection and coincides for Type I (thin blue) and Type II (thicker blue) neurons in antisaccade trials. At the moment marked by SRT in antisaccade trials the representation of the singleton decreases, and the representation of the location opposite the singleton, the endpoint of the antisaccade increases (indicated by the weaker spotlight on the singleton and growing spotlight on the saccade endpoint). At this same time in prosaccade trials the representation of the saccade endpoint is enhanced by the selection that occurs in the Type II neurons (indicated by the highlighted spotlight on the singleton). Subsequently, in antisaccade trials the endpoint of the saccade becomes selected more than the location of the singleton by Type I (thin, red, dashed) and Type II (thicker red, dashed) neurons (indicated by the highlighted spotlight on the antisaccade endpoint). The time taken to select the endpoint of the saccade predicts some of the delay and variability of RT. Reprinted from *Neuron*, **38**(4) Takashi R. Sato, Jeffrey D. Schall, Effects of Stimulus-Response Compatibility on Neural Selection in Frontal Eye Field pp. 637–648, Copyright (2003), with permission from Elsevier.

This experiment revealed a sequence of processes that can be distinguished in the modulation of different populations of neurons in FEF. The time course of these processes can be measured and compared across stimulus-response mapping rules (Fig. 19.4C). More details about the relationship of singleton selection time, endpoint selection time, and response time are described in Sato and Schall (2003). To summarize, Type I neurons selected the singleton earlier than did Type II neurons. In the population of Type I neurons the time of selection of the singleton in prosaccade and antisaccade trials did not vary with stimulus response mapping or account for the difference in RT. However, the singleton selection time of Type II neurons in prosaccade trials was less synchronized with array presentation and more related to the time of saccade initiation. In antisaccade trials the time of endpoint selection by Type I neurons was significantly later than that of Type II neurons. This result is as if the endpoint of a saccade must be identified before attention can shift to the location. The endpoint selection time of Type I neurons in antisaccade trials was too late to explain the increase in RT relative to prosaccade trials. In contrast, the endpoint selection time of Type II neurons in antisaccade trials, like the singleton selection time in prosaccade trials, accounted for some but not all of the delay and variability of RT.

This visual search task with prosaccades and antisaccades provided a powerful test of the pemotor theory of attention (Juan et al., 2004). The premotor theory of attention states that shifting visual spatial attention corresponds to preparing a saccade. The focus of attention was dissociated momentarily from the endpoint of a saccade by training monkeys to perform visual search for an attention-capturing colour singleton and then shift gaze either toward (prosaccade) or opposite (antisaccade) this colour singleton according to its orientation. Saccade preparation was probed by measuring the direction of saccades evoked by intracortical microstimulation of the frontal eye field at different times following the search array. Eye movements evoked on prosaccade trials deviated progressively toward the singleton that was the endpoint of the saccade. Eye movements evoked on antisaccade trials deviated not toward the singleton but only toward the saccade endpoint opposite the singleton. These results are interpreted in relation to previous work showing that on antisaccade trials most visually responsive neurons in frontal eye field initially select the singleton while attention is allocated to distinguish its shape. In contrast, preliminary data indicates that movement neurons are activated but do not produce a directional signal after the saccade endpoint is selected. Evidence consistent with these observations has been obtained in a study of human participants using transcranial magnetic stimulation (Juan et al., 2008), and in a study probing explicitly the locus of attention (Smith and Schenk, 2007). Thus, the brain can covertly orient attention without preparing a saccade to the locus of attention. The premotor theory should be revised to accommodate these results.

To produce arbitrary responses to specific stimuli requires a mechanism to encode the rules and context of the task. This brings us to areas in prefrontal cortex rostral to the FEF.

Prefrontal cortex

Rostral to the FEF are areas of ventrolateral and dorsolateral prefrontal cortex that have been the focus of extensive investigation and theory (e.g. Fuster, 2008). Before proceeding, we should note that the FEF is certainly an area in prefrontal cortex defined by the presence of a granular layer and afferents from the mediodorsal nucleus of the thalamus. Nevertheless, to simplify and summarize the function of the more rostral areas, we can state that they contribute to enacting flexible stimulus-response rules through time. According to the hypothesis that attentional selection and saccade production are accomplished by different neural circuits, then dorsolateral prefrontal cortex could enact this flexibility by modulating either the salience map represented by the visually responsive neurons or by modulating the timing of the saccade preparation process. Clear evidence for task-related modulation of the target selection process has been obtained in FEF (e.g. Bichot & Schall, 1999; 2002). Equally clear evidence for task-related modulation of the timing of saccade preparation process has also been obtained in FEF (Woodman et al., 2007). Further research is needed to understand how the flexible representations afforded by prefrontal cortex influence saccade target selection.

Recent lesion and microstimulation studies have established a general role of macaque dorsolateral prefrontal cortex in attention and saccade target selection (Opris et al., 2005; Rossi et al., 2007). However, we must note that the conditions of the experiments investigating prefrontal cortex were not typical of the visual search experiments reviewed above. For example, in one study, monkeys discriminated the orientation of a coloured target grating among distractor gratings. When the cue indicating which stimulus was the target was held constant across trials, monkeys with prefrontal cortex lesions were unimpared. When the cue switched frequently across trials, however, monkeys with prefrontal cortex lesions were severely impaired in attending to the target.

The activity of neurons in prefrontal cortex areas rostral to FEF has been described during tasks that required different forms of visual target selection (Boussaoud and Wise, 1993; Buschman and Miller, 2007; Constantinidis et al., 2001; Everling et al., 2006; Ferrera et al., 1999; Hasegawa et al., 2000; Kim and Shadlen, 1999; Rainer et al., 1998). In some of these studies the selection of the target appeared as effectively an all-or-none activation, largely because the responses began after the selection process was completed in visual areas of the cortex.

A common feature of neurons recorded in dorsolateral prefrontal cortex is the presence of activity during enforced delay periods in which monkeys must remember specific aspects of the stimuli to guide the eventual response. The characteristics of this delay period activation have been described in numerous studies. For example, one study presented monkeys with two stimuli, a bright target and a distractor with brightness that was varied across trials from that of the dim background to that of the bright target (Constantinidis et al., 2001). In this way the discriminability of the target from the distractor was varied. After an instructed delay in which the stimuli had been removed, monkeys shifted gaze to the location occupied by the brighter stimulus. The activation during the delay period varied according to the brightness of the stimulus in the receptive field and the performance of the monkeys. Neurons remained active during the delay period even if the stimulus in the receptive field had been the distractor. This affords an opportunity for the properties of the non-selected stimuli to influence subsequent performance. Also, the magnitude of the activation varied such that if the distractor was more similar to the target, the activation evoked by the distractor was more similar to the activation evoked by the target.

To summarize, the studies of dorsolateral prefrontal cortex have indicated that neurons may not participate directly in the target selection process but can encode the properties of selected and non-selected stimuli. Further work is needed to discover how the function of dorsolateral prefrontal cortex influences target selection in the more caudal parts of the brain.

Summary

Vision occurs naturally in a continuous cycle of fixations interrupted by gaze shifts. The guidance of these eye movements requires information about what is where in the image. The identity of objects is derived mainly from their visible features. Single neurons in the visual pathway represent the presence of specific features by the level of activation. Each point in the visual field is represented by populations of neurons activated by all types of features. Topographic representations are found throughout the visual and oculomotor systems; neighbouring neurons tend to represent similar visual field locations or saccades.

When confronted by an image with many possible targets, the visual system compares the features of elements across the visual field. The retinotopic maps of the visual field facilitate local interactions to implement such comparisons; in particular, a network of lateral inhibition can extract the locations of the most conspicuous stimuli in the visual field. The process of these comparisons can be influenced by knowledge so that inconspicuous but important elements in the image can be the focus of gaze. This selection process results in a state of activation in which neurons with potential targets in their receptive field are more active, and neurons with non-targets in their receptive field are less active.

The outcome of this selection process can be represented at a level of abstraction distinct from the representation of the features themselves. This is why the hypothetical construct of a salience map is useful. The state of neural selection of a salient target relative to surrounding non-target elements amounts to the covert allocation of attention that usually precedes overt shifts of gaze. The time taken for the brain to achieve an explicit representation of the location of a target varies predictably according to how distinct the target appears in relation to non-target elements.

Coordinated with this visual processing is activation in a network including FEF and superior colliculus that is responsible for producing the eye movement. A saccade is produced when the activation at one location within the motor map reaches a critical threshold. One job of visual processing influenced by memory and goals, is to insure that only one site—the best site—within the map of movements becomes activated. This is done when the neurons signalling the location of the desired target develop enhanced activation while the neurons responding to other locations are attenuated. When confronted with ambiguous images having multiple potential targets, partial activation can occur in parts of the motor map representing saccades to non-target elements that resemble the target. Saccade target selection converts an initially ambiguous pattern of neural activation into a pattern that reliably signals one target location in a winner-take-all fashion. However, the representation of likely targets for orienting does not automatically and unalterably produce a saccade. Sometimes potential targets are perceived without an overt gaze shift or gaze can shift to locations not occupied by salient stimuli. The explanation of this flexible coupling between target selection and saccade production requires separate stages or modules that select a target for orienting and that produce gaze shifts. The flexible relationship between target selection and saccade production also affords the ability to emphasize speed or accuracy. Accuracy in fixating correctly can be emphasized at the expense of speed by allowing the visual selection process to resolve alternatives before producing a saccade. On the other hand, accuracy can be sacrificed for speed, allowing the visuomotor system to produce a saccade that may be inaccurate because it is premature relative to the target selection process.

Obviously, many questions remain, but looking back just 20 years it is gratifying to note the progress that has been made describing how the brain selects the targets for saccades.

Acknowledgements

Research in Schall's laboratory has been supported by the National Eye Institute, the National Institute of Mental Health, the National Science Foundation, the McKnight Endowment Fund for Neuroscience, the Air Force Office of Scientific Research and by Robin and Richard Patton through the E. Bronson Ingram Chair in Neuroscience.

References

Andersen, R.A. and Buneo, C.A. (2002). Intentional maps in posterior parietal cortex. *Annual Review of Neuroscience*, **25**, 189–220.

Armstrong, K.M., and Moore, T. (2007). Rapid enhancement of visual cortical response discriminability by microstimulation of the frontal eye field. *Proceedings of the National Academy of Sciences U S A*, **104**, 9499–9504.

Armstrong, K.M., Fitzgerald, J.K., and Moore, T. (2006). Changes in visual receptive fields with microstimulation of frontal cortex. *Neuron*, **50**, 791–798.

Balan, P.F., Oristaglio, J., Schneider, D.M., and Gottlieb, J. (2008). Neuronal correlates of the set-size effect in monkey lateral intraparietal area. *PLoS Biology*, **6**, e158.

Barone, P., Batardiere, A., Knoblauch, K., and Kennedy, H. (2000). Laminar distribution of neurons in extrastriate areas projecting to visual areas V1 and V4 correlates with the hierarchical rank and indicates the operation of a distance rule. *Journal of Neuroscience*, **20**, 3263–81.

Basso, M. A. and Wurtz, R.H. (1998). Modulation of neuronal activity in superior colliculus by changes in target probability. *Journal of Neuroscience*, **18**, 7519–7534.

Behrmann, M., Geng, J.J., and Shomstein, S. (2004). Parietal cortex and attention. *Current Opinion in Neurobiology*, **14**, 212–217.

Bichot, N.P. and Schall, J.D. (1999a). Effects of similarity and history on neural mechanisms of visual selection. *Nature Neuroscience*, **2**, 549–554.

Bichot, N.P. and Schall, J.D. (1999b). Saccade target selection in macaque during feature and conjunction visual search. *Visual Neuroscience*, **16**, 81–89.

Bichot, N.P. and Desimone, R. (2006). Finding a face in the crowd: parallel and serial neural mechanisms of visual selection. *Progress in Brain Research*, **155**, 147–56.

Bichot, N.P., Schall, J.D., and Thompson, K.G. (1996). Visual feature selectivity in frontal eye fields induced by experience in mature macaques. *Nature*, **381**, 697–699.

Bichot, N.P., Rao, S.C., and Schall, J.D. (2001a). Continuous processing in macaque frontal cortex during visual search. *Neuropsychologia*, **39**, 972–982.

Bichot, N.P., Rossi, A.F., and Desimone, R. (2005). Parallel and serial neural mechanisms for visual search in macaque area V4. *Science*, **308**, 529–534.

Bichot, N.P., Thompson, K.G., Rao, S.C., and Schall, J.D. (2001b). Reliability of macaque frontal eye field neurons signaling saccade targets during visual search. *Journal of Neuroscience*, **21**, 713–725.

Boussaoud D. and Wise, S.P. (1993). Primate frontal cortex: neuronal activity following attentional versus intentional cues. *Experimental Brain Research*, **95**, 15–27.

Bruce, C.J. and Goldberg, M.E. (1985). Primate frontal eye fields I: Single neurons discharging before saccades. *Journal of Neurophysiology*, **53**, 603–635.

Bruce, C.J., Goldberg, M.E., Bushnell, C., and Stanton, G.B. (1985). Primate frontal eye fields II: Physiological and anatomical correlates of electrically evoked eye movements. *Journal of Neurophysiology*, **54**, 714–734.

Buschman, T.J. and Miller, E.K. (2007). Top-down versus bottom-up control of attention in the prefrontal and posterior parietal cortices. *Science*, **315**, 1860–1862.

Bushnell, M.C., Goldberg, M.E., and Robinson, D.L. (1981). Behavioral enhancement of visual responses in monkey cerebral cortex. I. Modulation in posterior parietal cortex related to selective visual attention. *Journal of Neurophysiology*, **46**, 755–772.

Camalier, C.R., Gotler, A., Murthy, A., Thompson, K.G., Logan, G.D., Palmeri, T.J., et al. (2007). Dynamics of saccade target selection: race model analysis of double step and search step saccade production in human and macaque. *Vision Research*, **47**, 2187–2211.

Carello, C.D. and Krauzlis, R.J. (2004). Manipulating intent: Evidence for a causal role of the superior colliculus in target selection. *Neuron*, **43**, 575–583.

Carpenter, R.H.S., (1995). Neural computation of log likelihood in control of saccadic eye movements. *Nature*, **377**, 59–62.

Caspi, A., Beutter, B.R., and Eckstein, M.P. (2004). The time course of visual information accrual guiding eye movement decisions. *Proceedings of the National Academy Sciences U S A.* **101**, 13086–13090.

Chelazzi, L., Duncan, J., Miller, E.K., and Desimone, R. (1998). Responses of neurons in inferior temporal cortex during memory-guided visual search. *Journal of Neurophysiology*, **80**, 2918–2940.

Chelazzi, L., Miller, E.K., Duncan, J., and Desimone, R. (2001). Responses of neurons in macaque area V4 during memory-guided visual search. *Cerebral Cortex*, **11**, 761–772.

Cohen, J.Y., Heitz, R.P., Schall, J.D., and Woodman, G.F. (2009a). On the origin of event-related potentials indexing covert attentional selection during visual search. *Journal of Neurophysiology* **102**, 2375–2386.

Cohen, J.Y., Heitz, R.P., Woodman, G.F., and Schall, J.D. (2009b). Neural basis of the set-size effect in the frontal eye field: Timing of attention during visual search. *Journal of Neurophysiology* **101**, 1699–1704.

Cohen, J.Y., Crowder, E.A., Heitz, R.P., Subraveti, C.R., Thompson, K.G., Woodman, G.F., et al. (2010). Cooperation and competition among frontal eye field neurons during visual target selection. *Journal of Neuroscience* **30**, 3227–3238.

Constantinidis, C. (2006). Posterior parietal mechanisms of visual attention. *Reviews in Neuroscience*, **17**, 415–427.

Constantinidis, C. and Steinmetz, M.A. (2001a). Neuronal responses in area 7a to multiple-stimulus displays: I. neurons encode the location of the salient stimulus. *Cerebral Cortex*, **11**, 581–591.

Constantinidis, C. and Steinmetz, M.A. (2001b). Neuronal responses in area 7a to multiple stimulus displays: II. responses are suppressed at the cued location. *Cerebral Cortex*, **11**, 592–597.

Constantinidis C., Franowicz, M.N., and Goldman-Rakic, P.S. (2001). The sensory nature of mnemonic representation in the primate prefrontal cortex. *Nature Neuroscience*, **4**, 311–316.

Connor, C.E., Preddie, D.C., Gallant, J.L., and Van Essen, D.C. (1997). Spatial attention effects in macaque area V4. *Journal of Neuroscience*, **17**, 3201–3214.

Crawford, T.J. and Muller, H.J. (1992). Spatial and temporal effects of spatial attention on human saccadic eye movements. *Vision Research*, **32**, 293–304.

David, S.V. Hayden, B.Y., Mazer, J.A., and Gallant, J.L. (2008). Attention to stimulus features shifts spectral tuning of V4 neurons during natural vision. *Neuron*, **59**, 509–521.

Desimone, R. and Duncan, J. (1995). Neural mechanisms of selective visual attention, *Annual Review of Neuroscience*, **18**, 193–222.

Desimone, R. and Schein, S.J. (1987). Visual properties of neurons in area V4 of the macaque: Sensitivity to stimulus form, *Journal of Neurophysiology*, **57**, 835–868.

Deubel, H. (2008). The time course of presaccadic attention shifts. *Psychological Research*, **72**, 630–640.

Deubel, H. and Schneider, W.X. (1996). Saccade target selection and object recognition: Evidence for a common attentional mechanism. *Vision Research*, **36**, 1827–1837.

DiCarlo, J.J. and Maunsell, J.H.R. (2000). Form representation in monkey inferotemporal cortex is virtually unaltered by free viewing. *Nature Neuroscience*, **3**, 814–821.

Donders, F.C. (1868). *On the speed of mental processes, in Attention and Performance II* (W.G. Koster, trans., 1969) (pp. 412–431). Amsterdam: North-Holland Publishing Co.

Dorris, M.C., Paré, M, and Munoz, D.P. (1997). Neuronal activity in monkey superior colliculus related to the initiation of saccadic eye movements. *Journal of Neuroscience*, **17**, 8566–8579.

Eckstein, M.P., Beutter, B.R., and Stone, L.S. (2001). Quantifying the performance limits of human saccadic targeting during visual search. *Perception* **30**, 1389–1401.

Eriksen, C.W. and Hoffman, J.E. (1972). Temporal and spatial characteristics of selective encoding from visual displays. *Perception & Psychophysics*, **12**, 201–204.

Everling, S. and Munoz, D.P. (2000). Neuronal correlates for preparatory set associated with pro-saccades and anti-saccades in the primate frontal eye field. *Journal of Neuroscience*, **20**, 387–400.

Everling, S., Dorris, M.C., Klein, R.M., and Munoz, D.P. (1999). Role of primate superior colliculus in preparation and execution of anti-saccades and pro-saccades. *Journal of Neuroscience*, **19**, 2740–2754.

Everling, S., Tinsley, C.J., Gaffan, D., and Duncan, J. (2006). Selective representation of task-relevant objects and locations in the monkey prefrontal cortex. *European Journal of Neuroscience*, **23**, 2197–2214.

Fecteau, J.H. and Munoz, D.P. (2006). Salience, relevance, and firing: a priority map for target selection. *Trends in Cognitive Sciences*, **10**, 382–390.

Fecteau, J.H. and Munoz, D.P. (2007). Warning signals influence motor processing. *Journal of Neurophysiology*, **97**, 1600–1609.

Ferrera, V.P., Cohen, J.K., and Lee, B.B. (1999). Activity of prefrontal neurons during location and color delayed matching tasks. *Neuroreport*, **10**, 1315–1322.

Findlay, J.M. (1997). Saccade target selection during visual search. *Vision Research*, **37**, 617–631.

Findlay, J.M. and Walker, R. (1999). A model of saccade generation based on parallel processing and competitive inhibition. *Behavioral and Brain Sciences*, **22**, 661–674.

Fischer, B. and Boch, R. (1981). Enhanced activation of neurons in prelunate cortex before visually guided saccades of trained rhesus monkeys. *Experimental Brain Research*, **44**, 129–137.

Fuster J. (2008). *The Prefrontal Cortex*, 4th edn. London: Academic Press.

Gallant, J.L., Connor, C.E., and Van Essen, D.C. (1998). Neural activity in areas V1, V2 and V4 during free viewing of natural scenes compared to controlled viewing. *Neuroreport*, **9**, 85–90.

Glimcher, P.W. and Sparks, D.L. (1992). Movement selection in advance of action in superior colliculus. *Nature*, **355**, 542–545.

Goldberg, M.E. and Wurtz, R.H. (1972). Activity of superior colliculus in behaving monkey, II. Effect of attention on neuronal responses. *Journal of Neurophysiology*, **35**, 560–574.

Gottlieb, J., (2007). From thought to action: The parietal cortex as a bridge between perception, action, and cognition. *Neuron*, **53**, 9–16.

Gottlieb, J.P., Kusunoki, M., and Goldberg, M.E. (1998). The representation of visual salience in monkey parietal cortex. *Nature*, **391**, 481–484.

Hamker, F.H. and Zirnsak, M. (2006). V4 receptive field dynamics as predicted by a systems-level model of visual attention using feedback from the frontal eye field. *Neural Networks*, **19**, 1371–1382.

Hanes, D.P. and Schall, J.D. (1996). Neural control of voluntary movement initiation. *Science*, **274**, 427–430.

Hanes, D.P., Patterson, W.F., and Schall, J.D. (1998). The role of frontal eye field in counter-manding saccades: Visual movement and fixation activity. *Journal of Neurophysiology*, **79**, 817–834.

Hasegawa, R.P., Matsumoto, M., and Mikami, A. (2000). Search target selection in monkey prefrontal cortex. *Journal of Neurophysiology*, **84**, 1692–1696.

Hayden, B.Y. and Gallant, J.L. (2005). Time course of attention reveals different mechanisms for spatial and feature-based attention in area V4. *Neuron*, **47**, 637–643.

Heitz, R.P., Cohen, J.Y., Woodman, G.F., and Schall, J.D. (2010). Neural correlates of correct and errant attentional selection revealed through N2pc and frontal eye field activity. *Journal of Neurophysiology*, **104**, 2433–2441.

Henderson, J.M. (1991). Stimulus discrimination following covert attentional orienting to an exogenous cue. *Journal of Experimental Psychology: Human Perception and Performance*, **17**, 91–106.

Henderson, J.M. and Graham, P.L. (2008). Eye movements during scene viewing: evidence for mixed control of fixation durations. *Psychonomic Bulletin and Review* **15**, 566–573.

Hoffman, J.E., and Subramaniam, B. (1995). The role of visual attention in saccadic eye movements, *Perception and Psychophysics*, **57**, 787–795.

Hooge, I.T.C. and Erkelens, C.J. (1996). Control of fixation duration in a simple search task. *Perception and Psychophysics*, **58**, 969–976.

Hooge, I.T. and Erkelens, C.J. (1999). Peripheral vision and oculomotor control during visual search. *Vision Research*, **39**(8), 1567–75.

Hooge, I.T. and Erkelens, C.J. (1998). Adjustment of fixation duration in visual search. *Vision Research*, **38**(9), 1295–302.

Hopf, J.M., Luck, S.J., Girelli, M., Hagner, T., Mangun, G.R., Scheich, H., *et al.* (2000). Neural sources of focused attention in visual search. *Cerebral Cortex*, **10**, 1233–1241.

Horwitz G.D. and Newsome, W.T. (2001). Target selection for saccadic eye movements: prelude activity in the superior colliculus during a direction-discrimination task. *Journal of Neurophysiology*, **86**, 2543–2558.

Huerta, M.F., Krubitzer, L.A., and Kaas, J.H. (1986). Frontal eye field as defined by intracortical microstimulation in squirrel monkeys, owl monkeys and macaque monkeys: I. Subcortical connections. *Journal of Comparative Neurology*, **253**, 415–439.

Hunt, A.R. and Kingstone, A. (2003). Covert and overt voluntary attention: linked or independent? *Cognitive Brain Research*, **18**, 102–105.

Ignashchenkova, A., Dicke, P.W., Haarmeier, T., and Their, P. (2004). Neuron-specific contribution of the superior colliculus to overt and covert shifts of attention. *Nature Neuroscience*, **7**, 56–64.

Ipata, A.E., Gee, A.L., Goldberg, M.E., and Bisley, J.W. (2006). Activity in the lateral intraparietal area predicts the goal and latency of saccades in a free-viewing visual search task. *Journal of Neuroscience*, **26**, 3656–3661.

Itti, L. and Koch, C. (2001). Computational modelling of visual attention. *Nature Reviews Neuroscience*, **2**, 194–203.

Jacobs, A.M., (1987). Toward a model of eye movement control in visual search. In J. K. O'Regan and A. Levy-Schoe (eds.) *Eye Movements: From Physiology to Cognition* (pp. 275–284). North-Holland: Elsevier Science Publishers B.V.

Jonides, J., (1980). Towards a model of the mind's eye's movement. *Canadian Journal of Psychology*, **34**, 103–112.

Jouve, B., Rosenstiehl, P., and Imbert, M. (1998). A mathematical approach to the connectivity between the cortical visual areas of the macaque monkey. *Cerebral Cortex*, **8**, 28–39.

Juan, C.H., Shorter-Jacobi, S.M., and Schall, J.D. (2004). Dissociation of spatial attention and saccade preparation. *Proceeding of the National Academy of Science U S A*, **101**, 15541–15544.

Juan, C.H., Muggleton, N.G., Tzeng, O.J., Hung, D.L., Cowey, A., and Walsh, V. (2008). Segregation of visual selection and saccades in human frontal eye fields. *Cerebral Cortex*, **18**, 2410–2415.

Kim, B. and Basso, M.A. (2008). Saccade target selection in the superior colliculus: a signal detection theory approach. *Journal of Neuroscience*, **28**, 2991–3007.

Kim, M.S. and Cave, K.R. (1995). Spatial attention in search for features and feature conjunctions. *Psychonomic Science*, **6**, 376–380.

Kim J.N. and Shadlen, M.N. (1999). Neural correlates of a decision in the dorsolateral prefrontal cortex of the macaque. *Nature Neuroscience*, **2**, 176–185.

Klein, R. (1980). Does oculomotor readiness mediate cognitive control of visual attention? In R. Nickerson (ed.) *Attention and performance* (pp. 259–276). New York: Academic Press.

Klein, R.M. and Pontefract, A. (1994). Does oculomotor readiness mediate cognitive control of visual attention? Revisited! In C. Umilta and M. Moscovitch (eds.) *Attention and Performance XV: Conscious and Nonconscious Information Processing* (pp. 333–350). Cambridge, MA: MIT Press.

Klein, R., Kingstone, A., and Pontefract, A. (1992). Orienting of visual attention. In K. Rayner (ed.) *Eye Movements and Visual Cognition: Scene Perception and Reading* (pp. 46–65). New York: Springer-Verlag.

Knierim, J.J. and Van Essen, D.C. (1992). Neuronal responses to static texture patterns in area V1 of the alert macaque monkey. *Journal of Neurophysiology*, **67**, 961–980.

Kowler, E., Anderson, E., Dosher, B., and Blaser, E. (1995). The role of attention in the programming of saccades. *Vision Research*, **35**, 1897–1916.

Knierim, J.J. and Van Essen, D.C. (1992). Neuronal responses to static texture patterns in area V1 of the alert macaque monkey. *Journal of Neurophysiology*, **67**, 961–980.

Krauzlis, R.J., Liston, D., and Carello, C.D., (2004). Target selection and the superior colliculus: goals, choices and hypotheses. *Vision Research*, **44**, 1445–1451.

Kustov, A.A., and Robinson, D.L. (1996). Shared neural control of attentional shifts and eye movements. *Nature*, **384**, 74–77.

Kusunoki, M., Gottlieb, J., and Goldberg, M.E. (2000). The lateral intraparietal area as a salience map: the representation of abrupt onset, stimulus motion, and task relevance. *Vision Research*, **40**, 1459–1468.

Li, X. and Basso, M.A. (2005). Competitive stimulus interactions within single response fields of superior colliculus neurons. *Journal of Neuroscience*, **25**, 11357–11373.

Lovejoy, L.P. and Krauzlis, R.J. (2010). Inactivation of primate superior colliculus impairs covert selection of signals for perceptual judgments. *Nature Neuroscience*, **13**, 261–266.

Luck, S.J. and Hillyard, S.A. (1994). Electrophysiological correlates of feature analysis during visual search. *Psychophysiology* **31**, 291–308.

Ludwig, C.J., Gilchrist, I.D., McSorley, E., and Baddeley, R.J. (2005). The temporal impulse response underlying saccadic decisions. *Journal of Neuroscience*, **25**, 9907–9912.

Lynch, J.C., Graybiel, A.M., and Lobeck, L.J. (1985). The differential projection of two cytoarchitectural subregions of the inferior parietal lobule of macaque upon the deep layers of the superior colliculus. *Journal of Comparative Neurology*, **235**, 241–254.

Maljkovic, V. and Nakayama, K. (1994). Priming of pop-out: I. Role of features. *Memory and Cognition*, **22**, 657–672.

Maljkovic, V. and Nakayama, K. (1996). Priming of pop-put: II. The role of position. *Perception and Psychophysics*, **58**, 977–991.

Mazer, J.A. and Gallant, J.L. (2003). Goal-related activity in V4 during free viewing visual search: Evidence for a ventral stream visual salience map. *Neuron*, **40**, 1241–1250.

McPeek, R.M. (2006). Incomplete suppression of distractor-related activity in the frontal eye field results in curved saccades. *Journal of Neurophysiology*, **96**, 2699–2711.

McPeek, R.M. (2008). Reversal of a distractor effect on saccade target selection after superior colliculus inactivation. *Journal of Neurophysiology*, **99**, 2694–2702.

McPeek, R.M. and Keller, E.L. (2002a). Saccade target selection in the superior colliculus during a visual search task. *Journal of Neurophysiology*, **88**, 2019–2034.

McPeek, R.M. and Keller, E.L. (2002b). Superior colliculus activity related to concurrent processing of saccade goals in a visual search task. *Journal of Neurophysiology*, **87**, 1805–1815.

McPeek, R.M., and Keller, E.L. (2004). Deficits in saccade target selection after inactivation of superior colliculus. *Nature Neuroscience*, **7**, 757–763.

McPeek, R.M., Maljkovic, V., and Nakayama, K. (1999). Saccades require focal attention and are facilitated by a short-term memory system. *Vision Research*, **39**, 1555–1566.

McPeek, R.M., Han, J.H., and Keller, E.L. (2003). Competition between saccade goals in the superior colliculus produces saccade curvature. *Journal of Neurophysiology*, **89**, 2577–2590.

Miller, J.O. (1988). Discrete and continuous models of human information processing: theoretical distinctions and empirical results. *Acta Psychologica*, **67**, 191–257.

Mirabella, G., G. Bertini, I. Samengo, B.E. Kilavik, D. Frilli, C.D. Libera, L. Chelazzi, (2007). Neurons in area V4 of the macaque translate attended visual features into behaviorally relevant categories. *Neuron*, **54**, 303–318.

Mohler, C.W., Goldberg, M.E., and Wurtz, R.H. (1973). Visual receptive fields of frontal eye field neurons. *Brain Research*, **61**, 385–389.

Monosov, I.E. and Thompson, K.G. (2009). Frontal eye field activity enhances object identification during covert visual search. *Journal of Neurophysiology* **102**, 3656–3672.

Monosov, I.E., Sheinberg, D.L., and Thompson, K.G. (2010). Paired neuron recordings in the prefrontal and inferotemporal cortices reveal that spatial selection precedes object identification during visual search. *Proceedings of the National Academy of Sciences U S A*. **107**, 13105–13110.

Monosov, I.E., Trageser, J.C., and Thompson, K.G. (2008). Measurements of simultaneously recorded spiking activity and local field potentials suggest that spatial selection emerges in the frontal eye field. *Neuron*, **57**, 614–625.

Moore, T. (1999). Shape representations and visual guidance of saccadic eye movements. *Science*, **285**, 1914–1917.

Moore, T. and Armstrong, K.M. (2003). Selective gating of visual signals by microstimulation of frontal cortex. *Nature*, **421**, 370–373.

Moore, T. and Chang, M.H. (2009). Presaccadic discrimination of receptive field stimuli by area V4 neurons. *Vision Research*, **49**(10), 1227–1232.

Motter, B.C., (1994a). Neural correlates of attentive selection for color or luminance in extrastriate area V4. *Journal of Neuroscience*, **14**, 2178–2189.

Motter, B.C. (1994b). Neural correlates of feature selective memory and pop-out in extrastriate area V4. *Journal of Neuroscience*, **14**, 2190–2199.

Motter, B.C. and Belky, E.J. (1998). The guidance of eye movements during active visual search. *Vision Research*, **38**, 1805–1815.

Mountcastle, V.B., Andersen, R.A., and Motter, B.C. (1981). The influence of attentive fixation upon the excitability of the light-sensitive neurons of the posterior parietal cortex, *Journal of Neuroscience*, **1**, 1218–1235.

Muggleton, N.G., Juan, C.H., Cowey, A., and Walsh, V. (2003). Human frontal eye fields and visual search. *Journal of Neurophysiology*, **89**, 3340–3343.

Murthy, A., Ray, S., Shorter, S.M., Schall, J.D., and Thompson, K.G. (2009). Neural control of visual search by frontal eye field: Effects of unexpected target displacement on visual selection and saccade preparation. *Journal of Neurophysiology*, **101**(5), 2485–2510.

Murthy, A., Ray, S., Shorter, S.M., Priddy, E.G., Schall, J.D., and Thompson, K.G. (2007). Frontal eye field contributions to rapid corrective saccades. *Journal of Neurophysiology*, **97**, 1457–1469.

Najemnik J, Geisler WS. (2009). Simple summation rule for optimal fixation selection in visual search. *Vision Research*, **49**(10), 1286–1294.

Ogawa, T. and Komatsu, H. (2004). Target selection in area V4 during a multidimensional visual search task. *Journal of Neuroscience*, **24**, 6371–6382.

Ogawa, T. and Komatsu, H. (2006). Neuronal dynamics of bottom-up and top-down processes in area V4 of macaque monkeys performing a visual search. *Experimental Brain Research*, **173**, 1–13.

Ogawa, T. and Komatsu, H. (2009). Condition-dependent and condition-independent target selection in the macaque posterior parietal cortex. *Journal of Neurophysiology*, **101**, 721–736.

Ogawa, T. and Komatsu, H. (2010). Differential temporal storage capacity in the baseline activity of neurons in macaque frontal eye field and area V4. *Journal of Neurophysiology*, **103**, 2433–2445.

Opris, I., Barborica, A., and Ferrera, V.P. (2005). Microstimulation of the dorsolateral prefrontal cortex biases saccade target selection. *Journal of Cognitive Neuroscience*, **17**, 893–904.

Orban, G.A., (2008). Higher order visual processing in macaque extrastriate cortex. *Physiological Reviews*, **88**, 59–89.

O'Shea, J., Muggleton, N.G., Cowey, A., and Walsh, V. (2004). Timing of target discrimination in human frontal eye fields. *Journal of Cognitive Neuroscience*, **16**, 1060–1067.

Ottes, F.P., van Gisbergen, J.A.M., and Eggermont, J.J. (1987). Collicular involvement in a saccadic colour discrimination task. *Experimental Brain Research*, **66**, 465–478.

Phillips, A.N. and Segraves, M.A. (2010). Predictive activity in macaque frontal eye field neurons during natural scene searching. *Journal of Neurophysiology*, **103**, 1238–1252.

Platt, M.L. and Glimcher, P.W. (1997). Response of intraparietal neurons to saccadic targets and visual distractors. *Journal of Neurophysiology*, **78**, 1574–1589.

Port, N.L. and Wurtz, R.H. (2009). Target selection and saccade generation in monkey superior colliculus. *Experimental Brain Research*, **192**, 465–477.

Posner, M. (1980). Orienting of attention. *Quarterly Journal of Experimental Psychology*, **32**, 3–25.

Pouget, P., Stepniewska, I., Crowder, E.A., Leslie, M.W., Emeric, E.E., Nelson, M.J., and Schall, J.D. (2009). Visual and motor connectivity and the distribution of calcium-binding proteins in macaque frontal eye field: implications for saccade target selection. *Frontiers in Neuroanatomy*, **3**, 2.

Powell, K.D. and Goldberg, M.E. (2000). Response of neurons in the lateral intraparietal area to a distractor flashed during the delay period of a memory-guided saccade. *Journal of Neurophysiology*, **84**, 301–310.

Purcell, B.A., Heitz, R.P., Cohen, J.Y., Logan, G.D., Schall, J.D., Palmeri, T.J. (2010) Neurally constrained modeling of perceptual decision making. *Psychological Review*, **117**(4), 1113–1143.

Rainer, G., Asaad, W.F., and Miller, E.K. (1998). Selective representation of relevant information by neurons in the primate prefrontal cortex. *Nature*, **393**, 577–579.

Ratcliff, R., Cherian, A., and Segraves, M. (2003). A comparison of macaque behavior and superior colliculus neuronal activity to predictions from models of two-choice decisions. *Journal of Neurophysiology*, **90**, 1392–1407.

Ray, S., Schall, J.D., and Murthy, A. (2004). Programming of double-step saccade sequences: modulation by cognitive control. *Vision Research*, **44**, 2707–2718.

Reddi, B.A.J. and Carpenter, R.H.S. (2000). The influence of urgency on decision time. *Nature Neuroscience*, **3**, 827–830.

Reddi, B.A.J., Asrress, K.N., and Carpenter, R.H.S. (2003). Accuracy, information, and response time in a saccade decision task. *Journal of Neurophysiology*, **90**, 3538–3546.

Remington, R.W. (1980). Attention and saccadic eye movements. *Journal of Experimental Psychology: Human Perception and Performance*, **6**, 726–744.

Reuter-Lorenz, P. and Fendrich, A.R. (1992). Oculomotor readiness and covert orienting: Differences between central and peripheral precuts. *Perception and Psychophysics*, **52**, 336–344.

Reynolds, J.H. and Chelazzi, L. (2004). Attentional modulation of visual processing. *Annual Review of Neuroscience*, **27**, 611–647.

Richmond, B.J. and Sato, T. (1987). Enhancement of inferior temporal neurons during visual discrimination. *Journal of Neurophysiology*, **58**, 1292–1306.

Rizzolatti, G. (1983). Mechanisms of selective attention in mammals. In J. Ewert, R.R. Capranica and D.J. Ingle (eds.) *Advances in vertebrate neuroethology* (pp. 261–297). New York: Elsevier.

Robinson, D.L., Bowman, E.M., and Kertzman, C. (1995). Covert orienting of attention in macaques II. Contributions of parietal cortex. *Journal of Neurophysiology*, **74**, 698–712.

Robinson, D.L., Goldberg, M.E., and Stanton, G.B. (1978). Parietal association cortex in the primate: Sensory mechanisms and behavioral modulations. *Journal of Neurophysiology*, **41**, 910–932.

Rodriguez-Sanchez, A.J., Simine, E., and Tsotsos, J.K. (2007) Attention and visual search. *International Journal of Neural Systems*, **17**(4), 275–88.

Rolls, E.T., Aggelopoulos, N.C., and Zheng, F. (2003). The receptive fields of inferior temporal cortex neurons in natural scenes. *Journal of Neuroscience*, **23**, 339–348.

Rossi, A.F., Desimone, R., and Ungerleider, L.G. (2001). Contextual modulation in primary visual cortex of macaques. *Journal of Neuroscience*, **21**, 1698–709.

Rossi, A.F, Bichot, N.P., Desimone, R., and Ungerleider, L.G. (2007). Top down attentional deficits in macaques with lesions of lateral prefrontal cortex. *Journal of Neuroscience*, **27**, 11306–11314.

Saito, H., Yukie, M., Tanaka, K., Kikosaka, K., Fukada, Y., and Iwai, E. (1986). Integration of direction signals of image motion in the superior temporal sulcus of the macaque monkey. *Journal of Neuroscience*, **6**, 145–157.

Sato, T., (1988). Effects of attention and stimulus interaction on visual responses of inferior temporal neurons in macaque. *Journal of Neurophysiology*, **60**, 344–364.

Sato, T., Murthy A., Thompson, K.G., and Schall, J.D. (2001). Search efficiency but not response interference affects visual selection in frontal eye field. *Neuron*, **30**, 583–591.

Sato, T.R. and Schall, J.D. (2003). Effects of stimulus-response compatibility on neural selection in frontal eye field. *Neuron*, **38**, 637–648.

Schall, J.D. (1991). Neuronal activity related to visually guided saccades in the frontal eye fields of rhesus monkeys: Comparison with supplementary eye fields. *Journal of Neurophysiology*, **66**, 559–579.

Schall, J.D. (1997). Visuomotor areas of the frontal lobe In K. Rockland, A. Peters, and J.H. Kaas (eds.) *Extra striate Cortex of Primates. Cerebral Cortex*, **12**, 527–638.

Schall, J.D., (2003). Selection of targets for saccadic eye movements. In L.M. Chalupa, J.S. Werner (eds.) *The Visual Neurosciences* (pp. 1369–1390). Cambridge, MA: The MIT Press.

Schall, J.D. (2004a). On building a bridge between brain and behavior. *Annual Review of Psychology*, **55**, 23–50.

Schall, J.D. (2004b). On the role of frontal eye field in guiding attention and saccades. *Vision Research*, **44**, 1453–1467.

Schall, J.D. and Hanes, D.P. (1993). Neural basis of saccade target selection in frontal eye field during visual search. *Nature*, **366**, 467–469.

Schall, J.D. and Thompson, K.G. (1999). Neural selection and control of visually guided eye movements. *Annual Review of Neuroscience*, **22**, 241–259.

Schall, J.D., Hanes, D.P., Thompson, K.G., and King, D.J. (1995a). Saccade target selection in frontal eye field of macaque I Visual and premovement activation. *Journal of Neuroscience*, **15**, 6905–6918.

Schall, J.D., Morel, A., King, D.J., and Bullier, J. (1995b). Topography of visual cortical afferents to frontal eye field in macaque: Functional convergence and segregation of processing streams. *Journal of Neuroscience*, **15**, 4464–4487.

Schall, J.D., Thompson, K.G., Bichot, N.P., Murthy, A., and Sato, T.R. (2003) Visual processing in the frontal eye field. In J. Kaas, C. Collins (eds.) *The Primate Visual System* (pp. 205–230). Boca Raton, FL: CRC Press.

Schiller, P.H. and Chou, I.H. (2000). The effects of anterior arcuate and dorsomedial frontal cortex lesions on visually guided eye movements: 2. Paired and multiple targets. *Vision Research* **40**, 1627–1638.

Schiller P.H. and Kendall, J. (2004). Temporal factors in target selection with saccadic eye movements. *Experimental Brain Research*, **154**, 154–159.

Schiller P.H. and Tehovnik, E.J. (2005). Neural mechanisms underlying target selection with saccadic eye movements. *Progress in Brain Research*, **149**, 157–171.

Schmolesky, M.T., Wang, Y., Hanes, D.P., Thompson, K.G., Leutgeb, S., Schall, J.D., *et al.* (1998). Signal timing across the macaque visual system. *Journal of Neurophysiology*, **79**, 3272–3278.

Segraves, M.A. (1992). Activity of monkey frontal eye field neurons projecting to oculomotor regions of the pons. *Journal of Neurophysiology*, **68**, 1967–1985.

Segraves, M.A. and Goldberg, M.E. (1987). Functional properties of corticotectal neurons in the monkey's frontal eye fields. *Journal of Neurophysiology*, **58**, 1387–1419.

Sharika, K.M., Ramakrishnan, A., and Murthy, A. (2008). Control of predictive error correction during a saccadic double-step task. *Journal of Neurophysiology*, **100**, 2757–2770.

Sheinberg, D.L. and Logothetis, N.K. (2001). Noticing familiar objects in real world scenes: The role of temporal cortical neurons in natural vision. *Journal of Neuroscience*, **21**, 1340–1350.

Sheliga, B.M., Riggio, L., and Rizzolatti, G. (1994). Orienting of attention and eye movements. *Experimental Brain Research*, **98**, 507–522.

Sheliga, B., Riggio, M.L., and Rizzolatti, G. (1995). Spatial attention and eye movements. *Experimental Brain Research*, **105**, 261–275.

Shen, K. and Paré, M. (2007). Neuronal activity in superior colliculus signals both stimulus identity and saccade goals during visual conjunction search. *Journal of Vision*, **7**, 15.1–13.

Shepherd, M., Findlay, J.M., and Hockey, R.J. (1986). The relationship between eye movements and spatial attention. *Quarterly Journal of Experimental Psychology*, **38A**, 475–491.

Smith, P.L. and Ratcliff, R. (2004). Psychology and neurobiology of simple decisions. *Trends in Neurosciences*, **27**, 161–168.

Smith, D.T. and Schenk, T. (2007). Enhanced probe discrimination at the location of a colour singleton. *Experimental Brain Research* **181**, 367–375.

Sommer, M.A. and Wurtz, R.H. (2000). Composition and topographic organization of signals sent from the frontal eye field to the superior colliculus. *Journal of Neurophysiology*, **83**, 1979–2001.

Sommer, M.A. and Wurtz, R.H. (2001). Frontal eye field sends delay activity related to movement, memory, and vision to the superior colliculus. *Journal of Neurophysiology*, **85**, 1673–85.

Stanton, G.B., Goldberg, M.E., and Bruce, C.J. (1988). Frontal eye field efferents in the macaque monkey: I. Subcortical pathways and topography of striatal and thalamic terminal fields. *Journal of Comparative Neurology*, **271**, 473–492.

Steinmetz, M.A. and Constantinidis, C. (1995). Neurophysiological evidence for a role of posterior parietal cortex in redirecting visual attention. *Cerebral Cortex*, **5**, 448–456.

Steinmetz, M.A., Connor, C.E., Constantinidis, C., McLaughlin, J.R. Jr. (1994). Covert attention suppresses neuronal responses in area 7a of the posterior parietal cortex. *Journal of Neurophysiology*, **72**, 1020–1023.

Sternberg, S. (1969). The discovery of processing stages: Extensions of Donders' method. *Acta Psychologica*, **30**, 276–315.

Theeuwes, J.A., Kramer, F., Hahn, S., and Irwin, D.E. (1998). Our eyes do not always go where we want them to go: Capture of the eyes by new objects. *Psychological Science*, **9**, 379–385.

Theeuwes, J. (1991). Cross dimensional perceptual selectivity. *Perception and Psychophysics*, **50**, 184–193.

Thomas, N.W.D. and Paré, M. (2007). Temporal processing of saccade targets in parietal cortex area LIP during visual search. *Journal of Neurophysiology*, **97**, 942–947.

Thompson, K.G. and Bichot, N.P. (2005). A visual salience map in the primate frontal eye field. *Progress in Brain Research*, **147**, 251–262.

Thompson, K.G., Bichot, N.P., and Schall, J.D. (1997). Dissociation of target selection from saccade planning in macaque frontal eye field. *Journal of Neurophysiology*, **77**, 1046–1050.

Thompson, K.G., Bichot, N.P., and Schall, J.D. (2001). From attention to action in frontal cortex. In J. Braun, C. Koch, J. Davis (eds.) *Visual Attention and Cortical Circuits* (pp. 137–157). Cambridge, MA: MIT Press.

Thompson, K.G., Hanes, D.P., Bichot, N.P., and Schall, J.D. (1996). Perceptual and motor processing stages identified in the activity of macaque frontal eye field neurons during visual search. *Journal of Neurophysiology*, **76**, 4040–4055.

Tolias, A., Moore, S.T., Smirnakis, S.M., Tehovnik, E.J., Siapas, A.G., and Schiller, P.H. (2001). Eye movements modulate visual receptive fields of V4 neurons. *Neuron*, **29**, 757–67.

Trageser, J.C., Monosov, I.E., Zhou, Y., and Thompson, K.G, (2008). A perceptual representation in the frontal eye field during covert visual search that is more reliable than the behavioral report. *European Journal of Neuroscience*, **28**, 2542–2549.

Treisman, A. and Sato, T. (1990). Conjunction search revisited. *Journal of Experimental Psychology: Human Perception and Performance*, **16**, 459–478.

Van Loon, E.M., Hooge, I.T., and Van den Berg, A.V. (2002). The timing of sequences of saccades in visual search. *Proceedings of the Royal Society B: Biological Science*, **269**(1500), 1571–9.

Wade, N.J. and Brožek, J. (2001). *Purkinje's Vision: The Dawning of Neuroscience*. Mahwah NJ: Lawrence Erlbaum Associates.

Wardak, C., Olivier, E., and Duhamel, J.-R. (2002). Saccadic target selection deficits after lateral intraparietal area inactivation in monkeys. *Journal of Neuroscience*, **22**, 9877–9884.

Wardak, C., Olivier, E., and Duhamel, J.-R. (2004). A deficit in covert attention after parietal cortex inactivation in the monkey. *Neuron*, **42**, 501–508.

Wardak, C., Ibos, G., Duhamel, J.-R., and Olivier, E. (2006). Contribution of the monkey frontal eye field to covert visual attention. *Journal of Neuroscience*, **26**, 4228–4235.

White, B.J., Boehnke, S.E., Marino, R.A., Itti, L., and Munoz, D.P. (2009). Color-related signals in the primate superior colliculus. *Journal of Neuroscience* **29**, 12159–12166.

Wolfe, J.M. (2007). Guided search 4.0: Current progress with a model of visual search. In W. Gray (ed.) *Integrated Models of Cognitive Systems* (pp. 99–119). New York: Oxford University Press.

Wolfe, J.M. and Horowitz, T.S. (2004). What attributes guide the deployment of visual attention and how do they do it? *Nature Reviews Neuroscience*, **5**, 1–7.

Woodman, G.F. and Luck, S.J. (1999). Electrophysiological measurement of rapid shifts of attention during visual search. *Nature*, **400**, 867–869.

Woodman, G.F., Kang, M.S., Rossi, A.F., and Schall, J.D. (2007). Nonhuman primate event-related potentials indexing covert shifts of attention. *Proceedings of the National Academy of Sciences U S A*, **104**, 15111–15116.

Woodman, G.F., Kang, M.S., Thompson, K., and Schall, J.D. (2008). The effect of visual search efficiency on response preparation: neurophysiological evidence for discrete flow. *Psychological Science* **19**, 128–136.

Wurtz, R.H. and Mohler, C.W. (1976). Organization of monkey superior colliculus: Enhanced visual response of superficial layer cells. *Journal of Neurophysiology*, **39**, 745–765.

Zelinsky, G.J. and D.L. Sheinberg, (1997). Eye movements during parallel-serial search. *Journal of Experimental Psychology: Human Perception and Performance*, **23**, 244–262.

Zhou, H.H. and Thompson, K.G. (2009). Cognitively directed spatial selection in the frontal eye field in anticipation of visual stimuli to be discriminated. *Vision Research*, **49**(10), 1205–1215.

Zipser, K.V., Lamme, A.F., and Schiller, P.H. (1996). Contextual modulation in primary visual cortex, *Journal of Neuroscience*, **16**, 7376–7389.

CHAPTER 20

Testing animal models of human oculomotor control with neuroimaging

Clayton E. Curtis

Abstract

We know more about the primate oculomotor system than any other motor system. From numerous studies that have measured electrical activity in single neurons, applied electrical microstimulation, characterized the behavioural sequelae of lesions, and mapped the afferent and efferent connections in oculomotor areas, exquisite animal models of human oculomotor control have evolved. In this chapter, I review studies that have begun to test these animal models in humans using neuroimaging techniques. I hope to highlight the importance of this form of translational research by describing several successes involving our understanding of the roles of the frontal and parietal cortex in saccade control. Moreover, I will discuss several problematic methodological issues that have proven challenging to our efforts of translation.

The primate oculomotor network

The superior colliculus (SC) is a phylogenetically ancient midbrain structure whose neural activity is synonymous with the conversion of sensory signals to commands used to control gaze (Robinson and McClurkin, 1989; Sparks and Hartwich-Young, 1989; see also White and Munoz, Chapter 11, this volume). Indeed, there are both visual and motor topographic maps within the SC's laminated intermediate and superficial layers, respectively. The SC is thought to reflect a convergence point where a variety of afferent cortical and subcortical signals are weighed, averaged, and compared to produce saccade commands (Krauzlis et al., 2004; Moschovakis, 1996; Munoz and Fecteau, 2002). The SC is particularly well positioned anatomically in the primate brain to integrate such signals (May, 2006). Importantly, in addition to visual signals from striate cortex that target the SC, a number of other cortical areas are known to influence neural activity in the SC. The frontal cortex contains over four distinct areas whose monosynaptic connections with the SC are thought to influence gaze programming. David Ferrier first reported that electrical stimulation of the monkey dorsal frontal cortex evoked contraversive eye movements (Ferrier, 1886). A dorsolateral portion of the large region he described has become known as the frontal eye field (FEF). With microstimulation, the

FEF has been more precisely localized to the anterior bank of the arcuate sulcus in Brodmann's area 8 (Bruce et al., 1985, 2004; Bruce and Goldberg, 1985; Robinson and Fuchs, 1969; Schall, 1991), where saccades can be elicited with very low current thresholds (<50 μA). However, the boundaries of the functionally defined monkey FEF remain unclear and may extend into Brodmann's area 6 and Walker's area 45 (Petrides and Pandya, 2002; Tehovnik et al., 2000). The FEF contains an organized map of mostly contralateral visual space defined in eye-centred coordinates (Bruce et al., 1985; Sommer and Wurtz, 2000). A rough progression of cells that code for large to short amplitude saccades can be found as one moves along the long axis of the FEF from dorsomedial to dorsolateral arcuate sulcus. Indeed, the dorsal and ventral visual streams in extrastriate cortex send topographical projections to the dorsomedial and dorsolateral FEF, respectively, that are thought to be used for orienting to extrafoveal space and visually exploring objects near the fovea (Schall et al., 1995). Several types of FEF neurons have been described, including ones that respond prior to and during the generation of saccades (i.e. saccade or motor neurons), ones that pause during saccades but are active during fixation (i.e. fixation neurons), and ones that respond when a behaviourally relevant stimulus is in its receptive field (i.e. visual neurons) (Bruce et al., 2004; Schall, 2002). However, the most common FEF neuron responds to both visual stimulation and motor plans (i.e. visuomotor neurons). Several cortical areas adjacent to the FEF in the premotor and prefrontal cortex often show saccade related neural activity (e.g. Fujii et al., 1998; Funahashi et al., 1989a; Schlag and Schlag-Rey, 1987). These areas, although are not involved in generating saccade commands, are thought to contribute to gaze control. For example, neural activity in the lateral prefrontal cortex (PFC), in and around the principal sulcus, is related to cognitive factors that affect gaze (see also Johnston and Everling, Chapter 15, this volume). For example, neurons in PFC fire persistently during the maintenance of endogenous saccade plans (Funahashi et al., 1989a, 1991). The contributions of neurons in the supplementary eye field (SEF) and dorsal anterior cingulate cortex (dACC) are less well understood, but in general are thought to involve higher cognitive processes that influence gaze. For example, neurons in these dorsomedial frontal areas track factors upon which eye movements are conditional (Olson and Gettner, 2002; Roesch and Olson, 2003), encode the learning of arbitrary visuomotor transformations (Chen and Wise, 1995a, 1995b, 1996; Parton et al., 2007) and sequences of eye movements (Isoda and Tanji, 2002, 2003; Lu et al., 2002), and monitor performance or decision variables associated with eye movements (Ito et al., 2003; Schall et al., 2002; Stuphorn et al., 2000). In the parietal cortex, the lateral intraparietal (LIP) area is known to play an important role in oculomotor behaviour (Gottlieb et al., 1998; Mazzoni et al., 1996; see also Paré and Dorris, Chapter 14, this volume) and is sometimes referred to by a functional label, the 'parietal eye field.' In many respects, LIP mimics the functions that have been ascribed to the FEF because almost identical patterns of neural activity have been found in LIP and FEF neurons during a wide variety of oculomotor behaviours. One main difference is that saccades are not reliably evoked with microstimulation of LIP neurons until current levels are quite high (<120 μA) (Mushiake et al., 1999) and therefore are not defined with stimulation. Recent evidence suggests that LIP neurons represent not only the sensory evidence favouring an eye movement, but the expected values of potential eye movements (Coe et al., 2002; Curtis and Lee, 2010; Glimcher, 2003; Glimcher and Rustichini, 2004; Platt and Glimcher, 1999; Seo et al., 2009). In summary, a variety of cortical areas provide inputs to the SC allowing our gaze to be controlled by visual, motor, cognitive, and motivational factors.

Translating monkey electrophysiology to human neuroimaging

Findings from monkey electrophysiological studies of the oculomotor system have been used to develop rich models of oculomotion and cognition. These models have guided the hypotheses and interpretations of data in neuroimaging research. In return, neuroimaging research has the potential to translate these findings from monkey to human. The importance of this step should not be underestimated. Until researchers test candidate animal models of human oculomotor control in humans, the efforts and contributions to neuroscience that the animal researchers are making are undermined. Translation, however, is not easy for several reasons, most notably the differences in the methodologies available and inherent differences in the species themselves. In the rest of this section I describe both the successes researchers have made as well as the problems that challenge the field.

Localizing oculomotor areas

If we are to translate and test animal models in humans, as a starting point we must first confirm that we can reliably localize homologous regions across the species. As mentioned above, monkey areas FEF and LIP can be localized using electrical microstimulation and a characteristic pattern of neural firing during memory-guided saccade tasks, respectively. Recently, functional magnetic resonance imaging (fMRI) studies of monkeys performing saccade tasks provided strong evidence that FEF and LIP defined by fMRI corresponds very well to electrophysiological methods (Baker et al., 2006; Ford et al., 2009; Koyama et al., 2004) (see Fig. 20.1A, B). Saccade production evoked BOLD activation along the monkey arcuate sulcus in FEF and intraparietal sulcus in area LIP. This is important because it shows, at least within species, that localizing oculomotor structures using BOLD imaging agrees with electrophysiological methods.

What homologies might we expect in humans? Although the SC is the most studied node in the oculomotor network in non-human primates, it has not been well studied in humans using brain imaging because of its small size (i.e. not much bigger than a few standard size MRI voxels) and the artefacts arising from pulsating vasculature near the SC. Instead, the most intensive work attempting to find human homologues of oculomotor areas have focused on FEF and LIP.

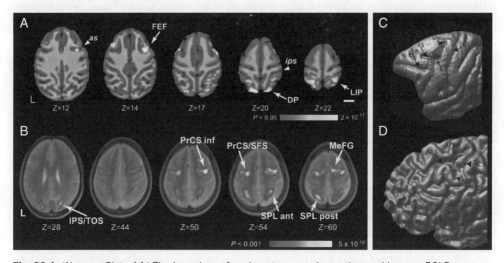

Fig. 20.1 (Also see Plate 14.) The homology of oculomotor areas in monkey and human. BOLD responses evoked by saccades in (A) monkeys and (B) humans using fMRI (Koyama et al., 2004) show promising homology. The monkey areas FEF and LIP appear to have putative homologies in human dorsal precentral and intraparietal sulci, respectively. Note that in humans, activation can be seen in the superior and inferior branches of the precentral sulcus making it difficult to localize the FEF in humans. Reprinted from *Neuron* **41**(5), M. Koyama, I. Hasegawa, T. Osada, Y. Adachi, K. Nakahara, and Y. Miyashita, Functional magnetic resonance imaging of macaque monkeys performing visually guided saccade tasks: comparison of cortical eye fields with humans, pp.795–807, © 2007 with permission from Elsevier. C) These two areas may correspond to the monkey dorsal premotor cortex (blue) and FEF (red). D) In humans, saccades evoke activation all along the precentral sulcus. However, the portion of the precentral sulcus that is dorsal to the junction of the superior frontal sulcus (blue) shows relatively greater hand movement related activity, while the portion ventral to the junction (red) shows relatively greater eye movement related activity (Amiez et al., 2006).

Intraoperative electrical stimulation of the human dorsal frontal cortex evokes contraversive eye movements (Blanke and Seeck, 2003; Blanke et al., 2000; Lobel et al., 2001; Penfield and Boldrey, 1937). Such invasive procedures, however, are not practical for most investigations into the functions of the FEF. Transcranial magnetic stimulation (TMS) does not evoke eye movements (Zangemeister et al., 1995) like electrical microstimulation does. Therefore, functional imaging will be key to localizing and studying the human oculomotor network. Early positron emission tomography (PET) studies localized the putative human homologue of the monkey FEF in the precentral sulcus (Paus, 1996; Sweeney et al., 1996). This was surprising given that it places the FEF in agranular cortex (Rosano et al., 2002, 2003), within Brodmann's area 6, and far caudal than would be predicted by the location of the monkey FEF. Subsequent fMRI studies that have imaged saccade production have supported the localization of the FEF in the dorsal precentral sulcus near its junction with the superior frontal sulcus (Brown et al., 2004; Connolly et al., 2000; Cornelissen et al., 2002; Curtis, 2006; DeSouza et al., 2003; Grosbras et al., 2001; Heide et al., 2001; Kimmig et al., 2001; Luna et al., 1998; Petit et al., 1997; Postle et al., 2000; Rosano et al., 2002).

Animal researchers have benefited tremendously from having a reliable method to define the FEF (<50 μa stimulation evokes saccade). With similar goals in mind, human fMRI researchers have used 'saccade localizers' to identify the same oculomotor areas across subjects and across labs. In particular, saccade localizers have been used to identify the putative human FEF. This typically involves scanning subjects as they make visually guided saccades interleaved with central fixation. Compared to central fixation, saccades do indeed evoke activation in the superior portion of the precentral sulcus, the putative human homologue of the monkey FEF (see Fig. 20.1B).

However, several other areas in the precentral, superior frontal, and inferior frontal sulci also activate during saccade production making it difficult to determine which of these are the homologues of monkey FEF. Moreover, defining the boundaries of the candidate FEF is an unreliable procedure because it depends on the statistical threshold used. Too low a threshold, even if statistically significant, and the entire precentral sulcus is often active. Too high a threshold, and the only statistically significant voxels that survive might be ones that are not in the superior precentral sulcus. The consequence is that researchers often use their judgement to decide which voxels to include in their FEF region-of-interest (ROI). Many studies label any activation in the precentral sulcus as FEF, regardless of its location. Additionally, other behaviours besides saccade production are invoked during performance of saccade localizer tasks, including visual, attentional, and motivational factors that may evoke spurious activations. For example, visual cortex is often activated by saccade localizer tasks. Despite their widespread use, the lesson here is that typical saccade localizers do not identify saccade-specific areas. Nonetheless, a small number of putative FEF candidates can readily be defined with functional imaging such that one can compare the physiological responses of different portions in and around the precentral sulcus during tasks that require different sensory, motor, and cognitive processes. Here is a great example from Michael Petrides' lab. Amiez et al. (2006) reported that both conditional eye and hand movements evoked BOLD responses in the superior precentral sulcus. However, greater responses to hand compared to eye were found in the segment of the precentral sulcus dorsal to the junction with the superior frontal sulcus. Conversely, greater responses to eye compared to hand were found in the segment of the superior precentral sulcus just ventral of the junction with the superior frontal sulcus. These findings appear to be homologous to the geometric relationship between the monkey FEF and dorsal premotor areas (Fig. 20.1C, D). These results make two important points. First, they suggest that researchers cannot assume that activation in the superior precentral sulcus is synonymous with FEF activation. Hand movements evoke activation strongly in the dorsal segment of the superior precentral sulcus and even in the ventral segment thought to be the FEF (Astafiev et al., 2003; Connolly et al., 2007; Levy et al., 2007). Second, these putative functional areas are yoked to an anatomical fiducial, the junction with the superior frontal sulcus, which is variable in shape and folding across individuals. Therefore, group studies that simply normalize the anatomy of subjects in volume space without constraining the registration to align the junction of the superior and precentral sulci across subjects could lead to misregistration and Type II error.

An exercise in testing our assumptions for translation

The ability to localize homologous areas between humans and monkeys through non-invasive imaging techniques has been a major breakthrough. Nonetheless, before researchers can confidently begin to test and translate models between the species, we must ask how do we translate between electrophysiological methods and neuroimaging methods. For example, because researchers have shown that neurons in the monkey FEF increase in spike rate prior to the execution of saccades, one might predict that BOLD activity should increase prior to saccades in human FEF. However, as has been much discussed in the last 10 years, the relationship between spiking and BOLD remains controversial (Logothetis, 2002; Nir et al., 2007). BOLD is an indirect measure of neural physiology. Local BOLD signal can be affected by the spiking of large pyramidal neurons, whose activity is largely thought to reflect the output of local computation, the spiking of small interneurons, whose activity is thought to reflect local computation, and a variety of metabolic processes in postsynaptic neurons, whose activity is thought to reflect incoming signals used in the local computations (Logothetis and Wandell, 2004). Several compelling lines of evidence suggest that BOLD is most strongly coupled with local field potentials (LFPs), which are strongly coupled with postsynaptic neural effects (Goense and Logothetis, 2008; Kayser et al., 2004; Kim and Ugurbil, 1997; Logothetis, 2002; Maier et al., 2008; Masamoto et al., 2008; Rauch et al., 2008a, 2008b). Frankly, this presents a problem for researchers trying to translate monkey electrophysiology studies that use spike rate as a dependent variable and human studies that use BOLD as a dependent variable. Fortunately, from a very practical standpoint much translational work can proceed even in the absence of complete parity in the methods. Spike rate and BOLD are significantly correlated (although not quite as strongly as with LFPs) (Logothetis et al., 2001), and spike rate and LFPs are highly correlated and these correlations will get stronger as one integrates over periods that match the timescale of BOLD (i.e. on the order of seconds). Therefore, electrophysiology data can be used by BOLD imaging studies to guide predictions.

Assuming, however, that BOLD is synonymous with spike rate is fallible and studies should build into their research checks on this assumption. Since this is one of the biggest challenges to human imaging researchers, I would like to illustrate how this can be done. First, let us assume we have identified the putative human FEF (see above). Second, let us take a set of findings from electrophysiological monkey studies that we believe should no doubt exist in the human homologue of the FEF. In this exercise, we will consider recordings from monkey FEF during memory-guided saccade tasks. Here is what we know. In FEF neurons, persistent activity (i.e. tonically increased spike rate): 1) is observed during the memory delay (Bruce and Goldberg, 1985; Funahashi et al., 1989a, 1993; Goldberg and Bruce, 1990; Lawrence et al., 2005; Segraves and Goldberg, 1987; Sommer and Wurtz, 2000, 2001; Takeda and Funahashi, 2002, 2004; Umeno and Goldberg, 2001), 2) is greater in neurons in the hemisphere contralateral to the memoranda (Bruce and Goldberg, 1985; Funahashi et al., 1993; Goldberg and Bruce, 1990; Lawrence et al., 2005; Sommer and Wurtz, 2000, 2001), 3) scales with the length of the memory delay (S. Funahashi et al., 1989b), and 4) correlates with performance accuracy (Funahashi et al., 1989b). BOLD changes should show a similar pattern if researchers intend to base their interpretations on monkey electrophysiological data. Indeed, BOLD signal in the putative human FEF changes in ways that would be predicted from the spike data from monkey FEF. Several studies from different laboratories have shown that BOLD signal in the FEF persists above pretrial baseline throughout the memory delay (Brown et al., 2004; Curtis, 2006; Curtis and D'Esposito, 2006; Curtis et al., 2004; Srimal and Curtis, 2008). Moreover, the persistent activity shows a contralateral bias, scales with the length of the delay, and correlates with performance accuracy (Fig. 20.2). The electrophysiological data in the monkey and the BOLD data in the human converge in this case and strongly suggest that the FEF play an important role in the maintenance of saccade goals. The activity appears to be mnemonic in nature because it persists until the memory-guided saccade is made and its level of activity correlates with the fidelity of the later memory-guided saccade. Its activity provides the bridge across time that links the visually cued location and contingent delayed response. The neural mechanism of spatial working memory may be persistent activity

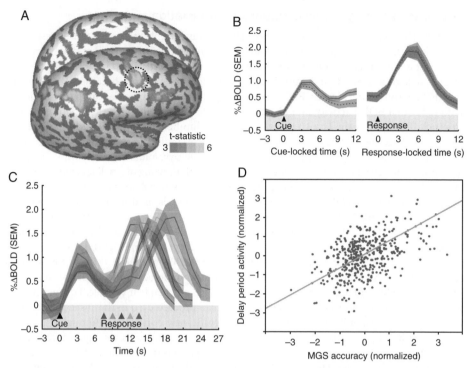

Fig. 20.2 (Also see Plate 15.) The functional homologies between monkey area FEF and putative human area FEF during a spatial memory-guided saccade task (MGS). A) BOLD activity during a memory delay period localizes to the precentral sulcus, the putative human FEF (circled). B) The time course of FEF BOLD activity persists above pretrial baseline during the delay period and is greater in the hemisphere contralateral (solid line) compared to ipsilateral (dashed line) to the location of the memoranda. C) FEF BOLD activity persists above baseline for the duration of the memory delay. Each coloured line is a different delay length, ranging from 7–13.5 s. (A–C). Reprinted from *NeuroImage*, **39**(1), R. Srimal and C.E. Curtis, Persistent neural activity during the maintenance of spatial position in working memory, Copyright (2008), with permission from Elsevier. D) The magnitude of the delay period activity predicts the later accuracy of the memory guided saccade; greater BOLD predicts greater accuracy. Reprinted from *Journal of Neuroscience*, **24**(16), 3944–52. Curtis, C. E., Rao, V. Y. & D'Esposito, M. (2004). Maintenance of spatial and motor codes during oculomotor delayed response tasks.

in neurons that code for contralateral space or contraversive eye movements. Moreover, these results strongly suggest that BOLD data from humans can be predicted from spiking data from monkeys at least under these simple controlled circumstances. Notice, however, there are a few striking differences between the monkey spike data and the human BOLD data that are worth noting. The timescales between the two are very different. Spikes can be recorded at a millisecond resolution, but haemodynamic responses are sluggish and take several seconds to resolve. Therefore, the experiments have to be designed very differently with more severe constraints on the BOLD designs where the resolution of subtrial events (e.g. cue, delay, response epochs) necessitate both temporal spacing and jittering of spacing (e.g. in the example, the cue and response was spaced apart from one another by long and variable length delays). One must always be wary that these modifications may change the nature of the task and behavioural data can be used to test this possibility. More importantly, notice that the contralateral BOLD responses are only slightly (i.e. ~10%) greater than the ipsilateral responses. From the spike data, we would predict that this difference would be much greater. The probable reason is that BOLD responses are driven by both spiking, that is highly contralateralized, and postsynaptic activity, that is not. Specifically, inhibitory postsynaptic potentials may cause increased BOLD responses in the ipsilateral FEF. Indeed, transcollosal homotopic projections from the contralateral to the ipsilateral FEF may be the source of the inhibitory postsynaptic potentials (Schlag et al., 1998). In any event, researchers should not assume, but instead measure the ways in which their BOLD data is similar to and different from existing monkey electrophysiology data. Testing this assumption is the first step in translational research.

Translation in action

In the exercise above, one can appreciate the successes made in translating and testing animal models of spatial working memory based upon electrophysiology studies in monkeys to the human using neuroimaging. Now let us turn to another example of successful translation, the inhibition of an unwanted saccade. A major goal of systems neuroscience is to understand the mechanisms by which we voluntarily control our actions. Control is necessary when the optimal response is uncertain or when prepotent responses must be inhibited. The well-characterized oculomotor system has been used to test several hypotheses about motor control. Two laboratory analogues of behavioural inhibition have been most successful at uncovering the neural mechanisms of saccade control, the antisaccade task and the stop-signal task.

Antisaccade and stop-signal tasks

In an antisaccade task (Hallett, 1978), subjects make a saccade (i.e. shift their gaze with a rapid ballistic eye movement) to the opposite hemifield, away from a visually-cued location. Correct performance requires that the subject first, inhibit the 'reflex-like' prepotent tendency to shift their gaze to the visual cue and second, generate a saccade to the mirror imaged location of the cue. Prosaccade trials, where gaze is simply shifted to the visual cue, are commonly performed in separate blocks or randomly intermixed with antisaccade trials. Compared to prosaccades, antisaccades are slower due to the extra time required to inhibit the automatic saccade plus the time to program the antisaccade. Errors on antisaccade trials are characterized by hypometric saccades generated towards the visual cue. These errors are thought to reflect inhibitory failures because a corrective antisaccade is almost always generated, indicating an awareness of the task demands.

Stop-signal or countermanding tasks (Logan, 1994), as they are called, require the voluntary control over the production of movements because an imperative stop signal is infrequently presented instructing the subject that the planned movements should be withheld. In a stop-signal task, subjects make a speeded response, for example, an eye movement, upon the presentation of a visual go cue. On rare trials, just after the presentation of the go cue, an imperative stop signal is presented instructing the subject to withhold the planned movement. Intuitively, as the stop signal is delayed, the motor plan has more time to evolve toward execution, and the probability that the subject will be able to inhibit the response decreases.

Both tasks require withholding a prepotent response, but they differ in terms of when in the perception-action cycle inhibition is thought to begin. During a stop-signal task, inhibition begins late, after the go cue has been presented and therefore during the planning of the motor response. During an antisaccade task, before a block or before a trial the subject must be instructed whether the trial is an antisaccade or prosaccade trial. Therefore, inhibition can begin early, as soon as the subject is cued that the trial is an antisaccade trial.

Background: electrophysiology of monkey FEF

To understand what we might expect from neuroimaging studies of antisaccade and stop-signal task performance, we will first briefly review what we know from monkey electrophysiological studies. Then, we will discuss how well these findings have translated to humans using functional imaging.

Electrophysiological studies of the monkey FEF have yielded promising clues to the neural mechanisms of saccade control (see also Johnston and Everling, Chapter 15, this volume). As reviewed in the chapter by Johnston and Everling, FEF neurons are traditionally thought to play a critical role in transforming visual information into saccade commands (Bruce et al., 2004). FEF *saccade-type* neurons respond just prior to the execution of a saccade into the neuron's response field. Electrical microstimulation of FEF saccade neurons evoke saccades with specific movement vectors. Moreover, the stochastic variability in saccade initiation is proportional to the time it takes the firing rate of these FEF neurons to reach a fixed threshold (Thompson et al., 1997). Therefore, FEF saccade neurons control the production of saccades (Schall, 2002). Another class of FEF neurons, *fixation-type*, are active when a monkey is actively fixating gaze on a stationary position. Microstimulation of FEF fixation neurons during the course of smooth pursuit or saccadic eye movements immediately halts oculomotion (Burman and Bruce, 1997). In summary, saccades are produced when activity in FEF saccade neurons increases and activity in FEF fixation neurons decreases (Everling and Munoz, 2000; Hanes and Schall, 1996; Munoz and Fecteau, 2002).

Antisaccade task

With these two different types of FEF neurons in mind, now let us consider the behaviour of FEF saccade and fixation neurons during prosaccade compared to antisaccade trials. Saccade neurons in the monkey FEF exhibit a greater firing rates prior to prosaccades compared to antisaccades (Everling and Munoz, 2000). Moreover, the difference in firing rate can be seen as early on well before the peripheral target even appears. Fixation neurons in the FEF exhibit a greater firing rate just prior to antisaccades compared to prosaccades, again hundreds of milliseconds before the appearance of the target. Therefore, on antisaccade trials when the animal anticipates that he will need to inhibit the prepotent reflex-like saccade, the firing rate of FEF saccade neurons decreases while the firing rate of fixation neurons increases. These changes are thought to bias the oculomotor system towards a less motile state where the onset of the target and its associated capture of attention is less likely to result in an unwanted saccade (Munoz and Everling, 2004). If activity in saccade neurons can be kept below a critical threshold just long enough for the voluntary antisaccade to be programmed and initiated, then the decision to make a correct antisaccade is likely to be achieved. Indeed, activity in FEF saccade neurons is greater on trials in which the animal failed to inhibit the saccade towards the target (Everling and Munoz, 2000).

Therefore, with these observations we can posit a simple neuronal mechanism that determines the ability to inhibit an unwanted saccade. At the time when the peripheral visual target stimulus appears, competition between FEF gaze-holding and gaze-shifting mechanisms determines whether a reflexive saccade is triggered or not. Moreover, the difference in firing rate between prosaccade and antisaccade trials, and the difference in firing rate between successful and failed antisaccades trials, can be seen several hundred milliseconds before the visually guided saccade must be inhibited. These competitive interactions may give rise to a psychological preparatory set that primes the oculomotor system towards a gaze holding or shifting state. Stochastic fluctuations in the firing rates of FEF neurons may destabilize the preparatory state leading to failures in the ability to inhibit the unwanted prosaccade.

Functional MRI studies have provided critical support in humans for the findings from monkey electrophysiology. First let us consider fMRI studies of antisaccades. Replicated many times now, the production of antisaccades compared to prosaccades causes *greater* BOLD activation in the human FEF (Brown et al., 2006, 2007; Cornelissen et al., 2002; Curtis and Connolly, 2008; Curtis and D'Esposito, 2003; Ettinger et al., 2005; Ford et al., 2005; Matsuda et al., 2004; McDowell and Clementz, 2001; O'Driscoll et al., 1995; Sweeney et al., 1996). This may seem counter to what one might predict since the monkey electrophysiology has shown that firing rates are *lower* in FEF prior to antisaccades compared to prosaccades (Everling and Munoz, 2000). However, fMRI does not have the spatial resolution to measure activity from saccade and fixation neurons independently. Therefore, the increase is presumably due to the co-activation of saccade and fixation neurons in the FEF just prior to and during saccade production. BOLD signal in FEF is thought to be higher during antisaccade trials compared to prosaccade trials because of the increased activity of fixation neurons. Additionally, the processes related to inverting the saccade vector to the visual cued location may also contribute to increased BOLD activity during antisaccade trials. Finally and in general, saccades that are endogenously guided (i.e. antisaccades and memory-guided saccades) evoke greater BOLD activation than exogenous or visually-guided saccades. For all of these reasons, it has been challenging for researchers to unambiguously identify the neural mechanisms underlying the BOLD signal changes during antisaccade tasks.

To address these ambiguities, researchers have turned to event-related fMRI designs that can estimate BOLD signal arising from preparation epochs separate from saccade generation epochs. Recall that inhibition related processes can be marshalled as soon as the antisaccade instruction is given. These processes are thought to prepare the oculomotor system for the forthcoming conflict between the automatic programming of a saccade towards the impending visual stimulus and the controlled programming of an antisaccade. The human FEF and supplementary eye field (SEF; located in the anterior bank of the paracentral sulcus) have both been shown to increase in activity more during a preparation interval following an antisaccade instruction compared to a prosaccade instruction (Brown et al., 2006, 2007; Cornelissen et al., 2002; Curtis and Connolly, 2008; Curtis and D'Esposito, 2003; Ford et al., 2005) (Fig. 20.3A). Importantly, the amount of SEF activity in the preparation interval prior to antisaccades predicts if the subject will later be successful at inhibiting the unwanted saccade to the prepotent visual target (Curtis and D'Esposito, 2003; Ford et al., 2005) (Fig. 20.3B). An identical pattern of results has been found using electrophysiological recordings from neurons in the monkey SEF (Schlag-Rey et al., 1997). Moreover, BOLD signal in the human SEF is greater in advance of antisaccades compared to prosaccades whether or not the location of the visual cue is known to the subject during the preparatory interval (Curtis and Connolly, 2008). Therefore, advance knowledge of the precise metrics of the forthcoming saccade does not abolish the need for inhibitory control. The putative roles of the FEF and SEF in the antisaccade task are different as evidenced by different patterns of BOLD activity. Activity in the FEF is consistent with neural changes tied to the competition between saccade and fixation neurons, the determinants of eventual behaviour. Activity in the SEF is consistent with a higher level role in oculomotor control. For instance, SEF neurons may reduce the excitability of the oculomotor system through its connections with saccade and fixation neurons in the FEF (Lu et al., 1994; Luppino et al., 1993; Parthasarathy et al., 1992; Schall et al., 1993; Shindo et al., 1995); more on this below).

Stop-signal task

The voluntary control of behaviour, of which withholding an action is a critical demonstration, can be exerted at any point along the series of processes that evolve over time from sensation to action. In the context of a stop-signal task, inhibition takes place far downstream in this evolution, after the movement has been planned. Inhibiting or cancelling a planned movement following an imperative stop signal can be modelled as a race between independent GO and STOP mechanisms (Hanes and Carpenter, 1999; Logan and Cowan, 1984). Which process first reaches a critical threshold, or finish line, determines whether the planned response is generated or not. By adjusting the time between the presentation of the stimulus that initiates the GO response processes and the presentation of the stop stimulus, an interval known as the stop signal delay, the probability that either one of the two possible responses will win the race can be adjusted (Logan, 1994). Cancelling is easier when the stop signal delay is short because one has more time to cancel the movement. Importantly, using the saccadic response time distribution for GO trials and the probability of successful saccade cancellation at different stop signal delays, one can estimate the time needed to cancel a planned saccade once the stop signal had been given; this time is referred to as the *stop signal reaction time* (SSRT).

The presaccadic growth of activity in FEF saccade neurons is correlated with saccade production while the growth of activity in FEF fixation neurons is correlated with saccade withholding during the performance of stop-signal tasks (Schall, 2001). FEF saccade neurons show a phasic burst of activity within 100 ms following the appearance of the visual target, while FEF fixation neurons

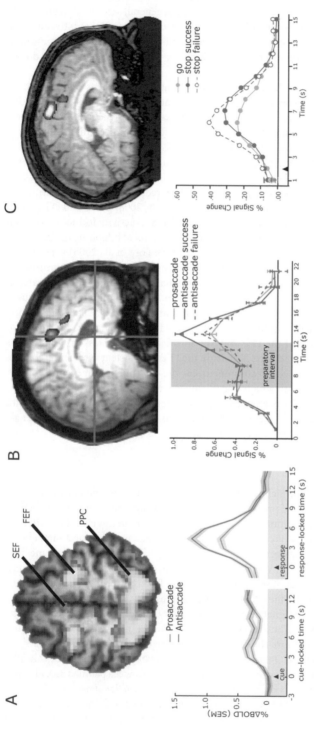

Fig. 20.3 (Also see Plate 16.) Functional imaging of saccade inhibition. A) Performance of antisaccade trials evokes greater BOLD activation than prosaccades in the FEF, SEF, and posterior parietal cortex (PPC). Top: significant antisaccade greater than prosaccade activation is overlaid on an axial slice through dorsal cortex. Bottom: BOLD time course from FEF during antisaccade and prosaccade trials. The task instruction (trial type) was given at the 'cue' period prompting the subject to prepare to make a prosaccade or antisaccade from a visual target presented at the 'response' period. Notice that BOLD signal increased to a greater extent for antisaccades compared to prosaccades shortly after the cue was given. Reprinted from *Journal of Neurophysiology*, **98**, Brown, MEG, Villis, T., and Everling, S., Frontoparietal activation with preparation for antisaccades. Copyright (2007) used with permission from The American Physiological Society. B) Saccade production activates the SEF (and anterior cingulate) as shown in the sagittal image (top). The time course of SEF BOLD activity ramps up during the preparatory period and is greater prior to correct than incorrect antisaccades, which are similar to prosaccades (bottom). Form C.E. Curtis and M. D'Esposito, Success and Failure Suppressing Reflexive Behavior, *Journal of Cognitive Neuroscience*, **15**(3) (April, 2003) (April), pp. 409–418. © 2003 by the Massachusetts Institute of Technology. Figure 3b. C) The SEF, depicted in the top sagittal image, show BOLD activation during the performance of an oculomotor stop-signal task. Time courses from the SEF show that activity is enhanced during stop trials when inhibition is successful and unsuccessful compared to go trials. From C.E. Curtis, M.W. Cole, V.Y. Rao, M. D'Esposito, Canceling planned action: an fMRI study of countermanding saccades, *Cerebral Cortex*, 2005, **15**, by permission of Oxford University Press.

activity declines rapidly (Schall and Hanes, 1998). These early changes in neuronal firing reflect the planning and preparation of the visually guided saccade. When no stop-signal is emitted (i.e. GO trials) the firing rate of saccade neurons continues to build until the critical threshold is reached and a saccade is finally generated. When a stop-signal is emitted (i.e. STOP trials) and the animal is successful at inhibiting the planned saccade, fixation neurons exhibit a burst of firing that coincides with a sharp decrease in the firing rate of saccade neurons. However, if these changes in firing invoked by the stop signal do not occur quickly enough, or to be more precise, do not occur within the SSRT, then the animal is not able to withhold the movement and a failure of inhibition occurs. Overall, the activity pattern of FEF saccade and fixation neurons corresponds very well with the hypothetical GO and STOP processes of the race model where the outcome of a race between saccade and fixation neurons determines whether or not a saccade is generated.

Functional imaging studies of oculomotor stop-signal task performance have been supportive of these animal models (Curtis et al., 2005; Leung and Cai, 2007). The successful cancellation of a planned saccade (i.e. STOP trial) causes greater human FEF activation than the generation of a saccade on no-stop signal, or GO, trials (Curtis et al., 2005; Leung and Cai, 2007) (Fig. 20.3B). Similar to the reasoning used to understand the increased activation during antisaccade compared to prosaccade trials, the increased activation likely reflects the coactivation of saccade and fixation neurons on STOP trials, which would evoke great BOLD signal than trials in which there were no stop signal. Above, it was suggested that the SEF plays a critical role in preparing the oculomotor system for conflict prior to antisaccades. Additionally, there must be a mechanism that allows animals to monitor their performance such that strategic changes can be implemented. Detecting the production of errors is necessary for one to make adaptive changes in future behaviour. Neurons in the monkey SEF show a pattern of activity during stop-signal tasks that suggest that they may play an important role in monitoring performance. Some SEF neurons show a burst of activity following errors on STOP trials and some show a burst of activity following successfully cancelled STOP trials (Stuphorn et al., 2000; Stuphorn and Schall, 2002). Note that the onset of the activity is after the SSRT so these signals are too late to be critically involved in the act of inhibition. Instead, they signal how successful or not the animal is performing the required task. From fMRI studies of humans, we know that BOLD activity in the human SEF is greater for both successful and unsuccessful STOP trials compared to GO trials (Curtis et al., 2005). This suggests that the human SEF contains the requisite signals for monitoring performance that could be used in feedback learning. Presumably, these signals cause changes in the oculomotor system by biasing the activity of saccade and fixation neurons on the next trial similar to the way in which it might bias activity when preparing to make an antisaccade.

As we can see from these studies, during oculomotor tasks that require inhibiting unwanted saccades, neurons in the FEF that code for mutually exclusive gaze shifts may compete for expression. Moreover, the SEF may provide control signals that can be used to optimize performance. These include increased activity when one anticipates and prepares for conflicting oculomotor responses and activity that signals both successes and failures inhibiting the unwanted responses.

Conclusions

In this review, I described both the challenges to and the successes in using fMRI to test models of oculomotor control. Imaging studies have provided key evidence in support of several models of saccade control that were developed with electrophysiological data recorded in monkey oculomotor areas. Testing these animal models of human cognition in humans is a necessary translational step whose importance cannot be underestimated.

References

Amiez, C., Kostopoulos, P., Champod, A.S., and Petrides, M. (2006). Local morphology predicts functional organization of the dorsal premotor region in the human brain. *Journal of Neuroscience,* **26**(10), 2724–2731.

Astafiev, S.V., Shulman, G.L., Stanley, C.M., Snyder, A.Z., Van Essen, D.C., and Corbetta, M. (2003). Functional organization of human intraparietal and frontal cortex for attending, looking, and pointing. *Journal of Neuroscience,* **23**(11), 4689–4699.

Baker, J.T., Patel, G.H., Corbetta, M., and Snyder, L.H. (2006). Distribution of activity across the monkey cerebral cortical surface, thalamus and midbrain during rapid, visually guided saccades. *Cereb Cortex,* **16**(4), 447–459.

Blanke, O. and Seeck, M. (2003). Direction of saccadic and smooth eye movements induced by electrical stimulation of the human frontal eye field: effect of orbital position. *Experimental Brain Research,* **150**(2), 174–183.

Blanke, O., Spinelli, L., Thut, G., Michel, C.M., Perrig, S., Landis, T., *et al.* (2000). Location of the human frontal eye field as defined by electrical cortical stimulation: anatomical, functional and electrophysiological characteristics. *Neuroreport,* **11**(9), 1907–1913.

Brown, M.R., Vilis, T., and Everling, S. (2007). Frontoparietal activation with preparation for antisaccades. *Journal of Neurophysiology,* **98**, 1751–176.

Brown, M.R., Goltz, H.C., Vilis, T., Ford, K.A., and Everling, S. (2006). Inhibition and generation of saccades: rapid event-related fMRI of prosaccades, antisaccades, and nogo trials. *Neuroimage,* **33**(2), 644–659.

Brown, M.R., DeSouza, J.F., Goltz, H.C., Ford, K., Menon, R.S., Goodale, M.A., *et al.* (2004). Comparison of memory- and visually guided saccades using event-related fMRI. *Journal of Neurophysiology,* **91**(2), 873–889.

Bruce, C.J. and Goldberg, M.E. (1985). Primate frontal eye fields. I. Single neurons discharging before saccades. *Journal of Neurophysiology,* **53**(3), 603–635.

Bruce, C.J., Goldberg, M.E., Bushnell, M.C., and Stanton, G.B. (1985). Primate frontal eye fields. II. Physiological and anatomical correlates of electrically evoked eye movements. *Journal of Neurophysiology,* **54**(3), 714–734.

Bruce, C.J., Friedman, H.R., Kraus, M.S., and Stanton, G.B. (2004). The primate frontal eye field. In L. M. Chalupa and J. S. Werner (eds.) *The Visual Neurosciences* (Vol. 1, pp. 1428–1448). Cambridge, MA: The MIT Press.

Burman, D.D. and Bruce, C.J. (1997). Suppression of task-related saccades by electrical stimulation in the primate's frontal eye field. *Journal of Neurophysiology,* **77**(5), 2252–2267.

Chen, L.L. and Wise, S.P. (1995a). Neuronal activity in the supplementary eye field during acquisition of conditional oculomotor associations. *Journal of Neurophysiology,* **73**(3), 1101–1121.

Chen, L.L. and Wise, S.P. (1995b). Supplementary eye field contrasted with the frontal eye field during acquisition of conditional oculomotor associations. *Journal of Neurophysiology,* **73**(3), 1122–1134.

Chen, L.L. and Wise, S.P. (1996). Evolution of directional preferences in the supplementary eye field during acquisition of conditional oculomotor associations. *Journal of Neuroscience,* **16**(9), 3067–3081.

Coe, B., Tomihara, K., Matsuzawa, M., and Hikosaka, O. (2002). Visual and anticipatory bias in three cortical eye fields of the monkey during an adaptive decision-making task. *Journal of Neuroscience,* **22**(12), 5081–5090.

Connolly, J.D., Goodale, M.A., Cant, J.S., and Munoz, D.P. (2007). Effector-specific fields for motor preparation in the human frontal cortex. *Neuroimage,* **34**(3), 1209–1219.

Connolly, J.D., Goodale, M.A., Desouza, J.F., Menon, R.S., and Vilis, T. (2000). A comparison of frontoparietal fMRI activation during anti-saccades and anti-pointing. *Journal of Neurophysiology,* **84**(3), 1645–1655.

Cornelissen, F.W., Kimmig, H., Schira, M., Rutschmann, R.M., Maguire, R.P., Broerse, A., *et al.* (2002). Event-related fMRI responses in the human frontal eye fields in a randomized pro- and antisaccade task. *Experimental Brain Research,* **145**(2), 270–274.

Curtis, C.E. (2006). Prefrontal and parietal contributions to spatial working memory. *Neuroscience,* **139**(1), 173–180.

Curtis, C.E., and Connolly, J. D. (2008). Saccade preparation signals in the human frontal and parietal cortices. *Journal of Neurophysiology,* **99**(1), 133–145.

Curtis, C.E. and D'Esposito, M. (2003). Success and failure suppressing reflexive behavior. *J Cogn Neurosci,* **15**(3), 409–418.

Curtis, C.E. and D'Esposito, M. (2006). Selection and maintenance of saccade goals in the human frontal eye fields. *Journal of Neurophysiology,* **95**(6), 3923–3927.

Curtis, C.E. and Lee, D. (2010). Beyond working memory: the role of persistent activity in decision making. *Trends in Cognitive Science,* **14**(5), 216–222.

Curtis, C.E., Rao, V.Y., and D'Esposito, M. (2004). Maintenance of spatial and motor codes during oculomotor delayed response tasks. *Journal of Neuroscience,* **24**(16), 3944–3952.

Curtis, C.E., Cole, M.W., Rao, V.Y., and D'Esposito, M. (2005) Canceling planned action: an FMRI study of countermanding saccades. *Cerebral Cortex,* **15**, 1281–1289.

DeSouza, J.F., Menon, R.S., and Everling, S. (2003). Preparatory set associated with pro-saccades and anti-saccades in humans investigated with event-related FMRI. *Journal of Neurophysiology,* **89**(2), 1016–1023.

Ettinger, U., Antonova, E., Crawford, T.J., Mitterschiffthaler, M.T., Goswani, S., Sharma, T., *et al.* (2005). Structural neural correlates of prosaccade and antisaccade eye movements in healthy humans. *Neuroimage,* **24**(2), 487–494.

Everling, S. and Munoz, D.P. (2000). Neuronal correlates for preparatory set associated with pro-saccades and anti-saccades in the primate frontal eye field. *Journal of Neuroscience,* **20**(1), 387–400.

Ferrier, D. (1886). *The Functions of the Brain* (2nd. edn.). London: Smith, Elder, and Co.

Ford, K.A., Goltz, H.C., Brown, M.R., and Everling, S. (2005). Neural processes associated with antisaccade task performance investigated with event-related FMRI. *Journal of Neurophysiology,* **94**(1), 429–440.

Ford, K.A., Gati, J.S., Menon, R.S., and Everling, S. (2009). BOLD fMRI activation for anti-saccades in nonhuman primates. *Neuroimage*, **45**(2), 470–476.

Fujii, N., Mushiake, H., and Tanji, J. (1998). An oculomotor representation area within the ventral premotor cortex. *Proceedings of the National Academy of Sciences U S A*, **95**(20), 12034–12037.

Funahashi, S., Bruce, C.J., and Goldman-Rakic, P.S. (1989a). Mnemonic coding of visual space in the monkey's dorsolateral prefrontal cortex. *Journal of Neurophysiology*, **61**(2), 331–349.

Funahashi, S., Bruce, C.J., and Goldman-Rakic, P.S. (1989b). Mnemonic coding of visual space in the monkey's dorsolateral prefrontal cortex. *Journal of Neurophysiology*, **61**, 331–349.

Funahashi, S., Bruce, C.J., and Goldman-Rakic, P.S. (1991). Neuronal activity related to saccadic eye movements in the monkey's dorsolateral prefrontal cortex. *Journal of Neurophysiology*, **65**(6), 1464–1483.

Funahashi, S., Bruce, C.J., and Goldman-Rakic, P.S. (1993). Dorsolateral prefrontal lesions and oculomotor delayed-response performance: evidence for mnemonic 'scotomas'. *Journal of Neuroscience*, **13**(4), 1479–1497.

Glimcher, P.W. (2003). The neurobiology of visual-saccadic decision making. *Annual Review of Neuroscience*, **26**, 133–179.

Glimcher, P.W. and Rustichini, A. (2004). Neuroeconomics: the consilience of brain and decision. *Science*, **306**(5695), 447–452.

Goense, J.B. and Logothetis, N.K. (2008). Neurophysiology of the BOLD fMRI signal in awake monkeys. *Current Biology*, **18**(9), 631–640.

Goldberg, M.E. and Bruce, C.J. (1990). Primate frontal eye fields. III. Maintenance of a spatially accurate saccade signal. *Journal of Neurophysiology*, **64**(2), 489–508.

Gottlieb, J.P., Kusunoki, M., and Goldberg, M.E. (1998). The representation of visual salience in monkey parietal cortex. *Nature*, **391**(6666), 481–484.

Grosbras, M.H., Leonards, U., Lobel, E., Poline, J.B., LeBihan, D., and Berthoz, A. (2001). Human cortical networks for new and familiar sequences of saccades. *Cerebral Cortex*, **11**(10), 936–945.

Hallett, P. (1978). Primary and secondary saccades to goals defined by instructions. *Vision Research*, **18**, 1279–1296.

Hanes, D.P. and Carpenter, R.H. (1999). Countermanding saccades in humans. *Vision Research*, **39**(16), 2777–2791.

Hanes, D.P. and Schall, J.D. (1996). Neural control of voluntary movement initiation. *Science*, **274**(5286), 427–430.

Heide, W., Binkofski, F., Seitz, R.J., Posse, S., Nitschke, M.F., Freund, H.J., *et al*. (2001). Activation of frontoparietal cortices during memorized triple-step sequences of saccadic eye movements: an fMRI study. *European Journal of Neuroscience*, **13**(6), 1177–1189.

Isoda, M. and Tanji, J. (2002). Cellular activity in the supplementary eye field during sequential performance of multiple saccades. *Journal of Neurophysiology*, **88**(6), 3541–3545.

Isoda, M. and Tanji, J. (2003). Contrasting neuronal activity in the supplementary and frontal eye fields during temporal organization of multiple saccades. *Journal of Neurophysiology*, **90**(5), 3054–3065.

Ito, S., Stuphorn, V., Brown, J.W., and Schall, J.D. (2003). Performance monitoring by the anterior cingulate cortex during saccade countermanding. *Science*, **302**(5642), 120–122.

Kayser, C., Kim, M., Ugurbil, K., Kim, D. S., and Konig, P. (2004). A comparison of hemodynamic and neural responses in cat visual cortex using complex stimuli. *Cerebral Cortex*, **14**(8), 881–891.

Kim, S.G. and Ugurbil, K. (1997). Comparison of blood oxygenation and cerebral blood flow effects in fMRI: estimation of relative oxygen consumption change. *Magnetic Resonance in Medicine*, **38**(1), 59–65.

Kimmig, H., Greenlee, M.W., Gondan, M., Schira, M., Kassubek, J., and Mergner, T. (2001). Relationship between saccadic eye movements and cortical activity as measured by fMRI: quantitative and qualitative aspects. *Experimental Brain Research*, **141**(2), 184–194.

Koyama, M., Hasegawa, I., Osada, T., Adachi, Y., Nakahara, K., and Miyashita, Y. (2004). Functional magnetic resonance imaging of macaque monkeys performing visually guided saccade tasks: comparison of cortical eye fields with humans. *Neuron*, **41**(5), 795–807.

Krauzlis, R.J., Liston, D., and Carello, C.D. (2004). Target selection and the superior colliculus: goals, choices and hypotheses. *Vision Research*, **44**(12), 1445–1451.

Lawrence, B.M., White, R.L., 3rd, and Snyder, L.H. (2005). Delay-period activity in visual, visuomovement, and movement neurons in the frontal eye field. *Journal of Neurophysiology*, **94**(2), 1498–1508.

Leung, H.C. and Cai, W. (2007). Common and differential ventrolateral prefrontal activity during inhibition of hand and eye movements. *Journal of Neuroscience*, **27**(37), 9893–9900.

Levy, I., Schluppeck, D., Heeger, D.J., and Glimcher, P.W. (2007). Specificity of human cortical areas for reaches and saccades. *Journal of Neuroscience*, **27**(17), 4687–4696.

Lobel, E., Kahane, P., Leonards, U., Grosbras, M., Lehericy, S., Le Bihan, D., *et al*. (2001). Localization of human frontal eye fields: anatomical and functional findings of functional magnetic resonance imaging and intracerebral electrical stimulation. *J Neurosurg*, **95**(5), 804–815.

Logan, G.D. (1994). On the ability to inhibit thought and action: a user's guide to the stop signal paradigm. In D. Dagenbach and T.H. Carr (eds.) *Inhibitory processes in attention, memory, and language*. San Diego, CA: Academic.

Logan, G.D. and Cowan, W.B. (1984). On the ability to inhibit thought and action—a theory of an act of control. *Psychological Review*, **91**(3), 295–327.

Logothetis, N.K. (2002). The neural basis of the blood-oxygen-level-dependent functional magnetic resonance imaging signal. *Philosophical Transactions of the Royal Society B: Biological Science*, **357**(1424), 1003–1037.

Logothetis, N.K. and Wandell, B.A. (2004). Interpreting the BOLD signal. *Annual Reviw in Physiology*, **66**, 735–769.

Logothetis, N.K., Pauls, J., Augath, M., Trinath, T., and Oeltermann, A. (2001). Neurophysiological investigation of the basis of the fMRI signal. *Nature*, **412**(6843), 150–157.

Lu, M.T., Preston, J.B., and Strick, P.L. (1994). Interconnections between the prefrontal cortex and the premotor areas in the frontal lobe. *Journal of Comparative Neurology*, **341**(3), 375–392.

Lu, X., Matsuzawa, M., and Hikosaka, O. (2002). A neural correlate of oculomotor sequences in supplementary eye field. *Neuron*, **34**(2), 317–325.

Luna, B., Thulborn, K.R., Strojwas, M.H., McCurtain, B.J., Berman, R.A., Genovese, C.R., *et al.* (1998). Dorsal cortical regions subserving visually guided saccades in humans: an fMRI study. *Cerebral Cortex*, **8**(1), 40–47.

Luppino, G., Matelli, M., Camarda, R., and Rizzolatti, G. (1993). Corticocortical connections of area F3 (SMA-proper) and area F6 (pre- SMA) in the macaque monkey. *Journal of Comparative Neurology*, **338**(1), 114–140.

Maier, A., Wilke, M., Aura, C., Zhu, C., Ye, F.Q., and Leopold, D.A. (2008). Divergence of fMRI and neural signals in V1 during perceptual suppression in the awake monkey. *Nature Neuroscience*, **11**(10), 1193–1200.

Masamoto, K., Vazquez, A., Wang, P., and Kim, S.G. (2008). Trial-by-trial relationship between neural activity, oxygen consumption, and blood flow responses. *Neuroimage*, **40**(2), 442–450.

Matsuda, T., Matsuura, M., Ohkubo, T., Ohkubo, H., Matsushima, E., Inoue, K., *et al.* (2004). Functional MRI mapping of brain activation during visually guided saccades and antisaccades: cortical and subcortical networks. *Psychiatry Research*, **131**(2), 147–155.

May, P.J. (2006). The mammalian superior colliculus: laminar structure and connections. *Prog Brain Research*, **151**, 321–378.

Mazzoni, P., Bracewell, R.M., Barash, S., and Andersen, R.A. (1996). Motor intention activity in the macaque's lateral intraparietal area. I. Dissociation of motor plan from sensory memory. *Journal of Neurophysiology*, **76**(3), 1439–1456.

McDowell, J.E. and Clementz, B.A. (2001). Behavioral and brain imaging studies of saccadic performance in schizophrenia. *Biological Psychology*, **57**(1–3), 5–22.

Moschovakis, A.K. (1996). The superior colliculus and eye movement control. *Curr Opin Neurobiol*, **6**(6), 811–816.

Munoz, D.P. and Everling, S. (2004). Look away: the anti-saccade task and the voluntary control of eye movement. *Nature Reviews Neuroscience*, **5**(3), 218–228.

Munoz, D.P. and Fecteau, J.H. (2002). Vying for dominance: dynamic interactions control visual fixation and saccadic initiation in the superior colliculus. *Progress in Brain Research*, **140**, 3–19.

Mushiake, H., Fujii, N., and Tanji, J. (1999). Microstimulation of the lateral wall of the intraparietal sulcus compared with the frontal eye field during oculomotor tasks. *Journal of Neurophysiology*, **81**(3), 1443–1448.

Nir, Y., Fisch, L., Mukamel, R., Gelbard-Sagiv, H., Arieli, A., Fried, I., *et al.* (2007). Coupling between neuronal firing rate, gamma LFP, and BOLD fMRI is related to interneuronal correlations. *Current Biology*, **17**(15), 1275–1285.

O'Driscoll, G.A., Alpert, N.M., Matthysse, S.W., Levy, D.L., Rauch, S.L., and Holzman, P.S. (1995). Functional neuroanatomy of antisaccade eye movements investigated with positron emission tomography. *Proceedings of the National Academy of Sciences U S A*, **92**(3), 925–929.

Olson, C.R. and Gettner, S.N. (2002). Neuronal activity related to rule and conflict in macaque supplementary eye field. *Physiology & Behavior*, **77**(4–5), 663–670.

Parthasarathy, H.B., Schall, J.D., and Graybiel, A.M. (1992). Distributed but convergent ordering of corticostriatal projections: analysis of the frontal eye field and the supplementary eye field in the macaque monkey. *Journal of Neuroscience*, **12**(11), 4468–4488.

Parton, A., Nachev, P., Hodgson, T.L., Mort, D., Thomas, D., Ordidge, R., *et al.* (2007). Role of the human supplementary eye field in the control of saccadic eye movements. *Neuropsychologia*, **45**(5), 997–1008.

Paus, T. (1996). Location and function of the human frontal eye-field: a selective review. *Neuropsychologia*, **34**(6), 475–483.

Penfield, W., and Boldrey, E. (1937). Somatic motor and sensory representation in the cerebral cortex of man as studied by electrical stimulation. *Brain*, **60**, 389–443.

Petit, L., Clark, V., Ingeholm, J., and Haxby, J. (1997). Dissociation of saccade-related and pursuit-related activation in human frontal eye fields as revealed by fMRI. *Journal of Neurophysiology*, **77**, 3386–3390.

Petrides, M. and Pandya, D.N. (2002). Comparative cytoarchitectonic analysis of the human and the macaque ventrolateral prefrontal cortex and corticocortical connection patterns in the monkey. *Europen Journal of Neuroscience*, **16**(2), 291–310.

Platt, M.L. and Glimcher, P.W. (1999). Neural correlates of decision variables in parietal cortex. *Nature*, **400**(6741), 233–238.

Postle, B.R., Berger, J.S., Taich, A.M., and D'Esposito, M. (2000). Activity in human frontal cortex associated with spatial working memory and saccadic behavior. *Journal of Cognitive Neuroscience*, **12**(Suppl 2), 2–14.

Rauch, A., Rainer, G., and Logothetis, N.K. (2008b). The effect of a serotonin-induced dissociation between spiking and perisynaptic activity on BOLD functional MRI. *Proceedings of the National Academy of Sciences U S A*, **105**(18), 6759–6764.

Rauch, A., Rainer, G., Augath, M., Oeltermann, A., and Logothetis, N.K. (2008a). Pharmacological MRI combined with electrophysiology in non-human primates: effects of lidocaine on primary visual cortex. *Neuroimage*, **40**(2), 590–600.

Robinson, D.A. and Fuchs, A.F. (1969). Eye movements evoked by stimulation of frontal eye fields. *Journal of Neurophysiology*, **32**(5), 637–648.

Robinson, D.L. and McClurkin, J.W. (1989). The visual superior colliculus and pulvinar. *Reviews of Oculomotor Research*, **3**, 337–360.

Roesch, M.R., and Olson, C.R. (2003). Impact of expected reward on neuronal activity in prefrontal cortex, frontal and supplementary eye fields and premotor cortex. *Journal of Neurophysiology*, **90**(3), 1766–1789.

Rosano, C., Sweeney, J.A., Melchitzky, D.S., and Lewis, D.A. (2003). The human precentral sulcus: chemoarchitecture of a region corresponding to the frontal eye fields. *Brain Research*, **972**(1–2), 16–30.

Rosano, C., Krisky, C.M., Welling, J.S., Eddy, W.F., Luna, B., Thulborn, K.R., *et al.* (2002). Pursuit and saccadic eye movement subregions in human frontal eye field: a high-resolution fMRI investigation. *Cerebral Cortex*, **12**(2), 107–115.

Schall, J.D. (1991). Neuronal activity related to visually guided saccades in the frontal eye fields of rhesus monkeys: comparison with supplementary eye fields. *Journal of Neurophysiology*, **66**(2), 559–579.

Schall, J.D. (2001). Neural basis of deciding, choosing and acting. *Nature Reviews Neuroscience*, **2**(1), 33–42.

Schall, J.D. (2002). The neural selection and control of saccades by the frontal eye field. *Philosophical Transactions of the Royal Society B: Biological Science*, **357**(1424), 1073–1082.

Schall, J.D. and Hanes, D.P. (1998). Neural mechanisms of selection and control of visually guided eye movements. *Neural Networks*, **11**(7–8), 1241–1251.

Schall, J.D., Morel, A., and Kaas, J.H. (1993). Topography of supplementary eye field afferents to frontal eye field in macaque: implications for mapping between saccade coordinate systems. *Visual Neuroscience*, **10**(2), 385–393.

Schall, J.D., Stuphorn, V., and Brown, J.W. (2002). Monitoring and control of action by the frontal lobes. *Neuron*, **36**(2), 309–322.

Schall, J.D., Morel, A., King, D.J., and Bullier, J. (1995). Topography of visual cortex connections with frontal eye field in macaque: convergence and segregation of processing streams. *Journal of Neuroscience*, **15**(6), 4464–4487.

Schlag, J. and Schlag-Rey, M. (1987). Evidence for a supplementary eye field. *Journal of Neurophysiology*, **57**(1), 179–200.

Schlag, J., Dassonville, P., and Schlag-Rey, M. (1998). Interaction of the two frontal eye fields before saccade onset. *Journal of Neurophysiology*, **79**(1), 64–72.

Schlag-Rey, M., Amador, N., Sanchez, H., and Schlag, J. (1997). Antisaccade performance predicted by neuronal activity in the supplementary eye field. *Nature*, **390**(6658), 398–401.

Segraves, M.A. and Goldberg, M.E. (1987). Functional properties of corticotectal neurons in the monkey's frontal eye field. *Journal of Neurophysiology*, **58**(6), 1387–1419.

Seo, H., Barraclough, D.J., and Lee, D. (2009). Lateral intraparietal cortex and reinforcement learning during a mixed-strategy game. *Journal of Neuroscience*, **29**(22), 7278–7289.

Shindo, K., Shima, K., and Tanji, J. (1995). Spatial distribution of thalamic projections to the supplementary motor area and the primary motor cortex: a retrograde multiple labeling study in the macaque monkey. *Journal of Comparative Neurology*, **357**(1), 98–116.

Sommer, M.A. and Wurtz, R.H. (2000). Composition and topographic organization of signals sent from the frontal eye field to the superior colliculus. *Journal of Neurophysiology*, **83**(4), 1979–2001.

Sommer, M.A. and Wurtz, R.H. (2001). Frontal eye field sends delay activity related to movement, memory, and vision to the superior colliculus. *Journal of Neurophysiology*, **85**(4), 1673–1685.

Sparks, D.L. and Hartwich-Young, R. (1989). The deep layers of the superior colliculus. *Review of Oculomotor Research*, **3**, 213–255.

Srimal, R. and Curtis, C.E. (2008). Persistent neural activity during the maintenance of spatial position in working memory. *Neuroimage*, **39**(1), 455–468.

Stuphorn, V. and Schall, J.D. (2002). Neuronal control and monitoring of initiation of movements. *Muscle & Nerve*, **26**(3), 326–339.

Stuphorn, V., Taylor, T.L., and Schall, J.D. (2000). Performance monitoring by the supplementary eye field. *Nature*, **408**(6814), 857–860.

Sweeney, J.A., Mintun, M.A., Kwee, S., Wiseman, M.B., Brown, D.L., Rosenberg, D.R., *et al.* (1996). Positron emission tomography study of voluntary saccadic eye movements and spatial working memory. *Journal of Neurophysiology*, **75**(1), 454–468.

Takeda, K. and Funahashi, S. (2002). Prefrontal task-related activity representing visual cue location or saccade direction in spatial working memory tasks. *Journal of Neurophysiology*, **87**(1), 567–588.

Takeda, K. and Funahashi, S. (2004). Population vector analysis of primate prefrontal activity during spatial working memory. *Cerebral Cortex*, **14**(12), 1328–1339.

Tehovnik, E.J., Sommer, M.A., Chou, I.H., Slocum, W.M., and Schiller, P.H. (2000). Eye fields in the frontal lobes of primates. *Brain Research. Brain Research Reviews*, **32**(2–3), 413–448.

Thompson, K.G., Bichot, N.P., and Schall, J.D. (1997). Dissociation of visual discrimination from saccade programming in macaque frontal eye field. *Journal of Neurophysiology*, **77**(2), 1046–1050.

Umeno, M.M. and Goldberg, M.E. (2001). Spatial processing in the monkey frontal eye field. II. Memory responses. *Journal of Neurophysiology*, **86**(5), 2344–2352.

Zangemeister, W.H., Canavan, A.G., and Hoemberg, V. (1995). Frontal and parietal transcranial magnetic stimulation (TMS) disturbs programming of saccadic eye movements. *Journal of the Neurological Sciences*, **133**(1–2), 42–52.

CHAPTER 21

Eye movements and transcranial magnetic stimulation

René M. Müri and Thomas Nyffeler

Abstract

Transcranial magnetic stimulation (TMS) is a technique which allows interference with cortical processing during planning, preparation, and execution of eye movements. The main application of TMS in eye movement research is to study the chronometry and the functional role of a given cortical oculomotor region. TMS is not able to elicit saccades directly, but the most consistent effect of single-pulse TMS is inhibitory on oculomotor function. This chapter gives an overview of published studies that tried to facilitate saccade triggering by TMS or to influence inhibition of saccades in the antisaccade task. Furthermore, studies that used TMS for spatial mapping of cortical oculomotor regions, spatial memory, and memory-guided saccades are presented. Finally, studies using TMS and double-step saccades and vergence are discussed.

Introduction

Transcranial magnetic stimulation (TMS) is based on the principle of electromagnetic induction (for a general review, see Hallett (2007)). According to Faraday's law, a changing electrical field produces a changing magnetic field that induces an electrical field in a nearby conducting material such as the brain. TMS is applied by a stimulation coil, which is held over the subject's head. The brief pulse of current flowing through the coil of wires generates a magnetic field with lines of flux passing perpendicularly to the plane of the coil. The magnetic field passes through the subject's scalp and skull with negligible attenuation (only decaying by the square of the distance). The voltage of the field itself may excite neurons, but more important are the induced currents in the brain. Neuronal elements are activated by two mechanisms. If the field is parallel to the neuronal element, then the field will be most effective where the intensity changes as a function of distance. If the field is not completely parallel, activation will occur at bends in the neural element (Hallett, 2007). Magnetic coils may have different shapes: round coils are relatively powerful; 'figure-of-eight' shaped coils are more focal, producing maximal current at the intersection of the two round components. Depending on the TMS machine, the magnetic field can reach up to about 2 Tesla and typically lasts for about 100 ms. In contrast to transcranial electrical stimulation of the brain, TMS application is almost without pain.

The technique of TMS was rapidly utilized in order to study the physiology of the motor cortex in humans, since single-pulse TMS applied over the motor cortex evokes motor potentials, and, when applied with suprathreshold intensity, elicits motor twitches. The exact underlying physiological mechanism of TMS interference is not completely understood. Most insight comes from stimulation of the hand area of the motor cortex. With stimulation strengths below the motor threshold TMS tends to act trans-synaptically, with higher stimulation strength the axon is directly stimulated. There are two main possibilities of TMS application: the online approach and the offline approach. In the online approach, TMS is applied during the performance of a saccade task, e.g. TMS may be applied during target presentation or during a memory delay, or just before saccade execution. Since the duration of a TMS pulse is in the range of several microseconds, the advantage of the online approach is to study the temporal organization and functional relevance of a cortical region. The offline approach is used in combination with repetitive TMS (rTMS). Some rTMS protocols have behavioural effects which last minutes or longer (Nyffeler et al., 2006) allowing time-consuming experiments. For instance, it is possible to analyse the neuronal oculomotor network when a cortical area is functionally inhibited over a longer time period (Hubl et al., 2008).

In summary, there are two major contributions of TMS to the understanding of ocular motor control: 1) the transient disruption of focal cortical activity to establish the causal role and the timing of the contribution of a given cortical region in ocular motor behaviour, and 2) the application of rTMS to study functional brain connectivity.

Studies trying to elicit saccades

The initial use of TMS in ocular motor research was delayed, since it was not possible to elicit eye movements by single-pulse TMS. Wessel and Kömpf (1991) tried to elicit eye movements by stimulating frontal, precentral, parietal, occipital, and temporal cortices. Even using intensities up to the maximal stimulator output, they were not able to elicit any eye movements during rest, during reflexive saccades, or during smooth pursuit.

Another study had similar negative results (Meyer et al., 1991). The authors stimulated the region of the frontal eye-field (FEF) on both hemispheres and did not elicit any eye movements. Clockwise or counterclockwise coil currents made no difference. With higher stimulator output eye blinks were observed in about 30% of the trials when the frontal region was stimulated. The blinks were associated with small vertical eye movements as part of the magnetically-induced blink reflex. The second region they investigated without success was the occipital cortex.

Müri and co-workers (Müri et al., 1991) applied TMS over the right FEF by means of a figure-of-eight coil. For the first time it could be shown that TMS is able to interfere with intentional saccade triggering. In the antisaccade task, a volitional saccade is performed to the side opposite of the target. They found that FEF stimulation using a focal coil significantly increased the latency of antisaccades after the visual target was presented. The vulnerable time window during which TMS had an effect on antisaccade latency was found to vary from subject to subject, lying between 60 and 100 ms. Interestingly, TMS did not increase the percentage of errors, i.e. the number of unwanted reflexive saccades towards the visual target, which may be an argument against an inhibitory role of the FEF on reflexive saccade control. Furthermore, TMS did not influence reflexive saccade latency or amplitude (see also Johnston and Everling, Chapter 15, this volume).

Elkington and colleagues (Elkington et al., 1992) stimulated over the posterior parietal cortex 80 ms after the appearance of the visual target. The authors observed an increase of divergence of the eyes, an increase in saccade latency, and a tendency to undershoot the visual target, which was more pronounced for contralateral targets. The general conclusion from these studies is that single-pulse TMS has an inhibitory effect on ocular motor control but is not able to directly elicit saccades.

Studies trying to facilitate saccade triggering

Other studies tried to facilitate saccade triggering. Theoretically, TMS may act in two different ways: a stimulation of structures that are involved in saccade triggering (in this case, TMS should also have

facilitatory effects) or stimulation of structures that are involved in the inhibition of saccade triggering (the inhibition of inhibitory function results in facilitation). Furthermore, it is important to
differentiate between specific facilitatory effects of TMS (e.g. shortening of saccade latencies by interfering with the cortical region) and the non-specific effect of shortening saccade latencies due to, for
example, increased arousal by intersensory facilitation (Nickerson, 1973). That intersensory facilitation may be relevant was shown in a recent study (Nagel et al., 2008). The researchers stimulated the
dorsolateral prefrontal cortex (DLPFC), the FEF, and the supplementary eye field (SEF) of the right
hemisphere and found increased saccade latency after stimulation. However, sham stimulation,
which provokes auditory and somatosensory stimulation without stimulating the cortex, provoked a
non-specific shortening of saccade latencies.

Müri and colleagues (Müri et al., 1999) have shown that facilitation of saccade triggering may also
be obtained by an inhibition of a region that is able to inhibit saccade triggering. Patients with lesions
of the DLPFC (Guitton et al., 1985; Pierrot-Deseilligny et al., 1991a) show an increased frequency of
express saccades, especially in the gap task. Müri and colleagues applied single-pulse TMS over the
right DLPFC in five subjects with two different time intervals during the gap paradigm: one stimulation was applied at 100 ms, i.e. half time of the gap, and the other stimulation at 200 ms, i.e. end of
the gap. TMS applied at the end of the gap induced in all subjects a significant increase of contralateral express saccades. Stimulation at half time of the gap had no significant influence on express
saccades. The control stimulation over the posterior parietal cortex (PPC) with the same time intervals had no significant effect on the percentage of express saccades. The authors interpreted the
results of DLPFC stimulation as a transient inhibition of the inhibitory function of the DLPFC
region, resulting consequently in a decreased inhibition of the superior colliculus (SC), which is
strongly connected with the prefrontal cortex (Johnston and Everling, 2006; Leichnetz et al., 1981;
see also White and Munoz, Chapter 11, this volume). Such a mechanism may then facilitate the triggering of express saccades. Furthermore, the described effect was only observed during stimulation
at the end of the gap, which is consistent with data from monkey experiments (Dorris and Munoz,
1995), indicating that the occurrence of express saccades is correlated with the activity of buildup
neurons of the SC at the end of the gap.

Further indications that TMS may also have facilitatory effects on ocular motor regions come
from rTMS and double-pulse TMS (dTMS) experiments. Li and colleagues (Li et al., 1997) used
short trains of rTMS over the premotor frontal cortex during double-step saccades (see also section
'Double-step saccades and saccade sequences'). rTMS was not capable of eliciting saccades, but
could, under certain circumstances, facilitate saccade triggering. They used the first saccade of the
double-step paradigm to trigger the stimulus train and found short-latency multistep saccades in
three out of nine subjects when rTMS was delivered over the premotor cortex. The intervals
between evoked saccades were proportional to the intervals between the TMS pulses delivered at
different frequencies. The authors concluded that TMS does not invariably have an inhibitory
effect on cortical structures involved in saccade control but is also capable of facilitating saccade
triggering.

The dTMS technique also seems to have the ability to trigger saccades. Double pulses may have the
advantage of intensifying the stimulus effect without losing the temporal resolution to the extent that
rTMS does. Furthermore, depending on the stimulus parameter used, contrasting effects are also
possible. Wipfli et al. (2001) stimulated the right FEF in 12 healthy subjects during memory-guided
saccades. They tested different interstimulus intervals (ISIs) of 35, 50, 65, or 80 ms. dTMS with identical strengths were applied, the first always simultaneously with the go-signal (i.e. the extinguishing
of the central fixation point), the second with the above mentioned variable ISIs. Only dTMS with an
ISI of 50 ms reduced memory-guided saccade latency of contralateral saccades significantly.
Stimulation over the occipital cortex had no significant effect indicating that the reduced saccade
latency was not due to intersensory facilitation. These results show that by using an appropriate ISI,
dTMS is able to facilitate saccade triggering. The authors speculated that dTMS may interfere with
the processing of presaccadic movement cells (Bruce and Goldberg, 1985) or may provoke an inhibition of suppression cells in the FEF (Burman and Bruce, 1997). It has been shown in monkeys

(Everling and Munoz, 2000) that saccade latency is closely correlated with the increasing activity of these cells (see also Johnston and Everling, Chapter 15, this volume).

Spatial mapping of cortical oculomotor regions

Several studies have focused on localization and spatial mapping of cortical regions involved in eye movement control. Thickbroom and colleagues (Thickbroom et al., 1996) mapped the FEF using single-pulse TMS during acoustically triggered saccades. The authors stimulated with a focal coil placed in relation to the vertex and the interaural line using 110–120% of the individual motor threshold. TMS was applied 50 ms before mean reaction time of saccades without stimulation. Typically, the greatest increase in saccade latency provoked by TMS was observed at stimulus sites on or 2 cm anterior to the interaural line, at a distance from the vertex of approximately 6 cm. By placing the coil away from this site, saccade latency decreased to values without stimulation. Furthermore, the study determined the anatomical spatial relationship of the cortical maps of the abductor pollicis brevis muscle and the orbicularis oculi muscle. All three maps lie close together, the centres of each map being separated only by about 5–10 mm. Ro et al. (1999) mapped the FEF by single-pulse TMS in two subjects in relation to the cortical hand area. They mapped the region anterior to the hand area during a saccade task. TMS was applied 50 ms before the onset of the go-signal. The researchers found a region where TMS produced an increase of contralateral saccade latencies. By combining the results with anatomical magnetic resonance imaging (MRI) of the subjects, the critical region was localized 2 cm anterior to the hand area on the middle frontal gyrus. In a follow-up study (Ro et al., 2002) the location of the FEF was defined in 10 subjects. They stimulated with 110% of the motor threshold and defined a location as FEF if TMS induced contralateral saccade latency increase. This functionally defined FEF across subjects was approximately 1.5 cm anterior to the motor hand area. In three subjects, they were not able to find an effect with this stimulation strength. Another study (Hubl et al., 2008) combined single-pulse TMS and functional MRI (fMRI). They were interested to evaluate the correlation between the localization of the FEF, defined by TMS and the centre of gravity activation of the FEF by fMRI in seven healthy subjects. The FEF was localized by TMS according the following procedure (Müri et al. 1991). First, the optimal site and individual resting motor threshold for each subject's related small hand muscles were determined by stimulating the right motor cortex. Second, the coil was moved on average 2 cm anterior to the motor hand area. Third, this location of the presumed FEF was marked with a vitamin-E capsule. fMRI was performed in a 3-T whole-body MRI system. The results are shown in Fig. 21.1.

Furthermore, they calculated the distance (i.e. the vector of the x and y Talaraich coordinates) between the location of the TMS application and the centre of gravity of the right FEF. This distance varied from 0.4–2.5 cm (mean 1.5 cm) showing that this simple localization method is valuable.

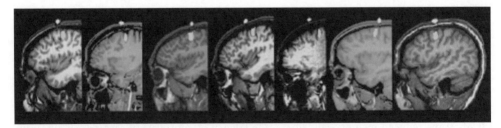

Fig. 21.1 (Also see Plate 17.) Individual localization of the FEF by TMS and fMRI. White mark: vitamin-E capsule Reprinted from *Neuroscience*, **151**(3), D. Hubl, T. Nyffeler, P. Wurtz, S. Chaves, T. Pflugshaupt, M. Lüthi, *et al.* Time course of blood oxygenation level–dependent signal response after theta burst transcranial magnetic stimulation of the frontal eye field, pp. 921–928. Copyright (2008), with permission from Elsevier.

Antisaccades and inhibition of saccades

The ability of the antisaccade task to suppress reflexive saccades towards the visual target critically depends on the integrity of a circumscribed region of the DLPFC, corresponding to Brodmann area 46 (Pierrot-Deseilligny et al., 2003; Ploner et al., 2005). This region projects through the anterior part of the internal capsule to the SC (Johnston and Everling, 2006; Leichnetz et al., 1981). Patients with lesions involving the DLPFC (Guitton et al., 1985; Pierrot-Deseilligny et al., 1991a, 2003; Ploner, et al., 2005; Walker et al., 1998), or the projections to the SC via the internal capsule (Gaymard et al., 2003) show an increased percentage of reflexive saccades towards the visual target, i.e. an increased percentage of antisaccade errors. Furthermore, it has been suggested that the FEF is responsible for the triggering of the correct antisaccades (Rivaud et al., 1994). Rivaud and colleagues found in patients with acute, small lesions restricted to the FEF that latencies of correct antisaccades were increased with no increase of the percentage of antisaccade errors.

Nyffeler et al. (2007a) studied the critical time interval at which the inhibition of the DLPFC influences the performance of antisaccades. They applied single-pulse TMS over the right DLPFC in 15 healthy subjects, either 100 ms before the onset of the visual target (i.e. −100 ms), at target onset (i.e. 0 ms), or 100 ms after target onset (i.e. +100 ms). TMS application 100 ms before target onset significantly increased the percentage of antisaccade errors to both directions, whereas stimulation at target onset, or 100 ms later had no significant effect. Latencies of correct antisaccades did not change in the three TMS conditions. The findings show that the critical time interval at which the DLPFC controls the suppression of a reflexive saccade in the antisaccade paradigm is before target onset. Furthermore, the results support the view that the triggering of correct antisaccades is not under direct control of the DLPFC. The results support electrophysiological findings in the monkey where the activity of DLPFC neurons projecting to the SC was recorded during pro- and antisaccades (Johnston and Everling, 2006). The authors showed that the activity in the pre-target period was higher for antisaccades than for prosaccades. Furthermore, the model of antisaccade control (Munoz and Everling, 2004) postulates that errors in the antisaccade paradigm are provoked due to an insufficient DLPFC-mediated inhibition of the saccade neurons in the SC prior to visual target onset: an insufficient inhibition of the saccade neurons of the SC provokes an increase of their pre-target activity which sums up with the visual response of the target provoking the triggering of a reflexive express saccade. Thus, whether a correct or an incorrect antisaccade is performed critically depends on the pre-target activity of SC saccade neurons, which is under the control of the DLPFC (Everling et al., 1998a; Johnston and Everling, 2006). Furthermore, Nyffeler and colleagues showed that the latencies of antisaccade errors after TMS are most in the range of express saccades, i.e. saccades with latencies as low as 100 ms (Fischer and Ramsperger, 1984).

Interestingly, TMS of the DLPFC resulted in a bilateral increase of antisaccade errors. In patients with lesions of the DLPFC the percentage of antisaccade errors may either be increased for both sides (Pierrot-Deseilligny et al., 2003; Walker et al., 1998) or the error rate may be higher when the target is presented in the contralesional hemifield (Gaymard et al., 2003; Ploner et al., 2005). Results from monkey studies suggest two different ways of DLPFC top-down inhibition: first, a connection to the rostral pole of the colliculus superior (Johnston and Everling, 2006) enhancing the activity of fixation neurons, and a second connection to the caudal SC (Goldman and Nauta, 1976; Leichnetz et al., 1981) which probably activates inhibitory interneurons. The fact that TMS induced interference with DLPFC top-down inhibition resulted in bilaterally increased percentage of errors suggest that the control by the first route might take place early, time-locked to the instruction period and thus before target onset.

In a further study Nyffeler and colleagues were interested in the control of visual vector inversion during the antisaccade paradigm (Nyffeler et al., 2008). To perform a correct amplitude of an antisaccade, the brain has to inverse the amplitude of the visual saccade amplitude from one hemifield to the other. Results from human and monkey studies suggest that the posterior parietal cortex plays a role in visual vector inversion (Everling et al., 1998b; Medendorp et al., 2005; Nyffeler et al., 2007b; Zhang and Barash, 2000, 2004). These studies suggested that the vector of the visual stimulus amplitude is perceived and inverted in the PPC contralateral to the visual stimulus and then transferred to the PPC ipsilateral to the stimulus for the motor program of the antisaccade. By applying single-pulse TMS over the right PPC at different time intervals during a delayed antisaccade task, Nyffeler and colleagues (Nyffeler et al., 2008) aimed to investigate the dynamics of vector inversion. They hypothesized that early TMS application should impair the process of vector inversion and late TMS application should impair the inverted visual vector signal that is stored to perform the antisaccades. This was exactly what they found (Fig. 21.2). TMS was applied over the right PPC 100, 217, 333, and 450 ms after target onset. For rightward antisaccades, i.e. the visual target was presented in the left screen-half, TMS had a significant effect on antisaccade gain 100 ms after presentation of the target, suggesting that the process of inversion of the visual vector was impaired. Gain of leftward antisaccades was significantly reduced when TMS was applied late, i.e. 333 ms or 450 ms after target presentation, suggesting that the stored inverted signal was impaired.

Thus, the double dissociation of the TMS effect on antisaccade gain suggests that the visual vector inversion takes place between 100 and 333 ms after target presentation. The results are in line with electrophysiological studies in monkeys. Zhang and Barash (2000, 2004) found cells in the lateral intraparietal area that were activated early when the visual stimulus matched the contralateral receptive field. Theses cells exhibited also a paradoxical activity later in the delay, when the visual target was presented ipsilaterally. In monkeys, the mean time delay between target onset and the onset of paradoxical activity which reflects the time to perceive, invert, and transfer the visual signal, seems to be in the order of 285 ms. See also Johnston and Everling, Chapter 15, and Curtis, Chapter 20, this volume.

Spatial memory and memory-guided saccades

Spatial memory allows memorization of the locations of diverse types of sensory stimuli occurring in the environment and to guide after their disappearance a correct motor response toward the remembered locations of these stimuli. Spatial memory has been studied for either short delays (of a few

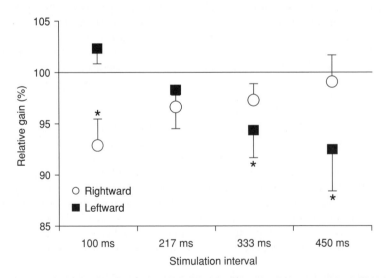

Fig. 21.2 Mean relative gain of antisaccades (SEM) for the four stimulation conditions. TMS had a significant effect on rightward antisaccade gain when applied 100 ms after target onset (p=0.002), but not for later conditions. For leftward antisaccades, a significant TMS effect was found at 333 ms (p=0.002) and 450 ms (p=0.002), but not for earlier conditions. Reprinted from *Progress in Brain Research*, **171**, T. Nyffeler, M. Hartmann, C.W. Hess, R.M. Müri. Copyright (2008), with permission from Elsevier.

seconds) or long delays (more than a few minutes). However, memory is continuously reorganizing (McGaugh, 2000; Squire and Kandel, 1999) and only few studies addressed intermediate delays (i.e. delay between a few seconds and a few minutes). Short-term spatial memory is the working memory used for current, ongoing behaviour. The memory delay of memory-guided saccades used in animal or human experiments usually vary from 1–6 s. Human lesions affecting the DPFC or the PPC result in an impairment of memory-guided saccades (Pierrot-Deseilligny et al., 1991b) and in the monkey sustained neuronal activity is found in both regions during the memory delay (Funahashi et al., 1989, 1990; Gnadt and Andersen, 1988). However, neither single-cell recordings nor lesion studies could determine the precise time interval at which the PPC and the DLPFC exert their influence during memory-guided saccades. Furthermore, functional imaging shows a large network of frontoparietal areas active during memory-guided saccades (O'Sullivan et al., 1995; Srimal and Curtis 2008; Sweeney et al., 1996). The memory-guided paradigm consists of three successive phases: 1) a phase of perception, during which the visual stimulus (a peripheral flashed target) is presented, 2) a memorization phase, and 3) an execution phase where the memory-guided saccade is performed. Therefore, single-pulse TMS is adequate to study the different stages of the paradigm. Müri et al. (1996) applied TMS over the PPC or the DLPFC on either hemisphere using a non-focal coil. TMS was delivered in relation to the appearance of the visual target whose location had to be memorized during a 2-s memory delay. TMS was applied 1) during the early phase (stimulation at 160, 260, and 360 ms after the presentation of the flashed target), 2) during a mid-memorization phase (TMS between 700 and 1500 ms), and 3) within the saccade latency before the execution of the saccade (i.e. 100 ms after the extinguishing of the central fixation point). Depending on the stimulated region, TMS affected the accuracy of the amplitude of contralateral memory-guided saccades at precise time intervals. Right PPC stimulation decreased the accuracy of contralateral saccades when applied in the early phase, i.e. 260 ms after the appearance of the visual target. The effect may be interpreted as interference of TMS with sensorimotor integration which is performed in the PPC (Andersen, 1997). TMS over the DLPFC had different effects: stimulation at 260 ms after the visual target presentation had no influence on the amplitude, but there was a significant decrease of the accuracy when TMS was applied during the mid-memorization period (700–1500 ms). Interestingly, there was no TMS effect after left-sided PPC stimulation at the same time interval (Müri et al., 2000), indicating a hemispheric asymmetry of the PPC for eye movement control. Such a hemispheric asymmetry of memory-guided saccade deficits was also found in patients with PPC lesions (Pierrot-Deseilligny et al., 1991b). No hemispheric asymmetry was found for DLPFC stimulation. Left-sided DLPFC stimulation during the mid-memorization delay also reduced accuracy of memory-guided saccades. Further studies (Nyffeler et al., 2002, 2004) examined the effect of TMS over the DLPFC during delays of 3 or 30 s. In the first study (Nyffeler et al., 2002) they used dTMS with an interstimulus interval of 100 ms and a stimulation strength of 120–140% of the resting motor threshold. In the first study, early stimulation, i.e. 1 s after presentation of the flashed target, significantly decreased the accuracy of the amplitude of contralateral memory-guided saccades compared to the control experiment without stimulation. However, TMS applied late, i.e. 27 s after the presentation of the flashed target, over the DLPFC had no significant effect on the accuracy of the saccade amplitude. A second important finding was that the effect of early stimulation in the long-delay paradigm was smaller than in the short-delay paradigm. The results indicate a functional dominance of DLPFC during the early memorization period and a serial processing of memory information is suggested, since DLPFC stimulation disturbed the saccades irrespective of the duration of the preceding delay. However, there is also a strong evidence for an additional parallel information processing component since the degrading effect of TMS on the memory-guided saccades was significantly greater in the short delay. The working memory might have access to other more stable representations of saccade parameters. This view is also supported by a recently published study in normal subjects (Ploner et al., 1998). They found that the time-course of saccade amplitude errors reverse significantly beyond memorization delays of about 20 s, and postulated parallel generated mental representations of spatial memory-guided behaviour. Such parallel information processing might be directly conveyed by parietotemporal anatomical connections, which in fact exist (Ding et al., 2000; Seltzer and Pandya, 1984; Seltzer and van Hoesen, 1979). On the other hand, both DLPFC are connected by callosal fibres (Goldman-Rakic and Schwartz, 1982; Schwartz and Goldman-Rakic, 1982). Therefore, the contralateral DLPFC could also contribute to the information transfer. In the second study (Nyffeler et al., 2004), single-pulse TMS was applied simultaneously over the left and right DLPFC to exclude memory information transfer by the contralateral DLPFC. They found that simultaneous stimulation early (i.e. after 1 s) resulted in a significantly greater degradation of memory-guided saccade amplitude in short- than in long-memory delay saccades. Thus, an additional information transfer to the MTL, probably from the PPC, has to be assumed, indicating a parallel processing component for long memorization periods.

Double-step saccades and saccade sequences

To have a constant visual world during exploration of the visual world by saccades, the brain has to update visual space across saccades, and visual information about the retinal position of objects has to be combined with extraretinal information about the actual eye position. The neural mechanisms underlying the craniotopic updating are not completely understood, and many cortical regions participate in the control (Andersen, 1997; Duhamel et al., 1992; Heide et al., 1995; Schall et al., 1993; Sommer and Tehovnik, 1999; Rivaud et al. 1994; Tobler and Müri, 2002). The role of extraretinal information processing can be studied by the double-step saccade paradigm where two visual targets are successively presented within the latency of the first saccade. The brain calculates the amplitude of both saccades from the retinal positions of the visual targets. To perform a correct amplitude of the second saccade, the intrinsic variability of the first retinotopic saccade amplitude requires extraretinal information about the actual position after completion of the first saccade. If the brain calculates the amplitude of the second saccade in craniotopic coordinates, it will be able to compensate for any variability of the metrics of the first saccade. In this case, a linear regression for the relationship between gain of the first and second saccade will result in a positive slope. If the central nervous system calculates the amplitude of the second saccade in retinotopic coordinates, the slope of the linear regression should be near zero. A single-pulse study (Van Donkelaar and Müri, 2002) examined the role of the PPC in the control of double-step saccades. They stimulated the PPC just after the first saccade (i.e. at 0 ms), 100 ms after, or 150 ms after the first saccade, i.e. before the second saccade. Craniotopic updating became no longer possible when TMS was applied just before the second contralateral saccade, i.e. stimulation 150 ms after the first saccade. TMS provoked a slope near to retinotopic calculation.

Another study (Tobler and Müri, 2002) examined the influence of FEF and SEF stimulation on the performance of double-step saccades. They stimulated the right FEF and the region of the SEF before executing the first saccade. Right FEF stimulation significantly affected the amplitude of the contralateral second saccade as compared to no stimulation. The effect was due to an interference with retinotopic but not craniotopic amplitude calculation. There was no influence on the first contralateral saccade. Stimulation of the SEF interfered with saccade ordering by increasing the errors in the sequence of the double-step saccades. They concluded that the FEF may be important for target memorization and that the SEF may be important for coding ordering information for sequential saccades, even for a simple order such as the double-step saccade paradigm. From studies in humans with focal lesions of the SEF (Gaymard et al., 1990, 1993), it is known that such patients have difficulties to perform saccade sequences in the correct order. Two studies (Müri et al., 1994, 1995) examined the effect of TMS application over the region of the supplementary motor area (SMA) during a memorized sequence of saccades task. The paradigm had four subsequent phases: 1) presentation phase of the visual targets, during which the subject had to learn the chronological order of the saccade sequence; 2) memorization phase to hold the information about the order online in the brain; 3) preparation phase of the motor programmes; and finally 4) the execution phase of the saccade sequence.

In the first study (Müri et al., 1990), TMS was applied by a non-focal coil over the SMA region including the SEF and pre-SEF at different times during the preparation phase of the saccade sequence, i.e. around the go-signal, which corresponded to the extinguishing of the central fixation point. With TMS being moved closer to the go-signal, the number of errors in order increased and TMS applied 80 ms before or 60 ms after the go-signal produced a significant increase of errors in the sequences of saccades. In the control stimulation over the occipital cortex there was no influence on the number of erroneous sequences. The increase of errors around the go-signal suggests that the movement preparation and possibly also the initiation of the sequence are controlled by the SMA region. Single cell recordings in the SEF and the SMA (Schall, 1991; Schlag and Schlag-Rey, 1987; Mushiake et al., 1991) revealed that more than 50% of theses neurons may be active during the pre-movement phase of internally guided movements, and sequence-specific neurons of the SMA are activated before a specific, learned sequence (Mushiake et al., 1991). Such neurons cease their activity before movement onset, which may explain why TMS over the SEF close to the execution of the sequence is no longer able to influence sequence performance. Furthermore, TMS increased the percentage of errors only if applied during the presentation of the visual targets, i.e. during the learning phase of the chronological order (Müri et al., 1995). During the memorization delay or the execution of the saccade sequence TMS did not increase the percentage of errors of memorized saccade sequences. In conclusion, the studies suggest that the SEF region, including the pre-SEF, is important during the learning phase of the chronological order of saccade sequences. In line with this interpretation are two fMRI studies (Grosbras et al., 2001; Heide et al., 2001) which have shown that the pre-SEF may be specifically involved in learning of saccade sequences.

Vergence

The cortical substrate of the control of eye vergence movements is not well known in humans. Results from monkey studies (Gnadt and Mays, 1995) suggest that stimulation of widely distributed cortical regions such as frontal, parietal, and occipital areas elicit vergence components of eye movements. Furthermore, neurons in the lateral intraparietal (LIP) are also sensitive for visual disparity and depth (Gnadt and Mays, 1995).

There are only a few studies investigating vergence eye movements by TMS. Kapoula et al. (2001) stimulated the right PPC during reflexive saccades or during vergence movements in a gap paradigm. TMS was applied 80 ms after the appearance of the visual target. Stimulation significantly increased latencies of saccade and vergence movements in both directions. The similarity of the observed TMS effect on both saccade and vergence movements support the idea of a common circuitry controlling both types of eye movements in the PPC. In a follow-up study, right prefrontal stimulation at the time of target onset in a gap task, a pure vergence task, and a combined saccade vergence task were performed (Coubard et al., 2003). The main finding was that TMS at that time interval significantly reduced latencies for contralateral pure saccades, i.e. provoked express saccades. The effect was less pronounced for combined saccade and vergence movements, and there was no influence of TMS on latencies of pure vergence movements, suggesting that the inhibitory role of the prefrontal cortex is saccade-specific.

References

Andersen, R.A. (1997). Multimodal integration for the representation of space in the posterior parietal cortex. *Proceedings of the Royal Society B: Biological Sciences*, **352**, 1421–1428.

Bruce, C.J., and Goldberg, M. (1985). Primate frontal eye fields: I. Single neurons discharge before saccades. *Journal of Neurophysiology*, **53**, 603–635.

Burman, D.D. and Bruce, C.J. (1997). Suppression of task-related saccades by electrical stimulation in the primate's frontal eye field. *Journal of Neurophysiology*, **77**, 2252–2267.

Coubard, O., Kapoula, Z., Müri, R.M., and Rivaud-Pechoux, S. (2003). Effects of TMS over the right prefrontal cortex on latency of saccades and convergence. *Investigative Ophthalmology and Visual Sciences*, **44**, 600–609.

Ding, S.L., Van Hoesen, G., and Rockland, K.S. (2000). Inferior parietal lobule projections to the presubiculum and neighboring ventromedial temporal cortical areas. *Journal of Comparative Neurology*, **425**, 510–530.

Dorris, M.C. and Munoz, D.P. (1995). A neural correlate for the gap effect on saccadic reaction times in monkey. *Journal of Neurophysiology*, **73**, 2558–2562.

Duhamel, J.R., Goldberg, M.E., Fitzgibbon, E.J., Sigiru, A., and Grafman, J. (1992). Saccadic dysmetria in a patient with a right frontoparietal lesion. The importance of corollary discharge for accurate spatial behaviour. *Brain*, **115**, 1387–1402.

Elkington, P., Kerr, G., and Stein, J. (1992). The effect of electromagnetic stimulation of the posterior parietal cortex on eye movements. *Eye*, **6**, 510–514.

Everling, S., Spantekow, A., Krappmann, P., and Flohr, H. (1998). Event-related potentials associated with correct and incorrect responses in a cued antisaccade task. *Experimental Brain Research*, **118**, 27–34.

Everling, S., Dorris, M.C., and Munoz, D.P. (1998). Reflex suppression in the anti-saccade task is dependent on prestimulus neural processes. *Journal of Neurophysiology*, **80**, 1584–1589.

Everling, S. and Munoz, D.P. (2000). Neuronal correlates for preparatory set associated with pro-saccades and antisaccades in the primate frontal eye field. *Journal of Neuroscience*, **20**, 387–400.

Fischer, B. and Ramsperger, E. (1984). Human express saccades: extremely short reaction times of goal directed eye movements. *Experimental Brain Research*, **57**, 191–195.

Funahashi, S., Bruce, C.J., and Goldman-Rakic, P.S. (1989). Mnemonic coding of visual space in the monkey's dorsolateral prefrontal cortex. *Journal of Neurophysiology*, **61**, 331–349.

Funahashi, S., Bruce, C.J., and Goldman-Rakic, P.S. (1990). Visuospatial coding in primate prefrontal neurons revealed by oculomotor paradigms. *Journal of Neurophysiology*, **63**, 814–831.

Gagnon, D., Paus, T., Grosbras, M.-H., Pike, B., and O'Driscoll, G.A. (2006). Transcranial magnetic stimulation of frontal oculomotor regions during smooth pursuit. *Journal of Neuroscience*, **26**, 458–466.

Gaymard, B., Pierrot-Deseilligny, C., and Rivaud, S. (1990). Impairment of sequences of memory-guided saccades after supplementary motor area lesions. *Annals of Neurology*, **28**, 622–626.

Gaymard, B., Rivaud, S., and Pierrot-Deseilligny, C. (1993). Role of the left and right supplementary motor areas in memory-guided saccade sequences. *Annals of Neurology*, **34**, 404–406.

Gaymard, B., Francois, C., Ploner, C.J., Condy, C., and Rivaud-Pechoux, S. (2003). A direct prefrontotectal tract against distractability in the human brain. *Annals of Neurology*, **53**, 542–545.

Gnadt, J.W. and Andersen, R.A. (1988). Memory related motor planning activity in posterior parietal cortex of macaque. *Experimental Brain Research*, **70**, 216–220.

Gnadt, J.W. and Mays, L.E. (1995). Neurons in monkey parietal area LIP are tuned for eye-movement parameters in three-dimensional space. *Journal of Neurophysiology*, **73**, 280–297.

Goldman, P.S. and Nauta, W.J.H. (1976). Autoradiographic demonstration of a projection from prefrontal association cortex to the superior colliculus in the rhesus monkey. *Brain Research*, **116**, 145–149.

Goldman-Rakic, P.S. and Schwartz, M.L. (1982). Interdigitation of contralateral and ipsilateral columnar projections to frontal association cortex in primates. *Science*, **216**, 755–757.

Grosbras, M.H., Leonards, U., Lobel, E., Poline, J.B., LeBihan, D., and Berthoz, A. (2001) Human cortical networks for new and familiar sequences of saccades. *Cerebral Cortex*, **11**, 936–945.

Guitton, D., Buchtel, H.A., and Douglas, R.M. (1985). Frontal lobe lesions in man cause difficulties in suppressing reflexive glances and in generating goal-directed saccades. *Experimental Brain Research*, **58**, 455–472.

Hallett, M. (2007). Transcranial magnetic stimulation: a primer. *Neuron*, **55**, 187–199.

Hashimoto, M. and Ohtsuka, K. (1995). Transcranial magnetic stimulation over the posterior cerebellum during visually guided saccades in man. *Brain*, **118**, 1185–1193.

Heide, W., Blankenburg, M., Zimmermann, E., and Kömpf, D. (1995). Cortical control of double step saccades: implications for spatial orientation. *Annals of Neurology*, **38**, 739–748.

Heide, W., Binkofski, F., Seitz, R.J., Posse, S., Nitschke, M.F., Freund, H.J., *et al.* (2001). Activation of frontoparietal cortices during memorized triple-step sequences of saccadic eye movements: an fMRI study. *European Journal of Neuroscience*, **13**, 1177–1189.

Hubl, D., Nyffeler, T., Wurtz, P., Chaves, S., Pflugshaupt, T., Lüthi, M., *et al.* (2008). Time course of blood oxygenation level-dependent signal response after theta burst transcranial magnetic stimulation of the frontal eye field. *Neuroscience*, **151**, 921–928.

Johnston, K. and Everling, S. (2006). Monkey dorsolateral prefrontal cortex sends task-selective signals directly to the superior colliculus. *Journal of Neuroscience*, **26**, 12471–12478.

Kapoula, Z., Isolato, E., Müri, R.M., Bucci, M.P., and Rivaud-Péchoux, S. (2001). Effects of transcranial magnetic stimulation of the posterior parietal cortex on saccades and vergence. *NeuroReport*, **18**, 4041–4046.

Leichnetz, G.R., Spencer, R.F., Hardy, S.G.P., and Astrue, J. (1981). The prefrontal corticotectal projection in the monkey: an anterograde and retrograde horseradish peroxidase study. *Neuroscience*, **6**, 1032–1041.

Li, J., Olson, J., Anand, S., and Hotson, J. (1997). Rapid-rate transcranial magnetic stimulation of human frontal cortex can evoke saccades under facilitating conditions. *Electroencephalography and Clinical Neurophysiology*, **105**, 246–254.

McGaugh, J.L. (2000). Memory—a century of consolidation. *Science*, **287**, 248–251.

Medendorp, W.P., Goltz, H.C., and Vilis, T. (2005). Remapping the remembered target location for anti-saccades in human posterior parietal cortex. *Journal of Neurophysiology*, **94**, 734–740.

Meyer, B., Diehl, R., Steinmetz, H., Britton, C., and Benecke, R. (1991). Magnetic stimuli applied over motor and visual cortex. Influence of coil position and field polarity on motor responses, phosphenes, and eye movements. *Electroencephalography and Clinical Neurophysiology*, Suppl **43**, 121–134.

Munoz, D.P. and Everling, S. (2004). Look away: the antisaccade task and the voluntary control of eye movement. *Nature Review Neuroscience,* **5**, 218–228.

Müri, R.M., Hess, C.W., and Meienberg, O. (1991). Transcranial stimulation of the human frontal eye field by magnetic pulses. *Experimental Brain Research,* **86**, 219–223.

Müri, R.M., Rösler, K.M., and Hess, C.W. (1994). Influence of transcranial magnetic stimulation on the execution of memorized sequences of saccades in man. *Experimental Brain Research,* **101**, 521–524.

Müri, R.M., Rivaud, S., Vermersch, A.I., Léger, J.M., and Pierrot-Deseilligny, C. (1995). Effects of transcranial magnetic stimulation over the region of the supplementary motor area during sequences of memory-guided saccades. *Experimental Brain Research,* **104**, 163–166.

Müri, R.M., Vermersch, A.I., Rivaud, S., Gaymard, B., Pierrot-Deseilligny, C. (1996). Effects of single-pulse transcranial magnetic stimulation over the prefrontal and posterior parietal cortices during memory-guided saccades in humans. *Journal of Neurophysiology,* **76**, 2102–2106.

Müri, R., Rivaud, S., Gaymard, B., Ploner, C., Vermersch, A.I., Hess, C.W. *et al.* (1999). Role of the prefrontal cortex in the control of express saccades. A transcranial magnetic stimulation study. *Neuropsychologia,* **37**, 199–206.

Müri, R.M., Gaymard, B., Rivaud, S., Vermersch, A.I., Cassarini, F., Hess, C.W., *et al.* (2000). Hemispheric asymmetry in cortical control of memory-guided saccades. A transcranial magnetic stimulation study. *Neuropsychologia* **38**, 1105–1111.

Mushiake, H., Inase, M., and Tanji, J. (1991). Neuronal activity in the primate premotor, supplementary, and precentral motor cortex during visually guided and internally determined sequential movements. *Journal of Neurophysiology,* **66**, 705–718.

Nagel, M., Sprenger, A., Lencer, R., Kömpf, D., Siebner, H., and Heide, W. (2008). Distributed representations of the 'preparatory set' in the frontal oculomotor system: a TMS study. *BMC Neuroscience,* **9**, 89.

Nickerson, R.S. (1973). Intersensory facilitation of reaction time: energy summation or preparation enhancement? *Psychological Review,* **80**, 489–509.

Nyffeler, T., Rivaud-Pechoux, S., Wattiez, N., and Gaymard, B. (2008a). Involvement of the supplementary eye field in oculomotor predictive behavior. *Journal of Cognitive Neurosciences,* **20**, 1583–1594.

Nyffeler, T., Hartmann, M., Hess, C.W., and Müri, R.M. (2008b). Visual vector inversion during memory antisaccades – a TMS study. *Progress of Brain Research* **171**, 429–32.

Nyffeler, T., Rivaud-Pechoux, S., Pierrot-Deseilligny, C., Diallo, R., and Gaymard, B. (2007b). Visual vector inversion in the posterior parietal cortex. *NeuroReport,* **18**, 917–920.

Nyffeler, T., Pierrot-Deseilligny, C., Felblinger, J., Mosimann, U.P., Hess, C.W., and Müri, R.M. (2002). Time-dependent hierarchical organization of spatial working memory: a transcranial magnetic stimulation study. *European Journal of Neuroscience,* **16**, 1823–1827.

Nyffeler, T., Pierrot-Deseilligny, C., Pflugshaupt, T., von Wartburg, R., Hess, C.W., and Müri, R.M. (2004). Information processing in long delay memory-guided saccades: further insights from TMS. *Experimental Brain Research,* **154**, 109–112.

Nyffeler, T., Wurtz, P., Lüscher, H.R., CHess, .W., Senn, W., Pflugshaupt, T., *et al.* (2006). Extending lifetime of plastic changes in the human brain. *European Journal of Neuroscience,* **24**, 2961–2966.

Nyffeler, T., Müri, R.M., Bucher-Ottiger, Y., Pierrot-Deseilligny, C., Gaymard, B., and Rivaud-Pechoux, S. (2007a). Inhibitory control of the human dorsolateral prefrontal cortex during the anti-saccade paradigm: a transcranial magnetic stimulation study. *European Journal of Neuroscience,* **26**, 1381–1385.

Ohtsuka, K., and Enoki, T. (1998). Transcranial magnetic stimulation over the posterior cerebellum during smooth pursuit eye movements in man. *Brain,* **121**, 429–435.

O'Sullivan, E.P., Jenkins, I.H., Henderson, L., Kennard, C., and Brooks, D.J. (1995). The functional anatomy of remembered saccades: a PET study. *Neuroreport,* **16**, 2141–2144.

Pierrot-Deseilligny, C., Rivaud, S., Gaymard, B., and Agid, Y. (1991a). Cortical control of reflexive visually-guided saccades. *Brain,* **114**, 1473–1485.

Pierrot-Deseilligny, C., Rivaud, S., Gaymard, B., and Agid, Y. (1991b). Cortical control of memory-guided saccades in man. *Experimental Brain Research,* **83**, 607–617.

Pierrot-Deseilligny, C., Müri, R.M., Ploner, C.J., Gaymard, B., Demeret, S., and Rivaud-Pechoux, S. (2003). Decisional role of the dorsolateral prefrontal cortex in ocular motor behaviour. *Brain,* **126**, 1460–1473.

Ploner, C.J., Gaymard, B., Rivaud-Pechoux, S., and Pierrot-Deseilligny, C. (2005). The prefrontal substrate of reflexive saccade inhibition in humans. *Biological Psychiatry,* **57**, 1159–1165.

Ploner, C.J., Gaymard, B., Rivaud, S., Agid, Y., and Pierrot-Deseilligny, C. (1998). Temporal limits of spatial working memory in humans. *European Journal of Neuroscience,* **10**, 794–797.

Rivaud, S., Müri, R.M., Gaymard, B., Vermersch, A.I., and Pierrot-Deseilligny, C. (1994). Eye movement disorders after frontal eye field lesions in humans. *Experimental Brain Research,* **102**, 110–120.

Ro, T., Farne, A., and Chang, E. (2002). Locating the human frontal eye fields with transcranial magnetic stimulation. *Journal of Clinical and Experimental Neuropsychology,* **24**, 930–940.

Ro, T., Cheifet, S., Ingle, H., Shoup, R., and Rafal, R.D. (1999). Localization of the human frontal eye fields and motor hand area with transcranial magnetic stimulation and magnetic resonance imaging. *Neuropsychologia,* **27**, 225–231.

Schall, J.D. (1991). Neuronal activity related to visually guided saccadic eye movements in the supplementary motor area of rhesus monkeys. *Journal of Neurophysiology,* **66**, 530–558.

Schall, J.D., Morel, A., and Kaas, J.H. (1993). Topography of supplementary eye field afferents to frontal eye field in macaque: implications for mapping between saccade coordinate systems. *Visual Neuroscience,* **10**, 385–393.

Schlag, J. and Schlag-Rey, M. (1987). Evidence of a supplementary eye field. *Journal of Neurophysiology,* **57**, 179–200.

Schwartz, M.L. and Goldman-Rakic, P.S. (1982). Single cortical neurones have axon collaterals to ipsilateral and contralateral cortex in fetal and adult primates. *Nature,* **299**, 154–155.

Seltzer, B. and Pandya, D.N. (1984). Further observations on parieto-temporal connections in the rhesus monkey. *Experimental Brain Research,* **55**, 301–312.

Seltzer, B. and Van Hoesen, G.W. (1979). A direct inferior parietal lobule projection to the presubiculum in the rhesus monkey. *Brain Research,* **179**, 157–161.

Sommer, M.A. and Tehovnik, E.J. (1999). Reversible inactivation of macaque dorsomedial frontal cortex: effects on saccades and fixations. *Experimental Brain Research,* **124**, 429–446.

Squire, L.R., and Kandel, E.R. (1999). *Memory.* New York: Freeman.

Srimal, R. and Curtis, C.E. (2008). Persistent neural activity during the maintenance of spatial position in working memory. *NeuroImage,* **39**, 455–468.

Sweeney, J.A., Mintun, M.A., Kwee, M., Wiseman, M.B., Brown, D.L. Rosenberg, D.R., *et al.* (1996). Positron emission tomography study of voluntary saccadic eye movements and spatial working memory. *Journal of Neurophysiology,* **75**, 454–468.

Thickbroom, G., Stell, R., and Mastaglia, F. (1996). Transcranial magnetic stimulation of the frontal eye field. *Journal of Neurological Sciences,* **144**, 114–118.

Tobler, P.N. and Müri, R.M. (2002). Role of human frontal and supplementary eye fields in double step saccades. *NeuroReport,* **13**, 253–255.

van Donkelaar, P. and Müri, R.M. (2002). Craniotopic updating of visual space across saccades in the human posterior parietal cortex. *Proceedings of the Royal Society B: Biological Sciences,* **269**, 735–739.

Walker, R., Husain, M., Hodgson, T.L., Harrison, J., and Kennard, C. (1998). Saccadic eye movement and working memory deficits following damage to human prefrontal cortex. *Neuropsychologia,* **36**, 1141–1159.

Wessel, K. and Kömpf, D. (1991). Transcranial magnetic brain stimulation: lack of oculomotor response. *Experimental Brain Research,* **86**, 216–218.

Wipfli, M., Felblinger, J., Mosimann, U.P., Hess, C.W., Schlaepfer, T.E. and Müri, R.M. (2001). Double-pulse transcranial magnetic stimulation over the frontal eye field facilitates triggering of memory-guided saccades. *European Journal Neuroscience,* **14**, 571–575.

Zhang, M. and Barash, S. (2000). Neuronal switching of sensorimotor transformations for antisaccades. *Nature,* **408**, 971–975.

Zhang, M. and Barash, S. (2004). Persistent LIP activity in memory antisaccades: working memory for a sensorimotor transformation. *Journal of Neurophysiology,* **91**, 1424–1441.

PART 3

Saccades and attention

CHAPTER 22

Determinants of saccade latency

Petroc Sumner

Abstract

How long it takes the brain to initiate a saccade has been a fundamental measure in sensorimotor research. Yet key questions remain about what determines saccade latency, even in the simplest of circumstances. In this chapter I discuss what makes some saccades fast while others are slow, and also briefly outline some established ways of manipulating saccade latency. A central question is why saccade latency varies so much even when all the stimuli and task requirements are kept the same. A related question is why most saccades to simple stimuli seem slower than they need to be. The chapter limits itself to simple cases of making saccades to onset targets, and does not examine latency or fixation duration in more complex visual search tasks, image viewing, or reading.

Introduction

The saccade latency distribution

Response time (RT) for manual, vocal, or oculomotor responses is one of the cornerstone measures of experimental psychology. The vast majority of studies compare mean or median RT in different conditions, but behind these means or medians are RT distributions that generally have a wide spread of values, often from around 200 ms to up to 1 s for relatively simple button-press tasks (e.g. Exner, 1873). These RT distributions also tend to have a characteristic shape (Fig. 22.1). Eye movements are no exception. Even for the simplest of tasks such as making a saccade to a single onset stimulus, untrained participants produce latencies that may vary as much as fivefold (e.g. from about 100 ms to 500 ms). Trained participants can often deliver shorter mean latency and less variance, however, they still make many saccades that are more than twice as long as others, and their distributions still show the characteristic shape (Fig. 22.1).

Thus the latency distribution appears to be a fundamental property of how our brains produce responses. When reporting mean or median latency (or RT) we take the underlying distribution for granted, and often forget that we do not fully understand it. In the case of eye movements, simply looking at a stimulus as soon as it appears would seem to be a very simple task, entailing exactly the same processing steps on every occasion. So if some saccades can be initiated in around 100 ms, why can't most saccades be initiated this quickly? Why do many saccades take twice, or even four times as long?

Modelling saccade latency—rise-to-threshold

A family of quantitative models have been developed that successfully capture the latency distributions of saccades to single target onsets (e.g. Carpenter, 1981; Godijn and Theeuwes, 2002; Kopecz, 1995;

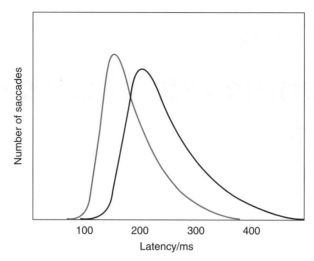

Fig. 22.1 The saccade latency distribution. The two distributions are typical of practised (grey) vs. novice (black) participants making saccades to simple onset targets. The illustrated distributions differ in their means and variances, but not in shape (skew). They could also represent the difference between stimulus-driven saccades (grey) and goal driven saccades (black), for example. Latency distributions with this kind of shape seem to be a fundamental property of most animal response systems.

Ludwig et al., 2007; Ratcliff, 2001; Smith and Ratcliff, 2004; Trappenberg et al., 2001). These models are discussed in more detail by Ludwig (Chapter 23 this volume), but an outline here will help frame some of the discussion below. The models envisage activity in a decision unit, or a motor unit, rising from a baseline activity level towards a threshold, and when that threshold is reached, the saccade is executed. This can also be seen as an accumulation of evidence in favour of one response or other, starting from the state of prior expectancy. In such models, the key determinant of saccade latency is rate of rise (or 'drift' or 'stochastic accumulation'), relative to the distance between starting activity and threshold (or 'boundary'). There is also a 'non-decisional delay' or 'dead time', which can be split into sensory delay (time from stimulus onset until the accumulation starts, ~60–100 ms) and execution delay (time from reaching threshold to saccade onset, ~20–30 ms).

Interestingly, even elegantly simple versions of these models, in which sensory and execution delays are constant and the rise rate is linear and just varies according to a Gaussian distribution (e.g. Carpenter, 1981), or the rise is a random walk with mean drift (e.g. Ratcliff, 2001), produce variation in saccade latency that fits very closely with the characteristic shape of the latency distribution. The skew in the distribution arises because small changes in fast rise rates make little difference to the time threshold is reached, but small changes in slow rise rates make much larger differences to the time threshold is reached (Fig. 22.2). The key concept of a rise-to-threshold can therefore explain the shape of the latency distribution, given random variability in the rise rate. But it does not remove the fundamental question of why this variability should be so large even on the simplest of tasks. We will return to this question below. First we will discuss other factors that affect latency, and how these are accounted for in oculomotor models.

Main factors determining mean latency

Endogenous versus exogenous saccades

Saccades that are driven primarily by the onset of a new stimulus are referred to as exogenous (generated from outside). Saccades that are driven primarily in a goal-directed manner, in the absence of a stimulus

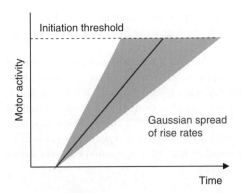
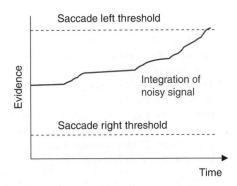

Fig. 22.2 Saccade initiation is thought to occur when activity representing a particular saccade rises or accumulates to a threshold level. If the rise rate has a Gaussian distribution, left, this can account for the basic shape of the saccadic latency distribution (e.g. Carpenter, 1981). A simple diffusion model (right) captures a similar idea (e.g. Ratcliff, 2001). Here the variability is produced by stochastic accumulation within a trial. See Ludwig, Chapter 23, this volume, for further discussion of rise-to-threshold models.

onset at the saccade destination, are called endogenous (generated inside). Both types produce latency distributions of the characteristic shape, but endogenous saccades are nearly always slower on average, with a wider distribution (e.g. Walker et al., 2000a). This difference is accounted for in the rise-to-threshold (or diffusion) models because stimuli at the saccade destination are assumed to drive faster rise rates and/or elicit quicker rise onset. For example, if an endogenous saccade is directed by an arrow at fixation, in a strictly serial model this central stimulus must be perceptually processed before the motor rise can start. In a more plausible cascading model, sensory evidence would start eliciting motor activity well before perceptual processing is complete, but it still takes time for the perceptual evidence to arrive. In all cases, a simple onset at the saccade destination is much simpler and quicker to translate into a motor signal. In more natural viewing conditions saccades are normally a mixture of exogenous and endogenous, purposely being directed to a certain stimulus location or stimulus change. Generally, saccades are highly goal directed, but any salient stimulus will speed saccades in that direction, because it helps drive the motor accumulation for that 'response field' (see Chapter 11, this volume; see also Chapters 19 and 23 for related discussion), and an onset is more efficient than a steady stimulus.

Stimulus strength and sensory delay

Just as the presence or absence of stimuli at the saccade destination strongly affects saccade latency, the strength and type of that stimulus can also have a major impact. High-contrast stimuli are expected to drive motor accumulation more efficiently than low-contrast stimuli, and their signals are also known to travel through the sensory system more quickly, resulting in shorter sensory delay before the rise-to-threshold can start (e.g. Bell et al., 2006; Carpenter, 2004; Wheeless et al., 1967). Similarly, latency to chromatic stimuli tends to be longer than to luminance stimuli, which can be attributed, at least partly, to the known delays in chromatic signals compared to luminance signals in the visual system (see Bompas and Sumner, 2008, for a review). However the minimum sensory delay—the time from stimulus onset until the earliest rise in motor activity occurs, which is about 60 ms in intermediate layers of superior colliculus (SC)—appears longer than necessary from neural transmission times along the shortest route from the retina. Thus it appears that the fastest sensory route is not the main driver of saccadic activity (see also Bompas and Sumner, 2009a; Sumner et al., 2006). We return to this point below.

Retinal eccentricity also affects latency. Generally there is an increase in latency the further the target is from the fovea, but the function is actually U-shaped with the lowest latencies between about 2° and 10°, with relatively long latencies for targets within 1° or 2° from the fovea (Kalesnykas and Hallett, 1994). This is possibly due to activation of fixation neurons by near-fovea targets (see later discussion of competition).

The influence of visual processes on latency is not purely 'bottom-up' (stimulus-driven). Perceptual attention is known to speed up visual signals and to increase their effective amplitude, both of which will lower saccade latency as outlined earlier (e.g. Kowler et al., 1995; Pashler, 1998). Interestingly, however, the neural systems controlling visual attention appear to overlap with those controlling eye movements (e.g. Kustov and Robinson, 1996; Rizzolatti et al., 1987; Shipp, 2004), so it may not be possible to attend to a location without also readying the oculomotor system to saccade there (see chapters 24–27, this volume). Clearly in such a linked system, attention would be a very strong determinant of saccade latency.

Expectancy, readiness, and warning

It is taken for granted throughout sensorimotor behavioural research that response latency is reduced when participants know when or where stimuli are likely to occur, or when and which response will be required. Such 'top-down' endogenous effects are generally referred to as spatial and temporal attention when acting on the sensory systems, and expectancy or readiness when affecting motor mechanisms. The latter are generally modelled by baseline shifts, which can also be viewed as changing the prior likelihood (expectancy) in the Bayesian stochastic decision process (Carpenter and Williams, 1995). Ludwig (Chapter 23, this volume) discusses expectancy in the context of saccade models, but in brief, spatial expectancy of where targets are likely to appear would raise the baseline activity in the decision units (or motor units) associated with those locations, and lower the baseline activity in units representing regions of low expectancy. Temporal expectancy of *when* a target will appear is envisaged to ramp up baseline activity just before the time the target is expected. Interestingly, while spatial expectancy is more often discussed, there is much more evidence that temporal expectancy has a large effect on latency than that spatial expectancy does (Findlay and Walker, 1999a; Walker et al., 2006). Such temporal expectancy can be created by almost any warning signal that is correlated in time with target appearance, or simply by any regularities in target onset times. In all natural and lab situations, some combination of spatial and temporal expectancy operates—there is never a case when every possible location and every possible time is an equal candidate for the next saccade. However we know relatively little about how and where these endogenous signals are generated, except that the frontal eye fields (FEFs), supplementary eye fields (SEFs), and prefrontal cortex in general are involved (see Chapter 15, this volume).

Criterion and speed–accuracy trade-off

Related to baseline shifts are criterion shifts—raising or lowering the threshold (or 'boundary' or 'confidence criterion'), that must be reached to initiate a saccade (e.g. Ratcliff, 2001; Reddi and Carpenter, 2000). Lowering the criterion will obviously speed saccades, but it comes at the cost of reduced accuracy: the classic speed–accuracy trade-off. Error may come in two forms, a saccade to a completely different location than the saccade target, or a saccade to the target that undershoots, overshoots, or goes a little wide. The former possibility is unlikely unless there are other stimuli at different locations to attract saccades (see competition discussion, below). The latter is thought to occur because the rise-to-threshold process becomes more spatially precise as the rise progresses (see discussion of field models by Ludwig, Chapter 23, this volume). At first a population of neurons representing locations near the target get activated, which can be imagined as a low broad hill on the motor map of potential saccade directions. As the activation hill rises, it becomes narrower, because local inhibitory connections cause the neurons at the edge to drop out (see Chapters 11 and 23, this volume). The higher the hill must become to reach threshold, the narrower it will be when it gets there, and therefore the more spatially precise the resultant saccade will be.

It is not known how criterion shifts are implemented neurally, but it could be achieved via the omnipause neurons that hold saccade initiation in check (see Chapters 9–12, this volume). Alternatively, or additionally, it could be effected through the mechanisms involved in baseline shifts. It is important to note that in the basic models outlined above (e.g. Figure 22.2), threshold shifts and baseline shifts have the same effect: they both simply change the required rise height. So although expectancy and criterion are conceptually distinct, they may not be neurally distinct.

Competition and inhibition

In everyday life, of course, saccades are made in the context of multiple stimuli. In this case, different potential saccade plans are thought to compete with each other, racing to reach threshold first and trigger a saccade (e.g. Leach and Carpenter, 2001; Theeuwes et al., 1998). However, if saccade plans simply raced, then latency would on average be faster when there are more possible targets, because there is more chance that one of the saccade plans would rise quickly. There would be no very slow saccades, because slow rises would always be beaten by an alternative plan. But in fact, mean latency tends to increase the more potential targets there are. To explain this, there must be mutual inhibition between alternative saccade plans, so that it takes longer for saccades to become activated in the context of competing plans (e.g. Findlay and Walker, 1999b; Godijn and Theeuwes, 2002; Kopecz, 1995; Leach and Carpenter, 2001; Trappenberg et al., 2001). Competition and inhibition have been investigated in a number of paradigms, the simplest of which are outlined below.

The gap paradigm

Even saccades to single stimuli seem to be subject to a basic push-pull competition with the alternative possibility of not making a saccade at all. Stimuli at fixation generally inhibit saccade activation. The simplest demonstration of this is the gap paradigm (Reuter-Lorenz et al., 1991; Saslow, 1967), in which saccades are faster if the fixation stimulus is turned off about 200 ms before target onset (the gap condition) compared to when the fixation stimulus is left on (the overlap condition). Some of this speeding can be accounted for by the warning signal given by fixation offset, but this is not the whole story. For example luminance increments at fixation give the same warning as luminance decrements, but the former slow saccades, while the latter speed them (e.g. Pratt et al., 2000). Thus the gap effect (or fixation offset effect) has been attributed to inhibitory connections between cells responsive to fixation stimuli and cells representing saccade plans (e.g. Findlay and Walker, 1999b; Kopecz, 1995). Such fixation-related inhibition is mainly associated with the SC (e.g. Dorris et al., 1997; Munoz and Fecteau, 2002; Munoz and Wurtz, 1992), but may have more than one source (Sumner et al., 2006).

The distractor paradigm

A second well-established phenomenon illustrating saccadic competition is the remote distractor effect (RDE), in which saccades are delayed when an irrelevant stimulus appears elsewhere in the visual field (e.g. Bompas and Sumner, 2009b; Honda, 2005; Lévy-Schoen, 1969; Ludwig et al., 2005a; Walker et al., 1997). Like the gap effect, the RDE is thought to be essentially automatic since it occurs even when the direction of the saccade target is known in advance and distractors always appear in the opposite hemifield and thus should be easy to voluntarily ignore (Benson, 2008; Walker et al., 1995, 2000b). The RDE has been hypothesized to involve long-range lateral inhibition between cell populations coding for the saccades to target and distractor (Fig. 22.3), either at the level of the SC (e.g. Olivier et al., 1999) or within the cortical eye fields (see discussion in Dorris et al., 2007). When the distractor is presented at or near fixation, competition between 'fixate' and 'move' subsystems in the SC has also been suggested as a source (Findlay and Walker, 1999b; Walker et al., 1997), although these views may be unified if the 'fixation neurons' in rostral SC in fact code for very small saccades, and thus are not categorically distinct from the 'move neurons' located caudally (Hafed et al., 2009). However, a simple interpretation of the RDE in terms of lateral inhibition is not without its problems (Walker et al., 1997).

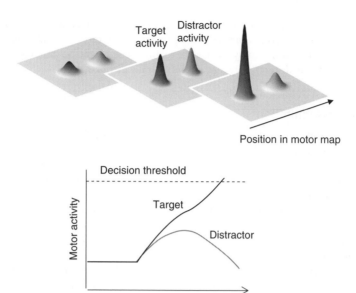

Fig. 22.3 Saccade competition: signals corresponding to different potential saccade endpoints, for instance a target and a distractor, are thought to compete in a race while mutually inhibiting each other (e.g. Godijn and Theeuwes, 2002; Trappenberg et al., 2001). By slowing the rise of target activity, the presence of a distractor delays saccades to the target. Competition between saccade targets and fixation stimuli is thought to operate in a similar way (e.g. Kopecz, 1995).

The antisaccade paradigm

A favourite tool for investigating competition between exogenous (reflexive) and purely endogenous (goal-directed) saccade plans has been the 'antisaccade' task, in which the participant is required to make an eye movement away from a visual onset, instead of a 'prosaccade' towards it (Hallet, 1978; Munoz and Everling, 2004). The saccadic latency for antisaccades is generally longer than that for prosaccades, because antisaccades require resolution of the conflict between the reflexive urge to look at the stimulus and the endogenous plan to saccade away. This 'antisaccade cost' is lessened if the participant knows that an antisaccade will be required before the stimulus arrives, relative to the case in which the type of stimulus (green or red, say) signals whether to make a prosaccade or antisaccade. Note that the participant does not know where the stimulus will occur, so cannot start to prepare any specific saccade plan in advance. Nevertheless, it appears that the brain can prepare some general top-down inhibition of the saccadic reflex, wherever it might come from (Everling et al., 1999; Everling and Munoz, 2000). Such top-down influence is generally thought to involve frontal areas, especially SEF and FEF (DeSouza et al., 2003). However, even with full preparation some antisaccade cost still exists, so it seems that, as in the distractor paradigm, top-down preparation cannot fully compensate for the automatic effects of stimulus onsets, and further inhibition is required after stimulus onset (E.J. Anderson et al., 2008; Everling and Munoz, 2000).

Modelling competition

In all cases outlined, the presence of a visual stimulus is thought to automatically produce a signal in some saccadic decision or planning area (e.g. SC), which slows down the activity rise needed to make the required saccade. To model this, three main ingredients are needed (e.g. Godijn and Theeuwes, 2002; Kopecz, 1995; Trappenberg et al., 2001). First, stimulus-driven activity must enter the motor competition even when those stimuli are known to be irrelevant for the task (i.e. there is some degree of automatic activation in motor areas even by irrelevant stimuli). Second, this activity has to be able to inhibit activity related to making other saccades, in order to delay the time saccade initiation threshold is reached. Third, there must be some component of goal-directed inhibition that helps overcome the irrelevant activity, so that most of the time the desired saccade is actually performed. Otherwise, for example, the distractor would often inhibit the target to the point of winning the race, which would result in many more errors than are typically measured. Likewise, in the antisaccade task, there would be many more erroneous prosaccades than typically occur. Thus there appear to be at least two types of inhibition: automatic mutual inhibition between competitors, and flexible inhibition that can bias the race for and against different types of stimuli.

Determinants of latency variation

Express saccades

Figure 22.4 shows a latency distribution of saccades to a simple onset. Comparing it to the schematic characteristic distribution in Fig. 22.1, there is a clear early bump that appears to represent an extra distribution of very fast saccades. These have become known as express saccades (e.g. Fischer and Boch, 1983; Fischer and Ramsperger, 1984) and are quite common in simple saccade experiments, especially when conditions favour rapid saccades, such as in the gap paradigm outlined above (e.g. Fischer and Boch, 1983; Fischer and Ramsperger, 1984; Munoz and Wurtz, 1992) or when urgency is encouraged over accuracy (e.g. Reddi and Carpenter, 2000). Why are express saccades able to be so much faster than other saccades given the same stimulus conditions? One possibility is that they are not true stimulus-driven saccades, but are correct guesses, initiated just before the stimulus actually appears (e.g. A.J. Anderson and Carpenter, 2008). However, one can correct for this by measuring erroneous saccades with short latency—anticipations that were wrong guesses—and usually a population of express saccades survives. Another possibility is that they are saccades triggered by very rapid visual information coming down a different pathway than the primary visual routes used for saccades (e.g. Schiller et al., 1987). The natural candidate pathway has been the retinotectal route, the direct pathway from retina to SC. However, express saccades still occur to chromatic targets (Bompas and Sumner, 2008; Weber et al., 1991), to which the retinotectal route is thought to be blind (Sumner et al., 2002).

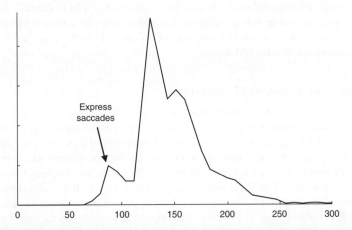

Fig. 22.4 When conditions favour fast saccades, there is often an extra 'bump' (mode) of very early saccades in the latency distribution. These have become known as express saccades (Fischer and Boch, 1983), and demonstrate that the saccade system is capable of producing saccades in under 100 ms. The reasons for the bimodal distribution, and the why most saccades are much slower, remain debated, but are presumably fundamental to understanding the mechanisms of saccade programming.

The conclusion that express saccades are not the product of a special visual pathway has also been reached by Carpenter (2001), who found that they occurred mostly on trials in which the target appeared on the opposite side from the preceding trial. Carpenter suggested that express saccades are a product of facilitation when saccades have the same direction as the return saccade from the preceding trial (see also A.J. Anderson et al., 2008). This cannot be the whole explanation because in other studies express saccades have not been restricted to particular trial-to-trial sequences (e.g. Bompas and Sumner, 2008). Nevertheless, the idea that express saccades rely on the state of the system before stimulus onset is probably correct (see e.g. Part 6, this volume; Dorris et al., 1997; Munoz et al., 2000). Thus it appears that express saccades occur only when inter-trial variations in attention, expectancy, readiness, criterion and motor priming (due to previous saccades) all coincide to favour a saccade to a particular location, and this is where the stimulus appears.

An evolutionary perspective

The existence of express saccades brings into sharp focus the question set out in the introduction to this chapter: if some saccades can be that fast, why are many saccades so slow? The system is clearly capable of making saccades with latencies below 100 ms, why can't the factors that allow this be applied for the majority of saccades when the task is very simple? From an evolutionary point of view, there are two possible classes of reason for a system appearing to be suboptimal: 1) there are biological limits that stop the system being any better than it is, 2) some property of the system actually gives an overall adaptive advantage that outweighs the apparent drawbacks (and the drawbacks are a necessary consequence of having the advantage).

Let us briefly examine possible biological limits. Clearly neural transmission and synaptic communication times cannot be the limit because saccades can be very fast. Variability in these times— unavoidable neural noise in the arrival times of signals at the SC for example—is not high enough to account for the large variability in saccadic latency (e.g. Bell et al., 2006). The most likely limit is that to initiate a saccade very quickly, the system must be in a very favourable state, and this state cannot be indefinitely maintained. This in turn may be due to factors such as the energetic cost of maintaining high baseline activity. However, if this is an important limit for the human saccade system, it is not a biological limit in the absolute sense: why should the system need high baseline activity in order to produce fast saccades? The reason why our saccadic system normally does not produce express saccades appears to be tonic inhibition, such as that from basal ganglia to the SC (see Chapter 12, this volume). Thus we must turn to possible adaptive advantages for a system whose default is to be in an inhibited state that cannot be easily turned off, and which therefore generally produces relatively slow saccades with large variability.

Procrastination as an agent of cleverness

One plausible argument is that the system has not been selected to be fast, but to be efficient in a complex environment, and this requires some degree of procrastination (e.g. Carpenter, 1999). There is in fact a striking discrepancy between our understanding of how simple saccades in laboratory experiments appear to be governed by saliency maps, and where most saccades are directed during natural viewing in real environments. Most natural saccades are simply not well predicted by bottom-up visual salience—the locations of the brightest, fastest, most contrast stimuli (e.g. Henderson, 2003; see Chapter 33, this volume). Instead the system seems to be much cleverer— directing saccades to places likely to yield the most important information for the current task (e.g. Findlay and Gilchrist, 2001; Land et al., 1999). In other words, saccade target selection depends more on relevance (or 'priority') than on bottom-up salience (Fecteau and Munoz, 2006; Treue, 2003).

For this reason the fastest routes by which the brain could produce saccades may have been purposely down-regulated to allow guidance by slower and more in-depth perceptual processing. This may be the reason for having tonic inhibition, and also why the sensory layers of the SC, which receive input directly from the retina as well as from primary visual cortex, do not appear to strongly activate the motor layers of SC, despite being arranged in corresponding maps (Isa, 2002; Moschovakis et al., 1988; Schiller and Stryker, 1972). Perhaps in the evolutionary past, these collicular layers communicated more strongly and saccade latency was generally shorter, but also more likely to be driven by simple visual changes. Through evolution the route may have become relatively 'turned off' and fast saccades discouraged, in favour of allowing more complex perceptual information to drive saccades. Thus inhibition became intrinsic to the system and cannot simply be taken away when not required during laboratory saccade tasks with simple stimuli. However, while this could explain why saccades seem unnecessarily delayed, it does not explain why they should be so variable even with simple stimuli.

Perceptual processing as the source of variance?

One possibility is that the variability comes from perceptual processing. In the simple case of saccading to a visual onset, this would mean that the brain takes a very variable amount of time to simply know whether the stimulus is there, rather than taking a variable amount of time to initiate a saccade to a stimulus it knows it there.

A perceptual source of latency variation fits the data when the perceptual task is not straightforward, for example when the stimuli are very hard to see (near-threshold), or when a difficult motion judgement is needed (e.g. Carpenter, 2004; Gold and Shadlen, 2001; Reddi et al., 2003). Even across simple and identical target onsets, there is variation in the time that sensory signals reach SC and other visuomotor areas (Bell et al., 2006; Bullier, 2001; Schmolesky et al., 1998). However, the measured sensory variation is of the order of 50 ms, which is not large enough to account for the wide variation is saccade latency. Likewise, in tasks where monkeys must distinguish between target and distractor stimuli, the time taken for cells in FEF to signal the distinction does not vary nearly enough to account for saccade latency variation, and has been found not to predict latency (Sato and Schall, 2003; Thompson et al., 1996). Similar conclusions—that the main source of latency variation is within the motor decision systems not in sensory processing—have been reached by modelling human saccade data (Carpenter, 2004; Ludwig and Gilchrist, 2006; see also Ludwig et al., 2005b; Taylor et al., 2006).

Latency variation as an agent of choice

Carpenter (e.g. Carpenter, 1999) has argued that variability is not a failing of the system, but has been directly selected for during evolution, because variability in simple decision mechanisms is an essential pre-requisite of choice—the ability not to always do the same thing given the same circumstances. For example, some element of randomness in motor decisions might initially prove beneficial simply so that an animal's behaviour cannot be easily predicted by predators. Since in race models, choices are a consequence of which plan reaches threshold first, choice is strongly related to rise rate. To achieve variability in action choices, the system must contain variability in rise rates. From this beginning we can speculate that the whole repertoire of human decision systems has emerged, with variability in rate as a core property from the start, which allows flexibility, creativity and discovery (see also Schall and Thompson, 1999).

Following the argument that variability in rate is not a by-product of motor systems, but is directly beneficial for creating variability in choice, it follows that procrastination (being unexpectedly slow on average) is necessary in order to allow sufficient variability. To achieve outcome variability (different choices) in a system in which different plans race to threshold, the variability in rise rates must be larger than the likely differences in mean signal strengths of the different alternatives. Otherwise the strongest signal would always win. Similarly, the race must run long enough that signals starting at a higher baseline can be overtaken, otherwise pre-stimulus activity would govern every choice. Thus in Carpenters view, variability in latency is the outcome of having variability in the rise rate of decision signals, which is needed to ensure variability in choice. Procrastination is essential both to allow sufficient variability, and to allow rise-rate differences to be translated into different choices, because some signals will start at a higher baseline.

Conclusions

The determinants of saccade latency can be treated in two main classes: 1) how different conditions change mean latency, and 2) factors that produce the wide latency distribution even when conditions are apparently constant. The former has been extensively studied, and the review provided above lays out the bare outline of some of the key factors. The reasons behind the latency distribution are much less investigated and understood, and so much of the above discussion is just plausible speculation. What is beyond dispute is that most saccades are relatively slow because the system is set up in a default state of inhibition. The likely reason for this is that it enables saccades to be directed by a combination of sophisticated perceptual processing and internal goals, rather than by simple visual salience. However, this still leaves the question of why latency distributions should be so broad. Of course, any factor that affects mean latency may also contribute to latency distributions if it varies within the trial category used to measure the distribution (for example, expectancy and priming from previous saccades). But these factors are normally modelled as baseline shifts, whereas the latency distribution is best accounted for by variation in the rate of a rise-to-threshold. This has led some to suggest that there is deliberate randomness in the rates of motor decision mechanisms because this leads to unpredictability in behaviour. But in sum, one of the most fundamental facts of animal behaviour—the distribution of response latencies—has no consensual explanation and remains partly mysterious.

References

Anderson, A.J. and Carpenter, R.H. (2008). The effect of stimuli that isolate S-cones on early saccades and the gap effect. *Proceedings Biological Sciences*, **275**(1632), 335–344.

Anderson, A.J., Yadav, H., and Carpenter, R.H. (2008). Directional prediction by the saccadic system. *Current Biology*, **18**(8), 614–618.

Anderson, E.J., Husain, M., and Sumner, P. (2008). Human intraparietal sulcus (IPS) and competition between exogenous and endogenous saccade plans. *Neuroimage*, **40**, 838–851.

Bell, A.H., Meredith, M.A., Van Opstal, A.J., and Munoz, D.P. (2006). Stimulus intensity modifies saccadic reaction time and visual response latency in the superior colliculus. *Experimental Brain Research*, **174**(1), 53–59.

Benson, V. (2008). A comparison of bilateral versus unilateral target and distractor presentation in the Remote Distractor Paradigm. *Experimental Psychology*, **55**, 334–341.

Bompas, A. and Sumner, P. (2008). Sensory sluggishness dissociates saccadic, manual, and perceptual responses: An S-cone study. *Journal of Vision*, **8**(8), 1011–13.

Bompas, A. and Sumner, P. (2009a). Oculomotor distraction by signals invisible to the retinotectal and magnocellular pathways. *Journal of Neurophysiology*, **102**, 2387–2395.

Bompas, A. and Sumner, P. (2009b). Temporal dynamics of saccadic distraction. *Journal of Vision*, **9**(9), 11–14.

Bullier, J. (2001). Integrated model of visual processing. *Brain Research Reviews*, **36**(2–3), 96–107.

Carpenter, R.H.S. (1981). Oculomotor procrastination. In D.F. Fisher, R.A. Monty, and J.W. Senders (eds.) *Eye movements: cognition and visual perception* (pp. 237–246). Hillsdale, NJ: Lawrence Erlbaum.

Carpenter, R.H.S. (1999). A neural mechanism that randomises behaviour. *Journal of Consciousness Studies*, **6**, 13–22.

Carpenter, R.H.S. (2001). Express saccades: is bimodality a result of the order of stimulus presentation? *Vision Research*, **41**(9), 1145–1151.

Carpenter, R.H.S. (2004). Contrast, probability, and saccadic latency: Evidence for independence of detection and decision. *Current Biology*, **14**(17), 1576–1580.

Carpenter, R.H.S. and Williams, M.L.L. (1995). Neural computation of log likelihood in control of saccadic eye-movements. *Nature*, **377**(6544), 59–62.

DeSouza, J.F., Menon, R.S., and Everling, S. (2003). Preparatory set associated with pro-saccades and anti-saccades in humans investigated with event-related FMRI. *Journal of Neurophysiology*, **89**(2), 1016–1023.

Dorris, M.C., Paré, M., and Munoz, D.P. (1997). Neuronal activity in monkey superior colliculus related to the initiation of saccadic eye movements. *Journal of Neuroscience*, **17**, 8566–8579.

Dorris, M.C., Olivier, E., and Munoz, D.P. (2007). Competitive integration of visual and preparatory signals in the superior colliculus during saccadic programming. *Journal of Neuroscience*, **27**(19), 5053–5062.

Everling, S. and Munoz, D.P. (2000). Neuronal correlates for preparatory set associated with pro-saccades and anti-saccades in the primate frontal eye field. *Journal of Neuroscience*, **20**(1), 387–400.

Everling, S., Dorris, M.C., Klein, R.M., and Munoz, D.P. (1999). Role of primate superior colliculus in preparation and execution of anti-saccades and pro-saccades. *Journal of Neuroscience*, **19**(7), 2740–2754.

Exner, S. (1873). Experimentelle Untersuchung der einfachsten psychischen Processe. Translated in W. James *The Principles of Psychology* (p. 92.). New York: Dover.

Fecteau, J.H. and Munoz, D.P. (2006). Salience, relevance, and firing: a priority map for target selection. *Trends in Cognitive Science*, **10**(8), 382–390.

Findlay, J.M. and Gilchrist, I.D. (2001). Visual attention: The active vision perspective. In M. Jenkins and L. Harris (eds.) *Vision and attention* (pp. 83–103). New York: Springer-Verlag.

Findlay, J.M. and Walker, R. (1999a). A model of saccade generation based on parallel processing and competitive inhibition. *Behavioral and Brain Sciences*, **22**(4), 661–721.

Findlay, J.M. and Walker, R. (1999b). A model of saccade generation based on parallel processing and competitive inhibition. *Behavioral and Brain Sciences*, **22**(4), 661–674; discussion 674–721.

Fischer, B. and Boch, R. (1983). Saccadic eye movements after extremely short reaction times in the monkey. *Brain Research*, **260**, 21–26.

Fischer, B. and Ramsperger, E. (1984). Human express saccades: Extremely short reaction times of goal directed eye movements. *Experimental Brain Research*, **57**, 191–195.

Godijn, R. and Theeuwes, J. (2002). Programming of endogenous and exogenous saccades: Evidence for a competitive integration model. *Journal of Experimental Psychology - Human Perception and Performance*, **28**(5), 1039–1054.

Gold, J.I. and Shadlen, M.N. (2001). Neural computations that underlie decisions about sensory stimuli. *Trends in Cognitive Science*, **5**(1), 10–16.

Hafed, Z.M., Goffart, L., and Krauzlis, R.J. (2009). A neural mechanism for microsaccade generation in the primate superior colliculus. *Science*, **323**(5916), 940–943.

Hallet, P.E. (1978). Primary and secondary saccades to goals defined by instructions. *Vision Research*, **18**, 1279–1296.

Henderson, J.M. (2003). Human gaze control during real-world scene perception. *Trends in Cognitive Science*, **7**(11), 498–504.

Honda, H. (2005). The remote distractor effect of saccade latencies in fixation-offset and overlap conditions. *Vision Research*, **45**(21), 2773–2779.

Isa, T. (2002). Intrinsic processing in the mammalian superior colliculus. *Current Opinion in Neurobiology*, **12**, 668–677.

Kalesnykas, R.P. and Hallett, P.E. (1994). Retinal eccentricity and the latency of eye saccades. *Vision Research*, **34**(4), 517–531.

Kopecz, K. (1995). Saccadic reaction times in gap/overlap paradigms: a model based on integration of intentional and visual information on neural, dynamic fields. *Vision Research*, **35**(20), 2911–2925.

Kowler, E., Anderson, E., Dosher, B., and Blaser, E. (1995). The role of attention in the programming of saccades. *Vision Research*, **35**(13), 1897–1916.

Kustov, A.A. and Robinson, D.L. (1996). Shared neural control of attentional shifts and eye movements. *Nature*, **384**, 74–77.

Land, M., Mennie, N., and Rusted, J. (1999). The roles of vision and eye movements in the control of activities of daily living. *Perception*, **28**(11), 1311–1328.

Leach, J.C.D. and Carpenter, R.H.S. (2001). Saccadic choice with asynchronous targets: evidence for independent randomisation. *Vision Research*, **41**(25–26), 3437–3445.

Lévy-Schoen, A. (1969). Détermination et latence de la réponse oculomotrice à deux stimulus simultanés ou successifs selon leur excenticité relative. *L'Anneé Psychologique*, **69**, 373–392.

Ludwig, C.J.H. and Gilchrist, I.D. (2006). The relative contributions of luminance contrast and task demands on saccade target selection. *Vision Research*, **46**(17), 2743–2748.

Ludwig, C.J.H., Gilchrist, I.D., and McSorley, E. (2005a). The remote distractor effect in saccade programming: channel interactions and lateral inhibition. *Vision Research*, **45**(9), 1177–1190.

Ludwig, C.J.H., Mildinhall, J.W., and Gilchrist, I.D. (2007). A population coding account for systematic variation in saccadic dead time. *Journal of Neurophysiology*, **97**(1), 795–805.

Ludwig, C.J.H., Gilchrist, I.D., McSorley, E., and Baddeley, R.J. (2005b). The temporal impulse response underlying saccadic decisions. *Journal of Neuroscience*, **25**(43), 9907–9912.

Moschovakis, A.K., Karabelas, A.B., and Highstein, S.M. (1988). Structure-function relationships in the primate superior colliculus. II. Morphological identity of presaccadic neurons. *Journal of Neurophysiology*, **60**(1), 263–302.

Munoz, D.P. and Everling, S. (2004). Look away: The anti-saccade task and the voluntary control of eye movement. *Nature Reviews Neuroscience*, **5**(3), 218–228.

Munoz, D.P. and Fecteau, J.H. (2002). Vying for dominance: dynamic interactions control visual fixation and saccadic initiation in the superior colliculus. *Progress in Brain Research*, **140**, 3–19.

Munoz, D.P. and Wurtz, R.H. (1992). Role of the rostral superior colliculus in active visual fixation and execution of express saccades. *Journal of Neurophysiology*, **67**(4), 1000–1002.

Munoz, D.P., Dorris, M.C., Paré, M., and Everling, S. (2000). On your mark, get set: Brainstem circuitry underlying saccadic initiation. *Canadian Journal of Physiology and Pharmacology*, **78**(11), 934–944.

Olivier, E., Dorris, M.C., and Munoz, D.P. (1999). Lateral interactions in the superior colliculus, not an extended fixation zone, can account for the remote distractor effect. *Behavioral and Brain Sciences*, **22**, 694–695.

Pashler, H.E. (1998). *The psychology of attention*. Cambridge, MA: MIT Press.

Pratt, J., Bekkering, H., and Leung, M. (2000). Estimating the components of the gap effect. *Experimental Brain Research*, **130**(2), 258–263.

Ratcliff, R. (2001). Putting noise into neurophysiological models of simple decision making. *Nature Neuroscience*, **4**(4), 336–337.

Reddi, B.A.J. and Carpenter, R.H.S. (2000). The influence of urgency on decision time. *Nature Neuroscience*, **3**(8), 827–830.

Reddi, B.A.J., Asrress, K.N., and Carpenter, R.H.S. (2003). Accuracy, information, and response time in a saccadic decision task. *Journal of Neurophysiology*, **90**(5), 3538–3546.

Reuter-Lorenz, P.A., Hughes, H.C., and Fendrich, R. (1991). The reduction of saccadic latency by prior offset of the fixation point: an analysis of the gap effect. *Perception & Psychophysics*, **49**(2), 167–175.

Rizzolatti, G., Riggio, L., Dascola, I., and Umiltá, C. (1987). Reorienting attention across the horizontal and vertical meridians: evidence in favor of a premotor theory of attention. *Neuropsychologia*, **25**, 31–40.

Saslow, M.G. (1967). Effects of components of displacement-step stimuli upon latency for saccadic eye movements. *Journal of the Optical Society of America*, **57**, 1024–1029.

Sato, T.R., and Schall, J.D. (2003). Effects of stimulus-response compatibility on neural selection in frontal eye field. *Neuron*, **38**(4), 637–648.

Schall, J.D. and Thompson, K.G. (1999). Neural selection and control of visually guided eye movements. *Annual Review of Neuroscience*, **22**, 241–259.

Schiller, P.H. and Stryker, M. (1972). Single-unit recording and stimulation in superior colliculus of the alert rhesus monkey. *Journal of Neurophysiology*, **35**, 915–924.

Schiller, P.H., Sandel, J.H., and Maunsel, J.H.R. (1987). The effect of frontal eye field and superior colliculus lesions on saccadic latencies in the rhesus monkey. *Journal of Neurophysiology*, **57**(4), 1033–1049.

Schmolesky, M.T., Wang, Y., Hanes, D.P., Thompson, K.G., Leutgeb, S., Schall, J.D., *et al.* (1998). Signal timing across the macaque visual system. *Journal of Neurophysiology*, **79**(6), 3272–3278.

Shipp, S. (2004). The brain circuitry of attention. *Trends in Cognitive Sciences*, **8**(5), 223–230.

Smith, P.L. and Ratcliff, R. (2004). Psychology and neurobiology of simple decisions. *Trends in Neurosciences*, **27**(3), 161–168.

Sumner, P., Adamjee, T., and Mollon, J.D. (2002). Signals invisible to the collicular and magnocellular pathways can capture visual attention. *Current Biology*, **12**(15), 1312–1316.

Sumner, P., Nachev, P., Castor-Perry, S., Isenman, H., and Kennard, C. (2006). Which visual pathways cause fixation-related inhibition? *Journal of Neurophysiology*, **95**, 1527–1536.

Taylor, M.J., Carpenter, R.H., and Anderson, A.J. (2006). A noisy transform predicts saccadic and manual reaction times to changes in contrast. *Journal of Physiology*, **573**(Pt 3), 741–751.

Theeuwes, J., Kramer, A.F., Hahn, S., and Irwin, D.E. (1998). Our eyes do not always go where we want them to go: Capture of the eyes by new objects. *Psychological Science*, **9**(5), 379–385.

Thompson, K.G., Hanes, D.P., Bichot, N.P., and Schall, J.D. (1996). Perceptual and motor processing stages identified in the activity of macaque frontal eye field neurons during visual search. *Journal of Neurophysiology*, **76**(6), 4040–4055.

Trappenberg, T.P., Dorris, M.C., Munoz, D.P., and Klein, R.M. (2001). A model of saccade initiation based on the competitive integration of exogenous and endogenous signals in the superior colliculus. *Journal of Cognitive Neuroscience*, **13**(2), 256–271.

Treue, S. (2003). Visual attention: the where, what, how and why of saliency. *Current Opinion in Neurobiology*, **13**(4), 428–432.

Walker, R., Kentridge, R.W., and Findlay, J.M. (1995). Independent contributions of the orienting of attention, fixation offset and bilateral stimulation on human saccadic latency. *Exp. Brain Res.*, **103**, 294–310.

Walker, R., McSorley, E., and Haggard, P. (2006). The control of saccade trajectories: Direction of curvature depends on prior knowledge of target location and saccade latency. *Perception and Psychophysics*, **68**(1), 129–138.

Walker, R., Deubel, H., Schneider, W.X., and Findlay, J.M. (1997). Effect of remote distractors on saccade programming: evidence for an extended fixation zone. *Journal of Neurophysiology*, **78**, 1108–1119.

Walker, R., Walker, D.G., Husain, M., and Kennard, C. (2000a). Control of voluntary and reflexive saccades. *Experimental Brain Research*, **130**(4), 540–544.

Walker, R., Mannan, S., Maurer, D., Pambakian, A.L.M., and Kennard, C. (2000b). The oculomotor distractor effect in normal and hemianopic vision. *Proc. R. Soc. Lond. B*, **267**, 431–438.

Weber, H., Fischer, B., Bach, M., and Aiple, F. (1991). Occurence of express saccades under isoluminance and low contrast luminance conditions. *Visual Neuroscience*, **7**, 505–510.

Wheeless, L.L., Cohen, G.H., and Boynton, R.M. (1967). Luminance as a parameter of eye-movement control system. *Journal of the Optical Society of America*, **57**(3), 394–396.

CHAPTER 23

Saccadic decision-making

Casimir J.H. Ludwig

Abstract

The generation of a saccade may be considered the outcome of some decision-making process. Functional models of saccadic decision-making are based on the accumulation of sensory evidence in favour of various alternative movement programmes in a race to a decision threshold. The outcome of this race is affected by a number of decision-related variables such as the quality of sensory evidence, the prior probability of alternative movements, and the reward associated with the different movements. I review a selection of behavioural and neurophysiological studies on the influence of these variables on saccadic decisions, and relate these variables to the distinct mechanisms posited by models of decision-making.

Decision-making may be regarded as that internal process which produces behaviour, as manifest in the motor output of an organism (Glimcher, 2003b, 2003a). Behaviour may be in response to sensory stimulation, triggered by non-sensory factors or, most typically, some combination of the two. Motor responses to sensory stimulation may be anything from what are often thought of as primitive reflexes—indeed, these were the starting point of the physiological study of decision-making—to more complex patterns of motor output that are less deterministically linked to the sensory input.

Clearly saccadic eye movement generation is a long way removed from what may be regarded as 'volitional' decision-making that we typically associate with human behaviour. Nevertheless, it is appropriate to view these movements as the consequences of some decision-making process that is more complicated than those underlying the most direct sensory-motor responses. That is, saccades may be internally generated on the basis of non-sensory factors (e.g. I can choose to look to the right and up even in absence of any sensory stimulation), may be withheld altogether even when presented with a highly salient stimulus, and may be triggered in response to sensory stimulation. The mapping between sensory stimulation and saccadic eye movement response may be direct (such as in a typical visually guided saccade task) or more arbitrary and symbolic. Regardless of the complexity of the sensory-motor mapping, a decision is made: 1) to move the eyes, 2) where to move the eyes to, and 3) when to move the eyes. The limited resolution of human vision dictates that such decisions are made at regular, relatively short intervals (around 3 or 4 times every second).

In this sense, any chapter in this volume on saccadic eye movements may be regarded as being about saccadic decision-making. As a result, there will inevitably be some overlap between the topics addressed in this chapter and issues reviewed elsewhere in the volume. I will restrict the focus of this review to a discussion of: 1) the functional mechanisms that serve saccadic decision-making; 2) the representation within the saccadic system of decision-related variables such as sensory evidence, prior probability and reward; and 3) whether and how these variables impinge on the mechanisms identified in models of saccadic decision-making.

Models of saccadic decision-making

Over the past two decades both behavioural and neurophysiological research on the saccadic system has started to address how saccade targets are selected in situations in which the system is confronted with a number of possible objects to look at (reviewed in Fecteau and Munoz, 2006; Schall and Thompson, 1999). Selectivity is studied by examining the accuracy and latency of target selection, as well as more dynamic variables such as saccade trajectories. The logic is straightforward: a more difficult selection process will be evidenced by less accurate saccades, triggered with longer latencies, and executed with more biased trajectories (either towards or away from the competing object location; see Chapter 5, this volume, as well as McSorley et al., 2006). Single-cell recordings from primate superior colliculus (SC) (McPeek et al., 2003; McPeek and Keller, 2002b, 2002a) and frontal eye fields (FEF) (Bichot et al., 2001; Schall et al., 1995; Thompson et al., 2005) in such paradigms have reinforced a view of target selection as a competitive process that is gradually resolved over time. Neurons with visual and/or motor responses in these structures will typically respond to any item that falls within their receptive or movement field. Over time, responses to non-selected items are suppressed in favour of neurons coding the selected, target location. This competitive process has been formalized at the functional level in the form of decision-field models.

Decision-field models

Decision-field models assume that the relevant parameters of movements towards the various response alternatives are coded in a continuous and dynamic activation field (Arai and Keller, 2005; Arai et al., 1999; Erlhagen and Schoner, 2002; Kopecz, 1995; Kopecz and Schoner, 1995; Ludwig et al., 2007; Trappenberg et al., 2001; Wilimzig et al., 2006). For instance, a generic saccadic 'motor map' may be conceptualized as a one or two-dimensional topographic representation of visual space (e.g. the amplitudes and directions of all different possible eye movements; see Fig. 23.1). Maps in which neighbouring units code nearby movement vectors are found throughout the saccadic eye movement system (e.g. in SC and FEF). An input into the system, which may be a localized visual stimulus or an internally generated movement plan, results in a broadly distributed pattern of activity. The peak of activity is centred on the movement vector associated with the input, but neighbouring vectors are also activated in the population code (e.g. Ottes et al., 1986; Goossens and Van Opstal, 2006; C.K. Lee et al., 1988; McIllwain, 1986). Fig. 23.1 illustrates a simple, two-item input which gives rise to two separate, broadly distributed activation patterns on the motor map.

The activity on the map evolves over time. For instance, the activity associated with one pattern may rise faster than that associated with the other, perhaps because of experimental instructions which may render one type of pattern more relevant than the other (e.g. 'look for squares'). Such computations are captured by the $f(input)$ term in Fig. 23.1, where f may represent anything from a simple linear transducer to more complicated and non-linear transformations of the sensory input. Units representing distant portions of space may mutually inhibit each other and nearby units may activate each other, in accordance with neurophysiological evidence from SC (Munoz and Istvan, 1998). In addition, units may 'leak' a certain proportion of the activity they are accumulating, which may be countered by some degree of recurrent self-excitation (Usher and McClelland, 2001; Wang, 2002; Wong and Wang, 2006). Regardless of the precise dynamics, the competition may be thought of as a parallel race to a response threshold. The saccade is executed soon after the threshold is reached, its target corresponding to the vector that won the race.

For such models to produce realistic variability in choice, latency and landing position, one or more sources of noise need to be assumed. For example, the input into the decision field may vary upon repeated presentation of the same stimulus configuration, as a result of internal noise in the transformation of the input. Additional noise is often added to the gradual evolution of activity on

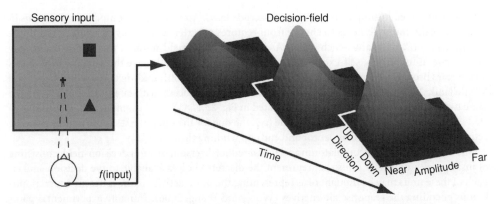

Fig. 23.1 Decision-field model of saccadic decision-making. An observer is presented with a test display and told to saccade to the square. The two potential saccade targets are represented by broadly distributed populations in a two-dimensional decision-field (r,θ). Due to the prioritization of squares over triangles (an operation assumed to occur in *f(input)*), the units representing the location of the square receive a stronger input. Over time the activity associated with the non-target is completely suppressed. The activity distributions in the decision field are based on a mapping of a 0.5-mm Gaussian activity profile in collicular coordinates to polar coordinates, according to the model of Ottes et al. (1986). Note that only the right visual field is represented.

the motor map over time. Together, this set of assumptions can account for an impressive array of data from a range of simple saccade target selection paradigms (Trappenberg et al., 2001). Decision-field models can provide an excellent functional description of the competitive interactions that take place throughout the saccadic eye movement system.

Evidence integration models

More abstract evidence integration models are based on a similar principle of the gradual evolution of noisy activity towards a response threshold (Luce, 1986; Ratcliff and Smith, 2004; Smith and Ratcliff 2004). Such models have been widely used in cognitive psychology to account for relatively simple decisions such as whether a string of letters is a word or non-word, whether a test item featured on a study list presented earlier, etc. Models in this class include a variety of sequential sampling models that are characterized by temporally dynamic noise (often referred to as 'wiener noise' in the continuous time domain) that is added to each sample. Examples of sequential sampling models are random walk models (Laming, 1969; Link and Heath, 1975), the widely used diffusion model (Ratcliff, 1978; Ratcliff and Rouder, 1998; Ratcliff and Smith, 2004), and accumulator models (Usher and McClelland, 2001; Vickers, 1970). Other evidence integration models do not assume that the temporal samples themselves are noisy (Brown and Heathcote, 2005, 2008; Carpenter and Williams, 1995). These models are often also referred to as accumulator models, but they are technically not in the same class as the sequential sampling models. The feature that unites both noisy and ballistic accumulator models is their absolute stopping rule: the decision process finishes as soon as an accumulator reaches a criterion amount of evidence. In the random walk and diffusion models, the criterion is a relative one: it corresponds to a certain amount of *net* evidence in favour of one particular alternative, relative to the other alternative(s).

In the saccadic domain one particularly simple model is the LATER (linear accumulation to threshold with ergodic rate; Carpenter and Williams, 1995) model developed by Roger Carpenter and colleagues (see also Sumner, Chapter 22, this volume). LATER assumes that activity associated with a particular saccade programme (i.e. movement vector) rises gradually towards a threshold. Importantly, the accumulation rate is assumed to vary randomly from one saccade to the next, according to a Gaussian distribution. This single noise source is sufficient to account for the latency variability observed in simple visually guided saccade tasks. Application to competitive situations in which there are multiple items to choose from requires an extension of this basic idea to multiple accumulators racing against each other. As in the dynamic field models, this competition may involve lateral inhibition, self-excitation, and leakage, which would make the accumulation paths non-linear (Brown and Heathcote, 2005; Leach and Carpenter, 2001; Ludwig et al., 2005a; Usher and McClelland, 2001). Fig. 23.2A illustrates this competitive process, with lateral inhibition, for the same two-alternative decision that was illustrated in Fig. 23.1. As in that example, the activity associated with one particular saccade programme (e.g. the one for the square) rises more rapidly than the activity associated with the competitor and ends up winning the race.

One way to view this accumulator model is as a reduced version of a full decision-field, consisting of just a small number of units that represent the discrete choices available to the decision-maker. Each of these units may be thought of as representing the mean activity of the different neural populations encoding the response alternatives (Wong and Wang, 2006). In many experimental paradigms the different potential saccade targets are well separated, so that the movements can be clearly and discretely classified as being directed towards one pattern or another. To model choice and latency variability in such paradigms then, this simplified representation is sufficient.

Finally, it should be noted that models involving competitive accumulation towards an absolute threshold are difficult to distinguish empirically from the noisy accumulation of net evidence towards a relative criterion, as assumed by the bounded diffusion model (Bogacz et al., 2006; Ratcliff and Smith, 2004). In the diffusion model, as applied to two-choice tasks, there is only a single 'accumulator' which moves through a decision space (analogous to the Brownian motion of a particle) towards one of two boundaries which represent the available response alternatives. The consequence is that motion towards one particular alternative necessarily implies a shift away from the competing alternative. The same inhibitory dynamics may be achieved through lateral inhibition between multiple accumulators that race to a single, common threshold.

Representation of decision-related variables

Evidence integration models suggest what functional mechanisms may underlie selection from multiple competing peripheral targets. I will now turn to the question of whether the saccadic eye

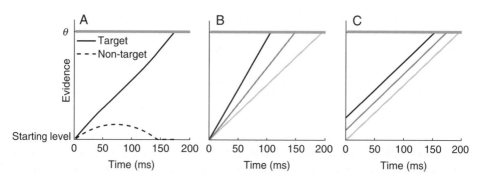

Fig. 23.2 Accumulator model of saccadic decision-making. A) Competition between two potential saccade targets is resolved over time through lateral inhibition, just as in Fig. 23.1. A saccade is initiated when one accumulator reaches threshold. The saccade target is determined by the winning accumulator. B) As reviewed in the 'Representation of decision-related variables' varying the quality of sensory evidence is best represented by changing the rate of accumulation. Weaker evidence is indicated by the lighter shaded, slower accumulators. C) The effect of varying the prior probability of a particular movement vector is best represented by changing the starting level of accumulation. Less probable responses are represented by lower initial levels of activation, as indicated by the lighter shaded accumulators.

movement system is capable of representing information that a sensible decision-maker would take into account. Neurophysiological, and to some extent behavioural, work has focused on three decision-related variables: strength of sensory evidence, prior probability, and reward (or, more precisely, relative expected utility). I will discuss each of these three variables in turn and attempt to link them to the functional mechanisms described in the previous section.

Sensory evidence

Evidence refers to the extent to which the sensory data provide support for one hypothesis relative to one or more competing hypotheses. In the context of saccadic decisions, the hypotheses correspond to the different possible saccade targets. The question is then whether the sensory evidence calls for a saccade to one potential target in favour of the others, and whether the strength of that evidence affects the decisions made in a predictable and adaptive manner.

Possibly the most straightforward manipulation of sensory evidence is simply to vary the visibility of a peripheral target (Ludwig et al., 2004; White et al., 2006). Unsurprisingly, in visually guided saccades to a single target the latency of the saccade decreases as the luminance contrast of the peripheral target increases. This is consistent with the idea that improving the sensory evidence enhances the rate of accumulation, which results in a shorter decision latency (see Fig. 23.2B). However, the visually guided saccade paradigm does not involve a decision between multiple competing response alternatives.

To examine saccadic decision-making in such competitive conditions, Ludwig et al. (2005a) (see also Caspi et al., 2004) presented human observers with two peripheral luminance patterns. The luminance contrast of both patterns was re-sampled every 25 ms, independently from partly overlapping probability distributions, so that one of the patterns had a slightly higher average contrast. Observers were asked to saccade to this higher contrast pattern. As a result of the temporal noise in the stimulus sequence, the sensory evidence provided in this paradigm is uncertain. Under these conditions, temporal integration of the evidence is a good strategy to decide which pattern to look at.

The sensory uncertainty introduced by the external noise enabled Ludwig et al. (2005a) to identify over what time window the sensory evidence was taken into account. Imagine a trial on which, through random sampling, the designated 'non-target' pattern (i.e. the one with the lower average contrast) happened to be a little brighter than the actual target for some brief period of time, shortly after the onset of the two patterns. If the observer chose to fixate the non-target pattern on that trial, this would indicate that the sensory evidence provided in this period of time was taken into account in the decision process. Over the course of many trials, this type of regression of the decisions against the noise in the stimulus reveals the temporal window of evidence integration.

Surprisingly, given average saccade latencies on the order of ~300 ms, this window was restricted to approximately the first 100 ms of stimulus presentation. Subsequently, Ludwig (2009) has demonstrated that the results from this study can be accounted for using the evidence integration framework. In this instance, the evidence is represented by temporally blurred versions of the sequence of luminance contrast values. The net evidence is computed as the difference between these temporally filtered internal responses. This difference is integrated over time to one of two boundaries, corresponding to the two decision alternatives. As a result, temporary variations in the strength and direction of sensory evidence result in corresponding temporary, blurred variations in the rate of accumulation. This model could account for the overall accuracy of the saccadic decisions, the latency distributions of correct and error decisions, as well as results from a different experiment in which the temporal availability of *useful* sensory evidence was manipulated systematically (Ludwig et al., 2005b, experiment 2).

Newsome, Shadlen, and colleagues have examined the neural mechanisms underlying the integration of sensory evidence during perceptual decisions about visual motion (Britten et al., 1992; Ditterich et al., 2003; Gold and Shadlen, 2003, 2000; Kim and Shadlen, 1999; Newsome et al., 1989; Palmer et al., 2005; Roitman and Shadlen, 2002). Figure 23.3 illustrates the classic paradigm.

The observer (mostly non-human primates) fixates a point on the screen and is presented with a central random dot kinematogram (RDK). This is a pattern consisting of a number of randomly moving dots. A subset of the dots, however, moves in the same direction. For instance, 10% of the dots may move coherently to the left, in which case the observer has to make a saccade to the marker object located left of the central RDK pattern. By varying the proportion of coherently moving dots (the motion coherence), the strength of the sensory evidence is manipulated. The evidence in favour of either option is weak when the coherence is close to 0%, but less and less ambiguous for higher coherence values.

Note that although the task calls for a saccadic decision, the mapping between the available saccade targets and the sensory evidence used to make the saccadic decision is symbolic and rather arbitrary. The main focus of these studies is on *perceptual* decision-making, but saccadic responses are used because the basic neurophysiological mechanisms underlying saccade generation are relatively well understood. In terms of the definition of decision-making provided at the start of this chapter, the saccadic system is treated as a model system to study the neural signature(s) of 'that internal process which produces behaviour'. It is important to bear in mind that in more naturalistic conditions, the sensory evidence in favour of a peripheral saccade target is typically bound to that peripheral location. In that regard, it could be argued that the decision-making task of Ludwig et al. (2005b) has greater ecological validity.

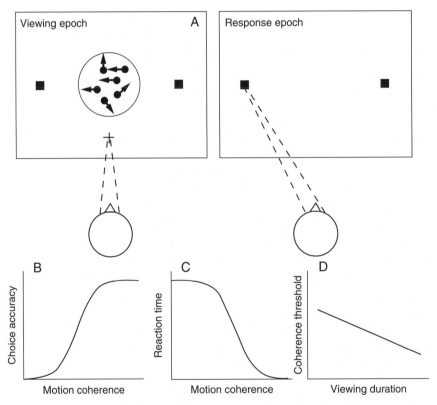

Fig. 23.3 Visual-saccadic decisions about perceptual motion. A) The observer views a RDK pattern in which only a subset of the dots move coherently in one direction. After a delay (determined by the experimenter or by the observer) the motion direction is signalled with a saccade to one of the two peripheral markers. B–D)Fictitious data showing how choice accuracy (B) and reaction time (C) vary as a function of motion coherence, and how motion coherence thresholds (D) for direction discrimination improve with viewing time.

In the RDK task observers do clearly adjust their behaviour in accordance with various manipulations of the sensory evidence. Their choice accuracy improves monotonically as a function of motion coherence (see Fig. 23.3B for a hypothetical example). For a typical viewing duration, performance ranges smoothly from close to chance for weak coherence to nearly perfect for high coherence (typically >25%; Gold and Shadlen, 2003). More interestingly, accuracy improves with increasing viewing duration in that motion coherence thresholds decrease as a function of viewing time (see Fig. 23.3C). This finding suggests strongly that the observers are taking advantage of the increase in viewing time by collecting more sensory evidence. Finally, in a reaction time version of the task (in which the viewing epoch is terminated by the observer's saccadic response) the decision time decreases with increasing coherence (Roitman and Shadlen, 2002; see Fig. 23.3B). This result indicates that when the evidence is weak, observers elect to wait longer and collect more data in order to make a more informed decision. Behaviourally then, it is clear that the saccadic system is capable of taking sensory evidence into account.

In terms of the underlying physiological mechanism, it is well established that directionally selective neurons in primate brain area MT respond to such motion patterns (Britten et al., 1992). A pool of MT neurons with the same direction preference (say leftward) then provides an ongoing, momentary estimate of the sensory evidence in favour of responding to the marker object that corresponds to this direction. Of course, a pool with the opposing directional selectivity will encode the evidence in favour of the alternative choice option. It is important to note that this evidence is momentary: due to the stochastic nature of the RDK pattern the evidence in favour of one or the other alternative will fluctuate over time.

Two pieces of evidence suggest very strongly that brain structures that are involved in saccade generation perform a gradual accumulation of the fleeting sensory evidence. First, micro-stimulation of the frontal eye fields results in evoked saccades with endpoints that are biased in the direction of the ensuing target-directed saccade (Gold and Shadlen, 2000). This bias indicates that the evoked saccade is some weighted combination of the vector coded by the stimulated site and the decision-related vector (i.e. to the marker that corresponds to the perceptual decision). Critically, the magnitude of this bias increases with viewing duration and motion coherence in a similar manner as behavioural choice accuracy, suggesting that the decision to make a saccade to the peripheral marker evolved gradually over time. Second, single cell recordings from LIP show that the activity of neurons coding the decision-related movement gradually increases over time (Gold and Shadlen, 2003; Huk and Shadlen, 2005; Roitman and Shadlen, 2002). The rate of increase is systematically related to the motion coherence so that strong evidence results in a faster increase than weak evidence. In the reaction time version of the task it appears that, when aligned to movement onset, neural activity reaches a critical level that is independent of motion coherence (see also Horwitz and Newsome, 2001; Kim and Shadlen, 1999, for similar signals in SC and in dorsolateral pre-frontal cortex).

These data can be modelled by assuming that LIP neurons integrate sensory evidence over time up to a criterion threshold, where evidence is the *difference* in the sensory response of pools of MT neurons coding the alternative directions used in the experiment (Ditterich, 2006b, 2006a; Mazurek et al., 2003). This variable is closely related to the optimal decision variable, namely the (log) likelihood ratio (Gold and Shadlen, 2001; Green and Swets, 1966). Human data from this paradigm are also successfully modelled under the assumption that the strength of sensory evidence affects the (mean) rate of evidence accumulation up to a decision threshold (Reddi et al., 2003).

Prior probability

The prior probability of an event or state is the probability of that event occurring, regardless of the momentary evidence. Consider the domain of medical diagnosis. A set of symptoms (evidence) may typically be attributed to various different possible underlying causes (hypotheses). Unless the evidence overwhelmingly points to one particular condition over any other, a sensible diagnosis takes into account how likely the various conditions are to occur in the first place. This idea is formalized in Bayes rule, which combines the current evidence (likelihood) with the prior probability of some event. In the present context, the question is whether the prior probability of a particular movement vector being required plays a role in saccadic decision making.

In this domain, a straightforward manipulation has been to vary target location (un)certainty. For instance, in a simple visually guided saccade task variation in the probability of the target appearing in one location results in a strong modulation of the saccade latency (Carpenter, 2004; Carpenter and Williams, 1995). Unsurprisingly, saccade latency increases with greater target uncertainty. Using LATER, the change in the reaction time distributions was best accounted for as a change in the separation between the starting point of accumulation and the threshold (Carpenter and Williams, 1995): increased target uncertainty results in an increase in this separation. Note that such a change may be brought about either by decreasing the starting point or increasing the threshold. However, in the context of a probabilistic interpretation of this kind of model, it is most natural to assume that variations in prior probability affect the starting point (see Fig. 23.2C). Saccade vectors that are unlikely to be called for will start off from a lower level, compared to movement programmes that are relatively more likely to be executed. It is distinctly possible that this modulation represents a purely local effect (Walthew and Gilchrist, 2006), in that every time one particular saccade (say leftward) is executed the starting point for that (left) programme is increased for the next trial. Over the course of a whole experiment then, this would result in a relatively decreased (mean) starting point for less likely saccade vectors.

Another way to vary target uncertainty is to manipulate the number of choice alternatives. Hick's law states that (manual) reaction time increases logarithmically with the number of choice alternatives (Hick, 1952). Hick's law has been observed with saccadic responses, provided that the task involves a transformation between the stimulus and saccadic response (e.g. antisaccades in Kveraga et al., 2002; mapping a colour cue to a location in K.-M. Lee et al., 2005). The latency distributions from K.-M. Lee et al. (2005) (where the number of alternatives varied from 1–8) were fit with the LATER model. These fits were—again—more consistent a change in the starting point of accumulation with varying numbers of alternatives.

Basso and Wurtz (1998, 1997) performed a series of similar experiments while recording from SC. Monkeys were presented with an array of objects arranged around a central fixation point. The size of the array ranged from 1–8. After a delay one of the items dimmed; this item was the saccade target. When the central fixation point extinguished the monkey was required to make the target-directed saccade. The critical interval in this paradigm is that between array onset and target specification. Build-up neurons in the intermediate layer of the SC showed a reduction in their activity as target uncertainty increased. Once the target was specified these neurons increased their activity more when target uncertainty was high, presumably to cover the extra ground needed to reach the common saccade trigger threshold. Indeed, the immediate, presaccadic burst of both build-up and burst neurons was not affected by target uncertainty. A similar modulation of activity may be seen in LIP neurons when a central cue signals which of two targets to saccade to and the prior probability of one or the response is varied (Platt and Glimcher, 1999).

Both modelling of behavioural results and neurophysiological evidence then suggest that effects of prior probability are mediated by varying the separation between the starting point of evidence integration and the decision criterion (see K.-M. Lee and Keller (2008) for tentative evidence for an effect of prior probability on the threshold of FEF visual-movement neurons). However, a recent study by Liston and Stone (2008) suggests that prior probability may also affect the sensory response that, presumably, forms the input into the oculomotor system. In this study, observers performed a two-AFC saccadic contrast discrimination task. A bias in the location of the higher contrast target influenced the saccadic decisions in a predictable fashion: choice was biased towards the more probable location and saccade latency was shorter. After completing the saccade a test disc appeared and observers were asked to indicate whether the previously fixated saccade target or the subsequent test stimulus was brighter. The perceptual decision task essentially probed the perceived contrast of the saccade target. If the bias induced by the prior probability variation affects the sensory response to the target, this should be manifest in the perceptual judgement. Indeed, Liston and Stone (2008) reported that increased estimates of contrast gain and internal noise for the more likely target location. These results are consistent with a multiplicative weighting mechanism that amplifies the noisy internal sensory response, before being transmitted to the oculomotor system. In the context of accumulating sensory evidence, this scheme is more consistent with an effect of prior probability on the rate of accumulation.

Finally, even in the absence of any real variation in the prior probability of certain locations becoming behaviourally relevant, humans (Anderson et al., 2008; Carpenter, 2001) and monkeys (Fecteau and Munoz, 2003) frequently develop idiosyncratic motor biases in that a particular response is favoured (e.g. a preference for successive movements in the same direction; Anderson et al., 2008). Such biases may be interpreted as internally generated, misguided estimates of prior probability and seem to be best accounted for in terms of an offset in the starting point of accumulation (Gold et al., 2008). Again, it is possible this offset is the result of a purely local mechanism that generates trial-by-trial adjustments of the starting point.

Reward

As with movements that are a priori more likely to be commanded, responses that are associated with larger expected rewards may also be expected to be weighted more heavily in the saccadic decision-making process. Indeed, the effect of reward magnitude on LIP activity is very similar to that of prior probability in the cued saccade paradigm of Platt and Glimcher (1999). Early activity (i.e. before specification of the movement target and the associated pre-motor ramp to threshold) is higher for neurons representing higher value choices, even when the prior probability of both responses is equal (see also Dorris and Glimcher, 2004).

These neurons also appear to be involved in tracking local variations in reward in a free-choice paradigm (Sugrue et al., 2004). In this paradigm the monkey is presented with two choice alternatives of different colours and is free to choose to look at either target. In blocks of 100–200 trials the response alternatives were associated with different rewards, which changed unpredictably. Behaviourally, the challenge is to match choice to the relative rewards. The monkey's performance was modelled by computing the expected relative reward from the different options, through leaky integration of the recent reward history (see also Corrado et al., 2005). This quantity, termed 'local fractional income', guides decision-making on the current trial. Importantly, LIP activity during the delay between the onset of the targets and a subsequent 'go' signal was correlated on a trial-by-trial basis with local fractional income: activity was higher for the option that was more generously rewarded in a relatively short window of recent choices. Interestingly, unlike in the cued saccade paradigm (Platt and Glimcher, 1999) this modulation evolved gradually over time during the delay period. That is, the LIP response to the onset of the two targets was independent of local fractional reward (perhaps because the reward was related to the colour of the peripheral target, rather than the location), but this dependency manifested itself gradually and lasted up to the onset of the saccade.

Reward-related modulations of neural activity can be found in a variety of brain areas (Sugrue et al., 2005), but in the context of saccadic decision-making the basal ganglia are a structure of particular interest. The basal ganglia are important for motor control in general. The caudate nucleus (CN) in the dorsal striatum and the substantia nigra pars reticulara (SNr) are involved in saccade generation. Briefly, the SNr tonically inhibits the SC motor map. For a saccade to occur the SC needs to be disinhibited, which is mediated by the inhibitory projection from CN to SNr (Hikosaka and Wurtz, 1989; Hikosaka et al., 2006). Activation of the CN, in turn, is achieved through cortical inputs from a variety of areas, including the FEF and LIP. The modulation of SC build-up neurons with prior probability reviewed above (Basso and Wurtz, 1998, 1997) appears to be preceded by a pause in SNr activity, the extent of which is also related to the level of target uncertainty (Basso and Wurtz, 2002).

In a similar vein, CN neurons are responsive to reward magnitude in that larger rewards trigger greater levels of CN activity (Lauwereyns et al., 2002). In a visually guided saccade task with unequal rewards associated with different target locations, the CN neurons coding 'richer' target locations showed elevated levels of activity before the target is presented (i.e. in the delay between fixation point onset and target presentation). Given the inhibitory connection between CN and SNr, it appears that the increase in CN activity would manifest itself as increased oculomotor readiness at the collicular level, similar to that seen in manipulations of prior probability. Indeed, the latency of saccades to the high-reward target location is typically reduced. It has been hypothesized that the reward-modulation of CN neurons is shaped through dopaminergic inputs into the CN that modulate the synaptic efficacy of the cortical inputs (Hikosaka et al., 2006). These dopamine neurons appear to encode a quantity related to the difference between predicted and obtained rewards (Hollerman and Schultz, 1998): a larger obtained reward than expected results in an increased response and a smaller than expected reward results in response suppression. As a result, these neurons may be regarded as computing a prediction error term that enables learning of the reward structure of an environment (Nakahara et al., 2004; Schultz, 1998).

These physiological data seem to point towards reward affecting the oculomotor readiness, which corresponds to the functional mechanism of the starting point of evidence accumulation. However, human behavioural evidence on this issue is scarce. The study reviewed in the previous section by Liston and Stone (2008) also included a manipulation of reward frequency to induce a saccadic motor bias. Like the variation in prior probability in that study, the bias in reward frequency associated with different locations affected the internal perceptual response, which a priori is more consistent with an effect on the rate of accumulation.

Conclusions

It should be noted that many of the reviewed studies on decision-related variables in the oculomotor system are not so much concerned with the saccadic system itself, but use the system in order to learn about more general principles of decision-making that may apply to more complex decision-problems and more complex patterns of motor behaviour. Nevertheless, what these studies show is that variables such as evidence, prior probability and (expected) reward are represented in neural mechanisms that play a role in saccade planning and generation. Moreover, the behavioural effects of these variables can be mapped onto functional mechanisms posited by decision-field and evidence integration models of saccadic decision-making. These models are based on the idea of accumulating sensory evidence up to a response threshold. Neurophysiological and behavioural work indicates that the (momentary) strength of sensory evidence acts upon the rate at which activity rises to the response threshold. Variations in prior probability and reward appear to act predominantly upon the starting level of accumulation, giving more likely and rewarding saccade targets a head-start in the race to threshold.

Acknowledgements

The author is supported by EPSRC fellowship EP/E054323/1. I thank Ray Klein and Petroc Sumner for their helpful comments on an earlier draft of this chapter.

References

Anderson, A.J., Yadav, H., and Carpenter, R.H.S. (2008). Directional prediction by the saccadic system. *Current Biology*, **18**, 614–618.

Arai, K. and Keller, E.L. (2005). A model of the saccade-generating system that accounts for trajectory variations produced by competing visual stimuli. *Biological Cybernetics*, **92**, 21–37.

Arai, K., Das, S., Keller, E.L., and Aiyoshi, E. (1999). A distributed model of the saccade system: simulations of temporally perturbed saccades using position and velocity feedback. *Neural Networks*, **12**, 1359–1375.

Basso, M.A. and Wurtz, R.H. (1997). Modulation of neuronal activity by target uncertainty. *Nature*, **389**, 66–69.

Basso, M.A. and Wurtz, R.H. (1998). Modulation of neuronal activity in superior colliculus by changes in target probability. *Journal of Neuroscience*, **18**, 7519–7534.

Basso, M.A. and Wurtz, R.H. (2002). Neuronal activity in substantia nigra pars reticulata during target selection. *Journal of Neuroscience*, **22**, 1883–1894.

Bichot, N.P., Thompson, K.G., Rao, S.C., and Schall, J.D. (2001). Reliability of macaque frontal eye field neurons signaling saccade targets during visual search. *Journal of Neuroscience*, **21**, 713–725.

Bogacz, R., Brown, E., Moehlis, J., Holmes, P., and Cohen, J.D. (2006). The physics of optimal decision making: A formal analysis of models of performance in two-alternative forced-choice tasks. *Psychological Review*, **113**, 700–765.

Britten, K.H., Shadlen, M.N., Newsome, W.T., and Movshon, J.A. (1992). The analysis of visual motion: A comparison of neuronal and psychophysical performance. *Journal of Neuroscience*, **12**, 4747–4765.

Brown, S.D. and Heathcote, A. (2005). A ballistic model of choice response time. *Psychological Review*, **112**, 117–128.

Brown, S.D. and Heathcote, A. J. (2008). The simplest complete model of choice reaction time: Linear ballistic accumulation. *Cognitive Psychology*, **57**, 153–178.

Carpenter, R.H.S. (2001). Express saccades: is bimodality a result of the order of stimulus presentation? *Vision Research*, **41**, 1145–1151.

Carpenter, R.H.S. (2004). Contrast, probability, and saccadic latency: Evidence for independence of detection and decision. *Current Biology*, **14**, 1576–1580.

Carpenter, R.H.S. and Williams, M.L.L. (1995). Neural computation of log likelihood in control of saccadic eye movements. *Nature*, **377**, 59–62.

Caspi, A., Beutter, B.R., and Eckstein, M.P. (2004). The time course of visual information accrual guiding eye movement decisions. *Proceedings of the National Academy of Sciences of the United States of America*, **101**, 13086–13090.

Corrado, G.S., Sugrue, L.P., Seung, H.S., and Newsome, W.T. (2005). Linear-Nonlinear-Poisson models of primate choice dynamic. *Journal of the Experimental Analysis of Behavior*, **84**, 581–617.

Ditterich, J. (2006a). Evidence for time-variant decision making. *European Journal of Neuroscience*, **24**, 3628–3641.

Ditterich, J. (2006b). Stochastic models of decisions about motion direction: Behavior and physiology. *Neural Networks*, **19**, 981–1012.

Ditterich, J., Mazurek, M.E., and Shadlen, M.N. (2003). Microstimulation of visual cortex affects the speed of perceptual decisions. *Nature Neuroscience*, **6**, 891–898.

Dorris, M.C. and Glimcher, P.W. (2004). Activity in posterior parietal cortex is correlated with the relative subjective desirability of action. *Neuron*, **44**, 365–378.

Erlhagen, W. and Schoner, G. (2002). Dynamic field theory of movement preparation. *Psychological Review*, **109**, 545–572.

Fecteau, J.H. and Munoz, D.P. (2003). Exploring the consequences of the previous trial. *Nature Reviews Neuroscience*, **4**, 435–443.

Fecteau, J.H. and Munoz, D.P. (2006). Salience, relevance, and firing: a priority map for target selection. *Trends in Cognitive Sciences*, **10**, 382–390.

Glimcher, P.W. (2003a). *Decisions, Uncertainty, and the Brain: The Science of Neuroeconomics*. Cambridge, MA: The MIT Press.

Glimcher, P.W. (2003b). The neurobiology of visual-saccadic decision making. *Annual Review of Neuroscience*, **26**, 133–179.

Gold, J.I. and Shadlen, M.N. (2000). Representation of a perceptual decision in developing oculomotor commands. *Nature*, **404**, 390–394.

Gold, J.I. and Shadlen, M.N. (2001). Neural computations that underlie decisions about sensory stimuli. *Trends in Cognitive Sciences*, **5**, 10–16.

Gold, J.I. and Shadlen, M.N. (2003). The influence of behavioral context on the representation of a perceptual decision in developing oculomotor commands. *Journal of Neuroscience*, **23**, 632–651.

Gold, J.I., Law, C.T., Connolly, P., and Bennur, S. (2008). The relative influences of priors and sensory evidence on an oculomotor decision variable during perceptual learning. *Journal of Neurophysiology*, **100**, 2653–2668.

Goossens, H. and Van Opstal, A.J. (2006). Dynamic ensemble coding of saccades in the monkey superior colliculus. *Journal of Neurophysiology*, **95**, 2326–2341.

Green, D.M. and Swets, J.A. (1966). *Signal Detection Theory and Psychophysics*. New York: Wiley.

Hick, W.E. (1952). On the rate of gain of information. *The Quarterly Journal of Experimental Psychology*, **4**, 11–26.

Hikosaka, O. and Wurtz, R.H. (1989). The basal ganglia. In R.H. Wurtz and M.E. Goldberg (Eds), *The neurobiology of saccadic eye movements* (pp. 257–282). Amsterdam: Elsevier.

Hikosaka, O., Nakamura, K., and Nakahara, H. (2006). Basal ganglia orient eyes to reward. *Journal of Neurophysiology*, **95**, 567–584.

Hollerman, J.R. and Schultz, W. (1998). Dopamine neurons report an error in the temporal prediction of reward during learning. *Nature Neuroscience*, **1**, 304–309.

Horwitz, G.D. and Newsome, W.T. (2001). Target selection for saccadic eye movements: Prelude activity in the superior colliculus during a direction-discrimination task. *Journal of Neurophysiology*, **86**, 2543–2558.

Huk, A.C. and Shadlen, M.N. (2005). Neural activity in macaque parietal cortex reflects temporal integration of visual motion signals during perceptual decision making. *Journal of Neuroscience*, **25**, 10420–10436.

Kim, J.N. and Shadlen, M.N. (1999). Neural correlates of a decision in the dorsolateral prefrontal cortex of the macaque. *Nature Neuroscience*, **2**, 176–185.

Kopecz, K. (1995). Saccadic reaction times in gap overlap paradigms: A model based on integration of intentional and visual information on neural, dynamic fields. *Vision Research*, **35**, 2911–2925.

Kopecz, K. and Schoner, G. (1995). Saccadic motor planning by integrating visual Information and pre-information on neural dynamic fields. *Biological Cybernetics*, **73**, 49–60.

Kveraga, K., Boucher, L., and Hughes, H.C. (2002). Saccades operate in violation of Hick's law. *Experimental Brain Research*, **146**, 307–314.

Laming, D.R.J. (1969). Subjective probability in choice-reaction time experiments. *Journal of Mathematical Psychology*, **6**, 81–120.

Lauwereyns, J., Watanabe, K., Coe, B., and Hikosaka, O. (2002). A neural correlate of response bias in monkey caudate nucleus. *Nature*, **418**, 413–417.

Leach, J.C.D. and Carpenter, R.H.S. (2001). Saccadic choice with asynchronous targets: evidence for independent randomisation. *Vision Research*, **41**, 3437–3445.

Lee, C.K., Rohrer, W.H., and Sparks, D.L. (1988). Population coding of saccadic eye movements by neurons in the superior colliculus. *Nature*, **332**, 357–360.

Lee, K.-M. and Keller, E.L. (2008). Neural activity in the frontal eye fields modulated by the number of alternatives in target choice. *Journal of Neuroscience*, **28**, 2242–2251.

Lee, K.-M., Keller, E.L., and Heinen, S.J. (2005). Properties of saccades generated as a choice response. *Experimental Brain Research*, **162**, 278–286.

Link, S.W. and Heath, R.A. (1975). A sequential theory of psychological discrimination. *Psychometrika*, **40**, 77–105.

Liston, D.B., and Stone, L.S. (2008). Effects of prior information and reward on oculomotor and perceptual choices. *Journal of Neuroscience*, **28**, 13866–13875.

Luce, D.R. (1986). *Response Times: Their Role in Inferring Elementary Mental Organization*. Oxford: Oxford University Press.

Ludwig, C.J.H. (2009). Temporal integration of sensory evidence for saccade target selection. *Vision research*, **49**, 2764–2773.

Ludwig, C.J.H., Gilchrist, I. D., and McSorley, E. (2004). The influence of spatial frequency and contrast on saccade latencies. *Vision Research*, **44**, 2597–2604.

Ludwig, C.J.H., Gilchrist, I.D., and McSorley, E. (2005). The remote distractor effect in saccade programming: channel interactions and lateral inhibition. *Vision Research*, **45**, 1177–1190.

Ludwig, C.J.H., Mildinhall, J.W., and Gilchrist, I.D. (2007). A population coding account for systematic variation in saccadic dead time. *Journal of Neurophysiology*, **97**, 795–805.

Ludwig, C.J.H., Gilchrist, I.D., McSorley, E., and Baddeley, R. J. (2005). The temporal impulse response underlying saccadic decisions. *Journal of Neuroscience*, **25**, 9907–9912.

Mazurek, M.E., Roitman, J.D., Ditterich, J., and Shadlen, M.N. (2003). A role for neural integrators in perceptual decision making. *Cerebral Cortex*, **13**, 1257–1269.

McIllwain, J.T. (1986). Point images in the visual system: new interest in an old idea. *Trends in NeuroScience*, **9**, 354–358.

McPeek, R.M., and Keller, E.L. (2002a). Saccade target selection in the superior colliculus during a visual search task. *Journal of Neurophysiology*, **88**, 2019–2034.

McPeek, R.M., and Keller, E.L. (2002b). Superior colliculus activity related to concurrent processing of saccade goals in a visual search task. *Journal of Neurophysiology*, **87**, 1805–1815.

McPeek, R.M., Han, J.H., and Keller, E.L. (2003). Competition between saccade goals in the superior colliculus produces saccade curvature. *Journal of Neurophysiology*, **89**, 2577–2590.

McSorley, E., Haggard, P., and Walker, R. (2006). Time course of oculomotor inhibition revealed by saccade trajectory modulation. *Journal of Neurophysiology*, **96**, 1420–1424.

Munoz, D.P. and Istvan, P.J. (1998). Lateral inhibitory interactions in the intermediate layers of the monkey superior colliculus. *Journal of Neurophysiology*, **79**, 1193–1209.

Nakahara, H., Itoh, H., Kawagoe, R., Takikawa, Y., and Hikosaka, O. (2004). Dopamine neurons can represent context-dependent prediction error. *Neuron*, **41**, 269–280.

Newsome, W.T., Britten, K.H., and Movshon, J.A. (1989). Neuronal correlates of a perceptual decision. *Nature*, **341**, 42–52.

Ottes, F., Van Gisbergen, J., and Eggermont, J. (1986). Visuomotor fields of the superior colliculus: A quantitative model. *Vision Research*, **26**, 857–873.

Palmer, J., Huk, A.C., and Shadlen, M.N. (2005). The effect of stimulus strength on the speed and accuracy of a perceptual decision. *Journal of Vision*, **5**, 376–404.

Platt, M.L. and Glimcher, P.W. (1999). Neural correlates of decision variables in parietal cortex. *Nature*, **400**, 233–238.

Ratcliff, R. (1978). Theory of memory retrieval. *Psychological Review*, **85**, 59–108.

Ratcliff, R. and Rouder, J.N. (1998). Modeling response times for two-choice decisions. *Psychological Science*, **9**, 347–356.

Ratcliff, R. and Smith, P.L. (2004). A comparison of sequential sampling models for two-choice reaction time. *Psychological Review*, **111**, 333–367.

Reddi, B.A.J., Asrress, K.N., and Carpenter, R.H.S. (2003). Accuracy, information, and response time in a saccadic decision task. *Journal of Neurophysiology*, **90**, 3538–3546.

Roitman, J.D. and Shadlen, M.N. (2002). Response of neurons in the lateral intraparietal area during a combined visual discrimination reaction time task. *Journal of Neuroscience*, **22**, 9475–9489.

Schall, J.D., Hanes, D.P., Thompson, K.G., and King, D.J. (1995). Saccade target selection in frontal eye field of macaque 1: Visual and premovement activation. *Journal of Neuroscience*, **15**, 6905–6918.

Schall, J.D. and Thompson, K.G. (1999). Neural selection and control of visually guided eye movements. *Annual Review of Neuroscience*, **22**, 241–259.

Schultz, W. (1998). Predictive reward signal of dopamine neurons. *Journal of Neurophysiology*, **80**, 1–27.

Smith, P.L. and Ratcliff, R. (2004). Psychology and neurobiology of simple decisions. *Trends in Neurosciences*, **27**, 161–168.

Sugrue, L.P., Corrado, G.S., and Newsome, W.T. (2004). Matching behavior and the representation of value in the parietal cortex. *Science*, **304**, 1782–1787.

Sugrue, L.P., Corrado, G.S., and Newsome, W.T. (2005). Choosing the greater of two goods: Neural currencies for valuation and decision making. *Nature Reviews Neuroscience*, **6**, 363–375.

Thompson, K.G., Bichot, N.P., and Sato, T.R. (2005). Frontal eye field activity before visual search errors reveals the integration of bottom-up and top-down salience. *Journal of Neurophysiology*, **93**, 337–351.

Trappenberg, T.P., Dorris, M.C., Munoz, D.P., and Klein, R.M. (2001). A model of saccade initiation based on the competitive integration of exogenous and endogenous signals in the superior colliculus. *Journal of Cognitive Neuroscience*, **13**, 256–271.

Usher, M. and McClelland, J.L. (2001). The time course of perceptual choice: The leaky, competing accumulator model. *Psychological Review*, **108**, 550–592.

Vickers, D. (1970). Evidence for an accumulator model of psychophysical discrimination. *Ergonomics*, **13**, 37–58.

Walthew, C. and Gilchrist, I.D. (2006). Target location probability effects in visual search: An effect of sequential dependencies. *Journal of Experimental Psychology Human Perception and Performance*, **32**, 1294–1301.

Wang, X.J. (2002). Probabilistic decision making by slow reverberation in cortical circuits. *Neuron*, **36**, 955–968.

White, B.J., Kerzel, D., and Gegenfurtner, K.R. (2006). The spatio-temporal tuning of the mechanisms in the control of saccadic eye movements. *Vision Research*, **46**, 3886–3897.

Wilimzig, C., Schneider, S., and Schoener, G. (2006). The time course of saccadic decision making: Dynamic field theory. *Neural Networks*, **19**, 1059–1074.

Wong, K.F. and Wang, X.J. (2006). A recurrent network mechanism of time integration in perceptual decisions. *Journal of Neuroscience*, **26**, 1314–1328.

CHAPTER 24

Models of overt attention

Wilson S. Geisler and Lawrence K. Cormack

Abstract

Formal models of overt attention have played an important role in motivating and interpreting studies of visual search and other tasks. This chapter briefly summarizes some general principles of attention, some general distinctions between models of overt attention, and some examples of existing models of overt attention in visual search, reading, free viewing, and interactive behaviours. Although many of these models have provided new insight into the factors that contribute to task performance, many are still in a formative stage. In the future, the most useful models will likely be those that take images as input, produce eye movements and decisions as output, apply to well-defined tasks, and explicitly represent the variation in early visual processing across the visual field.

Introduction

Humans and most other animals perform a wide array of tasks including navigating through the environment and manipulating objects. These, in turn, involve subtasks such as determining shapes and distances of surfaces, recognizing objects, etc. Each specific task depends on particular kinds of information from the immediate environment and from memory, on particular kinds of neural computations, and on particular kinds of motor control signals. Attention research is concerned with understanding the brain mechanisms that actively select the specific task-relevant information, neural computations, and motor control signals from among the myriad possibilities.

Attention research is enormously diverse and hence there is no entirely satisfactory definition of what would constitute an attention mechanism. The requirement of selectivity alone is not sufficient because every part of the nervous system is selective (e.g. the photoreceptors are selective to light and the hair cells to sound). What is usually meant by an attention mechanism is a neural mechanism that can perform (or modulate) selection dynamically, in a task dependent way, often under the control of learned cues or instructions. In other words, attention mechanisms are conceptualized as mechanisms that can flexibly control the flow of information from the environment to the organism and through the organism's various stages of neural processing.

This chapter concerns models of *overt attention*. An overt attention mechanism selects specific kinds of neural processing by physically moving the sensory organs. For example, the visual system has finer spatial neural processing at the centre of gaze (fovea) and the auditory system has finer spatial neural processing along the midline between the two ears. Thus, the brain has attention mechanisms that can dynamically select where to direct the high resolution circuits of the visual and auditory systems. *Covert attention* concerns attention mechanisms that do not involve explicit

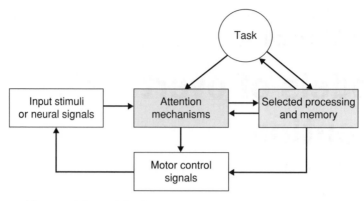

Fig. 24.1 General framework for models of overt attention.

movement of the sensory organs. Thus, an obvious advantage of modelling overt attention is that it is possible to test the models by measuring where the sensory organs are directed and hence where the organism has decided to apply (or not apply) its special processing. Currently, this is most commonly done by tracking the orientation of the eyes while a subject, whose head is held still, performs a visual search task on a computer monitor.

Most models of attention can be subsumed under a general framework such as the one in Fig. 24.1. A given task activates attention mechanisms as well as certain processing mechanisms and memory systems. The attention mechanisms select input signals or select specific processing to be applied to the input signals. Conversely, the attention mechanisms may be affected by the input signals (bottom-up effects) or by the output of the selected processing and memory systems (top-down effects). Overt attention is implemented by modulating motor-control signals (e.g. eye movement or head movement signals). Of course, there are mechanisms, such as vestibulo-ocular reflexes, that modulate the motor control signals but would generally not be considered attention mechanisms.

Many specific models of overt attention have been proposed in the literature, and thus it is not possible here to mention more than a representative subset. This chapter emphasizes quantitative models of performance in visual tasks involving eye movements. However, before discussing specific models we briefly list a few general principles of selective attention that are important to keep in mind and briefly describe a few general distinctions between overt attention models.

Some general principles of attention

Attention is required for efficient performance in almost all tasks, independent of any capacity limitations in the selected neural processing

The point here is simply that essentially all tasks involve active selection of neural processing. It is often suggested or implied in the attention literature that attention mechanisms exist because of limited neural processing resources, and thus that the purpose of attention is to allocate these precious resources in the best way possible. While this is sometimes true (e.g. directing the fovea to regions of interest), it is far from given. For example, consider the task of finding a target that may be at one of a few possible locations in a complex background. Efficient performance requires an attention mechanism that selects features from the possible locations and suppresses features from irrelevant locations, because features from irrelevant locations can lead to false detections of the target and potentially other pattern recognition problems. Such an attention mechanism is critical whether or not there is some capacity limitation in how many selected clusters of features can be simultaneously matched against a stored representation of the target.

The observation of less than perfect performance in a task does not automatically imply limitations in the attention mechanisms or in the capacity of the selected processing

Often, especially in natural tasks, the requirements of the task and the randomness and complexity of stimuli (or their representations in the early sensory pathways) make perfect performance impossible. Sometimes computational analysis, such as derivation of Bayesian optimal estimators or decision rules (i.e. ideal observers), can help determine the baseline performance that would be attainable with perfect attention and selected processing. This can help identify what aspects of performance cannot be explained by the task requirements and the properties of the input signals.

The flexibility, precision, and speed of an attention mechanism may each be limited

In addition to the effects of the task requirements and stimuli, performance may be limited by the properties of the relevant attention mechanisms. For example, an attention mechanism may not be able to select or suppress information from arbitrary spatial regions or along arbitrary feature dimensions. For overt attention, the relevant motor systems themselves will place upper bounds on all three of these aspects.

The amount or complexity of selected inputs may exceed the capacity of selected neural processing

Even if an attention mechanism is able to isolate information from appropriate regions and along appropriate feature dimensions, the selected neural processing may not be able to optimally process that information. Returning to the example above, an attention mechanism may be able to simultaneously select features from all relevant potential target regions and suppress all irrelevant features, but not be able to process in parallel (for target recognition) the features from all the selected locations.

Thus, in general, task performance is limited by task requirements and stimuli, and it may be limited by the flexibility, precision, or speed of the selective attention mechanisms, by the capacity or precision of the selected neural processing, or some combination thereof. Which of these factors dominates depends on the particular task and stimuli. Quantitative models of attention can play an important role in determining which factors are dominant in a given case and in determining the details of specific attention and selected-processing mechanisms.

Some general distinctions between models of overt attention

Strongly-specified versus weakly-specified tasks

Most models of overt attention are proposed for a specific kind of task. Some models are proposed for tasks with well-defined goals such as visual search for a specific target whereas other models are proposed for tasks with poorly-defined goals such as free viewing of natural images. Both kinds of task arise under natural conditions and are worthy of study. An advantage of a strongly-specified task is that it is possible to determine objectively how well the organism is performing and hence potentially evaluate the efficiency of the attention mechanisms. In a weakly-specified task, an organism probably has one or more specific goals, but exactly what they are is more hidden from the experimenter and is likely to be more variable, both within and across experiments.

Explicit versus implicit representation of the variable-resolution sensory system

In most natural tasks, the primary reason for moving the sensory organs (e.g. the eyes) is to bring the high resolution circuits onto stimuli of interest. For example, if the pinnae (outer ears) of a dog were structured to provide uniform sensitivity in all directions, there would be no need for the dog to be able to move its pinnae and, hence, no overt attention. Obviously, the same argument applies to the foveated nature of the human visual system; nonetheless, many models of overt visual attention do not explicitly represent the variable resolution of the sensory system. Explicit representation is not essential for predicting performance in some circumstances but, obviously, any model of overt attention must correctly specify the input and embody the reason for overt attention in the first place, both of which are accomplished by incorporating an appropriate foveated model of early visual processing (and a moment's reflection should confirm that an appropriate foveated model of early visual processing is also essential for models of covert attention).

Optimal versus suboptimal mechanisms

Traditionally, models of attention have been directed at predicting the organism's performance in specific tasks. More recently, there have also been efforts to develop normative (ideal observer) models. The goal of these models is to determine how an optimal attention mechanism should work and how well it would perform in the task. These models play an important role because they rigorously reveal the computational requirements of the task, they provide an appropriate baseline to compare with real performance and with measured neural responses, and they provide principled hypotheses for the underlying attention and selected-processing mechanisms.

Motor movements versus task performance

Models of overt attention also vary in what aspects of performance they predict. Some are designed to predict only the overt motor movements in a task (e.g. the patterns of eye movements), some only the performance speed (time to task completion), some only the performance accuracy, and some all three aspects (which is the ultimate goal of course). These differences can make it difficult to compare and test models.

Information-processing versus neurophysiological models

In recent years there has been much progress in understanding the neurophysiology and functional anatomy of attention mechanisms in the mammalian nervous system. The overall picture that emerges is of a heavily interconnected cortical network that relies on V1 for its primary (but not only) input, and the superior colliculus (SC) via the frontal eye fields (FEFs) for its primary (but not only) output. Subsequent to V1, the information forks into two streams. One is the ventral stream that is retinotopic but largely concerned with the identification of objects potentially relevant for a given task, and the other is the dorsal stream concerned with movement and object location, though there is also some sensitivity to form. The apexes of these pathways (that is, the anteriormost unarguably 'visual' areas of the two forks) are heavily interconnected, presumably to bind objects of interest with potential movement commands via their shared retinotopic representations. These areas also project to (and are heavily innervated by) the FEF, which represents the first stage in the final common pathway required for normal overt attention to occur. In addition to serving as an output stage, however, the FEF is heavily interconnected with both the ventral and dorsal visual processing streams, making it likely that it is a very dynamic component of a larger cortical network that actually embodies the purported 'salience map'. Additional interconnections with other cortical areas are probably responsible for learning, memory, and switching between different tasks requiring overt attention, as well as the more visceral and emotional factors that contribute in certain circumstances. These studies have led to quantitative models of how attention affects neural activity in various brain areas (for a review see Reynolds and Chelazzi, 2004), and informed the development of quantitative information-processing models of task performance, which is our focus here.

Tasks

Overt attention mechanisms are engaged in most natural and laboratory tasks, and thus there is no obvious taxonomy of overt-attention tasks, and no limit to the range of tasks that could be modelled in the context of studying the mechanisms of overt attention. Here, we focus on some well-known classes of overt attention task for which there has been some attempt to develop formal quantitative models. These include visual search tasks, visual recognition tasks (reading and shape recognition), free viewing tasks, and visual-motor tasks.

Visual search

Using the eyes to actively search the environment for specific objects or classes of object is a central subtask in most natural tasks performed by humans and nonhuman primates. Thus, not surprisingly, visual search is the most studied and modelled overt-attention task. In a common form of visual search task, a single target (known to the subject) is randomly located within a display having a well-defined search region that contains some sort of complex background (e.g. a texture of distracter objects, a texture of filtered or unfiltered noise, or a natural image). The subject's task is to locate the target as rapidly as possible. (Of course, real world search tasks can be much more complicated, e.g. search for 'human-made objects' or 'anything unusual'.)

A number of overt visual search models are based on the concept of a 'conspicuity area', which is defined to be the spatial region around the centre of gaze (assumed to be the centre of the fovea) where the target can be detected or identified in the background, within a single 'glimpse' (Bloomfield, 1972; Engel, 1971; 1977; Geisler and Chou, 1995; Toet et al., 1998; 2000).[1] The conspicuity area can vary dramatically depending on the specific target and background, from a fraction of a degree to many degrees of visual angle across. An example conspicuity area measured by Engel (1971) is shown in Fig. 24.2A.

Intuitively, the smaller the conspicuity area, the longer it should take for the subject to find the target, and indeed there is a strong correlation between search time and conspicuity area for simple targets in texture backgrounds (Geisler and Chou, 1995) and for real targets in natural images (Toet et al., 1998; Fig. 24.2B, C). This implies that the variable resolution of the visual system has a profound affect on search performance and that accurate modelling of target visibility as a function of retinal location is essential for developing general models of visual search in laboratory and natural conditions.

The simplest models of visual search based on the concept of conspicuity area postulate a strong top-down attention mechanism that selects fixation locations primarily on the basis of covering the search area rather than being driven by features in the periphery (Bloomfield, 1972; Engel, 1977; Geisler and Chou, 1995). In these models, feature detection, feature interaction (e.g. masking and crowding), and covert attention can affect the conspicuity area, but do not guide the fixation selection per se. Rather fixation selection is modelled as a random draw of a two-dimensional location either with or without replacement. If the target happens to fall into the conspicuity area it is detected and the search ends; otherwise the search continues. These random-fixation models can (with certain parameter values) predict approximately the relationship between conspicuity area and search time. However, models in this family that attempt to predict search times directly from images using a model of the conspicuity area are not yet very accurate on natural images (e.g. see Toet et al., 2000). Also, these models are not designed to (and do not adequately) predict eye movement statistics in visual search. There appear to be three major factors contributing to the shortcomings

---

[1] Although there has not been a consistent definition of what constitutes a glimpse, a sensible one is a period of retinal stimulation, with stable fixation, that is somewhat less than the average fixation duration in the search task (e.g., 250 ms).

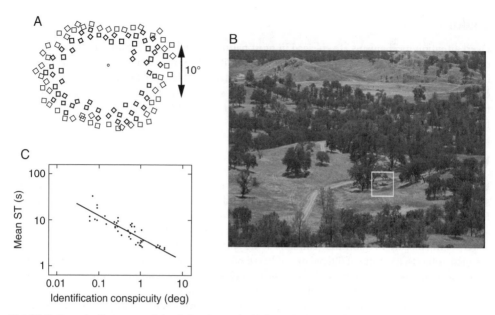

Fig. 24.2 Conspicuity-area models of visual search. A) Conspicuity area for a box target in random-line backgrounds. The bold boxes represent locations where the box could be detected in a random-line background, the thin boxes where it could not, with fixation at the small circle. The conspicuity area is the boundary between bold and thin boxes. Reprinted from *Vision Research*, **11**(6) F.L. Engel, Visual conspicuity, directed attention and retinal locus, pp. 563–575, Copyright (1971), with permission from Elsevier. B) Natural image containing vehicle target (in white box). C) Mean search time (for 60 subjects) as function of the radius of the conspicuity area (the average for two subjects). Reprinted from: A. Toet, F.L. Kooi, P. Bijl and J.M. Valeton, Visual conspicuity determines human target acquisition performance, *Optical Engineering*, **37**, © 1998.

of these models: 1) inadequate specification of the conspicuity area (or more generally of target detectability as a function of retinal position and background context), 2) no role for peripheral features in guiding fixation selection, and 3) no role for prior knowledge in guiding fixation selection (other than the confining of fixations to image regions where the target could be located or to select fixation locations without replacement).

In another general class of search model, the search process is driven largely by feature properties detected during the course of the search (Itti and Koch, 2000; Pomplun et al., 2003; Rao et al., 2002; Triesman and Gelade, 1980; Wolfe, 1994, 2007; Zelinsky, 2008). Strictly speaking, some of these models (e.g. Triesman and Gelade, 1980; Wolfe, 1994, 2007) were developed for covert search. They are often applied, however, to search tasks where reaction times are on the order of 500–2000 ms, which is sufficient time for saccadic eye movements, and thus they can and should be compared (in these tasks) with overt search models. There is a great deal of evidence demonstrating that eye movements in visual search tasks tend to be directed toward image locations containing features similar to those of the search target (Findlay, 1997; Motter and Belky, 1998), supporting the general notion of top-down, feature-based guidance in visual search (Wolfe 1994, 2007). For example, Fig. 24.3A shows the sequence of fixations of a monkey who is searching for a solid black bar that is tilted to the left (Motter and Belky, 1998). The fixations tend to occur at locations where the colour (black) matches that of the target. Similar results are obtained for search in more complex naturalistic backgrounds of Gaussian noise having the amplitude spectrum of natural images (i.e. $1/f$ noise). The maps at the bottom of Fig. 24.3B show the average features in the naturalistic noise backgrounds that tend to attract fixations in search tasks where the targets are low contrast versions of the patterns shown above the maps (Rajashekar et al., 2006). These maps (classification images) were obtained by

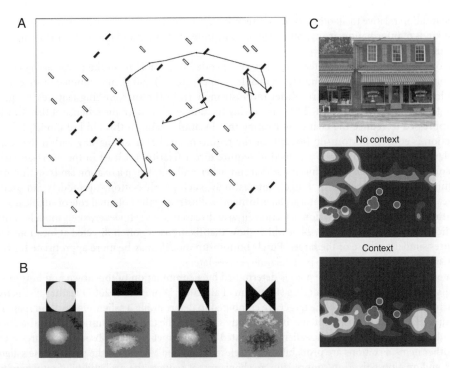

Fig. 24.3 Effect of feature properties and context on fixation selection during visual search. A) Sequence of fixations by a monkey searching for a solid black bar that is titled to the left. Reprinted from *Vision Research*, **38**(12), B.C. Motter and E.J. Belky, The guidance of eye movements during active visual search, pp. 1805–1815, Copyright (1998), with permission from Elsevier. B) Classification images (below) obtained by averaging the background noise at all the fixation locations of a human searching for targets (above) in a Gaussian noise background having an amplitude spectrum that falls inversely with spatial frequency. Rajashekar, U., Bovik, A.C., and Cormack, L. K. (2006). Visual search in noise: revealing the influence of structural cues by gaze-contingent classification image analysis. *Journal of Vision*, **6**, 379–386. Reproduced with permission by the Association for Research in Vision and Ophthalmology. C) Comparison of salience maps that do and do not take scene context into account. The circles are human fixations recorded when the task is to search for people in the street scene at the top. (Adapted from Torralba et al. 2006).

averaging the background noise across all fixations that were not on the target location. If fixations were not being directed at task-relevant features on a substantial proportion of saccades, then these maps would be unstructured. There is also evidence that local features that differ strongly from the features that surround them can attract fixations in free-viewing tasks, suggesting that under some circumstances bottom-up (i.e. non-task-specific), feature-based mechanisms may contribute to fixation selection in visual search (Ludwig and Gilchrist, 2002; Theeuwes et al., 1998).

The above findings are clearly not predicted by the random-fixation models that emphasize the role of a conspicuity area. Of course, it is possible that a random-fixation model that accurately models the conspicuity area could still be of practical value in predicting search time and accuracy, even if does not predict the correct patterns of eye movements.

Most models that emphasize the role of feature properties in guiding eye movements during visual search are structured around the intuitive concept of a 'salience map' (Koch and Ullman, 1985), which represents the instantaneous attractiveness of each possible fixation location. The salience map is updated over time as information is collected. If the salience becomes sufficiently high at some location relative to all other locations, then the eye is directed to that location. Models differ in what kinds of information are hypothesized to contribute to the map and in how the map is updated over time.

In one type of model, local feature maps are encoded in parallel from the image along certain stimulus dimensions (e.g. orientation, spatial frequency, colour) and then combined in such a way that locations where the features differ more strongly from the surrounding features are given stronger salience (Itti and Koch, 2000). Following fixation at a location, the salience at that location is suppressed to reduce the chance of fixating that location again. In this kind of model, fixation selection is entirely bottom-up (except for the requirement that fixations stay within the search display). Target recognition is assumed to require direct fixation (at least in the overt-attention versions of these models), and thus the search ends when and only when a fixation lands on the target (within some predefined error range). Interestingly, such purely bottom-up models can predict some qualitative aspects of visual search performance, illustrating the potential role of simple feature contrasts in determining fixation selection in visual search tasks. However, such models cannot predict results like those in Fig. 24.3, which show that fixations are often directed at locations with features similar to those of the target. Purely bottom-up models may be more appropriate for free-viewing tasks, where there is no particular target (see later).

In other models, the salience map is determined by a combination of top-down and bottom-up inputs. In the 'guided search' models (Pomplun et al., 2003; Wolfe 1994, 2007) feature distinctive-ness and feature similarity to the target are combined in determining a salience/activation map. For example, if a subset of 'display items' is sufficiently similar to the target and sufficiently distinct from the other display items, then the salience is boosted for the target-similar subset and suppressed for the other items. Fixations are probabilistically selected ('guided') based on the peaks of the salience map, and on a post-fixation suppression mechanism that reduces the probability of returning to a location after it has been fixated. Target recognition occurs (in the overt versions of these models) only if the fixation lands on the target or nearer to the target than any other item (Pomplun et al., 2003). Importantly, for determining the saliency map, the feature similarity is only computed for a very limited set of simple encoding dimensions such as orientation and 'colour' (Triesman and Gelade, 1980). With appropriate parameters, these models can qualitatively account for a range of search results obtained with simple displays (e.g. search patterns like those in Fig. 24.3A). However, the current versions of the models are limited because display items and feature dimensions are defined in a relatively simplistic way that limits generalization across experiments and prevents application to natural or naturalistic images. Crucially, they are not 'pixels-in/behaviour-out', so their predictive power is very limited. For example, these models are not designed to predict search in naturalistic noise backgrounds and hence cannot generate predictions that could be compared with the classification images in Fig. 24.3B.

More complete feature-based models of visual search take images as input and generate predicted fixation sequences (Rao et al., 2002; Zelinsky, 2008). Like Itti and Koch (2000), they generate a sali-ence map from feature maps obtained by filtering the input image along various dimensions at vari-ous scales; however, the salience at an image location is determined by the correlation between the feature values at that location and those defining the search target. Unlike the guided-search models, the salience map is not restricted to a small set of encoding dimensions. An important property of these models is that fixations are selected on the basis of a weighted average of the salience map (see also, Pomplun et al., 2003). This property is based on evidence that humans often fixate locations that are at the approximate 'centre-of-gravity' of possible target locations rather than directly at a specific target location (Findlay, 1987; He and Kowler, 1989; Zelinsky et al., 1997). Recent mathe-matical analyses show that similar fixation selection strategies are consistent with optimal search performance (Najemnik and Geisler, 2005, 2008, 2009). This behaviour may seem counterintuitive, but if two targets are similar and separated by some amount, less information might be gained by putting the central fovea on one target and relegating the other to the periphery than if the fovea is placed between them, thus affording at least an intermediate resolution of processing to both targets. The early model (Rao et al., 2002) has only been explored for a limited range of search tasks and it includes an unrealistic assumption about the role of course-to-fine spatial processing on fixation selection. The more recent version (Zelinsky, 2008) is more elaborate and realistic, and has been tested against a wider range of search tasks.

The models of visual search described so far have evolved in an effort to predict behavioural data in visual search tasks and to be roughly consistent with certain neurophysiological properties of the primate visual system. A conceptually different approach is to first ask: What kind of overt attention mechanism would a rational (optimal) organism—an ideal observer—use in search tasks, given the properties of natural stimuli and the properties of its sensory and motor systems? The answer to this question (if it can be obtained) can then provide a rigorous basis for formulating and testing more principled models of overt attention. Bayesian statistical decision theory provides a proper theoretical framework for addressing this question, and hence there have been recent attempts to develop Bayesian models of visual search (Najemnik and Geisler, 2005, 2008, 2009; Torralba, 2003; Torralba et al., 2006; Vincent et al., 2009). These models have their roots in signal detection theory (Green and Swets, 1968) and in applications of signal detection theory to covert visual search (e.g. Eckstein, 1998; Eckstein et al., 2001; Palmer et al., 2000; Vincent et al., 2009).

Torralba and colleagues (Torralba, 2003; Torralba et al., 2006) developed a Bayesian model in order to understand how a rational observer would combine natural scene statistics and scene context information when searching for objects. The structure of the model is represented by the following formula, which gives the posterior probability that the target object is present at image location x, given the feature values $F(x)$ at that location, and the global features values of the scene G (i.e. the context):

$$p\big(X = x | F(x), G\big) = \frac{1}{p\big(F(x) | G\big)} p\big(X = x | G\big) p\big(F(x) | X = x, G\big) \tag{1}$$

where X is the (random) location of a target object. This formula follows directly from Bayes' rule and other rules of conditional probability. (This version of the formula is equivalent to the one in Torralba et al. if we let $X = \varnothing$ represent the event of no target object in the scene.) The key assumption of the Torralba et al. model is that global scene features and local features are encoded rapidly in parallel when a scene is presented, and that together they define a salience map defined by the first two terms on the right side of equation (1), which are estimated from a statistical analysis of natural scenes:

$$s(x) = \frac{1}{p\big(F(x) | G\big)} p\big(X = x | G\big) \tag{2}$$

The global scene features G determine what kind of scene is being viewed (e.g. a forest scene, a city street scene, an office scene). Thus, the first term in equation (2) asserts that the more unlikely the encoded features at a location, given the type of scene, then the greater the salience. This is similar to the bottom-up definition of salience described earlier. The middle panel of Fig. 24.3C shows a salience map obtained with this component alone for the street scene in the upper panel. The second term asserts that the more likely a target location, given the type of scene, the greater the salience. This term represents the main effect of scene context. The lower panel in Fig. 24.3C shows the salience map obtained with both terms, for the case where the global context is a street scene and people are the targets. In agreement with intuition, the salient locations are now restricted to the sidewalk/ street level where people are most likely to be located. (For simplicity we do not show here how salience is updated across fixations.) The third term in equation (1) is the likelihood of the features at a location given that the target object is at that location in the scene with global features G. This is the object recognition component of a rational observer's search strategy, and Torralba et al. assume this component requires fixation on the location of interest. Thus, in the model, fixation locations are based on the salience map, and local recognition processing occurs during each fixation.

To implement this model, Torralba et al. start with feature maps similar to those of Itti and Koch (2000). These maps are used both for object recognition and for estimating the kind of scene being viewed. To estimate the kind of scene, the magnitudes of the feature map values are pooled into a small vector of global feature values. A classifier, trained on a large set of natural images, then takes these values as input and returns an estimate of the kind of scene.

The circles in Fig. 24.3c show human fixation locations when searching for people in the street scene. This example and many others demonstrate the importance of global context information for optimizing visual search performance and they demonstrate that humans make use of the context information.

While conceptually very similar (in that they are captured by equation (1)), the Bayesian models of visual search explored by Najemnik and Geisler (2005, 2008, 2009) differ from that of Torralba et al. in several important ways. The first major difference is that they consider the performance of a full Bayesian ideal observer. In other words, they consider a model where all three terms in equation (1), including the recognition process, are computed in parallel during a fixation. This means, in effect, that the 'salience map' is actually a surface giving the posterior probability (following each fixation) that the target is at each scene location:

$$s(x) = p(X = x|\mathbf{F}, G) \tag{3}$$

In equation (3), $F(x)$ has been replaced by $\mathbf{F} = \langle F(1), F(2), 1 \rangle$, where the integers are simply indexes to all possible locations (i.e. pixels), because in some search tasks the posterior probability at a given location depends on the features encoded at multiple locations.

The second major difference is that the variation in visual processing with retinal location is represented explicitly. In terms of equation (3), this means that the features encoded from the scene depend on both the content of the scene and the current fixation location x_0; in other words, $\mathbf{F}$ in equation (3) is replaced by $\mathbf{F}(x_0)$, which just means that now the set of feature values at each location are computed after accounting for the perceptual resolution of the image at that location given fixation at x_0. This adds a great deal of computational complexity to the model, but is essential because the variation in visual processing with retinal location is the very reason eye movements are made (and thus the reason that a chapter on overt attention exists), and because the variation has a huge effect on search performance in many tasks (e.g. see Figs. 24.2C and 24.4A, B). None of the models described above attempt to explicitly represent the effects of retinal location, except for the conspicuity-area models and the models of Zelinsky (2008) and Rajashekar et al. (2008), nor do they have a sufficient representation for determining what would be optimal search strategies and optimal search performance.

The local image features extracted by the visual system limit how detectable (salient) a target is in its background, and thus ultimately, a general model of visual search should include a model for the feature information extracted at each retinal location. Unfortunately, there remains much uncertainty about low-level feature encoding in the visual system as a function of retinal location. Najemnik and Geisler avoided specifying this component of the model by directly measuring the detectability of the target in the search backgrounds (in their case $1/f$ noise) at various retinal locations, in a two-alternative forced choice task, where the target location was cued on each trial. This allowed them to focus on the selective attention mechanisms and eliminate all free parameters. Figure 24.4A shows the measured detectability as function of retinal eccentricity (averaged across direction from the fovea) for low and high contrast backgrounds, with the target contrast set so the detectability was the same in the centre of the fovea ($d' = 3$). The widths of these functions at some criterion height would correspond to the classic definition of a conspicuity area (also note, perhaps surprisingly, that these would be larger at higher noise contrasts). However, it turns out that the shape of the whole distribution, especially the tails of the distribution, are important for determining optimal search performance and for understanding human search performance.

The third major difference is that they considered various non-optimal and optimal strategies for fixation selection. As we have seen, a common fixation selection strategy proposed by many visual search models is to fixate the location with the highest value in the salience map, which is not what

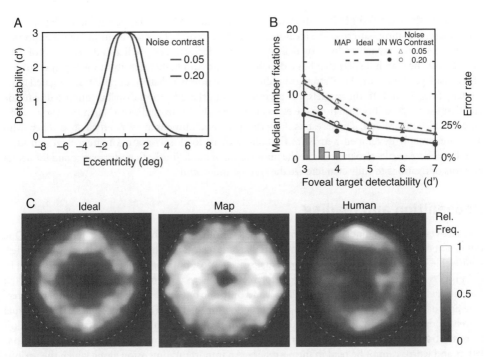

Fig. 24.4 Ideal and human visual search in naturalistic ($1/f$) noise backgrounds. A) Target detectability as a function of retinal eccentricity for two contrast levels of the noise background (target contrast was set to produce the same detectability at the point of gaze). B) Data and curves show the median number of fixations (left axis) to find a target randomly located in noise backgrounds of two different contrasts, as a function of the target detectability in the fovea. Grey bars show error rates (right axis) for model searchers and white bars for the human searchers. C) Distribution of fixation locations across all search trials for model and human searchers, with the first fixation at the centre of the display excluded. Reprinted by permission from Macmillan Publishers Ltd: *Nature*, Optimal eye movement strategies in visual search, J. Najemnik and W.S. Geisler, **434**(7031), copyright 2005.

the ideal observer would do (although some authors have assumed otherwise). This non-optimal strategy corresponds to fixating the location with the maximum a posteriori (MAP) probability after the previous fixation (the location x that maximizes the right side of equation (3)). The dashed curves in Fig. 24.4B show the predicted number of fixations to find a target (randomly located in a background of $1/f$ noise), as a function of the detectability of the target in the centre of the fovea, for two levels of background noise contrast.

The optimal strategy, however, is to fixate the location where the probability of identifying the target location will be greatest *after* the eye movement is made. In other words, the optimal eye movement is the one that will produce the biggest gain in information about where the target is located, which is not necessarily the single most likely target location. The solid curves show the performance of the ideal fixation selection strategy, and it is only slightly better than the MAP strategy. The symbols show the performance of two practised observers. Human performance is similar to the parameter free predictions of the ideal and MAP searchers. (The random fixation selection strategies of the conspicuity area models are completely inadequate because they are not capable of reaching human performance levels.) Notice the importance of the detectability functions—the modest differences in the functions shown in Fig. 24.4A produce big differences in the search performance of the ideal, MAP, and human searchers.

Although the ideal and MAP fixation selection strategies yield similar performance they predict very different fixation patterns. The ideal strategy makes 'centre of gravity fixations' when appropriate; the MAP strategy never does (by definition). The ideal strategy predicts a distribution of fixations across the search display that has a doughnut shape with higher density at the top and bottom of the display, whereas the MAP strategy predicts a more uniform distribution that is elongated horizontally (Fig. 24.4C). In the models, the asymmetries in these fixation distributions are due to the fact that the detectability functions are elongated along the horizontal axis (Najemnik and Geisler, 2008; see also Fig. 24.2A). These results show that practised humans are very efficient searchers who have presumably developed heuristics that allow them to closely approximate a Bayesian ideal searcher. These results also underscore the importance of modelling both performance and the actual patterns of fixations to fully characterize the system under study.

Recognition and reading

Formal overt attention models have been proposed for other tasks involving object recognition. One important case is the task of reading, for which there are a large number of formal models (for review see Reichle et al. 2003). As in the case of visual search, most of these models have been designed in the process of trying to predict reading performance and eye movement data (Engbert et al., 2002; Reichle et al., 2003; Reilly and Radach, 2003), and only one or two have taken the conceptually alternate approach of first trying to derive a ideal observer for the task (Legge et al., 2002). Unlike visual search models, essentially all formal models of reading include an explicit representation of the falloff in resolution of the visual system, perhaps because it is so obvious in typical printed text that letters and words cannot be read in the periphery. An important dimension along which the various models differ is the degree to which eye fixations are driven by the output of linguistic processing versus visual/oculomotor factors, such as word length and font, peripheral acuity, and noise in saccadic eye movement control. Many recent models include both kinds of factors to some extent.

There is not space to review the reading models in any detail, but we briefly describe the ideal reader model of Legge et al. (2002), for comparison with the ideal searcher models described above. We feel that this is important because, while the reading literature on the one hand and the visual search and attention literature on the other are largely separate and distinct, the way in which these particular models are formulated provides an opportunity to examine the two domains from a common perspective. The Legge et al. ideal reader: 1) knows its own visual acuity along a line of text (a centre region with perfect letter identification and a surrounding region where it can discriminate between character and blank space), 2) has a large lexicon of words and knows the marginal probability that each word will appear in the text (based on word frequency counts), and 3) knows the variability of its own saccadic landing points as a function saccade length. With these constraints it then picks fixations that minimize uncertainty (the expected entropy) about each word in sequence, with the goal of maximizing reading speed while correctly identifying each word. Legge et al. (2002) find that the ideal reader quantitatively predicts a number of statistical properties of human eye movement patterns in reading (e.g. frequency of words skipped), qualitatively predicts a number of other properties (e.g. saccade position with words), but does not predict some properties very well (e.g. percentages of refixations). Nonetheless, in all cases, the model provides real insight because all the parameters are specified by independently known facts about the lexicon and the visual and oculomotor systems. One way that the ideal reader model differs from the ideal searcher models is that it picks fixations to minimize expected entropy rather than maximize accuracy. However, these measures are closely related, and in fact, Najemnik and Geisler (2009) show that they yield similar performance and eye movement statistics.

Entropy minimization models have also been proposed for shape recognition tasks (Arbel and Ferrie, 2001; Renninger et al., 2005, 2007) and scene encoding/recognition tasks (Raj et al., 2005). Renninger et al. (2007) model a task in which observers are given a fixed amount of time to inspect the silhouette of a complex shape before being asked to pick that shape from a test pair of silhouettes place side by side. Using vernier acuity measurements as a function of eccentricity to estimate the falloff in shape boundary detectability, they determined the fixation pattern that maximally reduces the global shape uncertainty (global entropy). They found that these entropy-minimization fixations better capture human fixation locations than do bottom-up salience models (Itti and Koch, 2000), but that a local entropy minimization strategy (like the MAP strategy of visual search) also does well when coupled with a local centre-of-gravity rule. Because of the computational complexity of the shape recognition problem, the entropy estimates used in these models are not yet as rigorous as in the reading and visual search models, but they nonetheless demonstrate the useful insights that can be gained with the ideal observer approach.

Free viewing

There are many situations (e.g. gazing out the window between writing sentences, inspecting a friends vacation photos or videos) where humans actively direct their eyes to various locations in a visual scene without having an obvious goal or task. A common hypothesis is that under such circumstances attention and hence gaze is attracted by image features that stand out perceptually in some way from the other image features. A number of such models have been proposed for predicting eye movements in free viewing tasks. As mentioned earlier, Itti and Koch (2000) propose that fixations are directed at 'salient' image locations where the local feature values (along certain assumed dimensions) differ markedly from those of the surrounding features. Rajashekar et al. (2008) further incorporated a realistic model of foveation, and found marked improvement over uniform resolution predictions.

Several more recent models are similar in concept, but based on principles from information theory (Bruce and Tsotsos, 2006, 2009; Gao and Vasconcelos, 2009; Itti and Baldi, 2006; Zhang et al., 2008;). The central idea is that the current image (or perhaps a larger set of images) is used by the brain to estimate a statistical model of local image features, and that salience is based on how unusual the local image features are given the statistical model. Bruce and Tsotsos (2006, 2009) and Zhang et al. (2008) define salience as 'self-information'—essentially the first term in equation (2) above. Gao and Vasconcelos (2009) define salience as the discriminability of a location from its surroundings. Itti and Baldi (2005) are interested in predicting fixations during the free viewing of video, and they define the salience ('surprise') as the relative entropy (Kullback-Leibler divergence) of the posterior probability distributions over the space of possible image-feature models before and after the current video frame. The critical step in specifying these models of free viewing is specifying either how the statistical models of the image features might be estimated by a rational (optimal) system, or how they might be estimated by the brain.

Although many of recent models of free viewing are computationally interesting and can be applied to arbitrary images (or videos) they are still in a formative state and are difficult to test. One limitation is that the models do not explicitly represent the variation in feature detectability with retinal location; again, this is critically important—features not detected in the periphery cannot attract gaze. A second limitation is that the models make the strong implicit assumption that the task is to fixate (focus neural resources on) statistically unusual locations. Perhaps this is a useful low-level task performed on occasion, but there are other plausible low-level tasks that might drive fixations such as maximally reducing uncertainty about the features in the image (Raj et al., 2005). Furthermore, free-viewing probably involves a wide range of high-level tasks generated internally that vary across individuals and over time within an individual: Are there any birds out there? What kinds of trees are those? Where was that picture taken? What are the people in this video doing and what are they thinking?

Models of free viewing have been evaluated by comparing the average distribution of human fixations with the models' fixations on the same images or videos. These comparisons go some way toward discriminating between models, but the variability within and across individuals resulting from the unconstrained nature of the task is likely to limit what can be learned about the mechanisms of overt attention. Nonetheless, such models might be of practical value in predicting where people tend to fixate in still images and video.

Interactive behaviours

Overt attention mechanisms play an important role in every-day tasks where the organism is physically interacting with the environment. There is strong evidence that the eyes are directed toward critical locations in the environment just before the next step in an action sequence is executed (for reviews see Land and Hayhoe, 2001: Findlay and Gilchrist, 2003: Hayhoe and Ballard, 2005). For example, in making a peanut butter and jelly sandwich, humans first make an overt visual search of the scene to find relevant objects (e.g. knife, bread, peanut butter jar, etc.), then they sequentially fixate the objects (or locations within the objects) that are crucial for each step in the action sequence, often moving the eyes to the next step while the hands finish executing the current step. Developing and testing formal models of such visual-motor tasks is hard because of the difficulty in obtaining the necessary data (recording both eye movements and the other motor movements under controlled conditions), and because of the complexity of the tasks (e.g. visual search tasks are already complex and they are just one subtask of such interactive behaviours). Not surprisingly there are few formal models of eye movements in such complicated tasks. One potentially promising approach has been explored by Sprague and Ballard (2003). They consider a task where a walker (a model agent) is required to stay on a sidewalk, avoid obstacles, and pick up trash. The key assumptions of the model are that: 1) obtaining information about the edge of the sidewalk, the obstacles and the items of trash requires direct fixation, 2) internal noise (uncertainty) about the locations of the observer and relevant scene objects grows over time until there is an appropriate fixation, and 3) the walker uses an optimal fixation selection strategy (based on Kalman filtering) to reduce uncertainty during the task. An interesting aspect of this model is that is makes predictions for the variation in fixation duration, a dimension of behaviour not considered by most other models of overt attention. More mature versions of this type of model may produce eye movement predictions that can be usefully compared against human eye movements in everyday tasks.

Covert and overt attention

In most natural tasks, overt and covert attention processes operate in a highly intertwined fashion, and indeed the same cortical areas are consistently implicated in both processes, both at the cellular and systems level (e.g. Corbetta and Shulman, 1998). A key functional difference between covert and overt attention is that the actual input information is changed drastically after each shift in overt attention. The importance of feedback and updating is therefore greatly amplified, and it is thus likely that the attentional circuit(s) of overt attention, to the degree that they are distinct, reflect this fundamental difference. The close connection between covert and overt attention means that realistic models of overt attention must include a model of covert attention. In fact, overt visual attention (i.e. the use of volitional eye movements) probably has its origins in covert attention for the following reasons. As we pointed out earlier, attention mechanisms are necessary for optimal performance regardless of capacity limitations or a non-uniform sensor (such as a foveated retina). Foveation is not universal among vertebrates (e.g. Walls, 1963), and thus many species must have covert but not overt attention mechanisms. A contemporary example is the frog, which has a well-developed oculomotor system (following the standard six-muscle vertebrate plan) used for reflexive eye movements, but makes no spontaneous eye movements and thus has no overt attention (Lettvin et al. 1959; Walls, 1963). The frog does, however, have experimentally observable covert attention (Ingle, 1975). Assuming a similar situation existed at some point in our evolutionary ancestry, it is plausible that a mutation resulting in a non-uniform retina survived and thrived because the existing mechanisms of covert attention and the oculomotor system were already there to be exploited - both (reflexive) eye movements and covert attention are valuable in and of themselves, but a fovea is not very useful unless it can be moved voluntarily.

Conclusion

In recent years there has been much progress in developing formal models of overt attention. Many of these models have provided new insight into the factors that limit or contribute to task performance and into the underlying neural mechanisms. Some models also hold promise of practical application in predicting performance in real-world tasks. Nonetheless, because of the complexity of many overt attention tasks, the models are still largely in the formative stage. A major deficit in many models is lack of an explicit representation (and understanding) of the variation in early visual processing with location in the visual field, and thus there is great need for better general models of early vision. Progress in modelling and understanding overt attention is likely to be most rapid for tasks with well-defined goals, where it is possible to determine optimal performance, or at least determine the general principles of optimal performance.

Acknowledgements

Supported by NIH grant EY02688 to W.S.G. and NSF-IIS-0917175 to L.K.C.

References

Arbel, T. and Ferrie, F.P. (2001). Entropy based gaze planning. *Image and Vision Computing*, **19**, 779–786.

Bloomfield, J.R., (1972). Visual search in complex fields: size differences between target disc and surrounding discs. *Human Factors*, **14**, 139–148.

Bruce, N. and Tsotsos, J. (2006). Saliency based on information maximization. In Y. Weiss, B. Scholkopf, and J. Platt (eds.) *Advances in neural information processing systems* vol. 18 (pp. 155–162). Cambridge, MA: MIT Press.

Bruce, N.D.B. and Tsotsos, J.K. (2009). Saliency, attention, and visual search: An information theoretic approach. *Journal of Vision*, **9**(3), 1–24.

Corbetta, M. and Shulman, G.L. (1998). Human cortical mechanisms of visual attention during orienting and search. *Philosophical Transactions of the Royal Society of London, Series B: Biological Sciences*, **353**, 1353–1362.

Eckstein, M.P. (1998). The lower visual search efficiency for conjunctions is due to noise and not serial attentional processing. *Psychological Science*, **9**, 111–118.

Eckstein, M. and Abby, C. (2001). Model observers for signal-known-statistically tasks (SKS). *Proceedings of SPIE*, **4324**, 91–102.

Engbert, R., Longtin, A., and Kliegl, R. (2002). A dynamic model of saccade generation in reading based on spatially distributed lexical processing. *Vision Research*, **42**(5), 621–636.

Engel, F. (1971). Visual conspicuity, directed attention and retinal locus. *Vision Research*, **11**, 563–576.

Engel, F. (1977). Visual conspicuity, visual search and fixation tendencies of the eye. *Vision Research*, **17**, 95–108.

Findlay, J. (1987). Visual computation and saccadic eye movements: a theoretical perspective. *SpatialVision*, **2**(3), 175–89.

Findlay, J.M. (1997). Saccade target selection in visual search. *Vision Research*, **37**, 617–631.

Findley, J.M. and Gilchrist, I.D. (2003). *Active Vision*. New York: Oxford University Press.

Gao, D. and Vasconcelos, N. (2009). Decision-theoretic saliency: computational principles, biological plausibility, and implications for neurophysiology and psychophysics. *Neural Computation*, **21**(1), 239–271.

Geisler, W.S. and Chou, K.-L. (1995). Separation of low-level and high-level factors in complex tasks: visual search. *Psychological Review*, **102**(2), 356–1378.

Green, D.M. and Swets, J.A. (1966). *Signal detection theory and psychophysics*. Los Altos, CA: Peninsula Publishing.

Hayhoe, M. and D. Ballard (2005). Eye movements in natural behavior. *Trends in Cognitive Sciences*, **9**(4), 188–94.

He, P. and Kowler, E. (1989). The role of location probability in the programming of saccades: Implications for "center-of-gravity" tendencies. *Vision Research*, **29**(9), 1165–1181.

Ingle, D. (1975). Focal attention in the frog: behavioral and physiological correlates. *Science*, **188**(4192), 1033–1035.

Itti, L. and Baldi, P. (2005). A principled approach to detecting surprising events in video. *Computer Vision and Pattern Recognition*, **1**, 631–63.

Itti, L. and Baldi, P. (2006). Bayesian surprise attracts human attention. In Y. Weiss, B. Scholkopf, and J. Platt (eds.) *Advances in neural information processing systems* vol. 18 (pp. 1–8). Cambridge, MA: MIT Press.

Itti, L. and Koch, C. (2000) A saliency-based search mechanism for overt and covert shifts of visual attention. *Vision Research*, **40**, 1489–1506.

Koch, C. and Ullman, S. (1985). Shifts in selective visual attention: towards the underlying neural circuitry. *Human Neurobiology*, **4**, 219–227.

Land, M. and Hayhoe, M. (2001). In what ways do eye movements contribute to everyday activities? *Vision Research*, **41**, 3559–3566.

Legge, G.E., Hooven, T.A., T.S., Klitz, Mansfield, J.S., and Tjan, B.S. (2002). MrChips 2002: new insights from an ideal-observer model of reading. *Vision Research*, **42**, 2219–2234.

Lettvin, J., Maturana, H., McCulloch, W., and Pitt, W. (1959). What the frog's eye tells the frog's brain. *Proceedings of the IRE*, **47**(11), 1940–1951.

Ludwig, C.J.H. and Gilchrist, I.D. (2002). Stimulus-drive and goal-driven control over visual selection. *Journal of Experimental Psychology: Human Perception and Performance*, **28**, 902–912.

Motter, B.C., and Belky, E.J. (1998). The guidance of eye movements during active visual search. *Vision Research*, **38**, 1805–1815.

Najemnik, J. and Geisler, W.S. (2005). Optimal eye movement strategies in visual search. *Nature*, **434**, 387–391.

Najemnik, J. and Geisler, W.S. (2008). Eye movement statistics in humans are consistent with an optimal strategy. *Journal of Vision*, **8**, 1–14.

Najemnik, J. and Geisler W.S. (2009) Simple summation rule for optimal fixation selection in visual search. *Vision Research*. **49**, 1286–1294.

Palmer, J., Verghese, P., and Pavel, M. (2000). The psychophysics of visual search. *Vision Research*, **40**, 1227–1268.

Pomplun, M., Reingold, E. M., and Shen, J. (2003). Area activation: A computational model of saccadic selectivity in visual search. *Cognitive Science*, **27**, 299–312.

Raj, R., Geisler, W.S., Frazor, R.A. and Bovik, A.C. (2005). Contrast statistics for foveated visual systems: Fixation selection by minimizing contrast entropy. *Journal of the Optical Society of America A*, **22** (**10**), 2039–2049.

Rajashekar, U., Bovik, A.C. and Cormack, L.K. (2006). Visual search in noise: revealing the influence of structural cues by gaze-contingent classification image analysis. *Journal of Vision*, **6**, 379–386.

Rajashekar, U., Van der Linde, I., Bovik, A., and Cormack, L. (2008). GAFFE: A gaze-attentive fixation finding engine. *IEEE Transactions on Image Processing*, **17**(4), 564–573.

Rao, R.P.N., Zelinsky, G.J., Hayhoe, M.M. and Ballard, D.H. (2002). Eye movements in iconic visual search. *Vision Research*, **42**, 1447–1463.

Reichle, E.D., Rayner, K., and Pollatsek, A. (2003). The E-Z Reader model of eye movement control in reading: Comparisons to other models. *Behavioral and Brain Sciences*, **26**, 445–476.

Reilly, R. and Radach, R. (2003). Foundations of an interactive activation model of eye movement control in reading. In J. Hyona, R. Radach and H. Deubel (eds.) *The mind's eye: Cognitive and applied aspects of eye movements*. Amsterdam: Elsevier.

Renninger, L.W., Verghese, P., and Coughlan, J. (2007). Where to look next? Eye movements reduce local uncertainty. *Journal of Vision*, **7**(3), 1–17.

Renninger, L.W., Coughlan, J., Verghese, P., and Malik, J. (2005). An information maximization model of eye movements. *Advances in Neural Information Processing Systems*, **17**, 1121–1128.

Reynolds, J.H. and Chelazzi, L. (2004). Attentional modulation of visual processing. *Annual Review of Neuroscience*, **27**, 611–647.

Sprague, N. and Ballard, D. (2003). Eye movements for reward maximization. In S. Thrun, L.K. Saul and B. Scholkopf (eds.) *Advances in Neural Information Processing Systems* (Vol. 16) (pp. 1467–1474). Boston, MA: MIT Press.

Theeuwes J., Kramer A.F., Hahn S. and Irwin, D.E. (1998). Our eyes do not always go where we want them to go: capture of the eyes by new objects. *Psychological Science*, **9**, 379–385.

Toet, A., Bijl, P. and Valeton, J.M. (2000). Tests for three visual search and detection models. *Optical Engineering*, **39**, 1344–1353.

Toet, A., Kooi, F.L., Bijl, P., and Valeton, J.M. (1998). Visual conspicuity determines human target acquisition performance. *Optical Engineering*, **37**, 1969–1975.

Torralba, A. (2003). Modeling global scene factors in attention. *Journal of the Optical Society of America A*, **20**, 1407–1418.

Torralba, A., Oliva, A., Castelhano, M. and Henderson, J.M. (2006). Contextual guidance of attention in natural scenes: the role of global features on object search. *Psychological Review*, **113**(4), 766–786.

Treisman, A.M. and Gelade, G. (1980). A feature integration theory of attention. *Cognitive Psychology*, **12**, 97–136.

Vincent, B.T., Baddeley T.J., Troscianko T. and Gilchrist I.D. (2009). Optimal feature integration in visual search. *Journal of Vision*, **9**, 1–11.

Walls, G.L. (1963). *The vertebrate eye and its adaptive radiation*. New York: Hafner.

Wolfe, J.M. (1994). Guided Search 2.0: A revised model of visual search. *Psychonomic Bulletin and Review*, **1**, 202–238.

Wolfe, J.M. (2007). Guided Search 4.0: Current Progress with a model of visual search. In W. Gray (ed.), *Integrated Models of Cognitive Systems* (pp. 99–119). New York: Oxford.

Zhang L., Tong M.H., Marks T.K., Shan H., and Cottrell G.W. (2008) SUN: A Bayesian framework for saliency using natural statistics. *Journal of Vision*, **8**, 1–20.

Zelinsky, G.J. (2008) A theory of eye movements during target acquisition. *Psychological Review*, **115**, 787–835.

Zelinsky, G., Rao, R., Hayhoe, M., and Ballard, D. (1997). Eye movements reveal the spatio-temporal dynamics of visual search. *Psychological Science*, **8**, 448–453.

CHAPTER 25

The intriguing interactive relationship between visual attention and saccadic eye movements

Árni Kristjánsson

Abstract

We normally find it difficult to attend to a stimulus of interest in our visual field without shifting our gaze towards it. It is almost as if we have an urge to shift our gaze to where we attend to. This has often been interpreted as indicating that attending to a particular area in the visual field involves preparation for an eye movement to that location. The relationship between attention and eye movements has been investigated in many studies in recent years and the evidence suggests that before a saccadic eye movement is made, attention shifts to the upcoming saccade landing point. In addition, eye movements and attention share the same neural resources, at least to a considerable extent.

Introduction

We are all well aware of the fact that we can pay attention to things that fall outside our centre of gaze. Our 'mind's eye' may roam to other locations even though the centre of our gaze may fall somewhere else. The philosopher John Locke talked about this in his *Essay on human understanding* (1689/1975):

> How often may a Man observe in himself, that whilst his Mind is intently employ'd in the contemplation of some Objects; and curiously surveying some *Ideas* that are there, it takes no notice of Impressions of sounding Bodies, made upon the Organ of Hearing. [. . .]
>
> A sufficient impulse there may be on the Organ; but it not reaching the Observation of the Mind, there follows no Perception [. . .]
>
> Want of Sensation in this case, is not through any defect in the Organ, or that the Man's Ears are less affected, than at other times, when he does hear [. . .]
>
> (Locke, 1689/1975, p. 144.)

What Locke describes is usually referred to as *selective attention*. A stimulus may go unnoticed if it is not attended to, even though there is no 'defect in the organ' responsible for sensing the stimulus.

The 19th-century German scientist Hermann von Helmholtz is often credited with being among the first to study such attentional orienting in a systematic way. He constructed a box where he could illuminate an array of letters very briefly with a spark. He found that by preselecting a region of the array of letters while they were invisible because of the darkness, without moving his centre of gaze, he could identify the letters in this region, but not letters at a similar distance from the centre of gaze, or even the letters actually at the centre of gaze, during the brief period that they were illuminated (see Nakayama and Mackeben, 1989 and Wright and Ward, 2008, for a detailed discussion).

These observations of Helmholtz are commonly thought to reflect the operation of *selective* or *focal* attention (see e.g. Kristjánsson, 2006; Neisser, 1967; Pashler, 1998; Posner, 1980; Nakayama and Mackeben, 1989; Treisman and Sato, 1990; Wang et al., 2005) and a common subdistinction is between *covert* attentional orienting, where we do not look towards the locus of interest (by moving our heads, or shifting our gaze), and *overt* attentional orienting, where we, for example, move our eyes toward the location of interest. The topic of the current chapter is how *covert* attending interacts with saccadic eye movements.

This topic has been studied intensely over the last two or three decades, and it turns out that covert attention and saccadic eye movements have an intriguing interactive relationship. The general aim of such research has been to distinguish between a number of different possibilities regarding this relationship. Firstly, it is quite possible that the two do not interact at all—that they are simply independent of one another. A second possibility is that attention simply goes where the eyes go, although the observations of Locke and Helmholtz mentioned above, certainly suggest that this possibility is unlikely. A third possibility is that an attention shift precedes a gaze shift, and may even be necessary for the gaze shift. A fourth possibility is that the relationship is more complex than this and that the relationship may be modulated by the task demands or the immediate circumstances in each case. As we will see, the research on this relationship indicates that the answer is, most likely, a conglomeration of the third and fourth options.

Does an attention shift precede a shift of gaze?

While we can attend to a given location in space without shifting our gaze to that location, as Hermann von Helmholtz showed, we also intuitively know that some effort is required to *prevent* ourselves from shifting our gaze to where we have focused our attention. In fact it may sometimes feel as if we have something of an urge to look where we choose to attend. Anyone who has tried to attend to something of interest without looking there knows this. So while we can clearly attend to something without fixing the centre of our gaze upon it, this is not effortless.

This suggests that attentional orienting partly involves preparation for moving our centre of gaze to where we attend (see e.g. Klein, 1980; Posner, 1980). In the early 1990s a number of scientists designed experiments to study the question of whether attention precedes a shift of gaze to a particular location. Their basic question was whether when we perform a saccade to a particular location we start by shifting our attention there (as previously reasoned by Klein, 1980; see later section 'The premotor theory of attention'). They investigated what would occur in discrimination tasks when the task was presented at the location of an upcoming saccade target. The experimental question was whether attention is allocated to the landing point of an upcoming saccade, and if so, is this coupling obligatory?

Hoffman and Subramaniam, (1995) asked their observers to saccade to a specified location following a tone that indicated that the saccadic eye movement should be initiated, in addition to identifying a target letter presented 0, 50, or 100 ms before the trigger signal for saccade initiation (the target of the detection task was thus always presented before the saccade onset). At all stimulus onset asynchronies target recognition was by far the best at the upcoming landing point of the saccade, compared with other locations. In a second experiment Hoffman and Subramaniam tried to directly dissociate attention shifts and saccadic eye movements by instructing observers to attend to a certain location and then make either a saccade towards that location or to another one. In spite of this, target recognition was far superior at the saccade landing point than the attended location.

This result suggested that the coupling of attention and saccades is obligatory, that the observers have trouble *avoiding* shifting attention to the landing point of the saccade.

Deubel and Schneider (1996) asked their observers to perform a perceptual discrimination task while also making a saccadic eye movement to a location to the left or right of a fixation point at the centre of the display. The discrimination task was to decide whether an 'E' or an inverted 'E' had been presented (note that the target stimulus disappeared before the centre of gaze settled on the target following the saccade). They found that performance on the discrimination task improved as the distance decreased between the target and the landing point of the saccade and reasoned that since summoning attention to the location of a discrimination target (for example, following a spatial attentional cue) is known to improve performance compared to a discrimination task presented at an unattended location (cf. Carrasco et al., 2002; Kristjánsson and Nakayama, 2003, Kristjánsson and Sigurdardottir, 2008; Posner, 1980), attention had shifted to the locus of the landing point before the saccade was made and improved performance on the secondary task. Like Hoffman and Subramaniam they also observed that even when the observers knew in advance the location of the discrimination target and attempted to attend to this location, performance was better when the discrimination target occurred at the location of upcoming saccade, compared to the location they were instructed to attend to.

Kowler et al. (1995) reached similar conclusions, finding that requiring observers to saccade to one particular location facilitated letter discrimination at that precise location. Furthermore, Kowler et al. found that perceptual discrimination at the location of a saccade target was better than at other locations, and that it was difficult or impossible to make challenging perceptual judgements at a particular location while simultaneously preparing a saccadic eye movement to another location.

Other results of interest in this context are those of Shepherd et al. (1986). Their observers had to detect a flash presented in their visual periphery while making saccades to the left or right (dictated by a central arrow). The flash and saccade target either coincided spatially or appeared at opposite locations. The observers were faster at detecting flashes on the same side as the saccadic target even when targets were more likely to appear at the opposite side of the display. Shepherd et al. concluded that observers responded faster to peripheral stimuli both when they knew in advance where they were most likely to appear, and also when they prepared to make a saccade to that position, Overall their results indicated that while 'it is possible to make attention movements without making corresponding eye movements, it is not possible to make an eye movement (in the absence of peripheral stimulation) without making a corresponding shift in the focus of attention' (p. 475).

Overall, the consensus from studies of the relationship between saccadic eye movements and attention is that visual attention appears to precede the centre of gaze to the saccade landing point. These studies have in general supported a *premotor* conception of attention which in essence states that an attention shift entails a plan to move the centre of gaze to that location (see further discussion in the section 'The premotor theory of attention').

Of special note in this context is the study of Peterson and colleagues (Peterson et al., 2004). Their observers fixated on a central marker surrounded by six white circles which contained figure-8 premasks (see e.g. Yantis and Jonides, 1984). Five of the six circles then turned red and the premasks changed into letters. The task of the observers was to saccade as quickly as they could toward the single remaining white circle, while also identifying the letter on the target. In a critical manipulation a seventh circle appeared simultaneous to this change, but *never* contained a target, and was thus totally unrelated to the task. In spite of this, the observers frequently made saccades to this stimulus even though this contradicted the task instructions. Peterson et al. found that when this sudden onset led to an erroneous saccade towards it, a response compatibility/incompatibility effect was observed, in that the identity of this stimulus interfered with the letter identification task when it suggested a response incongruent with the correct response. This result suggests that 'reflexive' saccadic eye movements made in violation of task instructions also involve a shift of attention to the saccade landing point. In the words of the authors, the result indicates that 'the route that covert attention takes mimics the path that the eyes will take' (Petersson et al., 2004, p. 403).

Sequences of multiple saccades

Evidence which may be even more dramatic for a tight coupling between covert attention shifts and saccadic eye movements comes from studies of sequences of multiple saccades. Baldauf and Deubel (2008) asked their participants to perform a sequence of saccades to two or three letter targets arranged around a circle centred on a fixation point at screen centre, one after another on a single trial. The observers also had to perform a discrimination task either at required saccade locations or at other positions on the array. Baldauf and Deubel found that discrimination performance was good at *all* the required saccade locations while it was essentially at chance at all other locations, even those that were close to the saccade targets. The authors argued that this reflected that attention is allocated *in parallel* to all three of the saccade targets in the sequence, what might in essence be termed parallel programming of multiple saccades. During a sequence of saccades attention does not move to the next target location right before the saccade, but the basic saccade sequence is planned in total beforehand, and all locations in the sequence are attended to before the first saccade is initiated.

A finding along the same lines was reported by Godijn and Theeuwes (2003) who studied sequences of two speeded saccades. Identification of targets presented very briefly at the saccade landing points for both the first and second saccade was good, and far better than at other locations. Their results indicate that before the initiation of such sequences both the targets were attended in parallel, consistent with the findings of Baldauf and Deubel (2008).

Results from Gersch et al. (2004) were, however, seemingly not consistent with the conclusion that multiple saccades are programmed beforehand, as the results of Baldauf and Deubel and Godijn and Theeuwes suggested. There are some important methodological differences between the studies however. For one there was no cue as to the saccade sequence the observers were required to perform, so cue interpretation was not required and, Gersch et al. measured attentional performance *during* the saccade sequence whereas both Baldauf and Deubel and Godijn and Theeuwes measured attentional performance immediately *preceding* the first saccade in the sequence, which may explain the discrepancy in results.

When does attention move to the saccade target location?

If we concur that there is strong evidence that attention shifts to the landing point of an upcoming saccade that is being planned, an obvious question is *when* does this attention shift occur, relative to when the saccade is performed.

Findings from a study by Dore-Mazars et al. (2004) indicate that visual attention shifts to the saccade target, with a corresponding lack of attentional resources at other locations, at the time when the motor programme for the saccade is ready, and that the saccadic eye movement follows (see also Kowler et al., 1995).

In contrast to this, Deubel (2008) has shown that the temporal relationship between attention shifts and saccades may be more complex and dynamic than this might indicate. Deubel found that attention can shift to a location peripheral to fixation and that it can be sustained there *without* immediate saccade execution (even though the observers are supposed to make a saccade). But Deubel also found that saccades are in some cases executed immediately after attention has shifted. What this result indicates is that the temporal relationship between saccade execution and attention shifts may be more flexible and modulable by task demands or strategies than the results of Dore et al. suggest.

Note also that this result from Deubel (2008) is a seeming challenge to the premotor theory of attention (see the following section) since if attention shifts *necessarily* entail a motor plan, as the premotor theory states, the time courses of attention shifts and saccades should be tightly linked. The findings in Deubel (2008) raise, at the very least, some qualifications with regard to the premotor theory of attention (see further discussion below).

The overall conclusion to be drawn from this overview of the research on the relationship between attention shifts and saccadic eye movements is that a shift of attention to a particular location in space also entails a movement plan to shift gaze to that location, and this is essentially independent of whether the eye movement is actually executed or not (Schneider, 1995; Schneider and Deubel, 2002).

Some of the results reviewed indicate that this coupling is not quite compulsory, however, and that the temporal relationship between the two can be quite flexible.

The premotor theory of attention

If there is indeed a strong link between attention and saccadic eye movements, this supports an influential theory of attentional function, the *premotor* theory of attention (see Craigher and Rizzolatti, 2005; Rizzolatti, 1987). The basic tenet of the premotor theory is that attention and movement planning are two sides of the same coin, an attention shift to a particular target is essentially a result of a plan to shift our gaze to that location. Klein (1980) tested a similar conception which should predict that if an observer attends to a particular location, eye movements to that location should be facilitated and that discrimination at that location should also be facilitated. These predictions were not confirmed in Klein's studies leading him to reject this hypothesis. Some more recent evidence has, however, been more favourable to premotor conceptions of attention.

An important component of the theory is that the same neural machinery is assumed to be involved in both processes. The following is perhaps the essence of the theory:

> attention does not result from, nor require a control system separated from sensorimotor circuits. Attention derives from activation of the same circuits that under other conditions, determine perception and motor activity.
>
> (Craigher and Rizzolatti, 2005, p. 181.)

A fundamental claim of the premotor theory then is that there is a processing stage where motor commands are prepared but not executed (such as in covert attention shifts). Activation of maps in the nervous system which transform spatial information into movement plans leads to both an increase in motor readiness, and also facilitated processing of stimuli at the landing point of the upcoming movement (in the present discussion an eye movement, although this logic applies to other movement types as well). Further evidence for such a conception of attention comes from the results of Sheliga et al. (1994). Observers were instructed to attend to a location in space and additionally to perform vertical or horizontal saccades in response to the onset of a trigger signal. Sheliga et al. found that the trajectories of saccades in response to visual or auditory signals deviated in the direction of the attended location, even though the task did not require any saccades to these attended locations. Sheliga et al. argued that this result shows that allocation of spatial attention leads to activations of neural mechanisms concerned with the control of saccadic eye movements.

The strongest support for a premotor notion of attention is perhaps evidence that overlapping neural mechanisms are involved in saccade generation and attention (Beauchamp et al., 2001; Corbetta et al., 1998; Kustov and Robinson, 1996; Moore and Fallah, 2001; see also discussion by Schall and Thompson, 1999). For example, Kustov and Robinson tested the way shifts of attention were linked to the generation of saccadic eye movements while simultaneously recording from single neurons in the superior colliculi in macaque monkeys. They found that each attentional shift was closely related to eye movement preparation, but note that Klein (2004) argues that motor preparation and covert attending may have been confounded in that study. Moore and Fallah (2001) then found that by microstimulation of neurons in the frontal eye fields of monkeys they could enhance attentional performance, but only when the object to be attended was in the position that the cortical stimulation site represented.

The results reviewed above show how attending to a particular location can facilitate saccade execution to that location. The obvious flipside is withdrawing attention from the saccade target in some way. If attention is *required* for saccades, withdrawing attention should then by necessity interfere with the generation of the saccade. A number of studies have followed this logic and have indeed found results supporting this. Pashler et al. (1993) observed that when an auditory discrimination task was presented concurrently to the target, saccades to peripheral targets were slower than when no such discrimination was required. Stuyven et al. (2000) observed similar results, this time for pro- and antisaccade (see section 'Antisaccades and attention') latencies as such saccades were performed concurrently to a simultaneous tapping task. There is further discussion of effects of withdrawing attention from the saccade target below (see section 'Express saccades and attentional disengagement').

A strict interpretation of the premotor theory entails that stimulus detection should be facilitated at the locus of an intended eye movement and saccades should be faster to the locus of a discrimination requiring attention. However, there are some notable exceptions to this (Hunt and Kingstone, 2003; Klein, 1980). Recent evidence from neurophysiological studies has suggested that the relationship between saccades and attention is indeed not as tight and immediate as many had thought. Sato and Schall (2003) recorded from single cells in the frontal eye fields of Macaque monkeys. They trained the monkeys to perform antisaccades or prosaccades based on whether a singleton target bar in a search array was oriented horizontally or vertically. Sato and Schall were able to distinguish between two different types of frontal eye field neurons, in terms of their response patterns during an antisaccade versus prosaccade task. They found that while two-thirds of the neurons that they recorded from selected the singleton stimulus regardless of task instruction, and then subsequently the locus of the saccade endpoint (a result essentially consistent with a premotor conception of attention), approximately one-third of the neurons were *only* selective for the saccade endpoint, and *not* for the stimulus that instructed the monkey what to do (the horizontal or vertical singleton target bar). This result is quite important since it means that saccade target selection and visual selection are not quite as unitary as some previous findings had indicated. A subset of neurons in the frontal eye fields does not exhibit response patterns consistent with the predictions of a premotor theory of attention. Schall (2004) produced further results supporting this, finding such a dissociation in selectivity between response patterns of FEF neurons even when no saccade was made.

Juan et al. (2004) used microstimulation of the frontal eye fields of macaque monkeys who were trained on a task similar to that studied by Sato and Schall (2003). The monkeys had to perform antisaccades or prosaccades based on whether a singleton target bar in a search array was oriented horizontally or vertically. They found that even though attention was bound to the instruction stimulus (as inferred from accurate performance in the absence of FEF stimulation), on antisaccade trials the electrically-elicited saccades deviated in the direction of the to-be-fixated location rather than the attended singleton. Again this indicates that 'saccade preparation is not an obligatory or immediate outcome of visual selection and so challenges the premotor theory of attention' to use the words of Juan et al. (2004, p. 15544).

Other studies, where behavioural measures were used, have yielded results which are not quite consistent with a premotor theory of attention. A case in point are the results of Hunt and Kingstone (2003), who studied the inhibition of return phenomenon (Posner and Cohen, 1984; see Klein, 2000 for review) where an attention shift to a precued location is slower than to uncued locations when a certain amount of time (e.g. >~300 ms) have passed since the cue was presented. They were able to demonstrate that a double dissociation existed between an *attentional* component of inhibition of return, and a *motor* component, again arguing against a tight, necessary link between attention and eye movement generation.

The evidence that has been reviewed up until now shows that the relationship between attention and saccadic eye movements is tight, but it is probably not completely obligatory. Perhaps a good way to think of this relationship is as Findlay, 1995 wrote: 'covert attention operates in *conjunction* with eye movements' (Findlay, 1995 p. 461; see also Findlay and Gilchrist, 2003). Findlay's claim is in essence that covert attention co-evolved with saccadic eye movements for the support of active visual perception, but the view does not entail that an attention shift is *necessarily* in preparation of a motor movement of the eyes, although it certainly can be. The immediate task circumstances in each case dictate the exact nature of this relationship.

Express saccades and attentional disengagement

An influential conception of the relationship between attention and saccadic eye movements has been the idea that attentional engagement and disengagement are crucial concepts for the understanding of how saccades are generated (see e.g. Fischer and Weber, 1993). The core idea is that for attention to shift from one location to another we must first *disengage* our attention from its current locus of engagement (see e.g. Corbetta and Shulman, 2002; Posner et al., 1988; and Wright and Ward, 2008, for an excellent up-to-date discussion). The primary support for this concept are the so-called *express saccades*.

Express saccades were first described by Saslow (1967). The behavioural manifestation of express saccades is as follows. When the central fixation point in a typical saccade task is extinguished, shortly before a prosaccade is to be executed (e.g. by 100–200 ms), a large portion of the saccades are quite a bit faster than if no such gap were introduced before the saccade should be initiated (Fischer and Boch, 1983, Fischer and Weber, 1993; Ross and Ross, 1980, 1981; Saslow, 1967).

There has been some controversy over whether such saccades constitute a qualitatively distinct type of saccade from the 'regular' prosaccade, or whether they are simply fast prosaccades. Some authors have observed bimodal distributions of latencies in such a gap paradigm, lending support to the concept that express saccades are a special type of saccadic eye movement (Carpenter, 2001; Fischer and Ramsperger, 1984; Fischer and Weber, 1993; Jüttner and Wolf, 1992), while others have observed generally unimodal latency distributions which are more consistent with express saccades simply being fast regular prosaccades (Kalesnykas and Hallett, 1987; Kingstone and Klein, 1993; Reuter-Lorenz et al., 1991; Wenban-Smith and Findlay, 1991).

Further support for this conjecture, from the domain of studies on visual attention, comes from the finding that attention shifts from the location of a central fixation point to a peripheral target are speeded if the fixation point disappears from ~100 to 200 ms before target appearance (Mackeben and Nakayama, 1993; see also Pratt and Nghiem, 2000 for some related findings). Mackeben and Nakayama termed this express *attention* shifts. What is especially remarkable is the similarity in the time courses of such benefits, measured with percent correct performance on a challenging acuity discrimination, to the latency distributions for so-called *express saccades* (Mayfrank et al., 1986; see discussion in Mackeben and Nakayama, 1993).

The fact that saccades performed without the gap have longer latencies is thought to reflect a tendency to maintain gaze on the currently fixated stimulus, which competes with the signal to make a prosaccade, this conception has been supported by neurophysiological studies (Edelman and Keller, 1996, 1998; Fischer and Weber, 1993; Munoz and Wurtz, 1995a, 1995b). If this engagement to the central fixation point is not present anymore, since the fixation point is no longer visible on the screen, such inhibition is not required and the saccade can take place more quickly. This general conception is explained in Fig. 25.1.

Express saccades are thought to be the most reflexive of saccadic eye movements, and have sometimes been thought to be the purest manifestation of the visuomotor grasp reflex, the tendency to shift gaze to a stimulus that suddenly appears in the visual field.

A number of researchers have concluded from the results of studies of the gap effect that when a regular saccade is made (and there is no gap between fixation offset and presentation of the saccade target), disengagement from the fixated stimulus is required before the saccade can be executed (see, e.g. Fischer and Weber, 1993, as shown in Fig. 25.1). Many of these same authors have assumed that this disengagement is effortful and requires attention. This is the reason that saccade latencies, when there is no gap, are increased relative to such latencies when there is a gap. In the gap task, such disengagement is no longer needed to perform the saccade. This, in turn, results in faster saccades towards the target, which is the essence of the so-called gap effect, and the corresponding express saccades.

While express saccades are thought to be quite reflexive, recent results of Edelman and colleagues (Edelman et al., 2007) indicate that even these most reflexive types of saccadic eye movement can be modulated by intertrial history. Edelman et al. investigated the effects of learning in shifts of transient attention (see e.g. Kristjánsson, 2006 for review) and found that the landing points of express saccades could be modulated by between trial learning of cue-target consistencies. The results of Edelman et al. (2007) showed that 'high-level cognitive processes can influence the most reflexive of saccadic eye movements' (p. 1), even though the cognitive processes did not appear to be under voluntary control.

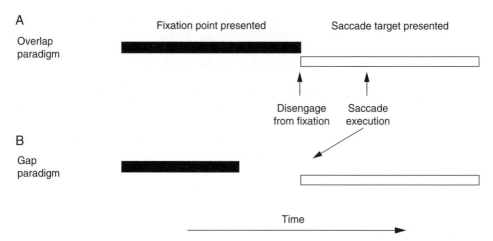

Fig. 25.1 The logic of the disengagement account of saccade generation. Panel A shows how this is conceived of for saccades in the overlap situation while panel B shows how in the gap paradigm saccade execution is speeded since disengagement from the fixation point is no longer needed before the saccade can be executed.

Antisaccades and attention

The so-called *antisaccade* task involves a saccadic eye movement in the direction *opposite* to where a trigger stimulus appears (Amador et al., 1998; Everling and Fischer, 1998; Funahashi et al., 1993; Hallett, 1978). Antisaccades may be contrasted with 'regular' saccades (or 'prosaccades', see Fig. 25.2) which would involve saccading to the location of the stimulus onset. In the prosaccade task the observer is required to shift his gaze from the current centre of fixation to the locus of a peripherally presented trigger stimulus. The antisaccade task, in contrast, requires a shift of gaze of the same size (or *amplitude*) in the exact opposite direction to the trigger stimulus.

Research on the antisaccade task has shown that saccades made away from stimulus onsets are overall less accurate than prosaccades (Krapmann et al., 1998), that antisaccades have lower maximum velocities (often called 'peak velocities') during the saccade (Leigh and Zee, 1999), and that they have higher response latencies, and very often higher error rates than prosaccades (Hallet, 1978, see e.g. Everling and Fischer, 1998, for a review of the basic findings of the antisaccade literature).

Many authors have argued that one essential component of the antisaccade task is *disengagement* (as explained in the section 'Express saccades and attentional disengagement' and Fig. 25.2) from the current locus of fixation before the saccade can be generated (Everling et al., 1998; Funahashi et al, 1993; Forbes and Klein, 1996; Schlag-Rey et al., 1997), and this has sometimes been called the *competition account* of pro- versus antisaccade generation (see e.g. Kristjánsson, 2007). Disengagement from the currently fixated target is also often mentioned as an explanation for the lower prosaccade latencies observed in the 'overlap' than the 'gap' paradigm (where express saccades tend to be observed, see previous section).

In summary, experimental results have indicated that for successful saccade generation, disengagement from the current locus of fixation is first required, and then if an antisaccade is required, competition between the two incompatible responses occurs. Another way to think of this is that antisaccades require that the so-called visuomotor-grasp reflex be overcome, and in fact pro- and antisaccades have often been thought of in terms of a race between the two processes during the antisaccade task—and when the prosaccade reflex wins the race an erroneous prosaccade is made (see e.g. Hutton, 2009 for review). This has been termed the competition account of pro- and antisaccade generation. In this conception visual attention plays a key role, since a central part of the explanation for the observed results involves disengagement of attention from fixation.

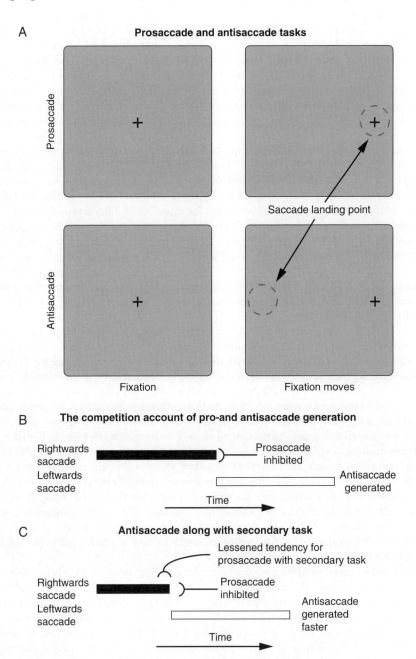

Fig. 25.2 The prosaccade and antisaccade tasks and the competition account of pro- and antisaccade generation. Panel A shows the typical pro and antisaccade tasks; the broken-line circles denote the intended landing point of the saccade. Panel B shows the standard competition account of saccade generation, where it is assumed that before an antisaccade is executed a reflexive prosaccade must be inhibited. Panel C shows an account of how speeded antisaccades in the studies of Kristjánsson et al. (2001a) might come about under this scenario.

Antisaccades may not only require attention but also seem to lead to demands upon working memory (Roberts et al., 1994). There is, in fact, evidence that when working memory is taxed in some way, antisaccades become harder to execute. Mitchell et al. (2002) asked observers to perform a so-called n-back task involving keeping letters in working memory for different amounts of time concurrently to performing an antisaccade task. Mitchell et al. found that errors on the antisaccade task were greatly increased with difficulty of the n-back task, and importantly, also that this inhibitory effect did not affect the saccade execution itself but rather the inhibitory component of the task.

Antisaccades have been found to be an important diagnostic tool with regard to various neurological disorders. Guitton et al. (1985) studied patients with lesions of the frontal lobes and found that they had great difficulty inhibiting reflexive prosaccades to the trigger stimulus when asked to perform a saccade in the opposite direction to the trigger stimulus (an antisaccade). Such difficulty in inhibiting the reflexive saccade has been found for a number of different conditions, all sharing the symptoms of prefrontal cortical dysfunction. This has been found for patients with schizophrenia (Fukushima et al., 1988; Sereno and Holzman, 1995) patients with Alzheimer's disease (Currie et al., 1991); Parkinson patients (Crevits and De Ridder 1997); a subset of patients with attention-deficit hyperactivity disorder (Cairny et al., 2001; Munoz et al., 2003), and patients with obsessive–compulsive disorder (Maruff et al., 1999; Rosenberg et al., 1997). This general pattern of results is quite consistent with effects of working memory tasks upon saccades found for normal observers (Mitchell et al., 2002).

The involvement of visual attention in the antisaccade task may lead to a somewhat counterintuitive prediction, however. If attention is required for the inhibition of the reflexive saccade, and dual task studies show that a secondary task interferes with prosaccade generation (see e.g. Pashler et al, 1993, Stuyven et al., 2000; see section 'The premotor theory of attention'), we might observe speeded antisaccades when the tendency for a prosaccade is lessened. Less effort would be needed for the suppression of the prosaccade reflex, which might then consequently speed up the antisaccade. Note that this should only occur if the secondary task would be presented sufficiently early with respect to the saccade trigger stimulus, around the time when the reflexive saccade is being inhibited.

Kristjánsson and colleagues (Kristjánsson et al., 2001a) designed experiments to address this exact question, asking: What would the effects of a secondary attentionally demanding task be on prosaccades and antisaccades? Their reasoning was that if an attentionally demanding secondary task is presented at a critical time relative to a saccade trigger stimulus, thus withdrawing attention, this might actually reduce the tendency for a prosaccade (see Fig. 25.2C). The secondary task was thus presented at various times before, after or simultaneously to the presentation of the saccade trigger stimulus (at the left or right of fixation) which indicated the time at which a prosaccade or antisaccade was to be made.

In light of the so-called competition account of prosaccade versus antisaccade generation, and the strong links between shifts of attention and saccadic eye movements, a secondary attentionally demanding task, presented concurrently to the saccade target at various times relative to the onset of the saccade target (prior to, simultaneous to and subsequent to the target onset) might lead to differential effects depending on when, relative to the trigger stimulus, this secondary task was presented.

Three different discrimination tasks were presented at different stimulus onset asynchronies relative to the displacement of the fixation cross (which was the saccade trigger stimulus) before, simultaneous to or following the saccade trigger. Prosaccades and antisaccades were to be performed on different blocks. When the secondary discrimination tasks preceded the presentation of the saccade trigger stimulus by 100–500 milliseconds, antisaccades were *faster* than antisaccades performed when the observers were simply instructed to ignore the secondary stimulus (which the results indicated that they were able to do very effectively). On the other hand when the secondary task was presented simultaneous to, or following the saccade trigger stimulus, antisaccades were slowed considerably, and were much slower than when the observers were asked to simply ignore the secondary stimulation.

The results of Kristjánsson et al. (2001a) indicated that when the tendency for a reflexive prosaccade is lessened (through the withdrawal of attention) antisaccades are speeded. This seemed then to be a classic 'trade-off' relationship where one process is speeded at the expense of the other and this result was thus quite consistent with the competition account of pro- and antisaccade generation. Neurally this conception is tractable since it can be thought of as reflecting competitive activity between fixation neurons and saccade burst neurons in the superior colliculus and frontal eye fields (Dorris and Munoz, 1995; Edelman and Keller, 1996; Everling and Munoz, 2000; Everling et al., 1999).

Kristjánsson et al. argued that this reflects that when attention is withdrawn (by the secondary task) less effort is needed to suppress a reflexive saccade towards the saccade trigger stimulus. A key assumption is that there is competition between the two mutually exclusive responses.

Kristjánsson et al. (2004) further investigated this competition account and followed the simple logic that any factor that may affect the latency of a prosaccade may have a converse effect upon antisaccade latencies. With this simple prediction in mind they tested performance on various tasks manipulating factors that are known or suspected to influence prosaccade latencies, asking whether such a manipulation would have similar or opposite effects on the latency of antisaccades.

One way to think of this relationship between prosaccades and antisaccades is in terms of processing stages. We would expect that a stimulus manipulation that has an adverse effect on prosaccade latencies would delay antisaccades if (but only if) the delay reflects effects at a stage of processing which is for example at the sensory stage that precedes the initiation of the motor response. Kristjánsson et al. reasoned that a given factor shown to influence prosaccade latencies could in principle lead to either speeded or slowed antisaccades, but this would depend on the processing stage that was affected (see Donders, 1864/1984, and subsequently Sternberg, 1969, for some applications of this general logic). So, for example, if a given manipulation has a slowing effect upon prosaccade latencies, this might then reflect that such influences could specifically strengthen a prosaccade reflex, influencing the mechanisms that would on average generate a reflexive prosaccade tendency.

But note again that if both antisaccades and prosaccades would be influenced in a similar way, this would argue that the manipulations had *similar* effects on pro- and antisaccades (i.e. speeding or slowing both), which would then be interpreted as influencing processing stages which affect both eye-movement types in a similar manner. Such a pattern of results would indicate no competition between the two processes, on this particular task, but rather effects upon processing stages preceding or following the stage of saccade planning and execution.

In light of this reasoning, Kristjánsson et al. (2004) made use of various manipulations that have been found to affect prosaccade latencies to investigate whether effects which may speed prosaccades might delay antisaccades, in other words producing opposite effects upon the two types of saccade. The first example used was a well-known effect of a nasal/temporal asymmetry effect for attention shifts.

Previous research has shown that manual responses are faster to stimuli presented in the temporal hemifield compared to the nasal hemifield when stimulus presentation is monocular (see e.g. Rafal et al., 1991). Kristjánsson et al. reasoned that if attention shifts are slowed to the nasal hemifield, the same might apply to saccadic eye movements, especially in light of the demonstrated strong link between attention and saccadic eye movements. This is indeed what was found, saccades were faster to targets presented in the temporal hemifield (which projects to the nasal hemiretina). More interestingly, though, Kristjánsson et al. found that the slower prosaccades towards a nasal hemifield target corresponded with faster antisaccades in the opposite direction to the saccade trigger in response to that target. It should be noted however, that there is some debate over whether the attentional nasal versus temporal asymmetry effects actually do result in slower prosaccades (see e.g. Bompas et al., 2008), although such effects were indisputably observed in the studies of Kristjánsson et al. (2004).

When saccades are triggered by somatosensory rather than visual stimulation, prosaccade latencies are typically slowed by about 50 ms for humans (Neggers and Bekkering, 1999). Such saccades tend, furthermore, to be less accurate than visually triggered saccades (Groh and Sparks, 1996a; see also Amlôt et al., 2003), so might, according to the general logic applied in Kristjánsson et al. (2004), lead to faster antisaccades. Kristjánsson et al. found that for the haptically triggered saccades the latencies for prosaccades and antisaccades were overall quite similar, while the normal latency difference between prosaccades and antisaccades was observed for the visual saccade triggers. These results show a case where prosaccades are slowed while the antisaccades are not slowed to the same degree as other types of antisaccade, since the somatosensory antisaccades have similar latencies as the somatosensory prosaccades. This is consistent with the prediction that delaying prosaccades may lead to speeded antisaccades measured against the prosaccade latencies.

In another manipulation Kristjánsson et al. tested pro- and antisaccade performance with a saccade target of varying contrast. Doma and Hallett (1988a, 1988b; see also Reuter-Lorenz et al., 1991) found that saccades tend to be faster with higher contrast of saccade target against the background. As the prosaccades became slower the antisaccades grew gradually faster, with the exception that this did not occur at very low contrast levels, where difficult detection of the saccade trigger stimulus most likely limits the quickness of both saccade types.

An exception to this pattern of results in Kristjánsson et al. (2004) was found, however, when an auditory stimulus, (a *nonspatial* alerting stimulus, Posner 1978; Posner and Petersen 1990) was used to trigger the saccade. Such a stimulus produced a speeding effect upon both saccade types, perhaps affecting a stage of processing that is common to the two types of saccade (see e.g. Sternberg, 1969). Overall, however, the studies in Kristjánsson et al., 2004 argue for the competition account of pro- and antisaccades but also showing that this competition may not occur when certain processing stages which are common to the two saccade types are affected.

Conclusions

Saccadic eye movements and attention seem to interact in profoundly interesting ways. They may at times appear completely tied together, while other research results indicate that when particular task demands call for it, they may in fact be dissociated. A lot of evidence suggests that the neural mechanisms subserving the two overlap to a large extent, while some notable exceptions to this have certainly been found.

While research on shifts of covert visual attention has attempted to exclude effects of eye movements, and those researchers studying eye movements have tried to study those without any contaminating influence of observers internal biases, the two seem desperately intertwined, while they may be dissociable under certain (maybe even very limited) conditions. Clearly, both fields of research benefit from the increased understanding of each process and their interaction.

References

Amador, N., Schlag-Rey, M. and Schlag, J. (1998). Primate antisaccades. I. Behavioral characteristics. *Journal of Neurophysiology*, **80**, 1775–1786.

Amlôt, R., Walker, R., Driver, J. and Spence, C. (2003). Multimodal visual-somatosensory integration in saccade generation. *Neuropsychologia*, **41**, 1016–1023.

Baldauf, D. and Deubel, H. (2008). Properties of attentional selection during the preparation of sequential saccades. *Experimental Brain Research*, **184**, 411–425.

Beauchamp, M.S., Petit, L., Ellmore, T.M., Ingeholm, J. and Haxby, J.V. (2001). A parametric fMRI study of overt and covert shifts of visuospatial attention. *Neuroimage*, **14**, 310–321.

Bompas, A., Sterling, T., Rafal, R.D. and Sumner, P. (2008). Naso-temporal asymmetry for signals invisible to the retinotectal pathway. *Journal of Neurophysiology*, **100**, 412–421.

Cairney, S., Maruff, P., Vance, A., Barnett, R., Luk, E. and Currie J. (2001). Contextual abnormalities of saccadic inhibition in children with attention deficit hyperactivity disorder. *Experimental Brain Research*, **141**, 507–518.

Carpenter, R.H. (2001). Express saccades: is bimodality a result of the order of stimulus presentation? *Vision Research*, **41**, 1145–1151.

Carrasco, M., Williams, P.E. and Yeshurun, Y. (2002). Covert attention increases spatial resolution with or without masks: Support for signal enhancement. *Journal of Vision*, **2**, 467–479.

Corbetta, M. and Shulman, G.L. (2002) Control of goal-directed and stimulus-driven attention in the brain. *Nature Reviews Neuroscience*, **3**, 215–229

Corbetta, M., Akbudak, E., Conturo, T.E., Snyder, A.Z., Ollinger, J.M., Drury, H.A., *et al.* (1998). A common network of functional areas for attention and eye movements. *Neuron*, **21**, 761–773.

Craigher, L. and Rizzolatti, G. (2005). The premotor theory of attention. In L. Itti, G. Rees and J. Tsotsos (eds.) *Neurobiology of Attention* (pp. 181–186). Burlington, MA: Elsevier.

Crevits, L. and De Ridder, K. (1997). Disturbed striatoprefrontal mediated visual behavior in moderate to severe Parkinsonian patients. *Journal of Neurology, Neurosurgery and Psychiatry*, **63**, 296–299.

Currie, J., Ramsden, B., McArthur, C. and Maruff, P. (1991). Validation of a clinical antisaccadic eye movement test in the assessment of dementia. *Archives of Neurology*, **48**, 644–648.

Deubel, H. (2008). The time course of presaccadic attention shifts. *Psychological Research*, **72**, 639–640.

Deubel, H. and Schneider, W.X. (1996). Saccade target selection and object recognition: Evidence for a common attentional mechanism. *Vision Research*, **36**, 1827–1837.

Doma, H. and Hallett, P.E. (1988a). Rod-cone dependence of saccadic eye movement latency in a foveating task. *Vision Research*, **28**, 899–913.

Doma, H. and Hallett, P.E. (1988b). Dependence of saccadic eye movements on stimulus luminance, and an effect of task. *Vision Research*, **28**, 915–924.

Donders, F.C. (1864/1984). *Accommodation and Refraction of the Eye* (trans. W.D. Moore). Birmingham, AL: The Classics of Ophthalmology Library.

Doré-Mazars, K., Pouget, P. and Beauvillain, C. (2004). Attentional selection during preparation of eye movements. *Psychological Research*, **69**, 67–76.

Dorris, M.C., Munoz, D.P. (1995). A neural correlate for the gap effect on saccadic reaction times in monkey. *Journal of Neurophysiology*, **73**, 2558–2562.

Edelman, J.A. and Keller, E.L. (1996). Activity of visuomotor burst neurons in the superior colliculus accompanying express saccades. *Journal of Neurophysiology*, **76**, 908–926.

Edelman, J., Kristjánsson, Á. and Nakayama, K. (2007). The influence of object-relative visuomotor set on express saccades. *The Journal of Vision*, 7(6), 12.1–13.

Everling, S. and Fischer, B. (1998). The antisaccade: A review of basic research and clinical studies. *Neuropsychologia*, **36**, 885–899.

Everling, S. and Munoz, D.P. (2000). Neuronal correlates for preparatory set associated with pro-saccades and anti-saccades in the primate frontal eye field. *Journal of Neuroscience*, **20**, 387–400.

Everling S., Dorris, M.C. and Munoz, D.P. (1998). Reflex suppression in the antisaccade task is dependent on prestimulus neural processes. *Journal of Neurophysiology*, **80**, 1584–1589.

Everling, S., Dorris, M.C., Klein, R.M. and Munoz, D.P. (1999) Role of primate superior colliculus in preparation and execution of anti-saccades and pro-saccades. *Journal of Neuroscience*, **19**, 2740–2754.

Munoz, D.P. and Everling S. (2004). Look away: the anti-saccade task and the voluntary control of eye movement. *Nature Reviews Neuroscience*, **5**, 218–228.

Findlay, J.M. (1995). Visual search: eye movements and peripheral vision. *Optometry and Vision Science*, **72**, 461–466.

Findlay, J.M. and Gilchrist, I.D. (2003). *Active Vision: The Psychology of Looking and Seeing*. Oxford: Oxford University Press.

Fischer, B. and Boch, R. (1983). Saccadic eye movements after extremely short reaction times in the monkey. *Brain Research*, **260**, 21–26.

Fischer, B. and Ramsperger, E. (1984). Human express saccades: extremely short reaction times of goal directed eye movements. *Experimental Brain Research*, **57**, 191–5.

Fischer, B. and Weber, H. (1993). Express saccades and visual attention. *Behavioral and Brain Sciences* 16, 553–610.

Forbes, K. and Klein, R.M. (1996). The magnitude of the fixation offset effect with endogenously and exogenously controlled saccades. *Journal of Cognitive Neuroscience*, **8**, 344–352.

Fukushima, J., Fukushima, K., Chiba, T., Tanaka, S., Yamashita, I. and Kato, M. (1988). Disturbances of voluntary control of saccadic eye movements in schizophrenic patients. *Biological Psychiatry*, **23**, 670–677.

Funahashi, S., Chafee, M.V. and Goldman-Rakic, P.S. (1993). Prefrontal neuronal activity in rhesus monkeys performing a delayed antisaccade task. *Nature*, **365**, 753–756.

Gersch, T.M., Kowler, E. and Dosher, B. (2004). Dynamic allocation of visual attention during the execution of sequences of saccades. *Vision Research*, **44**, 1469–1483.

Godijn, R., and Theeuwes, J. (2003). Parallel allocation of attention prior to the execution of saccade sequences. *Journal of Experimental Psychology: Human Perception and Performance*, **29**, 882–896.

Groh, J.M. and Sparks, D.L. (1996). Saccades to somatosensory targets. I. Behavioral characteristics. *Journal of Neurophysiology*, **75**, 412–427.

Guitton, D., Buchtel, H.A. and Douglas, R.M. (1985). Frontal lobe lesions in man cause difficulties in suppressing reflexive glances and in generating goal directed saccades. *Experimental Brain Research*, **58**, 455–472.

Hallett, P.E. (1978). Primary and secondary saccades to goals defined by instructions. *Vision Research*, **18**, 1279–1296.

Hutton, S.B (2008) Cognitive control of saccadic eye movements, *Brain and Cognition*, **68**, 327–833.

Hoffman, J.E. and Subramaniam, B. (1995). The role of visual attention in saccadic eye movements. *Perception and Psychophysics*, **57**, 787–795.

Hunt, A.R. and Kingstone, A. (2003). Inhibition of return: Dissociating attentional and oculomotor components. *Journal of Experimental Psychology: Human Perception and Performance*, **29**, 1068–1074.

Juan, C.H., Shorter-Jacobi, S.M. and Schall, J.D. (2004). Dissociation of spatial attention and saccade preparation. *Proceedings of the National Academy of Sciences U S A*, **101**, 15541–15544.

Jüttner, M. and Wolf, W. (1992) Occurrence of human express saccades depends on stimulus uncertainty and stimulus sequence. *Experimental Brain Research*, **89**, 678–681.

Kalesnykas, R.P. and Hallett, P.E. (1987). The differentiation of visually guided and anticipatory saccades in gap and overlap paradigms. *Experimental Brain Research*, **68**, 115–121.

Kingstone A. and Klein, R.M. (1993). What are human express saccades? *Perception and Psychophysics*, **54**, 260–273.

Klein, R.M. (1980). Does oculomotor readiness mediate cognitive control of visual attention. In R. Nickerson (ed.) *Attention and Performance VIII* (pp. 259–276). Hillsdale, NJ: Erlbaum.

Klein, R. (2000). Inhibition of return. *Trends in Cognitive Sciences*, **4**, 138–147.

Klein, R.M. (2004). On the control of orienting. In M.I. Posner (ed.) *Cognitive Neuroscience of Attention* (pp. 29–44). New York: Guilford Press.

Kowler, E., Anderson, E., Dosher B. and Blaser, E. (1995). The role of attention in the programming of saccades. *Vision Research*, **35**, 1897–1916.

Krappmann, P., Everling, S. and Flohr, H. (1998). Accuracy of visually and memory-guided antisaccades in man. *Vision Research*, **38**, 2979–2985.

Kristjánsson, Á. (2006). Rapid learning in attention shifts–a review. *Visual Cognition*, **13**, 324–362.

Kristjánsson, Á. (2007). Saccade landing point selection and the competition account of pro- and antisaccade generation: The involvement of visual attention–A review. *Scandinavian Journal of Psychology*, **48**, 97–113.

Kristjánsson, Á. and Nakayama, K. (2003). A primitive memory system for the deployment of transient attention. *Perception and Psychophysics*, **65**, 711–724.

Kristjánsson, Á. and Sigurðardóttir, H.M. (2008). On the benefits of transient attention across the visual field. *Perception*, **37**, 747–764

Kristjánsson, Á., Chen, Y. and Nakayama, K. (2001a). Less attention is more in the preparation of antisaccades, but not prosaccades. *Nature Neuroscience*, **4**, 1037–1042.

Kristjánsson, Á., Mackeben, M. and Nakayama, K. (2001b). Rapid, object-based learning in the deployment of transient attention. *Perception*, **30**, 1375–1387.

Kristjánsson, Á., Vandenbroucke, M.W. and Driver, J. (2004). When pros become cons for anti-versus prosaccades: Factors with opposite or common effects on different saccade types. *Experimental Brain Research*, **155**, 231–244.

Kustov, A.A. and Robinson, D.L. (1996). Shared neural control of attentional shifts and eye movements. *Nature*, **384**, 74–77.

Leigh, R.J. and Zee, D.S. (1999). *The Neurology of Eye Movements* (3rd edn.). Oxford: Oxford University Press.

Locke, J. (1689/1975) *An Essay concerning Human Understanding*. Oxford: Oxford University Press.

Mayfrank, L., Mobashery, M., Kimmig, H. and Fischer B. (1986). The role of fixation and visual attention in the occurrence of express saccades in man. *European Archives of Psychiatry and Neurological Science*, **235**, 269–275.

Mackeben, M. and Nakayama, K. (1993). Express attentional shifts. *Vision Research*, **33**, 85–90.

Maruff, P., Purcell, R., Tyler, P., Pantelis, C. and Currie, J. (1999). Abnormalities of internally generated saccades in obsessive-compulsive disorder. *Psychological Medicine*, **9**, 1377–1385.

Mitchell, J.P., Macrae, C.N. and Gilchrist I.D. (2002). Working memory and the suppression of reflexive saccades. *Journal of Cognitive Neuroscience*, **14**, 95–103.

Moore T. and Fallah, M. (2001). Control of eye movements and spatial attention. *Proceedings of the National Academy of Sciences USA*, **98**, 1273–1276.

Munoz, D.P. and Wurtz, R.H. (1995a). Saccade-related activity in monkey superior colliculus. I. Characteristics of burst and build-up cells. *Journal of Neurophysiology*, **73**, 2313–2333.

Munoz, D.P. and Wurtz, R.H, (1995b). Saccade-related activity in monkey superior colliculus. II. Spread of activity during saccades. *Journal of Neurophysiology*, **73**, 2334–2348.

Munoz, D.P., Armstrong, I.T., Hampton, K.A. and Moore, K.D. (2003). Altered control of visual fixation and saccadic eye movements in attention-deficit hyperactivity disorder. *Journal of Neurophysiology*, **90**, 503–514.

Nakayama, K. and Mackeben, M. (1989). Sustained and transient components of visual attention. *Vision Research*, **29**, 1631–1647.

Neggers, S.W.F. and Bekkering, H. (1999). Integration of visual and somatosensory target information in goal-directed eye and arm movements. *Experimental Brain Research*, **125**, 97–107.

Neisser, U. (1967). *Cognitive psychology*. New York: Appleton-Century-Crofts.

Pashler, H. (1998). *The Psychology of Attention*. Cambridge, MA: The MIT Press.

Pashler, H., Carrier, M. and Hoffman, J. (1993). Saccadic eye movements and dual-task interference. *Quarterly Journal of Experimental Psychology A*, **46**, 51–82.

Peterson, M.S., Kramer, A.F. and Irwin, D.E. (2004). Covert shifts of attention precede involuntary eye movements. *Perception and Psychophysics*, **66**, 398–405.

Posner, M.I. (1978). *Chronometric explorations of mind*. Hillsdale, NJ: Erlbaum.

Posner, M.I. (1980). Orienting of attention. *Quarterly Journal of Experimental Psychology*, **32**, 3–25.

Posner, M.I. and Cohen, Y. (1984) Components of visual orienting. In H. Bouma and D. Bouwhuis (eds.) *Attention and Performance* (Vol. X) pp. 531–556. Hillsdale, NJ: Erlbaum.

Posner, M.I. and Petersen, S.E. (1990). The attention system of the human brain. *Annual Review of Neuroscience*, **13**, 25–42.

Posner, M.I., Petersen, S.E., Fox, P.T. and Raichle, M.E. (1988). Localization of cognitive operations in the human brain. *Science*, **240**, 1627–1631.

Pratt, J. and Nghiem, T. (2000). The role of the gap effect in the orienting of attention: Evidence for express attentional shifts. *Visual Cognition*, **5**, 629–644.

Rafal, R., Henik, A. and Smith, J. (1991). Extrageniculate contributions to reflex visual orienting in normal humans: A temporal hemifield advantage. *Journal of Cognitive Neuroscience*, **3**, 322–328.

Reuter-Lorenz, P.A., Hughes, H.C. and Fendrich, R. (1991). The reduction of saccadic latency by prior offset of the fixation point: an analysis of the gap effect. *Perception and Psychophysics*, **49**, 167–175.

Rizzolatti, G., Riggio, L., Pascola, I. and Umilta, C. (1987). Reorienting attention across the horizontal and vertical medians: Evidence in favor of a premotor theory of attention. *Neuropsychologia*, **25**, 31–40.

Roberts, R.J., Hager, L.D. and Heron, C. (1994) Prefrontal cognitive-processes: Working-memory and inhibition in the antisaccade task. *Journal of Experimental Psychology: General*, **123**, 374–393.

Rosenberg, D.R., Averbach, D.H., O'Hearn, K.M., Seymour, A.B., Birmaher, B. and Sweeney, J.A. (1997). Oculomotor response inhibition abnormalities in pediatric obsessive-compulsive disorder. *Archives of General Psychiatry*, **54**, 831–838.

Ross, L.E. and Ross, S.M. (1980). Saccade latency and warning signals: Stimulus onset, offset, and change as warning events. *Perception and Psychophysics*, **27**, 251–257.

Ross, L.E. and Ross, S.M. (1981). Saccade latency and warning signals: Effects of auditory and visual stimulus onset and offset. *Perception and Psychophysics*, **29**, 429–437.

Saslow, M.G. (1967). Effects of components of displacement-step upon latency for saccadic eye movements. *Journal of the Optical Society of America A*, **57**, 1024–1029.

Sato, T.R. and Schall, J.D. (2003). Effects of stimulus-response compatibility on neural selection in frontal eye field. *Neuron*, **38**, 637–648.

Schall, J.D. (2004). On the role of frontal eye field in guiding attention and saccades. *Vision Research*, **44**, 1453–1467.

Schall, J.D. and Thompson, K.G. (1999). Neural selection and control of visually guided eye movements. *Annual Review of Neuroscience*, **22**, 241–259.

Schlag-Rey, M., Amador, N., Sanchez, H. and Schlag, J. (1997). Antisaccade performance predicted by neuronal activity in the supplementary eye field. *Nature*, **390**, 398–401.

Schneider, W.X. (1995). VAM: A neuro-cognitive model for visual attention control of segmentation, object recognition and space based motor action. *Visual Cognition*, **2**, 331–375.

Schneider, W.X. and Deubel, H. (2002). Selection-for-perception and selection-for-spatial-motor-action are coupled by visual attention: A review of recent findings and new evidence for stimulus driven saccade control. In W. Prinz and B. Hommel (eds.) *Common Mechanisms in Perception and Action: Attention and Performance XIX*, (pp. 609–627). New York: Oxford University Press.

Sereno, A.B. and Holzman, P.S. (1995). Antisaccades and smooth pursuit eye movements in schizophrenia. *Biological Psychiatry*, **37**, 394–401.

Sheliga, B.M., Riggio, L. and Rizzolatti, G. (1994). Orienting of attention and eye movements. *Experimental Brain Research*, **98**, 507–522.

Shepherd, M., Findlay, J.M. and Hockey, R.J. (1986). The relationship between eye movements and spatial attention. *Quarterly Journal of Experimental Psychology Section A Human Experimental Psychology*, **38**, 475–491.

Sternberg, S. (1969). The discovery of processing stages: Extension of Donders' method. *Acta Psychologica*, **30**, 276–315.

Stuyven, E., Van der Goten, K., Vandierendonck, A., Claeys, K. and Crevits, L. (2000). The effect of cognitive load on saccadic eye movements. *Acta Psychologica*, **104**, 69–85.

Treisman, A. and Sato, S. (1990). Conjunction search revisited. *Journal of Experimental Psychology: Human Perception and Performance*, **16**, 459–478.

Yantis, S. and Jonides, J. (1984). Abrupt visual onsets and selective attention: evidence from visual search. *Journal of Experimental Psychology: Human Perception and Performance*, **10**, 601–621.

Wang, D., Kristjánsson, Á. and Nakayama, K. (2005). Efficient visual search without top-down or bottom-up guidance. *Perception and Psychophysics*, **67**, 239–253.

Wenban-Smith, M.G. and Findlay, J.M. (1991). Express saccades: is there a separate population in humans? *Experimental Brain Research*, **87**, 218–222.

Wright, R.D and Ward, L.M. (2008). *Orienting of Attention*. Oxford: Oxford University Press.

CHAPTER 26

Oculomotor inhibition of return

Raymond M. Klein and Matthew D. Hilchey

Abstract

A mechanism referred to as inhibition of return (IOR) was proposed by Michael Posner and colleagues (Posner and Cohen, 1984; Posner et al., 1985) to account for delayed responses to stimuli presented in previously attended regions or on previously attended objects. This increase in response times is intricately linked to the orienting machinery of the oculomotor system and, as such, it was proposed that IOR plays a crucial role in facilitating search behaviour. Properties of IOR that have been identified using a simple cuing paradigm (e.g. IOR can be coded in environmental and object coordinates) are consistent with this functional interpretation. The interaction of IOR with oculomotor phenomena is reviewed with an emphasis on how orienting behaviour is modulated by IOR. Studies using a wide variety of methods demonstrate that fixations that return gaze to a recently fixated region (even when these refixations occur more frequently than chance) suffer a temporal cost, no doubt because whatever processes encourages the return of attention must overcome the inhibitory traces left behind by prior orienting.

In the laboratories of Michael Posner (Cohen, 1981) and Giovanni Berlucchi (Berlucchi et al., 1981) it was independently discovered that humans have a tendency toward slower response times (RT) to targets at locations toward which attention had been previously oriented. Posner and colleagues (Posner et al., 1985) later coined the phrase 'inhibition of return' (IOR) to describe this phenomenon but it subsequently began to appear in the literature with various plays on this phrase: including 'inhibitory aftereffect' (Tassinari et al., 1987), 'inhibitory tagging' (Fuentes et al., 1999; Klein, 1988), and when affecting oculomotor behaviour, 'inhibition of saccade return' (e.g. Hooge and Frens, 2000). Despite these variations in nomenclature, these examples of what is typically called IOR are all characterized by negative consequences for subsequent processing that is caused by spatial stimulation or spatial orienting. The seminal investigations conducted by Posner and Cohen (1984) used a variant of the spatial orienting paradigm (Posner, 1980) to generate and measure IOR. This pioneering work laid a foundation for much of the research that has emerged since the discovery of IOR.

Model task: early findings

In the model task used by Posner and Cohen (1984), observers were instructed to keep their eyes fixated on a central box flanked by two equi-eccentric peripheral boxes. Eye-movements were recorded and trials in which participants made a detectable eye-movement were excluded from analysis. A trial was initiated by a 150-ms brightening of the outline of one of the peripheral boxes. A bright target in one of the three potential boxes followed the peripheral stimulus. In one version of the experiment, the target most often appeared in the centre box (0.6 probability) but would occasionally (0.1 probability for each side) appear in one of the peripheral boxes at variable intervals (0, 50, 100, 200, 300, or 500 ms) after the onset of the cue. The participant was required to make a speeded manual response upon detection of a target stimulus. The remaining trials (occurring with a probability of 0.2) contained no target and served to deter any anticipatory responses. The underlying logic behind the high frequency of central target onsets was to encourage observers to maintain attention at the centre box or to endogenously return attention to that location if it was captured by the peripheral cue. Coupled with the knowledge that eye movements were being monitored, participants had ample incentive to maintain centre fixation and attention. In an alternative version, attention was returned to fixation exogenously by a second cue there prior to a peripheral target. At short stimulus onset asynchronies (SOAs less than approximately 150 ms), RTs to targets at the cued location were markedly faster than RT to targets at the uncued location. In contrast, when the SOA exceeded approximately 250 ms this pattern reversed and RTs became slowest at the cued location. Importantly, this inhibitory aftereffect was not observed following a shift of attention generated endogenously in response to an informative, centrally presented arrow.

Although this traditional methodology for exploring IOR focused entirely on manual responses to a peripheral target, from early on it was postulated that IOR was profoundly linked to the oculomotor system. This possibility was examined by introducing experimental manipulations that gauged the performance of oculomotor behaviour in similar paradigms. Posner and Cohen (1984), for example, demonstrated that saccadic latency was elevated when attention, by way of an eye movement (overt attentional shift), was reoriented toward a location that had previously been fixated. Additionally, the effect was relatively long-lasting (at least 1.5 s). Vaughan (1984) replicated the temporal effect of IOR on saccades and found, moreover, that there was an inhibitory gradient at the location of the previous fixation. The gradient extended a minimum of 1.5° vertically from the destination of the last saccade and the saccadic latencies became indistinguishable from all other regions in the visual field when 3.2° or more separated the last fixation from the next one (see also Hooge and Frens, 2000, and Fig. 26.3, later in this chapter).

Posner et al. (1985) provided converging evidence that the superior colliculus (SC, a subcortical structure responsible for saccadic eye movements) might play an important role in generating IOR. They tested patients with progressive supranuclear palsy (PSP), a degenerative neurological condition affecting the SC and consequently the ability to generate saccades (especially vertically-directed saccades) in the model task described above. Their performance was compared to normal and patient controls with lesions in various cortical regions. If the detection of a stimulus was somehow linked to prior oculomotor activity, one would expect that disruption of the superior colliculus would impact the expression of IOR. They found, in line with their hypotheses, that IOR was absent in PSP patients for vertically oriented stimuli while it was normal for all controls, a pattern that became the spark for further neuropsychological research on IOR. Sapir et al. (1999), for example, extended this finding by demonstrating that a patient with localized damage to the right SC showed early facilitation but failed to exhibit IOR to peripheral targets presented to the affected left visual field (see also Sereno et al. 2006). A telling double dissociation is revealed by combining these findings with those from a unique patient (Smith et al., 2004) who suffered from a congenital ophthalmoplegia and who, as a result, had never made a saccadic eye movement. This patient showed normal IOR despite showing no evidence of early facilitation in response to uninformative peripheral cues.

Mapping: oculocentric, environmental, and object-based

Some of the earliest investigative work centred on identifying the spatial distribution of IOR. Evidence that IOR was not mapped simply in oculocentric (or retinotopic) coordinates was first demonstrated by having participants make a saccadic eye movement after the cue and before the appearance of the target (Posner and Cohen, 1984; Vaughan, 1984; Maylor and Hockey, 1985). In such a situation it is possible to probe for inhibition at either the oculocentric or the environmental location that had been stimulated. Using variants of this method, both Posner and Cohen (1984) and Maylor and

Hockey (1985) found that the inhibitory effect was present for cues and targets that occupied the same environmental but not the same retinal location (but for evidence of oculocentric mapping following a smooth pursuit eye movement, see Abrams and Pratt (2000), Souto & Kerzel (2009)). By moving the objects in a display after one of them had been cued, Tipper et al. (1991) later discovered that IOR was liable to follow the movement of a previously attended object (an object-centred form of IOR) within a scene. These findings had profound implications for the role of the superior colliculus. Because the SC is a subcortical structure that controls gaze direction using oculocentric coordinates (Robinson, 1972), the findings that IOR could be mapped in environmental and/or object coordinates, implied that higher cortical processing must also have been involved. This was confirmed when Tipper et al. (1997) demonstrated that object-based IOR does not cross the vertical midline in split brain patients. Subsequently, Sapir and colleagues (Sapir et al., 2004) discovered that environmental IOR was abolished by lesions to the parietal lobe (more specifically the intraparietal sulcus). Using trans-cranial magnetic stimulation to generate a temporary lesion, van Koningsbruggen et al. (2010) provided converging evidence for this attribution and a more confident localization of spatiotopic coding of IOR to the right intraparietal sulcus.

Recording from single neurons in the parietal lobe of monkeys while they searched an array of targets and distractors, Mirpour et al. (2009), found neurophysiological evidence for an inhibitory tagging system in the lateral intraparietal area. Thus, while it is clear that the SC plays a substantial role in generating IOR, it is almost certainly operating in concert with other brain regions.

Function: IOR as a novelty-seeking mechanism

Posner and Cohen (1984) proposed that by discouraging the return of attention to recently visited locations or objects, IOR was essentially a novelty-seeking mechanism:

> We believe that the inhibition effect evolved to maximize sampling of the visual environment. Once the eyes move away from the target location, events that occur at that environmental location are inhibited—with respect to other positions. This would reduce the effectiveness of a previously active area of space in summoning attention and serve as a basis for favouring fresh areas at which no previous targets had been presented. The long-lasting nature of inhibition (1.5 sec or more) seems to be about the right length to ensure that the next movement or two will have a reduced probability of returning to the former target position.
>
> (Posner and Cohen, 1984, p. 550.)

Klein (1988) applied this idea to visual search, suggesting that IOR could improve the efficiency of search by discouraging reinspections. The ecological validity of such a claim, if not readily apparent, can be conceptualized quite easily by imagining an animal scavenging for sustenance or a hunter searching for game. Having already inspected what appeared to be a region of high potential but finding nothing there, there would be good reason to avoid revisiting it. Yet, in the absence of some form of reinspection-discouraging mechanism there would presumably be nothing to deter the searching agent from perpetually returning to the promising site (Itti and Koch, 2001). Klein (1988) tested his proposal that IOR was such a mechanism by probing areas that either previously contained a stimulus (on) or did not (off) in serial search (in which all items of the visual scene are scanned until a target is detected) and used similar conditions from a pop-out search task (in which a basic feature of the target can be selected pre-attentively) to provide a baseline. Confirming the proposal, response times to on-probes were greater than to off-probes following serial search and this difference was greater than that following pop-out search. Although this proposal was briefly contested in the early 1990s, on the basis of empirical findings about the properties of IOR, the empirical challenges were subsequently rebuffed (see Klein and MacInnes, 1999, and Klein, 2000, for a discussion) and it has since been widely endorsed (e.g. Itti and Koch, 2001; Tipper et al., 1994; for a review, see Wang and Klein, 2010). More recently the foraging facilitator proposal has been challenged again, not on the basis of the properties of IOR, but rather on the basis of evidence from the sequence of fixations made when we are inspecting a scene. This evidence will be critically reviewed in later sections of this chapter.

IOR and oculomotor phenomena

In this section, we review studies that have explored how IOR interacts with variables that are known to affect oculomotor behaviour.

Saccadic averaging

Saccadic averaging (known alternatively as the 'global effect' or the 'centre of gravity effect') occurs when two or more stimuli are presented simultaneously within the peripheral region of the visual field. The resulting saccade, rather than landing at one of the stimulated locations, often arrives at the midpoint or 'centre of gravity' of the separate elements. To determine how IOR affects saccadic averaging, Watanabe (2001) presented participants with either no cue, a left cue, right cue or paired cues at the location(s) where a single or paired target might subsequently appear (see Fig. 26.1).

Participants made a speeded eye movement in response to the target or pair of targets as quickly and accurately as possible. Reflecting IOR's effect on the speed of processing, trials on which a single cue corresponded spatially with a single target yielded slower saccadic reaction times than trials on which the target was uncued. On paired target trials eye movements were subject to saccadic averaging with many saccades directed to the region midway between the two targets. Perhaps reflecting IOR's effect on saccade metrics, when only one cue was presented on a paired target trial, the landing position was biased away from the cued location (see bottom panel of Fig. 26.1). A similar effect of a previously presented onset distractor upon the direction of saccades toward uncued targets was observed by Godijn and Theeuwes (2002) in their study of oculomotor capture reviewed in the next section.

Using manual responses to onset targets following a single cue or the simultaneous presentation of two, three, or four cues, Klein et al. (2005) discovered that IOR following multiple cues was present not at the locations of the individual elements of an array of cues, but rather in the direction of the net vector or centre of gravity of the grouped array. All of the key findings from Klein et al. (2005) were replicated by Langley et al. (2011). They interpreted their findings in terms of oculomotor activation and saccade averaging noting that an overt (saccade) or covert (shift of attention) orienting response was programmed to the centre of gravity (McGowan et al., 1998; Melcher and Kowler, 1999) of the elements making up the cue. Then, when a target was subsequently presented in the same direction as this prior orienting response, orienting to the target was delayed and, hence, RTs lengthened. In addition, as the target's direction differed from the inhibited direction, RT improved, revealing a gradient of inhibition similar to that generated on trials with a single cue.

Oculomotor capture

It has been shown that the spontaneous presentation of a new item in the visual field often reflexively captures eye movements (oculomotor capture) even when that target is irrelevant to the task (e.g. Theeuwes et al., 1998). In Godijn and Theeuwes' (2002) modified oculomotor-capture paradigm, a fixation point flanked seven of eight equi-distant circles to form an imaginary circle. Following fixation and a warning signal, a distractor circle appeared suddenly at the previously vacant eighth position (at either a 0°, 90°, 180° or 270° angle). After 50 ms, a colour change within a circle (at either 45°, 135°, 225° or 315° angle) denoted the location to which a saccade had to be executed. Another 800 ms later, a second target to which a saccade had to be executed was indexed by a colour change at one of the four possible sudden onset locations. On half of the trials, the second target coincided with the location of the sudden onset or with a non-onset location that maintained the same angle and distance from the first target to ensure that saccadic amplitude was equated. The other half of the trials displayed the second target at one of the remaining possible locations. Trials on which the onset stimulus failed to capture an eye movement (approximately 60% of the trials) and on which the second target coincided spatially with the sudden onset produced an IOR effect that was identical in magnitude to the IOR observed on oculomotor capture trials

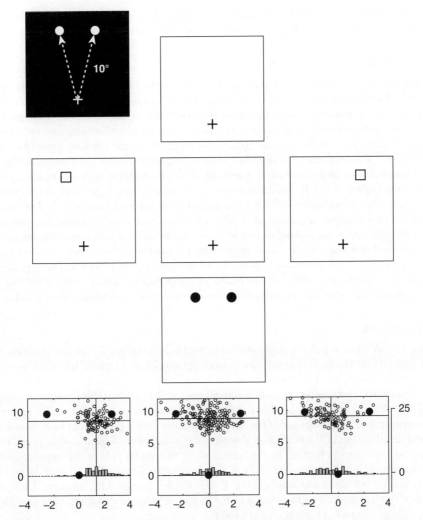

Fig. 26.1 Selected methods and results from Watanabe (2001). The upper left inset illustrates the white fixation + and circular targets as they were presented on a black background. The targets were 10° from fixation and 2.6° from the vertical midline. For convenience the contrast has been reversed in the remaining panels. The fixation display is shown on the top row. Three of the four possible cue conditions are shown on the next row (not shown was the cue condition in which both possible target locations were cued). Note that the fixation stimulus remained present when the cues appeared but was removed 100 ms prior to the appearance of the target display which contained either the left, right or both (as illustrated here) targets. Results from participant B on trials with the paired targets are shown in the bottom row in locations, from, left to right, corresponding to the cue conditions displayed two rows above. In the data panels the x-and y-axes represent horizontal and vertical positions (respectively) of the landing positions of saccades (in degrees). The solid circle displayed at y=0 represents the starting (fixation) position of each saccade while the solid circles at y=10 represent the locations of the simultaneously displayed targets. Vertical lines in each panel represent the mean horizontal and vertical landing positions and the horizontal landing positions are also represented by the histograms. With kind permission from Springer Science+Business Media: *Experimental Brain Research*, Watanabe, K. Inhibition of return in averaging saccades, **138**, 2001, 330–342.

(approximately 36% of the trials). Thus, covert activation of the oculomotor system generated the same amount of IOR as when an eye movement was actually executed.

Antisaccades

Several studies have examined IOR in the context of antisaccades (a saccadic response in the opposite direction of a peripheral onset). Rafal et al. (1994) were the first to use antisaccades in an IOR paradigm to investigate possible sensory (attentional/perceptual) versus oculomotor explanations for IOR. In two experiments, the sequence of experimental events was very much akin to what we have reviewed in the 'Model Task' section. Participants fixated a central element, ignored or made a prosaccade to a peripheral cue (first stimulus), observed centre brightening and responded by way of either a prosaccade or an antisaccade to a peripheral target (second stimulus). The basic rationale is relatively straightforward. If, following a peripheral cue, IOR affects primarily input processes, then reaction time should be delayed when the target repeats the cued location, whether the correct response is a prosaccade or an antisaccade. On the other hand, if IOR delays spatial responding, then targets calling for a response in the direction of the cue will suffer from inhibition, whether or not the target is presented in the cued location. Supporting a sensory/attentional locus of IOR's effect on processing both pro- and antisaccades were slowest when the cue and target had been presented at the same location (but see p. 480). Similar results were reported by Fecteau et al. (2004) in a target-target version of the model task in which pro- and antisaccades were randomly intermixed.

The gap effect

Whereas a stable fixation point is most commonly used in IOR studies, it is nonetheless known that the advance offset of the fixation point reduces saccadic latencies to peripheral targets (Saslow, 1967). Fixation removal just prior to the presentation of a target response is commonly referred to as a gap and the consequent reduction in saccadic reaction time (SRT) as the gap effect (Reuter-Lorenz et al., 1991). Behavioural studies suggest that the gap effect has at least two components (Taylor et al., 1998)—preparation induced by use of the fixation offset as a warning signal that a response is imminent and disinhibition of the oculomotor system, and neurophysiological studies reveal that the presence of a stimulus at fixation activates neurons in the rostral pole of the superior colliculus which, in turn, inhibit the remainder of the saccade-generating intermediate layer of the SC (Dorris and Munoz, 1995; Munoz and Wurtz, 1992, 1993a, 1993b). As noted by Taylor et al. (1998) this inhibition can be removed endogenously in the course of voluntary looking (Sommer, 1994) or exogenously by removal of the stimulus at fixation.

Abrams and Dobkin (1994a) were the first to explore whether IOR and removal of fixation affected common processing stages. They combined a peripheral cue to generate IOR with fixation removal to generate a gap effect. Applying additive factors logic (Sternberg, 1969), they reasoned that if IOR and the gap effect shared a common stage of processing then the two manipulations ought to have interactive effects on saccade latency whereas if they shared no stages of processing they ought to have additive effects. Although they found an interaction between the gap effect and IOR, two aspects of their pattern of results are anomalous. First, consider the direction of the interaction: IOR was less pronounced on the overlap trials than on those trials for which the fixation stimulus had been removed prior to the appearance of the target. If the superior colliculus were responsible for generating IOR then one might have imagined that this inhibition would be increased rather than decreased by the intracolliculus inhibition from its own fixation circuitry. Second, the effect of IOR generated on the overlap trials was alarmingly small (2–4 ms) considering that maintenance of fixation is the standard procedure in most studies of IOR. When Hunt and Kingstone (2003) repeated the strategy of combining IOR with the gap effect, they found the opposite interaction: IOR was more pronounced during fixation than after removal of fixation. To account for this opposite interaction, Hunt and Kingstone noted that in Abrams and Dobkin's experiment the cues, target and fixation stimulus were all so similar that there was a high potential for 'perceptual confusion' which may have impacted participants' response strategies and patterns.

Table 26.1 Dissociations reported when exploring properties of IOR using manual and saccadic responses

	Type of response	
	Manual	Saccadic
Effect of IOR on temporal order judgement (Maylor, 1985; Posner et al., 1985)	No	Yes
Target luminance and IOR (Hunt and Kingstone, 2003)	Interaction	Additive
Fixation removal (gap effect) and IOR (Hunt and Kingstone, 2003)	Additive	Interaction
S-Cone cues (Sumner et al., 2004)	IOR	No IOR
Effect of spatial working memory load on IOR (Zhang and Zhang, 2011)	Yes	No

Manual and saccadic response dissociation

One of the first dissociations (see Table 26.1) involving saccadic versus manual responses was demonstrated by Posner et al. (1985). Following a peripheral cue, a cue back to centre, and a long enough interval to measure IOR, they presented a pair of targets asynchronously (separated by 10, 25, 45, or 200 ms), with one at the previously cued location and one at the opposite location. When participants made saccadic responses in the 'most comfortable' direction there was a tendency to move opposite the cued location when the interval between the targets was short. Importantly, and replicating Maylor's (1985) findings, when a temporal order judgement was signalled by a manual response there was no effect of the cue upon perceived arrival times (for a review, see Klein et al., 1998).

When Hunt and Kingstone (2003) repeated the conditions described in the preceding section ('Gap effect') while using manual instead of saccadic responses, they found that the factors of fixation offset and cuing (IOR) were additive. Hunt and Kingstone (2003) also examined IOR as a function of the luminance of the target with manual and saccadic responses. Completing a conceptual double dissociation they found an additive pattern between cuing and target luminance when the responses were saccadic, and (replicating Reuter-Lorenz et al., 1996) an interaction (greater IOR with dimmer targets) when responses were manual.

A psychophysical manipulation was used by Sumner et al. (2004) to explore IOR using manual and saccadic responses by choosing stimuli that either bypassed or did not bypass the SC. Their method capitalized on the fact that the SC does not receive direct projections from short-wave-sensitive (S) cones. They reasoned that if the SC were solely responsible for generating IOR, one would expect that non-informative peripheral events that are processed via pathways that do not project directly to the SC might fail to generate the effect. In their experiments different cues were used to stimulate luminance or S-cone pathways and the participants detected or localized the luminance targets with manual or oculomotor responses, respectively. Manual detection responses showed evidence of IOR regardless of the nature of the cues while saccadic responses showed IOR with luminance cues but not with S-cone cues. Whereas the lesion studies reviewed earlier suggested that the SC plays an important role in generating IOR, Sumner et al. (2004), concluded that there must be separate IOR generators (see also Hunt and Kingstone, 2003): One mediated by the retino-tectal pathway that generates IOR in response to oculomotor activation, the other mediated cortically following attentional capture. The retinotectal generator causes saccadic IOR, while both generators contribute to traditional IOR, measured with a manual response.

Two 'flavours' of IOR

Noting the importance of distinguishing the causes of IOR from the effects of IOR on processing once IOR had been generated, Taylor and Klein (1998) considered a matrix of 24 combinations of experimental conditions that could be used to identify IOR's cause(s) and effects (see Fig. 26.2A). These conditions included whether the participant made manual or saccadic responses to the first of two target stimuli, or ignored this stimulus, made manual or saccadic responses to the second of two stimuli, and whether these stimuli were peripheral targets or central arrows that would elicit orienting exogenously or endogenously, respectively. At the time, only 10 of those 24 cells had been explored in the literature, with IOR being observed in nine and inferred to be present in the tenth. Taylor and Klein (1998) proposed a theory of IOR, consistent with the pattern of findings in the literature (Fig. 26.2A) in which IOR's effect is a response bias that is caused by prior oculomotor programming. According to this theory, IOR should be observed in all and only those conditions for which the vertical (IOR is caused by oculomotor activation) and horizontal arrows (IOR's motoric effect would impact performance) in Fig. 26.2A intersect. In her dissertation Taylor (1997; Taylor and Klein, 2000) conducted a parametric study explicitly testing this theory by exploring all 24 possible conditions illustrated in Fig. 26.2.

Every trial began with a 500-ms fixation period. A central box was flanked by two equidistant horizontally aligned peripheral boxes. Participants were required to fixate on the central box before the onset of an exogenous or endogenous stimulus (S1 or the first signal). The exogenous S1 consisted of a brightening of either the peripheral box, while the endogenous S1 consisted of a leftward or rightward pointing arrow appearing in the centre box. The four different S1s were equally probable and 300 ms in duration. The task in response to S1 (ignore, manual localization, or saccadic localization) varied across sessions. Following a 200-ms ISI, the centre box was illuminated for 300 ms and followed by another 200 ms ISI. In the Ignore-S1 and Manual-S1 blocks, feedback was provided to the participants if there was any evidence of an eye movement or failure to maintain fixation prior to the target, and any trial in which an eye movement was detected was discarded and recycled. On Saccade-S1 trials an eye-movement back to fixation was required. If participants failed to return to the centre box within 500 ms, the trial was flagged, discarded, and recycled.

The second stimulus (S2), appearing 1000 ms after the onset of the first one, was either a leftward or rightward central arrow or a peripheral dot centred in the left or right box for 1000 ms. All combinations were equally probable and designed to reveal the consequence of S1. The response was either manual or saccadic and was measured in accordance with the procedure for a response to S1. The results are shown in Fig. 26.2B. One encouraging aspect of the results from this study is that it replicated the finding of IOR in all 10 of the conditions for which IOR had previously been obtained or implied. Secondly, whereas IOR was obtained in all 12 conditions for which the unified account of IOR that Taylor and Klein were testing predicted it to occur, IOR was observed in four additional conditions where it was predicted not to occur.

Most importantly, the results can be organized into two strikingly different patterns. In sessions during which eye movements were not being executed at all (neither to the cue nor to the target, see bolded box in Fig. 26.2B) IOR was only observed in response to peripheral targets. Responses to central targets showed no evidence of IOR under these conditions. This suggests that when the oculomotor system is inactive, if not tonically inhibited (no-response manual and manual-manual cells), a perceptual/attentional flavour of IOR is generated. This conclusion follows from the finding that localization of cued peripheral targets was delayed while similar responses made in the cued direction in response to central arrows were not. In contrast to this pattern, in sessions for which the oculomotor system was active (either in response to the cue or to the target), whenever IOR was observed in response to a peripheral target it was also obtained in response to a central arrow. IOR in response to a centrally presented target is obviously not about a delay in the perception of, or orienting to, a peripheral stimulus; instead, it is about responding in the direction of the previous behaviour whether it was orienting, responding or both. Importantly, collapsed across these conditions the IOR in response to peripheral targets (17.1 ms) was no greater than the IOR in response to central arrows (22.4 ms) suggesting that there was no extra sensory/attentional component in those conditions not characterized by oculomotor inhibition.

Using an ignored peripheral cue to generate IOR and saccadic responses to measure it, Abrams and Dobkin (1994b) found, in conflict with Taylor and Klein (2000) a larger cued minus uncued

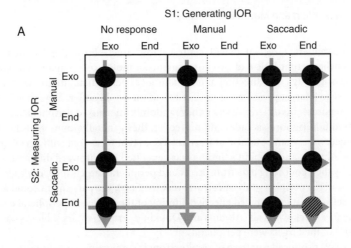

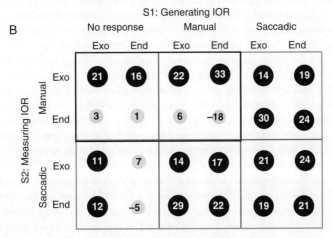

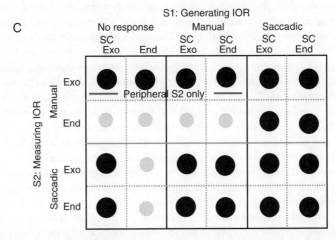

Fig. 26.2 Twenty-four possible conditions (A) reviewed by Taylor and Klein (1998) and (B) empirically measured by Taylor (1997; Taylor and Klein, 2000). In panel (B) the numbers represent uncued minus cued RT and all the black circles represent significant IOR (the 18 ms score represents significant facilitation in this condition). (C) Combining the implications of the two flavours of IOR (Taylor and Klein, 2000) as revealed in its effects with the S-cone finding (Sumner et al., 2004) that manual but not saccadic responses reflect IOR when the cues that generate it initially bypass the SC (see text for explanation). For this integration and the figure used to help represent it (Fig. 26.2C) we are grateful to Tracy Taylor (personal communication).

difference with peripheral targets than with central arrow targets. From this finding they concluded, incorrectly we believe, that IOR had two components: a motor component that would delay any response in the originally cued direction and an *additional* perceptual/attentional component from which a response to a target presented at the cued location would suffer. Note that Taylor and Klein (2000) did not replicate this difference when they randomly intermixed peripheral and central targets in the same condition (ignore-saccade) and moreover, they generally found that the IOR measured with arrow targets was, when obtained, at least as large as that measured with peripheral targets. We believe that the Abrams and Dobkin's finding was generated by untoward differences in mental set made possible by their collecting data from arrow and peripheral targets in *separate* blocks. When the target was never in the periphery (always an arrow at fixation), the participant could adopt an attentional control setting that encouraged effective filtering of the irrelevant peripheral cues. This would not be possible in a block when all (Abrams and Dobkin's peripheral target blocks) or some (Taylor and Klein, 2000) of the targets were peripheral.

Rafal et al. (1989) produced a pattern of results strongly supporting the proposition that oculomotor activation is the generator of IOR. Their participants were encouraged to direct attention toward, to foveate or to prepare to foveate a peripheral location in response to a peripheral cue or a central arrow. After attention or the eyes had returned to fixation or the preparation was cancelled, a target calling for a manual detection response was used to probe for IOR. Inhibition was found in all the conditions that involved a peripheral cue or an executed or prepared eye movement. The only condition in which IOR was not observed was in the aftermath of an endogenously generated shift of attention, which evidence suggests (for a review, see Klein, 2004) does not involve oculomotor preparation. Although this pattern of results from Rafal et al. (1989) has been frequently cited for strongly supporting the oculomotor activation proposal and contributed importantly to the unified theory put forward by Taylor and Klein (1998), recently Chica et al., 2010) convincingly failed to replicate the finding that endogenous preparation of an eye movement generates IOR. Although the failure to find IOR in this condition might be viewed as a challenge to the conventional view that oculomotor activation generates IOR, it is possible to escape this implication by rejecting the assumption that an endogenously prepared saccade activates the oculomotor system in the same way as does peripheral stimulation and actual saccade execution. Perhaps preparing a saccade endogenously while withholding its execution is accomplished by inhibition of the oculomotor machinery in the SC.

Findings reviewed earlier, in the section on antisaccades (Fecteau et al., 2004; Rafal et al., 1994), revealed that attention or input levels of processing or both, rather than motor responses are inhibited when participants are making antisaccades. The reader may wonder whether this finding from the antisaccade paradigm might challenge Taylor and Klein's (2000) inference that a motoric flavour is generated when the oculomotor system is engaged while a sensory/attentional flavour is generated when the oculomotor system is inhibited. Because eye movements are obviously made in an antisaccade task shouldn't the motor flavour be observed here? The answer may lie in the need to tonically inhibit the reflexive oculomotor machinery in the SC in order to perform correctly in an antisaccade task (Forbes and Klein, 1996; Rafal et al., 1994). Once the correct metrics are computed by cortical modules, this inhibition is released (Everling et al., 1999), but in the presence of this tonic inhibition, it would be the perceptual/attentional flavour that would have been generated.

The last issue we will consider in this section is how to integrate the two-flavours of IOR described here with the findings of Sumner et al. (2004) that manual but not saccadic responses are sensitive to IOR when it is generated by S-cone stimuli that bypass the colliculus of Sumner et al. (2004).

First consider only the conditions in which there was No Response made to S1 and a Manual or Saccadic response was made to a Peripheral S2. These conditions are the ones that map most clearly onto Sumner's cue-target paradigm. Since it is generally agreed that a peripheral S1 engages the SC, it should and does generate IOR for manual responses and saccadic responses to peripheral S2s. Next, consider that with manual responses IOR occurred for peripheral onset targets that followed non-predictive central arrow cues. While unexpected (because IOR is clearly not obtained in response to informative central arrow cues, Posner and Cohen, 1984; Rafal et al., 1989) this finding is also not a fluke as it was subsequently replicated by Taylor and Ivanoff (2005, expt. 2). On the assumption that uninformative and ignored arrows do not activate the SC, this finding is consistent with a non-SC generation of IOR. Taylor's dissertation used the different patterns produced by S2 responses to argue for a dissociation in what IOR measures (i.e. is IOR slowed responding to peripheral stimuli or is it slowed motor responding?). Sumner et al. used the different patterns produced by S2 responses following SC-blind cues to argue for a dissociation in how IOR is generated (i.e. by collicular or cortical pathways). Thus, the two studies are looking at two different sides of the generate-measure issue and can be integrated (Fig. 26.2C). Sumner suggests that SC-blind S1 stimuli should produce IOR for manual responses, while SC-visible S1 stimuli should produce IOR for saccadic and manual responses. Taylor (1997; Taylor and Klein, 2000) suggests that when the eyes are prevented from moving, IOR should reflect slowed responses to peripheral S2 stimuli but that when the eyes are free to move, IOR should reflect slowed responses to *all* S2 stimuli. These two views can be mapped onto the findings (Fig. 26.2B) from Taylor and Klein (2000) so long as one accepts the assumption that, through some sort of visuomotor mapping process, manual localization responses to central arrows engage SC mechanisms (for neuroscientific evidence supporting this possibility, see Krauzlis and Nummela (2008)). Under this assumption, the only condition for which the SC might not be involved in generating IOR is when No Response is made to a central S1. In this case, Sumner would predict IOR for manual response to S2 but not for saccadic responses to S2. This prediction is confirmed in our data. And, as described above, according to the two flavours of IOR's effects, when eye movements are prohibited IOR occurs only for peripheral S2 stimuli; when the reflexive eye movement system is not inhibited (because saccades are made to cues, targets or both), IOR occurs to both peripheral and central S2 stimuli so long as the SC in involved in generating IOR.

Sequences of overt orienting

IOR was discovered using the model task originally developed by Posner for exploring covert orienting. Yet, in our typical interactions with the real world, gaze direction is free to move in tandem with shifts of attention; rather than discrete trials with individualized cues and targets, these interactions are characterized by sequences of acts of orienting within visual scenes of varying complexity that may be static or dynamic and may be examined for a variety of reasons. If IOR is the novelty-seeking, foraging facilitator as described above, it should certainly be operating in situations that involve sequences of orienting behaviours. Although somewhat outside the scope of the present review it is worth noting that IOR has been directly observed at multiple locations following a sequence of exogenously generated covert shifts of attention (Snyder and Kingstone, 2000) and, using a probe-following-search paradigm (Klein, 1988), IOR has been inferred to be operating following a hypothetical sequence of covert shifts of attention during difficult search (for a review, see Wang and Klein, 2010).

Experimenter control of orienting

The first study to explicitly look for IOR following a sequence of saccades (overt orienting) was done by Posner and Cohen (1984). They used a 'look at a sequence of peripheral numerals' task to determine whether IOR was coded in oculocentric or environmental coordinates. A sequence of two digits, followed by a cue back to fixation, was carefully arranged so that a final detection target calling for a manual response could be presented either at a previously stimulated (oculocentric) or previously visited (environmental) location. In contrast to the facilitation that is present immediately after a peripheral cue captures attention, which is coded in oculocentric coordinates (Cohen, 1981; Golomb et al., 2008) Posner and Cohen found that IOR was coded in environmental coordinates (see section 'Mapping: oculocentric, environmental and object-based'). As noted earlier, environmental coding is essential for IOR to be useful as a foraging facilitator whenever foraging involves overt orienting.

In a departure from the typical procedure in which eye movements are purposefully initiated in response to peripheral (onsets) or central (arrows) stimuli, Hooge and Frens (2000) explored sequences of eye movements executed 'as rapidly as possible' between statically present and carefully

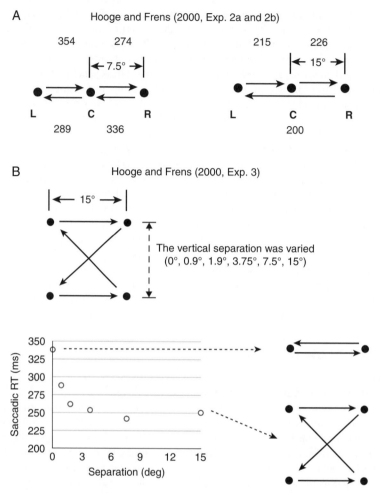

Fig. 26.3 Methods and results from Hooge and Frens (2000). Participants were instructed to saccade as rapidly as possible following the path (indicated by arrows) between statically displayed circles. A) Method and results from Experiment 2. Fixation durations are shown above or below the saccade (shown as an arrow) that terminated the fixation. B) Gradient of IOR is shown as a function the distance separating return saccade 'destinations'. Reprinted from *Vision Research*, **40**(24) I.T. Hooge and M.A. Frens, Inhibition of saccade return (ISR): spatio-temporal properties of saccade programming, pp. 3415–3426, © 2000 with permission from Elsevier.

arranged 'targets' (see Fig. 26.3). Fixation durations before saccades returning to the previously fixated position were considerably longer than to other locations. Based on some of their findings, Hooge and Frens (2000) rejected response conflict and a biomechanical difficulty associated with simply reversing direction (e.g. see the comparison of the findings from two experiments in Fig. 26.3A) as explanations for their findings. Although they called the delay prior to revisitations 'inhibition of saccade return,' we believe it is probably a manifestation of IOR and as such we will use that term when referring to it. By varying the distance between critical fixations they were able to measure the spatial properties of IOR in this paradigm. When a saccade immediately returned to or near the previous fixation IOR was dramatically large in their study and showed a relatively steep gradient (Fig. 26.3B).

Kramer and colleagues combined Posner and Cohen's *experimenter-driven sequence of saccades* method with Posner et al.'s (1985) *choose which target to foveate* task to provide evidence about the nature and capacity of the inhibitory tagging system. Their studies demonstrate that an inhibitory tendency to avoid fixating previously fixated objects and locations is relatively automatic and, like the inhibitory tags following covert orienting, can extend back several fixations. McCarley et al. (2003) presented a sequence of small stimuli (rotated Ls and Ts) with the task to indicate the orientation of any Ts detected. The stimuli were small enough that foveation was required to perform the task. After a sequence of several single items a pair of items was presented, essentially giving the participant a choice between fixating a new object or one that they had previously fixated (the 'old' item had either been removed during a previous saccade and then replaced during the most recent one or had simply remained in the display since its original presentation). Demonstrating some form of memory for previously inspected objects and locations participants correctly avoided the old items for lags up to four (that is, items that had been examined five fixations ago were still fixated significantly less than chance (0.5). Although old items that had not been removed were more successfully avoided than those that had been, the removed and then replaced items were, nevertheless, successfully avoided. Noting that IOR following search seems to depend on the presence of the search array (for a review see Wang and Klein, under review) McCarley et al. (2003) suggested that perhaps the memory their study demonstrated for items that had disappeared was different from IOR. However, based on the work of Tipper and colleagues, Klein (2004; see also Boot et al., 2004) suggested that the degree to which IOR might encode environmental locations versus objects in a scene will depend on the degree to which the display itself is scene-like: 'When a relatively rich scene is presented, the inhibition is more likely to be tagged to objects in the scene than to locations in space (Tipper et al., 1999), and hence removal of the search array is likely to remove the inhibitory tags.'

In a follow-up study (Boot et al., 2004, expt. 1), participants were instructed to follow a sequence of stimuli (+s) with each currently fixated stimulus removed during the saccade to the next. After the fourth + had been fixated two +s were presented in next frame: one was new while the other was presented at the location where, randomly selected, one of the first three +s had been presented. Participants were informed about such dual-target trials, and in different blocks were instructed to fixate the new item, the old item or either item (whichever they preferred) on these trials. The results from the fixate new and fixate either conditions were very similar to that from McCarley et al. (2003) demonstrating a strong avoidance of the old item when it had been most recently fixated (lag 1) with this avoidance diminishing but still remaining significant up to lag 3 (the longest lag tested). Demonstrating a highly automatic inhibitory tagging process participants were unable to follow the 'fixate the old' instructions. At lag 1 participants fixated the old item significantly more often than in the 'either' condition, but still failed to do so ~68% of the time, and at no lag tested was their rate of fixating the old item significantly greater than chance. Confirming that the effects in the 'follow the dots' paradigm are not due to decision processes related to the choice, but instead are due to inhibition of return, Boot et al. replicated the bias to orient to the new location when the task was to foveate an onset probe presented at a new or old location.

Ludwig et al. (2009) asked whether the IOR when measured in saccadic latencies was associated with a raised response criterion or a slower rate of activation of the inhibited response. They guided their observers through a sequence of saccades using endogenous (cues presented at fixation) or exogenous (cues presented in the periphery) means. After 1 or 2 saccades the next one signalled by the central or peripheral target might return gaze to a previously fixated location or a new one. When IOR was observed (curiously it was not consistently observed under all conditions) the emphasis was on the distribution of response times rather than simply the fact of or magnitude of the IOR effect. One novel feature of this study was the use of an explicit computational model of reaction time (the linear ballistic accumulator; Brown and Heathcote, 2008). The key finding was that the distributions of saccades directed at already visited locations as compared to new locations were better accounted for by a slower accumulation rate than an increased response criterion. At first blush, this finding might be interpreted as inconsistent with a response based account of IOR, and in favour of an attentional/perceptual account. Ludwig et al. (2009), however, construe the target-related accumulator as coding a movement vector to a specific location in the visual field. Consequently, it is not straightforward to unambiguously classify the source of this attenuation as perceptual or motor.

Observer control of orienting

If inhibitory tags were an obligatory consequence of orienting during free inspection of a scene, the probability of refixating previously inspected regions of a scene should be lower than chance. Using a variety of relatively open-ended instructions a number of studies have addressed this issue by having participants freely inspect scenes of varying complexity. The results from these studies have yielded somewhat inconsistent findings and claims. When a refixation occurs it is, by definition, a fixation of a region, item or object that had been inspected before. A key descriptor in this literature is how long ago (in number of inspections) the earlier fixation had been when the reinspection occurs. Because there are differences in the terminology used by different authors to refer to refixations of the same lag, it is important that we clearly define the terminology we are using here:

1	2	3	4	5	6	7	8	9	10	11
a	b	b	c	d	c	e	d	f	g	e

Consider a sequence of 11 fixations shown above (numbered from 1–11). The letters indicate the 5 different regions of a scene that might be foveated by each of these fixations. The 3rd fixation which represents the 2nd fixation of region (b) will be referred to as a 'successive fixation' of an item or region. The 6th fixation which represents a refixation of region (c) will be referred to as an 'immediate refixation' as this is the first opportunity to refixate (c) once it was no longer being fixated (this will also referred to as 'one-back'). The 8th and 11th fixation which represent refixation of regions (d) and (e) will simply be called non-immediate refixations (but in some studies a refixation like that of (e) would be referred to as 'two-back' because the two fixations of this region are separated by fixations on two different regions).

Gilchrist and Harvey's (2000) observers searched an array of letters for a target ('E') which was present among a number of distractor letters. Using elementary probability theory, they concluded that people return to a previously fixated item only a little more than would be expected if IOR were discouraging reinspections. However, when refixations did occur, their probability peaked at approximately 300 and 400 ms subsequent to the initial fixation. In the context of reading, such return saccades to a previously foveated item are often considered to be the result of inadequate information processing during the initial fixation (see Rayner, 1998 for a review). Consequently, Gilchrist and Harvey suggested that an indeterminate proportion of refixations were likely not failures of memory but rather reflected an effort to ameliorate the poor quality of information about an item that had sometimes been gathered during an original fixation.

Also monitoring eye movements during search, Peterson et al. (2001), while disagreeing with some of the conclusions of Gilchrist and Harvey, provided converging evidence for others. They found that the rate of non-immediate refixations was substantially less than would be predicted if there were no memory for which items had already been inspected. Indeed, most refixations were immediate (one-back) refixations and a large proportion of these were saccades back to the target rather than to a competing distractor. Peterson et al. (2001) concluded from their findings that the oculomotor system behaved as if there was some (but not perfect) memory of previous inspections. This memory operated to discourage refixations. The relatively high frequency of immediate refixations, in agreement with Gilchrist and Harvey (2000), was attributed to the need to gather further information about insufficiently processed targets or potential targets.

MacInnes and Klein's (2003) analysis of preprobe saccades during free search of complex stimulus array (see below) provides converging evidence that when observers saccade toward a just fixated item it is often because that item is being considered as a possible target. Their participants were instructed to inspect 'Where's Waldo?' pictures and to stop when they found something interesting. Prior to stopping and when search was resumed after having stopped, saccades were strongly directed away from the previously fixated location. In contrast, there was a strong tendency among the saccades that terminated search to be in the direction of the last fixated item (one-back).

Hooge et al. (2005) allowed observers to freely scan visual scenes of varying complexity and under two different attentional control settings. In one condition, observers were free to view complex, naturalistic, stimulus displays for which there were no explicit instructions to search or identify any particular target (Picture Viewing). Alternatively, there were two visual search conditions: One such condition required participants to search a series of identical, naturalistic, greyscale pictures for 0–7 little white crosses (the number of targets was variable) embedded within the image (Picture Search). In the final condition, similar targets (grey crosses) were placed in a uniform greyscale background (Uniform Search). Subjects were required to manually indicate whether they had detected a cross and the number of potential targets was concealed. Analyses of the eye movement data led Hooge et al. to conclude that observers made immediate refixations at above chance levels in the Picture Viewing and Picture Search conditions. Despite a general disagreement in the literature as to whether return saccades are occurring at above (Hooge et al., 2005; MacInnes and Klein, 2003; Peterson et al., 2001) or below (Gilchrist and Harvey, 2000; Klein and MacInnes, 1999; MacInnes and Klein, 2003; Peterson et al., 2001) chance levels (see next paragraph), the results are fairly unequivocal in illustrating that there can be a relatively high frequency of immediate refixations. Because immediate refixations in search and scene inspection, like those in reading, may be mediated by premature termination of a fixation (especially when, in search, the item happened to be the target) and the consequent need for further processing, it would be interesting to know whether Hooge et al.'s participants were making non-immediate refixations at above chance levels and what proportion of refixations in their search tasks were of targets. Whereas Hooge et al. (2005) found no evidence in their data for IOR in the form of what they considered to be below-chance refixation rates, they did find longer than average fixation durations prior to refixations, precisely what would be expected if IOR were present at previously inspected regions (see Fig. 26.4A).

Participants from Smith and Henderson (2009) were instructed to view a natural environment under the expectation that a memory test would later be administered. Analysis of successive eye movements revealed an elevated population of saccades that regressed in the direction of the previously examined location (one back). Yet, much like the results that we have highlighted from Hooge et al. (2005), there was nonetheless an accompanying temporal cost associated with such refixations (Fig. 26.4A). Both of these trends were observed, albeit in a somewhat weaker form, in relation to the two-back fixation. Although Smith and Henderson (2009) found evidence of what appears to be higher-than-chance revisitation rates in their memory task, it is unclear whether these rates can be generalized to search-related tasks (Dodd et al., 2009 found that IOR, in the form of refixations, is more pronounced in search tasks). Moreover, whether relatively high reinspection rates are an obligatory consequence of observing complex scenes or the aftermath of an attentional control setting that encourages enhanced processing of multiple stimuli within an environment will require further study.

In evaluating the claim from studies that have examined the rate of refixations and have concluded that they were occurring at a higher rate than would be expected by chance (leading to the assertion of a 'facilitation of return' mechanism), it is important to consider what is the 'chance' rate of a refixation. It is generally neglected that in real-world scenes and many experimenter defined arrays there are uncontrolled factors that may have caused the first fixation of an object or region—such as differences in bottom-up salience or top-down guidance based on the task, factors that continue to operate as inspection continues. As noted by Itti and Koch (2001), in the absence of an inhibitory damping of activity in the map that guides orienting, there will be perseverative orienting toward the most activated regions in this map. IOR, which has been proposed as a mechanism that temporarily reduces activity for previously inspected locations in this map, is not likely an all or none system. Rather, it is simply another source of input to the aforementioned map. It does not prevent reinspections; it simply discourages them by temporarily lowering the activation of previously visited regions. Consequently, when the other inputs to this map (say the need to reinspect a location when it might have been insufficiently processed on a previous fixation, cf. Henderson (1992)) call for a saccade to an inhibited region its execution will necessarily be delayed because the inhibition must be overcome to reach the threshold for action. It is important to note, in this context, that when these untoward factors are controlled (as they often were in previous sections) there is very clear evidence that the inhibitory tags that affect response times are also discouraging re-orienting (e.g. Boot et al., 2004; Godijn and Theeuwes, 2002).

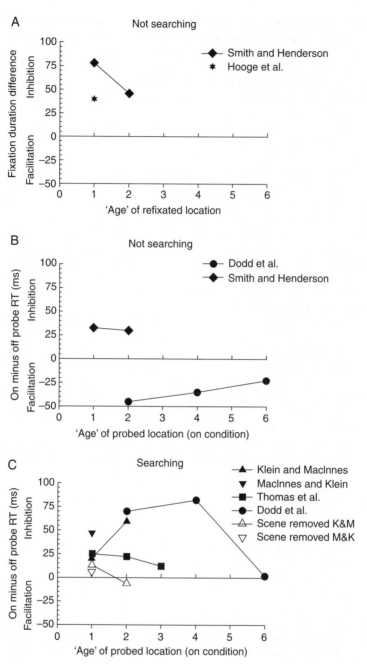

Fig. 26.4 Inhibition of return in the latency to respond (old minus new). A) Difference in fixation durations prior to eye movements that return gaze to the immediate or penultimate fixation (1- and 2-back, respectively) and those to new locations. B) Difference in saccadic response times to probes presented during non-search tasks (Smith and Henderson is from memorization; Dodd et al. is the average of their non-search tasks: memorization, pleasantness, free viewing). C) Differences in response times to probes presented a previously inspected versus new locations during and following search (see text for more details).

Hybrid control tasks

The probe-during or -following search paradigm initiated by Klein (1988) and extended by Klein and MacInnes (1999) to overt orienting (oculomotor search), represents a mixture of experimenter and participant control of orienting (for review see Wang and Klein, 2010). The participant examines a scene under their own control (though often with some sort of search instruction) and after some number of 'free' saccades a probe is placed into the scene with the instruction to foveate the probe as soon as you notice it. Klein and MacInnes's (1999) participants were looking for 'Waldo' in pictures selected from Martin Handford's series of 'Where's Waldo?' books when their search was occasionally interrupted by a probe target. The probe, the original fixation stimulus, was placed into the scene at a location that had just been fixated (1-back) or at the fixation just before the last one (2-back) or at one of five of equi-eccentric control locations that varied in angular distance from these previous fixations. In the 2-back condition, SRT to foveate the probe target was slowest when this was presented at the previously fixated location and decreased monotonically as the angular distance away from the previous fixation increased (the same vs. opposite difference was about 58 ms). A similar pattern was seen in the 1-back condition, except that SRTs directed to the location that had just been visited, while faster than SRTs in the opposite direction, were faster than expected.

Klein and MacInnes (1999) also reported that the saccades made when participants were performing their search task were more likely to be made away from than towards the previous fixation—a pattern others have referred to as 'saccadic momentum.' Because probes were delivered while the participant would be preparing their next search saccade Klein and MacInnes could not distinguish between two directions of causality: were inhibitory tags at previously fixated locations causing saccades to move away from these locations or was biased preparation within the oculomotor system responsible for the inhibitory gradient? In a subsequent study, MacInnes and Klein (2003) distinguished between these possibilities by changing the instructions ('look for something interesting and stop there') so that the probe was delivered after searching had stopped and it was, therefore, unlikely that a search saccade was being actively prepared. Only 1-back probes were presented in this experiment and they showed a monotonic gradient of declining SRTs as the distance between the probe and the previous fixation increased (the same vs. opposite difference was about 47 ms). Finding IOR when saccadic preparation would have been minimized led MacInnes and Klein (2003) to conclude that IOR was causing saccadic momentum rather than vice versa. It should be noted that whereas Klein and MacInnes viewed IOR and saccadic momentum as reciprocal processes (much like a see-saw) others (e.g. Smith and Henderson, 2009) have construed them as independent. It remains to be seen which view is correct.

Supporting the suggestion of Tipper et al. (1994) that IOR is coded in scene coordinates when there is a rich scene, in both studies there was no evidence of an inhibitory gradient around previously fixated locations when the scene was removed at the same time that the probe was presented. Thomas et al. (2006) collected data from a search task in which 'fruits' were concealed behind 'leaves' in a virtual environment that required arm, head, and eye movements. Confirming the 'IOR-during-search' finding from Klein's laboratory and extending it to a real-world foraging task, they found that manual detection responses to probes (flickering leaves) were slower for leaves that had previously been searched than for otherwise equivalent new leaves.

Recently, Dodd et al. (2009) used the Klein and MacInnes probe-during-scene-inspection paradigm probing at the 2-back, 4-back, and 6-back locations while varying the participant's task: Their participants viewed the scenes with search, memorization, pleasantness-ratings or freeviewing instructions Providing another replication of Klein and MacInnes's findings there was significant IOR in the search task in the 2-back location that remained significant in the 4-back location and was no longer significant in the 6-back condition. The probe-following-overt-search findings described so far in this section are summarized in Fig. 26.4C.

Importantly, Dodd et al. (2009) found no IOR in the other three conditions; quite the contrary: Participants were generally faster to respond to probes at previously fixated than at novel locations (Fig. 26.4B). Several other findings from this study support the uniqueness of search: The relative frequency of refixations was lower and the time between a fixation and refixation was longer in the search task than in the other tasks—precisely what would be expected if IOR were selectively operating during search. As noted by Dodd et al. (2009) their findings are compatible with the studies reviewed earlier demonstrating a higher than chance probability of refixations during inspection of scenes with no instruction or with memorization as the primary goal. And their findings are consistent with the proposal that IOR linked to overt orienting maybe flexibly turned on (search) or off (non-search tasks) depending on task requirements.

There is a problem, however, for this proposal. Firstly, IOR occurs ubiquitously in tasks for which—in contrast to search—it does not convey a net benefit to performance. This applies to cue-target and target-target tasks in which the first event's location is uninformative about the location of subsequent events. If IOR could be 'turned off' then surely it should be turned off in these situations. Secondly, consider the study by Boot et al. (2004) reviewed earlier, in which participants performed a sequence of orienting responses to stimuli presented by the experimenter and then, were given a choice between an old and a new location. When instructed to fixate the old location subjects were unable to do so. If IOR could be 'turned off' then surely it would have been in this situation. We will offer two possible explanations for escaping this conundrum.

In the situations for which IOR appears to be automatically generated the sequence of orienting behaviours is controlled by the experimenter, bottom-up as it were, through the presentation of a sequence of stimuli. In the situations for which IOR appears to be flexibly turned on or off, the observer is presented with a scene while their sequence of orienting behaviours is determined to a large degree top-down by their own, self-generated strategies (operating in collaboration, of course, with the bottom-up input in the scene). Perhaps, when orienting is captured primarily through bottom-up stimulation, IOR will be present whether it is needed or not, while when orienting is controlled by the observer, the observer can also control whether inspected regions and objects are associated with negative or positive tags, depending on the nature of their task. Under this view, whether IOR is automatic or under voluntary control depends on whether the orienting that might give rise to IOR is automatic or under voluntary control.

Another view takes advantage of Posner and Cohen's (1984) original suggestion that 'the inhibition builds up over the same time interval as facilitation but is simply masked by the larger facilitation resulting from covert orienting'. Perhaps IOR *is* an automatic consequence of orienting. In that case it would always be present, but would not necessarily be apparent when a behavioural measure is made because other processes that facilitate orienting toward previously attended and/or fixated locations might be operating.

While their participants were inspecting real-world scenes for a later memory test, Smith and Henderson (2009) presented irrelevant (to-be-ignored) onsets that were expected to occasionally result in oculomotor capture (Theeuwes et al., 1998). These probes were presented at the last (1-back) or penultimate (2-back) locations that had been fixated, or at new, distance-equated locations. Seemingly reflecting a facilitation effect, these 'irrelevant' onset probes were more likely to capture the oculomotor system when they were presented at old (previously inspected) locations. Yet, seemingly reflecting an inhibitory effect (Fig. 26.4B), there was a tendency for longer fixation durations prior to saccades to probes at old than at new locations(when tested across both the one-back and two-back conditions, this tendency was significant, $t(29)=2.558$, $p=0.016$, Smith, personal communication). Although further study will be required to confidently reconcile these apparently contradictory findings, we believe they may reflect the simultaneous presence of facilitation and inhibition, at different levels of processing, that Posner and Cohen (1984) hypothesized when they first discovered IOR (see also, Klein, 2004). Also requiring further study is the dramatic difference in probe reaction times between this non-search study (an inhibitory effect) and that of Dodd et al. (2009) (a facilitatory effect) which is highlighted in Fig. 26.4B. There are several noteworthy methodological differences between these studies. First, Smith and Henderson's probes were irrelevant onsets, participants were instructed to ignore but that, nevertheless, occasionally captured eye movements while Dodd et al.'s were task-relevant onsets, participants were instructed to fixate. The non-return probe locations in Dodd et al. were randomly selected with the sole restriction that they not have been among the past six fixation while Smith and Henderson's probes were distance matched to the 1- or 2-back fixation. Finally, probe delivery was early (Smith and Henderson, 2009) or late (Dodd et al., 2009) in the processing of the scene. Without further research, we can only speculate as to which of these might be responsible for the different results and why.

Summary and conclusions

IOR appears to be a consequence of exogenous orienting that has a negative impact on subsequent orienting. As originally proposed by Posner and Cohen (1984), IOR is a novelty seeking mechanism that facilitates foraging behaviour by discouraging reinspection of regions already determined to not to be what one is seeking (Klein, 1988). IOR is intricately linked to the oculomotor machinery in the brain. Although an intact superior colliculus is required for the generation of IOR, signals that do not directly project to the superior colliculus can nevertheless generate, presumably through cortical pathways, an inhibitory aftereffect. IOR that is generated in the context of an activated oculomotor system seems to be characterized by a bias against responses toward the inhibited region. IOR that is generated in the context of a quiescent, if not actively inhibited, oculomotor system is not motoric but rather seems to delay covert orienting to stimuli presented to the inhibited pathway. Cortical processes have been implicated in both environmental and object- or scene-based coding of IOR which have been demonstrated by movements of the eyes or a cued object between the cue and target. Whereas early work characterizing IOR was dominated by reaction times collected using the model task developed by Posner for exploring covert orienting, recent work has emphasized the operation of IOR during and upon the sequence of saccades made in more ecologically valid contexts such as when we are gathering information from a scene to find a target or for other purposes. Orienting, whether overt or covert, is likely controlled by a spatial representation or map that is the site of convergence of bottom-up signals from the environment, top-down signals based on task requirements, and the inhibitory tags left behind in the aftermath of our previous orienting behaviours. Our understanding of how these signals are integrated to guide our behaviour will be advanced through the development of computationally explicit models that can be confidently linked to the neural mechanisms that control orienting (e.g. Itti and Koch, 2001; Trappenberg et al., 2001).

Acknowledgements

The writing of this chapter was made possible by an NSERC Discovery grant to R. Klein and an NSERC Graduate Scholarship to M. Hilchey. We thank Dr Tracy Taylor-Helmick for her contributions to the manuscript and Casimir Ludvig and Thomas Geisler for their constructive suggestions.

References

Abrams, R.A. and Dobkin, R.S. (1994a). The gap effect and inhibition of return: Interactive effects on eye movement latencies. *Experimental Brain Research*, **98**, 483–487.

Abrams, R.A. and Dobkin, R.S. (1994b). Inhibition of return: Effects of attentional cuing on eye movement latencies. *Journal of Experimental Psychology: Human Perception and Performance*, **20**, 467–477.

Abrams, R.A. and Pratt, J. (2000). Oculocentric coding of inhibited eye movements to recently attended locations. *Journal of Experimental Psychology: Human Perception and Performance*, **26**(2), 776–788.

Berlucchi, G., Di Stefani, M., Marzi, C.A., Morelli, M. and Tassinari, G. (1981). Direction of attention in the visual field as measured by a reaction time paradigm. *Behavioral Brain Research*, **2**(2), 244–245.

Boot, W.R., McCarley, J.S., Kramer, A.R., and Peterson, M.S. (2004). Automatic and intentional memory processes in visual search. *Psychonomic Bulletin and Review*, **11**, 854–861.

Brown, S.D. and Heathcote, A.J. (2008). The simplest complete model of choice reaction time: Linear ballistic accumulation. *Cognitive Psychology*, **57**, 153–178.

Chica, A.B., Klein, R.M., Rafal, R.D., and Hopfinger, J.B. (2010). Endogenous saccade preparation does not produce inhibition of return: Failure to replicate Rafal, Calabresi, Brennan, and Sciolto (1989). *Journal of Experimental Psychology: Human Perception and Performance*, **36**(5), 1193–1206.

Cohen, Y. (1981). *Internal and external control of orienting*. Unpublished doctoral dissertation. University of Oregon.

Dodd, M.D., van der Stigchel, S., and Hollingworth, A. (2009). Novelty is not always the best policy: Inhibition of return and facilitation of return as a function of visual task. *Psychological Science*, **20**(3), 333–339.

Dorris, M.C. and Munoz, D.P. (1995). A neural correlate for the gap effect on saccadic reaction times in monkey. *Journal of Neurophysiology*, **73**, 2558–2562.

Everling S. and Fischer B. (1998). The anti saccade: a review of basic research and clinical studies. *Neuropsychologia*, 36, 885–899.

Fecteau, J.H., Au, C., Armstrong, I.T., and Munoz, D.P. (2004). Sensory biases produce alternation advantage found in sequential saccadic eye movement tasks. *Experimental Brain Research*, **159**, 84–91.

Forbes, K., and Klein, R. (1996). The magnitude of the fixation offset effect with endogenously andexogenously controlled saccades. *Journal of Cognitive Neuroscience*, **8**(4), 344–352.

Fuentes, L.J., Vivas, A.B., Humphreys, G.W. (1999). Inhibitory tagging of stimulus properties of inhibition of return: Effects on semantic priming and flanker interference. *Quarterly Journal of Experimental Psychology*, **52A**, 149–164.

Gilchrist, I.D. and Harvey, M. (2000). Refixation frequency and memory mechanisms in visual search. *Current Biology*, **10**(19), 1209–1212.

Godijn, R. and Theeuwes, J. (2002). Oculomotor capture and inhibition of return: Evidence for an oculomotor suppression account of IOR. *Psychological Research*, **66**(4), 234–246.

Golomb, J.D., Chun, M.M., and Mazer, J.A. (2008). The native coordinate system of spatial attention is retinotopic. *Journal of Neuroscience*, **28**, 10654–10662.

Henderson, J. M. (1992). Visual attention and eye movement control during reading and picture viewing. In K. Rayner (ed.) *Eye movements and visual cognition: Scene perception and reading* (pp. 261–283). New York: Springer-Verlag.

Hooge, I.T. and Frens, M.A. (2000). Inhibition of saccade return (ISR): Spatial-temporal properties of saccade programming. *Vision Research*, **40**, 3415–3426.

Hooge, I.T., Over, E.A., van Wezel, R.J., and Frens, M.A. (2005). Inhibition of return is not a foraging facilitator in saccadic search and free viewing. *Vision Research*, **45**, 1901–1908.

Hunt, A.R. and Kingstone, A. (2003). Inhibition of return: Dissociating attentional and oculomotorcomponents. *Journal of Experimental Psychology: Human Perception and Performance*, **29**(5), 1068–1074.

Itti, L. and Koch, C. (2001). Computational modelling of visual attention. *Nature Reviews Neuroscience*, **2**(3), 194–203.

Klein, R.M. (1988). Inhibitory tagging system facilitates visual search. *Nature*, **334**(6181), 430–431.

Klein, R.M. (2000). Inhibition of return. *Trends in Cognitive Sciences*, **4**(4), 138–147.

Klein, R. M. (2004). Orienting and inhibition of return. In M. S. Gazzaniga (ed.) *The CognitiveNeurosciences 3rd Edition* (pp. 545–559). Cambridge, MA: MIT Press.

Klein, R.M., and MacInnes, W.J. (1999). Inhibition of return is a foraging facilitator in visual search. *Psychological Science*, **10**, 346–352.

Klein, R.M., Schmidt, W.C., and Muller, H.J. (1998). Disinhibition of return: Unnecessary and unlikely. *Perception and Psychophysics*, **60**(5), 862–872.

Klein, R.M., Christie, J., and Morris, E.P. (2005). Vector averaging of inhibition of return. *Psychonomic Bulletin and Review*, **12**(2), 295–300.

Krauzlis, R. and Nummela, S. (2008). Superior colliculus inactivation biases target selection for smooth pursuit, saccades, and manual responses [Abstract]. Journal of Vision, **8**(6), 666a

Langley, L.K., Gayzur, N.D., Saville, A.L., Morlock, S.L. and Bagne, A.G. (2011). Spatial distribution of attentional inhibition is not altered in healthy aging. *Attention, Perception & Psychophysics*, **73**, 776–783.

Ludwig, C.J.H., Farrell, S., Ellis, L.A. and Gilchrist, I.D. (2009). The mechanism underlying inhibition of saccadic return. *Cognitive Psychology*, **59**, 180–202.

MacInnes, J.W. and Klein, R.M. (2003). Inhibition of return biases orienting during the search of complex scenes. *The Scientific World Journal*, **3**, 75–86.

Maylor, E.A. (1985). Facilitatory and inhibitory components of orienting in visual space. In M. I. Posner and O. S. Marin (eds.) *Attention and performance XI* (pp. 189–204). Hillsdale, NJ: Lawrence Erlbaum Associates Inc.

Maylor, E.A. and Hockey, R. (1985). Inhibitory component of externally controlled covert orienting in visual space. *Journal of Experimental Psychology: Human Perception and Performance*, **11**, 777–787.

McCarley, J.S., Wang, R.F., Kramer, A.F., and Irwin, D.E. (2003). How much memory does oculomotor search have? *Psychological Science*, **14**, 422–426.

McGowan, J.W., Kowler, E., Sharma, A., and Chubb, C. (1998). Saccadic localization of random dot targets. *Vision Research*, **38**, 895–909.

Melcher, D. and Kowler, E. (1999). Shapes, surfaces and saccades. *Vision Research*, **39**, 2929–2946.

Mirpour, K., Arcizet, F., Ong, W.S. and Bisley, J.W. (2009) Been there seen that: A Neural Mechanism for Performing Efficient, *Journal of Neurophysiology*, **102**, 3481–3491

Munoz, D.P. and Wurtz, R.H. (1992). Role of the rostral superior colliculus in active visual fixation and execution of express saccades. *Journal of Neurophysiology*, **67**, 1000–1002.

Munoz, D.P. and Wurtz, R.H. (1993a) Fixation cells in monkey superior colliculus. I. Characteristics of cell discharge. *Journal of Neurophysiology*, **70**(2), 559–575.

Munoz, D.P. and Wurtz, R.H. (1993b) Fixation cells in monkey superior colliculus. II. Reversible activation and deactivation. *Journal of Neurophysiology*, **70**(2), 576–589.

Peterson, M.S., Kramer, A.F., Wang, R.F., Irwin, D.E., and McCarley, J.S. (2001). Visual search has memory. *Psychological Science*, 12, 287–292.

Posner, M.I. (1980). Orienting of attention. *Quarterly Journal of Experimental Psychology*, 32, 3–25.

Posner, M.I. and Cohen, Y. (1984). Components of visual orienting. In H. Bouma and D. G. Bouwhuis (eds.) *Attention and performance X: Control of language processes* (pp. 531–556). Hove: Lawrence Erlbaum Associates Ltd

Posner, M.I., Rafal, R.D., Choate, L., and Vaughan, J. (1985). Inhibition of return: neural basis andfunction. *Cognitive Neuropsychologia*, 2, 211–228.

Rafal, R.D., Egly, R., and Rhodes, D. (1994). Effects of inhibition of return on voluntary and visually guided saccades. *Canadian Journal of Experimental Psychology*, 48, 284–300.

Rafal, R.D., Calabresi, P., Brennan, C., and Sciolto, T. (1989). Saccade preparation inhibits reorienting to recently attended locations. *Journal of Experimental Psychology: Human Perception and Performance*, 15, 673–685.

Rayner, K. (1998). Eye movements in reading and information processing: 20 years of research. *Psychological Bulletin*, 124(3), 372–422.

Reuter-Lorenz P.A., Hughes H.C., Fendrich R. (1991). The reduction of saccadic latency by prioroffset of the fixation point: an analysis of the gap effect. *Perception and Psychophysics*, 49, 167–175.

Reuter-Lorenz, P.A., Jha, A.P., and Rosenquist, J.N. (1996). What is inhibited in inhibition of return? *Journal of Experimental Psychology: Human Perception and Performance*, 22, 367–378.

Robinson, D.A. (1972). Eye movements evoked by collicular stimulation in the alert monkey. *Vision Research*, 12, 1795–1808.

Sapir, A., Soroker, N., Berger, A., Henik, A. (1999). Inhibition of return in spatial attention: direct evidence for collicular generation. *Nature Neuroscience*, 2(12), 1053–1054.

Sapir, A., Hayes, A., Henik, A. Danziger, S. and Rafal, R. (2004) Parietal lobe lesions disrupt saccadic remapping of inhibitory location tagging. *Journal of Cognitive Neuroscience*, 16, 503–509.

Saslow, M.G. (1967). Effects of components of displacement-step stimuli upon latency for saccadic eye movement. *Journal of the Optical Society of America*, 57, 1024–1029.

Sereno, A.B., Briand, K.A., Amador, S.C. and Szapiel, S.V. (2006) Disruption of reflexive attention and eye movements in an individual with a collicular lesion. *Journal of Clinical and Experimental Neuropsychology*, 28, 145–166.

Smith, D.T., Rorden, C., and Jackson, S.R. (2004). Exogenous orienting of attention depends upon the ability to execute eye movements. *Current Biology*, 14(9), 792–795.

Smith, T.J. and Henderson, J.M. (2009). Facilitation of return during scene viewing. *Visual Cognition*, 17(6–7), 1083–1108.

Snyder, J.J. and Kingstone, A. (2000). Inhibition of return and visual search: How many separate loci are inhibited? *Perception and Psychophysics*, 62, 452–458.

Sommer, M.A., (1994). Express saccades elicited during visual scan in the monkey. *Vision Research*, 15, 2023–2038.

Souto, D. and Kerzel, D. (2009). Involuntary cueing during smooth pursuit: facilitation and inhibition of return in oculocentric coordinates. *Experimental Brain Research*, 192, 25–31.

Sternberg, S. (1969). The discovery of processing stages: Extensions of Donders" method. In W. G. Koster (ed.) *Attention and performance II* (pp. 276–315). Amsterdam: North-Holland.

Sumner, P., Nachev, P., Vora, N., Husain, M., and Kennard, C. (2004). Distinct cortical and collicular mechanisms of inhibition of return revealed with S cone stimuli. *Current Biology*, 14(24), 2259–2263.

Tassinari, G., Aglioti, S., Chelazzi, L., Marzi, C.A., Berlucchi, G. (1987). Distribution in the visual-field of the costs of voluntarily allocated attention and of the inhibitory aftereffects of covert orienting. *Neuropsychologia*, 25(1A), 55–71.

Taylor, T.L. (1997). Generating and measuring inhibition of return. Unpublished doctoraldissertation. Dalhousie University.

Taylor, T.L. and Klein, R.M. (1998). On the causes and effects of inhibition of return. *Psychonomic Bulletin and Review*, 5, 625–643.

Taylor, T.L. and Klein, R.M. (2000). Visual and motor effects in inhibition of return. *Journal of Experimental Psychology: Human Perception and Performance*, 26, 1639–1656.

Taylor, T.L. and Ivanoff, J. (2005) Inhibition of return and repetition priming effects in localization and discrimination tasks. *Canadian Journal of Experimental Psychology*, 59, 75–89.

Taylor, T.L., Kingstone, A.F., and Klein, R.M. (1998). The disappearance of foveal and non-foveal stimuli: decomposing the gap effect. *Canadian Journal of Experimental Psychology*, 52, 192–200.

Theeuwes, J., Kramer, A.F., Hahn, S. and Irwin, D.E. (1998). Our eyes do not always go where wewant them to go: capture of the eyes by new objects. *Psychological Science*, 9, 379–385.

Thomas, L.E., Ambinder, M.S., Hsieh, B., Levinthal, B., Crowell, J.A., Irwin, D.E., *et al.* (2006). Fruitful visual search: Inhibition of returning a virtual foraging task. *Psychonomic Bulletin and Review*, 13(5), 891–895.

Tipper, S.P., Driver, J., and Weaver, B. (1991). Object-centered inhibition of return of visual attention. *Quarterly Journal of Experimental Psychology: Human Experimental Psychology*, 43A, 289–298.

Tipper, S.P., Jordan, H., and Weaver, B. (1999). Scene-based and object-centered inhibition of return: evidence for dual orienting mechanisms. *Perception and Psychophysics*, 61(1), 50–60.

Tipper, S.P., Weaver, B., Jarreat, L.M., Burak, A.L. (1994). Object-based and environmentbased inhibition of return of visual attention. *Journal of Experimental Psychology: Human Perception and Performance*, 20(3), 478–499.

Tipper, S.P., Rafal, R., Reuter-Lorenz, P.A., Starrveldt, Y., Ro, T., Egly, R., *et al.* (1997). Object-based facilitation and inhibition from visual orienting in the human split-brain. *Journal of Experimental Psychology: Human Perception and Performance*, **23**(5), 1522–1532.

Trappenberg, T.P., Dorris, M.C., Munoz, D.P., and Klein, R.M. (2001). A model of saccade initiation based on the competitive integration of exogenous and endogenous signals in the superior colliculus. *Journal of Cognitive Neuroscience*, **13**, 256–271.

van Koningsbruggen, M.G., Gabay, S., Sapir, A., Henik, A., and Rafal, R.D. (2010) Hemispheric asymmetry in the remapping and maintenance of visual saliency maps: a TMS study. *Journal of Cognitive Neuroscience*, **22**, 1730–1738.

Vaughan, J. (1984). Saccades directed at previously attended locations in space. In A.J. Gale and C.W. Johnson (eds.) *Theoretical and applied aspects of eye movement research* (pp. 143–150). North Holland: Elsevier.

Wang, Z. and Klein, R.M. (2010) Searching for inhibition of return in visual search: A review. *Vision Research*, **50**, 220–228.

Watanabe, K. (2001). Inhibition of return in averaging saccades. *Experimental Brain Research*, **138**, 330–342.

Zhang, Y. and Zhang, M. (2011) Spatial working memory load impairs manual but not saccadic inhibition of return. *Vision Research*, **51**, 147–153.

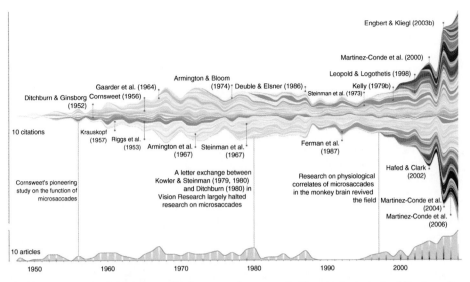

Plate 1 (Also see Fig. 6.2.) Impact of microsaccade research. The stacked graph at the top shows the impact of articles related to the function of microsaccades across time, from 1948 to 2008. Each stripe represents one of 253 articles for which data were available at the Web of Science. The height of the stripe shows the number of references to this article in a given year. Hence, the silhouette of the graph shows the overall impact of the field (685 citations in 2008). Stripe colours encode two dimensions: the age of an article (the warmer, the more recent) and its normalized impact (citations per year; the more saturated, the higher the impact; full saturation for >12 citations per year). The wiggle for each single stripe in the graph is minimized following the procedure proposed by Byron and Wattenberg (2008), ensuring best legibility. As time progresses, newer publications were evenly added at the rims, resulting in an inside-out (rather than bottom-to-top) layout and making the old literature the core of the graph. Labels highlight a selection of articles; both most cited and most neglected ones. The histogram at the bottom shows the number of items published in a given year; each dot is one article (same colour as in top panel). Reprinted from *Vision Research*, **49**(20), Martin Rolfs, Microsaccades: Small steps on a long way, 2415–2441. Copyright (2009), with permission from Elsevier.

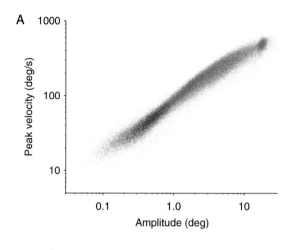

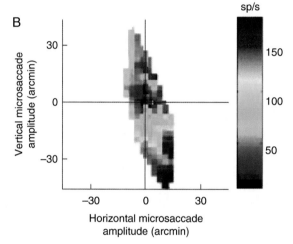

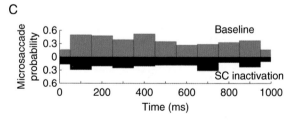

Plate 2 (Also see Fig. 6.6.) Microsaccade generation mechanisms. A) Microsaccades follow the saccadic main sequence, suggesting a common generator for microsaccades and saccades. Saccades and microsaccades recorded during free-viewing (blue) follow the same main sequence as those produced during fixation (red). (Note: some blue dots are obscured by the superimposed red dots.) N=159,874 saccades and microsaccades combined for 8 subjects. From Otero-Millan et al. (2008). Copyright held by Association for Research in Vision and Ophthalmology (ARVO). B) Peak discharge of a SC neuron during microsaccades, plotted as a function of their horizontal and vertical amplitudes. The neuron preferred microsaccades directed to the lower right quadrant. C) Microsaccade probability during one second of fixation before (grey) and after (black) SC inactivation. Inactivation reduced microsaccade production. (B, C) From *Science*, Z.M. Hafed, L. Goffart, and R.J. Krauzlis, A neural mechanism for microsaccade generation in the primate superior colliculus, copyright 2009. Reprinted with permission from AAAS.

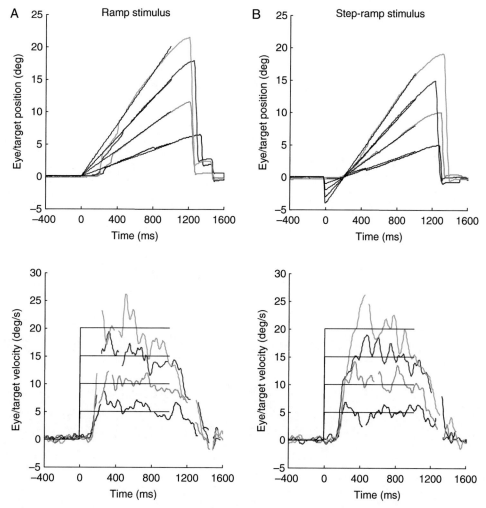

Plate 3 (Also see Fig. 7.1.) A) Typical eye position (upper) and smooth eye velocity (lower) responses to ramp target motion stimuli with velocity of 5 (blue), 10 (green), 15 (red) or 20(cyan) °/s. B) Typical eye position (upper) and eye velocity (lower traces) in response to step-ramp stimuli with velocity of 5-20°/s. Gaps in smooth eye velocity traces represent occurrence of saccades. Reprinted from *Brain and Cognition*, **68**(3), G.R. Barnes, Cognitive processes involved in smooth pursuit eye movements, copyright (2008), with permission from Elsevier.

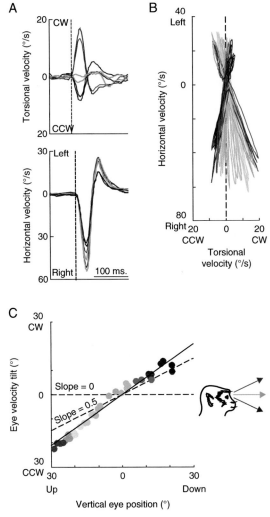

Plate 4 (Also see Fig. 8.3.) Characteristics of eye velocity during abducens nerve microstimulation. A) Temporal plots of eye velocity from different initial eye positions (green = straight ahead; red = 25° up; blue = 25° down) are similar in the horizontal domain (lower panel), but differ in the torsional domain (upper panel). B) Horizontal versus torsional velocity is plotted as the eye assumes different vertical positions. The eye's orientation when the stimulation was delivered is illustrated by a colour palette, ranging from 25° up (dark red) to 25° down (dark blue) in 5° intervals. The orientation of Listing's plane is indicated by the vertical dashed line at 0° torsion. C) Measures of eye velocity tilt angle are plotted against initial vertical eye position. A slope of 0 (indicating fixed axes of rotation and a zero-angle rule) and a slope of 0.5 (indicating eye position-dependent axes of rotation and proper implementation of the half-angle rule) are also shown (dashed lines). Replotted with permission from Klier et al. (2006).

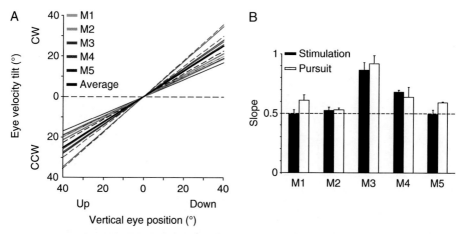

Plate 5 (Also see Fig. 8.4.) Stimulation-evoked eye movements have the same eye position-dependence as visually-guided pursuit. A) Slopes for all sites closely approximate the half-angle rule (slope = 0.5) and not a zero-angle rule (slope = 0) (black dashed lines). This finding is observed for both nerve (solid lines) and nucleus (dashed lines) stimulation. B) Comparison of median stimulation slopes (black bars) with half-angle rule slopes from pursuit (white bars), shown separately for each animal. Error bars illustrate 95% confidence intervals. Dashed line: half-angle rule slope of 0.5. Replotted with permission from Klier et al. (2006).

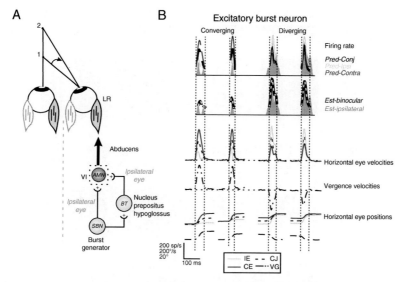

Plate 6 (Also see Fig. 9.5.) A) Schematic of the interaction that occurs between the vergence and saccadic premotor pathways during disconjugate saccades. When the lateral rectus is the agonist muscle the SBNs provide the abducens motoneurons with an integrated vergence/conjugate command (i.e. ipsilateral command) to drive the movement of the eye. B) Example discharges from an example EBN during (left) converging disconjugate saccades (contralateral eye moves more), and (right) diverging disconjugate saccades (ipsilateral eye moves more). The second row shows the same firing rate traces duplicated for clarity. Predicted model fits using conjugate, ipsilateral, and contralateral eye velocities as inputs to SBN model are shown in the top row in black, blue, and red respectively. Note the poor fits obtained when the conjugate and contralateral parameters are used to predict the firing rate of this neuron compared to the prediction using the ipsilateral eye (top row, red and black traces compared to blue trace). Estimated model fits using a binocular model (i.e. left eye and right eye as inputs) are shown in the second row (thick black curve). Estimated model fits using the reduced ipsilateral model are also shown (dashed grey curve). This finding is consistent with the hypothesis that burst neurons encode the movement of the ipsilateral eye rather than the conjugate component of the eye movements.

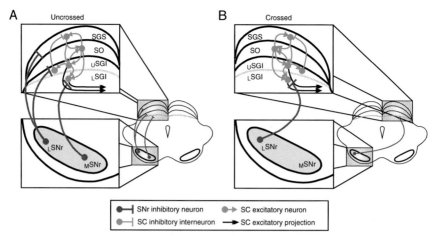

Plate 7 (Also see Fig. 12.3.) Schematic diagram of the connections between the SNr and the SC. A) A coronal section of the SC is shown with expanded views of the layers dorsally and the SNr ventrally indicated by the shaded portions in the inset. Uncrossed projections from the SNr to the SC arise from the lateral and medial SNr and target superficiale and intermediate layers of the SC. B) Crossed pathway from SNr to the SC. SGS, stratum griseum superficial; SO, stratum opticum; $_U$SGI, upper stratum griseum intermediale; $_L$SGI, lower stratum griseum intermediale; $_L$SNr, lateral substantia nigra pars reticulari; $_M$SNr, medial substantia nigra pars reticulata. Green arrows show excitatory SC connections; red lines show inhibitory SNr connections; blue lines show inhibitory SC connections; black arrows show excitatory projections.

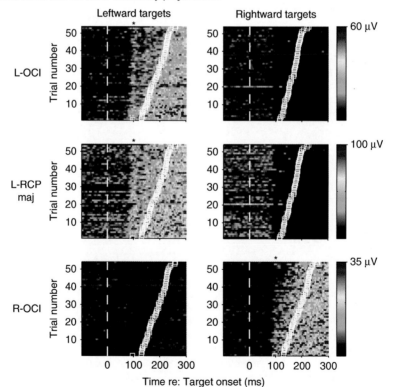

Plate 8 (Also see Fig. 16.3.) Representation of recruitment of bilateral OCI and left RCP maj muscles in a head-restrained monkey, aligned to the presentation of a visual target 27° to the left or right. Data segregated by side of target presentation (vertical dashed line), and sorted by saccadic reaction time (white square). Each row represents a different trial, with the colour conveying the magnitude of recruitment. Note the time-locked nature of recruitment following ipsilateral target presentation (asterisks), regardless of the time of initiation of the ensuing saccade. A prominent band of time-locked inhibition is also seen on left RCP maj following rightward target presentation. Such lateralized recruitment forms the core of the head turning synergy, despite head restraint.

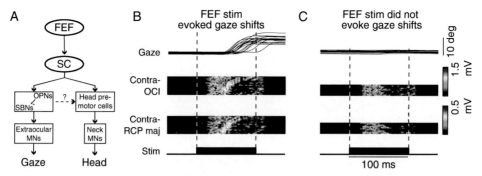

Plate 9 (Also see Fig. 16.4.) A) Conceptual schematic outlining role of various brainstem centres in eye-head gaze shifts. Descending commands from the dSC (superior colliculus), which receives converging information from a number of cortical areas including the FEF (frontal eye fields), is distributed to premotor centres governing gaze shifts and head movements. Gaze shifts are generated by saccadic burst neurons (SBNs), which are potently inhibited by omnipause neurons (OPNs). OPNs selectively inhibit the SBNs without exerting a similar influence on head premotor neurons. At the current time, it is unknown whether SBNs distribute a drive to the head when engaged ('?' in figure). Regardless, this schematic provides a plausible explanation for how head orienting can begin before, or in advance of, gaze orienting. B) Gaze shifts and neck muscle activity evoked by stimulation of the left FEF in a head-restrained monkey. Here, 100 ms of 50 μA of stimulation current evoked a 7° rightward gaze shift (upper traces), and recruitment of the contralateral (rightward) OCI and RCP maj muscles (same format as Fig. 16.3). Note how evoked neck muscle activity lead the evoked gaze shift. C) From the same FEF location, stimulation occasionally failed to evoke a gaze shift (top traces). However, evoked neck muscle activity persisted on such 'no gaze' trials. These results are consistent with the schematic in (A), whereby activity that was unable to engage the brainstem burst generator engaged an orienting drive on the head.

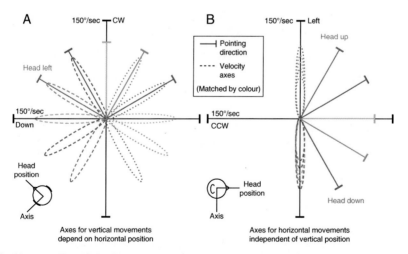

Plate 10 (Also see Fig. 18.2.) Schematic axes of rotation, and their dependence on orientation, in a Fick system, plotted in orthogonal Cartesian coordinates. Angular velocity (broken lines) is a vector parallel to the axis of rotation, scaled by the speed of rotation. The angular velocity of the eye and head generally follows the loops, starting at zero velocity, growing to maximum velocity, and then returning to zero. In each panel, five head pointing directions are shown (solid lines), each colour coded to two velocity loops in opposite directions (dashed vs. dotted lines). A) Velocity loops for vertical rotations at five horizontal positions, viewed from above. B) Velocity loops for horizontal rotations at five vertical positions, viewed from the side. Real head data follow the same pattern, but are never as symmetric. Reprinted from *Journal of Neurophysiology*, **97**, Klier, E.M., Wang, H., and Crawford, J.D., Interstitial nucleus of Cajal encodes three-dimensional head orientations in Fick-like coordinates, p. 604, figure 3 © 2007 The American Physiological Society, used with permission.

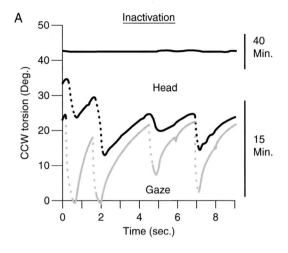

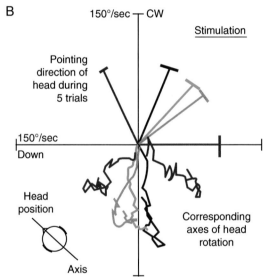

Plate 11 (Also see Fig. 18.5.) Evidence of a neural integrator for head orientation in the INC, organized in Fick coordinates. A) Head (dark line) and gaze/eye-in-space (grey line) torsion plotted against time following muscimol injection. Shortly after injection (15 min here) both drift away from the regular upright position, while rapid movements attempt to correct this. Later (40 min here) the head settles in a torsionally shifted position, i.e. corrective movements cease. From Klier et al., *Science* **295**, 1314 © 2002. Reprinted with permission from AAAS. B) During unilateral INC stimulation with the head free, the head rotates around vertical-torsional axes (clockwise for left INC; counterclockwise for right INC) that stay fixed relative to horizontal head orientation, as in a Fick gimbal. Conventions similar to Fig. 18.2A, but here real data are shown. Reprinted from *Journal of Neurophysiology*, **97**, Klier, E.M., Wang, H., and Crawford, J.D., Interstitial nucleus of cajal encodes three-dimensional head orientations in Fick-like coordinates, p 604, figure 5 © 2007 The American Physiological Society, used with permission.

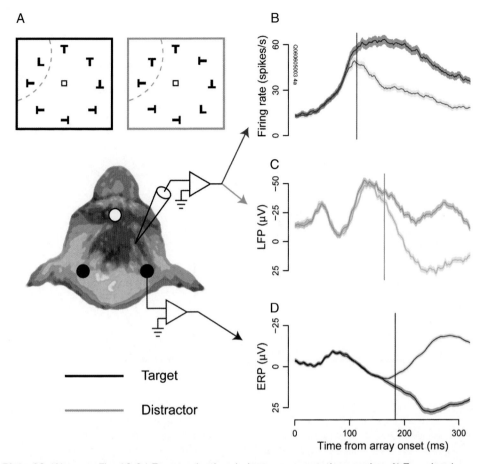

Plate 12 (Also see Fig. 19.2.) Target selection during a representative session. A) Top: visual search display (shown here with a set size of 8) with the target (L) inside the neuron's receptive field (indicated by the dashed arc) (left) and opposite the receptive field (right). Monkeys searched for a T or L target among 1, 3 or 7 L or T distractors. Bottom: schematic of recording sites and signals. Single unit discharges (blue) and local field potentials (green) were recorded intracranially from the frontal eye field. Event-related potentials were recorded from electrodes over extrastriate visual cortex (red). B) Average activity of one neuron when the search target was inside (dark) and opposite (light) its receptive field. Bands around average firing rates show time-varying standard error of the mean. Vertical line indicates target selection time when the two curves became statistically significantly different. C) FEF LFP with the target inside (dark) and opposite (light) the simultaneously recorded neuron's receptive field. D) ERP over extrastriate visual cortex from trials with the target inside (dark) and opposite (light) the receptive field of the concomitantly recorded FEF neuron. This component is the macaque homologue of the human N2pc (m-N2pc). Reprinted from *Journal of Neurophysiology*, **102**, Cohen, J.Y., R.P. Heitz, J.D. Schall, G.F. Woodman, On the origin of event-related potentials indexing covert attentional selection during visual search, pp. 2375–2386, figure 2 © 2009 The American Physiological Society, used with permission.

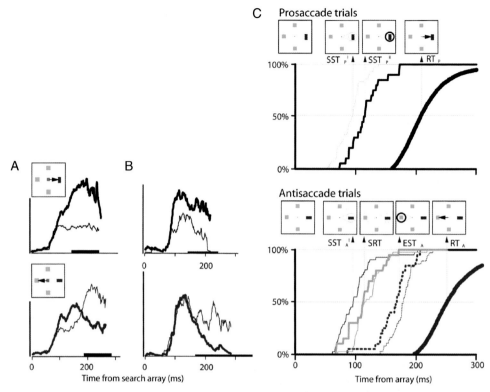

Plate 13 (Also see Fig. 19.4) Pattern and timing of neural activity in FEF when mapping between location of visual target and endpoint of saccade is varied. A) Activity of FEF neuron with activity that can be identified with the allocation of attention (Type I). Average spike density function when the singleton fell in the neuron's receptive field (thick line) and when the singleton was located opposite the receptive field (thin line) in prosaccade (top) and antisaccade (bottom) trials. Bracket on abscissa marks range of RT. Scale bar represents 100 spikes/s. B) Activity of FEF neuron with activity that can be identified with selection of the saccade endpoint (Type II). C) Cumulative distributions of modulation times in prosaccade (top) and antisaccade (bottom) trials for Type I (thin) and Type II (thicker) neurons with corresponding RT (thickest) (full caption available on p. 371).

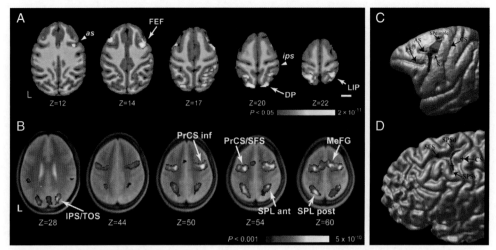

Plate 14 (Also see Fig. 20.1) The homology of oculomotor areas in monkey and human. BOLD responses evoked by saccades in (A) monkeys and (B) humans using fMRI (Koyama et al., 2004) show promising homology. The monkey areas FEF and LIP appear to have putative homologies in human dorsal precentral and intraparietal sulci, respectively. Note that in humans, activation can be seen in the superior and inferior branches of the precentral sulcus making it difficult to localize the FEF in humans. Reprinted from *Neuron* **41**(5), M. Koyama, I. Hasegawa, T. Osada, Y. Adachi, K. Nakahara, and Y. Miyashita, Functional magnetic resonance imaging of macaque monkeys performing visually guided saccade tasks: comparison of cortical eye fields with humans, pp.795–807, © 2007 with permission from Elsevier. C) These two areas may correspond to the monkey dorsal premotor cortex (blue) and FEF (red). D) In humans, saccades evoke activation all along the precentral sulcus. However, the portion of the precentral sulcus that is dorsal to the junction of the superior frontal sulcus (blue) shows relatively greater hand movement related activity, while the portion ventral to the junction (red) shows relatively greater eye movement related activity (Amiez et al., 2006).

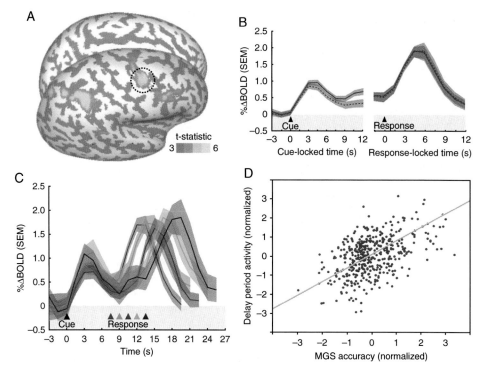

Plate 15 (Also see Fig. 20.2) The functional homologies between monkey area FEF and putative human area FEF during a spatial memory-guided saccade task (MGS). A) BOLD activity during a memory delay period localizes to the precentral sulcus, the putative human FEF (circled). B) The time course of FEF BOLD activity persists above pretrial baseline during the delay period and is greater in the hemisphere contralateral (solid line) compared to ipsilateral (dashed line) to the location of the memoranda. C) FEF BOLD activity persists above baseline for the duration of the memory delay. Each coloured line is a different delay length, ranging from 7–13.5 s. (A–C) Reprinted from *NeuroImage*, **39**(1), R. Srimal and C.E. Curtis, Persistent neural activity during the maintenance of spatial position in working memory, Copyright (2008), with permission from Elsevier. D) The magnitude of the delay period activity predicts the later accuracy of the memory guided saccade; greater BOLD predicts greater accuracy. Reprinted from *Journal of Neuroscience*, **24**(16), 3944–52. Curtis, C. E., Rao, V. Y. & D'Esposito, M. (2004). Maintenance of spatial and motor codes during oculomotor delayed response tasks.

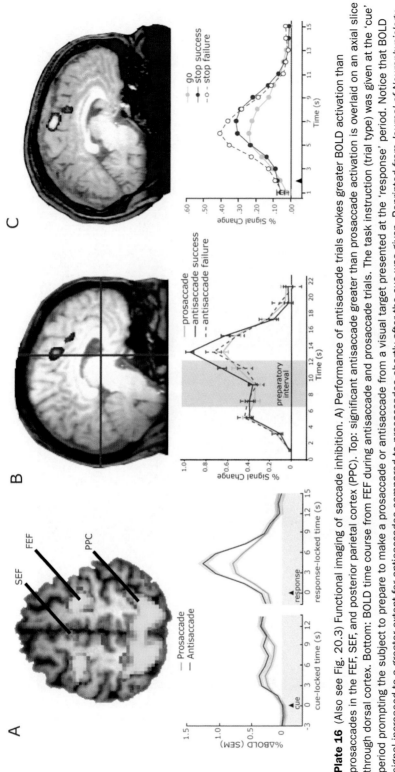

Plate 16 (Also see Fig. 20.3) Functional imaging of saccade inhibition. A) Performance of antisaccade trials evokes greater BOLD activation than prosaccades in the FEF, SEF, and posterior parietal cortex (PPC). Top: significant antisaccade greater than prosaccade activation is overlaid on an axial slice through dorsal cortex. Bottom: BOLD time course from FEF during antisaccade and prosaccade trials. The task instruction (trial type) was given at the 'cue' period prompting the subject to prepare to make a prosaccade or antisaccade from a visual target presented at the 'response' period. Notice that BOLD signal increased to a greater extent for antisaccades compared to prosaccades shortly after the cue was given. Reprinted from *Journal of Neurophysiology*, **98**, Brown, MEG, Villis, T., and Everling, S., Frontoparietal activation with preparation for antisaccades. Copyright (2007) used with permission from The American Physiological Society. B) Saccade production activates the SEF (and anterior cingulate) as shown in the sagittal image (top). The time course of SEF BOLD activity ramps up during the preparatory period and is greater prior to correct incorrect antisaccades, which are similar to prosaccades (bottom). Form C.E. Curtis and M. D'Esposito, Success and failure suppressing reflexive behavior, *Journal of Cognitive Neuroscience*, **15**(3) (April, 2003), pp. 409–418. © 2003 by the Massachusetts Institute of Technology. Figure 3b. C) The SEF, depicted in the top sagittal image, show BOLD activation during the performance of an oculomotor stop-signal task. Time courses from the SEF show that activity is enhanced during stop trials when inhibition is successful and unsuccessful compared to go trials. From C.E. Curtis, M.W. Cole, V.Y. Rao, M. D'Esposito, Canceling planned action: an fMRI study of countermanding saccades, *Cerebral Cortex*, 2005, **15**, by permission of Oxford University Press.

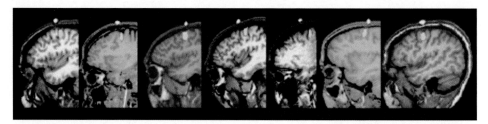

Plate 17 (Also see Fig. 21.1.) Individual localization of the FEF by TMS and fMRI. White mark: vitamin-E capsule Reprinted from *Neuroscience*, **151**(3), D. Hubl, T. Nyffeler, P. Wurtz, S. Chaves, T. Pflugshaupt, M. Lüthi, *et al*. Time course of blood oxygenation level–dependent signal response after theta burst transcranial magnetic stimulation of the frontal eye field, pp. 921–928. Copyright (2008), with permission from Elsevier.

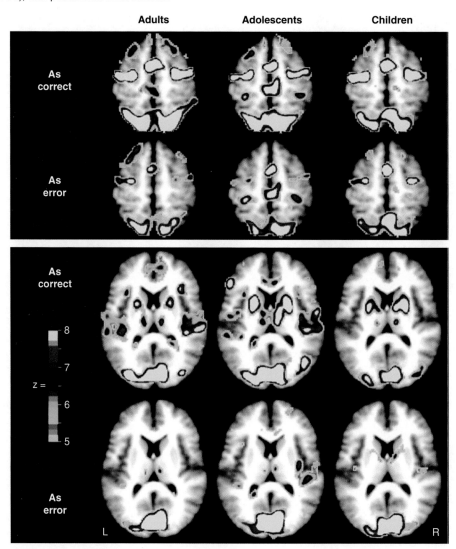

Plate 18 (Also see Fig. 35.4.) Mean group activation for a group of children, adolescents, and adults during correct and incorrect antisaccade task trials. Top panel) Horizontal sections at z = 54 show differing activity for correct and error trials, though similar activity across age groups in SMA/preSMA, FEF and PPC. Bottom panel) Horizontal sections at z = 12 show increased activity in putamen for correct versus error trials in all age groups. Reproduced from *Cerebral Cortex*, **18**, Katerina Velanova, Mark E. Wheeler, and Beatriz Luna, Maturational Changes in Anterior Cingulate and Frontoparietal Recruitment Support the Development of Error Processing and Inhibitory Control, 2008, with permission from Oxford University Press.

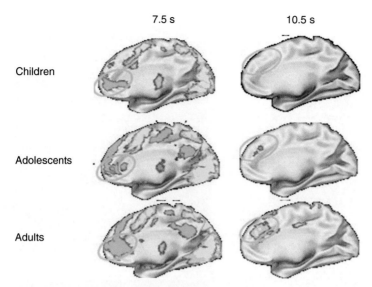

Plate 19 (Also see Fig. 35.5.) Mean group activation for antisaccade error trials in a group of children, adolescents, and adults overlaid on the partially inflated medial cortical surface of the right hemisphere. Activation is shown at two time points following trial onset—an 'early' time point at 7.5 s, and a 'late' time point at 10 s following trial onset. The approximate location of rostral ACC is circled in green and dorsal ACC in blue. Reproduced from *Cerebral Cortex*, **18**, Katerina Velanova, Mark E. Wheeler, and Beatriz Luna, Maturational Changes in Anterior Cingulate and Frontoparietal Recruitment Support the Development of Error Processing and Inhibitory Control, 2008, with permission from Oxford University Press.

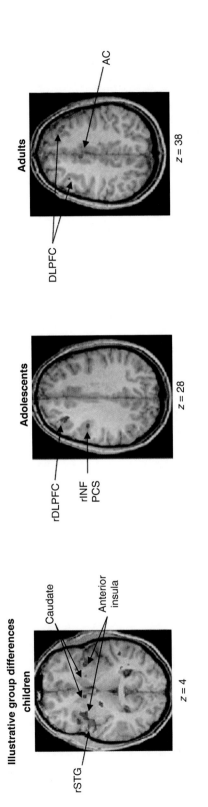

Illustrative group differences
children

Caudate

Anterior insula

rSTG

z = 4

Adolescents

rDLPFC

rINF PCS

z = 28

Adults

DLPFC

AC

z = 38

Proportion of total *active* voxels per ROI

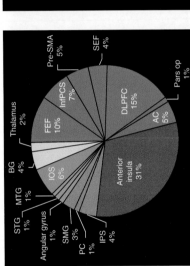

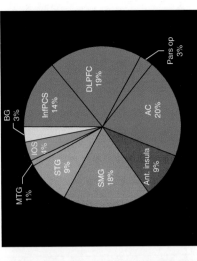

Plate 20 (Also see Fig. 35.7.) Mean group activation during a block memory-guided saccade task compared to prosaccade blocks for a group of children, adolescents, and adults overlaid on top of the structure of a representative subject. Each slice represents the location of primary activity for each group. Pie charts represent the proportion of total active voxels in each region of interest for each age group. From K.S. Scherf, J.A. Sweeney, B. Luna, Brain basis of developmental change in visuospatial working memory, *Journal of Cognitive Neuroscience*, **18**(7) (July, 2006), pp. 1045–1058. ©2006 by the Massachusetts Institute of Technology.

CHAPTER 27

Multisensory saccade generation

Richard Amlôt and Robin Walker

Abstract

Studies of saccadic eye movements have greatly informed our understanding of the processes involved in selection for action. As the primary function of saccades is to direct the fovea onto an object of interest there has been a natural tendency to regard them as a visually-guided behaviour. Saccades can, however, be directed to an auditory or even a somatosensory stimulus and combinations of stimuli in crossmodal situations. Neurophysiological studies have shown that neurons in structures such as the superior colliculus, involved in saccade-target selection and generation, respond to visual, auditory, and tactile stimuli. Combinations of stimuli can produce neural interaction effects depending on the spatial and temporal relationship between the stimuli. A number of studies have examined the behavioural consequences of crossmodal stimulus configurations on saccades and these will be reviewed in this chapter.

Introduction

Primates and humans are highly visual animals and rely on the visual system for the control of behaviour and visual guidance. The saccadic system has evolved in order to shift the high-resolution fovea onto objects, and to maintain fixation on them, thus enabling detailed visual processing and analysis (Carpenter, 1988; Findlay and Gilchrist, 2003). There has, therefore, been a natural tendency to regard saccades as a visual behaviour and much research has been restricted to investigating the characteristics and processes involved in the generation of visually-guided saccades (Schall, 1995; Wurtz, 2000). Although saccades are an essential component of our visual abilities they can also be guided by sounds (e.g. Zahn et al., 1978; Zambarbieri et al., 1995a), or somatosensory stimulation on the body surface (e.g. Groh and Sparks, 1996a; Grüsser, 1983). In natural environments, for example, different sensory stimuli can arise from the same object (the sight of a fly, the buzzing sound it makes and the tactile sensation of it landing on your hand) and the process of saccade target selection must operate in a multisensory context. Recent investigations have shown that visual, auditory and tactile stimuli have access to the same multisensory neurons in a number of brain regions including those located in the deeper layers of the superior colliculus (DLSC) and also neurons in cortical areas such as the anterior ectosylvian sulcus (AES) (Stein et al., 2004).

A number of studies have investigated the characteristics of saccades made with combinations of stimuli from more than one modality and have provided behavioural evidence of multisensory convergence and interactions. Such multisensory interactions appear consistent with neurophysiological evidence of multisensory effects in saccade-related brain regions which will be considered here.

In addition to the neural explanations, the modulation of saccade characteristics in multisensory situations may also be related to cognitive factors such as warning signal effects, and the 'mode' (endogenous or exogenous orienting) of saccade generation. This chapter will first describe some of the neurophysiological evidence of multisensory effects and will then discuss the findings from behavioural studies of saccades in terms of the neural and cognitive processes that may underlie multisensory saccade generation.

The selection of a saccade target and saccade generation involves a network of heavily interconnected cortical and subcortical brain regions (Schall, 1995). Some of these structures receive visual, auditory and somatosensory inputs for the control of eye movements (e.g. frontal eye fields: Meredith, 1999; posterior parietal cortex: Avillac et al., 2004). The superior colliculus (SC) is a midbrain structure that has a key role in the control and generation of saccades (Sparks and Hartwich-Young, 1989). The SC is a layered structure, the superficial layers principally contain maps of visual space, whereas the intermediate and deep layers contain burst and buildup neurons that fire in association with saccades of a particular amplitude or direction (Munoz and Wurtz, 1995a, 1995b). Importantly these sensory and motor maps are in spatial register (King, 2004), and therefore allow the visuomotor coordination of orienting (Schall, 1995). The SC provides one site where converging inputs from a number of different unimodal brain regions project onto 'multisensory' neurons for the control of orienting (Stein and Meredith, 1993). Neurons in the deep layers of the SC have multiple sensory receptive fields (e.g. visual and somatosensory) that are in close spatial alignment, so that if a stimulus falls within one sensory receptive field, it also falls in the other. In this way the combined input of the multisensory properties of a stimulus can excite the neuron. These multisensory neurons are also in close alignment with movement cells that are recruited for the generation of saccades; therefore the eyes can be efficiently moved to different locations in external space, allowing objects and events of interest to be foveated regardless of modality. The multisensory properties of a given stimulus can also significantly influence these movements. Saccades may be modified by the combined product of the convergence of information from separate sensory modalities onto multisensory neurons in the SC. Stimulus intensity and the relative spatial and temporal presentation of multisensory signals can influence the timing and size of neural responses, which are reflected in the subsequent behavioural characteristics of goal-driven saccadic responses (e.g. Frens and Van Opstal, 1998).

Studies of saccades made in response to combinations of multimodal stimuli have shown that basic behavioural characteristics, such as latency, amplitude, and peak velocity are sensitive to crossmodal stimulation. Saccade latency can be faster to combinations of visual and auditory stimuli, compared to saccades to each single modality alone (e.g. Frens et al., 1995; Hughes et al., 1994; Corneil and Munoz, 1996). Stimuli from different sensory modalities, at different locations in external space, can also modify saccade accuracy and trajectory (Doyle and Walker, 2002; Lueck et al., 1990). The majority of studies of non-visual and multisensory saccade generation have focused on visual and auditory stimuli and their interaction, while studies involving somatosensory stimuli are rare. Less still is known about visual-somatosensory interaction effects although a small number of pioneering studies have appeared in the past decade (Amlôt et al., 2003; Groh and Sparks, 1996b; Neggers and Bekkering, 1999) although direct comparisons with visual-auditory effects are even less prevalent (Doyle and Walker, 2002).

The neurophysiological basis of multisensory saccade generation

Neurons in the SC respond to a range of different sensory modalities and maps of visual, auditory and somatosensory space are aligned in topographical register, allowing for a range of different modality stimuli to elicit saccadic eye movements (Groh and Sparks, 1996b, 1996c; Bell et al., 2005). Perhaps the most notable property of some superior colliculus neurons is their ability to respond to combinations of sensory stimuli. Bi- and tri-modal cells have been identified with some unusual response properties and related behavioural consequences (Fig. 27.1A) (Meredith and Stein, 1983; Stein and Meredith, 1993; Wallace et al., 1996).

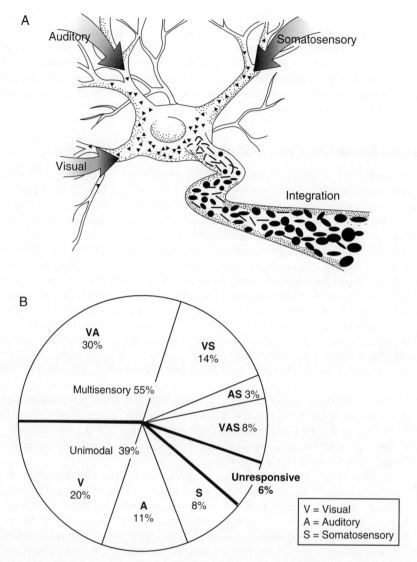

Fig. 27.1 A) The convergence of inputs from different senses onto a single neuron (after Stein and Meredith, 1993). Multisensory neurons are found in many areas of the brain including regions of the parietal lobe and frontal lobe and also subcortical structures such as the superior colliculus. B) Patterns of sensory convergence in deep-layer neurons of the cat superior colliculus. From B.E Stein and M.A. Meredith., *The Merging of the Senses*, figure 1b, © 1993 Massachusetts Institute of Technology, by permission of The MIT Press. Over half of the neurons studied in the samples (Meredith and Stein, 1985; 1986a) were classified as multisensory. Neurons with visual inputs were frequently observed and those responsive to visual-auditory multisensory stimuli were the most prevalent category—reflecting the cat's dependence on visual and auditory cues.

Estimates of the proportion of neurons involved in multisensory convergence vary across species and with the different neurophysiological methods employed to locate these stimuli. However, the most comprehensive investigations, performed in cats, suggest that up to 55% of neurons respond to a combination of different modality stimuli (Meredith and Stein, 1985, 1986a). Figure 27.1B shows the approximate proportion of multisensory, unimodal, and apparently unresponsive neurons identified in their studies of the cat SC. From Fig. 27.1B it is apparent that some modalities are represented more extensively than others, and this manifests as a bias for vision and visual-auditory combinations, which possibly reflects the dominant modalities employed by the cat to hunt and detect prey. Other combinations of stimulus modalities have been found to be more prevalent in different species, which is thought to reflect their different behavioural adaptations. For example, visual-somatosensory neurons predominate in rodent SC, reflecting the dependence on the whiskers for information from the external environment (Weldon and Best, 1992).

Stein and Meredith's rules of multisensory integration

Stein and Meredith (1993) identified several 'rules' that appear to govern the nature of the multisensory response properties of collicular neurons. These integrative rules have been supported by the existence of behavioural correlates supporting the functional relevance of these rules (Stein, 1998; Stein, et al., 1988). The rules are based on the unimodal receptive field characteristics and are determined by the spatial and temporal characteristics of the stimuli.

The spatial rule: multimodal neurons will show response enhancement for spatially coincident stimuli, while spatially non-aligned stimuli may cause response depression. This property of multisensory cells has been observed consistently in single cell recordings in the superior colliculus (Meredith and Stein, 1986a, 1986b; Perrault et al., 2005; Stein and Meredith, 1993) and is also supported by a number of behavioural studies. For example, the percentage of correct whole-body orienting movements by cats to a weakly effective visual stimulus was found to be increased when the target was accompanied by an additional auditory stimulus, but only when these stimuli were spatially coincident (Stein et al., 1988).

The temporal rule: describes the relatively long temporal 'window' during which stimuli from different sensory modalities can arrive and be integrated to influence the response properties of a neuron. Wallace et al. (1996) suggest that optimal enhancement of neural firing in visual-auditory multisensory neurons occurs when the stimulus onsets are within 150 ms of each other (Perrault et al., 2003; Wallace et al., 1996). The broad temporal window is thought to enable activity patterns from more than one sensory input to overlap given differences in the velocities and neural processing and conduction times for the different modalities.

The inverse effectiveness rule: the magnitude of multisensory interaction effects depends on the relative stimulus intensity of the combinations of sensory stimuli (Stein and Meredith, 1993). When stimulus intensity is high, the magnitude of the response enhancement seen to combinations of sensory stimuli is small. However, with weakly effective stimuli, the response enhancement is much greater. For example, as unimodal stimulus intensity was decreased so that progressively fewer neural discharges were evoked, the magnitude of the response enhancement evoked by auditory and visual stimuli in combination was as great as 450–500% (Meredith and Stein, 1986b).

The receptive field preservation rule: determines which stimuli can initiate multisensory integration, providing a consistent representation of the external world. For example, although the response properties of a multisensory neuron can be significantly modified by additional sensory stimulation, the stability of the individual receptive field properties will be maintained despite changes in responsiveness produced by the presence of a signal from a different modality. For example, the directional specificity shown by a neuron to a visual stimulus will not be changed by the increase in responsiveness following the introduction of a secondary auditory stimulus. Therefore, it is likely that a visual stimulus property will not be 'mis-perceived' in the presence of an auditory signal (Stein and Meredith, 1993).

Behavioural evidence of multisensory integration and interaction

Studies of non-visual and multisensory saccade generation have primarily been concerned with the visual and auditory modalities although there are notable exceptions which have included the somatosensory modality. In order to interpret the findings from crossmodal studies of saccade generation the characteristics of saccades made to unimodal visual, auditory, and somatosensory stimuli need to be considered. An issue that needs to be considered when making direct comparisons between saccades across stimulus modalities is that the relative level of salience of targets across modalities is difficult to estimate. Saccade latency is furthermore known to be sensitive to the spatial and temporal aspects of a task as well as to the level of cognitive control required for saccade generation. The combination of stimulus salience and also relevance (which depends on the goal of the observer) can be regarded as stimulus 'priority' (Fecteau and Munoz, 2006) which has yet to be considered in studies of multisensory saccade generation. Few studies have directly compared saccades across modalities, under the same conditions, adding a further confound. The interpretation of the experimental results suffers also from the fact that interactions between modalities may reflect interactions at the neural level, but could also be the result of differences in the way participants respond to stimuli from more than one modality. For example, if a tactile target and coincident visual (task-irrelevant) distractor are presented the participant may be generating a response to either stimulus modality rather than the 'sum' of both inputs.

Visual-auditory saccade generation

Unimodal response properties

Saccades to auditory targets generally have longer latency, lower peak-velocity and are less accurate than visually-guided saccades (e.g. Engelken and Stevens, 1989; Zahn et al., 1978; Zambarbieri et al., 1981, 1982). This relationship appears to depend on the intensity of the stimuli, the properties of the sound source and the eccentricity of the targets (Frens et al., 1995; Zambarbieri et al., 1995b). The latency of saccades made to visual targets can, however, be increased beyond that of auditory targets by reducing the intensity of the stimulus; however a similar reduction in intensity for auditory targets has little effect on latency (Frens et al., 1995). The latency of saccades to auditory targets is modulated by the eccentricity of the stimulus, such that sounds close to the body midline have a longer latency and this reduces with increasing eccentricity (Zambarbieri et al., 1982). This is in contrast to visual saccades where latency is found to increase with increasing eccentricity (Kalesnykas and Hallett, 1994). Figure 27.2 shows examples of saccades made to visual and auditory stimuli (under conditions

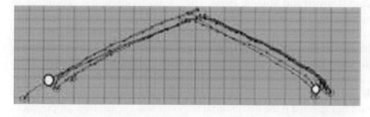

Saccades to visual targets. Mean endpoint deviation = 5.6° (±1.3°), mean latency = 206 ms

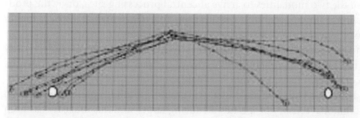

Saccades to auditory targets. Mean endpoint deviation = 10.6° (±1.8°), mean latency = 200 ms

Fig. 27.2 Example of unimodal visual and auditory saccades made by a single observer from a central fixation point to stimuli located in the lower visual field. Saccades made to auditory stimuli show wider variation in endpoint (polar coordinates). With kind permission from Springer Science+Business Media: *Experimental Brain Research*, Doyle, M. and Walker, R. Multisensory interactions in saccade target selection: curved saccade trajectories **142**(1) 2002, pp. 116–130.

of dim illumination) located in the lower visual field ($\pm 10.33°$ azimuth, $-7.1°$ elevation) (from Doyle and Walker, 1992). Saccades made to auditory stimuli appear more variable and are less accurate than visually guided saccades showing a much wider variation in saccade endpoint, although mean latency was broadly comparable (206 ms and 200 ms respectively).

The ability to accurately localize an auditory stimulus requires an interpretation of the arrival time and intensity at the two ears (interaural time and intensity difference) and an analysis of the component frequencies of the sound. Zambarbieri et al. (1982) proposed that smaller differences in these variables with auditory stimuli closer to the midline adds to the noise or 'uncertainty' in the early stages of target localization and saccade generation processes, thereby increasing saccade latency. However, more recently these researchers have shown that the pattern of latency effects for auditory stimuli exists relative to starting eye position, rather than just target position with respect to the midline (Zambarbieri et al., 1995b). These results suggest that for saccades to auditory targets, it is likely that in addition to sensory factors influencing the speed of saccadic response, modality-specific differences in the coordinate transformations and activation of the common motor pathway may be different when compared to saccades to visual targets.

Bimodal response properties

Early studies of bimodal stimulus presentation demonstrated that saccades to spatially aligned auditory and visual stimuli have a reduced latency compared to unimodal targets (Zahn et al., 1978, 1979). However in these studies participants were not instructed to respond to a specific modality in bimodal conditions, therefore it is not clear whether the facilitation of response was a product of a saccade being generated by the fastest modality or via the convergence and integration of the two stimuli. Later studies have confirmed the existence of latency facilitation effects with bimodal visual-auditory stimuli, under conditions where the participants were instructed to respond to the onset of a visual or auditory target in the presence of an irrelevant co-stimulus (Arndt and Colonius, 2003; Colonius and Arndt, 2001; Corneil and Munoz, 1996; Engelken and Stevens, 1989; Frens et al., 1995; Hughes et al., 1994). With increasing spatial disparity there is a gradual increase in saccade latency, until no facilitation is observed when stimuli are positioned in opposite hemifields (Frens et al., 1995; Harrington and Peck, 1998). An increase in saccade latency and directional error rates has been reported for visual targets with auditory distractors presented on the opposite-side of space (Corneil and Munoz, 1996). The latency facilitation is dependent on the simultaneous, or near simultaneous temporal presentation of the two stimuli (Corneil and Munoz, 1996; Frens et al., 1995; Hughes et al., 1994). In visual-auditory saccade studies, the most convincing evidence for latency facilitation via the integration of sensory signals comes from studies in which the upper limits of race model predictions are tested (Corneil and Munoz, 1996; Diederich and Colonius, 2004; Harrington and Peck, 1998; Hughes et al., 1994). In these studies the facilitation of saccade latency associated with spatially-coincident combinations of sensory stimuli is greater than would be expected if the behavioural response was elicited by a simple 'race', won by the first stimulus of the two modalities to arrive at central processing sites, or by the product of their combined response time probability distributions (e.g. Corneil et al., 2002; Hughes et al., 1994). As a result of these statistical analyses, the latency facilitation effects observed for combinations of visual and auditory saccades are thought to reflect the outcome of multisensory integration at the neural level rather than being attributed to the saccade being initiated by the modality with the fastest conduction rates.

The latency facilitation associated with bimodal visual and auditory stimulus presentation is also modulated by changes in unimodal sensory properties. Reducing target stimulus intensity has been found to increase the size of the latency facilitation effects observed with visual-auditory stimuli (Colonius and Arndt, 2001; Corneil et al., 2002), consistent with the principle of inverse effectiveness observed in neurophysiological studies (Stein and Meredith, 1993; Perrault et al., 2005). Visual and auditory stimuli can also combine to influence saccade trajectories. Lueck et al. (1990) examined saccades to simultaneous presentation of visual and auditory stimuli at increasing spatial disparities.

They found that saccades to visual targets with a close, but spatially disparate auditory co-stimulus produced saccade amplitudes with end points that represented an 'averaging' of the two saccade target positions. The effects observed here have also been found with two auditory stimuli (Zahn et al., 1979) and reflect a phenomenon first described in visually-elicited saccades as 'centre of gravity' or 'global' effects (e.g. Edelman et al., 2007; Findlay, 1982; He and Kowler, 1989). Here the amplitude of the saccade reflects the averaging or sum of the population of neurons encoding the stimuli locations in the superior colliculus. Frens et al. (1995) also report the phenomena of averaging for initial saccade trajectory under low stimulus intensity conditions with spatially separated auditory and visual stimuli, an effect that disappeared under higher intensity conditions.

Doyle and Walker (2002) investigated visual-auditory multimodal interactions, using a crossmodal distractor paradigm to investigate the influence of crossmodal distractors on saccade trajectory deviations. The distractor-related deviation of saccade trajectories has been widely used as a measure of inhibition involved in target selection in the visual modality (McSorley et al., 2006, 2009; Sheliga et al., 1994; Van der Stigchel et al., 2006) and was adopted as a method of investigating multimodal interaction effects. The trajectories of endogenous saccades (generated on the basis of the crossmodal distractor) deviated away from both visual and auditory distractors—although the greatest effect was observed for the visual distractor modality. The timing of the distractor onset in relation to the saccade target (or saccade initiation; McSorley et al., 2006) was found to be an important factor and the greatest effect on visually-guided saccade trajectories was observed when the distractor preceded the target by some 100 ms. Like the global effect, these multisensory trajectory effects can be explained in similar terms as the models used to account for the effects observed for visual distractors in unimodal studies (Van der Stigchel et al., 2006; Walker and McSorley, 2008).

Visual-somatosensory saccade generation

Unimodal response properties

Saccades to somatosensory targets in humans and monkeys have been found to be more variable and less accurate than saccades to visual stimuli at the same eccentricities (Amlôt et al., 2003; Blanke and Grüsser, 2001; Doyle and Walker, 2002; Groh and Sparks, 1996a; Grüsser, 1983; Neggers and Bekkering, 1999). Importantly however, this research has demonstrated that participants are able to localize the position of a somatosensory stimulus in the dark with no visual information regarding target location or hand position (see Amlôt et al., 2003; Doyle and Walker, 2002). This implies that the position of a somatosensory stimulus, initially encoded in a somatotopic frame of reference, can be transformed into oculomotor co-ordinates and recruit the same motor output pathways that produce visual or auditory saccades. Somatosensory saccades are also found to have longer latency, and lower peak-velocity than visually-guided saccades (Groh and Sparks, 1996a; Kristjánsson et al., 2004; Sullivan and Abel, 2000; Sullivan et al., 2004). Figure 27.3 shows examples of unimodal saccades made to visual and somatosensory stimuli (applied to fingers of left and right hands) which demonstrates the increased variability and latency of somatosensory saccades (from Amlôt et al., 2003). Differences in response time and accuracy may be attributed to differences in sensory processes such as neural transmission rates and the ability to localize a stimulus accurately in sensory space. However, differences in peak-velocity must be a reflection of a differential activation of the common motor output pathway (Groh and Sparks, 1996a). In order to reduce effects that could be attributed to differences in afferent processing time for visual and somatosensory stimuli, Groh and Sparks also included a delayed saccade task. They found that the difference between visual and somatosensory latency could be reduced but somatosensory saccade latency was still significantly greater than visual latency for two out of three monkeys tested. In addition, initial eye position could influence the accuracy of saccade landing position suggesting that the transformation from somatotopic to oculocentric coordinates may be imperfect. It seems therefore, that saccades to somatosensory stimuli are not simply substituted for their visual counterparts in a common oculomotor reference that elicits identical main-sequence saccades. Rather, there appears to be modality-specific differences in saccade

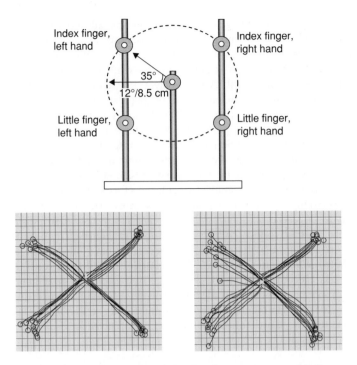

Top-diagram showing location of visual and somatosensory stimuli. Trajectories of saccades (made in semi-darkness) to visual targets (lower left) are more accurate than those made to somatosensory targets. Visual -mean endpoint deviation = 2.6°±0.4°, mean latency = 186 ms; Somatosensory mean endpoint deviation = 3.4°, ±0.8°, mean latency = 274 ms.

Fig. 27.3 Top) Schematic diagram showing visual and somatosensory stimulus configuration and sample trajectory plots of unimodal saccades made by a single observer. Somatosensory stimulation was applied to the fingertips of the index and little fingers of each hand at a distance of 40 cm. The trajectories of saccades to visual targets (lower left) are more accurate than those made to somatosensory targets (lower right). Reprinted from *Neuropsychologia*, **41**(1), R. Amlôt, R. Walker, J. Driver, and C. Spence, Multimodal visual-somatosensory integration in saccade generation, pp. 1–15, © 2003, with permission from Elsevier.

parameters as a consequence of the transformation of sensory representations and recruitment of saccade generation mechanisms (Neggers and Bekkering, 1999).

Although a number of factors are known to influence saccade latency (Carpenter, 1988; Findlay and Walker, 1999) a consistent finding is that somatosensory saccades have longer latency than comparable visually-guided saccades. The exact magnitude of the observed increase in latency varies from some 30 ms (Doyle and Walker, 2002; Groh and Sparks, 1996a), to 100 ms or more (Amlôt et al., 2003; Kristjánsson et al., 2004; Neggers and Bekkering, 1999). The increase in latency for somatosensory saccades may reflect differences in neural conduction rates: Groh and Sparks (Groh and Sparks, 1996b) showed that neurons in the SC took some 39 ms longer to respond to a somatosensory stimulus applied to the fingers of a monkey's paw than was required for a visual target at the same spatial location. However, sensory processing delays could not be the whole explanation as somatosensory saccade latency remains elevated in a delayed cueing task (Groh and Sparks 1996a). Groh and Sparks (1996a) attributed the increase in somatosensory saccade latency to modality-specific differences in the decision time to initiate a saccade. A similar sugges-tion was made by Amlôt et al. (2003) who noted that somatosensory saccades may be less similar to visually-guided saccades which can be regarded as being more 'reflexive' in nature than other forms of 'endogenous saccades' which rely more heavily on voluntary control processes for their generation. For example, endogenous saccades made on the basis of a symbolic arrow-cue and antisaccades directed away from a visual target have much longer latency than do visually-guided saccades (Walker et al., 2000). It is possible, therefore, that when an observer feels the tactile sensation somewhere on their body, a saccade may be made on the basis of an endogenous signal ('what's that touching my hand, must look at it') rather than it being comparable to a stimulus-elicited 'reflexive' saccade.

In order to test this idea we examined pro and antisaccades made to either visual or tactile targets (Amlôt and Walker, 2006). We reasoned that if somatosensory saccades are a form of endogenous saccade then there would be no difference in the latency of somatosensory pro- and antisaccades and that few prosaccade errors would be observed. This is because there is little difference in the level of *interpretation* required to translate a somatosensory stimulus into an instruction to look either towards, or away, from that finger. If, however, somatosensory saccades are generated in a similar way to exogenous (reflexive) saccades then there may be an increase in saccade latency when an antisaccade is required and prosaccade errors may be observed on a proportion of trials as is the case for the visual modality. Both visual and somatosensory antisaccades had longer latency than prosaccades. Erroneous prosaccades, made to the target, were observed for both visual and somatosensory targets on some 11–13% of antisaccade trials. The increase in latency for somatosensory antisaccades and the presence of prosaccade errors indicates that a somatosensory stimulus can elicit a form of reflexive saccade comparable to prosaccades made in the visual modality and that the increase in latency for somatosensory saccades is not entirely due to them depending on greater endogenous control processes. Our findings are in contrast with those of Kristjánsson, et al. (2004) who reported no difference in the latency of somatosensory pro and anti-saccades. We attribute the difference between these two studies to the long latency for prosaccades (some 416 ms) and high incidence of directional errors in the Kristjánsson study.

Bimodal response properties

Groh and Sparks (1996a) were the first to examine saccades made to combinations of visual and somatosensory stimuli (in monkeys only). These saccades had a shorter latency compared to unimodal somatosensory saccades although this difference was not always statistically significant. As previously mentioned, an issue that needs to be considered when interpreting multimodal effects, where a target from one modality is presented along with a distractor from another modality, is that it is not always possible to know which modality elicited the saccade. As some of the basic characteristics of saccades made to different stimulus modalities vary, measures such as peak-velocity can be used to inform the interpretation of the results (see Amlôt et al., 2003). Groh and Sparks found that the peak-velocity of somatosensory saccades made with coincident visual distractors was equivalent to that of visually-guided saccades, suggesting that it is possible that saccades in these conditions were actually elicited by the visual stimulus rather than the somatosensory target. However, several subsequent studies have also now reported multimodal visual-somatosensory saccades (Amlôt et al., 2003; Diederich and Colonius, 2004, 2006; Diederich et al., 2003; Rach and Diederich, 2006). Each of these studies provide evidence that visual-somatosensory interactions are observed in saccade generation, where spatially and temporally coincident visual-somatosensory stimuli result in a reduction in saccade latency when compared to unimodal visual saccades and saccades to more disparate combinations of bimodal visual-somatosensory stimuli. Each of these studies have focused primarily on visual target saccades with somatosensory distractors (Diederich et al., 2003; Rach and Diederich, 2006) or have used a 'redundant target' paradigm, where participants make saccades to combinations of different sensory stimuli, without a specific saccade target (Diederich and Colonius, 2004). The data could well be described by a model assuming that there is a fixed temporal window (cf. Stein and Meredith, 1993) in which multisensory stimuli can interact such as the TWIN 'Time Window of Integration' model (Diederich and Colonius, 2007b).

Studies in which participants made visually elicited saccades in the presence of visual distractors have shown that the spatial and temporal relationship between target and distractor (spatial separation, and stimulus onset asynchrony or SOA, respectively) strongly affected saccade latency (Walker et al., 1995, 1997). Using a similar paradigm, we (Amlôt et al., 2003) examined multisensory interactions between the visual and somatosensory modalities. In our study distractors from the non-target modality could appear coincident with the target, or in the opposite visual field and the SOA of target/distractor onset was varied. The latency of saccades made to visual targets was substantially reduced when a task-irrelevant somatosensory distractor was presented prior to target onset. Unlike the unimodal situation, the latency reduction was observed with both coincident and opposite field (remote) distractors. The reduction in latency observed when distractors appeared before the target, might in part arise from a temporal warning-signal effect (Ross and Ross, 1980; Ross and Ross, 1981). To test whether such warning effects could account fully for the faster response times an additional auditory warning signal was incorporated into the paradigm. In this situation coincident somatosensory distractors reduced saccade latency, but unlike the unimodal situation opposite side distractors did increase latency. The somatosensory target condition produced a different pattern of results: coincident visual distractors reduced saccade latency and remote visual distractors increased latency. However, a high proportion of directional errors was observed with opposite-side visual distractors and the peak velocity of saccades made with coincident visual distractors was increased (similar to that of visual saccades) indicating a bias for the visual modality for saccade generation. The motivation behind this study was to examine crossmodal distractor effects that would be predicted from the neurophysiological 'rules' of neural integration described above. The reduction in the latency of visually-guided saccades, when a coincident somatosensory distractor was presented, and when an additional temporal warning signal was included, are the most consistent evidence of a behavioural correlate of a neural summation effects. The study also highlighted how visual stimuli appear to be dominant in the saccadic system (as revealed by the high numbers of directional errors with opposite side visual distractors and the increase in peak velocity with spatially-coincident distractors) and we suggested that somatosensory stimuli may be less salient possibly because they activate fewer collicular neurons than do visual or auditory stimuli (Stein and Meredith, 1993).

The observed differences in saccade metrics between visual and somatosensory saccades may be due to differences in the activation of the common motor output pathway, and that proprioceptive position sense could also play an important role in the accuracy of somatosensory saccades (Amlôt et al., 2003; Groh and Sparks, 1996a). It remains for future research to determine more precisely the nature of the multisensory integration between somatosensation, proprioception, and vision that appears to be important (but not essential) for the localization of a somatosensory stimulus on the fingertip. Manipulating the relative contributions of these sensory inputs could be achieved by updating proprioceptive information on a trial-by-trial basis, via moving the arms and/or providing visual feedback during the inter-trial interval. Changes in somatosensory saccade accuracy would reflect the role of direct or indirect proprioceptive feedback on the localization accuracy of somatosensory stimuli. In the future, models of somatosensory saccade generation will need to account for both the control processes involved in saccade generation, as well as the modality-specific differences in oculomotor structures, to achieve a neurophysiologically-plausible model of saccade generation that can account for the properties of saccades to visual, auditory, somatosensory, and multimodal stimuli.

The behavioural studies reviewed here provide evidence of interaction effects in saccade generation that are consistent with the neurophysiological evidence of multisensory neuronal interactions observed in the SC. The reduction in saccade latency with spatially and temporally coincident multimodal stimuli, but conversely an increase in latency as the spatial separation between target and distractor increases, appears consistent with the neuronal enhancement or depression observed when one stimulus falls within or outside of the receptive field of another respectively. Models of multisensory interactions in saccade generation have drawn heavily upon the evidence of topographic representations of non-visual and multisensory space in the SC and the integration observed at the level of the single cell. Two such models with implications for the interaction of multisensory stimuli in the generation of saccades will now be reviewed.

Models of multisensory interactions in saccade generation

Frens et al. (1995) proposed a neurophysiologically plausible model of visual-auditory interactions in saccade generation (see Fig. 27.4). Visual and auditory signals arrive at the SC, and depending on their spatial and temporal configuration within a multisensory 'salience map', are able to more quickly inhibit the fixation cells at the rostral pole of the colliculus than either stimulus alone. These fixation cells are known to excite omnipause neurons in the brain stem that are active during fixation, and pause during saccades. Combinations of sensory stimuli aligned in time and space result in enhanced firing rates in presaccadic neurons in the deep layers of the colliculus, which are able to inhibit fixation-related activity and therefore reduce saccade latency. Also, as a result of the properties of the multisensory neurons in the SC, visual and auditory stimuli separated in space and time will not result in latency facilitation. However, an auditory stimulus arriving sometime before a

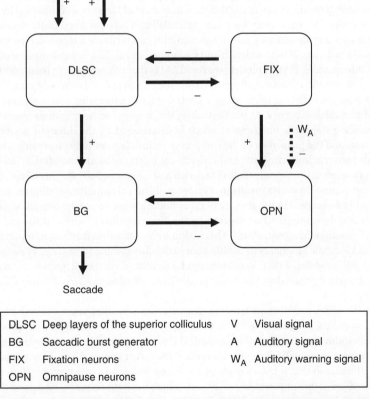

DLSC	Deep layers of the superior colliculus	V	Visual signal
BG	Saccadic burst generator	A	Auditory signal
FIX	Fixation neurons	W_A	Auditory warning signal
OPN	Omnipause neurons		

Fig. 27.4 Proposed mechanism for multimodal saccade facilitation (from Frens et al., 1995). Visual (V) and auditory (A) signals project to saccade-related burst neurons in the deep layers of the superior colliculus. Based on the spatiotemporal relationship between multisensory combinations of signals, the stimuli can facilitate the inhibition of fixation cells in the rostral pole of the colliculus. In this model, the auditory signal (W_A) can also act as a generalized warning signal, inhibiting omnipause neurons, which release their inhibitory control on the saccadic burst generator in the brainstem.

visual stimulus may also exert a non-specific inhibitory effect on brain stem omnipause neurons, resulting in a reduction in saccade latency. This warning signal effect may account for the absence of a remote distractor effect on saccade latency with spatially disparate visual and auditory stimuli (Frens et al., 1995).

This model affords similar predictions when considering saccades to combinations of visual and somatosensory stimuli. The spatial and temporal alignment of somatosensory and visual stimuli may result in similar latency facilitation effects as a result of the existence of visual-somatosensory multisensory neurons in the SC (e.g. Meredith and Stein, 1986b) which encode saccades in eye-centred coordinates (Groh and Sparks, 1996a and 1996b). However, there are fewer of these neurons, and firing rates are lower relative to other multisensory stimulus combinations (Stein and Meredith, 1993). Also, the representation of a somatosensory stimulus must be transformed from somatotopic coordinates to eye-centred coordinates, a calculation that is likely to be more complex and time-consuming than that required for an auditory or visual stimulus. Therefore, these factors may play an important role in the nature and presence of multisensory interaction effects with visual and somatosensory stimulus combinations. However, the broad temporal window observed for multi-sensory interactions at the neural level (Wallace et al., 1996) may allow multisensory enhancement even under these conditions, despite relatively long separations in arrival time for somatosensory and visual stimuli at the SC.

Colonius and Arndt (2001) have proposed a two-stage model to account for visual-auditory inter-actions in saccade generation, under conditions where a visual target is accompanied by an auditory non-target stimulus. More recently they have extended this account to consider conditions where either a somatosensory or auditory non-target stimulus can facilitate a target-driven visual saccade (Colonius and Diederich, 2004; Diederich and Colonius, 2007a). The key assumption of their 'Time Window of Integration' (TWIN) model (see Fig. 27.5) is that the process of visual-auditory saccade generation must include at least two distinguishable stages, a peripheral processing stage where initial sensory processes are separate, followed by a central stage of processing where sensory integration and saccade preparation occurs. At the first stage, the different sensory stimuli 'race' to reach the central processing stage, the outcome of which is determined by the different peripheral neural processing rates and the properties of the competing stimuli (e.g. stimulus intensity). At the second stage, signals converge and integrate, and crossmodal interactions are manifest by an increase (or decrease) in processing time at this stage (Diederich and Colonius, 2007a). This distinction between peripheral and central processes means that under multimodal stimulus conditions, a reduction in latency can still be observed in the absence of crossmodal integration at the central processing stage, as responses may in some part be triggered by the first stimulus to arrive at the second stage of processing (Colonius and Arndt, 2001). This is akin to the statistical facilitation reported in studies of manual and saccadic responses to multisensory stimulus combinations (e.g. Forster et al., 2002; Hughes et al., 1994; Miller, 1982). Responses can be facilitated via the integration of sensory signals at the second stage of processing, but this crucially depends upon the arrival time of the target and distractor stimuli.

In the TWIN model, it is the non-target or distractor stimulus that determines whether multimo-dal integration occurs. If a non-target stimulus (Fig. 27.5) (a) arrives at the central processing stage first, a 'time window of integration' is opened. If the target stimulus arrives within this window, multisensory integration will occur (b), however if the target arrives first (c), or too long after the non-target stimulus so that it falls outside of the time window (d), integration will not occur. The estimated duration of this time window is 200 ms, which has been shown to be a good fit to the data observed with visual-auditory stimulation (Arndt and Colonius, 2003) and visual-somatosensory stimulation (Diederich and Colonius, 2007b). This estimate is plausible, as it is similar to the time window observed for multisensory interactions at the single neuron level in the superior colliculus (± 100 ms), reported in neurophysiological studies (e.g. Wallace et al., 1996). A further property of this model is that the relative spatial position of the incoming stimuli will also determine the nature of subsequent interactions, and this occurs at the second stage of processing, and is independent of the stimulus onset asynchrony. This postulation of separate mechanisms governing the spatial and

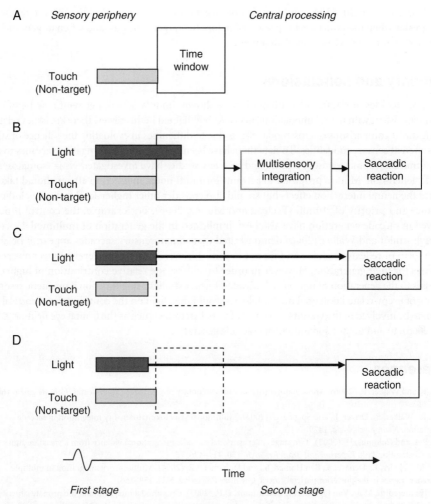

Fig. 27.5 The TWIN model of multisensory integration (Diederich and Colonius, 2007b). In (A) the temporal integration window is opened by the non-target stimulus winning the 'race' in the first peripheral stage. If the target stimulus (Light) falls within this window, multisensory integration occurs (B). If the target stimulus arrives ahead of the non-target, the time window is not opened (C), or if the window is opened by the non-target stimulus but the target stimulus arrives so late that the window is already closed (D), no integration occurs. With kind permission from Springer Science+Business Media: *Experimental Brain Research*, Diederich, A. and Colonius, H. Why two 'Distractors' are better than one: modelling the effect of non-target auditory and tactile stimuli on visual saccadic reaction time, **179**(1) 2007, pp. 43–54.

temporal relationship between stimulus combinations, allows for interactions to occur even for stimuli separated in space (such as the opposite-side distractor conditions in Amlôt et al., 2003), as long as they fall within the time window for integration (Colonius and Diederich, 2004). Finally, the model takes into account the individual stimulus characteristics (such as stimulus intensity), in so far as they can affect the outcome of the 'race' at the first stage of processing. Diederich and Colonius propose that the elements of the TWIN model reflect the underlying neurophysiology of saccade-related structures such as the SC. The predictions afforded by this model have been tested with combinations of visual targets with auditory and somatosensory saccades, and have provided a good fit to their data and previous reports of visual-auditory interactions (Diederich and Colonius, 2007a, 2007b).

Saccade latency is reduced to combinations of target and non-target stimuli, with the facilitation effect greater when the non-target is presented before the target stimulus, and when targets and non-targets are presented in close spatial alignment.

Summary and conclusions

Studies of saccades in multimodal situations have shown modulations of behaviour, some of which appears consistent with neural interaction effects. As highlighted in this review there are issues related to making direct comparisons of crossmodal effects due to difficulties in evaluating the salience of stimuli from different sensory modalities. To date there have been more studies investigating saccades to auditory stimuli than somatosensory stimuli and very few studies have investigated visual-somatosensory saccade generation. Models proposed to account for multimodal interaction effects should take into account the neural interaction effects but should also consider other higher-level factors including the relevance and priority of stimuli (Fecteau and Munoz, 2006). For example, the control processes involved in saccade generation have also been implicated in the generation of multimodal saccades, although Amlôt and Walker (2006) demonstrated that somatosensory saccades appear to be able to elicit a form of reflexive saccade and do not depend exclusively on higher-level endogenous control processes for their generation. However in order to address the relative contribution of higher level processes to the generation of non-visual saccades, further studies using functional magnetic resonance imaging or event-related potential methodologies would shed light on the contribution of cortical areas known to be involved in the voluntary control of visual saccades (such as the frontal eye fields; e.g. Mort et al., 2003), to auditory or somatosensory saccade generation.

References

Amlôt, R. and Walker, R. (2006). Are somatosensory saccades voluntary or reflexive? *Experimental Brain Research*, **168**, 557–565.

Amlôt, R., Walker, R., Driver, J., and Spence, C. (2003). Multimodal visual-somatosensory integration in saccade generation. *Neuropsychologia*, **1479**, 1–15.

Arndt, P.A. and Colonius, H. (2003). Two stages in crossmodal saccadic integration: evidence from a visual-auditory focused attention task. *Experimental Brain Research*, **150**, 417–426.

Avillac, M., Olivier, E., Denève, S., Ben Hamed, S., and Duhamel, J.R. (2004). Multisensory integration in multiple reference frames in the posterior parietal cortex. *Cognitive Processing*, **5**(3), 159–166.

Bell, A.H., Meredith, M.A., Van Opstal, A.J., and Munoz, D.P. (2005). Crossmodal integration in the primate superior colliculus underlying the preparation and initiation of saccadic eye movements. *Journal of Neurophysiology*, **93**, 3659–3673.

Blanke, O. and Grüsser, O.J. (2001). Saccades guided by somatosensory stimuli. *Vision Research*, **41**, 2407–2412.

Carpenter, R.H.S. (1988). *Movements of the eyes* (2nd edn.). London: Pion.

Colonius, H. and Arndt, P. (2001). A two-stage model for visual-auditory interaction in saccadic latencies. *Perception and Psychophysics*, **63**, 126–147.

Colonius, H. and Diederich, A. (2004). Multisensory interaction in saccadic reaction time: A time-window-of-integration model. *Journal of Cognitive Neuroscience*, **16**(6), 1000–1009.

Corneil, B.D. and Munoz, D.P. (1996). The influence of auditory and visual distractors on human orienting gaze shifts. *Journal of Neuroscience*, **16**(24), 8193–8207.

Corneil, B.D., van Wanrooij, M., Munoz, D.P., and van Opstal, A.J. (2002). Auditory-visual interactions subserving goal-directed saccades in a complex scene. *Journal of Neurophysiology*, **88**, 438–454.

Diederich, A. and Colonius, H. (2004). Bimodal and trimodal multisensory enhancement: effects of stimulus onset and intensity on reaction time. *Perception and Psychophysics*, **66**(8), 1388–1404.

Diederich, A. and Colonius, H. (2007a). Modelling spatial effects in visual-tactile saccadic reaction time. *Perception and Psychophysics*, **69**(1), 56–67.

Diederich, A., and Colonius, H. (2007b). Why two 'Distractors' are better than one: modelling the effect of non-target auditory and tactile stimuli on visual saccadic reaction time. *Experimental Brain Research*, **179**(1), 43–54.

Diederich, A., Colonius, H., Bockhorst, D., and Tabeling, S. (2003). Visual-tactile spatial interaction in saccade generation. *Experimental Brain Research*, **148**(3), 328–337.

Doyle, M. and Walker, R. (2002). Multisensory interactions in saccade target selection: curved saccade trajectories. *Experimental Brain Research*, **142**, 116–130.

Edelman, J.A., Kristjánsson, A., and Nakayama, K. (2007). The influence of object-relative visuomotor set on express saccades. *Journal of Vision*, 7(6), 12.1–13.

Engelken, E.J. and Stevens, K.W. (1989). Saccadic eye-movements in response to visual, auditory, and bisensory stimuli. *Aviation Space and Environmental Medicine*, 60(8), 762–768.

Fecteau, J.H. and Munoz, D.P. (2006). Salience, relevance and firing: a priority map for target selection. *Trends in Cognitive Sciences*, 10(8), 382–390.

Findlay, J.M. (1982). Global visual processing for saccadic eye movements. *Vision Research*, 22(8), 1033–1045.

Findlay, J.M. and Gilchrist, I.D. (2003). *Active vision: the psychology of looking and seeing*. Oxford: Oxford University Press.

Findlay, J.M. and Walker, R. (1999). A model of saccade generation based on parallel processing and competitive inhibition. *Behavioural and Brain Sciences*, 22, 661–721.

Forster, B., Cavania-Pratesi, C., Aglioti, S.M. and Berlucchi, G. (2002). Redundant target effect and intersensory facilitation from visual-tactile interactions in simple reaction time. *Experimental Brain Research*, 143, 480–487.

Frens, M.A. and Van Opstal, A.J. (1998). Visual-auditory interactions modulate saccade-related activity in monkey superior colliculus. *Brain Research Bulletin*, 46, 211–224.

Frens, M.A., Van Opstal, A.J., and Van der Willigen, R.F. (1995). Spatial and temporal factors determine auditory-visual interactions in human saccadic eye movements. *Perception and Psychophysics*, 57, 802–816.

Groh, J.M. and Sparks, D.L. (1996a). Saccades to somatosensory targets I. Behavioral characteristics. *Journal of Neurophysiology*, 75, 412–427.

Groh, J.M. and Sparks, D.L. (1996b). Saccades to somatosensory targets II. Motor convergence in primate superior colliculus. *Journal of Neurophysiology*, 75, 428–438.

Groh, J.M. and Sparks, D.L. (1996c). Saccades to somatosensory targets III. Eye-position dependent somatosensory activity in primate superior colliculus. *Journal of Neurophysiology*, 75, 439–453.

Grüsser, O.J. (1983). Multimodal structure of the extrapersonal space. In A. Hein and M. Jeannerod (eds.) *Spatially oriented behaviour* (pp. 327–352). New York: Springer-Verlag.

Harrington, L.K. and Peck, C.K. (1998). Spatial disparity affects visual-auditory interactions in sensorimotor processing. *Experimental Brain Research*, 122, 247–252.

He, P.Y., and Kowler, E. (1989). The role of location probability in the programming of saccades—implications for centre-of-gravity tendencies. *Vision Research*, 29(9), 1165–1181.

Hughes, H.C., Reuter-Lorenz, P.A., Nozawa, G., and Fendrich, R. (1994). Visual-auditory interactions in sensorimotor processing: saccades versus manual responses. *Journal of Experimental Psychology: Human Perception and Performance*, 20, 131–153.

Kalesnykas, R.P. and Hallett, P.E. (1994). Retinal eccentricity and the latency of eye saccades. *Vision Research*, 34, 517–531.

King, A.J. (2004). The superior colliculus. *Current Biology*, 14(9), R335–R338.

Kristjánsson, A., Vandenbroucke, M.W.G. and Driver, J. (2004). When pros become cons for anti- versus pro-saccades: factors with opposite or common effects on different saccade types. *Experimental Brain Research*, 155, 231–244.

Lueck, C.J., Crawford, T.J., Savage, C.J., and Kennard, C. (1990). Auditory-visual interaction in the generation of saccades in man. *Experimental Brain Research*, 82, 149–157.

McSorley, E., Haggard, P., and Walker, R. (2006). Time-course of oculomotor inhibition revealed by saccade trajectory modulation. *Journal of Neurophysiology.*, 96(3), 1420–1424.

McSorley, E., Haggard, P., and Walker, R. (2009). The spatial and temporal shape of oculomotor inhibition. *Vision Research*, 49, 608–614.

Meredith, M.A. (1999). The frontal eye fields target multisensory neurons in cat superior colliculus. *Experimental Brain Research*, 128(4), 460–470.

Meredith, M.A. and Stein, B.E. (1983). Interactions among converging sensory inputs in the superior colliculus. *Science*, 221(4608), 389–391.

Meredith M.A. and Stein B.E. (1985). Descending efferents from the superior colliculus relay integrated multisensory information. *Science*, 227(4687), 657–659.

Meredith, M.A. and Stein, B.E. (1986a). Visual, auditory, and somatosensory convergence on cells in superior colliculus results in multisensory integration. *Journal of Neurophysiology*, 56, 640–662.

Meredith, M.A. and Stein, B.E. (1986b). Spatial factors determine the activity of multisensory neurons in cat superior colliculus. *Brain Research*, 365, 350–354.

Miller, J. (1982). Divided attention: evidence for coactivation with redundant signals. *Cognitive Psychology*, 14, 247–279.

Mort, D.J., Perry, R.J., Mannan, S.K., Hodgson, T.L., Anderson, E., Quest, R., *et al.* (2003). Differential cortical activation during voluntary and reflexive saccades in man. *Neuroimage*, 18, 231–246.

Munoz, D.P. and Wurtz, R.H. (1995a). Saccade-related activity in monkey superior colliculus I. Characteristics of burst and buildup cells. *Journal of Neurophysiology*, 73(6), 2313–2333.

Munoz, D.P. and Wurtz, R.H. (1995b). Saccade-related activity in monkey superior colliculus II. Spread of activity during saccades. *Journal of Neurophysiology*, 73(6), 2334–2348.

Neggers, S.F.W. and Bekkering, H. (1999). Integration of visual and somatosensory target information in goal-directed eye and arm movements. *Experimental Brain Research*, 125, 97–107.

Perrault, T.J., Vaughan, J.W., Stein, B.E., and Wallace, M.T. (2003). Neuron-specific response characteristics predict the magnitude of multisensory integration. *Journal of Neurophysiology*, **90**, 4022–4026.

Perrault, T.J., Vaughan, J.W., Stein, B.E., and Wallace, M.T. (2005). Superior colliculus neurons use distinct operational modes in the integration of multisensory stimuli. *Journal of Neurophysiology*, **93**, 2575–2586.

Rach, S. and Diederich, A. (2006). Visual-tactile integration: does stimulus duration influence the relative amount of response enhancement? *Experimental Brain Research*, **173**, 514–520.

Ross, L.E. and Ross, S.M. (1980). Saccade latency and warning signals: stimulus onset, offset, and change as warning events. *Perception and Psychophysics*, **27**, 251–257.

Ross, S.M. and Ross, L.E. (1981). Saccade latency and warning signals: Effects of auditory and visual stimulus onset and offset. *Perception and Psychophysics*, **29**, 429–437.

Schall, J.D. (1995). Neural basis of saccade target selection. *Reviews in the Neurosciences*, **6**, 63–85.

Sheliga, B.M., Riggio, L., and Rizzolatti, G. (1994). Orienting of attention and eye movements. *Experimental Brain Research*, **98**, 507–522.

Sparks, D.L. and Hartwich-Young, R. (1989). The deep layers of the superior colliculus. In R.H. Wurtz and M.E. Goldberg (eds.) *The neurobiology of saccadic eye movements. Reviews of oculomotor research, volume 3* (pp.213–255). Amsterdam: Elsevier.

Stein, B.E. (1998). Neural mechanisms for synthesizing sensory information and producing adaptive behaviours. *Experimental Brain Research*, **123**, 124–135.

Stein, B.E. and Meredith, M.A. (1993). *The merging of the senses*. Cambridge, Mass: MIT Press.

Stein, B.E., Hunneycutt, W.S. and Meredith, M.A. (1988). Neurons and behaviour: The same rules of multisensory integration apply. *Brain Research*, **448**, 335–358.

Stein, B.E., Stanford, T.R., Wallace, M.T., Vaughan, W., and Jiang, W. (2004). Crossmodal spatial interactions in subcortical and cortical circuits. In C. Spence and J. Driver (eds.) *Crossmodal space and crossmodal attention* (pp. 25–50). Oxford: Oxford University Press.

Sullivan, A. and Abel, L.A. (2000). The effects of age on saccades made to visual, auditory and tactile stimuli. *Australian Orthoptic Journal*, **35**, 7–12.

Sullivan, A., Fitzmaurice, K. and Abel, L.A. (2004). Latency and accuracy of saccades to somatosensory targets. *Experimental Brain Research*, **154**, 407–410.

Van der Stigchel, S., Meeter, M., and Theeuwes, J. (2006). Eye movement trajectories and what they tell us. *Neuroscience and Biobehavioral Reviews*, **30**(5), 666–679.

Walker, R. and McSorley, E. (2008). The influence of distractors on saccade-target selection: saccade trajectory effects. *Journal of Eye Movement Research*, **2**(3), 1–9.

Walker, R., Kentridge R.W., and Findlay, J.M. (1995). Independent contributions of the orienting of attention, fixation offset and bilateral stimulation on human saccadic latency. *Experimental Brain Research*, **103**, 294–310.

Walker, R., Deubel, H., Schneider, W.X. and Findlay, J.M. (1997). Effect of remote distractors on saccade programming: evidence for an extended fixation zone. *Journal of Neurophysiology*, **78**, 1108–1119.

Walker, R., Walker, D. Husain, M. and Kennard, C. (2000). Control of voluntary and reflexive saccades. *Experimental Brain Research*, **130**, 540–544.

Wallace, M.T. Wilkinson, L.K. and Stein, B.E. (1996). Representation and integration of multiple sensory inputs in primate superior colliculus. *Journal of Neurophysiology*, **76**(2), 1246–1266.

Weldon, D.A. and Best, P.J. (1992). Changes in sensory responsivity in deep layer neurons of the superior colliculus of behaving rats. *Behavioural Brain Research*, **47**(1), 97–101.

Wurtz, R.H. (2000). Vision for the control of movement. In M.S. Gazzaniga (ed.) *Cognitive neuroscience: A reader* (pp. 341–365). Oxford: Blackwell.

Zahn, J.R., Abel, L.A. and Dell'Oso, L.F. (1978). The audio-ocular response characteristics. *Sensory Processes*, **2**, 32–37.

Zahn, J.R. Abel, L.A. and Dell'Oso, L.F. (1979). The audio-ocular response: intersensory delay. *Sensory Processes*, **3**, 60–65.

Zambarbieri, D., Beltrami, G. and Versino, M. (1995b). Saccade latency toward auditory targets depends on the relative position of the sound source with respect to the eyes. *Vision Research*, **35**(23/24), 3305–3312.

Zambarbieri, D., Schmid, R., Prablanc, C., and Magenes, G. (1981). Characteristics of eye movements evoked by the presentation of acoustic targets. In A.F. Fuchs and W. Becker (eds.) *Progress in oculomotor research* (pp. 559–566). Amsterdam: Elsevier/North Holland.

Zambarbieri, D., Schmid, R., Magenes, G., and Prablanc, C. (1982). Saccadic responses evoked by presentation of visual and auditory targets. *Experimental Brain Research*, **47**, 417–427.

Zambarbieri, D., Andrei, I., Beltrami, G., Fontana, L. and Versino, M. (1995a). Saccade latency towards auditory targets. In J.M. Findlay, R. Walker, and R.W. Kentridge (eds.) *Eye Movement Research: Mechanisms, Processes and Applications* (pp. 157–164). Amsterdam: Elsevier Science.

PART 4

Visual cognition and eye movements

CHAPTER 28

Visual stability

Bruce Bridgeman

Abstract

Space constancy, the perception that the visual world remains stable despite the fact that all visual information arrives through retinas that are in continuous motion, has historically been explained by an 'efference copy' of eye innervation that is subtracted from retinal image shifts. Quantitative work has found the efference copy to be too small and too slow to offer full compensation. A newer conception is that little is carried over from one fixation to the next; we do not build a visual world by pasting together samples calibrated with efference copy, but use what is currently available, plus a gist and a few previously attended objects. The stable, rich visual world of our perception is more promise than physiological reality.

Everyone takes visual stability for granted—the idea that the visual world should seem to jump or jiggle with each movement of the eyes or of the head seems bizarre. Yet all visual information arrives in the brain through the retinas, and the images projected on the retinas are in nearly continuous motion. They are displaced with each saccadic (jumping) eye movement, and the images of the visual background sweep across the retinas when we track visual targets.

How does the brain accomplish the stabilization? This problem defines one of the fundamental accomplishments of visual perception: space constancy, the perception that the world remains stable and in a fixed position even as the eyes scan across it. The perception seems paradoxical. Yet perceiving a stable visual world establishes the platform on which all other visual functions rest, making possible judgements about the positions and motions of the self and of other objects.

Historically the problem of visual stability has been simplified to address only the mechanisms involved in perceiving a fixed visual world despite saccadic eye movements with a fixed head. More recently considerations of stability have expanded to include situations of locomotion, of tracking eye movements, and of tiny eye movements that occur during normal visual fixation. The problem of space constancy across saccades will be considered first.

History

By the mid-20th century it seemed that the problem of space constancy had been solved; the basic mechanism was known, and it remained only to find the physical substrate and clean up the details. The solution was a signal emanating from motor areas of the brain to inform the visual system about when and where the eyes had moved. At the time of an eye movement this signal could be subtracted from the resulting shift of the retinal image, achieving visual space constancy. Because the idea requires that the visual centres receive a copy of the neural efference to the eye muscles, it was named efference copy. It is also called 'outflow', because a signal flows out from the oculomotor centres to compensate for retinal image motion (Teuber, 1960). An extraretinal signal (Matin, 1972), it affects vision but does not originate from the retina.

The solution was a long time in coming, for ideas about something coming out of the brain, complementing what was coming in, go back to the ancient Greeks (Grüsser, 1986). Their idea was very different, though; for Aristotle, some sort of energy emanated from the eyes to allow vision to take place. Thinking that the eyes of animals seeming to glow in the dark were visible manifestations of such emanations, they concluded that the emanations interacted with objects in the world to mediate vision. This was evidence enough for the Greeks, though we know now that the glow of animal eyes in the dark is actually a reflection from a highly reflective layer behind the retinas of nocturnal creatures. Arab scholars followed the Greek interpretation. Needless to say, such ideas did little to advance vision science. The first formal description of efference copy originated with the physiologist Charles Bell (1823/1974), who was already one of the era's leading authorities on neuroscience. At about the same time Jan Purkinje (1825) also described the idea, apparently independently.

Both descriptions are based in part on perceptions that occur when the side of an eye is pressed with a finger. If the eye is pressed in darkness with an afterimage on the retina, the afterimage does not appear to move. An active eye movement, though, will result in apparent movement of the afterimage. Experience with a real image is just the reverse—it appears to move when the eye is pressed, but does not move with a voluntary eye movement. The experiments are so simple that the reader can verify the results personally. These four observations could be explained if an active eye movement elicited an extraretinal signal to compensate for the eye movement, but the eyepress did not.

The explanation of these effects was taken as evidence for the efference copy. Failure of afterimage movement with the eyepress in darkness would be inevitable, for the afterimage would remain fixed on the retina while the eyepress did not elicit an extraretinal signal. The movement of the afterimage with an eye movement in otherwise dark surroundings could be explained only by an efference copy, for only the efference copy is changing in this condition. A normal eye movement in a normal environment would not elicit apparent motion because the efference copy would be matched by an equal and opposite retinal image motion. But the eyepress in a normal environment would elicit apparent motion because the resulting retinal image motion would not be compensated by an extraretinal signal. The four conditions and their results are summarized in Table 28.1. The conditions in bold type result in space constancy, either with both efference copy and active eye movement, or with neither efference copy nor active eye movement. The other two conditions represent failure of space constancy because of a mismatch between efference copy and image movement.

The evidence seemed so convincing that for more than a century after this, efference copy was the major mechanism assumed to mediate space constancy. Both Bell and Purkinje went further to conclude that gaze movement signals cancelled retinal image displacements to achieve space constancy. Somewhere in the brain, signals representing change in position of a retinal image were subtracted from signals representing change in oculomotor innervation. Ewald Hering (1861) further asserted that one should obtain compensation for voluntary eye movements but not for involuntary movements such as those generated during dizziness. These are the involuntary eye movements induced by continuing vestibular activity following sustained head rotation, accompanied by feelings of vertigo and perceived motion of the visual world. The breakdown in space constancy occurs because the eye movements are driven directly by the vestibular system, in a 3-neuron arc that does not activate the normal efference copy.

Hermann von Helmholtz assured the dominance of outflow mechanisms in explaining space constancy in his monumental *Physiological Optics* (1866), then and now the most influential work in

Table 28.1 Physical and perceptual conditions in eyepress and eye movement

	Retinal image motion	No retinal image motion
Efference copy	**Normal eye movement**	Afterimage with saccade
No efference copy	Eypress in normal field	**Eyepress in darkness**

the field. He expanded the empirical base for outflow theories with observations of neurological patients collected by Albrecht von Graefe. These patients had damage to one or more eye muscles, so that they could not use part of their oculomotor fields. When they attempted to look into the paralysed field, the world seemed to jump in the direction of the intended movement, and pointing to a target in that direction went too far in the direction of the intended movement. In analysing these observations Helmholtz extended the efference copy idea to include sensorimotor coordination as well as perception. The patient has two facts to evaluate, for example in pointing with a gaze that is paralysed for movements to the right:

1. I am looking toward the right.

2. There is an image on my fovea (the fixational area of the retina).

The reasonable conclusion is that there is an image to the patient's right, though (due to the failure of the eyes to move) the patient's gaze has actually remained straight ahead. Helmholtz called this reasoning an 'unconscious inference', analogous to the processes of formal logic but executed effortlessly and without training. Pointing too far in the direction of the paretic field ('past pointing'), to the right in this case, shows that the patient has no information from eye muscle proprioception or any other source that might inform him of the actual gaze position. It is only the intended gaze position that affects perception and action. Helmholtz called the intention to change gaze position a 'Willensanstrengung', an effort of will, pointedly avoiding a mathematical or physiological interpretation of the signal.

The explanation is similar for the perception of a jump of the world in the direction of an intended eye movement. Before the intended jump there is an image on the fovea and a Willensanstrengung straight ahead. After the intended jump the eyes have not moved because of the paralysis, but the Willensanstrengung is now directed toward the right, and the same image is still on the fovea. The patient's quite reasonable conclusion is that the image has now jumped to the right, because eye position (as reported by Willensanstrengung) has changed but the retinal image position has not.

Helmholtz also gave four observations in normal subjects supporting his outflow theory: first, moving the eye passively results in apparent motion; second, moving the eye passively does not result in apparent motion of an afterimage; third, image displacement is compensated in normal saccades (space constancy); and fourth, that adaptation to displacing prisms transfers intermanually.

Perhaps because Helmholtz saw his eye movement signal as related to the will, he did not analyse it mathematically. Ernst Mach (1906), another physicist-physiologist, made that step by hypothesizing that a neuronal copy of eye muscle innervation sums algebraically with the retinal signal to yield a position of viewed objects relative to the head.

In 1950 two papers appeared that defined efference copy theory for the next generation. In fact the term 'efference copy' first appeared in a paper in German by Erich von Holst and Horst Mittelstaedt (1950) as 'Efferenzkopie'. This paper describes the results of an experiment inverting the head of the blowfly *Eristalis* by rotating its neck 180° and holding it there with a bit of wax (the blowfly has a very flexible neck).

Von Holst and Mittelstaedt observed that the fly would circle continually. When the fly was in darkness, though, its locomotion seemed normal. With light restored, the fly would circle either in the original direction or in the opposite direction at random. These results were explained with the assumption that the fly monitored the output of its locomotor system and compared that output with the retinal flow field (since the *Eristalis* eye is fixed to the head, and in the experiment also fixed to the body, the locomotor system is also the oculomotor system). The copy of locomotor efference, the 'Efferenzkopie,' would normally be subtracted from the retinal signal to stabilize locomotion by negative feedback. Inverting the head converted the negative feedback to a positive feedback—a random nudge in one direction would feed back a signal to 'correct' in the same direction. That would result in a further deviation in the same direction, and continuous circling would result.

Von Holst and Mittelstaedt also contributed an engineering flow diagram and algebraic analysis, with the efference copy exactly cancelling the afferent retinal signal. This seminal paper also introduced the terms exafference, a retinal motion signal resulting from motion of objects in the world, and reafference, a retinal motion signal resulting from the organism's movements.

Roger Sperry (1950) independently made similar observations in a fish whose eye he inverted surgically. He concluded that his fish's normal swimming in the dark excluded the possibility of brain or nerve damage from the eye operation, and he introduced the term 'corollary discharge' to identify the efferent signal. These papers formalized the quantitative compensation idea that had dominated physiology and psychology for more than a century. The new evidence offered for the idea was motor rather than sensory in nature, an emphasis that would prove important in the coming decades, though some speculations about perception were made.

Visual stability across saccadic eye movements

Though compensation theories completely dominated thinking about space constancy up to this point, there had always been some problems with them. Considerations from control theory, which had made rapid progress during World War II, made these problems clear. First, the efference copy is feedforward, a signal that informs the brain of where the eyes ought to be rather than where they actually are. As such it cannot be exact—it should drift with time, and could not be corrected when it is in error. Yet the perception of space constancy is perfect—the world does not appear to jump in the slightest when the eyes move.

To the average person, the idea that the world should jump with each saccade seems bizarre at best. If perception is rock solid, but the efference copy is not, something else must be supplementing the feedforward signal. That something else might be all that is necessary to do the job, making the efference copy redundant for perception.

Ethyl Matin (1974), recognizing these arguments, proposed that saccadic suppression could mask the inevitable errors. It was known then that displacements of the entire visual world would not be detected perceptually if they occurred during saccadic eye movements (Mack, 1970; Wallach, 1965); if the imprecision of efference copy was less than the displacement thresholds during saccades, space constancy could be maintained despite small mismatches of efference copy and retinal displacement.

Though it was the best idea available at the time, Matin's solution didn't last long. The first parametric evaluation of saccadic suppression of displacement showed that at the optimal synchronization of image displacement and saccade, the perceptual threshold was nearly one-third as large as the saccade itself (Bridgeman et al., 1975). Clearly, any visual orientation mechanism that tolerated an error of one part in three had no idea where the visual world was, and could support neither perceptual space constancy nor any reasonable visual-motor calibration. This result along with similar observations should have led to a capitulation of the efference copy theory, but it did not. The reason why is that a theory cannot be abandoned because of evidence; it can only be replaced by another theory, and none was at hand. There was a realization, though, that efference copy would not be the answer to the space constancy question.

Other problems with the efference copy theory soon began to surface. One of them emerged from the technique of reverse modelling, applying an output (behaviour) to a linear model and running the equations backward to read the input (nerve signals to the muscles) that must have been necessary to drive the behaviour. Applied to the oculomotor system, reverse modelling was able to clarify the motor signals that drive 'voluntary nystagmus', a rapid oscillation of the eyes that can be performed by a small proportion of otherwise normal people. The oscillations are small in size, usually 3° or less, but high in frequency, up to 20 alternations of eye motion per second. The resulting rotatory accelerations of the eye are so great that the oculomotor driving signals can be generated only by the brain's saccadic controller. Even though the movements have a nearly sine-wave profile, they must be elicited by the pulse-step mechanism of saccades; the sinusoidal appearance is a result of temporal filtering by the eye itself and its motor apparatus.

All of this is relevant to the space constancy question because subjects experience oscillopsia, a back-and-forth fluttering of the visual world, during voluntary nystagmus. In short, space constancy

Table 28.2 Physical and perceptual conditions in voluntary nystagmus

	Retinal image motion	No retinal image motion
Space constancy	Normal saccade	Nystagmus with afterimage
No space constancy	Nystagmus in normal field	Saccade with afterimage

breaks down. But normally, space constancy survives saccades, which are accompanied by saccadic suppression. What is going on? The possibility that small saccades do not elicit saccadic suppression was disproved by comparing suppression during voluntary nystagmus to suppression during single voluntary saccades matching the amplitude of nystagmus in the same observer (Nagle et al., 1980). The suppression was virtually identical in both cases, demonstrating that space constancy does not necessarily accompany saccadic suppression. Further, an afterimage remained motionless during voluntary nystagmus (Table 28.2), showing that the changes of eye position failed to elicit changes in apparent position of a visible target fixed on the retina. Space constancy must use some other mechanism.

The voluntary nystagmus experiment showed that single isolated saccades were accompanied by space constancy, while rapidly alternating saccades of the same size were not. Perhaps the space constancy mechanism was still operating, but could not keep up with the rapidly alternating saccades of voluntary nystagmus. Grüsser et al. (1984) achieved a better temporal resolution of the constancy/frequency relationship in studies of the apparent movement of an afterimage with saccadic eye movements in darkness. They asked subjects to look from one loudspeaker to another, cued by tones from each speaker. After a bright light gave a lasting afterimage, eye movements were performed in darkness. The experimenters measured the subjects' estimates of the spatial separation of the afterimages when the eye was aimed at the left speaker versus the right speaker. As saccades became more frequent, the subjective separation of the afterimages decreased until at the highest eye movement frequency (about 3.8 saccades/s) the afterimage appeared to remain fixed in front of the subject. Space constancy had failed completely. The result showed that the voluntary nystagmus frequency was far higher than space constancy could handle, and that perceptual compensation is quite slow. Even for inter-saccade intervals well within the temporal range of eye movements accompanying normal perception, the compensation was smaller than the saccade amplitudes.

A few years later, temporal properties of space constancy were linked directly with efference copy in experiments exploiting the deceptively simple manoeuvre of pressing with a finger on the outer canthus of the eye. Explaining the method in these experiments requires a brief diversion into methodology. The consequences of a gentle press on the outer edge of the eyelid have been misunderstood for centuries, since Purkinje's 1825 assumption that the press resulted in a passive eye movement. Helmholtz (1866) made the same assumption, that pressing on the eye moves it passively, and that the resulting experience of apparent motion originates from retinal image movement without an efference copy.

Two observations support this interpretation: first, the entire visual world appears to move in the direction opposite the eyepress; and second, the eye of another person appears to move when it is observed during their eyepress. The two observations are consistent with one another, but both are misinterpretations. The apparent motion is based on the assumption that there is motion on the retina, but the two kinds of motion are not necessarily linked. The real situation is easily demonstrated—simply pick a fixation target, then close one eye while slowly pressing on the outer canthus of the other. You will be able to hold your gaze on your fixation target, even while the entire visual world, fixation target and all, appears to move. This means that the retina is not moving with respect the visual world.

Since motion is experienced despite lack of motion of the target on the retina, the motion must come from another source. That source originates with the activation of oculomotor tracking mechanisms, which cannot be turned off, keeping the eye on the fixation target despite the eyepress. The effort requires oculomotor innervation, and with it a change in efference copy. Thus, far from demonstrating the effect of passive eye movement, the eyepress actually demonstrates the effects of active compensation for oculomotor disturbance, and shows that efference copy alone can drive motion perception.

The observation that the eye of another person performing an eyepress appears to move is also misinterpreted. What the observer sees in another person is not an eye rotation but a lateral translation of the eye in the orbit. The eye is influenced by two rotational forces in opposite directions; one originates from the pressing finger producing a nasalward rotational force; the other is an equal and opposite force generated by the eye muscle that normally rotates the eye away from the nose. The oculomotor innervation is driven by a small retinal motion initiated from the finger but compensated by the involuntary object tracking system. Thus the two rotatory forces cancel, and the eye does not rotate.

But each of these forces also moves the eye sideways in the medial direction, the finger pushing the front part of the eye nasalward and the eye muscle pulling the back part of the eye nasalward. The translational forces sum to move the eye several millimeters in the orbit, as measured in the laboratory (Stark and Bridgeman, 1983). Because the cue that humans use to perceive movements of the eyes of others is the amount of sclera visible on the two sides of the iris, the translational motion is misinterpreted by observers as a rotation. The rotation of the covered fellow eye, whose rotation is not cancelled by the eyepress, provides an objective measure of the forces applied. We could now exploit the eyepress technique, which changes the efference copy without changing the position of the image on the retina, to measure the temporal aspects of efference copy. First, though, we needed some additional methods.

Normally eye movements are monitored by finding the position of the eye's pupil relative to the head, because the centre of rotation of the eye remains constant. These methods cannot be used for measuring eye movements during an eyepress, however, because the whole eye is translating in the orbit. The alternative method uses tiny coils of fine wire embedded in a contact lens that fits tightly over the border between the iris of the eye and the white sclera. It was possible to use scleral 'search coils' in both eyes simultaneously, and also to press on the eye without popping out the contact lens (the experiment is not for the faint-hearted). Again the non-pressed eye is covered, so that its movements are measured in darkness. In this experiment we pressed repeatedly on the viewing eye in a roughly sine-wave pattern (Ilg et al., 1989), using a force transducer on the fingertip to provide an objective record of the frequency and timing of the eyepresses.

At low temporal frequencies the viewing eye did not rotate, replicating Stark and Bridgeman (1983). Only the covered eye rotated, under its occluder, revealing the compensatory eye muscle innervation according to Hering's law (Hering, 1868), that innervation affects both eyes equally.

When we began pressing more rapidly on the eye, however, the compensation was no longer complete. At a rate of less than one eyepress per second the covered eye still rotated, but in addition the viewing eye rotated passively as it was repeatedly pressed and released. At the surprisingly low rate of two presses per second the covered eye ceased its rotation completely, and only the viewing eye rotated, in the passive manner that Purkinje and Helmholtz would have predicted.

These data implied that the motor compensation system ceases to function somewhere between these two rates. Thus any efference-copy based system that normally contributes to space constancy must cease to function at these rates, well within the temporal range of normal perception.

By 1989, then, evidence from a number of directions was converging on the idea that efference copy could not be responsible for space constancy. Its action was too slow, and its gain too low to support a perceptual compensation for eye movements. The theory continued to dominate, however, because no theory was available to replace it. Evidence of a more qualitative sort should also have eliminated efference-based theories from consideration, but did not, again because of the lack of an alternative theory.

One bit of evidence came from an experiment by Brune and Lücking (1969), who fed an eye movement signal into a mirror that moved an image with the eyes, but at variable gain (output/input). At low gains, when the image was moving one-tenth as far as the eye, the image appeared always to be stable, demonstrating saccadic suppression. But at a slightly higher gain, 'prominent objects' would seem to jump or jiggle with each saccade even while the world as a whole continued to appear stable. The efference copy theories, however, do not allow this possibility—the visual world is conceived as a monolithic object. The observation would seem to eliminate all efference copy and related theories in a single stroke. There are technical reasons, however, why this experiment might have resulted in dissociations for uninteresting reasons. The prominent objects might have been brighter than the background, for example, and therefore signals coding them would move through the visual system faster than the signals from dimmer parts of the image. In a continuously moving environment, prominent objects would then be perceived in different locations than the background.

These possibilities were eliminated in an extension of the study that used images by the Dutch artist Maurits Escher as the stimulus materials. Escher used two repeated shapes that interlocked to completely cover a surface. For instance, devils and angels might cover a plane. Some subjects could selectively concentrate on just the angels, or just the devils, at will. All of those subjects saw slight movement of the attended figure while the 'background' figure remained stable, at a near-threshold feedback gain from eye movement to image movement (Bridgeman, 1981). Because this perception occurred for either figure, without any change in the stimulus, all image variables were controlled. Something was very wrong with compensation theories—none of them could account for this result.

Another method stems from an illusory motion. Normally the visual world remains quite stable, but observing a small bright dot in darkness results in the dot beginning to appear to wander slowly through the dark field. Space constancy in the efference copy theory, however, requires an extraretinal signal that is compared to whatever comes in through the retina, regardless of its structure or extent. This 'autokinetic' motion is thought to originate from noise in the vestibular system affecting eye movements through a vestibulo-ocular reflex that is not registered in perception (Leibowitz et al., 1983). The noise drives the eye away from a target, and pursuit eye movements, which are registered in perception, are required to cancel the eye drifts. In a full field, however, another motor reflex, which is also not registered in perception, stabilizes the eye relative to the visual field.

The observations can be made consistent with efference copy theory only if one assumes that some kinds of eye movements are accompanied by an efference copy while others are not. It then becomes impossible for any brain mechanism comparing efference copy and retinal input to know what head-centred position to assign to the retinal input (Bridgeman, 1995).

If the extraretinal signal theories have so many problems, what use are they? An answer came from quantitative work on the gains of the efference copy and of proprioceptive signals, coming from sensors in the eye muscles that report muscle length to the brain. The work again exploited the static eyepress technique, but with an additional twist. Pressing on the side of the viewing eye changed efference without changing gaze position, but pressing on the covered eye should change only proprioception. The argument is that the covered eye when pressed will rotate under the eyelid, because the press does not result in any corrective signal from error feedback. Since the proprioceptive signals from the two eyes are summed in the brain, the resulting binocular gaze signal would equal half of the deviation of the covered eye.

As infrared techniques had already been developed to monitor this eye position in darkness, the proprioception could be measured, and its effect on behaviour could be assessed simultaneously by having subjects point to targets while eyepress deviates the covered eye. The situation in pressing the viewing eye is now more complicated, because the perceptual changes will result from a combination of two signals working in opposite directions. Proprioceptive signals will come from the deviated, covered eye, and altered efference copy will be driven by the active compensation for the press of the viewing eye (this analysis was suggested by Wenshun Li). With these improvements in the eyepress technique it became possible to quantify gains of both efference copy and proprioception. The internal signals could be recovered ay algebraic rearrangement of the measured signals.

Careful measurements of perceptual deviations with various magnitudes of eyepress on the viewing or the covered eye (Bridgeman and Stark, 1991) resulted in magnitudes of deviations that could be used to recover the internal proprioception and outflow signals. The resulting gains were 0.61 for efference copy and 0.26 for proprioception, a disturbing result because even with perfect summation of the two gains, the brain would underestimate how far the eye really moved. The efference copy gain is in general agreement with earlier estimates made with indirect methods.

There was still a 'missing' gain of 0.13. Where did it go? The answer came from data on perception of the deviation of an eccentric target from an observer's midline. Targets are perceived as more eccentric if their position is judged while looking at them through peripheral vision, with the eyes straight ahead, than if they are fixated with eccentric gaze (Morgan, 1978). This implies that eye deviations are registered as being smaller than the actual eccentricity of gaze. It was a simple matter to calculate the gain from Morgan's graph, and the result was 0.13, precisely the 'missing' gain from the eyepress experiments. Efference copy, proprioception and illusion gains sum to 1.00, closing the circle on the signals used in registering eye gaze position and the resulting perceptions.

We can draw two conclusions from this work. First, proprioception and outflow gains are summed in the brain's calculation of eye eccentricity. Two centuries of work on efference copy and proprioception had led to the conclusion that efference copy dominates; we can now see that the reason for the apparent domination is that the efference copy gain is about 2.4 times greater than the proprioceptive gain. Thus efference copy explains a wide range of results and clinical observations better than proprioceptive input. Second, proprioceptive deviations are not compensated in eye posture. Presses on the covered eye are passive, resulting in no oculomotor compensation. The role of efference copy and of extraretinal signals generally, then, appears to be to inform the brain about static eye position during visual fixation, the time between saccades when the retina is transducing the visual world reliably. It does not support space constancy.

The efference copy was finally discarded only recently as a mechanism for space constancy, with a new theory reanalysing the information that is carried over from one fixation to the next. The break came in 1992 when Kevin O'Regan asserted that it is not necessary to link successive images together—there need be no memory of the content of previous fixations, because the information remains in the world and can be re-acquired whenever the observer wants it. What the brain possesses is the presently available retinal information, and nothing more. This idea that memory across saccadic eye movements is in the world rather than in the brain turned out to be too radical, but not by much.

Two years later another reanalysis appeared, along with a critique of previous theories (Bridgeman et al., 1994). According to this analysis three information sources are traditionally used to achieve space constancy: proprioception from eye muscles, efference copy, and retinal information. The work reviewed above, in addition to other physiological studies, converges on the conclusion that none of these sources by itself provides adequate information. Physiologically, we were already certain by then that no brain area contained a panoramic, high-acuity representation that corresponds to our perceptual experience. The experience had to come from something else, something not coded in a topographic visual map in the brain. The alternative was a 'calibration' solution: correct spatiotopic positions are calculated anew from proprioception, outflow and retinal sources for each fixation. There is no need to take previous fixational positions into account; the world appears to be in the same place because nothing tells the brain that it isn't. The role of extraretinal signals during saccades, if any, is not to compensate the previous retinal position but to destroy it. Perception can then begin anew during the next fixation interval.

In a more specific elaboration of this idea, attention shifts to a reference object at the saccade target before a saccade is executed (Deubel et al., 2004). Due to the attention shift, location and visual attributes of the reference object and of surrounding objects are stored in transsaccadic memory. After the saccade, the visual system searches for the reference object within a restricted spatiotemporal 'constancy window' which is about 50 ms in duration, and is confined to a few degrees around the saccade target. If the object is found, the world is assumed to be stable. Spatial information from the previous fixation is discarded or ignored, and localization proceeds using the currently available information. If no other prominent objects are in the region of the saccade landing point, even an object quite dissimilar to the original saccadic goal object will be accepted as the target if it is in the right position. Other objects in the visual field are then localized in terms of the position of the reference object. Only if the object is not found do outflow and other information sources come to bear.

Extraretinal signals are used in static conditions, though, especially for controlling motor behaviour (Bridgeman and Stark, 1991).

Evidence for this new position comes from a number of sources, the most dramatic being the demonstrations of change blindness, the inability of observers to identify changes in naturalistic scenes if the change in images is masked by a brief blank of 100 ms or even less, a 'flicker' paradigm (Rensink et al., 1997; Simons, 1996). The interruption need not blank the entire image; if a few 'mud spashes' provide visual transients simultaneous with the image change, the change becomes equally invisible (O'Regan et al., 1999). Even the abrupt transient has been shown not to be necessary (Turatto et al., 2003); an image can be ramped down from normal contrast to zero contrast in 1 s, changed at the instant of zero contrast, and immediately ramped up again, the pattern repeating as in the flicker paradigm. Change blindness is just as strong as in the flicker paradigm, suggesting that it is the diversion of attention rather than abrupt image transients that underlie the effect.

The importance of change blindness for this review, then, is that a wilful inattention to previous images prevents their interfering with present perception. This reanalysis posits that little is carried over from one fixation to the next; we do not build a visual world by pasting together samples calibrated with efference copy, but simply use what is currently available, plus a gist and a few previously attended objects. The stable, rich visual world of our perception is more promise than physiological reality.

Visual stability across pursuit eye movements and locomotion

The achievement of apparent visual stability of the world is fundamentally different during self-motion, and during the continuous tracking of moving objects, from the achievement of stability across saccadic eye movements, because saccadic suppression of vision cannot aid the process. Further, stabilizing mechanisms must operate continuously, rather than in short bursts as in the case of saccadic eye movements with a fixed head. As a result, qualitatively different mechanisms are involved in the continuous case than in the saccadic case.

Several characteristics of physiological optics, however, make the problem easier than it seems at first. Unlike the saccade case, where abrupt translation of the visual field is the only consequence of eye movement, a rich variety of transformations provides information about self-motion and motions of objects in the world. The process of differentiating shifts of retinal images from object motions begins in the retinal ganglion cells, some of which respond to differences between motion in the receptive field center and periphery (Ovlczky et al., 2003). An example at higher levels is looming of the visual image, where all points in the image undergo a retinal motion away from a single point, which is the point toward which the observer is moving. Looming always specifies movement of the observer, never of the environment, and therefore is always interpreted by the brain as an indication of self-motion (Gibson, 1966). If the observer is fixating in the direction of locomotion, distance of objects in the world can also be inferred from looming because the sweep of objects across the retina is faster as they grow nearer. For a given retinal eccentricity of a target, the sweep speed on the retina also specifies the distance of that target once the distance to any point in the field (such as the distance to the feet) is known (Nakayama, 1990).

The looming situation becomes more complicated if the observer is tracking a target that is offset from the direction of motion. In that case the tracked target does not sweep across the retina (because of pursuit eye movements), but looming will occur for all other parts of the retinal array. The geometry of the looming pattern is slightly different from the case of looming from the direction of motion, but the differences are subtle if the target is not far from the direction of motion. In the extreme case of fixating sideways from the direction of motion the pattern of retinal sweep becomes a horizontal sweeping pattern rather than a diverging one, with objects nearer than the fixated target moving faster on the retina, and more distant objects moving more slowly. This sort of pattern is seen, for instance, when looking out of a train window. There is a controversy about whether an efference copy signal is necessary or is used to disambiguate the direction of motion for fixation on slightly eccentric targets.

The family of continuous image transformations that takes place does not specify whether motion belongs to the observer, the world, or some combination of the two. Looming, for instance, might originate from self-motion or from the entire visual world moving toward the observer. Because the latter condition occurs only in the laboratory, however, looming of the entire visual field is invariably interpreted by the visual brain as self-motion. This interpretation is the source of illusions of self-motion, for instance in films, video games, or amusement parks.

Similar illusions of motion occur for continuous unidirectional motion of the entire visual field, interpreted by the brain as translation of the body with respect to the visual texture. Using the algorithms reviewed here, the visual system is continually distinguishing motion of objects in the world from motion of the self. Space constancy is an achievement of the visual brain, not simply a lack of perception of motion of the world.

References

Bell, C. (1823). Idea of a new anatomy of the brain. In P. Cranefield (ed.) *Francois Magendie, Charles Bell and the Course of the spinal Nerves.* Mt. Kisco, NY: Futura, 1974.

Bridgeman, B. (1981). Cognitive factors in subjective stabilization of the visual world. *Acta Psychologia,* **48,** 111–121.

Bridgeman, B. (1995). Extraretinal signals in visual orientation. In W. Prinz and B. Bridgeman (eds.) *Handbook of Perception and Action Vol. 1: Perception* (pp. 191–223). London: Academic Press.

Bridgeman, B. and Stark, L. (1991). Ocular proprioception and efference copy in registering visual direction. *Vision Research,* **31,** 1903–1913.

Bridgeman, B., Hendry, D., and Stark, L. (1975). Failure to detect displacement of the visual world during saccadic eye movements. *Vision Research,* **15,** 719–722.

Bridgeman, B., van der Heijden, A.H.C., and Velichkovsky, B. (1994). Visual stability and saccadic eye movements. *Behavioral and Brain Sciences,* **17,** 247–258.

Brune, F. and Lücking, C. (1969). Okulomotorik, Bewegungswahrnehmung und Raumkonstanz der Sehdinge. *Der Nerverarzt,* **240,** 692–700.

Deubel, H. Bridgeman, B. & Schneider W.X. (2004). Different effects of eyelid blinks and target blanking on saccadic suppression of displacement. *Perception & Psychophysics,* **66,** 772–778.

Gibson, J.J. (1966). *The Senses Considered as Perceptual Systems.* Boston, MA: Houghton-Mifflin.

Grüsser, O.J. (1986). Interaction of efferent and afferent signals in visual perception. A history of ideas and experimental paradigms. *Acta Psychologica,* **63,** 3–21.

Grüsser, O.J., Krizic, A. and Weiss, L.-R. (1984). Afterimage movement during saccades in the dark. *Vision Research,* **27,** 215–226.

Helmholtz, H. von (1866). *Handbuch der physiologischen Optik.* Leipzig, Voss.

Hering, E. (1861). *Beiträge zur Physiologie, Erstes Heft: Vom Ortsinne der Netzhaut.* Leipzig: Engelmann.

Hering, E. (1868). *Die Lehre vom Binokularen Sehen* Leipzig: Engelmann/ *The Theory of Binocular Vision* (1977). (B. Bridgeman, Trans.). B. Bridgeman and L. Stark (Eds.). New York: Plenum.

Ilg, U., Bridgeman, B., and Hoffman, K.-P. (1989). Influence of mechanical disturbance on oculomotor behavior. *Vision Research,* **29,** 545–551.

Leibowitz, H.W., Shupert, C.L., Post, R.B. & Dichgans, J. (1983). Autokinetic drifts and gaze deviation. *Perception & Psychophysics,* **33,** 455–459.

Mach, E. (1906). *Die Analyse der Empfindungen und das Verhältnis des Physischen zum Psychischen,* 5th edition. Jena: Fischer.

Mack, A. (1970). An investigation of the relationship between eye and retinal image movement in the perception of movement. *Perception & Psychophysics,* **8,** 291–298.

Matin, E. (1974). Saccadic suppression: A review and an analysis. *Psychological Bulletin,* **81,** 899–917.

Matin, L. (1972). Eye movements and perceived visual direction. In D. Jameson and L. Hurvich (eds.) *Handbook of Sensory Physiology, vol. 7 part 3* (pp. 331–380). New York: Springer,

Morgan, C.L. (1978). Constancy of egocentric visual direction. *Perception and Psychophysics,* **23,** 61–68.

Nagle, M., Bridgeman, B., and Stark, L. (1980). Voluntary nystagmus, saccadic suppression, and stabilization of the visual world. *Vision Research,* **20,** 1195–1198.

Nakayama, K. (1990). Properties of early motion processing: Implications for the sensing of ego motion. In R. Warren and A.H. Wertheim (eds.) *The Perception and Control of Self Motion* (pp. 69–80). Hillsdale, NJ: Lawrence Erlbaum.

Olveczky, B., Baccus, S. and Meister, M. (2003). Segregation of object and background motion in the retina. *Nature,* **423,** 401–408.

O'Regan, J.K., Rensink, R.A., & Clark, J.J. (1999). Change-blindness as a result of 'mud-splashes'. *Nature,* **398,** 34.

Purkinje, J. (1825). Über die Scheinbewegungen, welche im subjectiven Umfang des Gesichtsinnes vorkommen. *Bulletin der naturwissenschaftlichen Sektion der Schlesischen Gesellschaft,* **4,** 9–10.

Rensink, R.A., O'Regan, J.K., & Clark, J.J. (1997). To see or not see: The need for attention to perceive changes in scene. *Psychological Science*, **8**, 368–373.

Simons, D.J. (1996). In sight, out of mind: when object representation fails. *Psychological Science*, **7**, 301–305.

Sperry, R. (1950). Neural basis of the spontaneous optokinetic response produced by visual inversion. *Journal of Comparative and Physiological Psychology*, **43**, 482–489.

Stark, L. and Bridgeman, B. (1983). Role of corollary discharge in space constancy. *Perception and Psychophysics*, **34**, 371–380.

Teuber, H.-L. (1960). Perception. In, J. Field and H. Magoun (eds.) *Handbook of Physiology, sect. 1; Neurophysiology, vol. 3* (pp. 1595–1668). Washington, DC: American Physiological Society,

Turatto, M., Betella, S., Umiltà, C. and Bridgeman, B. (2003). Perceptual conditions necessary to induce change blindness. *Visual Cognition*, **10**, 233–255.

von Holst, E., and Mittelstaedt, H. (1950). Das Reafferenzprinzip. Wechselwirkungen zwischen Zerntalnervensystem und Peripherie. *Naturwissenschaften*, **27**, 464–476.

Wallach, H. and Lewis, C. (1965). The effect of abnormal displacement of the retinal image during eye movements. *Perception & Psychophysics*, **81**, 25–29.

CHAPTER 29

Eye movements and visual expertise in chess and medicine

Eyal M. Reingold and Heather Sheridan

Abstract

The chapter highlights the theoretical and applied contributions of eye movement research to the study of human expertise. Using examples drawn from the domains of chess and medicine, the chapter demonstrates that eye movements are particularly well-suited for studying two hallmarks of expert performance: the superior perceptual encoding of domain related patterns, and experts' tacit (or implicit) domain related knowledge. Specifically, eye movement findings indicate that expertise is associated with a greater ability to process domain related visual information in terms of larger patterns of features rather than isolated features. Furthermore, in support of the role of tacit knowledge in expertise, there is evidence that the eye movements of experts may contain information that is not consciously accessible.

Introduction

To assess the usefulness of eye movement measurement for the study of expertise one need look no further than the pivotal role played by eye movement paradigms in the study of reading skill (see Rayner, 1998 for a review; Part 5 of this volume). However, there is a rapidly growing literature employing eye movement monitoring to study expertise in domains other than reading. Our survey of this literature found over 1000 relevant publications, in over a dozen skill domains. In addition to chess and medicine, which are the focus of the present chapter, these domains include art (e.g. Kozbelt and Seeley, 2007; Locher, 2006; Nodine et al., 1993), aviation (e.g. Ahlstrom and Friedman-Berg, 2006; Sarter et al., 2007), driving (e.g. Hills, 1980; Shinar, 2008; Underwood, 2007), forensics and security (e.g. Bond, 2008; Dyer et al., 2006; McCarley et al., 2004), music reading (e.g. Goolsby, 1989; Madell and Hébert, 2008; Rayner and Pollatsek, 1997), sports (e.g. Land and McLeod, 2000; Mann et al., 2007; Vickers, 1992), scientific knowledge (e.g. Jarodzka et al., 2010; Tai et al., 2006; Van Gog et al., 2005), teaching (e.g. Behets, 1996; Petrakis, 1993), and typing (e.g. Butsch, 1932; Inhoff and Gordon, 1997).

A review of these studies is beyond the scope of the present chapter. Instead we illustrate the unique contributions of eye movement studies to the study of skilled performance by reviewing findings from two domains of expertise: chess and medicine. The domain of chess was selected due to its crucial historical significance for expertise research, while the domain of medicine was chosen because of the extensive and productive use of eye movement paradigms in this domain during the past four decades. In addition, the present chapter is focused on two fundamental aspects of skilled performance for which eye movement techniques are uniquely suited: 1) the superior perceptual encoding of domain related patterns by experts and 2) the exploration of tacit, or implicit knowledge, which constitutes a hallmark of human expertise. In the remainder of this chapter, we introduce these topics and review related studies followed by a brief concluding section.

Expertise and superior perceptual encoding of domain related patterns

Introductory textbooks to cognitive science typically discuss perception in the early book sections and problem solving and expertise in the final book sections to reflect the progression from 'low-level perception' to 'high-level cognition'. However, one of the most fascinating and impressive aspects of skilled performance is the ability of the experienced eye to encode at a glance the essence of briefly presented stimulus material that is related to the domain of expertise (henceforth, domain related patterns). The most influential investigation of the perceptual aspects of skilled performance originated from pioneering work on expertise in chess by de Groot (1946/1965) and Chase and Simon (1973a, 1973b). Indeed, this research is often regarded as the origin of modern expertise research. Accordingly, we begin this section by briefly reviewing this work and its impact. We then review eye movement findings concerning both the superior perceptual encoding of chess related patterns by experts, and the unconscious processing of chess related patterns by experts. Later on in this chapter, the generality of these findings is assessed by reviewing related findings concerning eye movements and visual expertise in medicine.

Perception in chess

Chess research dates back to the beginning of modern experimental psychology during the late 1800s and early 1900s (e.g. Binet, 1894; Cleveland, 1907; Djakow et al., 1927). Simon and Chase (1973) argued that similar to the use of *Drosophila* (the fruit fly) as a model organism for the study of genetics, chess offers cognitive scientists an ideal task environment for the study of cognitive processes in general, and skilled performance in particular. Similarly, Newell and Simon (1972) selected chess as one of the three model tasks that they used in developing their highly influential information processing theory of human problem solving. Consistent with these suggestions, during the last century chess research has proven to be very instrumental in enhancing our understanding of human expertise and in contributing to the study of AI (for reviews see Charness, 1992; Ericsson and Charness, 1994).

Arguably, the most important contribution of chess research is in producing a major theoretical shift in the conceptualization of expertise in cognitive science away from viewing skilled performance as the product of superior general intelligence and innate talent, and toward the recognition that expertise largely reflects domain specific knowledge acquired through extensive and deliberate practice (for a review see Ericsson and Charness, 1994). This dramatic change in perspective originated from pioneering work on chess by de Groot (1946/1965) and Chase and Simon (1973a, 1973b). De Groot (1946/1965) presented chess positions briefly (2–15 s) and then removed them from view. Even after such a brief exposure the best chess players were able to reproduce the locations of the chess pieces almost perfectly (about 93% correct for positions containing about 25 pieces), and substantially better than less skilled players. In a classic study, Chase and Simon (1973a, 1973b) replicated and extended de Groot's findings by demonstrating that after viewing chess positions for only a few seconds, chess masters were able to reproduce these positions much more accurately than less skilled players. Chase and Simon also presented chess positions with randomly rearranged chess pieces. There was little difference as a function of expertise when random board configurations were used, which indicates that the superior immediate memory performance of the skilled players was not attributable to the general superiority or unique structure of their memory systems or processes. More recently, a very small but reliable advantage in recall for random configurations has been shown for expert players, though this is probably attributable to occasional presence of familiar configurations in random positions (Gobet and Simon, 1996a).

Taken together, the findings reported by de Groot and Chase and Simon suggest that chess grandmasters use efficient perceptual encoding of chess configurations to generate the most promising candidate moves and to restrict their reliance on the effortful and slow serial search through the space of possible moves. Consistent with this suggestion, both de Groot and Chase and Simon highlighted the importance of perceptual encoding of chess configurations as a key determinant of chess skill. For example, in a seminal paper entitled 'Perception in Chess', Chase and Simon (1973a) introduced their chunking theory of skilled performance in chess. Echoing an earlier conclusion by de Groot (1946/1965) that the efficiency of perceptual encoding processes was a more important differentiator of chess expertise than was the ability to think ahead in the search for good moves, Chase and Simon (1973a) argued 'that the most important processes underlying chess mastery are these immediate visual-perceptual processes rather than the subsequent logical-deductive thinking processes' (p. 215). Chase and Simon (1973a, 1973b) proposed that through extensive study and practice, expert players build up associations between perceptually recognizable chunks (i.e. groups of chess pieces related by type, colour, or role) and long-term memory structures that trigger the generation of plausible moves. Search for the best move is thereby constrained to the more promising branches in the space of possible moves from a given chess position. The size of an expert's vocabulary of chess related configurations was initially estimated to be 50,000–100,000 chunks (Simon and Gilmartin, 1973). However, a more recent estimate puts the number of chunks at approximately 300,000 (Gobet and Simon, 2000). In addition, small perceptual chunks are most likely supplemented by larger structures termed templates (Gobet and Simon, 1996b, 1998).

Eye movements in chess: predictions and studies

An important goal of the present review is to illustrate the potential role of eye movement measurement in supplementing traditional measures of performance such as reaction time (RT), accuracy, and verbal reports as a means for investigating the perceptual aspects of skilled performance in general, and chess skill in particular. One facilitating factor for using eye movement measurement in chess is that just like words and sentences, the chess board is easily, visually segmentable. In addition, if as suggested by Chase and Simon and de Groot, chess masters perceptually encode chess positions more efficiently by relying upon larger patterns of related pieces (i.e. chunks), then several predictions concerning the differences in eye movement patterns between expert and intermediate players can be made. Specifically, chess experts' encoding of chunks rather than individual pieces should result in fewer fixations, and fixations between rather than on individual pieces. This may also imply that in any given fixation that is produced while examining structured but not random chess configurations, experts process information about a larger segment of the chessboard than less skilled players constituting an increase in the visual span as a function of expertise (the term visual span is also referred to in the literature as the perceptual span or the span of effective vision, see Jacobs, 1986; Rayner, 1998). Such a visual span advantage should also mean that experts make greater use of peripheral and parafoveal processing to extract information from a larger portion of a chessboard during an eye fixation. In addition, experts may make greater use of automatic and parallel extraction of chess relations relative to intermediate players.

Several early studies employing eye movement measurement provided weak support for the idea that perception of chess related configurations improves with skill. Tikhomirov and Poznyanskaya (1966) and Winikoff (1967) both found evidence that when chess players fixate on a chess piece, they also extract information about other pieces near the point of gaze and often move to fixate on a related piece. Based on this general process, Simon and Barenfeld (1969) devised a computer model to simulate the initial scanning patterns chess players might use when encoding a chess position. Their simulation, PERCEIVER, produced eye movement patterns that resembled those of chess players.

Reynolds (1982) and Holding (1985) re-examined the eye movement data collected by Tikhomirov and Poznyanskaya (1966), and noted that many fixations did not fall on pieces, but on empty squares. There was no report of systematic variation in the proportion of fixations on empty squares as a function of skill.

Re-analysing the work of Jongman (1968), de Groot and Gobet (1996) reported no significant difference in the proportion of fixations on empty squares as a function of skill. These authors cautioned however that the negative results do not necessarily refute the chunking hypothesis. They pointed out that the crude frame-by-frame analysis of film records of eye movements and the transformation of gaze positions from a three-dimensional chessboard viewed by the players to a two-dimensional coordinate system may have resulted in the introduction of noise making it difficult to estimate the accuracy of the computed gaze position. Furthermore, de Groot and Gobet (1996) demonstrated that skilled players made more fixations along the edges of squares (28.7% of fixations) as compared with novices (13.7%), providing some indication that the skilled players may be able to encode two or more pieces in a single fixation. In addition, de Groot and Gobet (1996) concluded based on their analysis of retrospective verbal reports that the best players tended to perceive groups of pieces, rather than individual pieces.

More recently, a research programme by Reingold, Charness, and their colleagues (Charness et al., 2001; Reingold and Charness, 2005; Reingold et al., 2001a, 2001b) that employed more modern eye movement paradigms provided strong support for enhanced perceptual encoding as a function of chess expertise. Across studies Reingold, Charness, and their colleagues employed three different tasks: 1) a check detection paradigm, 2) a 'change blindness' flicker paradigm, and 3) a move-choice task. These tasks and the findings obtained will be discussed below.

The check detection task

Saariluoma (1985) has shown that master players can rapidly and accurately decide whether a chess piece is attacked, and do so more quickly than their less skilled counterparts. The rather simple chess relation of check detection (attack of a King) is highly salient and presents a good model for the extraction of chess-relevant relations among pieces. As shown in Fig. 29.1A, the check detection task employed by Reingold et al. (2001a) was performed using a minimized 3×3 chessboard containing a Black King and one or two potentially checking pieces. At the beginning of each trial, participants fixated the centre square of the board, a square that was always empty. A large visual span in this task may result in few if any saccades during a trial and in fixations between, rather than on individual pieces. To demonstrate that the encoding advantage of experts is related at least in part to their chess experience, rather than to a general perceptual superiority, Reingold et al. (2001a) manipulated the familiarity of the notation (symbol vs. letter) used to represent the chess pieces (see Fig. 29.2A). The symbol and letter notations were used to represent identical chess problems. However, the symbol representation is much more familiar than the letter representation. Consequently, if encoding efficiency is related to chess experience, any skill advantage should be more pronounced in the symbol than in the letter trials (i.e. a skill by notation interaction).

In order to compare the spatial distributions of gaze positions in the check detection task across the novice, intermediate and expert groups, Fig. 29.2B shows scattergrams with each dot representing an individual gaze position. An inspection of the scattergrams collapsing across all trial types (i.e. the spatial layout of chess pieces, check status, and notation), reveals a greater concentration of black pixels in the centre of the scattergram for the experts as compared to the intermediates and novices. This centre of gravity effect reflects a large disparity between skill groups in the proportion of trials without an eye movement (i.e. No-saccade trials). In such trials the gaze position remained in the centre square of the chessboard throughout the duration of the trial. For each skill group by notation type, Panel C of Fig. 29.2 displays the proportion of No-saccade trials. As can be clearly seen in this figure, only the expert group demonstrated a substantial proportion of No-saccade trials and the proportion of such trials was greater for the symbol notation than the letter notation in this group of players.

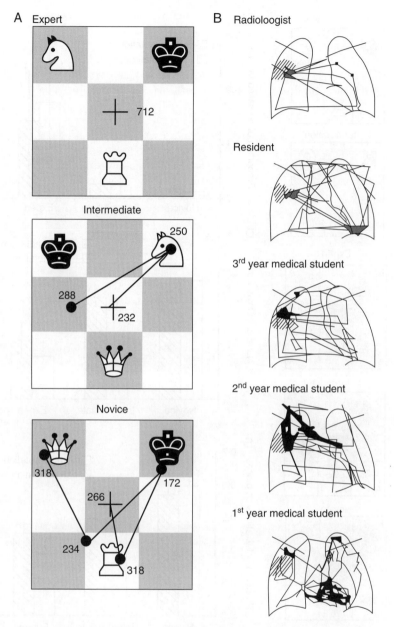

Fig. 29.1 Scan path efficiency as a function of expertise for chess players (A) and radiologists (B).

As shown in Fig. 29.2D, on trials in which eye movements occurred, experts made fewer fixations than intermediates and novices. In addition, compared to their less skilled counterparts, experts placed a smaller proportion of these fixations on pieces (Fig. 29.2E). More importantly, all skill related differences were more pronounced in the symbol than the letter notation. Thus, consistent with Chase and Simon's chunking hypothesis, in the check detection task chess experts made fewer fixations and placed a greater proportion of fixations between individual pieces, rather than on pieces. The magnitude of these effects was stronger for the more familiar symbol notation than for the letter notation, demonstrating that the experts' encoding advantage is related at least in part to their chess experience, rather than to a general perceptual superiority.

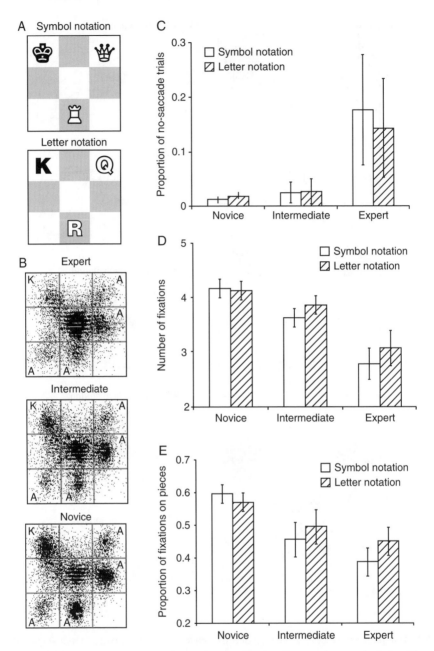

Fig. 29.2 The check detection task from Reingold et al. (2001a). The notation manipulation (A). Scattergrams of gaze positions in the check detection task (B) the capital letter 'A' represents the position of an attacker piece and 'K' represents the position of the King). Proportion of No-saccade trials (C), number of fixations (D), and proportion of fixations on pieces (Panel E). Eyal M. Reingold, Neil Charness, Marc Pomplun, and Dave M. Stampe, *Psychological Science*, **12**(1), copyright © 2001 by Sage Publications. Reprinted by Permission of SAGE Publications.

The change blindness flicker paradigm

The flicker paradigm was introduced by Rensink et al. (1997). Reingold et al. (2001a) used two types of configurations: chess configurations (with 20 chess pieces in each) selected from a large database of chess games, and random configurations, which were created by repeatedly and randomly exchanging pieces in the chess configurations. Thus, random positions maintained the same spatial configuration but destroyed the chess relation information. Each random or chess configuration was modified by changing the identity but not the colour of a single piece to create a modified display (see Fig. 29.3A). In each trial, images of the original and modified board configurations were displayed sequentially and alternated repeatedly with a blank interval between each pair of configurations. Each variant of the configuration (i.e. original, modified) was presented for 1000 ms, with the display blanking for 100 ms between each alternation. As soon as participants detected the changing piece (the target), they ended the trial by pressing a button and naming the alternating pieces. Previous research indicated that participants are surprisingly poor at change detection in the flicker paradigm, a phenomenon termed 'change blindness' (Rensink et al., 1997; for a review see Simons and

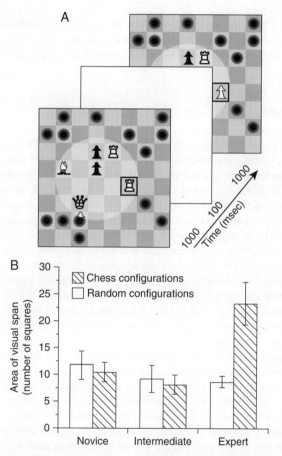

Fig. 29.3 Illustration of the gaze-contingent flicker paradigm from Reingold et al. (2001a). A) Shows an original (bottom left) and a modified (top right) chess configuration (with a box indicating the changed piece) and with chess pieces outside the window being replaced by blobs masking their identity and colour. B) Area of visual span (number of squares). Eyal M. Reingold, Neil Charness, Marc Pomplun, and Dave M. Stampe, *Psychological Science*, **12**(1), copyright © 2001 by Sage Publications. Reprinted by Permission of SAGE Publications.

Levin, 1997). It was predicted that when processing chess configurations, but not random configurations, chess experts would demonstrate larger visual spans than less skilled players.

In this task the visual span as a function of chess skill (novice vs. intermediate vs. expert) and configuration type (chess configuration vs. random configuration) was measured using a gaze-contingent window technique (e.g. McConkie and Rayner, 1975; see Rayner, 1998, for a review). As shown in Fig. 29.3A, a gaze-contingent window requires obscuring the identity of all chess pieces except those within a certain 'window' that is continually centred on the participant's gaze position. The pieces outside a circular, gaze-centred window were replaced with grey blobs masking the actual colours and shapes. The participant's visual span was measured by varying the size of the window over successive trials and determining the smallest possible window that did not significantly differ from the participant's normative RT criteria. These criteria were established separately for chess configuration and random configuration by using baseline trials in which the entire display was visible (i.e. No-window trials). Note that this change detection task required no chess knowledge and consequently Reingold et al. (2001a) were able to explore visual span across a broad range of chess skill stretching from novice to master. For each skill group by configuration type, Panel B of Fig. 29.3 displays the visual span results. Experts' span area for chess configurations was dramatically larger than all other skill group by configuration type cells, which in turn did not differ from each other. Thus, consistent with Chase and Simon's hypothesis, the increase in visual span area which characterizes expert performance on trials with chess, but not random configurations, clearly indicates an encoding advantage attributable to chess experience, rather than to a general perceptual or memory superiority.

The move-choice task

Given the strong support for enhanced perceptual encoding as a function of chess expertise obtained in the tasks reviewed above, Charness et al. (2001) and Reingold and Charness (2005), attempted to extend these findings to the more ecologically valid task of choosing the best move with full chessboard displays (henceforth, the move-choice task). Focusing on the perceptual encoding phase during move-choice trials, Charness et al. (2001) restricted their analysis to the first five fixations in each trial (approximately the first 1–2 s). Consistent with the check detection findings, experts produced a greater proportion of fixations on empty squares than intermediates (experts: M = 0.52; intermediates: M = 0.41). In addition, consistent with de Groot and Gobet (1996), among fixations on pieces, experts produced a greater proportion of fixations on salient pieces (i.e. active pieces that were relevant to generating the best move) than intermediates (experts: M = 0.80; intermediates: M = 0.64). Piece saliency was determined by asking two international masters to classify pieces in each position used in the experiment as salient or non-salient. Thus, as indicated by the spatial distribution of early fixations, experts processed larger patterns or chunks and such processing of global position information might have enabled them to be remarkably efficient in rapidly identifying task relevant pieces and configurations.

Whereas in Charness et al. (2001) the focus was on the first five eye fixations during the performance of the move-choice task, in the follow-up experiment Reingold and Charness (2005) recorded fixations during the first 10 s in each trial. They hypothesized that an examination of changes in the number and duration of fixations, which might occur as the trial progresses, would be potentially useful in distinguishing between perceptual encoding and problem solving or solution retrieval and evaluation. Specifically, perceptual encoding was expected to involve shorter fixations and consequently a greater number of fixations in a given time interval than problem solving. Reingold and Charness (2005) were also interested in the proportion of fixations with durations greater than 500 ms Such fixations have been identified previously as reflecting visual problem solving and evaluation (e.g. Nodine et al., 1978).

Fig. 29.4A shows scattergrams aggregating all fixations in the first 10 s for both intermediates (left panel) and experts (right panel) for one of the positions used in the experiment. Each circle represents an individual fixation, and the diameter of the circle increases as a function of an increase in

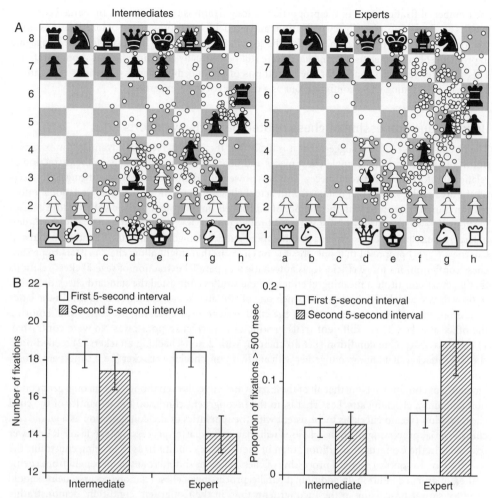

Fig. 29.4 Scattergrams aggregating all fixations in the first 10 s across intermediates (left) and experts (right) for one of the positions used in the move choice task in Reingold and Charness (2005) (A). Each circle represents an individual fixation, and the diameter of the circle increases as a function of an increase in fixation duration. Best move for this position = White Queen takes Pawn at h5 check, Black Rook takes White Queen, White Bishop moves to g6 mate. Number of fixations (left), and the proportion of fixations longer than 500 ms (right) in the move choice task by skill and interval (first 5-s interval vs. second 5-s interval) (B). Reproduced from G. Underwood, *Cognitive Processes in Eye Guidance*, 2005, with permission from Oxford University Press.

fixation duration. As can be clearly seen by comparing the scattergrams, consistent with the chunking hypothesis and the findings of Charness et al. (2001), experts produced a greater proportion of fixations on empty squares than intermediates (experts: M = 0.55; intermediates: M = 0.43). In addition, as indicated by a comparison of the relative size of the circles across scattergrams, experts clearly produced a higher proportion of longer fixations than intermediates. Reingold and Charness (2005) divided the 10-s period of eye movement recording in the beginning of each trial into two 5-s intervals. For each interval, the mean number of fixations and the proportion of fixations with durations greater than 500 ms were computed. Fig. 29.4B displays these two dependent variables by skill group and interval. As can be seen in this figure, the pattern of performance is qualitatively different across experts and intermediates. Specifically, for intermediates there was no difference across intervals in the number of fixations and in the proportion of long fixations (i.e. >500 ms). In marked contrast, experts produced substantially fewer fixations and a much greater proportion of long fixations as the trial progressed. This indicates that during the second 5-s interval in a trial experts started engaging in problem solving, whereas intermediates were still perceptually encoding the chess configurations. This provides further support for the hypothesis of enhanced efficiency of pattern recognition processes in encoding chess configurations as a function of chess expertise.

Unconscious processing of chess related patterns by experts

The results reviewed above suggest that it is likely that the main perceptual advantage for experts is not in the identification of single chess pieces and board locations, but rather in the extraction of relational information between pieces. This was powerfully demonstrated by the strong skill effects on the area of the visual span obtained with actual chess configurations (i.e. where relational information is intact), coupled with the absence of skill effects on span size obtained with random configurations (i.e. where relational information is broken down). Based on this dramatic demonstration of larger visual span in chess experts, in subsequent studies Reingold et al. (2001b) and Reingold and Charness (2005) proposed that one possible mechanism that might allow chess masters to process chess configurations more efficiently is automatic and parallel extraction of several chess relations that together constitute a meaningful chunk. These studies contrasted the standard check detection trials with two attackers with trials in which one of two attackers was cued (coloured). In the latter condition, the task was to determine if the cued attacker was checking the King while ignoring the other attacker. Three different trials in which the correct response was No were contrasted: 1) a standard No-Cue condition (i.e. no cueing), with 2 non-checking attackers, 2) a cued non-checking attacker that appeared together with another non-checking attacker (i.e. a congruent condition), and 3) a cued non-checking attacker that appeared together with a checking attacker (i.e. incongruent condition). Note that all of these trials are No trials even though the Incongruent condition contains a checking attacker. That is, in the Incongruent condition the semantics of the cued chess relation (i.e. no check) is inconsistent with the semantics of the configuration as a whole (i.e. check). Serial processing of chess relations will manifest as faster processing (e.g. faster RTs, fewer fixations) in the Congruent condition, than in the No-Cue condition, as the cueing constrains the search space. In contrast, parallel processing of chess relations should result in no benefit from cueing in the Congruent condition. In addition, if parallel processing of chess relations occurs, cueing should produce slower processing in the Incongruent, than in the Congruent condition, demonstrating Stroop-like interference. While novices and intermediates displayed serial processing of chess relations, experts showed a parallel processing pattern including a Stroop like interference effect. Such an interference effect constitutes the 'gold standard' for demonstrating automaticity and an absence of conscious control. In other words, the experts, but not their less skilled counterparts were unable to avoid processing the global pattern even when such processing was detrimental to task performance.

Eye movements have also revealed evidence of unconscious processing in a chess study concerning the Einstellung (set) effect (Bilalić et al., 2008). This effect refers to the finding that in many problem-solving situations, initially generating a less optimal solution can prevent a better solution from coming to mind. In the case of chess, Bilalić et al. (2008) observed that when expert players (Candidate Masters) are asked to find the fastest way to win a game, they might miss the best solution (checkmate in three moves) when a familiar, less optimal solution is also present (checkmate in five moves). To study the mechanisms underlying this effect, Bilalić et al. (2008) compared the percentage of time that players spent looking at the squares that were important for the optimal versus the less optimal solution. In retrospective reports, the players claimed that they had continued to search for a faster solution after discovering the five-move solution. However, their eye movement record showed that throughout the problem-solving period they spent a greater proportion of time looking at the squares associated with the less optimal than the optimal solution. This finding suggests that the Einstellung (set) effect may work by directing the problem-solvers' attention towards evidence which is consistent with their initial solution and preventing them from considering evidence that is consistent with new solutions. Furthermore, the inconsistencies between the retrospective reports given by the players and their pattern of eye movements suggest that their eye movements reflected information that was not accessible to awareness.

Superior perceptual encoding and visual expertise in medicine

In medical domains such as radiology, pathology, dermatology, and minimally invasive surgery, there is a growing reliance on imaging equipment and the development of specialized visual expertise. Like experts in other domains, medical experts exhibit superior performance as indicated by their faster decision times and greater accuracy on domain related tasks (for a review, see Nodine and Mello-Thoms, 2000). Importantly for the present context, the application of eye tracking to the study of visual expertise in medicine (primarily in the field of radiology) has revealed a number of differences between experts and novices. As indicated in the review below, although eye movement studies in chess and medicine constitute independent research efforts with almost no overlap or cross citation, there is substantial theoretical and empirical convergence across these two domains. Table 29.1 contains brief summaries (in chronological order) of studies that directly compared the eye movements of experts and novices in order to study medical expertise. Taken together, many of these studies suggest visual expertise in medicine involves superior encoding of domain related configurations (often referred to as a global processing advantage) by experts (see Fig. 29.1B for an illustration of increased efficiency of scan paths as a function of skill).

To explain the superior encoding of domain related patterns by medical experts, models, such as the global-focal search model (Nodine and Kundel, 1987) and the two-stage detection model (Swensson, 1980), have incorporated a global processing component. Both of these models postulate that experts have more efficient scan paths because they can simultaneously process visual information from across a wide field of vision (i.e. a larger visual span). According to the global-focal search model, upon viewing an image, experts quickly obtain a global impression, which consists of a comparison between the contents of the image and the expert's schema. The term schema refers to the expert's knowledge about the overall visual patterns that are associated with abnormal and normal radiographs. During the global impression, the expert makes note of both perturbations, which are deviations from the expert's schema, and of potential abnormalities. These perturbations and the potential abnormalities are then scanned with the fovea. Thus, the expert radiologist's knowledge about the visual patterns typically associated with normal and abnormal anatomic structures allows them to quickly pinpoint suspicious regions. As pointed out by Gunderman et al. (2001), this explanation of how prior experience shapes search patterns in radiology is similar to the concept of 'chunking' (Miller, 1956). As such the global-focal search model is also reminiscent of Chase and Simon's chunking theory of skilled performance in chess. Both models argue that given that experts have a vocabulary of domain specific visual patterns built up from their prior experiences in the domain, they are able to evaluate larger constellations of features, instead of only perceiving individual features.

Similarly, the two-stage detection model (Swensson, 1980) incorporates the idea that radiologists can quickly evaluate large regions of an image. This model assumes that expert radiologists have developed perceptual mechanisms, which act as an initial filter that automatically identifies features that require further examination. With experience, these visual mechanisms have been trained to filter out normal structures, in order to direct the radiologist's attention to structures that are likely to be abnormalities. Thus, the notion that experts engage in global processing in order to flag potential abnormalities is captured by both the global-focal model (Nodine and Kundel, 1987) and by the two-stage detection model (Swensson, 1980). As outlined below, a variety of evidence is consistent with these two models.

Early evidence that radiologists engage in global processing was provided by the brief exposure studies, which are sometimes referred to as 'flash studies'. When an image is presented for a brief period of time, radiologists can still identify a large number of abnormalities (Carmody et al., 1980a; 1981; Gale et al., 1990; Kundel and Nodine, 1975; Mugglestone et al., 1995; Oestmann et al., 1988).

Table 29.1 Summary table of studies of eye movements and medical expertise

Reference	Range of expertise	Task	Key findings
Kundel and La Follette (1972)	Laypersons, medical students, residents, radiologists	Lung nodules in chest radiographs	The radiologists showed more efficient scan paths and required fewer fixations to reach the abnormalities
Kundel (1974, 1983)	Laypersons, radiologists	Lung nodules in chest radiographs	The radiologists spent more time fixating the abnormalities in abnormal films, and more time fixating areas that were more likely contain abnormalities in the normal films
Carmody et al. (1984)	Radiology residents, radiology instructors	Lung nodules in chest radiographs	This study reports a discrepancy between verbal reports and eye movements: radiology experts reported that they frequently used bilateral comparison scans (alternating between the same sections on the two lungs). In contrast, radiologists' eye movements showed that this type of scanning occurred only 4% of the time
Krupinski (1996a, 1996b, 2000)	Radiology residents, Radiologists	Mammograms	Radiologists had shorter overall viewing times, faster times to first fixation on abnormality, more efficient scan patterns, covered less of the image, and had longer false-negative durations
Nodine et al., (1996a, 1996b)	Laypersons, residents, technologists, mammographers	Mammograms	Mammographers had faster times to first fixation on the abnormality, and longer fixation times on the lesion
Nodine and Kundel (1997); Nodine and Krupinski (1998)	Laymen, radiologists	Lung nodules in chest radiographs	Radiologists had faster times to first fixation on the abnormalities in the chest images, but not in control visual search tasks
Wooding et al. (1999)	Mean experience in months: 0 (laymen), 2.3 (novices), 16.5 (trainees), 90 (radiologists)	Lung nodules in chest radiographs	The fixation patterns of trainees show the least within-group consistency and the least amount of similarity to radiologists, suggesting that trainees go through a developmental phase characterized by more idiosyncratic patterns of attention allocation and eye movements
Krupinski (2000)	Residents, mammographers	Mammograms	Observers' eye movements were monitored before and after computer-aided detection (CAD) prompts, which identified locations containing suspicious features that were likely to be a lesion. Prior to the prompt, the mammographers had longer false-negative durations than the residents. After the prompt, the residents had longer durations for all four response outcomes
Nodine et al. (2002)	Trainees, mammographers	Mammograms	Mammographers were more likely to fixate on the lesion for 1000ms or greater. Both groups showed longer fixations for false-negative than for true-negative responses and this difference was numerically larger for the mammographers

Table 29.1 (continued) Summary table of studies of eye movements and medical expertise

Reference	Range of expertise	Task	Key findings
Mello-Thoms et al. (2002); Mello-Thoms (2003)	Residents, mammographers	Mammograms	Mammographers were more consistent than residents in terms of their visual search and decision-making strategies. For residents, but not mammographers, there were differences in local spatial frequency information between missed lesions that attracted visual attention, and those that did not, indicating that the residents' search strategy was more influenced by the local saliency of the lesions whereas the experts were better able to make use of global patterns
Manning et al. (2003, 2006a)	Novices, radiographers, radiologists	Lung nodules in chest radiographs	Increased experience resulted in longer saccades amplitudes, fewer fixations, less coverage of the image, and faster decision times
Law et al. (2004)	Novices, surgeons	Laparoscopic surgery simulation	While performing an aiming task that involved touching a small target with the tip of a tool, the experts spent more time fixating on the target, less time fixating on the tool, and had fewer saccades between the tool and the target
Kundel and Nodine (2004)	Residents, mammography fellows, mammographers	Mammograms	Mammographers had longer false-negative durations, were more likely to fixate on lesions, and had faster times to first fixation on abnormalities
Manning et al. (2004, 2006b)	Novices, radiographers, radiologists	Lung nodules in chest radiographs	All the groups showed longer fixation times for false-negative than true-negative responses, and this effect tended to be larger for the inexperienced groups. The experienced groups covered less of the image
Donovan et al. (2005)	Laymen, first-year students, third-year students, experts	Wrist fractures	Perceptual feedback about eye movements resulted in decreased performance by experienced observers and showed a trend towards improving the performance of less experienced observers
Kocak et al. (2005)	Novice, intermediate, expert	Laparoscopic surgery simulation	As expertise increased, there was a decrease in the saccadic rate and an associated increase in mean fixation times, and there was a trend towards larger saccadic amplitudes
Krupinski (2005)	Residents, mammographers,	Mammograms	The mammographers had faster times to first fixation on abnormality, and this effect was greater in magnitude for the more subtle lesions. For both groups, lesions associated with true-positive outcomes were fixated for longer than lesions associated with false-negative outcomes, and subtle lesions were fixated for longer than more obvious lesions

(continued)

Table 29.1 (continued) Summary table of studies of eye movements and medical expertise

Reference	Range of expertise	Task	Key findings
Krupinski et al. (2006)	Medical students, residents, pathologists	Telepathology virtual slides	The observers' task was to view a low magnification image, and to decide on the top three locations that they would zoom into if they were to continue to examine the slide. The pathologists showed a more efficient scan path with shorter overall viewing times, fewer fixations, fewer saccades and longer saccades. They did not fixate at all, significantly more frequently than the trainees, on some of their preferred zoom locations, indicating greater use of parafoveal and peripheral vision to extract global information
Burgert et al. (2007)	13 surgeons with varying levels of expertise	Neck dissection planning	Experienced surgeons showed fewer saccades and longer fixations on areas of interest, indicating more efficient integration of 3-dimensional global information
Kundel et al. (2007)	Observers varied in experience, and expertise was defined based on detection accuracy	Mammograms	The more accurate performers had faster times to first fixation on the abnormality, and were more likely to exhibit a long saccade towards the abnormality immediately upon viewing the image, indicating greater peripheral and parafoveal processing of global information
Leong et al. (2007)	Expertise varied widely from officers to surgeons and radiologists	Fracture detection (shoulder, hand, and knee)	For true-positive trials, the more experienced observers spent a smaller proportion of time fixating the fracture site but there was no difference between the groups on false-negative trials. The more experienced observers showed greater consistency in their search patterns. The experts, but not the novices, displayed distinct stages in eye movement search patterns
Donovan et al. (2008)	Laymen, level 1 students, level 2 students, experts	Lung nodules in chest radiographs	Perceptual feedback about eye movements produced improvement across all levels of expertise, with the greatest improvement shown by the level 1 group
Litchfield et al. (2008)	Novice radiographers, expert radiographers	Lung nodules in chest radiographs	Both novice and expert radiographers show improved performance after viewing the eye tracking record of another observer who had examined the same image, but the improvements were more pronounced for the novices than the experts

For example, after viewing chest films for 200 ms, expert radiologists were able to detect 70% of the abnormalities, compared with 97% true-positives with unlimited viewing conditions (Kundel and Nodine, 1975). Similarly, expert mammographers were above chance at identifying abnormalities under flash viewing conditions, although they tended to miss the more subtle abnormalities (Mugglestone et al., 1995). To determine the limits of performance under brief exposure conditions, Carmody et al. (1980a), systematically varied the distance between the observers' point of fixation and the location of a chest nodule. Although accuracy decreased as the distance increased, it was found that a radiologist could detect some nodules that were 15° away, and a less experienced film reader could detect some nodules that were 10° away. Given that brief exposure conditions preclude eye movements toward the abnormalities, it appears that radiologists can identify abnormalities without foveal vision.

The evidence from brief exposure studies was later supplemented by a variety of eye movement findings. One prominent finding is that expert radiologists exhibit more efficient scan paths than novices (e.g. Krupinski 1996a, 1996b, 2000; Krupinski et al., 2006; Kundel and La Follette 1972), suggesting that they can use information that is outside of the fovea to guide their search. Figure 29.1B (taken from Kundel and La Follette, 1972; see also Kundel, 2007) shows examples of the range of scan paths exhibited by medical students, residents, and expert radiologists. As shown in this figure, expert radiologists often exhibit a circumferential scan pattern (Kundel and Wright, 1969) that involves making a wide sweep around the image with long saccades and a small number of widely spaced fixations. An efficient scan path entails quickly discovering abnormalities while at the same time covering less area with the fovea. Relative to novices, experts exhibit a number of the characteristics associated with efficient scan paths, including fewer fixations (Krupinski et al., 2006; Manning et al., 2003, 2006a), fewer saccades (Burgert et al., 2007; Kocak et al., 2005; Krupinski et al., 2006; Law et al., 2004), longer saccades (Kocak et al., 2005; Krupinski et al., 2006; Manning et al., 2003; Manning et al., 2006a), less coverage of the image (Krupinski; 1996a, 1996b, 2000; Manning, et al., 2003, 2004, 2006a) arriving at the abnormality faster (Krupinski; 1996a, 1996b, 2000, 2005; Kundel and Nodine, 2004; Kundel et al., 2007; Nodine et al., 1996a, 1996b), and spending a greater proportion of time fixating on abnormalities (Kundel, 1974; Kundel and La Follette, 1972, Kundel and Nodine, 1983, 2004; Nodine et al., 1996a, 1996b, 2002; but see Leong et al., 2007).

In further support of the models, when the number of abnormalities reported is plotted against time, experts display a rapid reporting phase, followed by a more gradual reporting phase (Christensen et al., 1981; Nodine et al., 2002). This is because the expert can quickly identify many abnormalities with peripheral and parafoveal vision, before engaging in a slower search for the more subtle abnormalities that require foveal vision. In contrast, less experienced observers show a more constant rate of reporting instead of the rapid and slow reporting phases, because the global mode of processing is less developed for them. Given that novices are unable to identify as many abnormalities with their peripheral and parafoveal vision, they must instead examine a large proportion of the image with their fovea.

The rapid reporting phase shown by experts is consistent with eye movement findings that experts fixate many abnormalities within 1 second of viewing the image (e.g. Kundel et al., 2008). As 1 s is not enough time for the entire image to be scanned with foveal vision, the short times to the first fixation on the abnormality provide strong evidence experts use parafoveal and peripheral vision to locate abnormalities. Furthermore, relative to novices, experts have faster times to their first fixation on an abnormality (Krupinski 1996a, 1996b, 2000, 2005; Kundel and Nodine, 2004; Kundel et al., 2007; Nodine et al., 1996a, 1996b). For example, Kundel et al. (2007) showed that the time to fixate the abnormality decreased as the observer's accuracy increased, and the more accurate observers were more likely to exhibit a long saccade towards the abnormality immediately upon viewing the mammogram.

Gaze-contingent window experiments have strongly supported the role of global processing. As in chess research, the gaze-contingent window paradigm has been used to selectively vary the extent to which information is accessible by foveal, parafoveal and peripheral vision. Chest nodules were fixated faster when they were visible by parafoveal and peripheral vision, compared to a condition in which the nodule was only visible when fixated directly (within 3.5 or 5.25°) (Kundel et al., 1991). Similarly, when nodules are only visible within a central gaze-contingent window, the time it takes to first fixate the nodule decreases as the window size increases (Kundel et al., 1984). Thus, removing parafoveal and peripheral information decreases search efficiency, as indexed by the amount of time required to fixate the abnormality. Building on these findings, future research could employ the gaze-contingent window paradigm to directly compare the size of the perceptual span for medical experts and novices for both domain-relevant and non-relevant visual information.

The gaze-contingent window findings seem to be consistent with an earlier study that compared a full-image viewing condition to a segmented viewing condition, in which a chest image was divided into six segments that were viewed one at a time (Carmody et al., 1980b). The segmented condition resulted in lower accuracy, suggesting that experts benefited from global viewing conditions. Similarly, Carmody (1984) reported decreased accuracy in a constrained viewing condition that prevented participants from making visual comparisons between different regions of the image. In line with these findings, instructing radiologists to focus on particular regions or features diminishes accuracy in comparison to a free search condition (Swensson et al., 1982; 1985). Overall, these studies provide evidence that radiology experts perform best under free search conditions that allow them to use a wide field of view to guide their search. As discussed previously, a wide field of view may improve efficiency by directing observers to abnormalities in their peripheral and parafoveal vision. However, global processing may also improve accuracy by facilitating comparisons between different regions of the same image. It has been previously argued that comparison scans (alternating between different regions with foveal vision) play an important role in visual search (Carmody, 1984; Carmody et al., 1980b), but it is possible that some visual comparisons rely on global processing. In free search conditions, radiologists may use their parafoveal and peripheral vision to detect asymmetries between different parts of the radiograph, and segmented viewing conditions could interfere with this type of processing.

Similar to the above findings from the field of radiology, there is evidence that medical experts in other fields are able to use parafoveal and peripheral information to improve the efficiency of their performance. For example, a recent study examined the eye movements of medical students, pathology residents, and practicing pathologists while they viewed telepathology virtual slides (Krupinski et al., 2006). The observers' task was to select three locations that they would zoom into further if they were to continue to examine the slide. While selecting the three locations, the pathologists showed a more efficient scan path with fewer fixations and longer saccades. Furthermore, the experts did not fixate at all, significantly more frequently than the trainees, on some of their preferred zoom locations, suggesting that they used parafoveal and peripheral vision to extract global information.

These observations of pathology experts are consistent with reports that surgeons show fewer saccades than novices during laparoscopic surgery simulation tasks (Kocak et al., 2005; Law et al., 2004). For example, while performing a task that involved touching a small target with the tip of a tool, the experts spent more time fixating on the target, less time fixating on the tool, and had fewer saccades between the tool and the target (Law et al., 2004). This indicates that the expert surgeons were able to direct the tool using peripheral and parafoveal vision alone. Thus, the global processing advantage shown by medical experts seems to span a number of different fields, including radiology, pathology, and minimally invasive surgery.

Three main parallels can be drawn between the global processing advantage shown by medical experts, and the larger visual span shown by chess experts. First, in both cases the perceptual encoding advantage appears to be domain specific. Radiologists do not perform better than novices when tested with control visual search tasks that involved searching for the character WALDO and searching for the word NINA (Nodine and Krupinski, 1998; Nodine and Kundel, 1997), and a comparative visual search task that more closely mimics radiology tasks showed a similar pattern of results between radiologists and laymen (Moise et al., 2005). Second, chess expertise is analogous to expertise in medical diagnosis because both forms of expertise involve extensive, domain specific knowledge of visual configurations (Wood, 1999). This knowledge allows experts to 'chunk' together domain specific information such that they can recognize patterns instead of only seeing individual features (Gunderman et al., 2001). Furthermore, it is likely that it is necessary to build up this vocabulary of domain related visual knowledge in order to facilitate the global mode of processing. Third, for both chess players and medical experts, it is possible that not all of this knowledge is accessible to conscious awareness (Heiberg Engel, 2008; Norman et al., 1992). The remainder of this chapter will focus on eye movement findings that suggest that there is an unconscious component to expertise.

Expertise and tacit or implicit knowledge

One of the prominent modern philosophers to extensively theorise about implicit or tacit knowledge was Michael Polanyi. In describing the gradual acquisition of the skill with which a blind person uses a stick to navigate, Polanyi provides a very eloquent portrayal of non-analytic implicit learning generating implicit knowledge:

> Someone using a stick for the first time to feel his way in the dark, will at first feel its impact against his palm and fingers when the stick hits an object. But as he learns to use the stick effectively, a transformation of these jerks will take place into a feeling of the point of the stick touching an object; the user of the stick is no longer attending then *to* the meaningless jerks in his hand but attends *from* them to their meaning at the far end of the stick.
>
> (Italics in original; Polanyi, 1969, p.145.)

With practice there is a gradual shift from attending to the manipulation and placement of the stick, to focusing on the objects in the environment which are being probed by it. Just as we are only marginally aware of the movements of our limbs during a leisurely walk (our attention is focused on the sights and sounds around us), a blind person skilled at navigating with a stick might have only a subsidiary awareness of its placement and manipulation. In a sense, the stick is being assimilated as an extension of the skilled user's body.

As the above examples illustrate, implicit knowledge may be considered an integral part of expertise. This can be powerfully demonstrated by considering Expert systems, a subarea of artificial intelligence. Practitioners in this area attempt to create computer programs that mimic the performance of human experts. A prerequisite of such an enterprise is an explicit representation of the rules and strategies used by experts to achieve skilled performance (i.e. domain specific knowledge). However, extracting the knowledge of experts turned out to be much more difficult than first assumed. Basing the programs on rules experts claimed they were using resulted in inferior performance. It is not that experts were uncooperative; rather, they knew much more than they could verbalize. For the purpose of creating expert systems it is important to explicitly represent not only experts' declarative knowledge (i.e. knowing that), but also their procedural knowledge (i.e. knowing how). Unfortunately, such procedural knowledge is largely implicit (i.e. not easily verbalized or consciously accessed). To overcome this problem, designers of expert systems sometimes referred to as knowledge engineers interrogate experts as they undertake a variety of carefully selected skill related examples. Critics of expert systems point out that this effort is only partially successful at making the implicit knowledge of experts explicit. Accordingly, they argue that the performance of expert systems cannot rival that of the best human experts, and that there are restrictions on the nature and scope of the domains for which expert systems can be developed.

Eye movements have the potential to contribute to the study of expertise by revealing information about ongoing cognitive processing that is not consciously accessible to the expert. Previously, in the chess section of this chapter, we briefly discussed evidence for automatic and parallel extraction of chess related patterns in the absence of conscious control (Reingold and Charness, 2005; Reingold et al., 2001b) and evidence that chess players' eye movements provide information that is not contained in their retrospective reports (Bilali et al., 2008). We now focus on the case of medical expertise, in order to highlight the consistent finding that even when radiologists fail to report abnormalities, their eye movements still differentiate between the missed abnormalities and abnormality-free areas (for a reviews, see Krupinski et al., 1998; Krupinski and Borah, 2006). We will argue that both chess and medicine findings suggest that eye tracking is uniquely suited for studying the unconscious component of expertise.

Eye movements, implicit knowledge and radiology

In the field of radiology, it has been reported that inter-rater variability is high and abnormalities are missed as frequently as 30% of the time (e.g. Austin et al., 1992; Bird et al., 1992; Birkelo, Chamberlain et al., 1947; Guiss and Kuenstler, 1960). Eye tracking has been used to investigate why many abnormalities are missed even though they are visible in retrospect. Misses (referred to as false-negative responses) are frequently classified as either scanning errors, recognition errors, or decision-making errors (Kundel et al., 1978). Scanning errors occur when the radiologist does not fixate near the abnormality. Recognition errors occur when the region containing the abnormality is fixated for a short period of time, indicating a failure to recognize the presence of a potential abnormality. Decision-making errors occur when the abnormality was fixated for a long period of time, indicating that the observer might have recognized the presence of a potential abnormality, but they incorrectly decided that the region was normal. Typically, false-negative responses are categorized as recognition errors if the cumulative cluster duration on the abnormality is less than a threshold value and as decision-making errors if the cumulative cluster duration is above the threshold value. For example, Kundel et al., (1978) used an 800-ms threshold value and found that 30% of false-negative responses were considered scanning errors, 25% were recognition errors, and 45% were decision-making errors. Subsequent research has confirmed that a substantial proportion of false-negative responses can be categorized on this basis as a failure of decision-making (e.g. Berbaum et al., 1996, 2001; Krupinski and Nishikawa, 1997; Kundel et al., 1989; Manning et al., 2004; Manning et al., 2006b). Furthermore, an additional source of false-negative errors that has been investigated extensively is the satisfaction of search (SOS) effect (Berbaum et al., 2000; Berbaum et al., 1990, 2010), which is the finding that radiologists are less accurate at detecting subtle abnormalities if additional abnormalities are present on the same radiograph.

However, regardless of how false-negative errors are classified, it is clear that missed abnormalities are fixated for a prolonged period of time relative to abnormality-free regions. There are two reasons why this eye movement finding might constitute an example of implicit knowledge. First, radiologists adopt a lenient response criterion (Scheft, 1963) for detecting abnormalities because the costs associated with missed abnormalities (the critical importance of early detection in improving outcomes) far exceed the costs associated with false alarms (patient anxiety and the costs of additional testing). Due to this bias towards avoiding a miss, radiologists are taught to report any evidence that indicates the presence of a possible abnormality, even if this evidence is weak. Given that the knowledge reflected by the eye movement record on missed abnormalities was not reflected in the overt decision, it was likely that it was not consciously accessible at the time of the decision. Second, providing radiology experts with feedback about their eye movements has been shown to improve accuracy, suggesting that the eye movement record reflected information that was previously not consciously accessible to the expert (Kundel et al., 1990). As outlined below, although further work is required, this line of research has the potential to contribute to our understanding of implicit knowledge and expertise.

Given that radiology images do not have predefined interest areas, a set of procedures was developed for categorizing and grouping fixations. As detailed by Nodine et al. (1992), fixation clusters are formed by summing together nearby consecutive fixations. This is done by setting a spatial threshold (typically 2.5°) and then comparing the location of each new fixation to the mean location of all of the previous fixations in the current cluster. If the distance of the new fixation from the cluster mean is below a threshold of 2.5°, it is grouped with the previous fixations in that cluster, and if it exceeds the threshold, the new fixation marks the start of a new cluster. Given that regions are sometimes refixated, to compute the total time associated with a region throughout the trial (referred to as the cumulative cluster duration) clusters are summed whenever the centre of two or more clusters in a trial is closer than the threshold of 2.5°.

Cumulative clusters can be associated with four different response outcomes, depending on whether or not there was an abnormality in the fixated region, and whether or not an abnormality was reported. When the centre of a cumulative cluster is within 2.5° degrees of the centre of an abnormality, it is associated with a *true-positive* (TP) response (i.e. a hit) if the abnormality was later reported, and with a *false-negative* (FN) response (i.e. a miss) if the abnormality was not reported. For abnormality-free regions, cumulative clusters are associated with a *false-positive* (FP) response (i.e. a false alarm) if the observer had incorrectly reported an abnormality in a location that was less than 2.5° from the centre of the cumulative cluster. Cumulative clusters falling in unreported, abnormality-free regions are associated with *true-negative* (TN) responses (i.e. a correct rejection).

Subsequent research consistently documented that the longest cumulative cluster durations are associated with true-positive and false-positive responses, with somewhat lower durations for false-negative responses, and the lowest durations for true-negative responses. As can be seen from Fig. 29.5A,

A

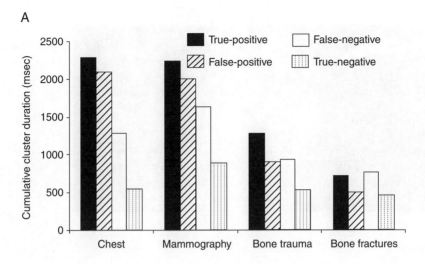

B

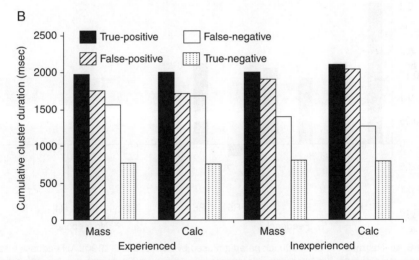

Fig. 29.5 Cumulative cluster duration as a function of response outcome and image type (Chest data from Kundel et al., 1990, Mammography data from Krupinski, 1996a, bone trauma data from Krupinski and Lund, 1997, bone fractures data from Hu et al. 1994) (A), and cumulative cluster duration as a function of response outcome and level of expertise in mass and microcalcification cluster (Calc) mammogram search tasks (from Krupinski, 1996a) (B). Reprinted from *Academic Radiology*, 3(2), Elizabeth A. Krupinski, Visual scanning patterns of radiologists searching mammograms, pp. 137–44, Copyright (1996), with permission from Elsevier.

the finding that cumulative cluster durations are longer for false-negative responses than true-negative responses is very general and was demonstrated for a variety of image types, including chest x-rays (e.g. Kundel et al., 1978, 1989, 1990; Krupinski and Roehrig, 2002; Manning et al., 2004, 2006b), mammography (e.g. Krupinski, 1996a, 1996b; Krupinski and Roehrig, 2000; Krupinski et al., 1999; Nodine et al., 2002; Nodine et al., 2001), bone trauma and fractures (e.g. Hu et al., 1994; Krupinski and Lund, 1997). As shown in Fig. 29.5B, this effect was also demonstrated across different levels of expertise (e.g. Krupinski 1996a, 1996b; Manning et al., 2006b).

The finding that eye movements consistently distinguish between false-negative and true-negative responses has been exploited by researchers in order to develop a visual feedback method for improving diagnostic accuracy (Kundel et al., 1990). The visual feedback method involves monitoring

A

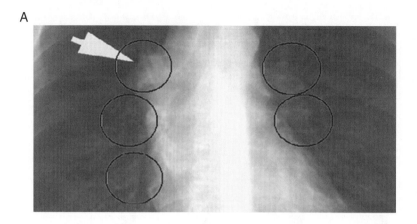

B

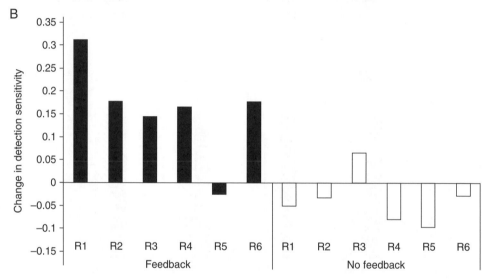

Fig. 29.6 An illustration of the feedback paradigm used by Kundel et al. (1990). A) Feedback was provided in the form of circles (5° in diameter) that were overlaid on top of an image to indicate the locations that were fixated for greater than a threshold duration that is typically set at 1000 ms. The white arrow (not shown in the study) indicates the location of an abnormality. B) Change in detection sensitivity (as measured by the area under the AFROC curve) for six observers by condition (feedback vs. no feedback).

radiologists' eye movements while they make an initial decision about the presence or the absence of an abnormality, and then providing them with feedback about the locations and durations of their eye movements. On the basis of this feedback, the radiologist may then either confirm or revise their initial decision. Typically, the feedback is provided in the form of circles (5° in diameter) that are overlaid on top of the image to indicate the locations that were fixated for greater than a threshold duration that is typically set at 1000 ms (see Fig. 29.6A).

Although earlier work had discussed the possibility of using perceptual feedback about eye movements to improve performance (Nodine and Kundel, 1987), the idea was first tested by Kundel et al. (1990). Six radiology residents examined chest images for lung nodules for 15 s while their eye movements were monitored. After making an initial decision about the locations containing nodules, they either received feedback about the regions that they looked at for 1000 ms or greater, or they were given another look without any feedback. In both conditions, they were given an unlimited amount of time during the second viewing, and they could either confirm or revise their initial decision. The same observers repeated the experiment 2 months later in order to counterbalance these two conditions. Importantly, in the feedback condition, performance improved by an average of 16% after the second view, relative to the initial view, while the no feedback condition led to an average decrease of 3% (see Fig. 29.6B). The performance benefit in the feedback condition reflected both an increase in the number of true-positives, and a decrease in the number of false-positives, and performance was measured by calculating the area under the AFROC curve (Chakraborty and Winter, 1990), which is a variant of the ROC analysis technique that is adapted for cases in which multiple responses are associated with a single image.

Building on the finding that visual feedback improves lung nodule detection, Barrett and Trainer (1997) suggested that local image enhancement (such as contrast adjustments) could be made in regions that received prolonged dwell times. Furthermore, it has been reported that both novice and expert radiographers show improved performance after viewing the eye tracking record of another observer who examined the same image, although the improvements were more pronounced for the novices than the experts (Litchfield et al., 2008). In addition to these eye tracking variations on the original method, researchers have proposed non-eye tracking feedback methods. These methods include the monitoring of interpretation times for mammograms (Saunders and Samei, 2006), and the pattern and duration of the zooming choices made by observers while using an interface that allows them to zoom in or out of particular regions (Mello-Thoms et al., 2000).

While the finding reported by Kundel et al. (1990) was replicated using another lung nodule detection task (Donovan et al., 2008), a 12% improvement in the case of mammography (Nodine et al., 2001) was not significant. In addition, for bone fractures feedback did not improve performance (Donovan et al., 2005). There are a number of factors that might influence the effectiveness of feedback, including the physical appearance of the cue itself (Krupinski et al., 1993a, 1993b), the experience of the observers and the complexity of the task (Donovan et al., 2005; Nodine, et al., 2001), the amount of time spent viewing the image (Krupinski, et al. 1998), and the threshold selected (Krupinski, et al. 1998). As shown in Figs. 29.7 and 29.8, survival curves can be used to make predictions about the efficacy of different feedback thresholds (Krupinski et al., 1998). Survival curves are created by plotting the proportion of cumulative cluster durations that were at least as long as (i.e. survived) certain duration cut-off points. The four response types (TP, FP, FN, TN) are plotted separately in order to compare their different time-courses. For example, as can be seen in Fig. 29.7, for all image types, a greater proportion of FN responses than TN responses survived the 1000-ms cut-off point. For the purpose of feedback, a cut-off point should be selected such that it maximizes the number of circles containing abnormalities, and minimizes the number of circles without abnormalities. An inspection of the survival curves in Fig. 29.7 reveals that for the case of chest images the 1000-ms threshold is the most effective. In contrast, for mammograms, it appears that a higher threshold might be more effective than 1000 ms at differentiating between FN and TN responses. Finally, for bone trauma and bone fractures, although there is still a difference between FN and TN responses, the difference is very small, suggesting that feedback would be less effective for these image types, which is consistent with empirical findings (Donovan et al., 2005). In considering the effectiveness of the feedback, in addition to considering the different image domains and detection tasks, it might be important to consider the characteristics of the observer. The few studies that looked at the effects of expertise revealed that the FN and TN difference is quite consistent across levels of expertise. Krupinski (1996a) reported no significant differences between groups, although the difference between FN and TN cumulative cluster durations was numerically larger for radiologists than residents (see Fig. 29.5B). In addition, as shown in Fig. 29.8, Manning et al. (2006b) reported that FN responses were significantly higher than TN responses for all levels of experience. FP responses were longer than TP responses for the three more experienced groups, while the reverse was true for novices. Importantly, at least in the case of mammography and chest nodules, it appears that feedback could be effective for a wide range of levels of expertise.

To sum up, eye movements consistently distinguish between missed abnormalities and abnormality-free areas and it is possible that radiologists are not always aware of their prolonged fixations on

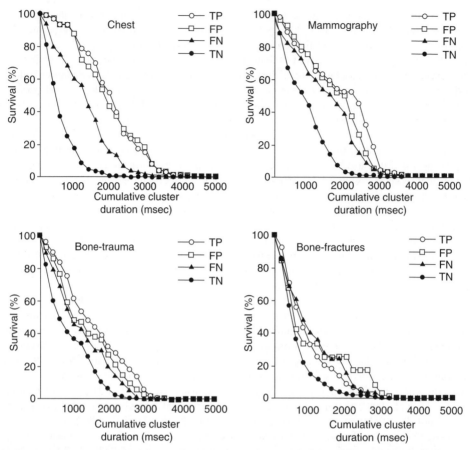

Fig. 29.7 Survival curves (created by plotting the percentage of cumulative clusters that are longer than certain threshold values) as a function of image type (Chest data from Kundel et al., 1990, Mammography data from Krupinski, 1996a, bone trauma data from Krupinski and Lund, 1997, bone fractures data from Hu et al. 1994).

missed abnormalities. There is evidence that radiologists cannot accurately report the pattern of eye movements that they use to examine an image (Carmody et al., 1984) and due to the lenient response criterion adopted by radiologists (Scheff, 1963), the fact that they do not make use of all of the information reflected in the eye movement record suggests that at least part of this information was not available to them at the time of the overt decision. Consistent with this notion, providing radiologists with feedback about their eye movements has been shown to improve accuracy in the case of lung nodule detection (Kundel et al., 1990). However, although the feedback paradigm seems promising, further research is needed to determine the factors that maximize its effectiveness and to determine the mechanisms through which feedback improves performance. It has been suggested that feedback works by focusing attention on specific locations containing abnormalities while at the same time reducing interference from the surrounding regions (Krupinski et al., 1993a, 1993b). However, as discussed above, feedback might also be effective because it provides an additional source of information that was previously not consciously accessible to the radiologists.

Conclusion

The present review illustrates that eye movement paradigms may prove invaluable in supplementing traditional measures of performance such as RT, accuracy, and verbal reports as a means for

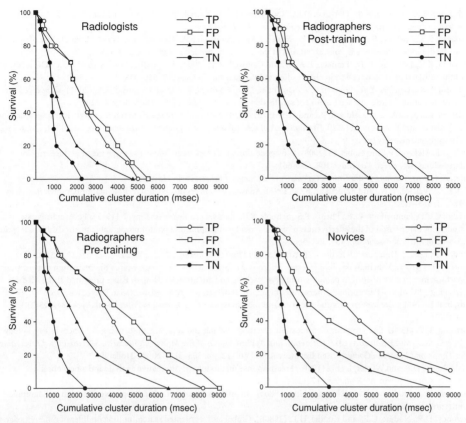

Fig. 29.8 Survival curves (created by plotting the percentage of cumulative clusters that are longer than certain threshold values) as a function of expertise. Based on data from Manning et al. (2006b).

understanding human expertise in general, and visual expertise in chess and medicine in particular. Specifically, by employing eye-movement methodology, the research reviewed here provided powerful and direct evidence for the suggestion of de Groot (1946/1965) and Chase and Simon (1973a, 1973b) that a perceptual advantage is a fundamental component of chess skill and that in line with the global-focal search model (Nodine and Kundel, 1987) a global processing advantage is a crucial aspect of visual expertise in medicine. In addition, evidence derived from eye movement studies suggests the occurrence of unconscious or implicit processing of domain related patterns by experts, and such findings might begin to illuminate this important but as of yet relatively unexplored topic. In addition to its theoretical significance, the study of expertise and eye movements could lead to practical applications, such as more effective training programmes, expert systems and tools for computer aided diagnosis.

References

Ahlstrom, U. and Friedman-Berg, F.J. (2006). Using eye movement activity as a correlate of cognitive workload. *International Journal of Industrial Ergonomics*, **36**(7), 623–636.

Austin, J.H.M., Romney, B.M., and Goldsmith, L.S. (1992). Missed bronchogenic carcinoma: radiographic findings in 27 patients with a potentially respectable lesion evident in retrospect. *Radiology*, **182**, 115–22.

Barrett, J.R. and Trainor, F. (1997). Eye movements can control localized image enhancement and analysis. *Radiographics*, **17**, 525–530.

Behets, D. (1996). Comparison of visual information processing between preservice students and experienced physical education teachers. *Journal of Teaching in Physical Education*, **16**(1), 79–87.

Berbaum K.S., Franken, E.A. Jr, Dorfman D.D., Rooholamini, S.A., Kathol, M.H., Barloon, T.J., *et al.* (1990). Satisfaction of search in diagnostic radiology. *Investigative Radiology*, **25**, 133–140.

Berbaum, K.S., Franken, E.A., Dorfman, D.D., Miller, E.M., Krupinski, E.A., Kreinbring, K., *et al.* (1996). Cause of satisfaction of search effects in contrast studies of the abdomen. *Academic Radiology*, **3**, 815–826.

Berbaum, K.S., Dorfman, D.D., Franken, E.A., Jr, and Caldwell, R.T. (2000). Proper ROC analysis and joint ROC analysis of the satisfaction of search effect in chest radiography. *Academic Radiology*, **7**, 945–958.

Berbaum, K.S., Brandser, E.A., Franken, E.A., Dorfman, D.D., Caldwell, R.T., and Krupinski, E.A. (2001). Gaze dwell times on acute trauma injuries missed because of satisfaction of search. *Academic Radiology*, **8**, 304–314.

Berbaum, K.S., Franken, E., Caldwell, R., and Schartz, K. (2010). Satisfaction of search in traditional radiographic imaging. In E. Samei and E. Krupinski (eds.) *The handbook of medical image perception and techniques* (pp. 107–138). Cambridge: Cambridge University Press.

Bilalić, M., McLeod, P., and Gobet, F. (2008). Why good thoughts block better ones: The mechanism of the pernicious Einstellung (set) effect. *Cognition*, **108**, 652–661.

Binet, A. (1894). *Psychologie des Grands Calculateurs et Joueurs d'Echecs*. Paris: Hachette.

Bird, R.E., Wallace, T.W., and Yankaskas, B.C. (1992). Analysis of cancers missed at screening mammography, *Radiology*, **184**(3), 613–617.

Birkelo, C.C., Chamberlain, W.E., Phelps, P.S., Schools, P.E., Zacks, D., and Yerushalmy, J. (1947). Tuberculosis case finding. A comparison of the effectiveness of various roentgenographic and photofluorographic methods. *Journal of the American Medical Association*, **133**, 359–366.

Bond, G.D. (2008). Deception detection expertise. *Law and human behavior*, **32**(4), 339–51.

Burgert, O., Örn, V., Velichkovsky, B.M., Gessat, M., Joos, M., Strauss, G., *et al.* (2007, March 8). Evaluation of perception performance in neck dissection planning using eye tracking and attention landscapes. Paper presented at the Medical Imaging 2007: Image Perception, Observer Performance, and Technology Assessment, San Diego, CA, USA.

Butsch, R.L. (1932). Eye movements and the eye-hand span in typewriting. *Journal of Educational Psychology*, **23**(2), 104–121.

Carmody, D.P. (1984). Lung tumour identification: Decision-making and comparison scanning-Advances in Psychology. In A.G. Gale, and F.Johnson (eds.) *Theoretical and Applied Aspects of Eye Movement Research, Selected/Edited Proceedings of The Second European Conference on Eye Movements* (Vol. **22**, pp. 305–312). North-Holland.

Chakraborty, D.P. and Winter, L.H.L. (1990), Free-response methodology: Alternative analysis and a new observer performance experiment. *Radiology*, **174**(3), 873–881.

Carmody, D.P., Nodine, C.F., and Kundel, H.L. (1980a). An analysis of perceptual and cognitive factors in radiographic interpretation. *Perception*, **9**, 339–344.

Carmody, D.P., Nodine, C.F., and Kundel, H.L. (1980b). Global and segmented search for lung nodules of different edge gradients. *Investigative Radiology*, **15**, 224–233.

Carmody, D.P., Nodine, C.F., and Kundel, H.L. (1981). Finding lung nodules with and without comparative visual scanning. *Perception and Psychophysics*, **29**, 594–598.

Carmody, D.P., Kundel, H.L., and Toto, L.C. (1984). Comparison scans while reading chest images: taught, but not practiced. *Investigative Radiology*, **19**(5), 462–466.

Charness, N. (1992). The impact of chess research on cognitive science. *Psychological Research*, **54**, 4–9.

Charness, N., Reingold, E.M., Pomplun, M., and Stampe, D.M. (2001). The perceptual aspect of skilled performance in chess: Evidence from eye movements. *Memory and Cognition*, **29**, 1146–1152.

Chase, W.G. and Simon, H.A. (1973a). Perception in chess. *Cognitive Psychology*, **4**, 55–81.

Chase, W.G. and Simon, H.A. (1973b). The mind's eye in chess. In W.G. Chase (ed.) *Visual information processing* (pp. 215–281). New York: Academic Press.

Christensen, E.E., Murry, R.C., Holland, K., Reynolds, J., Landay, M.J., and Moore, J.G. (1981). The effect of search time on perception. *Radiology*, **138**(2), 361–365.

Cleveland, A.A. (1907). The psychology of chess and of learning to play it. *American Journal of Psychology*, **18**, 269–308.

de Groot, A.D. (1946). *Het denken van den schaker*. Amsterdam: Noord Hollandsche.

de Groot, A.D. (1965). *Thought and choice in chess*. The Hague: Mouton.

de Groot, A.D. and Gobet, F. (1996). *Perception and memory in chess*. Assen (The Netherlands): Van Gorcum.

Djakow, I.N., Petrowski, N.W., and Rudik, P.A. (1927). *Psychologie des Schachspiels*. Berlin: de Gruyter.

Donovan, T., Manning, D.J., and Crawford, T. (2008, February 20). Performance changes in lung nodule detection following perceptual feedback of eye movements. Paper presented at the Medical Imaging 2008: Image Perception, Observer Performance, and Technology Assessment, San Diego, CA, USA.

Donovan, T., Manning, D.J., Phillips, P.W., Higham, S., and Crawford, T. (2005, February 15). The effect of feedback on performance in a fracture detection task. Paper presented at the Medical Imaging 2005: Image Perception, Observer Performance, and Technology Assessment, San Diego, CA, USA.

Dyer, A.G., Found, B., and Rogers, D. (2006). Visual attention and expertise for forensic signature analysis. *Journal of Forensic Sciences*, **51**(6), 1397–404.

Ericsson, K.A. and Charness, N. (1994). Expert performance: Its structure and acquisition. *American Psychologist*, **49**, 725–747.

Gale, A.G., Vernon, J., Miller, K., and Worthington, B.S. (1990). Reporting in a flash. *British Journal of Radiology*, **63**, S71.

Gobet, F. and Simon, H.A. (1996a). Recall of rapidly presented random chess positions is a function of skill. *Psychonomic Bulletin and Review*, **3**, 159–163.

Gobet, F. and Simon, H.A. (1996b). Templates in chess memory: A mechanism for recalling several boards. *Cognitive Psychology*, **31**, 1–40.

Gobet, F. (1998). Expert memory: a comparison of four theories, *Cognition*, **66**(2), 115–152.

Gobet, F. and Simon, H.A. (2000). Five seconds or sixty? Presentation time in expert memory. *Cognitive Science*, **24**, 651–682.

Goolsby, T. (1989). Computer applications to eye movement research in music reading. *Psychomusicology*, **8**(2), 111–126.

Guiss, L.W. and Kuenstler, P. (1960). A retrospective view of survey photofluorocarbons of persons with lung cancer. *Cancer*, **13**, 91–95.

Gunderman, R., Williamson, K., Fraley, R., and Steele, J. (2001). Expertise: implications for radiological education. *Academic Radiology*, **8**, 1252–6.

Heiberg Engel, P.J. (2008). Tacit knowledge and visual expertise in medical diagnostic reasoning: Implications for medical education. *Medical Teacher*, **30**, e184–e188.

Hills, B.L. (1980). Vision, visibility, and perception in driving. *Perception*, **9**, 183–216.

Holding, D.H. (1985). *The psychology of chess skill*. Hillsdale, N.J: Erlbaum.

Hu, C.H., Kundel, H.L., Nodine, C.F., Krupinski, E.A., and Toto, L.C. (1994). Searching for bone fractures: a comparison with pulmonary nodule search. *Academic Radiology*, **1**, 25–32.

Inhoff, A.W. and Gordon, A.M. (1997). Eye movements and eye-hand coordination during typing. *Current Directions in Psychological Science*, **6**(6), 153–157.

Jacobs, A.M. (1986). Eye movement control in visual search: How direct is visual span control? *Perception and Psychophysics*, **39**, 47–58.

Jarodzka, H., Scheiter, K., Gerjets, P., and Van Gog, T. (2010). In the eyes of the beholder: How experts and novices interpret dynamic stimuli. *Learning and Instruction*, **20**(2), 146–154.

Jongman, R.W. (1968). *Het oog van de meester* [The eye of the master]. Assen (The Netherlands): Van Gorcum.

Kocak, E., Ober, J., Berme, N., and Melvin, W.S. (2005). Eye motion parameters correlate with level of experience in video-assisted surgery: Objective testing of three tasks. *Journal of Laparoendoscopic and Advanced Surgical Techniques*, **15**, 575–580.

Kozbelt, A. and Seeley, W.P. (2007). Integrating art historical, psychological, and neuroscientific explanations of artists' advantages in drawing and perception. *Psychology of Aesthetics, Creativity, and the Arts*, **1**(2), 80–90.

Krupinski, E.A. (1996a). Visual scanning patterns of radiologists searching mammograms. *Academic Radiology*, **3**, 137–144.

Krupinski, E.A. (1996b). Influence of experience on scanning strategies in mammography. *SPIE*, **2712**, 95–101.

Krupinski, E.A. (2000, January 24). Medical image perception: Evaluating the role of experience. Paper presented at the Human Vision and Electronic Imaging V, San Jose, CA, USA.

Krupinski, E.A. (2005). Visual search of mammographic images: influence of lesion subtlety. *Academic Radiology*, **12**, 965–969.

Krupinski, E. and Borah, J. (2006). Eye tracking helps improve accuracy in radiology. *Biophotonics International*, **13**(6), 44–49.

Krupinski, E.A. and Lund, P.J. (1997). Differences in time to interpretation for evaluation of bone radiographs with monitor and film viewing. *Academic Radiology*, **4**, 177–182.

Krupinski, E.A. and Nishikawa, R.M. (1997). Comparison of eye position versus computer identified microcalcification clusters on mammograms. *Medical Physics*, **24**, 17–23.

Krupinski, E.A., Nodine, C.F., and Kundel, H.L. (1993a). Perceptual enhancement of tumor targets in chest X-ray images. *Perception and Psychophysics*, **53**, 519–526.

Krupinski, E.A., Nodine, C.F., and Kundel, H.L. (1993b). A perceptually based method for enhancing pulmonary tumor recognition. *Investigative Radiology*, **28**, 289–294.

Krupinski, E.A. Nodine, C.F., and Kundel, H.L. (1998). Enhancing recognition of lesions in radiographic images using perceptual feedback. *Optical Engineering*, **37**(3), 813–818.

Krupinski, E.A. and Roehrig, H. (2000). The influence of a perceptually linearized display on observer performance and visual search. *Academic Radiology*, **7**, 8–13.

Krupinski, E.A. and Roehrig, H. (2002). Pulmonary nodule detection and visual search: P45 and P104 monochrome versus color monitor displays. *Academic Radiology*, **9**, 638–645.

Krupinski, E., Roehrig, H., and Furukawa, T. (1999). Influence of film and monitor display luminance on observer performance and visual search. *Academic Radiology*, **6**, 411–418.

Krupinski, E.A., Tillack, A.A., Richter, L., Henderson, J.T., Bhattacharyya, A.K., Scott, K.M., *et al.* (2006). Eye-movement study and human performance using telepathology virtual slides. Implications for medical education and differences with experience. *Human Pathology*, **37**, 1543–1556.

Kundel, H.L. (1974). Visual sampling and estimates of the location of information on chest films. *Invest Radiol*, **9**, 87–93.

Kundel, H.L. (2007, February 21). How to minimize perceptual error and maximize expertise in medical imaging. Paper presented at the Medical Imaging 2007: Image Perception, Observer Performance, and Technology Assessment, San Diego, CA, USA.

Kundel, H.L. and La Follette, P.S. Jr (1972). Visual search patterns and experience with radiological images. *Radiology*, **103**, 523–528.

Kundel H.L. and Nodine, C.F. (1975). Interpreting chest radiographs without visual search. *Radiology*, **116**(3), 527–532.

Kundel, H.L. and Nodine, C.F. (1983). A visual concept shapes image perception. *Radiology*, **146**, 363–368.

Kundel, H.L. and Nodine, C.F. (2004, February 17). Modeling visual search during mammogram viewing. Paper presented at the Medical Imaging 2004: Image Perception, Observer Performance, and Technology Assessment, San Diego, CA, USA.

Kundel, H.L. and Wright, D.J. (1969). The influence of prior knowledge on visual search strategies during the viewing of chest radiographs. *Radiology*, **93**, 315–320.

Kundel, H.L., Nodine, C.F., and Carmody, D.P. (1978). Visual scanning, pattern recognition and decision making in pulmonary nodule detection. *Investigative Radiology*, **13**, 175–181.

Kundel, H.L., Nodine, C.F., and Krupinski, E.A. (1989). Searching for lung nodules: Visual dwell indicates location of false-positive and false-negative decisions. *Investigative Radiology*, **4**, 472–478.

Kundel, H.L., Nodine, C.F., and Krupinski, E.A. (1990). Computer-displayed eye position as a visual aid to pulmonary nodule interpretation. *Investigative Radiology*, **25**, 890–896.

Kundel, H.L., Nodine, C.F., Conant, E.F., and Weinstein, S.P. (2007). Holistic component of image perception in mammogram interpretation: Gaze-tracking study. *Radiology*, **242**, 396–402.

Kundel, H.L., Nodine, C.F., Krupinski, E.A., and Mello-Thoms, C. (2008). Using gaze-tracking data and mixture distribution analysis to support a holistic model for the detection of cancers on mammograms. *Academic Radiology*, **15**, 881–886.

Kundel, H.L., Nodine, C.F., and Toto, L. (1984). Eye movements and the detection of lung tumors in chest images – Advances in Psychology. In A.G. Gale, and F. Johnson (eds.) *Theoretical and Applied Aspects of Eye Movement Research, Selected/ Edited Proceedings of The Second European Conference on Eye Movements* (Vol. 22, pp. 297–304). Elsevier: North-Holland.

Kundel, H.L. Nodine, C.F., and Toto, L. (1991). Searching for lung nodules. The guidance of visual scanning. *Investigative Radiology*, **26**, 777–781.

Land, M.F. and McLeod, P. (2000). From eye movements to actions: how batsmen hit the ball. *Nature neuroscience*, **3**(12), 1340–5.

Law, B., Atkins, M.S., Kirkpatrick, A.E., Lomax, A.J., and Mackenzie, C.L. (2004). Eye gaze patterns differentiate novice and experts in a virtual laparoscopic surgery training environment. In A. Duchowski, and R. Vertegan (eds.) *Proceedings of the 2004 Symposium on Eye Tracking Research and Applications* (pp. 41–48). San Antonio, TX: Association for Computing Machinery.

Leong, J.J. H., Nicolaou, M., Emery, R.J., Darzi, A.W., and Yang, G.Z. (2007). Visual search behaviour in skeletal radiographs: A cross-speciality study. *Clinical Radiology*, **62**, 1069–1077.

Litchfield, D., Ball, L.J., Donovan, T., Manning, D.J., and Crawford, T. (2008, February 20). Learning from others: Effects of viewing another person's eye movements while searching for chest nodules. Paper presented at the Medical Imaging 2008: Image Perception, Observer Performance, and Technology Assessment, San Diego, CA, USA.

Locher, P. (2006). The usefulness of eye movement recordings to subject an aesthetic episode with visual art to empirical scrutiny. *Psychology Science*, **48**(2), 106–114.

Madell, J. and Hébert, S. (2008). Eye Movements and Music Reading: Where Do We Look Next? *Music Perception*, **26**(2), 157–170.

Mann, D.T., Williams, A.M., Ward, P., and Janelle, C.M. (2007). Perceptual-cognitive expertise in sport: a meta-analysis. *Journal of Sport and Exercise Psychology*, **29**(4), 457–78.

Manning, D., Ethell, S.C., and Crawford, T. (2003, February 18). An eye-tracking AFROC study of the influence of experience and training on chest x-ray interpretation. Paper presented at the Medical Imaging 2003: Image Perception, Observer Performance, and Technology Assessment, San Diego, CA, USA.

Manning, D., Ethell, S., and Donovan, T. (2004, February 17). Categories of observer error from eye-tracking and AFROC data. Paper presented at the Medical Imaging 2004: Image Perception, Observer Performance, and Technology Assessment, San Diego, CA, USA.

Manning, D., Ethell, S., Donovan, T., and Crawford, T. (2006a). How do radiologists do it? The influence of experience and training on searching for chest nodules. *Radiography*, **12**, 134–142.

Manning, D., Barker-Mill, S.C., Donovan, T., and Crawford, T. (2006b). Time-dependent observer errors in pulmonary nodule detection. *British Journal of Radiology*, **79**, 342–346.

McCarley, J.S., Kramer, A.F., Wickens, C.D., Vidoni, E.D., and Boot, W.R. (2004). Visual skills in airport-security screening. *Psychological Science*, **15**(5), 302–6.

McConkie, G.W. and Rayner, K. (1975). The span of the effective stimulus during a fixation in reading. *Perception and Psychophysics*, **17**, 578–586.

Mello-Thoms, C. (2003). Perception of breast cancer: Eye-position analysis of mammogram interpretation. *Academic Radiology*, **10**, 4–12.

Mello-Thoms, C., Nodine, C.F., and Kundel, H.L. (2002, February 26). Relating image-based features to mammogram interpretation. Paper presented at the Medical Imaging 2002: Image Perception, Observer Performance, and Technology Assessment, San Diego, CA, USA.

Mello-Thoms, C., Nodine, C.F., Weinstein, S.P., Kundel, H.L., and Toto, L.C. (2000, February 16). An unobtrusive method for monitoring visual attention during mammogram reading. Paper presented at the Medical Imaging 2000: Image Perception, Observer Performance, and Technology Assessment, San Diego, CA, USA.

Miller, G.A. (1956). The magic number seven, plus or minus two. *Psychological Review*, **63**, 81–87.

Moise, A., Atkins, M.S., and Rohling, R. (2005). Evaluating different radiology workstation interaction techniques with radiologists and laypersons. *Journal of Digital Imaging*, **18**(2), 116–130.

Mugglestone, M.D., Gale, A.G., Cowley, H.C., and Wilson, A.R.M. (1995). Diagnostic performance on briefly presented mammographic images. *SPIE*, **2436**, 106–115.

Newell, A. and Simon, H.A. (1972). *Human problem solving*. Englewood Cliffs, N. J.:Prentice Hall.

Nodine, C.F. and Krupinski, E.A. (1998). Perceptual skill, radiology expertise, and visual test performance with NINA and WALDO. *Academic Radiology*, **5**, 603–612.

Nodine, C.F. and Kundel, H.L. (1987). The cognitive side of visual search in radiology. In J.K. O'Regan and A. Levy-Schoen (eds.) *Eye movements: From physiology to cognition* (pp. 573–582). Amsterdam: Elsevier.

Nodine, C.F. and Kundel, H.L. (1997). Al Hirschfeld's NINA as a prototype search task for studying perceptual error in radiology. *SPIE*, **3036**, 308–312.

Nodine, C.F. and Mello-Thoms, C. (2000). The nature of expertise in radiology. In J. Beutel, H.L. Kundel, and R.L. Van Metter (eds.) *The handbook of medical imaging: Physics and psychophysics* (pp. 859–894). Bellingham, WA: SPIE Press.

Nodine, C.F., Carmody, D.P. and Kundel, H.L. (1978). Searching for Nina. In J.W. Sanders, D.F. Fisher, and R.A. Monty (eds.) *Eye movements and the higher psychological functions* (pp. 241–258). Hillsdale, NJ: Erlbaum.

Nodine, C.F., Kundel, H.L., Lauver, S.C., and Toto, L.C. (1996a). Nature of expertise in searching mammograms for breast masses. *Academic Radiology*, **3**, 1000–1006.

Nodine, C.F., Kundel, H.L., Lauver, S.C., and Toto, L.C. (1996b). The nature of expertise in searching mammograms for breast lesions. *SPIE*, **2712**, 89–94.

Nodine, C.F., Kundel, H.L., Mello-Thoms, C., and Weinstein, S.P. (2001, February 21). Role of computer-assisted visual search in mammographic interpretation. Paper presented at the Medical Imaging 2001: Image Perception and Performance, San Diego, CA, USA.

Nodine, C.F., Kundel, H.L, Toto, L.C., and Krupinski, E.A. (1992). Recording and analyzing eye-position data using a microcomputer workstation. *Behavior Research Methods, Instruments, & Computers*, **24**, 475–485.

Nodine, C.F., Locher, P.J., and Krupinski, E.A. (1993). The role of formal art training on perception and aesthetic judgment of art compositions. *Leonardo*, **26**(3), 219–227.

Nodine, C.F., Mello-Thoms, C., Kundel, H.L., and Weinstein, S.P. (2002). Time course of perception and decision making during mammographic interpretation. *American Journal of Roentgenology*, **179**, 917–923.

Norman, G.R., Coblentz, C.L., Brooks, L.R., and Babcook, C.J. (1992). Expertise in visual diagnosis: A review of the literature. *Academic Medicine*, **67**, S78–S83.

Oestmann, J.W., Greene, R., Kushner, D.C., Bourgouin, P.M., Linetsky, L., and Llewellyn, H.J. (1988). Lung Lesions: Correlation between viewing time and detection. *Radiology*, **166**, 451–453.

Petrakis, E. (1993). *Analysis of visual search patterns of tennis teachers*. In G. d'Ydewalle, and J. Van Rensbergen (eds.) *Perception and cognition: Advances in eye movement research* (Vol. 4, pp. 159–168). Amsterdam: Elsevier.

Polanyi, M. (1969). Knowing and being. In M. Grene (ed.) *Knowing and being: essays*. London: Routledge and K. Paul.

Rayner, K. (1998). Eye movements in reading and information processing: 20 years of research. *Psychological Bulletin*, **124**, 372–422.

Rayner, K. and Pollatsek, A. (1997). Eye movements, the eye-hand span, and the perceptual span during sight-reading of music. *Current Directions in Psychological Science*, **6**(2), 49–53.

Reingold, E.M. and Charness, N. (2005). Perception in chess: Evidence from eye movements. In G. Underwood (ed.) *Cognitive processes in eye guidance* (pp. 325–354). Oxford: Oxford University Press.

Reingold, E.M., Charness, N., Pomplun, M., and Stampe, D.M. (2001a). Visual span in expert chess players: Evidence from eye movements. *Psychological Science*, **12**, 48–55.

Reingold, E.M., Charness, N., Schultetus, R.S., and Stampe, D.M. (2001b). Perceptual automaticity in expert chess players: Parallel encoding of chess relations. *Psychonomic Bulletin and Review*, **8**, 504–510.

Rensink, R.A., O'Regan, J.K., and Clark, J.J. (1997). To see or not to see: The need for attention to perceive changes in scenes. *Psychological Science*, **8**, 368–373.

Reynolds, R.I. (1982). Search heuristics of chess players of different calibers. *American Journal of Psychology*, **95**, 383–392.

Saariluoma, P. (1985). Chess players' intake of task-relevant cues. *Memory and Cognition*, **13**, 385–391.

Sarter, N.B., Mumaw, R.J., and Wickens, C.D. (2007). Pilots' monitoring strategies and performance on automated flight decks: An empirical study combining behavioral and eye-tracking data. *Human Factors*, **49**(3), 347–357.

Saunders, R.S. and Samei, E. (2006). Improving mammographic decision accuracy by incorporating observer ratings with interpretation time. *The British Journal of Radiology*, **79**, S117–S122.

Scheff, T. (1963). Decision rules and types of error, and their consequences in medical diagnosis. *Behavioural Science*, **8**, 97–107.

Shinar, D. (2008). Looks are (almost) everything: where drivers look to get information. *Human Factors*, **50**(3), 380–384.

Simon, H.A., and Barenfeld, M. (1969). Information-processing analysis of perceptual processes in problem solving. *Psychological Review*, **76**, 473–483.

Simon, H.A. and Chase, W.G. (1973). Skill in chess. *American Scientist*, **61**(4), 394–403.

Simon, H.A. and Gilmartin, K. (1973). A simulation of memory for chess positions. *Cognitive Psychology*, **5**, 29–46.

Simons, D.J., and Levin, D.T. (1997). Change blindness. *Trends in Cognitive Sciences*, **1**, 261–267.

Swensson, R.G. (1980). A two-stage detection model applied to skilled visual search by radiologists. *Perception & Psychophysics*, **27**, 11–16.

Swensson, R.G., Hessel, S.J., and Herman, P.G. (1982). Radiographic interpretation with and without search: visual search aids the recognition of chest pathology. *Investigative Radiology*, **17**(2), 145–51.

Swensson, R.G., Hessel, S.J., and Herman, P.G. (1985). The value of searching films without specific preconceptions. *Investigative Radiology*, **20**(1), 100–114.

Tai, R., Loehr, J., and Brigham, F. (2006). An exploration of the use of eye-gaze tracking to study problem-solving on standardized science assessments. *International Journal of Research and Method in Education*, **29**(2), 185–208.

Tikhomirov, O.K. and Poznyanskaya, E. (1966). An investigation of visual search as a means of analyzing heuristics. *Soviet Psychology*, **5**, 2–15.

Underwood, G. (2007). Visual attention and the transition from novice to advanced driver. *Ergonomics*, **50**(8), 1235–1249.

Van Gog, T., Paas, F., and Van Merriënboer, J.J. (2005). Uncovering expertise-related differences in troubleshooting performance: combining eye movement and concurrent verbal protocol data. *Applied Cognitive Psychology*, **19**(2), 205–221.

Vickers, J.N. (1992). Gaze control in putting. *Perception*, **21**(1), 117–132.

Winikoff, A.W. (1967). Eye movements as an aid to protocol analysis of problem solving behavior. Unpublished doctoral dissertation. Carnegie-Mellon University, Pittsburgh, PA.

Wood, B.P. (1999). Visual expertise. *Radiology*, **211**, 1–3.

CHAPTER 30

Eye movements both reveal and influence problem solving

Michael J. Spivey and Rick Dale

Abstract

Within the context of the theory of embodied cognition, our most frequent motor movements—eye movements—are sure to play an important role in our cognitive processes. Not only do eye movements provide the experimenter with a special window into these cognitive processes, they provide the individual with a way to modify their cognitive processes. This chapter examines this dual role of eye movements (both revealing and modifying cognition) in a variety of problem solving tasks. Experimenters can better understand the underlying cognitive processes that are involved in problem solving by recording eye movement patterns, and individuals can better perform their problem solving when they produce the right eye movement patterns.

Introduction

A well known puzzle, known as the river-crossing problem, places missionaries in boats with cannibals and asks you to transit them across a river in a manner that ensures that no missionary is eaten. Consider one such dire scenario: 'Three missionaries and three cannibals want to get to the other side of a river. There is a small boat, which can fit only two. To prevent a tragedy, there can never be more cannibals than missionaries together.' If the reader is like this chapter's authors, this puzzle induces a flurry of dynamic imagery, including a visualization of the nervous missionaries, salivating cannibals, a boat, a river, and perhaps even irrelevant factors like the protagonists' appearance, or a sun in the sky. The reader, like us, may manipulate the visualization and begin moving its 'pieces' in seeking a solution.

General solutions to versions of this problem have been proposed since the 19th century (Pressman and Singmaster, 1989), and into the mid-20th century in a burgeoning field of artificial intelligence (Amarel, 1968). These solutions have never attempted to integrate the rich 'perceptual simulation' (Barsalou, 1999) noted in the previous paragraph. In general, they have had highly formal logical characteristics, translating relevant parts of these problems into variables and operators often dubbed 'amodal' because they lack the characteristics of sensorimotor modalities involved in imagery. This has been a general feature of 'classical' approaches to our cognitive system: treating our internal thought processes as governed by abstract symbols not much different from a digital computer's states and processes (e.g. Newell, 1990; Newell and Simon, 1961). To the uninitiated, this may seem like a very complex, mathematical way of approaching these issues as potential explanations for how we ourselves solve them. But in fact this strategy has been an influential simplification, allowing cognitive scientists to develop computer programs that perform human-like problem solving in a diverse range of problem spaces (see Poole et al., 1997, for many examples).

There has been considerable debate about the usefulness of these formalistic approaches to understanding human cognition in general (e.g. Dreyfus, 1979; Marcus, 2001; Searle, 1980; Spivey, 2007). One charge against the classical approach has been its lack of perceptual and motor detail that we seem richly to experience in day-to-day cognitive functioning, as the first paragraph of this chapter attempts to demonstrate (see, e.g. Clark, 1997, for review). In the past two decades, the view that cognitive scientists should integrate sensorimotor, or 'modal,' representations in our theories of cognition has been gaining traction. Often dubbed the 'embodiment of cognition,' the approach sees cognitive processes as directly involving modal sensorimotor systems, e.g. visual, somatosensory, and auditory perception, as well as oculomotor and skeletomotor planning. In other words, even during 'high-level' cognitive processes such as problem solving, the brain recruits 'low-level' sensorimotor neural subsystems to assist in the cognitive computations.

In this chapter, we review research showing that eye movements support the embodiment of problem solving. When facing many kinds of puzzles and problems, our cognitive system makes use of implicit perceptuomotor activities to search the problem space for solutions. In what follows, we present a selective review of evidence for embodiment especially relevant to eye movements and problem solving. This review motivates two key predictions: Eye movements should: 1) reveal problem solving processes as they unfold, and 2) potentially aid problem solving directly. We then showcase recent empirical support for both predictions. The chapter ends with theoretical discussion, and future directions in which eye movement and other dynamic, temporal methodologies could contribute to our understanding of high-level cognition.

The embodiment of cognition

Consider again the river-crossing problem. This type of problem has some basic properties that many puzzles and problems have in common. First, it is conveyed through linguistic means. Problem solvers are provided statements that lay out a set of premises, assumptions, arrangements, etc. that are intended to establish basic rules or constraints on a scenario. Second, a given scenario may have some spatiotemporal conditions that approximate arrangements of things in the natural world. The river-crossing problem has folks travelling in boats, while other problem spaces involve moving blocks about pegs (e.g. Tower of Hanoi problem: Simon, 1975), or connecting dots on a two-dimensional surface (e.g. nine-dot problem: MacGregor et al., 2001). Both of these qualities—linguistic transmission and spatiotemporal arrangement—invoke cognitive processes that have embodied sensorimotor qualities. Evidence for this has come directly from eye tracking experiments.

In an obvious way, concrete spatial language that explicitly mentions positions or directions of movement may invoke sensorimotor representations. But even abstract figurative language can generate embodied effects, evidenced in eye movement patterns. For example, Matlock and colleagues have investigated the processing of sentences that figuratively invoke motion, known as 'fictive motion' descriptions (Matlock, 2004). Matlock and Richardson (2004) conducted a passive viewing experiment in which participants saw a scene of objects and listened to sentences. Some scene/sentence pairs contained fictive motion. For example, a view of a desert with a road down the centre of the scene could be described with 'The road *runs through* the desert' (fictive motion) or simply 'The road is in the desert'. Participants spent more time fixating the path of motion when they heard fictive motion sentences than when they heard the literal control sentences. Richardson and Matlock (2007) further demonstrated that when the sentences described movement difficulty (e.g. '. . . the desert is rough'), participants' eye movement patterns covaried with this movement difficulty. Scanpaths exhibited enhanced focus on the region of the fictive motion (e.g. along the road) under conditions of more difficult movement. These and numerous other studies have shown that a diverse range of language processes make use of sensorimotor representations (for reviews, see Anderson and Spivey, 2009; Barsalou, 2008; Glenberg and Kaschak, 2003).

As for spatiotemporal arrangement, river-crossing and other problems may induce visual imagery of manipulating this arrangement, during which modal visual areas of cortex are activated (see Kosslyn and Thompson, 2003; Kosslyn et al., 2003 for review). If this visual system activation is functionally important to visual imagery, then oculomotor output is likely to correspond to the structure of imagery. Indeed, Spivey and Geng (2001, expt. 1) have shown that visual imagery elicits eye movements (while viewing a blank screen) that correspond to the locations and movement directions in the spoken descriptions (Altmann, 2004; Brandt and Stark, 1997; Laeng and Teodorescu, 2002; see also Altmann, Chapter 54, this volume).

There may be good reasons for this oculomotor enactment of cognition: memory systems make use of external spatial locations as anchors for encoded information. The eyes should thus reflect these external 'indexes' (Pylyshyn, 1989) for recalled information. Richardson and Spivey (2000) have shown that when participants learn new facts in association with spatial regions on a screen, participants look to those now-blank regions when recalling the facts. In a series of experiments, participants saw a 2×2 grid, and in different cells viewed a video of a face presenting various statements (e.g. 'Australia's capital is Canberra'). When participants were queried to verify a version of one of those statements, they frequently looked to the corresponding empty cell in the grid while they answered the query—even though they could easily tell in their peripheral vision that it was empty, and the statement has been delivered auditorily anyway!

A natural question that follows is whether these eye movements to those locations can improve memory for that object or event. That is, can recreating during recall the eye movement pattern that took place during encoding instigate at kind of pattern completion process? It has recently been hypothesized that if eye movements are systematically manipulated by the experimental task, e.g. turned into an independent variable instead of a dependent variable, then one might observe different memory performance for trials in which the eyes are fixating the correct location versus an incorrect location (Ferreira et al., 2008). Although this is certainly a logical possibility, the existing data are not consistent with it (Richardson et al., 2009). In every test for such an improvement in memory accuracy conducted so far, none has been found (Hoover and Richardson, 2008; Richardson and Kirkham, 2004; Richardson and Spivey, 2000; Spivey and Geng, 2001, expt. 2). Recently, there is evidence for a slight decrease in reaction time to memory probes when the eyes are fixating the correct location compared to when they are fixating the wrong location, but no evidence for improvements in memory accuracy (Theeuwes et al., in press; Vankov, 2009). For example, Vankov (2009) presented participants with four line drawings of objects and then presented a memory probe consisting of a single word that might refer to one of the objects. In some conditions, the word showed up in the same location as the now-absent object, and in other conditions, it showed up in a different location. Vankov observed some subtle reaction time differences between these conditions, but the accuracy of memory performance was not affected by the location of the memory cue. Thus, rather than these memory-induced eye movements being evidence for an embodiment of cognition solely inside the sensorimotor system (where pattern completion of neural patterns can take place), they may be better evidence for an embeddedness of cognition in the environment (e.g. O'Regan and Noë, 2002; Spivey et al., 2004), whereby a small bit of internal semantic information regarding an object or event is linked to a location in the visual field where 'the rest' of the information is expected to be accessible (O'Regan, 1992).

The selective review above supports the involvement of embodied representations in language processes and visual imagery, both likely components of naturalistic problem solving. Memory processes accompanying both of these can be anchored in spatial locations in the world, and eye-movement signatures reveal this. In the next section, we briefly provide a more mechanistic account of the deep connection between eye movements and cognition, which leads to two broad predictions about how eye movements should be involved in problem solving.

Eye movements are coextensive with cognition

The key reason why eye movement patterns are so informative about mental activity is that they are part and parcel of it. Rather than being a slave output system that patiently awaits discrete finalized commands from the cognitive system, oculomotor processing is coextensive with cognitive process-ing. The ongoing processes of cognition continuously 'spill over' (before a decision is final) into the oculomotor system, causing it to prepare partially-active movement plans that are consistent with the gradually accumulating perceptual evidence (Gold and Shadlen, 2007). This is due in part to the fact that the eyes tend to make saccadic movements about every 200–300 ms, whereas it takes about 400–500 ms for a neural population code that embodies the representation of a visual object to achieve its maximal activation (e.g. Rolls and Tovee, 1995). As a result, the eyes are often moving to fixate a new object before the previous object has been fully and completely recognized. This contin-uously flowing perception-action cycle (Neisser, 1976) becomes an autocatalytic causal loop, in which cognition emerges (Spivey, 2007). Before a cognitive decision to respond to the stimulus envi-ronment has reached completion, the eyes will often move to fixate a new object or location in the visual field. This newly foveated perceptual information then changes the cognitive processes which led to that eye movement—and which were on their way to one decision but now may be on their way to a different one! Cognition somehow manages to simultaneously be a major cause of eye-movement patterns and partly a result of them.

A concrete demonstration of this continuity between a cognitive process (such as a decision) and an eye movement comes from a study by Gold and Shadlen (2000). As perceptual input accumulates over time to produce an overt decision and motor response, the continuous evolution of that decision can be seen in eye movement data. That is, the network of brain systems in which a perceptual deci-sion is generated includes oculomotor nuclei, such as the frontal eye fields. Gold and Shadlen trained a monkey to respond to a pseudorandom dot-motion stimulus by looking at an upper response target when the central motion stimulus had upward motion in it, and at a lower response target when the central motion stimulus had downward motion in it. Then, just before a voluntary eye movement response was made, they microstimulated a region of the monkey's frontal eye fields (via mild electric current delivered through an electrode) to generate an involuntary rightward saccade. When the monkey was allowed only a couple hundred milliseconds to see the motion stimulus, the involuntary evoked saccade was a nearly pure rightward movement. However, with 300 or 400 or 500 ms to see the motion stimulus, the involuntary evoked saccade showed more and more vertical component in its direction. Essentially, the perceptual decision (of upward vs. downward motion) that was evolving over several hundred milliseconds was simultaneously generating a pattern of neural activity in the frontal eye fields that formed the beginnings of a voluntary upward or downward eye movement command. When the microstimulation caused the involuntary rightward saccade, the partly evolved voluntary eye movement command influenced the direction that the eyes actually went. Thus, rather than the oculomotor system waiting until a single confident perceptual decision was achieved, it was continuously 'listening to' and 'involved in' the gradual formation of that perceptual decision.

One might, in fact, wish to draw a distinction between the notions of the eye movement system continuously *listening* to cognition versus being continuously *involved in* cognition. This kind of distinction is often raised when discussing embodied cognition in general (Mahon and Caramazza, 2008), where some embodied cognition results may be best interpreted as a spreading of activation from cognitive to motor subsystems (e.g. Glenberg and Kaschak, 2002), and other embodied cogni-tion results clearly demonstrate a functional role for motor patterns feeding back into cognitive proc-esses (Pulvermüller et al., 2005). Accordingly, the next two sections in this chapter will address evidence for eye movements revealing certain cognitive processes related to problem solving tasks because those cognitive processes continuously spread their activation patterns into the oculomotor system, and also evidence for eye movements influencing the cognitive processes related to problem solving tasks because those eye movement patterns change the way the cognitive processes function.

Eye movements reveal problem solving

Mathematical problem solving

A number of studies have shown a relationship between the activity of the eyes and the activity of the mind during mathematical problem solving. Hess and Polt (1964) were the first to demonstrate that a person's pupils dilate when he or she is solving a difficult mathematical problem. As their multiplication problems got harder, pupil dilation steadily increased. It was a few years later that saccadic movements of the eyes were linked to problem-solving tasks. Yarbus (1967) showed that it is not merely visual input that determines eye movement patterns, but task constraints as well. In his experiment, the same painting (Ilya Repin's *An Unexpected Visitor*) elicited very different eye movement scanning patterns (scanpaths) when the viewer was probed with different queries, such as 'What are the ages of the people in the painting?,' 'What had the family been doing before the visitor arrived?', and 'How long had the visitor been away?' (For similar results in individuals with Asperger's syndrome, see Benson and Fletcher-Watson, Chapter 39, this volume.)

Using the record of saccadic eye movements to uncover the cognitive processes involved in mathematical problem solving was first systematically explored by Suppes et al. (1982). In testing their procedural theory of eye movements during addition and subtraction problems, they found that although arithmetic problems that require 'carrying' or 'borrowing' are more difficult and take longer than those that do not, actually 'carrying' or 'borrowing' values while solving the problem increases eye fixation durations only very slightly. When solving algebra problems, it is noteworthy that students do not simply fixate each number and symbol left-to-right. Instead, they will sometimes skip values (presumably perceiving them parafoveally) and other times they will refixate values (Salvucci and Anderson, 2001).

Where we can clearly observe the eyes spending substantially more time fixating difficult parts of a math problem is with word problems. Word problems can be written with inconsistent relational terms, such as 'Johnny has five cookies, which is three fewer than Mary has. How many cookies does Mary have?' This word problem is referred to as 'inconsistent' because the relational term 'fewer than' can trick students into using subtraction (instead of addition) to solve the problem. In fact, eye movement patterns (such as more regressive saccades back to the relational terms) suggest that this is exactly why students are sometimes unsuccessful with inconsistently worded problems (Hegarty et al., 1995; Verschaffel et al., 1992).

Eye movements during the linguistic delivery of math and logic problems have also been explored when there were no visual stimuli at all. For example, Demarais and Cohen (1998) presented participants with spoken recordings of transitive inference problems, such as 'a jar of pickles is below a box of tea bags; the jar of pickles is above a can of coffee; where's the can of coffee?' While staring at a completely blank display, participants tended to make more vertical (than horizontal) eye movements while hearing those above/below inference problems. When hearing inference problems where objects were aligned to the left and right of one another, participants made more horizontal (than vertical) eye movements. These results suggest that when people are solving transitive inference problems, with no external visual aids, they nonetheless generate some form of spatial mental model to assist their logical induction (Byrne and Johnson-Laird, 1989), and they perform eye movements consistent with the spatial characteristics of that mental model.

Eye movement patterns can also reveal the cognitive processes involved in solving geometry problems. Epelboim and Suppes (2001) tracked participants' eye movements while they looked at diagrams that had letters indexing the endpoints of lines and centroids of circles, and then some angles provided in degrees, and then a particular angle whose size (in degrees) was to be solved. The eye movement patterns exhibited a variety of interesting properties. For example, participants tended to look away from the diagram when they were performing mental arithmetic (as indicated by their verbal protocols). More importantly, the scanpaths revealed a great many redundant sequences consisting of many rescans of previously fixated diagram components throughout the solving of the problem. This observation is consistent with Epelboim and Suppes's model of geometry reasoning in which fixated components of a diagram tend to overwrite existing diagram components in visual working memory—suggesting that visual working memory may tend to store a surprisingly small amount of information at any one time (see also Ballard et al., 1997).

Mechanical problem solving

Carpenter and Just (1978; see also Just and Carpenter, 1985) were the first to show a relationship between eye movements and mental rotation. When participants compare a target shape to a set of alternative rotated shapes, to find the matching one, the eye movement patterns suggest that participants go through a few different procedures in sequence. They encode the target shape and *search* for a matching component among the shapes, then *transform* or rotate that component in one of the shapes, and then *confirm* whether the other components match those in the target shape after this mental transformation (Just and Carpenter, 1985). Interestingly, the eye movement data suggested that the increased latencies resulting from more complex shape comparisons appeared to have been due to longer encoding and confirmation phases, rather than longer transformation or rotation phases (Carpenter and Just, 1978).

While eyetracking a simplified version of the Tower of London problem, Hodgson et al. (2000) also found evidence for a search phase, followed by a transformation phase, and then a confirmation phase. Participants started each trial with multiple fixations of the target stack of balls, then multiple fixations of the stack of balls that they were to imagine manipulating to match the target, and then finishing with fixations of the target stack again. Interestingly, on trials where participants produced incorrect answers, their scanpaths were surprisingly conspicuously similar to those of the previous trial. Hodgson et al. suggested that participants sometimes get stuck from one trial to the next in an ocolumotor routine that may not be optimal for the new problem diagram.

Mental animation during mechanical reasoning can also be revealed in eye movement data. For example, Hegarty (1992; see also Hegarty and Just, 1993) recorded participants' eye movements while they looked at diagrams of pulley systems, and found evidence that when people mentally animate these diagrams, in order to verify/deny statements about them, their animations are piecemeal. Rather than imagining all the pulleys moving at once, as would actually happen when the rope threads its way through them, the eye movement patterns suggest that participants mentally animate small portions of the pulley system in sequential order, reflecting the causal chain of forces.

The same observation was made for eye movement patterns with more complex gear-and-belt diagrams. Rozenblit et al. (2002) tracked participants' eye movements while they looked at gear-and-belt diagrams in which the leftmost gear was specified to rotate in a particular direction, and it connected to several intermediate gears (which alternate the previous direction of rotation) and straight belts (which maintain the previous direction of rotation), culminating in a pendulum. The participant's task was to guess which direction the pendulum would swing. Practised eye movement coders could tell which directions a participant was mentally animating a set of connected gears and belts by watching the slow-motion video of the eye movement trace overlaid on the diagram. For example, a few fixations near the conjunction of two gears can reveal that the participant was mentally animating the left gear clockwise and the right gear counter-clockwise simply by the fact that the sequence of fixations went left-to-right on the *upper* portion of the left gear and then left-to-right on the *lower* portion of the right gear. The proof for this observation comes especially clear when that direction of animation is incorrect and thus allows the coder to accurately predict an incorrect guess from the participant on that trial. In fact, Rozenblit et al. showed that even unpractised coders— naïve experimental participants watching the slow-motion video of multiple trials (with their final portions edited out)—can use the eye movement traces to perform well above chance in predicting incorrect guesses. Thus, even when it is difficult to identity the specific properties of the eye-movement trace that reveal cognition, there is clearly information in those scanpaths that can nonetheless be used (even by non-experts) to infer cognitive processes.

Insight problem solving

So far, we have been discussing problem-solving tasks where the formulation of the solution plods along relatively linearly. With problems like that, participants tend to have accurate intuitions about how close they are to reaching the solution. With insight problems, by contrast, that is not the case at all. With insight problems—and there is a wide variety of them—participants usually reach a point partway through where they feel like they've run out of ideas, known as an *impasse*. When encouraged to keep trying anyway, some proportion of the participants will eventually achieve *insight*, in some cases even widening the eyes and declaring 'Aha!' Notably, on the way toward that 'Aha!'

moment, if they are asked to report how close to the solution they think they might be, their ratings do not correlate with their actual remaining time-to-solution. Insight problems tend to be difficult puzzles, so a substantial proportion of participants never find the solution at all (or they require guiding hints from the experimenter to get there). Participants typically describe the solution as having come to them 'suddenly out of nowhere.' Nonetheless, more subtle measures of performance, such as two-alternative forced-choice (Bowers et al., 1990), reaction-time priming (Bowden and Jung-Beeman, 1998), and eye-tracking (Knoblich et al., 2001), can often provide inklings of how the solution gradually emerges over time. This opacity to subjective reports makes insight problem solving particularly intriguing for theories of cognition, and a prime target of eye movement methodologies.

Before discussing the more standard insight problems, however, it might be useful to examine a kind of problem that falls somewhere in between non-insight problems and insight problems. This next eyetracking study that opens a window onto a mechanical problem-solving task is not typically considered an insight problem, per se, because it does not involve an impasse phase. Participants view a sequence of connected gears, are told that the leftmost gear will turn clockwise (or counter-clockwise), and then asked which direction the rightmost gear will turn. After several trials of solving these simple linear-gear-sequence problems, participants rather suddenly discover a new easy strategy for solving them. In fact, sometimes they even shout 'Aha!' when they suddenly realize that one need not mentally animate each gear to figure out which direction the last one rotates; one can just count whether there is an even or odd number of gears (Dixon and Bangert, 2004). If there is an even number of linearly-connected gears, then the last gear will rotate in the *opposite* direction of the first gear. If there is an odd number of gears, then the last gear will rotate in the *same* direction as the first gear. What is interesting about this discovery process is that the statistical structure of the eye-movement patterns presages that moment of discovery. That is, over the course of the two to five trials that precede the 'Aha' moment of figuring out the even-odd strategy, the eye-movement trace shows a statistically reliable increase in entropy, a measure of disorder in the data (Stephen et al., 2009). Stephen et al. interpret this as evidence that the mental animation strategy is becoming unstable, and is on the brink of yielding to the emerging even-odd strategy. On the one trial immediately preceding the trial on which they first use their new even-odd strategy, the eye-movement trace shows a statistically reliable *decrease* in entropy. This suggests that right before the new strategy is implemented, participants' scanning behaviour reveals a renewed stability and order reflecting the completion of the cognitive restructuring from the old mental animation strategy to the newly-adopted even–odd strategy. Thus, eye-movement patterns can provide a window into the gradual emergence of a new strategy during problem solving—even predicting when a new strategy is on its way.

This particular view on cognitive processes provided by eye-tracking can even be seen in genuine insight problems, which involve both an impasse and then an 'Aha' moment (for a more extensive review, see Knoblich et al., 2005). Knoblich et al. (2001) tracked participants' eye movements while they attempted to solve/repair Roman numeral arithmetic problems written with matchsticks. For example, reposition a single matchstick to make the following equation true: IV = III + III. (Note that all numerals and operators are formed with straight matchsticks.) In this non-insight example, one simply needs to change the 'IV' to a 'VI', and the equation is true. Participants tend to solve that one quickly and easily. However, more difficult problems, such as III = III + III, will often induce an impasse; and when the participant discovers the solution, they experience an 'Aha' moment. The solution for converting that false equation into a true one, involves relaxing an implicitly assumed constraint (that only matchsticks forming numerals can be modified).

Knoblich et al. (2001) found that, during the impasse phase with the difficult problems, mean fixation duration increased significantly. Basically, when participants had run out of ideas, they stared at the display without exploring new solution strategies. While that finding shows the impasse stage of insight problem solving, this next finding shows how eye movements can reveal the representational change that takes place right before achieving insight. As would be expected from an implicit (and incorrect) assumption that only matchsticks forming numerals can be modified, participants typically began the difficult problems fixating the numerals almost exclusively, rarely fixating the operators.

Over the course of attempting to solve these difficult 'constraint relaxation' problems, the participants who would soon discover the solution (e.g. changing the plus sign to an equal sign with a single movement of one matchstick) showed a steady gradual increase in proportion of fixations on operators prior to their 'Aha!' moment.

Similar evidence for eye movements revealing the emergent temporal dynamics of a seemingly-sudden insight comes from work by Jones (2003). Jones used a diagram-based car park problem, where the tricky insight is that, in addition to moving other cars out of the way to form an exit path, one's own car must move to make room for some of those other cars' movements. Jones operationalized the impasse as a looking time for a particular move that exceeded that participant's mean looking time by two standard deviations. He found that all 30 (out of 37) participants who solved the problem experienced at least one such impasse. Moreover, the bulk of that impasse was focused on the part of the problem that required realizing that one's own car needed to be moved. Mean looking time for that move was five times greater than the mean looking time for other moves. However, about one-third of the participants exhibited impasses (long gazes without making any moves) quite early on, suggesting that they may have been strategizing multiple moves in advance. In fact, those participants with early impasses solved the car park problem faster and with fewer moves than participants who did not exhibit early impasses.

Eye movements influence problem solving

In addition to providing cognitive scientists with a peek into the mental activity involved in problem solving, eye movements may themselves be able to instigate insight for a person attempting to solve a problem. For example, Grant and Spivey (2003, expt. 1) showed that fixating certain regions of a tumour-and-stomach diagram, for Duncker's classic radiation problem, was correlated with achieving insight. The schematic diagram consisted of a solid oval, representing the tumour, with a circumscribing oval representing the stomach lining. While viewing that display, participants were told, 'Given a human being with an inoperable stomach tumour, and lasers which destroy organic tissue at sufficient intensity, how can one cure the person with these lasers and, at the same time, avoid harming the healthy tissue that surrounds the tumour?'

All participants reported experiencing a period of impasse, where they had run out of ideas. Only about a third of the participants produced the correct solution (i.e. to use multiple low-intensity lasers, which are too weak to damage the skin, and converge their incident rays onto the tumour to combine their intensities and burn it away). These successful participants routinely blurted out an 'Aha!' (or some equivalent) when they discovered this solution. Although the eye movement patterns were somewhat similar for successful and unsuccessful participants, one key difference stood out. Successful solvers tended to spend more time looking at the stomach-lining portion of the diagram than unsuccessful solvers. In fact, the pattern of eye movements that was most closely associated with achieving insight with this problem was one in which one or two saccades were made from the external portion of the diagram inward to the tumour (often stopping at the stomach-lining) and then back out to another external region. This triangular sequence of saccades, which almost 'paints a sketch' of multiple incident rays converging on the tumour, was especially common prior to the participant achieving insight. Could it be that people who *happened to* produce eye movement patterns like that were steered toward the cognitive insight by their sensorimotor patterns priming a 'perceptual simulation' (Barsalou, 1999) of multiple incident rays? Or is it merely that their cognitive processes were gradually forming the correct solution anyway, and this caused their eye movements to reflect that nascent solution?

In a first step toward addressing this question, Grant and Spivey (2003) conducted a second experiment in which a computer display animated either the tumour or the stomach-lining, with a one-pixel increase in diameter flashing at about 3 Hz. With attention and eye movements drawn toward the animated tumour, only a third of those participants solved the radiation problem—the same as with the static diagram in their first experiment. However, of the participants whose diagrams had the stomach-lining flashing, two-thirds discovered the insight of converging multiple weak lasers onto the tumour. Thus, in this second experiment, attracting participants' attention toward the stomach-lining region of the diagram (which is where successful solvers were spontaneously looking in the first experiment) *doubled* the solution rate for this difficult insight problem. Note, however, that because Grant and Spivey did not track eye movements in this second experiment, it is not clear whether it is eye movements, per se, that jump-started this cognitive insight, or whether it might be covert spatial attention that did so.

Following up on this issue, Thomas and Lleras (2007) used a similar schematic diagram with Duncker's radiation problem and added to it a secondary visual-tracking task that, for some subjects, *just happened to* make their eyes move in the same triangular fashion that Grant and Spivey (2003) first noticed in their eye-movement data. Eye movements were recorded to ensure that participants adhered to the visual-tacking task. Importantly, participants whose eye movements were guided (by the visual-tracking task) to reproduce this triangular pattern were more than twice as likely to discover the solution than participants whose eye movements were driven in neutral or irrelevant patterns. Since participants reported not detecting any relationship between the visual-tracking task and the radiation problem, Thomas and Lleras (2007) concluded that the eye movements were influencing the formation of insight in this problem.

Interestingly, since covert allocation of spatial attention is often likened to programmed eye movements that simply aren't executed (e.g. Sheliga et al., 1994), one might expect that patterns of covert spatial attention—independent of eye movements—might be equally capable of influencing cognition in a diagram-based problem like this. Indeed, Thomas and Lleras (2009) found that when eye position was fixed on the tumour, but visual cues directed covert spatial attention to the external portion of the diagram and then back to the tumour again and again, the solution rate almost tripled—compared to central fixation without attentional cues. Essentially, preparing eye movements (with or without executing them) that are spatially compatible with the convergence solution to the radiation problem is sufficient to prime the perceptual simulation that embodies the cognitive insight. Thus, eye movement processes do more than simply *reveal* (to the experimenter) the temporal dynamics of cognition during problem solving. Eye movement processes can also *influence* (for oneself) the cognitive processes that go into an attempt to solve a problem.

Conclusion

Classical approaches to explaining problem solving, described in the introduction, neglect the perceptuomotor processes that are likely involved in problem solving. The eye-tracking work described above shows that embodied representations both reflect unfolding problem solving, and may directly aid in solving certain kinds of problems. Eye-tracking methodologies are extremely well suited to identifying these representations as they occur. For one, the eye-movement record is a semi-continuous real-time source of information about cognitive processes, in many ways out of conscious strategic control of participants (Liversedge and Findlay, 2000). In addition, as a motor system, it maps out spatial coding of the sensorimotor processes themselves (see Spivey et al., 2009, for further review).

These characteristics guarantee that eye movements will remain, well into the future, an important methodological window on high-level cognitive processes, such as problem solving. In conjunction with other near-continuous measures of cognition used recently, such as the dynamics of reaching and pointing movements (e.g. Spivey and Dale, 2006; Spivey et al., 2005; Stephen et al., 2009), it offers investigation into the time-course and fine-grained representational structure of problem solving. Spatially and temporally coarser techniques, such as coded video streams or think aloud protocols (Ericsson and Simon, 1993) are still applied extensively to complex cognitive processes, like knowledge acquisition, problem solving, metacognition, and so on. Advances in the analysis of semi-continuous methods continue to offer novel insights that those coarser methods cannot access, especially in these high-level contexts (e.g. Graesser et al., 2005).

Finally, the theoretical question regarding whether there can be a preferred account of problem solving, classical or embodied, is not at present resolvable. In many regards, classically formal approaches enjoy more currency in this domain (Poole et al., 1997). Recently, some artificial intelligence research has been integrating symbolic and spatial representations, and solutions to some problems come handily with both in operation, compared to either alone (e.g. Wintermute and Laird, 2008). This perhaps encourages one to consider that both theoretical schemes may be helpful for understanding what guides a problem solver. Such integration will depend on a number of important factors, such as the particular problem at hand, problem-solving context, and any potential expertise. Eye tracking and other semicontinuous methods will inevitably provide fine-grained explorations of these and other factors in the future, contributing to ongoing theoretical debate.

Acknowledgements

Work on this chapter was supported by a collaborative research grant from the NSF to both authors.

References

Altmann, G., and Kamide, Y.(2004). Now you see it, now you don't: Mediating the mapping between language and the visual world. In J. Henderson and F. Ferreira (eds.) *The interface of language, vision, and action: Eye movements and the visual world.* New York: Psychology Press.

Amarel, S. (1968). On representations of problems of reasoning about actions. In D. Michie (ed.) *Machine Intelligence 3* (Vol. 3) (pp. 131–171). Amsterdam: Elsevier/North-Holland.

Anderson, S.E. and Spivey, M.J. (2009). The enactment of language: Decades of interactions between linguistic and motor processes. *Language and Cognition*, **1**, 87–111.

Ballard, D.H., Hayhoe, M.M., Pook, P.K., and Rao, R.P.N. (1997). Deictic codes for the embodiment of cognition. *Behavioral and Brain Sciences*, **20**(4), 723–742.

Barsalou, L.W. (1999). Perceptions of perceptual symbols. *Behavioral and brain sciences*, **22**(4), 637–660.

Barsalou, L.W. (2008). Grounded cognition. *Annual Review of Psychology*, **59**, 617–45.

Bowden, E.M. and Beeman, M.J. (1998). Getting the right idea: Semantic activation in the right hemisphere may help solve insight problems. *Psychological Science*, **9**(6), 435–440.

Bowers, K.S., Regehr, G., Balthazard, C., and Parker, K. (1990). Intuition in the context of discovery. *Cognitive Psychology*, **22**(1), 72–110.

Brandt, S. and Stark, L. (1997). Spontaneous eye movements during visual imagery reflect the content of the visual scene. *Journal of Cognitive Neuroscience*, **9**, 27–38.

Byrne, R.M.J. and Johnson-Laird, P.N. (1989). Spatial reasoning. *Journal of Memory and Language*, **28**(5), 564–575.

Carpenter, P.A., and Just, M.A. (1978). Eye fixations during mental rotation. In J. Senders, R. Monty, and D. Fisher (eds.) *Eye movements and the higher psychological functions* (pp. 115–133). Hillsdale, NJ: Erlbaum.

Clark, A. (1997). *Being there: Putting brain, body, and world together again.* Cambridge, MA: MIT press.

Demarais, A.M. and Cohen, B.H. (1998). Evidence for image-scanning eye movements during transitive inference. *Biological Psychology*, **49**(3), 229–247.

Dixon, J.A. and Bangert, A.S. (2004). On the spontaneous discovery of a mathematical relation during problem solving. *Cognitive Science*, **28**(3), 433–449.

Dreyfus, H.L. (1979). *What computers can't do: The limits of artificial intelligence.* London: HarperCollins.

Epelboim, J. and Suppes, P. (2001). A model of eye movements and visual working memory during problem solving in geometry. *Vision Research*, **41**(12), 1561–1574.

Ericsson, K.A. and Simon, H.A. (1993). *Protocol analysis: Verbal reports as data.* Cambridge, MA: MIT Press.

Ferreira, F., Apel, J., and Henderson, J.M. (2008). Taking a new look at looking at nothing. *Trends in Cognitive Sciences*, **12**(11), 405–410.

Glenberg, A.M. and Kaschak, M.P. (2002). Grounding language in action. *Psychonomic Bulletin and Review*, **9**(3), 558–565.

Glenberg, A.M. and Kaschak, M.P. (2003). The body's contribution to language. *Psychology of Learning and Motivation*, **43**, 93–126.

Gold, J.I. and Shadlen, M.N. (2000). Representation of a perceptual decision in developing oculomotor commands. *Nature*, **404**(6776), 390–394.

Gold, J.I. and Shadlen, M.N. (2007). The neural basis of decision making. *Annual Review of Neuroscience*, **30**, 535–574.

Graesser, A.C., Lu, S., Olde, B.A., Cooper-Pye, E., and Whitten, S. (2005). Question asking and eye tracking during cognitive disequilibrium: Comprehending illustrated texts on devices when the devices break down. *Memory and Cognition*, **33**(7), 1235–1247.

Grant, E.R. and Spivey, M.J. (2003). Guiding attention guides thought. *Psychological Science*, **14**(5), 462–466.

Hegarty, M. (1992). Mental animation: inferring motion from static displays of mechanical systems. *Journal of experimental psychology. Learning, Memory, and Cognition*, **18**(5), 1084–1102.

Hegarty, M., and Just, M.A. (1993). Constructing mental models of machines from text and diagrams. *Journal of Memory and Language*, **32**(6), 717–742.

Hegarty, M., Mayer, R.E., and Monk, C.A. (1995). Comprehension of arithmetic word problems: A comparison of successful and unsuccessful problem solvers. *Journal of Educational Psychology*, **87**, 18–32.

Hess, E.H. and Polt, J.M. (1964). Pupil size in relation to mental activity during simple problem-solving. *Science*, **143**, 1190–1192.

Hodgson, T.L., Bajwa, A., Owen, A.M., and Kennard, C. (2000). The strategic control of gaze direction in the Tower of London task. *Journal of Cognitive Neuroscience*, **12**(5), 894–907.

Hoover, M.A., and Richardson, D.C. (2008). When facts go down the rabbit hole: Contrasting features and objecthood as indexes to memory. *Cognition*, **108**, 533–542.

Jones, G. (2003). Testing two theories of cognitive insight. *Journal of Experimental Psychology: Learning, Memory and Cognition*, **29**(5), 1017–1027.

Just, M.A. and Carpenter, P.A. (1985). Cognitive coordinate systems: Accounts of mental rotation and individual differences in spatial ability. *Psychological Review*, **92**, 137–172.

Knoblich, G., Ohlsson, S., and Raney, G.E. (2001). An eye movement study of insight problem solving. *Memory and Cognition*, **29**(7), 1000–1009.

Knoblich, G., Öllinger, M., and Spivey, M. (2005). Eye movements providing insight into insight problem solving. In G. Underwood (ed.) *Eye Guidance in Cognition* (pp. 355–375). Oxford: Oxford University Press.

Kosslyn, S.M. and Thompson, W.L. (2003). When is early visual cortex activated during visual mental imagery? *Psychological Bulletin*, **129**(5), 723–746.

Kosslyn, S.M. Ganis, G., and Thompson, W.L. (2003). Mental imagery: Against the nihilistic hypothesis. *Trends in Cognitive Sciences*, **7**(3), 109–111.

Laeng, B. and Teodorescu, D.S. (2002). Eye scanpaths during visual imagery reenact those of perception of the same visual scene. *Cognitive Science*, **26**(2), 207–231.

Liversedge, S.P. and Findlay, J.M. (2000). Saccadic eye movements and cognition. *Trends in Cognitive Science*, **4**, 6–14.

MacGregor, J.N., Ormerod, T.C., and Chronicle, E.P. (2001). Information processing and insight: A process model of performance on the nine-dot and related problems. *Journal of Experimental Psychology: Learning, Memory, and Cognition*, **27**(1), 176–201.

Mahon, B.Z. and Caramazza, A. (2008). A critical look at the embodied cognition hypothesis and a new proposal for grounding conceptual content. *Journal of Physiology (Paris)*, **102**(1–3), 59–70.

Marcus, G.F. (2001). *The Algebraic Mind: Integrating Connectionism and Cognitive Science*. Cambridge, MA: MIT Press.

Matlock, T. (2004). Fictive motion as cognitive simulation. *Memory and Cognition*, **32**(8), 1389–1400.

Matlock, T. and Richardson, D.C. (2004). Do eye movements go with fictive motion? *Proceedings of the 26th Annual Meeting of the Cognitive Science Society*. Mahwah, NJ: Erlbaum.

Neisser, U. (1976). *Cognition and reality*. San Francisco, CA: WH Freeman.

Newell, A. (1990). *Unified theories of cognition*. Cambridge, MA: Harvard University Press.

Newell, A. and Simon, H.A. (1961). Computer simulation of human thinking. *Science*, **134**(3495), 2011–2017.

O'Regan, J.K. (1992). Solving the 'real' mysteries of visual perception: the world as an outside memory. *Canadian Journal of Psychology*, **46**, 461–488.

O'Regan, J.K. and Noë, A. (2002). A sensorimotor account of vision and visual consciousness. *Behavioral and Brain Sciences*, **24**(5), 939–973.

Poole, D., Mackworth, A., and Goebel, R. (1997). *Computational intelligence: a logical approach*. Oxford: Oxford University Press.

Pressman, I. and Singmaster, D. (1989). ''The jealous husbands'' and ''the missionaries and cannibals''. *The Mathematical Gazette*, **73**(464), 73–81.

Pulvermüller, F., Hauk, O., Nikulin, V.V., and Ilmoniemi, R.J. (2005). Functional links between motor and language systems. *European Journal of Neuroscience*, **21**(3), 793–797.

Pylyshyn, Z. (1989). The role of location indexes in spatial perception: A sketch of the FINST spatial-index model. *Cognition*, **32**, 65–97.

Richardson, D.C. and Kirkham, N.Z. (2004). Multimodal events and moving locations: Eye movements of adults and 6-month-olds reveal dynamic spatial indexing. *Journal of Experimental Psychology: General*, **133**(1), 46–62.

Richardson, D.C. and Matlock, T. (2007). The integration of figurative language and static depictions: An eye movement study of fictive motion. *Cognition*, **102**(1), 129–138.

Richardson, D.C. and Spivey, M.J. (2000). Representation, space and Hollywood Squares: looking at things that aren't there anymore. *Cognition*, **76**(3), 269–295.

Richardson, D.C., Altmann, G., Spivey, M.J., and Hoover, M. (2009). Much ado about eye movements to nothing. *Trends in Cognitive Sciences*, **13**, 235–236.

Rolls, E.T. and Tovee, M.J. (1995). Sparseness of the neuronal representation of stimuli in the primate temporal visual cortex. *Journal of Neurophysiology*, **73**(2), 713–726.

Rozenblit, L., Spivey, M.J., and Wojslawowicz, J. (2002). Mechanical reasoning about gear-and-belt systems: Do eye movements predict performance? In M. Anderson, B. Meyer, and P. Olivier (eds.) *Diagrammatic representation and reasoning* (pp. 223–240). Berlin: Springer-Verlag.

Salvucci, D.D. and Anderson, J.R. (2001). Automated eye-movement protocol analysis. *Human-Computer Interaction*, **16**(1), 39–86.

Searle, J. (1980). Minds, brains, and programs. *Behavioral and Brain Sciences*, **3**(3), 417–457.

Sheliga, B.M., Riggio, L., and Rizzolatti, G. (1994). Orienting of attention and eye movements. *Experimental Brain Research*, **98**(3), 507–522.

Simon, H.A. (1975). The functional equivalence of problem solving skills. *Cognitive Psychology*, **7**(2), 268–288.

Spivey, M.J. (2007). *The continuity of mind*. Oxford: Oxford University Press.

Spivey, M.J. and Dale, R. (2006). Continuous dynamics in real-time cognition. *Current Directions in Psychological Science*, **15**(5), 207–211.

Spivey, M.J. and Geng, J.J. (2001). Oculomotor mechanisms activated by imagery and memory: Eye movements to absent objects. *Psychological Research*, **65**(4), 235–241.

Spivey, M.J., Richardson, D.C., and Fitneva, S.A. (2004). Thinking outside the brain: spatial indices to visual and linguistic information. In J.M. Henderson and F. Ferreira (eds.) *The interface of language, vision, and action: Eye movements and the visual world.* (pp. 161–189). New York, NY: Psychology Press.

Spivey, M., Grosjean, M., and Knoblich, G. (2005). Continuous attraction toward phonological competitors. *Proceedings of the National Academy of Sciences*, **102**, 10393–10398.

Spivey, M.J., Richardson, D., and Dale, R. (2009). The movement of eye and hand as a window into language and cognition. In E. Morsella, J. Bargh, and P.M. Gollwitzer (eds.) *The Psychology of Action* (Vol. 2) (pp. 225–249). New York: Oxford University Press.

Stephen, D.G., Boncoddo, R.A., Magnuson, J.S., and Dixon, J.A. (2009). The dynamics of insight: Phase transitions and entropy in mathematical discovery. *Memory and Cognition*, **37** *(8)*, 1132–1149.

Suppes, P., Cohen, M., Laddaga, R., Anliker, J., and Floyd, H. (1982). Research on eye movements in arithmetic performance. In R. Groner and P. Fraisse (eds.) *Cognition and eye movements* (pp. 57–73). North-Holland.

Theeuwes, J., Kramer, A.F., and Irwin, D.E. (in press). Attention on our mind: The role of spatial attention in visual working memory. *Acta Psychologica*. doi:10.1016/j.actpsy.2010.06.011

Thomas, L.E. and Lleras, A. (2007). Moving eyes and moving thought: On the spatial compatibility between eye movements. *Psychonomic Bulletin and Review*, **14**, 663–668.

Thomas, L.E. and Lleras, A. (2009). Covert shifts of attention function as an implicit aid to insight. *Cognition*, **111**(2), 168–174.

Vankov, I. (2009). Mind the gap: The cost of looking at nothing, or the performance implications of memory-induced attention shifts. *Proceedings of the 31st Annual Conference of the Cognitive Science Society* (pp. 1318–1323). Austin, TX: Cognitive Science Society.

Verschaffel, L., De Corte, E., and Pauwels, A. (1992). Solving compare problems: An eye movement test of Lewis and Mayer's consistency hypothesis. *Journal of Educational Psychology*, **84**(1), 85–94.

Wintermute, S. and Laird, J.E. (2008). Bimodal spatial reasoning with continuous motion. *Proceedings of the Twenty-Third AAAI Conference on Artificial Intelligence (AAAI-08)* (pp. 1331–1337). Chicago, IL: AAAI-08.

Yarbus, A. L. (1967). *Eye movements and vision*. New York: Plenum Press.

CHAPTER 31

Eye movements and change detection

James R. Brockmole and Michi Matsukura

Abstract

Despite stability in its global structure, the visual world is dynamic with respect to its local composition. Detection and appreciation of local changes to an environment are therefore important to a variety of visually-guided behaviours. In this chapter, we summarize how eye movements reveal both the failures and successes of change detection while we view our world. In terms of mechanisms, we consider the roles of low-level visual information, online scene memory, and long-term memory in change detection. Reciprocally, we describe the impact that change detection research has had on theory regarding these mechanisms.

Introduction

The visual world in which we live is a remarkably stable place. For example, each time we go to our neighbourhood park, we recognize the athletic fields, playground equipment, and pavilions as the same objects and features arranged in the same spatial configuration. Even movable objects appear in regular spatial arrangements; parents often congregate near the benches, and children's kites are in the air. Similar regularities exist at our homes, offices, gyms, churches, and grocery shops. The stability and predictability of the visual world enables observers to reduce the cognitive complexity of their environments and increase the efficiency of their behaviour (see Chun and Turk-Browne, 2008 for a thorough review and discussion). For example, a stable world can be easily re-referenced over time and, as a result, less cognitive effort needs to be devoted to the moment-to-moment storage of visual information (see Hayhoe, 2009 for a review). In addition, behaviourally-relevant information can be profitably stored in visual long-term memory for future use (see Jiang et al., 2009 for a review).

Despite stability in global scene structures across viewing encounters, the visual world is also dynamic and ever-changing with regard to its local compositions (see Fig. 31.1). While standing on a street corner, an observer may witness drastic changes in the composition of a scene including the objects in view (e.g. specific people and cars) as well as the visual properties of objects (e.g. the colour of the traffic lights, rate and direction of traffic flow, etc.). While some of these changes may be trivial to our hypothetical pedestrian, others must be appreciated in order for him or her to safely cross the street. The world's dynamic nature also means that our visual experience will not always meet our expectations or conform to our predictions. Drivers failing to stop at a red light are (fortunately) rare and unexpected but can clearly be important to one's health and well-being. Thus, the detection of changes in the environment can be as behaviourally relevant as an appreciation of the world's

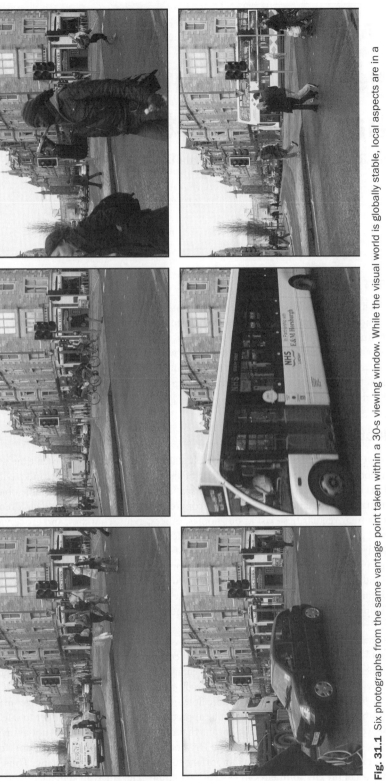

Fig. 31.1 Six photographs from the same vantage point taken within a 30-s viewing window. While the visual world is globally stable, local aspects are in a constant state of flux leading to unique and dynamically changing perceptual events.

relative stability. To vision scientists, therefore, the mechanisms by which, and the circumstances under which, changes are (and are not) detected in visual displays are important topics to study.

The use of change detection tasks to investigate the properties of visual attention and visual memory has a rich history in vision science, which is impossible to exhaustively review in this short chapter. In order to produce a succinct and tractable discussion of the mechanisms supporting change detection, in this chapter, we will restrict our discussion of the literature in two important ways. First, in keeping with the theme of this volume, we will centre our discussion on research that has combined eye movement recording and change detection tasks. Second, we will focus our discussion on studies which investigated change detection during real-world scene viewing. Of course, some commentary on research employing other paradigms and measures of change detection will be necessary, but the goal here is to summarize how eye movements—one of the most common behaviours we exhibit—reveal both the failures and successes of change detection while we view our world. This discussion is divided into three main sections which will, in turn, consider the roles of low-level visual factors, online scene memory, and long-term memory in the detection of changes in scenes.

Visual factors in change detection

The guidance of the eyes through a scene is an active process of sampling and processing the localized regions relevant to one's goals (e.g. Antes, 1974; Buswell, 1935; Hayhoe et al., 2003; Henderson et al., 2007; Henderson and Hollingworth, 1998; Mackworth and Morandi, 1967; Land et al., 1999; Torralba et al., 2006; Yarbus, 1967). However, in order to achieve a balance between the need to selectively focus on task-relevant stimuli against the need to be interrupted by other important events, such as changes in the visual world, the goal-directed control of gaze is not absolute and can be disrupted. In this section, we will describe a phenomenon known as *oculomotor capture* in which transient changes to visual displays reflexively attract gaze.

The first demonstrations of oculomotor capture concerned the effect of a suddenly appearing, but task-irrelevant, new object on gaze (Boot et al., 2005a; Godijn and Kramer, 2002, 2008; Irwin et al., 2000; Peterson et al., 2004; Theeuwes et al., 1998, 1999). For example, Theeuwes et al. (1998) presented observers with six grey circles surrounding a central fixation point. Five circles then turned red and letters were revealed in each circle. Observers were to move their eyes to the remaining grey circle and identify the letter presented within it. Critically, along with the revelation of the search target, an additional red item appeared in the display. Although this new item was never the target of search, observers' eyes moved to the onset on approximately 50% of trials. Fixations on the onset were atypically brief, suggesting that the saccade to the target was programmed, but before the eye movement could be executed to this target, the onset interrupted the goal-directed eye movement. Interestingly, observers were often unaware of this deviation. Thus, sudden changes to a visual display can influence the allocation of attention by influencing the eyes' scan pattern even when these changes are task-irrelevant and the observer is unaware of the change.

Similar oculomotor capture effects can be observed in somewhat more naturalistic situations where new objects appear in real-world scenes (Brockmole and Henderson, 2005a, 2005b, 2008; Matsukura et al., 2009). For example, while monitoring observers' eye movements, Brockmole and Henderson (2005a) added new objects to scenes after approximately 6 s of viewing. When care was taken to add the new object during a fixation (i.e. so that it was not masked by saccadic suppression), over half of the next four fixations were directed to the onset (the chance level was 11%), and approximately two-thirds of all first looks to the new object occurred with the fixation immediately following the onset. These results show that new objects can attract attention and gaze quickly and reliably in a natural scene and that oculomotor capture is not limited to simple and relatively homogeneous visual displays. Additional studies have shown that this effect is not dependent on the task-relevance of the onset (Brockmole and Henderson 2005a), the semantic identity of the new object (Brockmole and Henderson, 2008), or the visual salience of the new object within the scene (Matsukura et al., 2009). These results collectively suggest that the detection of new objects takes place independently of their semantic identification and that eye movements to scene changes under these viewing conditions may be reflexive, although stringent tests of this second conclusion have not been conducted.

While the examples of oculomotor capture discussed up to this point have involved the addition of objects to visual displays, the effect extends to other types of scene change as well. Both disappearing objects (Boot et al., 2005b; Brockmole and Henderson, 2005b) and changes to the surface features of existing objects such as their colour (Irwin et al., 2000; Matsukura et al., 2009) and luminance (Irwin et al., 2000) can also attract gaze, albeit at a somewhat lesser rate. Whereas 60% of the very first eye movements following an onset within a real-world scene are allocated to the new object, 35–40% of these saccades are allocated to those same objects following either their disappearance (Brockmole and Henderson, 2005b) or change in colour (Matsukura et al., 2009). In all of these cases, however, the majority of all first looks to the scene change occur at the observer's first opportunity to do so.

Clearly, new objects, disappearing objects, and changes to an object's surface features can attract attention swiftly, reliably, and frequently. To this point, however, we have left aside questions concerning the mechanism that underlies oculomotor capture. Why are such scene changes prioritized for viewing? In our view, a purely new-object based account (cf. Yantis, 1993, 1996, 2000; Yantis and Gibson, 1994; Yantis and Hillstrom, 1994; Yantis and Jonides, 1996) is insufficient because capture can be observed for changes that do not involve the appearance of a physically new object. Another possibility is that oculomotor capture is driven by the low-level transient motion signals that often accompany scene changes (cf., Boyce and Pollatsek, 1992; Brockmole and Henderson, 2005a; Franconeri et al., 2005). Such an explanation could account for capture by any number of scene changes. To test the validity of this possible explanation, researchers have contrasted the prioritization afforded to scene changes that occur with and without transient motion signals. To eliminate transient motion signals during scene changes, researchers have made changes either gradually (Wong et al., 2007), during brief occlusions (Franconeri et al., 2005), or during saccades which momentarily suppress visual perception (Brockmole and Henderson, 2005a, 2005b; Matsukura et al., 2009). Regardless of the methods used, the elimination of transient motion signals drastically reduces, and in some cases eliminates, the prioritization of changes within visual displays. Where prioritization is not eliminated, evidence suggests that a qualitatively different mechanism from oculomotor capture is at work. Namely, one that is less efficient, slower, and driven by observers' memory rather than a reflexive capture of attention (we will return to this *memory-guided prioritization* mechanism (Brockmole and Henderson, 2005a) in the next section).

From our discussion above, it appears that where transient motion signals are present, oculomotor capture is likely to follow. Given that the eyes are at fixation 90% of the time, most scene changes have the potential to generate transient motion signals that can be detected quite easily and quickly. The challenge of change detection arises when some visual disruption blocks these signals. Eye movements provide only one example. In a dynamic world composed of a myriad background elements, surfaces, structures, objects, and occlusions, perception of local scene elements can be frequently disrupted. In the next section, we consider change detection in the face of these visual disruptions.

Cognitive factors in change detection

The preceding section discussed change detection when low-level visual factors such as a transient motion signal can be used to signal the occurrence and location of a variety of scene changes. This section focuses on situations where such signals are absent, specifically, situations where changes occur to scenes during periods of visual disruption. We will begin by discussing the effect of relatively short disruptions (tens of milliseconds) on change detection before considering the effects of much longer disruptions (minutes or hours).

Effects of short disruptions to vision: a test of online scene memory

In this section, we discuss the effects of short disruptions to vision on change detection. We consider these short disruptions to be a challenge to online scene memory, broadly defined as an internal mental representation that is developed and maintained during the current perceptual episode. In this discussion, we are agnostic as to whether these online memory representations are limited by the capacity of a short-term or working memory storage (e.g. Irwin and Andrews, 1996), or if they also involve contributions of long-term memory (e.g. Hollingworth, 2004).

Change blindness

The line of research that is perhaps most closely associated with change detection across visual disruptions is *change blindness*, the tendency for an observer to fail to notice changes (especially unexpected ones) that are introduced to a visual display during a disruption in visual input (see Rensink, 2002; Simons, 2000; Simons and Rensink, 2005 for reviews). Anyone who has played 'spot the difference' puzzles (Fig. 31.2) in which one is to identify the few differences between two otherwise identical pictures understands this challenge (see Gajewski and Henderson, 2005 for an empirical examination of eye movements in 'spot the difference' tasks). As we look back and forth between the images, our eye movements serve to disrupt the continuity of vision. As a result, the differences between the images (which, in this case, can be considered changes to a scene across views) are difficult to detect. In fact, most observers are surprised as to how long it takes for them to notice that *anything* is different between the scenes, let alone actually locate *a* difference (see Levin et al., 2000, for discussion of some metacognitive beliefs people hold about their ability to detect changes in the visual world).

In controlled experiments, a variety of approaches have been used to demonstrate and evaluate the phenomenon of change blindness (for a different taxonomy than the one presented here, see Simons, 2000). The most common method has been to artificially occlude the observer's view of a scene during a change by using a 'flicker' or strobe-like effect which is intended to simulate blinks or eye movements. Using this method, a brief (e.g. 80-ms) blank interval is inserted between continuously alternating presentations of pre- and post-change displays on a computer screen (e.g. Rensink et al., 1997). Another approach has been to disrupt the continuity of visual input by occluding an observer's visual field in a more naturalistic way through the movement of objects (e.g. Simons and Levin, 1998) or a change in the observer's viewpoint (e.g. Levin and Simons, 1997). The third approach has been to introduce changes to a scene during a saccadic eye movement (e.g. Currie et al., 2000; Grimes, 1996; Henderson and Hollingworth, 1999; McConkie and Currie, 1996) so that saccadic suppression will serve as a naturally occurring, momentary, though subjectively imperceptible, disruption to visual input. In all three of these paradigms, the primary dependent variable is the rate (measured either in time required to localize a repeating change or the proportion of changes that are detected within a defined temporal window) with which the imposed changes are explicitly noticed by the observer.

Each of these methodological approaches has unequivocally demonstrated that colour alterations, object translations, object rotations, size scalings, object additions or deletions, and object token

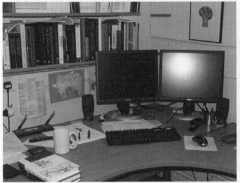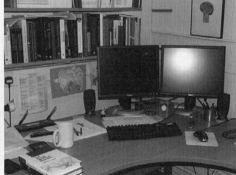

Fig. 31.2 How quickly can you locate the four differences between these two pictures?

substitutions can be missed at surprising rates—even when vision is disrupted for only tens of milliseconds during the change. For example, in Grimes' (1996) study where changes occurred during saccades, 100% of observers failed to detect a one-fourth increase in the size of a building in a city skyline, 92% failed to detect a one-third reduction in a flock of 30 birds, 58% failed to detect a change in a model's swimsuit from bright pink to bright green, 50% failed to detect two cowboys exchange their heads, and 25% failed to notice a 180° rotation of Cinderella's Castle at Disneyland! More recent work has shown that global changes to an entire scene, rather than to a single object, can also be missed when they occur during saccades. For example, shifts of scene backgrounds relative to a single saccade target are missed over 60% of the time (Currie et al., 2000), and substantial increments in a scene's luminance or contrast are missed up to 90% of the time (Henderson et al., 2008). Additionally, a shift in the position of a set of vertical occluders arranged over a scene, so that the visible portion is completely changed from one fixation to another, eludes observers' detection 97% of the time (Henderson and Hollingworth, 2003). Thus, even when every pixel in an image changes from one view to the next, massive failures in explicit detection of scene changes can be observed.

Change blindness and online scene memory

While demonstrations of change blindness are dramatic and surprising, the theoretical interpretation ascribed to them has been a subject of debate (see Hollingworth, 2008, 2009 for thorough reviews). At first blush, the systematic failure to explicitly detect such a wide array of scene changes across a variety of experimental paradigms might suggest that online visual representations of scenes are limited to the currently attended object (e.g. Rensink 2000, 2002) and that precise visual details from past views of a scene are not maintained in memory (e.g. O'Regan, 1992; O'Regan and Noe, 2001). Indeed, such an argument is consistent with an extensive literature demonstrating that little visual detail is accumulated across individual saccades (Bridgeman and Mayer, 1983; Henderson, 1997; Irwin, 1991; Irwin et al., 1983, 1988; McConkie, 1991; McConkie and Zola, 1979; O'Regan and Levy-Schoen, 1983; Rayner and Pollatsek, 1983) and that observers often resample scene regions as they become momentarily task-relevant (Ballard et al., 1995; Droll and Hayhoe, 2007; Gajewski and Henderson, 2005; Hayhoe et al., 1998; Land and Hayhoe, 2001; Triesch et al., 2003). However, evidence from change detection studies that involve eye movement recording demonstrates that change blindness is not predicated on absent, highly-limited, or low-quality online memory. By using change detection as a tool to study online scene memory, evidence gathered over the last decade has revealed a complex online memory system that supports visual behaviour. We will briefly review how the dynamics of scene viewing, the predictability of scene changes, the measurement of change detection, and the establishment of baseline rates for change detection are critical factors that one must take into account in assessing failures of change detection and the nature of online scene memory.

The dynamics of scene viewing During scene viewing, observers shift their gaze from place to place, with high-fidelity details obtained from relatively local aspects of the scene surrounding the point of fixation. Thus, the viewing history of an object may be very important in change detection. In order to detect local changes in scene features, an observer must first acquire detailed information about that area before the change takes place. Indeed, Hollingworth and Henderson (2002) showed that while changes to objects that have not yet been fixated are poorly detected (in fact, correct detections did not exceed false alarms), changes to objects that have been fixated are noticed at rates up to five times greater than false alarms (see also Grimes, 1996). Similarly, the accuracy of change detection is correlated with the distance between the scene change and the position of gaze immediately prior to the change (Grimes, 1996; Henderson and Hollingworth, 1999).

Change detection also depends on post-change viewing behaviour. In order to detect a change, the current view of the scene needs to be compared to a previous view of the scene. In order for this comparison to be successful, re-fixation on the now-changed object may be necessary. During normal unconstrained viewing, however, such re-fixation may not occur quickly. Thus, in tasks where speed of detection is taken as the measure of change blindness (e.g. the flicker paradigm), an observer's ability to detect a change may be underestimated. When change detection is examined in light of the eye movement record, however, once refixations on a post-changed object do occur, observers are quite good at detecting changes (Hollingworth and Henderson, 2002). Together, such findings indicate that high rates of change blindness can be, in part, an artefact of experimental and analytical design rather than a systemic failure to retain information about scenes in online memory.

Prediction and expectation Predictions and expectations clearly influence attentional control. For example, in visual search tasks, targets are found more readily when they appear at predictable locations (e.g. Brockmole and Henderson, 2006; Chun and Jiang, 1998; Geng and Behrmann, 2002; Walthew and Gilchrist, 2006) or times (e.g. Brady and Oliva, 2008; Fiser and Aslin, 2002; Kirkham et al., 2002). However, many of the scene changes we have described so far are arbitrary and would hardly be expected in the real world. Buildings do not change in size and people do not exchange their heads! In light of our previous discussion on the dynamics of scene viewing, any factor that influences the locus of gaze may also influence change detection. Hence, when reasonable expectations concerning changes exist, detection rates may improve.

Indeed, change detection rates are typically much improved in situations where changes are made to objects that are likely to change (e.g. the pedestrians and cars in the opening section of this chapter and Fig. 31.1). For example, Droll and colleagues (Droll et al., 2007) presented observers with object arrays in which a set of objects changed orientation across a flicker. Objects were repeatedly presented across trials and each object had either a 0%, 10%, 30%, or 60% chance of switching its orientation. Over the course of the experiment, a greater proportion of fixations and dwell time were afforded to objects undergoing frequent change. As a result, changes to these objects were detected more quickly and more often. This pattern of findings suggests that observers can determine which objects are likely to change and thereby concentrate their viewing on those objects in order to increase the likelihood that scene changes are detected. In the same vein, experience with a visual environment also leads to better detection as observers' gaze durations on changed objects are elevated in familiar scenes relative to novel ones (Karacan and Hayhoe, 2008). Thus, studies using arbitrary scene changes in unfamiliar environments may underestimate observers' ability to notice discontinuities in their visual world (see also Beck et al., 2004, 2008; Olson et al., 2005 for converging evidence from other experimental paradigms).

Implicit versus explicit awareness It is false to assume that explicit awareness provides a clear window through which to view and examine memory (Fernandez-Duque and Thornton, 2000). Even in the absence of explicit awareness, implicit measures of behaviour can reveal that a change is nevertheless detected. For example, fixations on changed objects are atypically long even when the change is 'missed' in terms of explicit report (Hayhoe et al., 1998; Henderson and Hollingworth, 2003; Hollingworth and Henderson, 2002; Hollingworth et al., 2001). To describe one result in detail, Hollingworth and colleagues (Hollingworth et al., 2001) made object-token substitutions during the first eye movement away from a critical object. Eighteen per cent of these changes were correctly reported by observers. However, among those changes that were missed in terms of explicit report, first-pass gaze durations on changed objects averaged 753 ms, relative to 419 ms on unchanged control objects. This near doubling in gaze duration reveals an implicit detection of changes, even when the changes fail to rise to conscious awareness (see also Beck et al., 2008).

Establishing baseline rates for detection To note that a particular change is missed by 100% of observers, or that it takes 30 s to detect a change, may be less of a comment on one's ability to detect changes as it is on the prominence (both visually and cognitively) of the changing object in the scene. It can be difficult to determine baseline levels of performance against which one can extract experimental effects. Undoubtedly, a set of scene changes could be created for which change detection is perfect, and likewise a set for which change blindness is absolute. For example, change blindness is reduced when changes are made to semantically informative objects (Hollingworth and Henderson, 2000) and to objects that are of central interest to observers compared to those of more marginal interest (Rensink et al., 1997). When proper baselines are established, however, there is now clear evidence that changes to scenes are *prioritized* for viewing, even as the detection rates remain modest. We turn to these studies next.

Memory-guided prioritization

In the first section of this chapter, we briefly contrasted the detection of scene changes both with and without a transient motion signal by inserting them into a scene either during a fixation or during a saccade. We noted that transient scene changes capture gaze very quickly (usually the very next fixation) and reliably (60–80% of the time). However, non-transient scene changes attract gaze more slowly and substantially less often than their transient counterparts, suggesting weaker change detection under these conditions (Brockmole and Henderson, 2005a, 2005b, 2008; Matsukura et al., 2009). For example, non-transient new objects tend to attract 30–40% of fixations immediately following their insertion into the scene while offsets attract 10–20% of fixations, and colour changes attract 25–30% of fixations. How should we interpret these values? In many respects, these values parallel those obtained in more traditional change blindness studies. Taking the probability of fixating the region of the scene change as a measure of change detection, non-transient scene changes are clearly 'missed' most of the time, and, from this, one could conclude that observers are generally blind to change. However, when one takes into account the baseline rates at which these same objects are fixated when they are constantly present in a scene and do not constitute changes, a different picture emerges. Under these baseline conditions, the critical objects in these experiments received approximately 10% of fixations. Thus, non-transient scene changes are fixated at rates two to four times what is expected by chance, indicating that they are prioritized for viewing over all other objects in the scene.

What mechanism can generate prioritization of changes in a scene in the absence of a transient motion signal? We have argued that one must appeal to memory mechanisms to account for this finding. First, we manipulated the viewing time afforded to observers prior to the appearance of a new object in a scene and have shown that reducing the viewing time prior to the appearance of a new object from 6000 ms to approximately 550 ms results in the effective elimination of prioritization (Brockmole and Henderson, 2005a). In contrast, transient onsets continue to be prioritized for viewing within this temporal window. This result is exactly predicted by the hypothesis that the prioritization of non-transient new objects is guided by scene memory built up over the course of viewing that includes object identities and details, a memory which is not required when transient motion signals accompany a change in a visual scene (see also Castelhano and Henderson, 2005; Henderson and Hollingworth, 2003; Hollingworth and Henderson, 2000, 2002; Hollingworth et al., 2001; Tatler et al., 2003).

In a second unpublished study we conducted with Walter Boot and John Henderson, we investigated the role of memory in the prioritization of non-transient scene changes using a dual-task paradigm. Observers' primary task was to study real-world scenes in which objects suddenly changed colour. Some observers additionally monitored an auditorily presented stream of digits and counted sequential item repetitions (see also Boot et al., 2005b; Boot et al., 2005; Matsukura et al., 2011) while viewing these scenes. Other observers ignored the auditory stream while viewing the scenes. In post-study recognition tests, observers in the single-task condition differentiated studied scenes and lures with 98% accuracy. For observers in the dual-task condition accuracy on the post-test was 74%. This disruption in scene memory was correlated with a disruption in change detection during the study phase. In the single-task condition, 47% of eye movements launched immediately after the colour change were directed toward the change. In the dual-task condition, this rate fell to 27%. Hence, limiting the quality of memory for a scene by reducing general attention resources has profound consequences on one's ability to detect changes within that scene when they occur during periods of brief visual disruption.

Summary comments

The body of work described above clearly shows that, when viewing the visual world around us, changes can often escape explicit visual detection. These 'failures' of change detection, however, are mediated by the temporal dynamics of visual exploration. When gaze-dependent and implicit measures of detection are employed, and when appropriate baselines for change detection are established, we see that observers are quite sensitive to changes in the visual world and, indeed, *change prioritization* can be observed. There is therefore no theoretical inconsistency between change blindness and the existence of relatively detailed online memory representations for visual information which span short delays in visual input. Even though rather robust online memory representations for scenes are generated as viewing progresses, failures of change detection can still result when changes are made to aspects of scenes that are not included in these representations. Unfortunately, due to the complexity of the visual world such failures can occur quite often. This discussion is just one example from a larger literature in which the analysis of eye movements reveals much richer mental representations of visual scenes than more traditional dependent measures such as manual response time and accuracy (see e.g. McCarley et al., 2003; Peterson et al., 2001).

What, then, explains the recursive viewing behaviours observed in real-world tasks? For example, when executing various natural actions such as comparing two pictures, making a sandwich, preparing tea, or sorting blocks, observers adopt a *just-in-time strategy* in that they only obtain and represent the minimum information needed to accomplish moment-to-moment subgoals of the action (e.g. Ballard et al, 1995; Gajewski and Henderson, 2005; Karn and Hayhoe, 2000; Land et al., 1999). For example, Karn and Hayhoe (2000) asked observers to arrange a random assortment of coloured blocks to match a model. Observers typically fixated a block in the model before picking up a block of the same colour only to then look back at the model before placing the selected block in their copy. Observers apparently only acquired colour information in the first fixation and had to re-fixate the model to obtain location information in the second fixation. Hence, in many situations, only specific momentarily relevant features of an object or scene are selectively attended and retained in memory even when the capacity of memory would clearly allow for additional future-relevant information to be encoded and retained. The degree of inconsistency between arguments for detailed online scene memory and arguments for minimal scene memory is a matter for continuing exploration. However, these positions may not be as incommensurate as one might initially suppose. A stable visual world is likely to provide a more accurate point of reference than a memory representation. Given the ease with which the world can be re-sampled, it may not be surprising that observers often behave in ways suggestive of more minimal memory representations or strategically choose to avoid the cognitive expenses associated with the encoding, maintenance, and retrieval of information in memory (see Henderson, 2008 for additional discussion).

Effects of long disruptions to vision: a test of long-term memory

The continuity of visual experience is not only broken by the short pauses associated with eye movements, blinks, and momentary visual occlusions. The environments in which humans live and work are massively large and, as a result, we cannot maintain constant perceptual contact with all aspects of the visual world. In this section, we describe studies in which changes occur between long delays in exposure to a visual scene. Because these changes span discrete perceptual experiences with a visual display, we consider them a challenge to long-term memory for scene details.

Comparing change detection across long and short delays

The first issue to consider when thinking about change detection after long disruptions to visual experience is the extent to which the duration of the disruption affects one's ability to notice changes to it. To address this question, Hollingworth and Henderson (2002) presented observers with three-dimensionally rendered illustrations of real-world scenes and tested their memory for a single critical object in each scene with a two alternative forced choice (2AFC) test. One alternative was an unaltered view of the previewed scene while the other alternative included either a change in the orientation of the critical object or an object-token substitution for the critical object. In one experiment, this memory test was given immediately after viewing each scene. In another experiment, this test was administered after viewing all of the scenes which imposed a delay of up to 30 min between preview and test. In both cases, eye movements were recorded to ensure that the critical object was fixated at least once during the preview period (see the section: 'The dynamics of scene viewing'). Astonishingly, discrimination performance was very similar in each case. When tested immediately, 87% of token discriminations and 82% of orientation discriminations were made correctly. When tested after a substantial delay (and interference from subsequently presented scenes), 81% of token discriminations and 82% of orientation discriminations were made correctly. Subsequent studies have shown that observers' sensitivity to changes of this type can remain above chance after delays of up to 24 h (Hollingworth, 2005). These results indicate that long-term memory for objects and scenes is as efficient at supporting change detection as is the online scene memory maintained during the original perceptual event.

The capacity of long-term scene memory in support of change detection

Observers are able to explicitly recognize thousands of previously novel scenes after a single exposure to them (Shepard, 1967; Standing, 1973; Standing et al., 1970). These long-term memories include global scene structure and object position information as observers are able to accurately discriminate the images they saw from mirror reversed lures in which the gist remains unchanged while visual details change (Standing et al., 1970). More recent studies have addressed the degree to which the visual details of individual objects are remembered long-term. For example, Hollingworth (2004) guided observers' eye movements through a series of scenes by asking them to follow a moving dot that shifted from object to object. After viewing each sequence, observers were tested on their memory for one of the viewed objects with a 2AFC test in which they had to discriminate a viewed object from a lure defined by an object-token substitution (observers were not aware which object would be tested during the study sequence). Not surprisingly, serial position effects were observed with increases in the number of intervening objects between the last viewed object and the tested object resulting in lesser change detection. What was surprising, however, was the modesty of these serial position effects. When the 2AFC task immediately followed fixation on the to-be-tested object, performance on this discrimination test, as measured by A' (a measure of non-parametric sensitivity where 0.5 indicates chance performance and 1.0 indicates perfect performance) was approximately 0.9. When the number of intervening objects increased to 10, A' only fell to approximately 0.85. Truly amazingly, when the number of intervening objects was increased to 402, A' still exceeded 0.75! Clearly, observers are able to discriminate fine details of objects very well even after substantial delays following their last view of those objects.

Incidental memory and change detection

In our discussion of long-term memory and change detection, we have thus far described experiments in which observers are aware that they are to detect changes in visual displays. To what extent can changes be detected in the absence of this intention? We briefly describe two studies designed to answer this question. First, Williams et al. (2005) engaged observers in a visual search task for a target item in an array of arbitrarily arranged real-world objects. In addition to the search target (e.g. a red apple), these arrays contained semantically related objects (e.g. a green apple), objects with shared visual features (e.g. a red truck), and unrelated objects (e.g. a brown stapler). During this search task, targets were fixated longer than distractors, but the related distractors were in turn fixated longer than unrelated distractors. Following the completion of the search task, observers were unexpectedly asked to perform a change-detection task using the same arrays employed in the search task. This task required observers to discriminate (through a 2AFC task) the objects presented in the search arrays from semantically-related foils. Discriminations were made for search targets as well as the semantically related and shared-feature distractors. Because observers did not know about this change-detection test in advance, it examined incidental memory for the objects in the search arrays. Discrimination accuracy mirrored the eye movement behaviour during search: Memory was graded in nature with best performance for search targets, intermediate performance for the related distractors, and worst performance for unrelated distractors.

In a second study, Castelhano and Henderson (2005) directly compared change detection ability following intentional (memorization) and incidental (search) using real-world scenes. Following these tasks, memory for objects in the scenes was tested with a 2AFC task in which the objects presented in the scenes had to be discriminated from object-token substitutions and mirror reversals (this analysis was again confined to objects fixated during the memorization and search tasks). As in Williams et al. (2005), change detection accuracy in both intentional and incidental conditions was above chance. What is more striking was that discrimination accuracy of previously viewed objects and object changes did not vary as a function of the prior task. In combination with the results described above, these studies demonstrate that accurate change detection (as measured via discrimination of previously viewed objects and lures that alter the visual features of previous objects) can be achieved even when observers do not intentionally attempt to remember the details of their visual world.

Change detection and contextual cueing

Throughout this chapter, we have described the degree to which observers are able to detect changes to specific objects within otherwise stable visual environments. In doing so, we have implicitly treated the stability of the visual world as a hindrance to performance. In the penultimate discussion of this section, we return to a point we made at the outset of this chapter: The stability of the visual world enables observers to *increase* the efficiency of many behaviours because task-relevant information can be profitably stored in visual long-term memory. One example of this is a phenomenon known as *contextual cueing*—a process by which visual search becomes progressively faster as specific arrangements of target and distractor items are repeatedly encountered (Chun and Jiang, 1998). For example, a can of beans is much easier to find in our local (familiar) grocery shop than in one we are visiting for the first time. It is important to ask what information in long-term memory is functional in guiding attention to known locations. One method of investigating this is to determine the effects of various unexpected alterations of the information available in a once-familiar display (e.g. Brady and Oliva, 2008; Brockmole and Henderson, 2006b; Brockmole and Võ, 2010; Brockmole et al., 2006; Crist et al., 1997; Ehinger and Brockmole, 2008; Jiang and Song, 2005; Jiang and Wagner, 2004; Turk-Browne and Scholl, 2009). Here, we discuss one of these studies that contrasted the role of a scene's basic-level category membership with its specific arrangement of visual properties in contextual cueing.

Brockmole and Henderson (2006b) showed observers photographs of scenes that contained arbitrarily positioned target letters. A subset of these scenes were repeated throughout the experiment. Because the target was consistently located in the same position with each repetition of a scene, target locations could be associated with scene content (Brockmole and Henderson, 2006a). As this association developed, search times for the target improved as the number of fixations and the total amplitude of eye movements required to find the target decreased (see also Peterson and Kramer, 2001). Learned scenes were then unexpectedly mirror reversed, which spatially translated visual features as well as the target across the display while preserving the scene's identity and concept. Mirror reversals produced a search cost as the eyes initially moved toward the position in the display in which the target had previously appeared, suggesting that the scene change was not detected by observers. The cost did not completely erase the benefits of learning, however; when initial search failed to locate the target, the eyes were quickly directed to the target's new position, which is a correction that could only be made if the change was subsequently detected. These results suggest that contextual cueing operates in real-world scenes by at least two recognition processes. First, the identity of the scene is recognized without reference to the specific arrangement of visual features.

Then, subsequent shifts are guided by more detailed information regarding scene and object layout. Interestingly, though, such additional information may not be used unless recognition of scene identity alone fails. More recent work suggests that the influences of identity and local detail cannot be entirely decoupled and that both levels of analysis interact to determine the deployment of attention (Brooks et al., 2010). Even if prior arguments for sequential influences (Brockmole et al., 2006) are relaxed, however, a bias to deploy attention according to scene identity persists (Brockmole and Vō, 2010; Brockmole et al., 2006; Brooks, et al., 2010; Ehinger and Brockmole, 2008) and may be a contributing factor in failures of change detection.

Summary comments

The work summarized in this section illustrates how long-term memory can be used in the service of change detection. Observers are able to discriminate current views of the world to previously experienced views accurately and as well as with online scene memory. Even after a single exposure to a scene and a delay of 24 h before test, observers are able to detect small changes in object details such as their orientation in the scene at above-chance levels. What is more startling is that this ability does not require intentional memorization of the scene on the part of the observer. Thus, observers are able to remember not only what scenes they've seen before but also many of the details of the objects within those scenes. Despite this ability, however, the guidance of attention through familiar scenes appears to be first guided by more semantic level memory representations as the functionality of more detailed object memory becomes apparent as viewing progresses.

Conclusion

In this chapter, we considered visual and cognitive mechanisms that underlie the detection of changes in real-world scenes. Considering visual factors, we have seen how display changes can be detected with high probability and rapidity when they are accompanied by transient motion signals that reveal the change. When these signals are eliminated by virtue of some disruption in visual continuity (such as an eye movement), change detection suffers dramatically. A great deal of investigation has been devoted to interpreting this 'change blindness' that occurs across visual disruptions. We have argued that a variety of factors are important in the detection of change including the temporal dynamics of scene viewing and the manner in which change detection is measured. Indeed, we have shown that when these factors are taken into account, change detection performance can be quite good and that changes are often prioritized for viewing. These results indicate that rather robust on-line memory representations for scenes are generated as viewing progresses, and that change detection failures occur when changes involve aspects of scenes that fall outside of these online memory representations (which, due to the complexity of the visual world, can occur quite often). We have also shown how change detection research has shed light on the properties of robust and detailed long-term memories for scenes. These long-term memories have a high capacity and support accurate change detection even after substantial delays and even when observers have no intension to memorize visual displays. In conclusion, the work we have reviewed throughout this chapter indicates that even though the global stability of the world serves as an external memory resource that can be re-sampled, by maintaining internal representations of the world—both online during scene viewing and in a long-term store after a viewing episode ends—local variability in visually and cognitively prominent aspects of the world can be detected and acted upon, if necessary.

References

Antes, J.R. (1974). The time course of picture viewing. *Journal of Experimental Psychology*, **103**, 62–70.

Ballard, D., Hayhoe, M., and Pelz, J. (1995). Memory representations in natural tasks. *Cognitive Neuroscience*, **7**, 66–80.

Beck, M.R., Angelone, B.L., and Levin, D.T. (2004). Knowledge about the probability of change affects change detection performance. *Journal of Experimental Psychology: Human Perception and Performance*, **30**, 778–791.

Beck, M.R., Angelone, B.L., Levin, D.T., Peterson, M.S., and Varakin, D.A. (2008). Implicit learning fro probably changes in a visual change detection task. *Consciousness and Cognition* **17**, 778–791.

Boot, W.R., Kramer, A.F., and Peterson, M.S. (2005a). Oculomotor consequences of abrupt object onsets and offsets: Onsets dominate oculomotor capture. *Perception and Psychophysics*, **67**, 910–928.

Boot, W.R., Brockmole, J.R., and Simons, D.J. (2005b). Attention capture is modulated in dual-task situations. *Psychonomic Bulletin and Review*, **12**, 662–668.

Boyce, S.J. and Pollatsek, A. (1992). Identification of objects in scenes: The role of scene background in object naming. *Journal of Experimental Psychology: Learning, Memory, and Cognition*, **18**, 531 543.

Bridgeman, B. and Mayer, M. (1983). Failure to integrate visual information from successive fixations. *Bulletin of the Psychonomic Society*, **21**, 285–286.

Brady, T.R. and Oliva, A. (2008). Statistical learning using real-world scenes: Extracting categorical regularities without conscious intent. *Psychological Science*, **19**, 678–685.

Brockmole, J.R., and Henderson, J.M (2005a). Prioritization of new objects in real-world scenes: Evidence from eye movements. Journal of Experimental Psychology: *Human Perception and Performance*, **31**, 857–868.

Brockmole, J.R., and Henderson, J.M. (2005b). Object appearance, disappearance, and attention prioritization in real-world scenes. *Psychonomic Bulletin and Review*, **12**, 1061–1067.

Brockmole, J.R., and Henderson, J.M. (2006a). Using real-world scenes as contextual cues for search. *Visual Cognition*, **13**, 99–108.

Brockmole, J.R., and Henderson, J.M. (2006b). Recognition and attention guidance during contextual cueing in real-world scenes: Evidence from eye movements. *Quarterly Journal of Experimental Psychology*, **59**, 1177–1187.

Brockmole, J.R., and Henderson, J.M. (2008). Prioritizing new objects for eye fixation in real-world scenes: Effects of object-scene consistency. *Visual Cognition*, **16**, 375–390.

Brockmole, J.R. and Võ, M.L.-H. (2010). Semantic memory for contextual regularities within and across scene categories: Evidence from eye movements. *Attention, Perception, and Psychophysics*, **72**, 1803–1813.

Brockmole, J.R., Castelhano, M.S., and Henderson, J.M. (2006). Contextual cueing in naturalistic scenes: Global and local contexts. *Journal of Experimental Psychology: Learning, Memory, and Cognition*, **32**, 699–706.

Brooks, D.I., Rasmussen, I.P., and Hollingworth, A. (2010). The nesting of search contexts within natural scenes: Evidence from contextual cuing. *Journal of Experimental Psychology: Human Perception and Performance*, **36**(6), 1406–1418.

Buswell, G.T. (1935). *How people look at pictures.* Chicago: University of Chicago Press.

Castelhano, M.S. and Henderson, J.M., (2005). Incidental visual memory for objects in scenes. *Visual Cognition*, **12**, 1017–1040.

Chun, M.M. and Jiang, Y. (1998). Contextual cueing: Implicit learning and memory of visual context guides spatial attention. *Cognitive Psychology*, **36**, 28–71.

Chun, M.M. and Turk-Browne, N.B. (2008). Associative learning mechanisms in vision. In S. Luck and A. Hollingworth (eds.) *Visual memory* (pp. 209–246). Oxford: Oxford University Press.

Crist, R.E., Kapadia, M.K., Westheimer, G., and Gilbert, C.D. (1997). Perceptual learning of spatial localization: Specificity for orientation, position, and context. *Journal of Neurophysiology*, **78**, 2889–2894.

Currie, C., McConkie, G., Carlson-Radvansky, L.A., and Irwin, D.E. (2000). The role of the saccade target object in the perception of a visually stable world. *Perception and Psychophysics*, **62**, 673–683.

Droll, J. and Hayhoe, M. (2007) Trade-offs between working memory and gaze. *Journal of Experimental Psychology: Human Perception and Performance*, **33**(6), 1352–1365.

Droll, J., Hayhoe, M. and Gigone, K. (2007) Learning where to direct gaze during change detection. *Journal of Vision*, **7**(14), 6.1–12.

Ehinger, K.A. and Brockmole, J.R. (2008). The role of color in visual search in real-world scenes: Evidence from contextual cueing. *Perception and Psychophysics*, **70**, 1366–1378.

Fernandez-Duque, D., and Thornton, I.M. (2000). Change detection without awareness: Do explicit reports underestimate the representation of change in the visual system? *Visual Cognition*, **7**, 323–344.

Fiser, J. and Aslin, R.N. (2002). Statistical learning of higher-order temporal structure from visual shape sequences. *Journal of Experimental Psychology: Learning, Memory, and Cognition*, **28**, 458–467.

Franconeri, S.L., Hollingworth, A., and Simons, D.J. (2005). Do new objects capture attention? *Psychological Science*, **16**, 275–281.

Gajewski, D.A. and Henderson, J.M. (2005). Minimal use of working memory in a scene comparison task. *Visual Cognition*, **12**, 979–1002.

Geng, J.J. and Behrmann, M. (2002). Probability cuing of target location facilitates visual search implicitly in normal participants and patients with hemispatial neglect. *Psychological Science*, **13**, 520–525.

Godijn, R. and Kramer, A.F. (2002). Oculomotor capture and inhibition of return: Evidence for an oculomotor suppression account of IOR. *Psychological Research*, **66**, 234–246.

Godijn, R. and Kramer, A.F. (2008). Oculomotor capture by surprising onsets. *Visual Cognition*, **16**, 279–298.

Grimes, J. (1996). On the failure to detect changes in scenes across saccades. In K. Atkins (ed.), *Vancouver studies in cognitive science* (Vol. 5) (pp. 89–110). New York: Oxford University Press.

Hayhoe, M.M. (2009). Visual memory in motor planning and action. In J.R. Brockmole (ed.) *The Visual World in Memory* (pp. 117–139). Hove: Psychology Press.

Hayhoe, M., Bensinger, D., and Ballard, D. (1998). Task constraints in visual working memory. *Vision Research*, **38**, 125–137.

Hayhoe, M.M., Shrivastava, A., Mruczek, R., and Pelz, J.B. (2003). Visual memory and motor planning in a natural task. *Journal of Vision*, **3**, 49–63.

Henderson, J.M. (1997). Transsaccadic memory and integration during real-world object identification. *Psychological Science*, **8**, 51–55.

Henderson, J.M. (2008). Eye movements and visual memory. In S. Luck and A. Hollingworth (eds.) *Visual memory* (pp. 87–121). Oxford: Oxford University Press.

Henderson, J.M. and Hollingworth, A. (1998). Eye movements during scene viewing: An overview. In G Underwood (Ed.), *Eye guidance while reading and while watching dynamic scenes.* (pp. 269–293). Oxford: Elsevier.

Henderson, J.M. and Hollingworth, A. (1999). The role of fixation position in detecting scene changes across saccades. *Psychological Science*, **10**, 438–443.

Henderson, J.M. and Hollingworth, A. (2003). Eye movements and visual memory: Detecting changes to saccade targets in scenes. *Perception and Psychophysics*, **65**, 58–71.

Henderson, J.M., Brockmole, J.R., and Gajewski, D.A. (2008). Differential detection of global luminance and contrast changes across saccades and flickers during active scene perception. *Vision Research*, **48**, 16–29.

Henderson, J.M., Brockmole, J.R., Castelhano, M.S., and Mack, M. (2007). Visual saliency does not account for eye movements during visual search in real-world scenes. In R. van Gompel, M. Fischer, W. Murray, and R. Hill (eds.) *Eye movements: A window on mind and brain* (pp. 537–562). Oxford: Elsevier.

Hollingworth, A. (2004). Constructing visual representations of natural scenes: The roles of short- and long-term visual memory. *Journal of Experimental Psychology: Human Perception and Performance*, **30**, 519–537.

Hollingworth, A. (2005). The relationship between online visual representation of a scene and long-term scene memory. *Journal of Experimental Psychology: Learning, Memory, and Cognition*, **31**, 396–411.

Hollingworth, A. (2008). Visual memory for natural scenes. In S. Luck and A. Hollingworth (eds.) *Visual memory* (pp. 123–162). Oxford: Oxford University Press.

Hollingworth, A. (2009). Memory for real-world scenes. In J.R. Brockmole (ed.) *The Visual World in Memory* (pp. 89–116). Hove: Psychology Press.

Hollingworth, A. and Henderson, J.M. (2000). Semantic informativeness mediates the detection of changes in natural scenes. *Visual Cognition*, **7**, 213–235.

Hollingworth, A. and Henderson, J.M. (2002). Accurate visual memory for previously attended objects in natural scenes. *Journal of Experimental Psychology: Human Perception and Performance*, **28**, 113–136.

Hollingworth, A., Williams, C.C., and Henderson, J.M. (2001). To see and remember: Visually specific information is retained in memory from previously attended objects in natural scenes. *Psychonomic Bulletin and Review*, **8**, 761–768.

Irwin, D.E. (1991). Information integration across saccadic eye movements. *Cognitive Psychology*, **23**, 420–456.

Irwin, D.E. and Andrews, R. (1996). Integration and accumulation of information across saccadic eye movements. In T. Inui and J.L. McClelland (eds.) *Attention and Performance XVI: Information Integration in Perception and Communication*. Cambridge, MA: MIT Press.

Irwin, D.E., Yantis, S., and Jonides, J. (1983). Evidence against visual integration across saccadic eye movements. *Perception and Psychophysics*, **34**, 49–57.

Irwin, D.E., Brown, J.S., and Sun, J.S. (1988). Visual masking and visual integration across saccadic eye movements. *Journal of Experimental Psychology: General*, **117**, 276–287.

Irwin, D.E., Colcombe, A.M., Kramer, A.F., and Hahn, S. (2000). Attentional and oculomotor capture by onset, luminance and color singletons. *Vision Research*, **40**, 1443–1458.

Jiang, Y.V. and Song, J.-H. (2005). Hyperspecificity in visual implicit learning: Learning of spatial layout is contingent on item identity. *Journal of Experimental Psychology: Human Perception and Performance*, **31**, 1439–1448.

Jiang, Y.V. and Wagner, L.C. (2004). What is learned in spatial contextual cuing—configuration or individual locations? *Perception and Psychophysics*, **66**, 454–463.

Jiang, Y.V., Makovski, T., and Shim, W.M. (2009). Memory for features, conjunctions, objects, and locations. In J. R. Brockmole (ed.) *The Visual World in Memory* (pp. 33–65). Hove: Psychology Press.

Karacan, H. and Hayhoe, M. (2008). Is attention drawn to changes in familiar scenes? *Visual Cognition*, **16**, 346–374.

Karn, K. and Hayhoe, M. (2000). Memory representations guide targeting eye movements in a natural task. *Visual Cognition*, **7**, 673–704.

Kirkham, N.Z., Slemmer, J.A., and Johnson, S.P. (2002). Visual statistical learning in infancy: Evidence for a domain general learning mechanism. *Cognition*, **83**, B35–B42.

Land, M. and Hayhoe, M. (2001). In what ways do eye movements contribute to everyday activities? *Vision Research*, **41**, 3559–3566.

Land, M., Mennie, N., and Rusted, J. (1999). The roles of vision and eye movements in the control of activities of daily living. *Perception*, **28**, 1311–1328.

Levin, D.T. and Simons, D.J. (1997). Failure to detect changes to attended objects in motion pictures. *Psychonomic Bulletin and Review*, **4**, 501–506.

Levin, D.T., Momen, N., Drivdahl, S.B., and Simons, D.J. (2000). Change blindness blindness: The metacognitive error of overestimating change-detection ability. *Visual Cognition*, 7, 397–412.

Mackworth, N.H., and Morandi, A.J. (1967). The gaze selects informative details within pictures. *Perception and Psychophysics*, 2, 547–552.

Matsukura, M., Brockmole, J.R., and Henderson, J.M. (2009). Overt attentional prioritization of new objects and feature changes during real-world scene viewing. *Visual Cognition*, 17, 835–855

Matsukura, M., Brockmole, J.R., Boot, W.R., and Henderson, J.M. (2011). Oculomotor capture during real-world scene viewing depends on cognitive load. *Vision Research*, 51, 546–552.

McCarley, J.S., Wang, R.F., Kramer, A.F., Irwin, D.E., and Peterson, M.S. (2003). How much memory does oculomotor search have? *Psychological Science*, 14, 422–426.

McConkie, G.W. (1991). Perceiving a stable visual world. In J. van Rensbergen, M. Deuijver, and G. d'Ydewalle (eds.) *Proceedings of the Sixth European Conference on Eye Movements* (pp. 5–7). Leuven, Belgium: Laboratory of Experimental Psychology.

McConkie, G.W. and Currie, C.B. (1996). Visual stability across saccades while viewing complex pictures. *Journal of Experimental Psychology: Human Perception and Performance*, 22, 563–581.

McConkie, G.W. and Zola, D. (1979). Is visual information integrated across successive fixations in reading? *Perception and Psychophysics*, 25, 221–224.

O'Regan, J.K. (1992) Solving the 'real' mysteries of visual perception: The world as an outside memory. *Canadian Journal of Psychology* 46, 461–488.

O'Regan, J.K. and Levy-Schoen, A. (1983). Integrating visual information from successive fixations: Does trans-saccadic fusion exist? *Vision Research*, 23, 765–768.

O'Regan, J.K. and Noe, A. (2001). A sensorimotor account of vision and visual consciousness. *Behavioral and Brain Sciences*, 24, 939–1011.

Peterson, M.S. and Kramer, A.F. (2001) Attentional guidance of the eyes by contextual information and abrupt onsets. *Perception and Psychophysics*, 63, 1239–1249.

Peterson, M.S., Kramer, A.F., and Irwin, D.E. (2004). Covert shifts of attention precede involuntary eye movements. *Perception and Psychophysics*, 66, 398–405.

Peterson, M.S., Kramer, A.F., Wang, R.F., Irwin, D.E., McCarley, J.S. (2001). Visual search has memory. *Psychological Science*, 12, 287–292.

Rayner, K. and Pollatsek, A. (1983). Is visual information integrated across saccades? *Perception and Psychophysics*, 34, 39–48.

Rensink, R.A. (2000). The dynamic representation of scenes. *Visual Cognition*, 7, 17–42.

Rensink, R.A. (2002). Change detection. *Annual Review of Psychology*, 53, 245–277.

Rensink, R.A., O'Regan, J.K., and Clark, J.J. (1997). To see or not to see: The need for attention to perceive changes in scenes. *Psychological Science*, 8, 368–373.

Shepard, R.N. (1967). Recognition memory for words, sentences, and pictures. *Journal of Verbal Learning and Verbal Behavior*, 6, 156–163.

Simons, D.J. (2000). Current approaches to change blindness. *Visual Cognition*, 7, 1–16.

Simons, D.J., and Levin, D.T. (1998). Failure to detect changes to people during real-world interaction. *Psychonomic Bulletin and Review*, 5, 644–649.

Simons, D.J., and Rensink, R.A. (2005). Change blindness: Past, present, and future. *Trends in Cognitive Sciences*, 9, 16–20.

Standing, L. (1973). Learning 10,000 pictures. *Quarterly Journal of Experimental Psychology*, 25, 207–222.

Standing, L., Conezio, J., and Haber, R.N. (1970). Perception and memory for pictures: Single-trial learning of 2500 visual stimuli. *Psychonomic Science*, 19, 73–74.

Talter, B.W., Gilchrist, I.D., and Rusted, J. (2003). The time course of abstract visual representation. *Perception*, 32, 579–592.

Theeuwes, J., Kramer, A.F., Hahn, S., and Irwin, D.E. (1998). Our eyes do not always go where we want them to go: Capture of the eyes by new objects. *Psychological Science*, 9, 379–385.

Theeuwes, J., Kramer, A.F., Hahn, S., Irwin, D.E., and Zelinsky, G.J. (1999). Influence of attentional capture on oculomotor control. *Journal of Experimental Psychology: Human Perception and Performance*, 25, 1595–1608.

Torralba, A., Oliva, A., Castelhano, M.S., and Henderson, J.M. (2006). Contextual guidance of eye movements and attention in real-world scenes: The role of global features in object search. *Psychological Review*, 113, 766–786.

Triesch, J., Ballard, D., Hayhoe, M., and Sullivan, B. (2003). What you see is what you need. *Journal of Vision*, 3, 86–94.

Turk-Browne, N.B., and Scholl, B.J. (2009). Flexible visual statistical learning: Transfer across space and time. *Journal of Experimental Psychology: Human Perception and Performance*, 35, 195–202.

Walthew, C. and Gilchrist, I.D. (2006). Target location probability effects in visual search: An effect of sequential dependencies. *Journal of Experimental Psychology: Human Perception and Performance*, 32, 1294–1301.

Williams, C.C., Henderson, J.M., and Zacks, R.T. (2005). Incidental visual memory for targets and distractors in visual search. *Perception and Psychophysics*, 67, 816–827.

Wong, J.H., Peterson, M.S., and Hillstrom, A.P. (2007). Are changes in semantic and structural information sufficient for oculomotor capture? *Journal of Vision*, 7(12), 1 10.

Yantis, S. (1993). Stimulus-driven capture and attentional control settings. *Journal of Experimental Psychology: Human Perception and Performance*, **19**, 676–681.

Yantis, S. (1996). Attentional capture in vision. In A. Kramer, M. Coles, and G. Logan (eds.) *Converging operations in the study of selective visual attention* (pp. 45–76). Washington, DC: American Psychological Association.

Yantis, S. (2000). Goal-directed and stimulus-driven determinants of attentional control. In S. Monsell and J. Driver (eds.) *Attention and Performance* (Vol. 18) (pp. 73–103). Cambridge, MA: MIT Press.

Yantis, S., and Gibson, B.S. (1994). Object continuity in motion perception and attention. *Canadian Journal of Experimental Psychology*, **48**, 182–204.

Yantis, S., and Hillstrom, A.P. (1994). Stimulus-driven attentional capture: Evidence from equiluminant visual objects. *Journal of Experimental Psychology: Human Perception and Performance*, **20**, 95 107.

Yantis, S., and Jonides, J. (1996). Attentional capture by abrupt visual onsets: New perceptual objects or visual masking? *Journal of Experimental Psychology: Human Perception and Performance*, **22**, 1505–1513.

Yarbus, A.L. (1967). *Eye movements and vision*. New York: Plenum Press.

CHAPTER 32

Eye movements and memory

Matthew S. Peterson and Melissa R. Beck

Abstract

Compared to other techniques used to study memory, recording eye movements can be relatively unobtrusive. In addition, recording eye movements also allows the investigator to ask questions that might not be answerable using conventional behavioural methods. In this chapter we present a brief history of the use of eye movement techniques to study scene memory and memory during visual search and discuss the theoretical frameworks that attempt to explain the interactions between attention, eye movements, and memory.

Eye movements and memory

At first glance, using eye movements to study memory might not seem like an obvious method to use—after all, wouldn't it be more efficient to simply ask individuals whether or not they remembered or recognized something that they had encountered earlier? But, as we shall see, eye movements allow us to explore questions about scene memory that are not readily available using other methods. For example, in a visual search experiment, in which the task is to determine whether or which target is present, a potential problem with manual responses is that they are indirect measures, and as indirect measures, there is the potential for processes other than search to drive the responses. The advantage of using eye movements is that because a covert shift of attention seemingly precedes an eye movement to the target of a saccade, eye movements can serve as a more direct measure of attentional shifts than manual responses (Deubel and Schneider, 1996; Henderson, 1992; Henderson and Hollingworth, 1999; Henderson et al., 1989; Hoffman and Subramaniam, 1995; Irwin and Gordon, 1998; Kowler et al., 1995; Peterson et al., 2004; Rayner et al., 1978). In addition, when properly designed, eye movement experiments allow attention to be tracked on an item-by-item basis. Therefore, eye tracking allows us to answer questions that are more difficult, if not sometimes impossible, to explore using traditional behavioural measures.

Eye movements and memory in change detection

Eye tracking has been used to study memory in tasks that involve intentional encoding and maintenance of information in memory (e.g. change detection tasks) and in tasks that do not necessarily involve intentional memory strategies (e.g. visual search tasks). First we will examine research employing eye movement methodology to change detection tasks as a way to investigate what is remembered across fixations (transsaccadic memory), what and how much is encoded into short-term memory (STM) and long-term memory (LTM), and when information from LTM is available for retrieval into STM or available to affect eye movement patterns without awareness. Later in this chapter, we will examine the use of eye movement methodology to investigate the roles of prospective and retrospective memory, memory for where and what in visual search, and the role of executive working memory in visual search tasks.

Transsaccadic memory

Traditionally it was thought that during each fixation, a complete visual representation was formed that was then combined with the next fixation to maintain a seamless representation of a scene (Jonides et al., 1982; McConkie and Rayner, 1975). However, recent research using measures of eye movements during change detection tasks suggests that the information retained from one fixation to the next is much less detailed than previously thought, and may contain predominantly information about the location of items in the scene (Henderson and Hollingworth, 1999; Henderson and Hollingworth, 2003; Henderson and Siefert, 2001).

Although, complete visual details are not maintained across fixations, the location and some identity information of the saccade target is maintained. Henderson and Hollingworth (1999) examined the role of memory for the saccade target using a change detection task in which the target of a saccade would either rotate or disappear. When the saccade target was deleted during the saccade, change detection rates were high, suggesting that memory for the presence of an object at the intended fixation location is maintained between fixations. Furthermore, the rate of detecting deletions of objects at the saccade target location was much higher than the rate of detecting object rotations, demonstrating that the location of the target object is maintained in memory across saccades more so than the visual detail of the target object. This is consistent with a study by McConkie and Zola (1979) in which while reading a sentence, participants rarely noticed that the case of every letter changed during each saccade. Together these results support the conclusion that the information retained across fixations includes the location of the saccade target object but not necessarily specific visual details of the target object.

Short-term memory

Change detection tasks have become the most popular methodology for examining visual memory across short retention intervals (see Luck, 2008), and monitoring eye movements during change detection tasks has proved to be instrumental in developing theories about STM (Beck et al., 2007; Henderson and Hollingworth, 1999; Hollingworth and Henderson, 2002; Chapter 31 this volume). In the typical change detection task a change occurs to a previously viewed scene during a brief disruption or a saccade. Participants' ability to detect the visual change is a measure of what was encoded and maintained in memory.

There are several stages of processing necessary for change detection to occur. The pre-change state of the object must be attended and encoded into memory. This representation must be maintained until the post-change information is attended. The pre-change information must then be available for comparison with the post-change information. Finally the results of the comparison process must be available to conscious awareness for a correct response to be given. A failure of processing at any of these stages could result in a failure to detect the change. In typical change detection tasks, it is difficult to determine at which stage the processing failure occurred when participants fail to detect the change. However, by tracking participants' eye movements during change detection tasks and by using saccade contingent techniques for timing the change, significant progress has been made in determining what types of failures contribute to change blindness.

The phenomenon of change blindness has been used to argue that nothing or only the most recently attended object is maintained in memory (O'Regan, 1992; O'Regan and Noë, 2001). However, this view has largely been unsupported by the research. Rather, it is generally agreed that up to three to four objects can be maintained in STM (Beck and Levin, 2003; Luck and Vogel, 1997; Pashler, 1988; Phillips, 1974; Simons, 1996). The locus of attention during scene viewing is a strong predictor of which objects in a scene are encoded into memory. Therefore, tracking participant's eye movements during change detection tasks has been a useful method for determining how attention during scene viewing is related to memory for visual information (Beck et al., 2007; Henderson and Hollingworth, 1999; Hollingworth and Henderson, 2002; Gajewski and Henderson, 2005). Beck et al. (2007) reported that the proportion of fixations on the pre-change region was higher for accurately detected changes than for missed changes. Therefore, the tendency to spend more time attending to the pre-change region leads to an increased probability of accurate change detection, presumably through increased encoding of the attended items.

Although attending to an object before the change is a strong predictor of change detection performance, changes to previously attended objects can be missed if the changed feature of the object is not encoded. This means that change detection tasks can be used to examine what information about an object is most likely to be encoded while the object is fixated. Henderson and Hollingworth (1999) measured change detection for object deletions and object rotations that occurred after the object had been previously fixated. Participants detected deletions at a high rate—much higher than target rotations. This suggests that during fixations, location information is more accurately encoded and maintained in memory compared to other types of information about the objects. This is consistent with what Beck et al. (2006a) found in a visual search task where changes to previously examined items were made (this is covered in more detail later in the chapter). If a previously examined item moved to a new location, participants were much more likely to refixate the item than if it changed identity. This demonstrates that participants were using memory for previously examined locations to guide eye movements and not using memory for previously examined identities. Therefore, attention to an object is necessary for encoding, and it appears that location information is more likely to be encoded and/or maintained in memory than identity information regardless of task demands (intentionally looking for changes or searching for a target).

Although it is generally agreed that attention to an object leads to the encoding of information about the object in STM, there is some debate about how many encoded objects are maintained in STM. Some theories argue that three to four items are maintained and as additional information is attended, information in STM is transferred into LTM (Hollingworth and Henderson, 2002). For example, Hollingworth and Henderson (2002) demonstrated that change detection performance remained above chance even when up to nine fixations intervened between when the change occurred and the last fixation on the object before the change. Other research suggests that only the information immediately needed for a task is maintained in STM. The later proposal is termed the 'just-in-time approach' to maintaining information in STM (Ballard et al., 1995; Droll and Hayhoe, 2007). Evidence to support the just-in-time approach has come primarily from interactive block sorting tasks, where the participant's task is to select bricks based on the value of a particular feature (e.g. the colour of the brick), and then to sort the bricks either based on the same feature or on a different feature (e.g. the width of the brick). During this sorting task, changes are occasionally made to the features of the brick being sorted. Eye movement data and change detection performance indicate that participants are only storing the information immediately needed for the task, and when additional information is needed, a fixation is made to the object to obtain the current task relevant information (this also provides evidence that people remember the locations, rather than the details of an object). Other research has supported the just-in-time approach using a spot-the-difference task (Gajewski and Henderson, 2005). This task is different from the traditional change detection task in that the images are presented simultaneously side-by-side rather than sequentially. Participants' eye movement patterns revealed that instead of encoding several items into memory from one image, participants encoded and compared one item at a time. This suggests that although participants may be able to store several items in STM they often prefer to only store what is needed. Again, this data suggests that although subjects may not have remembered all of the visual properties of the objects, they still remembered their locations and were able to successfully saccade back to the items.

Not only is it necessary to fixate (attend to) the pre-change object in order to detect a change, but it also appears to be necessary to fixate the post-change object (Beck et al., 2007; Hollingworth and Henderson, 2002). Beck et al. (2004) demonstrated that probable changes to objects (e.g. a lamp changing from on to off) are more likely to be detected than improbable changes to objects (e.g. a blue lamp changing into a green lamp). Beck et al. (2007) examined the stage at which the bias toward probable object changes occurred by monitoring participants' eye movements during the change detection task. The pattern of eye movements revealed that probable and improbable change objects were attended equally in the pre-change scene, demonstrating that probable change objects were not preferentially encoded. As expected both probable and improbable changes were attended for long durations in the post-change scene when a change was accurately detected. Detecting the change naturally leads to longer fixations; therefore, to accurately measure a bias during the retrieval/comparison process toward probable change objects, they examined fixation durations on trials when the participants failed to report the change. On these trials, participants fixated the probable change objects for longer durations than the improbable change objects. This demonstrates that changes that are more likely to be detected, are also more likely to be attended after the change. The tendency for observers to fixate a change object after the change when a change is accurately detected may be due to retrieval and comparison processes that are only possible once the post-change region has been fixated (Henderson et al., 2003) or it may be only necessary for confirmation of a change before a response is given (Parker, 1978; Zelinsky, 2001). This suggests that change detection requires not only attention to the pre-change feature, but attention to the post-change features as well.

Tracking eye movements in order to identify the locus of attention becomes more complicated when visual information is processed holistically. For example, the pattern of eye movements during a face change detection task is not necessarily related to change detection ability. Changes to own-race faces are generally detected faster than changes to other-race faces (Humphreys et al., 2005), suggesting that attention is preferentially directed to own-race faces. Hirose and Hancock (2007) examined this hypothesis by tracking participants' eye movements during a change detection task where own-race or cross-race faces changed identity. Although own-race face changes were detected more frequently than other-race face changes, there was no difference in the number or duration of fixations on own-race versus other-race faces. In contrast, chess experts detect meaningful changes to chess patterns more readily than novices, but they make fewer fixations while viewing the chess array and tend to focus in the centre of several pieces rather than on individual pieces (Reingold et al., 2001). Therefore, although tracking eye movements is a useful tool for determining the locus of attention during online viewing, it does not necessarily tell us what type of processing is occurring or what information about the attended object is being encoded during a fixation on an object.

Long-term memory

Examining eye movements is not only useful for investigating what is stored in STM but also for investigating what information is stored and retrieved from LTM. For example, Nelson and Loftus (1980) examined the role of fixation position during encoding on LTM. They found that objects within 2° of fixation were more likely to be accurately recognized on a later LTM test. Furthermore, Williams et al. (2005) demonstrated a similar relationship between eye movements during encoding and LTM. Participants completed a search task in which they had to count the number of instances of a particular target (e.g. yellow phone) among identity-related distractors (e.g. brown phone), colour-related distractors (e.g. yellow cat), and non-related distractors (e.g. brown cat). Following the search tasks, participants were given a surprise two-alternative forced choice recognition test that required discriminating the target or a distractor from a non-search item with the same verbal label (e.g. a yellow phone) but different visual features. Memory performance for targets was fairly high (approximately 85%), but performance for related distractors, although above chance, was much lower (approximately 60%), and performance for unrelated distractors, although still above chance, was even lower (approximately 55%). Although this was partially due to the task-relevance of the objects, fixations during encoding were also predictive of memory performance. Distractors that were fixated more frequently and for a longer total duration were more likely to be remembered. Specifically, as the number of fixations on a distractor increased during encoding, LTM memory performance increased as well (Williams et al., 2005).

Not only is the locus of attention important for encoding into LTM, it is also important for retrieval from LTM (Beck and van Lamsweerde, 2011; Beck et al., 2007; Hollingworth and Henderson, 2002). This is supported by demonstrations of higher change detection performance when attention and fixations are drawn to the change region after the change (Beck and van Lamsweerde, 2011; Beck et al., 2007; Hollingworth, 2003). Presumably if the information needed for detecting the change is in STM, then retrieval of change detection information from LTM should not be necessary. However, if the information no longer exists in STM and has been transferred to LTM, then a more effortful retrieval process is needed, which in turn increases the potential for missed changes due to retrieval failures. Beck and colleagues (2007) presented participants with a LTM task following a change detection task. The main difference between the tasks was that an arrow pointed at the potential change region in the LTM task, drawing attention and retrieval processes to the object of interest. Participants performed better on the LTM memory task (M = 77%) than on the change detection task (M = 45%), demonstrating the importance of retrieval processes in successful change detection (Beck, et al., 2007). Similarly, Beck and van Lamsweerde (2011) showed that providing a cue in the post-change scene during a change detection task improved change detection compared to a condition with no post-change cue. Participants monitored 2, 4, 7, or 10 objects for a change and reported whether or not an object changed identity on each trial. On half of the trials an arrow (post cue) indicated which of the monitored objects was the object that could have changed (see Fig. 32.1). As the number of objects competing for attention exceeded STM capacity, the effect of using a cue to draw attention to the post-change object increased. These results demonstrate that retrieval from LTM is more likely to be successful if a cue directs fixations and, therefore attention to the post-change object.

Studies employing eye movement tracking methodology provide further evidence that LTM for visual information is highly linked to fixation locations not only during encoding (Nelson and Loftus, 1980), but also during retrieval. For example, prior experience with a particular change in a scene influences the pattern of eye movements during later views of the scene (Ryan et al., 2000; Takahashi and Watanabe, 2008). Holm and Mantyla (2007) demonstrated a correspondence between the pattern of eye movements during encoding and retrieval when the scenes were accurately recognized. The authors concluded that reinstating the pattern of eye movements from encoding during retrieval increases the likelihood of accurate retrieval. In addition, knowledge of a change that previously occurred in a scene can bias fixations toward the previous change location during subsequent views of the scene (Takahashi and Watanabe, 2008). Participants completed a flicker change detection task during which the pre- and post-change images alternate back and forth repeatedly. When an old scene was presented in which a previous change was well known, participants looked repeatedly at the old change location even after sufficient looking time could lead to the awareness that the previous change was not occurring. Together, these studies demonstrate the strong effect of eye movements on LTM encoding and retrieval.

Eye movement measures have also been used to support the notion that information encoded into memory can influence viewing behaviour without conscious awareness. Specifically, evidence for implicit change detection occurs when participants fail to explicitly report detection of the change, but sensitivity to the change is revealed through measures such as eye movements (Beck et al., 2007; Hollingworth et al., 2001), reaction times (Fernandez-Duque and Thornton, 2003; Thornton and Fernandez-Duque, 2000; Williams and Simons, 2000), and event-related potential (Fernandez-Duque et al., 2003). Ryan and Cohen (2004) argue that implicit change detection is evidence of the role of LTM in online scene viewing, because information in STM would necessarily be available to conscious awareness. Implicit change detection was demonstrated by showing a change in the overall pattern of eye movements on the post-change scene for missed change trials. In addition, amnesic subjects showed the same eye movement pattern as normal subjects on explicit change detection trials (trials in which participants accurately reported the change), but revealed no evidence of

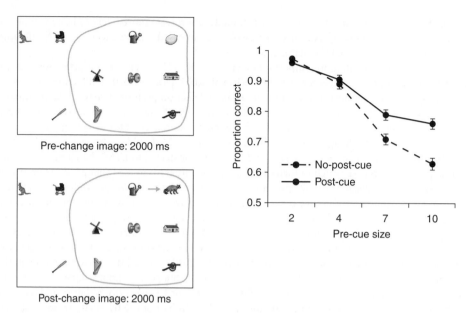

Fig. 32.1 Left side) Stimuli used in Beck and van Lamsweerde (2011). Participants completed a change detection task, on half of the trials a post-cue was provided in the post-change scene directing attention to the potential change object. In the pre- and post-change scenes 2, 4, 7, or 10 objects were circled. The circle indicated which objects needed to be encoded for the change detection trial. In this example, 7 items are circled (pre-cue size 7) and the lemon in the top right corner changes into a raccoon. The arrow pointing at the raccoon in the post-change image was only present in the post-cue block of trials. Right side) Results from Beck and van Lamsweerde (2011). Proportion correct (chance = 0.50) for each pre-cue size in the post-cue block and the no-post-cue block. Reproduced here from *Memory and Cognition*, **39**(3), Beck, M.R. and van Lamsweerde, A.E., Accessing long-term memory representations during visual change detection, © 2011, pp. 433–446, figures 1 and 2, with permission from Springer Science+Business Media.

implicit change detection as measured by the pattern of eye movements on missed change trails. The authors argue that this is evidence that implicit change detection is driven by LTM representations. In addition, this eye movement evidence demonstrates that both LTM and STM contribute to online scene viewing.

What sorts of memory guide our eye movements during visual search?

Tracking eye movements during change detection tasks has been fruitful in determining the role of transsaccadic memory, STM, and LTM in visual tasks that involve the intentional encoding of visual information. However, most visual tasks completed in the real world do not involve purposefully encoding visual information, but rather searching the visual environment for task-relevant information. Therefore, it is important to consider what eye movements can tell us about the role of memory in visual search tasks.

Although most theories of visual search assumed that memory played a role in guiding attention or otherwise played a role in controlling processing, it was only within the last decade that this assumption was tested directly. A classic assumption is serial self-terminating search (Sternberg, 1966), whereby items are examined one-at-a-time and search is terminated after either a target is found or every item has been examined. To examine whether memory plays a role in guiding attention during search, Horowitz and Wolfe (1998) used a task designed to prevent subjects from using memory to guide their attention. Performance in that task was compared to performance in a more conventional control condition, with the logic being that if memory does play a role, search performance should be more efficient in the task that allows for memory. In the experimental condition, the locations of the search items changed every 107 ms, and because search rates in their control condition were roughly 40 ms per item, it was unlikely that more than two to three items could be examined before a switch occurred. Because items were constantly disappearing and reappearing, if subjects did build a memory representation for the locations they had already visited, this memory would only be useful during the brief period of time between switches.

Much to the surprise of many, search efficiency in the experimental condition was as efficient as in the control condition. This suggested to Horowitz and Wolfe, that when people search a scene, they do not use memory to keep track of where they have been. Instead, search is amnesic, and the visual system is stuck 'in a sort of eternal present' (Horowitz and Wolfe, 1998).

To many, these results seemed counterintuitive, especially when compared to everyday subjective experiences. However, subjective impressions can often be misleading, as can be seen by the case of change blindness, in which we have the subjective impression of a rich perception of the world around us, yet our memory from one fixation to the next is quite poor. Nonetheless, these findings lead to a flurry of research to determine whether or not memory is used to guide attention during visual search.

Most of the research designed to address this question used response times (Kristjánsson, 2000) or response accuracy (Horowitz and Wolfe, 1998) as a measure of search efficiency. As discussed earlier, eye movements are often a more sensitive measure because they are less likely than response times to be contaminated by other processes, and tracking eye movements allows for a moment-by-moment examination of attention. Peterson et al. (2001) used eye tracking to measure attention and the role of memory in visual search. By using small search items that required foveation to identify, and by spacing them far enough apart that only one item could be identified at a time, this ensured that only one item could be identified during each fixation. In addition, because search items were small, visually similar (rotated T's and L's), and were all the same colour, this ensured that items in the periphery were indistinguishable from each other.

Because the nature of the displays prevented parallel processing (other than the localization of search items), search would have to ensue in a serial manner. One diagnosis of whether or not a system has memory is to examine the hazard function of completion times, or in this case, the number of eye movements needed to find the target (Luce, 1986). Because the reader may be unfamiliar with hazard function, it might be easier to show how they relate to more common distribution functions, such as the probability density function (PDF) and cumulative distribution function (CDF).

The reader may be familiar with PDF functions from statistics, with the bell-shaped (Gaussian) curve being perhaps the most common PDF. In our case, the PDF would be the probability of fixating the target as a function of the number of eye movements. In some instances, the subject may be lucky and the first item fixated would be the target. If there are 10 items in the display, the probability of finding the target on the first fixation is 1 in 10, or 10%. If an individual has perfect memory and never backtracks, then 10% of the time the target will be found on the second fixation, 10% the third fixation, and so on up to 10 fixations. In this instance, the graph of the PDF would look flat or rectangular ('boxcar'). The problem with just looking at this distribution is that the PDF is only diagnostic of memory when memory is perfect.

Related to the PDF is the cumulative distribution function. In the case of visual search, the CDF is the cumulative probability that the target is found. So, in an individual with perfect memory and 10 items to search through, the probability that the target was found by the first fixation is 10%, by the second fixation 20%, and so on. Whether a person has perfect memory or is amnesic, the CDF will always increase.

The hazard function is the probability of an event occurring given that it has not yet occurred. For example, over time, the probability that a disk drive will fail given that it has not already failed will increase. Mathematically, the hazard function is PDF/(1-CDF). In our above example, if 8 items have been examined without finding the target, the probability that the ninth item will be the target is 50% (2 unexamined items remain). Likewise, if 9 items have been examined without finding the target, then the probability that the tenth item is the target is 100%. Importantly, for any system that has memory, the hazard function will be increasing, and thus provides a diagnosis as to whether memory exists or not. This is exactly what Peterson and colleagues found: as the number of fixations increased, so did the hazard function. In contrast, a system with no memory will have a flat hazard function. Thus, visual search is guided by memory.

Revisitation rates

Although hazard functions are diagnostic of memory, they do little to tell us about the types of memory or the capacity of the memory that is guiding visual search. An alternative method is to look at revisitation rates, or the probability of revisiting an item as a function of when it was last examined. This allows us not only to compare the observed revisitation rates against the revisitation rates predicted by other models, but it also allows us to examine the types of items that are re-examined.

In the case of Peterson et al. (2001, but see also Beck et al., 2006a, 2006b; Gilchrist and Harvey, 2000), the overall revisitation rate was very low (5.7%) compared to that predicted by memoryless search (26.1%). Based on these results, it would be reasonable to conclude that search is far from memoryless, as the revisitation rates are much lower than predicted by memoryless search, yet memory is not perfect, as the revisitation rate is greater than zero.

However, when the revisitation rate is examined as a function of when an item was last visited, an interesting pattern emerges: the majority of refixations are to the last examined item. Interestingly, a majority (53.7%) of these immediate refixations were to the target. This suggested that these refixations were not due to a memory failure, but instead could be due to inadequate processing because attention moved away too soon (Gilchrist and Harvey, 2000). Indeed, a simple model (Miss+Realization) fit the pattern of revisitations remarkably well ($R^2 = 0.86$). This simple model assumed that on some proportion of fixations, people occasionally fixate but do not adequately process an item before leaving ('miss'), and that some of these misses are later realized, leading to immediate refixations.

Memory for where I am going?

Although the Miss+Realization model did a good job of fitting the observed data, there are other models that could fit the data equally as well—including models that assumed no memory! For example, if a person searched systematically using a simple set of rules, such as starting at the top, scanning from left to right, and moving downward, they could search the entire display without ever revisiting an item (Gilchrist and Harvey, 2006). Note that this would require no memory for past actions, a term we will call *retrospective memory*. Alternatively, a person could have memory, but that memory is for future actions—in other words, the ability to preplan a search path (*prospective memory*). Again, even without retrospective memory, perfect prospective memory would lead to no revisits.

To rule out the possibility that subjects were using simple rules to prevents revisits, McCarley et al. (2003) devised a task that would prevent the use of scanning rules or prospective memory. In this task, no more than three of the search items were visible: the currently fixated item and two potential saccade targets. As the subject moved their eyes to the new saccade target, the previously fixated item as well as the other potential saccade choice were replaced with two new items from the search set. Early in the search, the two new items that appeared during a saccade were always new items that had never been examined. However, after several saccades, one of the two potential saccade targets was always an old previously fixated item whereas the other was always a new item (see Fig. 32.2). At this point, if the subject has memory for previously fixated items, then the subject should choose the new item 100% of the time. Alternatively, if there is no memory, then the old item should be chosen 50% of the time. The key to this paradigm is that search items were not consistently visible, and therefore, subjects could plan no more than one saccade in advance.

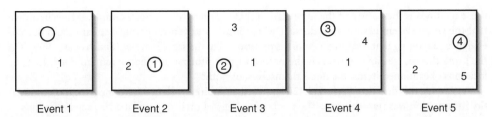

Event 1   Event 2   Event 3   Event 4   Event 5

Fig. 32.2 Schematic of displays used by McCarley et al. (2003). At the start of a trial, only a single member of the search set is visible (Event 1). During the first saccade, a new member of the search set becomes visible (Event 2). Starting with Event 3, one of the potential saccade targets is always an old item and the other is always a new item. Eyal M. Reingold, Neil Charness, Marc Pomplun, and Dave M. Stampe, *Psychological Science*, **12**(1), copyright © 2001 by Sage Publications. Reprinted by Permission of SAGE Publications.

Despite the strange nature of the search task (items were appearing and reappearing on the screen during saccades) and the impoverished nature of the search display (no more than three items were visible at any one time), subjects were able to successfully avoid refixating old items. However, this avoidance only lasted for approximately four items, suggesting that retrospective memory was limited to only the last four items or so (note that this is in line with the capacity limits of STM found using change detection tasks). Similar effects have been found using inhibition-of-return (IOR) type paradigms (Klein and McInnes, 1999; Snyder and Kingstone, 2000), and memory in this case might have been due to a simple IOR-type inhibitory mechanism. Nonetheless, this demonstrates that a lack of revisitations during search is due to a retrospective component, and is not just a by-product of strategic scanpath planning. However, as we'll see below, it is likely that other forms of memory other than simple inhibition play a role in guiding attention during search.

One potential problem with this task is the non-persistent nature of the stimuli. That is, although the task prevents scanpath planning, the disappearance of old items during saccades might interfere with tagging old locations, and in turn lead to a low estimate of the capacity of retrospective memory. To rectify this, Peterson et al. (2007) used a task that prevents scan-path planning but allowed full retrospective memory. In their task, old examined items remained static, but unexamined items (other than the current target of the saccade) moved to new locations during each saccade. This prevented subjects from planning more than one saccade in advance, but allowed for fuller memory representations to be generated for old items. Compared to a static condition, in which items remained in their places throughout the trial, the probability of revisiting an old item was consistently low, at least for the last four items examined. After that, revisitation rates increased compared to the static condition, suggesting that retrospective memory was able to prevent revisitations for only that last four items, with the lower revisitation rate found in the static condition being due to the addition of prospective memory.

This method can also be used to confirm whether scan-path planning can successfully prevent revisitations. By using a dynamic condition in which old examined items were repositioned during each saccade, subjects were prevented from using any form of retrospective memory, and some form of prospective memory (simple rules or more complex scanpath planning) would be needed to prevent revisitations. Like the static control condition, revisitations initially remained low and only started to diverge from the control condition after the last 4 to 11 items. Interestingly, subjects were able to delay revisitations for longer (last 11 items vs. last 4 items) when searching through the larger of the two set sizes used (16 vs. 8 items). This might reflect some form of coarse spatial encoding, with the larger set size packing more items into a given region (see Dickinson and Zelinsky, 2007; Kramer et al., 2006).

Memory for what or where?

As discussed in the previous sections, there are several ways to examine patterns of eye movements to determine whether or not a location has been remembered. One question we cannot answer using those methods is the nature of the information that is remembered. For example, it is well known that the visual system is split in to dorsal ('where/how') and ventral ('what') streams, and there is evidence suggesting that working memory is partitioned in the same manner (Smith et al., 1995). On the same theme, we can ask what is the nature of the information that is remembered: is it the locations of examined items, the items themselves, or both?

To examine this question Beck et al. (2006a) used an indirect task to determine if location or identity information was remembered. The underlying logic of their task was if a characteristic, such as location or identity, was remembered, then changing that characteristic should cause an old examined item to be treated like a new unexamined item. That is, if there is memory, then unexamined items should be fixated more often than previously examined items. Therefore, if a particular dimension is important for memory, then changing that dimension should lead to an increase in revisits.

As in previous research, the response features of the stimuli (whether a left or right rotated T was present) were made small enough such that direct fixation was necessary to perform the task. To make sure that items' identities were visible in peripheral vision, each response stimulus was embedded in a larger outlining shape (individuating feature). Each individuating feature was a unique shape (square, circle, triangle) and colour (red, blue, yellow, green) combination. This ensured that the individuating feature information as well as location information was available in peripheral vision, but response information was not.

After several items were examined in the display, the identity of one of the items (old or new) was randomly changed (e.g. red-triangle to blue-square) during a saccade. To examine whether or not identity information was used to keep track of examined items, the probability of visiting an item after the change was compared to chance. Both the changed and unchanged unexamined ("new") items were visited at a rate far higher than chance, illustrating a bias to fixate unexamined items. More importantly, the probability of visiting an old item was far less than chance—in fact, old items were rarely revisited—and this held for both the changed and unchanged old items. In other words, old items that changed their identity were still treated as old items, suggesting that identity information is not used.

The next question we can ask is whether location information is used during visual search. In a separate experiment, rather than changing the identity of items, the location of one item was changed during a saccade. Although the location changed, the identity stayed the same (e.g. a blue square). Again, after the change occurred, unexamined items were examined more often than predicted by chance, but this effect only held for unexamined items that had not moved. Likewise, old examined item that had not moved were revisited at a level lower than chance, indicating that memory biased saccades away for these items. However, this effect did not hold for those old examined items that had been moved. Instead, the probability that they would be examined after they changed locations was no different from chance, indicating that moving old examined items to a new location disrupted the memory representation. Taken as a whole, this suggests that location, rather than identity, is used to remember which items had been examined.

On the other hand, just because identity information is not used during search does not mean that the information is not remembered. To examine this possibility, Beck et al. (2006b) used a task in which on approximately 30% of the trials, search was stopped, and subjects were quizzed about the identity of an object that had occurred at a previously examined location. In one version of the experiment, when search was terminated, the locations of search items were replaced by masks, a specific location was circled, and subjects were ask which of two items had appeared at that location.

In a more stringent version, the alternative choice (foil) was an item that had been examined earlier in the trial. In other words, to respond correctly, a subject needed to know not just whether an item had recently been examined, as the foil was also a recently examined item, but also needed to explicitly remember which item had occurred at the probed location. Surprisingly, subjects were only 74% correct (chance was 50%) for correctly identifying the last examined item, and memory performance dropped to 56% for items that were examined four fixations prior. At first glance, this suggests that memory for the identities of examined items is quite poor.

On the other hand, it might very well be that successfully performing the search task does not require memory for the locations of rejected items, and therefore there was no reason for subjects to expend effort to encode the items. Indeed, when the memory test was changed, such that the foil was an item that had not occurred on that trial, memory increased to 85% for the last examined item and to 72% for items examined four fixations prior. This suggests that subjects did retain some information about examined items, but that this information was not necessarily tied to the locations where the items had occurred. Indeed, Williams et al. (2005) found similar memory performance using an incidental memory test 10 min after subjects performed visual search (see also Castelhano and Henderson, 2005). Taken as a whole, this suggests that although information about an item's identity is encoded during search, it does not appear that is used to guide attention.

Koerner and Gilchrist (2007) used a double search task to investigate subjects' memory for the identity and locations of examined items. In their task, subjects were auditorily presented with a target to search for, and were to respond with a keypress as to whether the target was present or absent. After this first search was completed, as indicated by a manual response from subject, the subject was then given a new target to search for. The key to this experiment is that the display for the second search was identical to that used in the first search. Therefore, if subjects are encoding and remembering the items that they examined, then they should be quicker to find the second target if it is present. Indeed, Koerner and Gilchrist (2007) found a benefit, but this benefit lasted for only the last three to five items examined in the first search. This suggests that although some information is retained about the locations and identities of rejected distractors, it is fleeting, and is only used to guide attention when it is relevant to the task at hand. Note, however, that Dickinson and Zelinksy (2007) suggest that there might be a higher capacity form of retrospective memory that codes coarse locations.

Do executive processes play a role in search memory?

Finally, the last question we will ask is whether or not executive processes play a role in search memory. For example, executive processes may be used to actively maintain representations, or executive processes may be used to act upon those memory representations.

An early suggestion that executive processes play a role in visual search comes from the work of Han and Kim (2004). When subjects were required to perform a task with a high-load executive component, such as counting backwards by 3 s, search took longer to complete compared to when subjects were simultaneously performing a low-load task, such as passively remembering a series of digits. More importantly, the search-slope (a measure of search efficiency) increased. However, because their task only measured response times, it was not possible to determine what lead to these increased search slopes. For example, search slopes could have increased because more time was needed to examine each item. But search slopes could have also increased if the executive load lead to an increased number of examinations.

To try to determine why loading executive working memory lead to a decrease in search efficiency, Peterson et al. (2008) tracked subjects' eyes while they simultaneously performed visual search and an auditory executive working memory task. As in Han and Kim (2004), performing the simultaneous executive working memory task lead to slower and less efficient search. Interestingly, some of this loss of efficiency was due to an increased number of fixations while performing the working memory task. More importantly, the increased number of fixations was due to higher revisitation rates compared to the no-load trials (search trials completed without doing the executive working memory task). At first glance, this suggests that executive functioning plays a role in preventing revisitations. However, a closer look at the fixation durations suggests that something else might be occurring.

Overall, performing the auditory working memory task lead to longer gaze durations, suggesting that the working memory task interfered with processes that occur during fixations, such as image processing or saccade planning. What is interesting is that in both conditions, gaze durations for items that were later revisited were significantly shorter than gaze durations on items that were never revisited. This suggests that revisits may occur when attention prematurely leaves an item, leaving it poorly processed. Prior evidence for this comes from studies showing that a disproportionately large number of revisitations are to targets (Peterson et al., 2001, 2008).

On the other hand, Koerner and Gilchrist (2008) have suggested that increased revisitations might be due to a loss of working memory capacity that could have been used to keep track of examined items. Unlike most search tasks, the goal of their task was to determine if only one target was present in the display, and this memory requirement might have caused subjects to reserve a portion of visual-working memory for remembering the target location. Another possibility they suggest is that because the task required subjects so be sure that no more than one target was present, this might have made subjects more cautious and more likely to wilfully reinspect old items. A final possibility they suggested is that the increased executive demands of the only-one-target task, at least compared to a conventional visual search, might have interfered with perceptual processing. However, given the complex nature of their task, it difficult to know what aspects of working memory might have been impacted.

Conclusions

The goal of this chapter is to illustrate some of the more recent research that uses eye movements to investigate memory. As shown throughout this chapter, monitoring eye movements can reveal aspects of memory that are not measurable through other means. Examples of this include many of the gaze-contingent paradigms used to examine scene memory, change detection, and visual search. Eye movements can also be more sensitive measures. An example of this is seen in the long-term scene memory experiments of Ryan and Cohen (2004), where eye movements suggested implicit change detection in instances in which subjects could not verbalize a change. Finally, monitoring eye movements can be less intrusive compared to alternative methods that might alter the task at hand. For example, several psychophysical studies using flashing displays have suggested that memory does not guide attention during search, whereas eye movement studies suggest otherwise. We hope that the reader finds this chapter useful, and that the many creative ways of using eye movements to investigate memory illustrated in this chapter might prove inspirational.

References

Ballard, D.H., Hayhoe, M., and Pelz, J.B. (1995). Memory representations in natural tasks. *Journal of Cognitive Neuroscience*, **7**, 66–80.

Beck, M.R. and van Lamsweerde, A.E. (2011). Accessing long-term memory representations during visual change detection. *Memory and Cognition*, **39**(3), 433–446.

Beck, M.R. and Levin, D.T. (2003). The role of representational volatility in recognizing pre- and postchange objects. *Perception and Psychophysics*, **65**(3), 458–468.

Beck, M.R., Angelone, B.A., and Levin, D.T. (2004). Knowledge about the probability of change affects change detection performance. *Journal of Experimental Psychology: Human Perception and Performance*, **30**(4), 778–791.

Beck, M., Peterson, M.S., and Vomela, M. (2006a). Memory for where, but not what, is remembered during visual search. *Journal of Experimental Psychology: Human Perception and Performance*. **32**, 235–250.

Beck, M.R., Peterson, M.S., and Angelone, B.A. (2007). The roles of encoding, retrieval, and awareness in change detection, *Memory and Cognition*, **35**(4), 610–620.

Beck, M.R., Peterson, M.S., Boot, W.R., Vomela, M., and Kramer, A.F. (2006b). Explicit memory for rejected distractors in visual search. *Visual Cognition*, **14**, 2, 150–174.

Castelhano, M.S., and Henderson, J.M. (2005). Incidental visual memory for objects in scenes. *Visual Cognition*, **12**, 1017–1040.

Deubel, H. and Schneider, W.X. (1996). Saccade target selection and object recognition: evidence for a common attentional mechanism. *Vision Research*, **36**, 1827–1837.

Dickinson, C.A. and Zelinsky, G.J. (2007). Memory for the search path: Evidence for a high-capacity representation of search history. *Vision Research*, **47**, 1745–1755.

Droll, J.A. and Hayhoe, M.M. (2007). Trade-offs between gaze and working memory use. *Journal of Experimental Psychology: Human Perception and Performance*, **33**(6), 1352–1365.

Fernandez-Duque, D., Grossi, G., Thornton, I.M., and Neville, H.J. (2003). Representation of change: Separate electrophysiological markers of attention, awareness, and implicit processing. *Journal of Cognitive Neuroscience*, **15**(4), 1–17.

Gajewski, D.A. and Henderson J.M. (2005). Minimal use of working memory in a scene comparison task. *Visual Cognition*, **12**, 979–1212.

Gilchrist, I.D. and Harvey, M. (2000). Refixation frequency and memory mechanisms in visual search. *Current Biology*, **10**(19), 1209–1212.

Gilchrist, I.D. and Harvey, M. (2006). Evidence for a systematic component within scanpaths in visual search. *Visual Cognition*, **14**, 704–71.

Grimes, J. (1996). On the failure to detect changes in scenes across saccades. In Akins, K., *Perception* (Vancouver Studies in Cognitive Science), 2 (pp. 89–110). New York: Oxford University Press.

Han, S.H. and Kim, M.S. (2004). Visual search does not remain efficient when executive working memory is working. *Psychological Science*, **15**, 623–628.

Henderson, J.M. (1992). Identifying objects across saccades: Effects of extrafoveal preview and flanker object context. *Journal of Experimental Psychology. Learning, Memory, and Cognition*, **18**, 521–530.

Henderson, J.M. and Hollingworth, A. (1999). The role of fixation position in detecting scene changes across saccades. *Psychological Science*, **10**, 438–443.

Henderson, J.M. and Hollingworth, A. (2003). Eye movements and visual memory: Detecting changes to saccade targets in scenes. *Perception and Psychophysics*, **65**(1), 58–71.

Henderson, J.M. and Siefert, A.B.C. (2001). Types and tokens in transsaccadic object identification: Effects of spatial position and left-right orientation. *Psychonomic Bulletin and Review*, **8**(4), 753–760.

Henderson, J.M., Pollatsek, A., and Rayner, K. (1989). Covert visual attention and extrafoveal information use during object identification. *Perception and Psychophysics*, **45**, 196–208.

Henderson, J.M., Williams, C.C., Castelhano, M.S., and Falk, R.J. (2003). Eye movements and picture processing during recognition. *Perception and Psychophysics*, **65**(5), 725–734.

Hirose Y. and Hancock, P.J.B. (2007). Equally attending but still not seeing: An eye-tracking study of change detection in own- and other-race faces. *Visual Cognition*, **15**(6), 647–660.

Hoffman, J.E. and Subramaniam, B. (1995). The role of visual attention in saccadic eye movements. *Perception and Psychophysics*, **57**, 787–795.

Hollingworth, A. and Henderson, J.M. (2002) Accurate visual memory for previously attended objects in natural scenes. *Journal of Experimental Psychology: Human Perception and Performance*, **28**(1), 113–136.

Hollingworth, A., Williams, C.C., and Henderson, J.M. (2001). To see and remember: Visually specific information is retained in memory from previously attended objects in natural scenes. *Psychonomic Bulletin and Review*, **8**, 761–768.

Holm, L. and Mantyla, T. (2007). Memory for scenes: Refixations reflect retrieval. *Memory and Cognition*, **35**(7), 1664–1674.

Humphreys, G.W., Hodsoll, J. and Campbell, C. (2005) Attending but not seeing: The 'other race' effect in face and person perception studied through change blindness. *Visual Cognition*, **12**, 249–262.

Horowitz, T.S. and Wolfe, J.M. (1998). Visual search has no memory. *Nature*, **394**, 575–577.

Irwin, D.E. and Gordon, R.D. (1998). Eye movements, attention, and trans-saccadic memory. *Visual Cognition*, **5**, 127–155.

Jonides, J., Irwin, D.E., and Yantis, S. (1982). Integrating visual information from successive fixations. *Science*, **215**, 192–194.

Klein, R.M. and MacInnes, W.J. (1999). Inhibition of return is a foraging facilitator in visual search. *Psychological Science*, **10**, 346–352.

Koerner, C. and Gilchrist, I.D. (2007). Finding a new target in an old display: Evidence for a memory recency effect in visual search. *Psychonomic Bulletin and Review*, **14**, 846–851

Koerner, C. and Gilchrist, I.D. (2008). Memory processes in multiple-target visual search. *Psychological Research*, **72**, 99–105.

Kowler, E., Anderson, E., Dosher, B. and Blaser, E. (1995) The role of attention in the programming of saccades. *Vision Research*, **35**, 1897–1916

Kramer, A.F, Boot, W.R., McCarley, J.S., Peterson, M.S., Colcombe, A.F., and Scialfa, C.T. (2006). Aging, memory, and visual search. *Acta Psychologica*, **122**, 288–304.

Kristjánsson, A. (2000). In search of remembrance: Evidence for memory in visual search. *Psychological Science*, **11**, 328–332.

Luce, R.D. (1986). *Response times: Their role in inferring elementary mental organization*. New York: Oxford University Press.

Luck, S.J. (2008). Visual short-term memory. In A. Hollingworth and S. J. Luck (eds.) *Visual Memory* (pp. 43–85). New York: Oxford, Press.

Luck, S.J. and Vogel, E.K. (1997). The capacity of visual working memory for features and conjunctions. *Nature*, **390**, 279–281.

McCarley, J.S., Wang, R.F., Kramer, A.F., Irwin, D.E., and Peterson, M.S. (2003). How much memory does oculomotor search have? *Psychological Science*, **14**, 422–426

McConkie, G.W. and Currie, C.B. (1996). Visual stability across saccades while viewing complex pictures. *Journal of Experimental Psychology: Human Perception and Performance*, **22**(3), 563–581.

McConkie, G.W. and Rayner, K. (1975). The span of the effective stimulus during a fixation in reading, *Perception and Psychophysics*, **17**, 578–586.

McConkie, G.W. and Zola, D. (1979). Is visual information integrated across successive fixations in reading? *Perception and Psychophysics*, **25**, 221–224.

Nelson, W.W. and Loftus, G.R. (1980). The functional visual field during picture viewing. *Journal of Experimental Psychology: Human Learning and Memory*, **6**, 391–399.

O'Regan, J.K. (1992). Solving the 'real' mysteries of visual perception: The world as an outside memory. *Canadian Journal of Psychology* **46**(3), 461–488.

O'Regan, J.K. and Noë, A. (2001). A sensorimotor account of vision and visual consciousness. *Behavioral and Brain Sciences*, **24**, 939–1031.

Parker, R.E. (1978). Picture processing during recognition, *Journal of Experimental Psychology: Human Perception and Performance*, **4**(2), 284–293.

Pashler, H. (1988). Familiarity and the detection of change in visual displays. *Perception and Psychophysics*, **44**, 369–378.

Peterson, M.S., Beck, M.R., and Wong, J.H. (2008). Were you paying attention to where you looked? The role of executive working memory in visual search. *Psychonomic Bulletin and Review*, **15**, 372–377.

Peterson, M.S., Kramer, A.F., and Irwin, D.E. (2004). Covert shifts of attention precede involuntary eye movements. *Perception and Psychophysics*, **66**, 398–405.

Peterson, M.S., Kramer, A.F., Wang, R.F., Irwin, D.E., and McCarley, J.S. (2001). Visual search has memory. *Psychological Science*, **12**, 287–292.

Phillips, W.A. (1974). On the distinction between sensory storage and short-term visual memory. *Perception and Psychophysics*, **16**(2), 283–290.

Rayner K., McConkie G.W., and Ehrlich S. (1978). Eye movements and integrating information across fixations. *Journal of Experimental Psychology: Human Perception and Performance*, **4**, 529–544.

Reingold, E.M., Charness, N., Pomplun, M., and Stampe, D.M. (2001). Visual span in expert chess players: Evidence from eye movements. *Psychological Science*, **12**(1), 48–55.

Ryan, J.D. and Cohen, N.J. (2004). The nature of change detection and online representations of scenes. *Journal of Experimental Psychology: Human Perception and Performance*, **30**(5), 988–1015.

Ryan, J.D. Althoff, R.R., Whitlow, S., and Cohen, N.J. (2000). Amnesia is a deficit in relational memory, *Psychological Science*, **11**, 454–461.

Simons, D.J. (1996). In sight, out of mind: When object representations fail. *Psychological Science*, **7**, 301–305.

Smith, E.E., Jonides, J., Koeppe, R.A., Awh, E., Schumacher, E.H., and Minoshima, S. (1995). Spatial versus object working memory: PET investigation. *Journal of Cognitive Neuroscience*, **7**(3), 337–356.

Snyder, J.J. and Kingstone, A. (2000). Inhibition of return and visual search: How many separate loci are inhibited? *Perception and Psychophysics*, **3**, 452–458.

Sternberg, S. (1966). High-speed scanning in human memory. *Science*, **153**, 652–654.

Takahashi, K. and Watanabe, K. (2008). Persisting effect of prior experience of change blindness. *Perception*, **37**, 324–327.

Thornton, I.M. and Fernandez-Duque, D. (2000). An implicit measure of undetected change. *Spatial Vision*, **14**, 21–44.

Williams, C.C., Henderson, J.M., and Zacks, R.T. (2005). Incidental visual memory for targets and distractors in visual search. *Perception and Psychophysics*, **67**(5), 816–827.

Williams, P. and Simons, D.J. (2000). Detecting changes in novel 3D objects: Effects of change magnitude, spatiotemporal continuity, and stimulus familiarity. *Visual Cognition*, **7**, 297–322.

Zelinsky G.J. (2001). Eye movements during change detection: Implications for search constraints, memory limitations, and scanning strategies. *Perception and Psychophysics*, **63**(2), 209–225.

CHAPTER 33

Eye movements and scene perception

John M. Henderson

Abstract

In human vision, acuity and colour sensitivity are greatest at the point of fixation and fall off rapidly as visual eccentricity increases. What we see, remember, and understand about a scene is tightly tied to fixation. The visual-cognitive system exploits the high resolution of central vision by actively controlling eye movements to direct fixation to important and informative scene regions in real time. Therefore, how gaze control operates over complex real-world scenes is of central concern in several core cognitive science disciplines including cognitive psychology, visual neuroscience, and machine vision. This chapter reviews current approaches and empirical findings in human gaze control during real-world scene perception.

Introduction

During human scene perception, high quality visual information is acquired only from a limited spatial region surrounding the centre of gaze (the *fovea*). Visual quality falls off rapidly and continuously from the centre of gaze into a low-resolution visual surround. We move our eyes about three times each second via rapid eye movements (*saccades*) to reorient the fovea through the scene. Pattern information is only acquired during periods of relative gaze stability (*fixations*) due to *saccadic suppression* during the saccades themselves (Matin, 1974; Thiele et al., 2002; Volkmann, 1986). Humans therefore direct fixation through a scene in real time in the service of ongoing perceptual, cognitive, and behavioural activity (Fig. 33.1).

This chapter provides an overview of what is known about saccadic eye movements during real-world scene viewing. Research in this area has been growing rapidly over the last decade and has become of interest across a wide variety of disciplines as eye movements are more commonly used to study an ever-larger number of topics in cognitive science, vision science, and cognitive neuroscience.

What is a scene?

Before beginning, it is useful to have a working definition of *scene*. A *scene* can be defined as a view of the real-world environment from a particular vantage point. Scenes typically comprise background elements and multiple discrete objects arranged in a spatially licensed and semantically coherent manner (Henderson and Ferreira, 2004b; Henderson and Hollingworth, 1999). Background elements are relatively large-scale, immovable surfaces and structures, and objects are smaller-scale discrete entities that move or can be moved (or more generally, that act or can be acted on) within the scene.

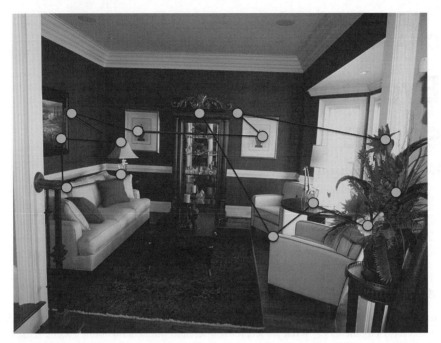

Fig. 33.1 Example scan pattern in photograph.

Real-world scenes have a hierarchical spatial structure in that smaller-scale scenes form parts of larger-scale scenes. For example, a desktop can be considered a scene but so can the entire office containing the desktop. Views of the environment can be further zoomed in and zoomed out. We use the notion of human scale to bound the definition of scene and rule out views that would not typically be encountered during normal interaction with the environment (Henderson and Ferreira, 2004b; Henderson and Hollingworth, 1999a). Objects in a real-world scene are spatially arranged according to the laws of physics and the constraints associated with the functions of that environment. Spatial licensing includes adherence to the physical constraints of the universe (*syntactic* constraints as defined by Biederman et al., 1982), including gravity, space, and time, and to the *semantic* constraints imposed by object identity and function. Examples of physical constraints include the fact that objects generally cannot float unsupported in the air and that two objects cannot occupy the same region of space at the same time. Examples of semantic constraint are that a dining room chair typically is not found on top of a china cabinet, and that stoves are not typically found outdoors (Biederman et al., 1982). These categories are not perfectly discrete (Henderson, 1992), but the critical point is that a well-formed scene must conform to a set of basic physical and semantic constraints that impose structure on the environment.

Another important concept is that a *scene* is a view from a particular vantage point of the environment within which the viewer is situated, whereas other biologically important classes of visual entities such as objects and faces are viewed from a vantage point outside of themselves. Because of this distinction, most objects can be rotated around an internal axis without changing the vantage point of the viewer with respect to that object. In contrast, if a scene within which the viewer is embedded rotates around an axis, then the viewer also rotates and/or translates too.

Real-world scenes differ in many ways from the types of visual stimuli that are often used in psychophysical experiments. For example, they produce specific wavelength, intensity, and spatial frequency profiles that are constrained by properties of the world (Field, 1987; Geisler, 2008; Simoncelli and Olshausen, 2001). Image regularities arise in part from semantic and spatial constraints that in turn give rise to the semantics of the scene as a whole. Real-world scenes and their depictions also appear to be supported by dedicated cortical hardware (e.g. Epstein and Kanwisher, 1998; Epstein et al., 1999, 2003; Henderson et al., 2008; O'Craven and Kanwisher, 2000). Succinctly, real-world scene perception involves sensory and cognitive processing of visual input that in some important sense is like that typically encountered during the natural course of everyday human activity.

In practice, most research on eye movements in scene perception is based on scene depictions (e.g. drawings, photographs, and computer-generated graphics) taken to be reasonable substitutes for views of the actual environment. The purpose of using depictions is to capture some of the important properties of scene perception by including those properties that are thought to be important, such as visual complexity, structural and semantic constraint, and meaning, while allowing for control over factors that would be difficult if not impossible to control in the real world. Scene depictions necessarily reduce the amount of information normally available to the visual system, such as non-pictorial depth cues (e.g. those involving stereopsis and motion parallax) and motion, as well as the size of the visual field. One reason for highlighting the difference between depictions and the real environment is that the answers to some questions about eye movements in scenes may depend on the nature of the image. It is therefore important to ensure that results obtained from a particular type of depiction generalizes to other types of depictions and ultimately to the visual world itself. Nevertheless, a good deal of information has been gained about eye movements from scene perception defined in this way.

Getting the gist

The gist of a real-world scene can be apprehended very rapidly, well within the duration of a single eye fixation (Biederman, 1972; Intraub 1979, 1980, 1981; Potter, 1975, 1976, 1999; Schyns and Oliva, 1994; Thorpe et al., 1996; VanRullen and Thorpe, 2001). This rapid 'gist' understanding in turn can influence various other visual and cognitive processes such as the tendency to report that a particular object is present in a scene (Biederman et al., 1974; 1982; Boyce and Pollatsek, 1992; Hollingworth and Henderson, 1998, 1999; Murphy and Wisniewski, 1989). *Gist* is an ill-defined term, but the apprehension of scene gist from an initial glimpse likely includes a representation of basic-level scene identity (Tversky and Hemenway, 1983), gross spatial layout (Sanocki and Epstein, 1997), and identities of at least some objects (e.g. large objects near fixation, Gareze and Findlay, 2007; Fei Fei et al., 2006). Gist apprehension also likely involves activation or retrieval of a related scene schema (Friedman, 1979; Lampinen et al., 2001; Mandler and Johnson, 1977). The rapid comprehension of scene gist can affect eye movements in a scene, with fixation directed toward informative scene regions after only a single gimpse (Antes, 1974; Castelhano and Henderson, 2007; Eckstein et al., 2006; Loftus and Mackworth, 1978; Mackworth and Morandi, 1967; Torralba et al., 2006).

In summary, *gist* typically refers to knowledge of the scene category (e.g. kitchen), spatial layout, and the schema information that can be retrieved from memory based on that category. Gist of a real-world scene can be apprehended well within the duration of a single eye fixation.

Eye movements

Given that scenes can be identified and their gist apprehended very rapidly, what function do eye movements serve? First, human vision is a dynamic process in which the perceiver actively seeks visual input as it is needed. Virtually all animals with developed visual systems actively control their visual input using eye, head, and/or body movements (Land, 1999). Eye movements ensure that high quality visual information is available when it is needed to support ongoing cognitive and behavioural activity. What we see and understand about the visual world is tightly tied to where our eyes are pointed. For example, close or direct fixation is typically needed to identify objects in scenes and to perceive their visual details (Henderson and Hollingworth, 1999a, Hollingworth et al., 2001a). Fixation is also tightly tied to memory encoding, both for short-term memory (Ballard et al., 1995) and long-term memory (Nelson and Loftus, 1980). Second, fixation provides a deictic pointer to entities in the world. Fixation can therefore simplify a large variety of otherwise difficult computational problems (Ballard, 1996; Ballard et al., 1997; Churchland et al., 1994). For example, targeting world entities for motor control may be simplified when the target is fixated (Land and Hayhoe, 2001). Similarly, fixation seems to facilitate language processing, both during language production (Meyer and Lethaus, 2004; Griffin, 2004) and language comprehension (Tanenhaus et al., 2004; see Henderson and Ferreira, 2004a). Third, because attention plays a central role in visual processing, and because eye movements are an observable behavioural expression of the allocation of attention in a scene, eye movements serve as a window into the operation of attention. Although a good deal has been learned by studying attention divorced from eye movements, the natural case is the one in which the eyes freely move and there is a tight link between fixation and internal attention. Fourth, eye movements provide an unobtrusive, sensitive, real-time behavioural index of ongoing visual and cognitive processing (Rayner, 1998). Cognitive scientist hoping to capitalize on the use of the eye movement record as a window into underlying cognitive processes in real-world vision will ultimately need to base their theories on an up-to-date understanding of how visual and cognitive processes are revealed by eye movements.

Where do we look?

Initial investigation of eye movements in scene perception demonstrated that empty, uniform, and uninformative scene regions are typically not fixated. Buswell was among the first investigators to measure both a viewer's direction of gaze and the duration of each fixation in a picture (Buswell, 1935). Buswell demonstrated that fixations are not randomly placed in a scene; instead, viewers tend to cluster fixations on informative image regions. Based on his observations, Buswell concluded that there is an important relationship between eye movements and visual attention: 'Eye movements are unconscious adjustments to the demands of attention during a visual experience' (Buswell, 1935, p. 9).

But what specifically determines where fixations are placed in a scene? A majority of the research on eye movements in scene perception can be seen as having focused on this question. Two potential answers have been pursued: image features generated bottom-up from the scene, and knowledge structures used to drive the eyes in a top-down manner (Henderson, 2007). Although early studies tended to emphasize the latter (e.g. Antes and Penland, 1981; Loftus and Mackworth, 1978; Yarbus, 1967), research over the past 10 years or so has tended to focus on the former (Itti and Koch, 2000; Parkhurst et al., 2002). Recently, the field has begun investigating how to integrate them (Navalpakkam and Itti, 2005; Torralba et al., 2006).

Eye movement control by image features

Do image features determine where viewers will fixate? Three general approaches have been used to investigate this question. In the first method, the image features at viewer-generated fixation locations are measured in a scene. The image features at these locations are compared to a control set of locations such as randomly selected locations from the same scenes (e.g. Henderson et al., 2007; Mannan et al., 1997b; Parkhurst and Neibur, 2003; Reinagel and Zador, 1999). A common result is that edges are preferentially fixated (Baddeley and Tatler, 2006; Henderson et al., 2009a).

A second method for determining the stimulus properties that control the placement of fixation involves building computational models that attempt to predict fixation locations. The dominant type of model computes a *saliency map* from basic image features like luminance, colour, and orientation (Itti and Koch, 2000, 2001; Itti et al., 1998, 2001; Koch and Ullman, 1985; see also Torralba, 2003; Torralba et al., 2006). In this approach, the image features present in a scene give rise in a bottom-up manner to a representation (the saliency map) that makes explicit the locations of the most visually distinct regions in the image. Saliency maps explicitly mark regions that are different from their surround over multiple spatial scales. The maps generated for each feature are then combined in some manner to create a single saliency map. The intuition behind this approach is that regions that are uniform in their features are uninformative, whereas regions whose features differ from neighbouring regions are potentially informative (Treisman and Gelade, 1980). Thus, these models attempt to capture the tendency to fixate things rather than empty regions as described earlier. Such models can generate specific quantitative predictions about the spatial distribution of eye fixations over a scene, and the predictions can be correlated with observed human fixations (Carmi and Itti, 2006; Parkhurst et al., 2002; Torralba et al., 2006).

A critical issue for saliency map models is how the salient points should be prioritized. For example, a single saliency map can be computed across the entire image, with fixation sites ordered on the basis of the ordered saliency derived from that single map. Inhibition of return (IOR) can then be applied to assure that the same sites are not re-selected for fixation, preventing oscillation among the most highly salient locations (Itti and Koch, 2000). An issue with this application of IOR is that the empirical evidence is weak that it operates to reduce the probability of refixating previously fixated sites. Recent evidence suggests that previously fixated locations are typically more rather than less likely to be fixated in both array search (Hooge et al., 2005; Motter and Belky, 1998) and in real-world scenes (Dodd et al., 2009; Smith and Henderson, 2009), contrary to the prediction that IOR should reduce the likelihood of such fixations.

Several additional issues arise with the visual salience approach. The first issue is whether a single saliency map is retained over multiple fixations, or whether instead a new saliency map is generated in each successive fixation. Using the latter option and weighting saliency by distance from the current fixation, Parkhurst and colleagues showed that better correlations were obtained with observed human fixation sites (Parkhurst et al., 2002). A second important issue involves determining which image properties should be taken into consideration in generating a saliency map. The model developed by Itti and colleagues (Itti and Koch, 2000; Itti et al., 1998, 2001) assumes that the saliency map is derived from a weighted linear combination of intensity, orientation, and colour, with motion recently added (Carmi and Itti, 2006), but other image properties including higher-order features (e.g. corners) could be considered (Krieger et al., 2000). A third issue concerns biological implementation: where in the brain is the saliency map computed and represented (Findlay and Walker, 1999; Gottlieb et al., 1998; Li, 2002)? Is there a single saliency map, or might there be multiple maps (Corbetta and Shulman, 2002; Li, 2002)?

A final related issue is whether computational models of visual saliency are to be taken as biologically and psychophysically plausible accounts of human perception of saliency, or whether instead they are meant to serve as testable hypotheses about how perceptual salience might be computed, or even simply as potential engineering solutions to the question of finding image differences. It is becoming common for investigators to use a specific implemented saliency model as a stand-in for perceptual salience, but this would appear to be a misuse of these models because to date there has been no strong test of the relationship between the models and perception. Casual inspection often reveals large discrepancies between model output and human judgements of visual salience. Appropriately used, these models serve as a hypothesis to be tested (against eye movement data or otherwise) about what determines visual salience. But they are sometimes taken instead as a proxy for visual salience itself as the human brain generates it and as the human mind perceives it. For example, the implemented Itti and Koch model is often used as a way to equate visual salience across experimental conditions. This use seems ill advised at best given that the ground-truth validity of the model, or even of the general approach, has not been established.

A shortcoming of both the scene statistics and saliency map approaches is that they rely on correlation techniques. However, an observed correlation of features (or saliency) with fixations does not allow a causal link to be established (Henderson, 2003). In a third method of investigating the influence of image features on fixation location, investigators have manipulated the nature of the scene images presented to viewers to try to establish a causal relationship. For example, Mannan et al. (1995, 1996) low-pass filtered scenes to remove all of the mid and high spatial frequency information in them, producing blurred versions of the original pictures. Over the first 1.5 s of viewing, viewers who inspected the low-pass filtered scenes fixated similar scene locations as those viewers presented the unfiltered images. Because the objects in many of the low-pass filtered scenes were not readily identifiable (though the gist of the scene may have been clear in some of the images and may have constrained image identities), these data suggest that eye movement control does not rely on object identification in the scene, consistent with the hypothesis that image features guide fixation. Studies directly manipulating image features have been rare, and more are needed to directly test hypotheses about their influence on eye movement control in scenes.

Investigation of the role of image features in eye movement control has generated important insights. However, the approach has several limitations. First, these approaches focus on stimulus-driven control of fixation placement at the expense of knowledge-based factors, even though image features do not seem strongly related to fixation placement for meaningful stimuli and active viewing tasks (Chen and Zelinsky, 2006; Einhäuser et al., 2008; Henderson et al., 2007; Henderson et al., 2009b; Jovancevic et al., 2006; Torralba et al., 2006; Turano et al., 2003; see also Land and Hayhoe, 2001; Pelz and Canosa, 2001). Most investigators working within the saliency framework are aware of the shortcoming of focusing only on stimulus influences and explicitly note that top-down factors will need to be incorporated into a complete model. The approach, though, is predicated on the assumption that top-down factors will modulate the fixation sites determined from bottom-up information. This is a reasonable first step, but substantial progress likely requires more emphasis on top-down information; for example, even initial saccades tend to take the eyes in the direction of a search target in a scene, presumably because information about the global scene gist and spatial layout generated from the first fixation provides important information about where a particular object is likely to be found (Castelhano and Henderson, 2007; Eckstein et al., 2006; Henderson et al., 1999; Oliva et al., 2003). Later fixations are even more likely to be based on knowledge about the identities and meanings of specific objects and their relationships to each other and to the scene (Henderson et al., 1999; Land and Hayhoe, 2001; Pelz and Canosa, 2001). In summary, perhaps the most important contribution of the bottom-up approach will be the demonstration that it does not do a very good job alone of predicting individual fixation positions.

Knowledge-driven control

The *looking at nothing* phenomenon highlights the active nature of scene perception: When a blank area of a scene becomes task-relevant, viewers will tend to fixate it (Ferreira et al., 2008). Intuitively, imagine trying to determine whether the colour of your wall is attractive. You can easily fixate a blank region of the wall to ponder its colour. In the laboratory, a strong tendency to fixate empty regions of a scene when they are task-relevant has been illustrated in several studies (e.g. Parker, 1978; Ryan et al., 2000; for other examples see Ferreira et al., 2008), providing direct evidence that top-down control can over-ride image features in guiding the eyes.

Human eye movement control clearly draws not only on currently available visual input, but also on a number of cognitive systems, including short-term memory for previously attended information in the current scene; stored long-term visual, spatial, and semantic information about other similar scenes; and the goals and plans of the viewer. Even the very first saccade in a scene can be strongly driven by scene knowledge, for example taking the eyes in the likely direction of a search target (Brockmole and Henderson, 2006; Castelhano and Henderson, 2007; Eckstein et al., 2006; Henderson et al., 1999; Torralba et al., 2006). These movements can be observed even when the search target is not actually present (Castelhano and Henderson, 2007).

Henderson and Ferreira (2004b) categorized the types of knowledge available to the eye movement control system (see Table 33.1). Information about a specific scene can be learned over the short term in the current perceptual encounter (short-term episodic scene knowledge) and over the long term across multiple encounters (long-term episodic scene knowledge). For example, knowing that you have recently placed your coffee cup on your desk to the right of your keyboard (short-term episodic knowledge), you would be in a position to more effectively direct your eyes when you are ready to pick it up again. Short-term knowledge ensures that objects are fixated when needed during motor interaction with the environment over the course of a complex visuomotor task (Hayhoe et al., 2003; Land et al., 1999) and also allows refixation of previously visited semantically interesting or informative scene areas. Short-term priming (e.g. Castelhano and Henderson, 2007) can also be considered a form of (very) short-term learning. In contrast, long-term episodic knowledge provides

Table 33.1 The types of knowledge available to direct eye movements

Knowledge sources influencing eye movements in scenes	Description	Example
Short-term episodic scene knowledge	Specific knowledge about a particular scene at a particular time	My cup is currently on my desk
Long-term episodic scene knowledge	Specific knowledge about a particular scene that is stable over time	My coffeemaker always sits on a shelf under the window.
Scene schema knowledge	Generic knowledge about a particular category of scene	Office computers are typically found on desks
Task knowledge	Generic knowledge about a particular category of task	Changing lanes while driving requires checking the side-view mirror

Modified from Henderson and Ferreira (2004b).

top-down information about aspects of specific scene instances that tend not to change. An example might be the knowledge that your coffeemaker always sits on a shelf under your office window.

A third important source of scene information is scene schema knowledge, generic semantic regularities in the environment of the sort that have traditionally been considered aspects of scene schemas (Biederman et al., 1982; Friedman, 1979; Mandler and Johnson, 1977). Scene schema knowledge arises from semantic regularities across multiple episodes with scenes instances from a common scene category. For example, in offices, computers are typically found on desks.

A fourth type of knowledge is task knowledge, that is, knowledge about how to move one's eyes in the service of a particular goal or set of goals. In a classic example of task effects on gaze control, Yarbus (1967) noted that viewers change their scan patterns over a scene depending on the specific viewing task they are engaged in. Under more controlled conditions, it has been shown that the distribution of fixations in a scene differs depending on whether a viewer is searching for an object or trying to memorize that scene (Castelhano et al., 2009; Henderson et al., 1999). More generally, specific tasks generate specific kinds of eye movement behaviour. Land et al. (1999) and Hayhoe et al. (2003) showed that when making tea or sandwiches, people had a strong tendency to fixate a task relevant object as the object became important in the task sequence. Pelz and Canosa (2001) reported in a hand-washing task that viewers sometimes produced what they called *look-ahead fixations* that were related to future actions associated with the high-level goals of the task rather than to the salience of the visual properties of the immediate environment. Eye movements also have particular patterns during other complex and well-learned activities such as driving (Land and Lee, 1994) and cricket batting (Land and McLeod, 2000).

Task related knowledge could potentially produce specific sequences of fixations, though the evidence for such patterns is currently weak (see Henderson, 2003). The study of eye movement sequences (*scan patterns*) has received less attention among scene researchers than perhaps it should (though see Foulsham and Underwood, 2008). One reason for this lack of interest is that the general concept of scan patterns became entangled with a specific theory that did not survive close empirical scrutiny. In *scan path theory*, the scan pattern produced during complex image viewing was assumed to be an integral part of the memory for that image (Noton and Stark, 1971a, 1971b). Learning a new image was taken to involve encoding both its visual features and the gaze sequence used to acquire it, with the motor pattern becoming part of an integrated memory representation. Recognition was assumed to require recapitulating the gaze sequence. Similarity in scan patterns across learning and recognition was taken to support the theory. However, it is not necessary for a viewer to make eye movements to recognize scenes that were learned using eye movements, as shown by studies of scene identification within a single fixation (e.g. see many of the references associated with scene gist above). Also, sequences of fixations through scenes are highly variable across and within viewers

(Groner et al., 1984; Mannan et al., 1997a; Walker-Smith et al., 1977; cf. Foulsham and Underwood, 2008). The nature of scan patterns in scenes is a relatively understudied issue, and future work may produce evidence for some consistency over scenes due either to feature-based or top-down factors (Foulsham and Underwood, 2008). Also, in dynamic scenes where motion may influence fixations, the *attentional synchrony* or time-locked similarity in scan patterns produced by viewers does tend to be stronger (Smith and Henderson, 2008).

In summary, although prior work has tended to focus either on image features or knowledge-based control, in the end image properties about potential fixation targets must somehow be combined with top-down constraints. How this is accomplished is a critical issue in the study of eye movements during scene viewing. One approach is to construct the initial stimulus-based saliency map taking relevant knowledge (e.g. visual properties of a search target) into account from the outset (Rao et al., 2002). Another approach is to compute a stimulus-based saliency map independently of other knowledge-based maps. For example, Torralba et al. (2006) combined an image-based saliency map with a separate knowledge-based map highlighting regions likely to contain a specific search target. A third method is to use visual saliency in an intermediate computational step on the way to generating a scene region map that does not represent saliency (Henderson et al., 2009). Other methods are certainly possible. How best to account for the combined influences of image and knowledge is an important current topic of investigation.

How long do we look?

Average fixation duration during scene viewing is about 300 ms, but there is significant variability around this mean both within an individual viewer and across individuals (Andrews and Coppola, 1999; Castelhano et al., 2009; see Henderson and Hollingworth, 1998; Rayner, 1998) (Fig. 33.2). Conclusions about the distribution of attention over a scene can differ markedly when fixation position is weighted by fixation duration because the distribution of processing time across a scene is a function of both the spatial distribution and duration of fixations (Henderson, 2003). This variability is at least partially controlled by visual and cognitive factors associated with the currently fixated scene. For example, individual fixation duration (the duration of each discrete fixation) is affected by scene luminance (Loftus, 1985), contrast (Loftus et al., 1992), and quality (van Diepen et al., 1995). Mean individual fixation duration is also longer for full colour photographs than black-and-white line drawings, though the distributions are very similar (Henderson and Hollingworth, 1998). Individual fixation durations are influenced by viewing task, with longer fixation durations during scene memorization than search (Castelhano et al., 2009; Henderson et al., 1999). Fixation durations are also related to the amplitude of related saccades (Unema et al., 2005). The influence of visual and cognitive factors on fixation duration is generally acknowledged in the eye movement control literature and has been explicitly incorporated in computational models of reading (Engbert et al., 2005; Reichle et al., 1998), but has generally been overlooked in the literature on eye movement control in scenes.

Stimulus and task can affect summed measures of fixation time even when individual fixation durations are unchanged. For example, first-pass gaze duration (the sum of all fixations in a region from first entry to exit) on an object in a scene is increased by a visual change to that object, even when the viewer does not notice the change (Henderson and Hollingworth, 2003; Hollingworth and Henderson, 2002; Hollingworth et al., 2001b; Hayhoe et al., 1998). Gaze durations are also influenced by object and scene semantics, with longer durations on semantically informative (i.e. less consistent) than uninformative (i.e. more consistent) objects (De Graef et al., 1990; Friedman, 1979; Henderson et al., 1999; Hollingworth et al., 2001b; Vō and Henderson, 2009).

An important issue is whether the durations of individual fixations are directly controlled by the immediately present information, or whether instead they're controlled by global parameters. For example, are fixation durations elevated for low-contrast images because a general parameter is set to delay all fixations, or because each fixation is individually affected by the lower contrast? Interestingly, up until recently it has been very difficult to find immediate effects of the current scene on fixation durations during scene viewing (see Henderson and Ferreira, 2004b, for discussion).

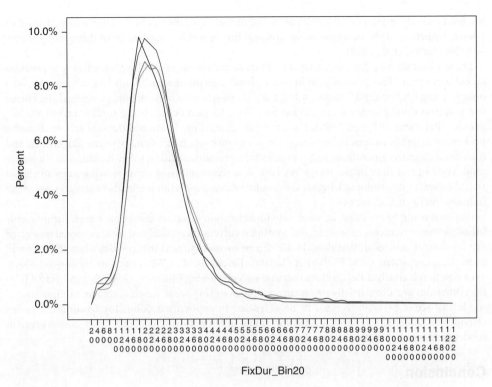

Fig. 33.2 Four example fixation duration distributions. Curves are based on histograms with 20 ms bins.

Two studies have recently investigated in a more direct manner the degree to which fixation duration variability is controlled by the immediately available visual input within a given fixation (Henderson and Pierce, 2006; Henderson and Smith, 2009). These studies used a scene onset delay paradigm in which the presence of the scene was delayed at the beginning of specific critical fixations. To implement the delay, a saccade-contingent display change technique was used to blank the scene during the saccade just prior to the critical fixation. Following a pre-specified delay period, the scene returned to view. The main question was how the duration of the critical fixation would be affected by the scene onset delay. The results showed that the distribution of fixation durations changed as a function of delay. A set of early fixation durations was little influenced by the duration of the delay. These fixations appeared to be insensitive to the current visual input. A second set of fixations increased in duration as a function of delay duration. These fixations appeared to be under immediate influence of the current visual input. This overall pattern held for delays filled with a noise mask or a grey field, was not due to the predictability of the delay period or to learning the nature of the delay, and generalized across visual search and memorization tasks.

The results are most consistent with a mixed control model of fixation duration in which an autonomous control component works to keep the eyes moving at a relatively constant rate independently of the current visual input, along with a process monitoring component that monitors current input and exerts an immediate influence on the current fixation duration. The autonomous component leads to a set of fixation durations that are unaffected by the currently available scene input. The process-monitoring component leads to another set of fixation durations that are lengthened with increasing delay of the current input.

One way to think about the interaction of an autonomous timer and process monitoring is in terms of an inhibitory signal generated by process monitoring that can override saccades that would otherwise be generated from the timer (Findlay and Walker, 1999; Yang and McConkie, 2001).

We have recently implemented a computational model based on this basic scheme as well as other known properties of the oculomotor system, and this model fits the data from this paradigm very well (Nuthmann et al., 2010).

The finding that stimulus onset delay can influence the durations of at least some fixations provides an existence proof that fixations can be under direct control in scenes. This fact in turn opens the door to using fixation durations as a subtle measure of attention and ongoing perceptual and cognitive processes during scene viewing, as has been done to great benefit in the reading and psycholinguistics literatures (Rayner, 1998). For example, in reading, fixation durations reflect stimulus properties as subtle as lexical frequency, more abstract representational systems like syntax, and high-level cognitive operations like semantic interpretation. The fact that fixation durations are modulated in real time by the image available in a fixation during scene viewing suggests that it would be worth determining whether more subtle scene properties might also exert an immediate influence on fixation durations.

It is interesting to note that because individual fixation duration effects have been firmly established for eye movements in reading, the dominant current theoretical and computational models of eye movement control in that domain are driven by mechanisms that predict when the eyes will move (e.g. Carpenter, 1988; Engbert et al., 2005; Reichle et al., 1998; Yang and McConkie, 2001). This situation is clearly different from that in the scene viewing literature. Given that individual fixation durations are also partially under direct control during scene viewing, current computational models of scene perception need to be extended to explicitly account for fixation durations (Henderson, 2003, 2007). Such an extension would potentially lead to an instructive convergence of models across scene viewing and reading.

Conclusion

Humans use knowledge about the world to guide gaze intelligently through a scene. Cognitive systems interact with each other and with the scene image to determine where the eyes fixate and how long they remain fixated at a particular location. Evolution has clearly favoured this active vision approach, and understanding why is of central concern in the study of natural scene perception.

References

Andrews, T.J. and Coppola, D.M. (1999). Idiosyncratic characteristics of saccadic eye movements when viewing different visual environments. *Vision Research*, **39**, 2947–2953.

Antes, J.R. (1974). The time course of picture viewing. *Journal of Experimental Psychology*, **103**, 62–70.

Antes, J.R. and Penland J.G. (1981). Picture context effect on eye movement patterns. In D. F. Fisher, R. A. Monty, and J.W. Senders (eds.) *Eye movements: Cognition and visual perception*. Hillsdale, NJ: Erlbaum.

Baddeley, R.J., and Tatler, B.W. (2006). High frequency edges (but not contrast) predict where we fixate: A Bayesian system identification analysis. *Vision Research*, **46**, 2824–2833.

Ballard, D.H. (1996). On the function of visual representation. In K. Akins (ed.) *Perception: Vancouver Studies in Cognitive Science*. Oxford: Oxford University Press.

Ballard, D.H., Hayhoe, M.M., and Pelz, J.B. (1995). Memory representations in natural tasks. *Journal of Cognitive Neuroscience*, **7**, 66–80.

Ballard, D.H., Hayhoe, M.M., Pook, P.K., and Rao, R.P. (1997). Deictic codes for the embodiment of cognition. *Behavioral and Brain Sciences*, **20**, 723–767.

Biederman, I. (1972). Perceiving real-world scenes. *Science*, **177**, 77–80.

Biederman, I., Mezzanotte, R.J., and Rabinowitz, J.C. (1982). Scene perception: Detecting and judging objects undergoing relational violations. *Cognitive Psychology*, **14**, 143–177.

Biederman, I., Rabinowitz, J.C., Glass, A.L., and Stacy, E.W. Jr (1974). On the information extracted from a glance at a scene. *Journal of Experimental Psychology*, **103**, 597–600.

Boyce, S.J. and Pollatsek, A. (1992). The identification of objects in scenes: The role of scene backgrounds in object naming. *Journal of Experimental Psychology: Learning, Memory, and Cognition*, **18**, 531–543.

Brockmole, J.R. and Henderson, J.M. (2006). Recognition and attention guidance during contextual cueing in real-world scenes: Evidence from eye movements. *Quarterly Journal of Experimental Psychology*, **59**, 1177–1187.

Buswell, G.T. (1935). *How People Look at Pictures*. Chicago, IL: University of Chicago Press.

Carmi, R. and Itti, L (2006). Visual causes versus correlates of attentional selection in dynamic scenes. *Vision Research*, **46**, 4333–4345.

Carpenter, R.H.S. (1988). *Movements of the eyes*. London: Pion.

Castelhano, M.S. and Henderson, J.M. (2007). Initial scene representations facilitate eye movement guidance in visual search. *Journal of Experimental Psychology: Human Perception and Performance*, **33**, 753–763.

Castelhano, M.S., Mack, M., and Henderson, J.M. (2009). Viewing task influences eye movement control during active scene perception. *Journal of Vision*, **9**(3), 6.1–15.

Chen, X., and Zelinsky, G.J. (2006). Real-world visual search is dominated by top-down guidance. *Vision Research*, **46**, 4118–4133.

Churchland, P.S., Ramachandran, V.S., Sejnowski, T.J. (1994). A critique of pure vision. In C. Koch and S. Davis (eds.) *Large scale neuronal theories of the brain*. (pp. 23–60). Cambridge MA: MIT Press.

Corbetta, M. and Shulman, G.L. (2002). Control of goal-directed and stimulus-driven attention in the brain. *Nature Reviews Neuroscience*, **3**, 201–215.

De Graef, P, Christiaens, D, d'Ydewalle, G. 1990. Perceptual effects of scene context on object identification. *Psychological Research*, **52**, 317–329.

Dodd, M.D., Van der Stigchel, S., and Hollingworth, A. (2009). Novelty is not always the best policy: Inhibition of return and facilitation of return as a function of visual task. *Psychological Science*, **20**, 333–339.

Eckstein, M.P., Drescher, B., and Shimozaki, S.S. (2006). Attentional cues in real scenes: saccadic targeting and Bayesian priors. *Psychological Science*, **17**, 973–980.

Einhäuser, W., Rutishauser, U., and Koch, C. (2008). Task-demands can immediately reverse the effects of sensory-driven saliency in complex visual stimuli. *Journal of Vision*, **8**(2), 2.1–19.

Engbert, R., Nuthmann, A., Richter, E. and Kliegl, R. (2005). SWIFT: A dynamical model of saccade generation during reading. *Psychological Review*, **112**, 777–813.

Epstein, R. and Kanwisher, N. (1998). A cortical representation of the local visual environment. *Nature*, **392**, 598–601.

Epstein, R., Graham, K.S., and Downing, P.E. (2003). Viewpoint-specific scene representations in human parahippocampal cortex. *Neuron*, **37**, 865–876.

Epstein, R., Harris, A., Stanley, D., and Kanwisher, N. (1999). The parahippocampal place area: Recognition, navigation, or encoding. *Neuron*, **23**, 115–125.

Fei-Fei, L., Iyer, A., Koch, C., and Perona, P. (2006). What do we perceive in a glance of a real-world scene? *Journal of Vision*, **7**(1), 10.1–29.

Ferreira, F., Apel, J., and Henderson, J.M. (2008). Taking a new look at looking at nothing. *Trends in Cognitive Sciences*, **12**, 405–410.

Field, D.J. (1987). Relations between the statistics of natural images and the response properties of cortical cells. *Journal of the Optical Society of America A*, **4**, 2379–2394.

Findlay, J.M. and Walker, R. (1999). A model of saccade generation based on parallel processing and competitive inhibition. *Behavioral and Brain Sciences*, **22**, 661–721.

Foulsham, T. and Underwood, G. (2008). What can saliency models predict about eye movements? Spatial and sequential aspects of fixations during encoding and recognition. *Journal of Vision*, **8**(2), 6.1–17.

Friedman, A. (1979). Framing pictures: The role of knowledge in automatized encoding and memory for gist. *Journal of Experimental Psychology: General*, **108**, 316–355.

Gareze, L. and Findlay, J.M. (2007). Absence of scene context effects in object detection and eye gaze capture. In R. van Gompel, M. Fischer, W. Murray, and R. Hill (eds.) *Eye movements: A window on mind and brain* (pp. 618–637). Oxford: Elsevier.

Geisler, W.S. (2008) Visual perception and the statistical properties of natural scenes. *Annual Review of Psychology*, **59**, 167–192.

Griffin, Z. (2004). Why look? Reasons for speech-related eye movements. In J.M. Henderson, and F. Ferreira (eds.) *The interface of language, vision, and action: Eye movements and the visual world*. New York: Psychology Press.

Gottlieb, J.P., Kusunoki, M., and Goldberg, M.E. (1998). The representation of salience in monkey parietal cortex. *Nature*, **391**, 481–484.

Groner, R., Walder, F., and Groner, M. (1984). Looking at face: Local and global aspects of scanpths. In A.G. Gale and F. Johnson (eds.) *Theoretical and applied aspects of eye movement research* (pp. 523–533). Amsterdam: Elsevier.

Hayhoe, M.M., Bensinger, D.G., and Ballard, D.H. (1998). Task constraints in visual working memory. *Vision Research*, **38**, 125–137.

Hayhoe, M.M., Shrivastava, A., Mruczek, R., and Pelz, J.B. (2003). Visual memory and motor planning in a natural task. *Journal of Vision*, **3**, 49–63.

Henderson, J.M. (1992). Object identification in context: The visual processing of natural scenes. *Canadian Journal of Psychology*, **46**, 319–341.

Henderson, J.M. (1993). Visual attention and saccadic eye movements. In G. d'Ydewalle and J. Van Rensbergen (eds.) *Perception and cognition: Advances in eye movement research* (pp. 37–50). Amsterdam: North Holland.

Henderson, J.M. (2003). Human gaze control in real-world scene perception. *Trends in Cognitive Sciences*, **7**, 498–504.

Henderson, J.M. (2007). Regarding scenes. *Current Directions in Psychological Science*, **16**, 219–222.

Henderson, J.M. and Ferreira, F. (eds.) (2004a). *The interface of language, vision, and action: Eye movements and the visual world*. New York: Psychology Press.

Henderson, J.M. and Ferreira, F. (2004b). Scene perception for psycholinguists. In J. M. Henderson and F. Ferreira (eds.) *The interface of language, vision, and action: Eye movements and the visual world* (pp. 1–58). New York: Psychology Press.

Henderson, J.M. and Hollingworth, A. (1998). Eye movements during scene viewing: An overview. In G. Underwood (ed.), *Eye Guidance in Reading and Scene Perception* (pp. 269–283). Oxford: Elsevier.

Henderson, J.M. and Hollingworth, A. (1999). High-level scene perception. *Annual Review of Psychology*, 50, 243–271.

Henderson, J.M. and Hollingworth, A. (2003). Eye movements, visual memory, and scene representation. In M. Peterson and G. Rhodes (eds.) *Perception of faces, objects, and scenes: Analytic and holistic processes*. Oxford University Press.

Henderson, J.M. and Pierce, G.L. (2008). Eye movements during scene viewing: Evidence for mixed control of fixation durations. *Psychonomic Bulletin & Review*, 15, 566–573.

Henderson, J.M. and Smith, T.J. (2009). How are eye fixation durations controlled during scene viewing? Further evidence from a scene onset delay paradigm. *Visual Cognition*, 17, 1055–1082.

Henderson, J.M., Weeks, P.A. Jr, and Hollingworth, A. (1999). Effects of semantic consistency on eye movements during scene viewing. *Journal of Experimental Psychology: Human Perception and Performance*, 25, 210–228.

Henderson, J.M., Larson, C.L., and Zhu, D.C. (2008). Full scenes produce more activation than close-up scenes and scene-diagnostic objects in parahippocampal and retrosplenial cortex: An fMRI study. *Brain and Cognition*, 66, 40–49.

Henderson, J.M., Chanceaux, M., and Smith, T.J. (2009a). The influence of clutter on real-world scene search: Evidence from search efficiency and eye movements. *Journal of Vision*, 9(1), 32.1–8.

Henderson, J.M., Malcolm, G.L., and Schandl, C. (2009b). Searching in the dark: Cognitive relevance drives attention in real-world scenes. *Psychonomic Bulletin and Review*, 16, 850–856.

Henderson, J.M., Brockmole, J.R., Castelhano, M.S., and Mack, M. (2007). Visual saliency does not account for eye movements during visual search in real-world scenes. In R. van Gompel, M. Fischer, W. Murray, and R. Hill (eds.) *Eye movements: A window on mind and brain* (pp. 537–562). Oxford: Elsevier.

Hollingworth, A. and Henderson, J.M. (1998). Does consistent scene context facilitate object perception? *Journal of Experimental Psychology: General*, 127, 398–415.

Hollingworth, A. and Henderson, J.M. (1999). Object identification is isolated from scene semantic constraint: Evidence from object type and token discrimination. *Acta Psychologica*, 102 (Special Issue on Object Perception and Memory), 319–343.

Hollingworth, A. and Henderson, J.M. (2002). Accurate visual memory for previously attended objects in natural scenes. *Journal of Experimental Psychology: Human Perception and Performance*, 28, 113–136.

Hollingworth, A., Schrock, G., and Henderson, J.M. (2001a). Change detection in the flicker paradigm: The role of fixation position within the scene. *Memory and Cognition*, 29, 296–304.

Hollingworth, A., Williams, C.C., and Henderson, J.M. (2001b). To see and remember: Visually specific information is retained in memory from previously attended objects in natural scenes. *Psychonomic Bulletin and Review*, 8, 761–768.

Hooge, I.T., Over, E.A., van Wezel, R.J., and Frens, M.A. (2005). Inhibition of return is not a foraging facilitator in saccadic search and free viewing. *Vision Research*, 45, 1901–1908.

Intraub, H. (1979). Presentation rate and the representation of briefly glimpsed pictures in memory. *Journal of Experimental Psychology: Human Learning and Memory*, 5, 78–87.

Intraub, H. (1980). The role of implicit naming in pictorial encoding. *Journal of Experimental Psychology: Human Learning and Memory*, 6, 1–12.

Intraub, H. (1981). Rapid conceptual identification of sequentially presented pictures. *Journal of Experimental Psychology: Human Perception and Performance*, 7, 604–610.

Itti., L. and Koch, C. (2000). A saliency-based search mechanism for overt and covert shifts of visual attention. *Vision Research*, 40, 1489–1506.

Itti, L. and Koch, C. (2001). Computational modeling of visual attention. *Nature Reviews: Neuroscience*, 2, 194–203.

Itti, L., Koch, C., and Niebur, E. (1998). A model of saliency-based visual attention for rapid scene analysis. *IEEE Transactions on pattern Analysis and Machine Intelligence*, 20, 1254–1259.

Itti, L., Gold, C., and Koch, C. (2001). Visual attention and target detection in cluttered natural scenes. *Optical Engineering*, 40, 1784–1793.

Jovancevic, J., Sullivan, B., and Hayhoe, M. (2006). Control of attention and gaze in complex environments. *Journal of Vision*, 6(12), 9.1431–1450.

Koch, C. and Ullman, S. (1985). Shifts in selective visual attention: towards the underlying neural circuitry. *Human Neurobiology*, 4, 219–227.

Krieger, G., Rentschler, I., Hauske, G., Schill, K., and Zetsche, C. (2000). Object and scene analysis by saccadic eye-movements: an investigation with higher-order statistics. *Spatial Vision*, 13, 201–214.

Land, M.F. (1999). Motion and vision: Why animals move their eyes. *Journal of Comparative Physiology A*, 185, 341–352.

Land, M.F. and Hayhoe, M. (2001). In what ways do eye movements contribute to everyday activities? *Vision Research*, 41, 3559–3565.

Land, M.F. and Lee, D.N. (1994). Where we look when we steer. *Nature*, 369, 742–744.

Land, M.F., and McLeod, P. (2000). From eye movements to actions: How cricket batsmen hit the ball. *Nature Neuroscience*, 3, 1340–1345.

Land, M.F., Mennie, N., and Rusted, J. (1999). Eye movements and the roles of vision in activities of daily living: making a cup of tea. *Perception*, **28**, 1311–1328.

Lampinen, J.M., Copeland, S.M., and Neuschatz, J.S. (2001). Recollections of things schematic: Room schemas revisited. *Journal of Experimental Psychology: Learning, Memory, and Cognition*, 27, 1211–1222.

Li, Z. (2002). A saliency map in primary visual cortex. *Trends in Cognitive Sciences*, **6**, 9–16.

Loftus, G.R. (1985). Picture perception: Effects of luminance on available information and information-extraction rate. *Journal of Experimental Psychology: General*, **114**, 342–356.

Loftus, G.R. and Mackworth, N.H. (1978). Cognitive determinants of fixation location during picture viewing. *Journal of Experimental Psychology: Human Perception and Performance*, **4**, 565–572.

Loftus, G.R., Nelson, W.W., and Kallman, H.J. (1983). Differential acquisition rates for different types of information from pictures. *Quarterly Journal of Experimental Psychology*, **35A**, 187–198.

Loftus, G.R., Kaufman, L., Nishimoto, T., and Ruthruff, E. (1992). Effects of visual degradation on eye-fixation durations, perceptual processing, and long-term visual memory. In K.Rayner (ed.) *Eye movements and visual cognition: Scene perception and reading* (pp. 203–226). New York: Springer.

Mackworth, N.H. and Morandi, A.J. (1967). The gaze selects informative details within pictures. *Perception and Psychophysics*, **2**, 547–552.

Mandler, J.M. and Johnson, N.S. (1977). Some of the thousand words a picture is worth. *Journal of Experimental Psychology: Human Learning and Memory*, **2**, 529–540.

Mannan, S., Ruddock, K.H., and Wooding, D.S. (1995). Automatic control of saccadic eye movements made in visual inspection of briefly presented 2-D images. *Spatial Vision*, **9**, 363–386.

Mannan, S.K., Ruddock, K.H., and Wooding, D.S. (1996). The relationship between the locations of spatial features and those of fixations made during visual examination of briefly presented images. *Spatial Vision*, **10**, 165–188.

Mannan, S.K., Ruddock, K.H., and Wooding, D.S. (1997a). Fixation sequences made during visual examination of briefly presented 2D images. *Spatial Vision*, **11**, 157–178.

Mannan, S.K., Ruddock, K.H., and Wooding, D.S. (1997b). Fixation patterns made during brief examination of two-dimensional images. *Perception*, **26**, 1059–1072.

Matin, E. (1974). Saccadic suppression: A review and an analysis. *Psychological Bulletin*, **81**, 899–917.

Meyer, A.S., and Lethaus, F. (2004). The use of eye tracking in studies of sentence generation. In J. M. Henderson, and F. Ferreira (eds.) *The interface of language, vision, and action: Eye movements and the visual world*. New York: Psychology Press, Taylor and Francis Group.

Motter, B.C. and Belky, E.J. (1998). The guidance of eye movements during active visual search. *Vision Research*, **38**, 1805–1815.

Murphy, G.L., and Wisniewski, E.J. (1989). Categorizing objects in isolation and in scenes: What a superordinate is good for. *Journal of Experimental Psychology: Learning, Memory, and Cognition*, **4**, 572–586.

Navalpakkam, V. and Itti, L. (2005). Modeling the influence of task on attention. *Vision Research*, **45**, 205–231.

Nelson, W.W., and Loftus, G.R. (1980). The functional visual field during picture viewing. *Journal of Experimental Psychology: Human Learning and Memory*, **6**, 391–399.

Noton, D. and Stark, L. (1971a). Scan paths in eye movements during pattern perception. *Science*, **171**, 308–311.

Noton, D. and Stark, L. (1971b). Scan paths in saccadic eye movements while viewing and recognizing patterns. *Vision Research*, **11**, 929–944.

Nuthmann, A., Smith, T.J., Engbert, R., and Henderson, J.M. (2010). CRISP: A computational model of fixation durations in scene viewing. *Psychological Review*, **117**, 382–405.

O'Craven, K.M. and Kanwisher, N. (2000). Mental imagery of faces and places activates corresponding stimulus-specific brain regions. *Journal of Cognitive Neuroscience*, **12**, 1013–1023.

Oliva, A., Torralba, A., Casthelano, M. and Henderson, J. (2003). Top-Down control of visual attention in object detection. Proceeding of the IEEE International Conference Image Processing, Vol 1 (pp 253–256).

Parker, R.E. (1978). Picture processing during recognition. *Journal of Experimental Psychology: Human Perception and Performance*, **4**, 284–293.

Parkhurst, D., Law, K., and Niebur, E. (2002). Modeling the role of salience in the allocation of overt visual attention. *Vision Research*, **42**, 107–123.

Parkhurst, D.J. and Niebur, E. (2003). Scene content selected by active vision. *Spatial Vision*, **6**, 125–154.

Pelz, J.B. and Canosa, R. (2001). Oculomotor behavior and perceptual strategies in complex tasks. *Vision Research*, **41**, 3587–3596.

Potter, M.C. (1975). Meaning in visual search. *Science*, **187**, 965–966.

Potter, M.C. (1976). Short_term conceptual memory for pictures. *Journal of Experimental Psychology: Human Learning and Memory*, **2**, 509–522.

Potter, M.C. (1999). Understanding sentences and scenes: The role of conceptual short-term memory. In V. Coltheart (ed.), *Fleeting memories* (pp. 13–46). Cambridge, MA: MIT Press.

Rao, R.P.N., Zelinsky, G.J., Hayhoe, M.M., and Ballard, D.H. (2002). Eye movements in iconic visual search. *Vision Research*, **42**, 1447–1463.

Rayner, K. (1998). Eye movements in reading and information processing: 20 years of research. *Psychological Bulletin*, **124**, 372–422.

Reichle, E.D., Pollatsek, A., Fisher, D.L., Rayner, K. (1998). Toward a model of eye movement control in reading. *Psychological Review*, **105**, 125–157.

Reinagel, P., and Zador, A.M. (1999). Natural scene statistics at the centre of gaze. *Network: Computer and Neural Systems*, **10**, 1–10.

Ryan, J.D., Althoff, R.R., Whitlow, S., and Cohen, N.J. (2000). Amensia is a deficit in relational memory. *Psychological Science*, **11**, 454–461.

Sanocki, T. and Epstein, W. (1997). Priming spatial layout of scenes. *Psychological Science*, **8**, 374–378.

Schyns, P. and Oliva, A. (1994). From blobs to boundary edges: Evidence for time- and spatial-scale-dependent scene recognition. *Psychological Science*, **5**, 195–200.

Simoncelli, E.P. and B.A. Olshausen (2001). Natural image statistics and neural representation. *Annual Review of Neuroscience*, **24**, 1193–1216.

Smith, T.J. and Henderson, J.M. (2008). Edit Blindness: The relationship between attention and global change blindness in dynamic scenes. *Journal of Eye Movement Research*, **2**(2):6, 1–17.

Smith, T.J. and Henderson, J.M. (2009). Facilitation of return during scene viewing. *Visual Cognition*, **17**, 1083–1108.

Tanenhaus, M.K., Chambers, C.G., and Hanna, J.E. (2004). Referential domains in spoken language comprehension: Using eye movements to bridge the product and action traditions. In J.M. Henderson and F. Ferreira (eds.) *The interface of language, vision, and action: Eye movements and the visual world*. New York: Psychology Press.

Thiele, A., Henning, M., Buischik, K., Hoffman, P. (2002). Neural mechanisms of saccadic suppression. *Science*, **295**, 2460–2462.

Thorpe, S.J, Fize, D., and Marlot, C. (1996). Speed of processing in the human visual system. *Nature*, **381**, 520–522.

Torralba, A. (2003). Modeling global scene factors in attention. *Journal of the Optical Society of America*, **20**, 1407–1418.

Torralba, A., Oliva, A., Castelhano, M.S., and Henderson, J.M. (2006). Contextual guidance of eye movements and attention in real-world scenes: The role of global features in object search. *Psychological Review*, **113**, 766–786.

Treisman, A. and Gelade, G. (1980). A feature integration theory of attention. *Cognitive Psychology*, **12**, 97–136.

Turano, K.A. Geruschat, D.R., and Baker, F.H. (2003). Oculomotor strategies for the direction of gaze tested with a real-world activity. *Vision Research*, **43**, 333–346.

Tversky, B. and Hemenway, K. (1983). Categories of environmental scenes. *Cognitive Psychology*, **15**, 121–149.

Unema, P.J.A., Pannasch, S., Joos, M., and Velichkovsky, B.M. (2005). Time course of information processing during scene perception: The relationship between saccade amplitude and fixation duration. *Visual Cognition*, **12**, 473–494.

van Diepen, P.M.J., De Graef, P., and d'Ydewalle, G. (1995). Chronometry of foveal information extraction during scene perception. In J.M. Findlay, R. Walker, and R.W. Kentridge (eds.) *Eye movement research: Mechanisms, processes and applications* (pp. 349–362). Amsterdam: Elsevier.

VanRullen, R. and Thorpe, S.J. (2001). Is it a bird? Is it a plane? Ultra-rapid visual categorisation of natural and artifactual objects. *Perception*, **30**, 655–668.

Volkmann, F.C. (1986). Human visual suppression. *Vision Research*, **26**, 1401–1416.

Võ, M.L.-H. and Henderson, J.M. (2009). Does gravity matter? Effects of semantic and syntactic inconsistencies on the allocation of attention during scene perception. *Journal of Vision* **9**(3), 24.1–15.

Walker-Smith, G.J., Gale, A.G., and Findlay J.M. (1977). Eye movements strategies involved in face perception. *Perception*, **6**, 313–326.

Yang, S.N. and McConkie, G.W. (2001). Eye movements during reading: a theory of saccade initiation times. *Vision Research*, **41**, 3567–3585.

Yarbus, A.L. (1967). *Eye movements and vision*. New York: Plenum Press.

CHAPTER 34

Mechanisms of gaze control in natural vision

Mary M. Hayhoe and Dana H. Ballard

Abstract

Recent developments in measurement of eye movements in unconstrained observers have led to a variety of insights that would be difficult to achieve in more constrained experimental contexts. This work shifts the focus away from the properties of the stimulus, toward a consideration of the behavioural goals of the observer. This insight has been accompanied by a growing understanding of the importance of reward in modulating the underlying neural mechanisms of eye movement control, and by theoretical developments using Reinforcement Learning models of sensorimotor behaviour. These developments provide us with the tools to understanding how tasks might control acquisition of information through use of gaze.

A central feature of natural vision is that information is dynamically acquired from the environment to guide ongoing actions and behavioural goals. Information from a scene is actively sampled by a sequence of gaze changes that reflect three fundamental constraints on the visual system. First, the limited acuity of the peripheral retina necessitates gaze changes that bring the high resolution fovea onto regions of interest. Second, attention limits the information that can be processed within a single fixation, and finally, working memory limits the information retained across gaze positions. Although the resolution limits are quite well understood, the consequences of attentional and memory limitations, and how they act to control the selective acquisition of visual information, are much less clear. Thus to understand vision we need to understand how the sequential sampling of visual information is controlled, in the context of these constraints. Recent research suggests that the concepts of *reward* (costs and benefits of the outcome of a gaze change), *uncertainty* (of both sensory state and outcome), and *prior knowledge* (probability distributions associated with world states) are all critical factors for understanding gaze allocation in the natural world.

The role of stimulus features

The traditional approach to understanding control of attention and gaze has been to assume that gaze is primarily controlled by properties of the stimulus itself. It is generally thought that some ongoing bottom-up, pre-attentive analysis of the visual image takes place, and that the products of this analysis attract the observer's attention to important or salient aspects of the image for further processing (Wolfe, 1994). There is evidence that image features such as high spatial frequency content, edge density, and local contrast play a role in attracting fixations (e.g. Henderson, 2003). It has also been demonstrated that visual saliency, based on image features such as colour, intensity, contrast, and edge orientation, can account for some of the variance in gaze distribution when viewing two-dimensional (2D) images (e.g. Itti and Koch, 2001; Torralba, 2003). In addition, sudden onset stimuli have considerable ability to capture attention even if the observer's attention is directed elsewhere (e.g. Gibson et al., 2008; Jonides and Yantis, 1988; Theeuwes and Godisn, 2001; Yantis, 1998;). Other stimuli, such as a unique colour or shape, or motion stimuli also capture attention or gaze (e.g. Franceroni and Simons, 2003; Irwin et al., 2000). Recent models of gaze in 2D images add a top-down component that reflects scene gist, or specification of a search target (Navalpakkam and Itti, 2005; Torralba et al., 2006; Zhang et al., 2008;) but rely on modulation of an initial stimulus saliency computation, and the concept of the saliency map has become a central organizing focus of models of gaze control.

The role of behavioural goals

Despite the large body of work on capture of attention and gaze by stimulus properties per se, it is unlikely that these mechanisms can explain gaze and attention in natural environments. Models based on stimulus saliency usually cannot predict the exact fixation points and can leave more than half of the fixations unaccounted for (e.g. Foulsham and Underwood, 2008). It seems likely that the central problem is that stimulus saliency is correlated with fixation behaviour, but is not actually causal (Einhauser et al., 2008; Henderson, 2007; Tatler, 2007). While high signal/noise ratio resulting from bottom-up signals is obviously important and will facilitate detection and discrimination, it is only one component of the general problem of gaze allocation. In natural behaviour the visual input is dynamic and contingent on the actions of the observer. However, almost all of the work showing stimulus-based effects of attentional or oculomotor capture has been done with 2D experimental displays and either simple geometric stimuli or photographic renderings of natural scenes that are much simpler than real, time-varying environments. Perhaps most critically, subjects need different information when negotiating real environments than when looking at a picture, and this information changes as a function of time. Paradigms where subjects view 2D images cannot capture these aspects of attention and gaze control. To address these complexities, and to understand the deployment of gaze, it is therefore necessary to directly examine natural visually guided behaviour in realistic 3D environments that capture the exigencies of the real world. Investigation of gaze allocation in these environments has revealed the importance of additional factors as follows:

Acquisition of visual information is goal driven

Since the development of head-mounted eye trackers, eye movements during a variety of natural behaviours such as driving, walking, various sports, and making tea or sandwiches have been investigated. The central finding is that gaze locations are very tightly linked to the task (Epelboim et al., 1995; Hayhoe et al., 2003; Land and Furneaux, 1997; Land and Lee, 1994; Land et al., 1999; Patla and Vickers, 1997; Pelz and Canosa, 2001). Observers rarely look at regions or objects that are irrelevant to the task at hand (Land, 2004; Hayhoe and Ballard, 2005). Figure 34.1 shows all the fixations that are made in the course of making a sandwich. When viewing a video replay from the subject's viewpoint, with eye position superimposed, it is clear that fixations are tightly linked, moment-by-moment, to the actions, such a grasping and manipulating objects, and move on to the next object when the needs of the current action have been met (Johanssen et al., 2001; Land et al., 1999; Rothkopf et al., 2007). Thus momentary cognitive goals account for many of the fixations in natural vision, including their sequence and timing.

Since many aspects of ordinary visually-guided behaviour are clearly dominated by the information that is required for the momentary visual operation, what is the potential role of examining the properties of the stimulus as a basis for gaze behaviour? One of the implicit rationales might be that tasks are special in some way, and that there is some body of visual processing that does not involve tasks. Consequently, many of the experiments involve what is called 'free viewing', with the goal of isolating task-free visual processing. It is possible that the global visual perception of a scene is distinct in some way from the kind of vision involved in tasks. Certainly humans need to extract information about the spatial structure of scenes and the identity of the objects, but is this qualitatively different from specific visual operations such as those involved in visual search, or extracting location information for grasping an object, operations that are performed in the context of a task such as making a sandwich? One possibility is that all vision can be conceptualized as a task of some kind. The issue is important and needs to be examined explicitly.

Acquisition of visual information is selective

Even at the point of fixation, multiple kinds of information are available. It seems likely that, in the context of natural behaviour, the task controls the specific information that is selected within a given fixation. For example, when first viewing the table-top scene in Fig. 34.1, subjects make a series of short duration fixations on the relevant objects, such as the peanut butter jar. In this case the fixation on the peanut butter is presumably for the purpose of recognition, and perhaps locating it for future use. Subsequent fixations on the jar will be for guiding the grasping action, or for removing the lid. In the absence of ongoing behaviour, we are inclined to think that the job of vision is primarily object recognition. These examples remind us of the complexity of the information that can be obtained while fixating an object, and the variety of operations that vision must perform. The specificity of visual operations is indicated not only by the ongoing actions and the point in the task, but also by the durations of the fixations, which may vary over a range from less than 100 ms to several seconds (Hayhoe et al., 2003). A large component of this variation appears to depend on the particular information required for that point in the task, fixation being terminated when the particular information is acquired (Henderson, 2003).

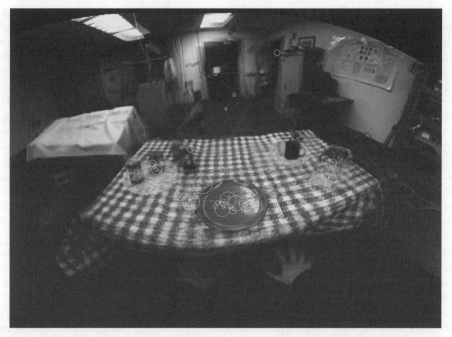

Fig. 34.1 The circles show the fixations made while a subject makes a peanut butter and jelly sandwich. Views from a video camera mounted on the subject's head have been superimposed to make a composite mosaic to compensate for the subject's head movements during the task using the method described by Rothkopf and Pelz (2004). The diameter of the circles indicates the duration of the fixations.

The hypothesis that very specific information is acquired within a fixation is, strictly, a hypothesis about neural mechanisms. That is, cortical state (including V1) is different when subjects are involved in different tasks, even when the retinal input is the same. However, it is possible to get supporting evidence psychophysically. Recent work by Droll, Triesch, and others, using virtual environments, has revealed that subjects use vision to extract information very selectively from an image (Droll et al., 2005; Triesch et al., 2003). In a task where subjects picked up and sorted coloured virtual blocks of different sizes, properties of the blocks, for example, the block colour, were artificially changed at unpredictable moments during the task. Subjects were twice as likely to notice these changes when that property was needed in order to perform the task as when it was irrelevant. For example, if subjects were instructed to pick up a tall brick, they would be more sensitive to a change in size than if they were required to pick up a red brick, when only the colour is relevant. Thus subjects are more aware of some visual properties of the blocks than others, even though the block is the focus of attention throughout the trial. Given the subjective coherence of an object's features, such selectivity or preferential representation is non-intuitive, but nonetheless it highlights the specialized nature of visual computations, even for such simple visual properties like size or colour.

It is commonly thought that the effect of fixating and attending to an object is to bind object properties together into a coherent representation, called an 'object file' (Treisman, 1993). Droll et al.'s experiment suggests that such binding does not always happen, even when the object is the focus of attention. Representations of objects where features are bound together might of course be stored in working memory, or in some longer-term memory representation of the scene.

Eye movements are learned

Implicit in much of the research on natural tasks is the finding that the observed pattern of eye movements is a consequence of learning at several levels (Chapman and Underwood, 1998; Land, 2004; Land and Furneaux, 1997). By implication, the sequential deployment of attention must also be learned. For example, in tea making and sandwich making, observers must have learnt what objects in the scene are relevant, since almost no fixations fall on irrelevant objects. In driving, Shinoda and colleagues (2001) showed that approximately 45% of fixations fell in the neighbourhood of intersections. As a consequence of this, subjects were more likely to notice Stop signs located at intersections as opposed to signs in the middle of a block. Thus it is likely that subjects have learnt that traffic signs are more likely around intersections. At a more detailed level, subjects must learn the optimal location for the information they need. For example, when pouring tea, fixation is located at the tip of the teapot spout. Presumably, flow from the spout is best controlled by fixating this location. Similarly, in walking, observers must learn where and when to look at locations critical for avoiding obstacles while controlling direction and balance. Subjects must learn not only the locations at which relevant information is to be found, but also the order in which the fixations must be made in order to accomplish the task. Thus, a subject must locate the peanut butter and the bread before picking them up, pick up the knife before spreading, and so on. This means that a complete understanding of vision in natural behaviour will require an understanding of the way that tasks are learnt and executed by the brain.

Another way in which learning is critical for deployment of gaze and attention is that observers must learn the dynamic properties of the world in order to distribute gaze and attention where they are needed. Much of the time, items remain in stable locations with stable properties. In a familiar room, the observer need only update the locations of items that are moved, or monitor items that are changing state (for example, water filling the kettle). In dynamic environments, such as driving, walking, or in sports, more complex properties must be learnt. In walking, humans need to know how pedestrians typically behave and how often to look at them. The fact that humans do indeed learn such statistics was demonstrated by Jovancevic and Hayhoe (2009). In a real walking setting, they were able to actively manipulate gaze allocation by varying the probability of potential collisions. Manipulation of the probability of a potential collision by a risky pedestrian was accompanied by a rapid change in gaze allocation. Subjects learn new priorities for gaze allocation within a few encounters, and look both sooner and longer at potentially dangerous pedestrians. Other evidence for such learning is the fact that saccades are often pro-active; that is, they are made to a location in a scene in advance of an expected event. In walking, subjects looked at risky pedestrians before they veered onto a collision course. In cricket, batsmen anticipated the bounce point of the ball, and more skilled batsmen arrived at the bounce point about 100 ms earlier than less skilled players (Land and MacLeod, 2000). The ability to predict where the ball will bounce depends on previous experience of the cricket ball's trajectory. These saccades were always preceded by a fixation on the ball as it left the bowler's hand, showing that batsmen use current sensory data in combination with prior experience of the ball's motion to predict the location of the bounce. This suggests that observers have learnt models of the dynamic properties of the world that can be used to position gaze in anticipation of a predicted event.

The role of reward

The role of learning in governing the selective acquisition of information via sequential deployment of gaze implicates mechanisms of reward. This suggestion is consistent with a number of findings on the neural basis of gaze control. Cells in the FEF reflect the learning of arbitrary stimulus-response associations, and change with experience to reflect the target selection processes involved in visual search (Bichot and Schall, 1999, 2002; Bichot et al., 1996). Similar behaviour is observed in prefrontal cortext (Miller and Cohen, 2001; Pasupathy and Miller, 2005). These dynamic changes in properties are consistent with other work that reveals sensitivity to expectation of reward in many of the regions involved in saccade target selection and generation. Saccade-related areas in the cortex (lateral intra-parietal, frontal eye field, supplementary eye field, and dorsolateral prefrontal cortex) all exhibit sensitivity to reward (Deaner et al., 2005; Dorris and Glimcher, 2004; Glimcher et al., 2009; Platt and Glimcher, 1999; Stuphorn et al., 2000; Sugrue et al., 2004). These areas converge on the caudate nucleus in the basal ganglia, and the cortical–basal ganglia–superior colliculus circuit appears to regulate the control of fixation and the timing of planned movements. Such regulation is a critical requirement for task control of fixations. Caudate cell responses reflect both the target of an upcoming saccade and the reward expected after making the movement (Hikosaka et al., 2000, 2006; Watanabe et al., 2003). Cells in the supplementary eye fields and anterior cingulate cortex also code expected reward and play an important role in monitoring the behavioural significance of saccades (Schall et al., 2002; Stuphorn and Schall, 2006).

Modelling eye movements using reward

The recent development of the mathematics of reinforcement learning (Sutton and Barto, 1998) has made it possible to understand how the neural reward circuitry might be involved in the control of eye movements, and in particular, the way that tasks are involved. The behaviour of cells in the substantia nigra pars compacta is consistent with that expected on the basis of reinforcement learning algorithms, and the pervasive sensitivity of the eye movement circuitry to reward opens the way to modelling gaze control using reinforcement learning (Montague et al., 2004; Schultz, 2000). In neurophysiological paradigms, usually a primary reward such a juice or a raisin is delivered after the animal performs an action. This, of course, does not happen in real life when one makes an eye movement. However, eye movements are for the purpose of obtaining information, and this information is used to achieve behavioural goals such as making a sandwich, that are ultimately important for survival. Thus visual information acquired during a fixation can be thought of as a secondary reward, and mediate learning of gaze patterns by virtue of its ultimate significance for adaptation and survival.

There have been few attempts to model the eye movements observed in complex behaviour, however, one such model, by Sprague et al. (2007) shows how a simulated agent in a virtual environment can learn to allocate gaze to avoid obstacles and control direction in walking (Fig. 34.2). The model assumes that visual computations required in the real world can be broken down into a set of subtasks, such as controlling direction, avoiding obstacles, and so on. Each subtask is associated with some reward value. For example, obtaining visual information that allows avoidance of an obstacle presumably provides secondary reward. The model provides a computational account of how to distribute attention and gaze between these visual subtasks in a dynamic environment. The model is implemented and tested on a human avatar walking along a virtual path with three tasks: stay on the path, avoid obstacles, and pick up 'litter'. The virtual agent can only attend to one location at any

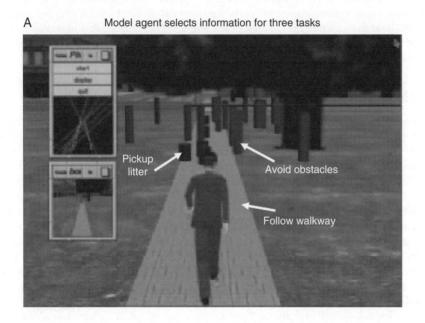

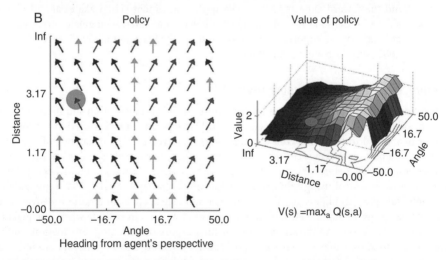

Fig. 34.2 The model of Sprague et al. (2007). A) A virtual agent in a simulated walking environment. The agent must extract visual information from the environment in order to do three subtasks: staying on the walkway, avoiding blue obstacles, and picking up purple litter objects (achieved by contacting them). The inset shows the computation for staying on the path. The model agent learns how to deploy attention/gaze at each time step. B) The agent learns a policy for choosing an action, given the current state information from gaze for a given task. Each action has an associated value, and the agent chooses the option with the highest value.

C   Sequence of fixations

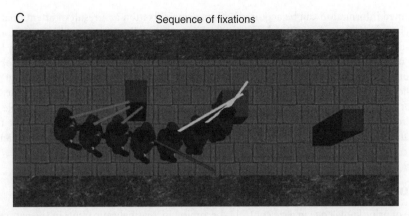

Fig. 34.2 (*continued*) C) Seven time steps after learning. The agent chooses the task that reduces uncertainty of reward the most. The red lines indicate that the agent is using visual information to avoid the obstacle. The blue line indicates that the agent is using information about position on the sidewalk, and the green lines show the agent using vision to intersect the purple litter object. *ACM Transactions on Applied Perception*, Sprague, N., Ballard, D., and Robinson, A., Modeling embodied visual behaviors, **4**(2), page 11© 2007 Association for Computing Machinery, Inc. Reprinted by permission.

moment in time and the agent's uncertainty about state relevant to unattended tasks grows over time. The decision about which task to attend to is based on the expected reward of switching attention to another task. To choose between ongoing competing tasks, in their model, uncertainty increases (together with an attendant cost) when gaze is withheld from an informative scene location. The model assumes that eye movements are selected to maximize reward by reducing uncertainty that could result in suboptimal actions.

Recent applications of statistical decision theory to understanding control of body movements also use the concepts of *reward* (costs and benefits of the outcome of the action), *uncertainty* (of both sensory state and outcome), and *prior knowledge* (probability distributions associated with world states) to model visually-guided reaching movements (e.g. Schlicht and Schrater, 2007; Tassinari et al., 2006). When reward is externally defined (e.g. by monetary reward), it has been shown that subjects making rapid hand movements learn a complicated spatially distributed target reward system and behave in a nearly optimal manner to maximize reward (e.g. Seydell et al., 2008; Trommershäuser et al., 2003). Thus it seems likely that reward (gains and losses) is critical factor in controlling eye movements in natural behaviour.

The role of uncertainty

Another important factor to consider in gaze control is uncertainty. While this factor is recognized in models of movement control (primarily reaching; cf. Todorov and Jordan, 2002; Wolpert, 2007) there is only limited consideration of the role of uncertainty in eye movements. Uncertainty is a critical factor in the Sprague et al. model described previously. Clearly humans need to deploy gaze to the most important regions of a scene, like an oncoming car, but this needs to be modulated by the information the observer already has. If the position of the car is precisely specified, little is gained by another fixation, and the observer is free to gather information on some other aspect of the scene. Recent work by Najemnik and Geisler (2005) shows that fixations in visual search for a simple pattern in noise appear to be chosen in order to reduce uncertainty, as opposed to going to the location that is most likely to be the target. A similar strategy predicts fixations in a simple shape learning and shape-matching task (Renninger et al., 2007). Although gaze changes are often driven by resolution that limits the information from the peripheral retina, other important determinants are cognitive.

Only limited information can be acquired within a single fixation as a result of attentional limitations. When gaze moves to another location, working memory limits the visual information that is retained. Thus, there are multiple sources of uncertainty in dynamic natural environments. In walking, the uncertainty might be about the specific visual information needed for detecting obstacles. Uncertainty about the state of the environment, such as location of obstacles, is likely to grow with time following a fixation, if the information were being held in visual short term memory, which decays or gets noisier over time. Other sources of uncertainty derive from the unpredictable state of the environment itself. Thus uncertainty reduction might be a common unifying principle that can explain fixation patterns in both very simple situations such as search for a contrast target, and more natural complex environments involving more specific behavioural goals.

The role of prior knowledge

The role of prior knowledge in gaze control is becoming increasingly apparent. In the natural world we might expect that prediction based on prior knowledge is pervasive, especially in dynamic environments such as driving or sports, where sensory delays place a purely reactive system at a disadvantage. It is well known that the pursuit system involves a predictive component (Becker and Fuchs, 1985; Kowler et al., 1984). This 'extraretinal' component incorporates visual memory (Barnes and Collins, 2008) and reflects the influence of previous trials (Tabata et al., 2008). There is evidence for the influence of previous trials and stimulus probability on saccadic reaction time and targeting (Basso and Wurtz, 1998; Emeric et al., 2007; Fecteau and Munoz, 2003; He and Kowler, 1989; McPeek et al., 1999). More recently, evidence is accumulating that saccades are often proactive; that is, they are made to a location in a scene in advance of an expected event. Such purely predictive movements reveal the properties of the subject's prior knowledge, because they are made in advance of the visual stimulus. In cricket, batsmen anticipated the bounce point of the ball, and more skilled batsmen arrived at the bounce point about 100 ms earlier than less skilled players (Land and MacLeod, 2000). Similarly, subjects anticipate the bounce point when catching a ball (Hayhoe et al., 2005). Measurements of eye movements in squash reveal predictive saccades of great precision (McKinney et al., 2008). For example, just before hitting the ball, the subject often makes a saccade to a location in (empty) space where the ball arrives about 200 ms later, with an accuracy of about 2.5°. This requires a very complex prediction suggesting subjects know both where it will hit the wall and the angle and speed with which it will bounce off the wall. The ability to predict where the ball will be in all these cases depends on previous experience with the way that balls with particular dynamic properties typically bounce, following a range of different trajectories, speeds, etc. This stored information can be thought of as an internal model, similar to those postulated in the control of aiming movements of the hand (Wolpert, 2007). This predictive aspect of gaze control deserves further investigation, as it is likely that a substantial proportion of human actions, including eye movements, are planned well in advance. This planning component of gaze has so far received relatively little attention.

Summary

Natural behaviour is distinctive, in that eye movements, attention, working memory, sensory decisions, and control of actions are all involved in the generation of even the simplest behaviours. In standard paradigms these issues are typically studied in isolation. Consideration of gaze behaviour *in situ* allows us to understand how these factors jointly contribute to the composition of natural behavioural sequences. Historically, the study of visual perception has followed a reductionist strategy, with the goal of understanding complex visually guided behaviour by separate analysis of its elemental components. Recent developments in monitoring behaviour, such as measurement of eye movements in unconstrained observers, have allowed investigation of the use of vision in the natural world. This has allowed a variety of insights that would be difficult to achieve in more constrained experimental contexts. In general it shifts the focus of vision away from the properties of the stimulus toward a consideration of the behavioural goals of the observer. It appears that behavioural goals are a critical factor in controlling the acquisition of visual information from the world. This insight has been accompanied by a growing understanding of the importance of reward in modulating the underlying neural mechanisms, and by theoretical developments using Reinforcement Learning models of complex behaviour. These developments provide us with the tools to understanding how tasks are represented in the brain, and how they control acquisition of information through use of gaze.

References

Basso, M. and Wurtz, R. (1998). Modulation of neuronal activity in superior colliculus by changes in target probability. *Journal of Neuroscience*, **18**, 7519–7534.

Becker, W. and Fuchs, A. (1985). Prediction in the oculomotor system: smooth pursuit during the transient disappearance of a visual target. *Experimental Brain Research*, **57**, 562–575.

Bichot, N., Schall, J., and Thompson, K. (1996). Visual feature selectivity in frontal eye fields induced by experience in mature macaques. *Nature*, **381**, 697–699.

Bichot, N. and Schall, J. (1999). Effects of similarity and history on neural mechanisms of visual selection. *Nature Neuroscience*, **2**, 549–554.

Bichot, N. and Schall, J. (2002). Priming in macaque frontal cortex during pop-out visual search: Feature-based facilitation and location-based inhibition of return. *Journal of Neuroscience*, **22**, 4675–4685.

Chapman, P. and Underwood, G. (1998). Visual search of dynamic scenes: event types and the role of experience in viewing driving situations. In G. Underwood (ed.) *Eye guidance in reading and scene perception* (pp. 369–394). Oxford: Elsevier.

Deaner, R.O., Khera, A.V. and Platt, M.L. (2005). Monkeys pay per view: Adaptive valuation of social images by rhesus macaques. *Current Biology*, **15**, 543–8.

Dorris, M.-C. and Glimcher, P.-W. (2004). Activity in posterior parietal cortex is correlated with the subjective desirability of an action. *Neuron*, **44**: 365–378.

Droll, J.A., Hayhoe, M.H., Triesch, J., and Sullivan, B.T. (2005). Task demands control acquisition and storage of visual information. *Journal of Experimental Psychology: Human Perception and Performance*, **31**(6), 1416–1438.

Einhauser, W., Rutishauser, U., and Koch. C. (2008). Task-demands can immediately reverse the effects of sensory-driven saliency in complex visual stimuli. *Journal of Vision*, **8**, 2:1–19.

Emeric, E.E., Brown, J.W., Boucher, L., Carpenter, R.H., Hanes, D.P., Harris, R., *et al.* (2007). Influence of history on saccade countermanding performance in humans and macaque monkeys. *Vision Research*, **47**(1), 35–49.

Epelboim, J., Steinman, R., Kowler, E., Edwards, M., Pizlo, Z., Erkelens, C., *et al.* (1995). The function of visual search and memory in sequential looking tasks. *Vision Research*, **35**, 3401–3422.

Fecteau, J.H. and Munoz, D.P. (2003). Exploring the consequences of the previous trial. *Nature Reviews Neuroscience*, **4**, 435–443.

Foulsham T. and Underwood, G. (2008). What can saliency models predict about eye movements? spatial and sequential aspects of fixations during encoding and recognition. *Journal of Vision*, **8**(6), 1–17.

Franconeri, S.L. and Simons, D.J. (2003). Moving and looming stimuli capture attention. *Perception and Psychophysics*, **65**, 999–1010.

Gibson, B., Folk, C., Theeuwes, J., and Kingstone, A. (2008). Introduction to Special Issue on Attentional Capture. *Visual Cognition*, **16**, 145–154.

Glimcher, P., Camerer, C., Fehr, E., and Poldrack, R. (2009). *Neuroeconomics: Decision Making and the Brain*. London: Academic Press.

Hayhoe, M. and Ballard, D. (2005). Eye movements in natural behavior. *Trends in Cognitive Sciences*, **9**(4), 188–193.

Hayhoe, M., Shrivastrava, A., Myruczek, R., and Pelz, J. (2003). Visual memory and motor planning in a natural task. *Journal of Vision*, **3**, 49–63.

Hayhoe, M., Mennie, N., Sullivan B., and Gorgos, K. (2005). The role of internal models and prediction in catching balls. *Proceedings of AAAI Fall Symposium Series*.

He, P. and Kowler, E. (1989). The role of location probability in the programming of saccades: implications for 'center-of-gravity tendencies. *Vision Research*, **29**, 1165–1181.

Henderson, J. (2003). Human gaze control during real-world scene perception. *Trends in Cognitive Science*, **7**, 498–504.

Henderson, J. (2007). Regarding scenes. *Current Directions in Psychological Science*, **16**, 219–227.

Hikosaka, O., Nakamura, K., and Nakahara, H. (2006). Basal ganglia orient eyes to reward. *Journal of Neurophysiology*, **95**(2), 567–84.

Itti, L. and Koch, C. (2001). Computational modeling of visual attention. *Nature Reviews Neuroscience*, **2**, 194–203.

Johansson, R., Westling, G., Backstrom, A., and Flanagan, J.R. (2001). Eye-hand coordination in object manipulation. *Journal of Neuroscience*, **21**, 6917–6932.

Jonides, J. and Yantis, S. (1988). Uniqueness of abrupt visual onset in capturing attention. *Perception and Psychophysics*, **43**, 346–354.

Jovancevic-Misic, J. and Hayhoe, M. (2009). Adaptive gaze control in natural environments. *Journal of Neuroscience*, **29**(19), 6234–6238.

Kowler, E., Martins, A., and Pavel, M. (1984). The effect of expectations on slow oculomotor control. IV Anticipatory smooth eye movements depend on prior target motions. *Vision Research*, **24**, 197–210.

Land, M. (2004). Eye movements in daily life. In L. Chalupa and J. Werner (eds.) *The Visual Neurosciences* (Vol. 2) (pp. 1357–1368). Cambridge, MA: MIT Press.

Land, M.F. and Lee, D.N. (1994). Where we look when we steer. *Nature* **369**, 742–744.

Land M. and Furneaux, S. (1997). The knowledge base of the oculomotor system. *Philosophical Transactions of the Royal Society B: Biological Science*, **352**, 1231–1239.

Land, M.F. and McLeod, P. (2000). From eye movements to actions: how batsmen hit the ball. *Nature Neuroscience*, **3**, 1340–1345.

Land, M., Mennie, N., and Rusted, J. (1999). The roles of vision and eye movements in the control of activities of daily living. *Perception*, **28**, 1311–1328.

McKinney, T., Chajka, K., and Hayhoe, M. (2008). Pro-active gaze control in squash. *Journal of Vision*, **8**, 111.

McPeek, R., Maljkovic, V., and Nakayama, K. (1999) Saccades require focal attention and are facilitated by a short-term memory system. *Vision Research*, **39**, 1555–1565.

Miller, E.K. and Cohen, J.D. (2001). An integrative theory of prefrontal cortex function. *Annual Review of Neuroscience*, **24**, 167–202.

Montague, P.R., Hyman, S.E., Cohen, J.D. (2004). Computational roles for dopamine in behavioral control. *Nature*, **431**, 760–767.

Najemnik, J. and Geisler, W.S (2005). Optimal eye movement strategies in visual search. *Nature*, **434**, 387–391.

Navalpakkam, V. and Itti, L. (2005). Modeling the influence of task on attention. *Vision Research*, **45**, 205–231

Pasupathy, A. and Miller, E. (2005). Different time courses of learning-related activity in the prefrontal cortex and striatum. *Nature*, **433**, 873–876

Patla, A.E. and Vickers, J.N. (1997). Where and when do we look as we approach and step over an obstacle in the travel path? *Neuroreport*, **8**, 3661–3665.

Pelz, J.B. and Canosa, R. (2001). Oculomotor behavior and perceptual strategies in complex tasks. *Vision Research*, **41**, 3587–3596.

Platt, M.-L. and Glimcher, P.-W. (1999). Neural correlates of decision variables in parietal cortex. *Nature*, **400**, 233–238.

Renninger, L.W., Verghese, P., and Coughlan, J. (2007). Where to look next? Eye movements reduce local uncertainty. *Journal of Vision*, **7**(3), 6.1–17.

Rothkopf, C.A. and Pelz, J.B. (2004). Head movement estimation for wearable eye tracker. In *Proceedings ACM SIGCHI: Eye Tracking Research and Applications* (pp. 123–130). ACM Press.

Rothkopf, C, Ballard, and Hayhoe, M. (2007). Task and scene context determines where you look. *Journal of Vision*, **7**(14), 16.1–20.

Schall, J.D., Stuphorn, V., and Brown, J.W. (2002). Monitoring and control of action by the frontal lobes. *Neuron*, **36**, 309–322.

Schlicht, E. and Schrater, P. (2007). Reach-to-grasp trajectories adjust for uncertainty in the location of visual targets. *Experimental Brain Research*, **182**, 47–57.

Schultz, W. (2000). Multiple reward signals in the brain. *Nature Reviews: Neuroscience*, **1**, 199–207.

Seydell, A., McCann, B.C., Trommershäuser, J., and Knill, D.C. (2008). Learning stochastic reward distributions in a speeded pointing task. *Journal of Neuroscience*, **28**(17), 4356–4367.

Shinoda, H., Hayhoe, M., and Shrivastava, A (2001). Attention in natural environments. *Vision Research*, **41**, 3535–3546.

Sprague, N., Ballard, D., and Robinson, A. (2007). Modeling embodied visual behaviors. *ACM Transactions on Applied Perception*, **4**(2), 11.

Stuphorn, V. and Schall, J.D. (2006). Executive control of countermanding saccades by the supplementary eye field. *Nature Neuroscience*, **9**, 925–931.

Sugrue, L.-P., Corrado, G.-S., and Newsome, W.-T. (2004) Matching behavior and the representation of value in the parietal cortex. *Science*, **304**(5678), 1782–1787.

Sutton, R. and Barto, A (1998). *Reinforcement Learning: An Introduction*. Cambridge, MA: MIT Press.

Tassinari, H., Hudson, T.E., and Landy, M.S. (2006). Combining priors and noisy visual cues in a rapid pointing task. *Journal of Neuroscience*, **26**(40), 10154–10163

Tabata, H. Muira, K., and Kawano, K (2008). Trial-by-trial updating of the gain in preparation for smooth pursuit eye movement based on past experience in humans. *Journal of Neurophysiology*, **99**, 747–758.

Tatler, B. (2007). The central fixation bias in scene viewing: selecting an optimal viewing position independently of motor biases and image feature distributions. *Journal of Vision*, **7**(4), 1–17.

Theeuwes, J. and Godisn, R. (2001). Attentional and oculomotor capture. In C. Folk and B. Gibson (eds.) *Attraction, distraction, and action: Multiple perspectives on attentional capture* (pp. 121–150). Amsterdam: Elsevier.

Todorov, E. and Jordan, M. (2002). Optimal feedback control as a theory of motor coordination. *Nature Neuroscience*, **5**(11), 1226–1235.

Torralba, A. (2003). Contextual priming for object detection. *International Journal of Computer Vision*, **53**, 169–91.

Torralba, A., Oliva, A, Castelhano, M., and Henderson, J.M. (2006). Contextual guidance of attention and eye movements in real world scenes: The role of global features on object search. *Psychological Review*, **113**(4) 766–786.

Treisman, A. (1993). The perception of features and objects. In A. Baddeley and L. Weiskrantz (eds.) *Attention: selection, awareness, and control. A tribute to Donald Broadbent* (pp. 5–35). Oxford: Clarendon Press.

Triesch, J., Ballard, D.H., Hayhoe, M.M., and Sullivan, B.T. (2003). What you see is what you need. *Journal of Vision*, **3**(1), 86–94.

Trommershäuser, J., Maloney, L.T., and Landy, M.S. (2003) Statistical decision theory and the selection of rapid, goal-directed movements. *Journal of the Optical Society of America*, **20**, 1419–1433.

Watanabe, K., Lauwereyns, J., and Hikosaka, O. (2003). Neural correlates of rewarded and unrewarded movements in the primate caudate nucleus. *Journal of Neuroscience*, **23**, 10052–10057.

Wolfe, J.M. (1994). Guided Search 2.0: A revised model of visual search. *Psychonomic Bulletin and Review*, **1**(2), 202–238.

Wolpert, D. (2007). Probabilistic models in human sensorimotor control. *Human Movement Science*, **26**, 511–524.

Yantis, S. (1998). Control of visual attention. In H. Pashler (ed.) *Attention* (pp. 233–256). Hove: Psychology Press.

Zhang, L., Tong, M.H., Marks, T.K., Shan, H., and Cottrell, G.W. (2008). SUN: A Bayesian framework for saliency using natural statistics. *Journal of Vision*, **8**, 1–20.

PART 5

Eye movement pathology and development

CHAPTER 35

Development from reflexive to controlled eye movements

Beatriz Luna and Katerina Velanova

Abstract

Reflexive, stimulus-driven eye movements mature early in development while voluntary, cognitively-driven eye movements continue to improve through adolescence. In this chapter, we describe developmental improvements in reflexively-guided eye movements, such as visually-guided saccades, fixation, and pursuit eye movements, and then developmental improvements in eye movements guided by voluntary control, such as antisaccades and memory-guided saccades. The latency to initiate both reflexive and voluntary eye movements decreases with age suggesting enhanced speed of information processing (e.g. Irving et al., 2006; Luna et al., 2004). The ability to voluntarily control eye movements, reflected in the ability to inhibit a reflexive eye movement and guide saccades using spatial working memory, continues to improve through adolescence (e.g. Fischer et al., 1997; Fukushima et al., 2000; Klein and Foerster, 2001; Luna et al., 2004). Further, neuroimaging studies demonstrate a transition to use of more distributed brain circuitries in adulthood that may support better cognitive control of eye movements (e.g. Luna et al., 2001; Scherf et al., 2006). Brain maturational processes such as myelination and synaptic pruning, which permit efficient top-down modulation of behaviour, may underlie age-related enhancements in the efficiency of eye movement control.

Introduction

The basic sensorimotor hardware that supports oculomotor function is mature early in development enabling even infants to generate a wide range of eye movements. The ability to *control* eye movements, however, continues to improve through adolescence as cognitive control of behaviour matures enabling purposeful interaction with the environment. Improved control of eye movements is reflected in a range of oculomotor measures including speed of response initiation, accuracy, and in withholding inappropriate but prepotent saccadic responses. Understanding the development of eye movements can inform us about broader domains of development, particularly the development of voluntary control, which is a foundation for adult-level decision-making. Further, characterizing the aspects of eye-movement control that emerge at different stages of development can help us specify the roles of the different brain regions that comprise the oculomotor system thus informing our understanding of basic systems.

The oculomotor system is an ideal system for investigating the neural basis of reflexive and voluntary behaviour and for characterizing their development. Oculomotor tasks are typically simple and can be readily performed by children as young as 4–6 years of age (Cohen and Ross, 1978; Ross et al., 1993). These tasks permit minimal use of verbal strategies which can confound developmental results in many neuropsychological tasks. Further, stimulus-response (visual stimulus-saccade) mappings are often direct in oculomotor tasks, in contrast to paper and pencil tests or tasks requiring manual responses where transformations are required to adapt to different input/output modalities. Additionally, eye-movement responses can be measured with extreme precision and are rich in derivable parameters. And, the oculomotor system's neurophysiology, neuroanatomy, and neurochemistry have been described to a greater degree than other systems (Bon and Lucchetti, 1990; Bruce and Goldberg, 1985; Leigh and Zee, 1991; Robinson et al., 1978). In human subjects, oculomotor tasks also produce robust brain activation in a distributed network including the frontal eye fields (FEF), posterior parietal cortex (PPC), the supplementary eye fields (SEF), dorsolateral prefrontal cortex (DLPFC), basal ganglia, thalamus, superior colliculus (SC), and cerebellum (Luna et al., 1998; Muri et al., 1996; Petit et al., 1997; Sweeney et al., 1996). The oculomotor system is thus particularly well-suited for functional neuroimaging studies and to test hypotheses about changes in brain systems during development.

When considering the processes underlying eye movements, the oculomotor system can be viewed as consisting of two major subsystems—the saccade system and the fixation system—with a pursuit system sometimes further distinguished from the fixation system. Saccades refer to rapid eye movements that are performed to redirect fixation to targets of interest. Fixation refers to the active retention of gaze on a stationary visual stimulus by correcting movements or drifts away from a foveated stimulus. Pursuit refers to smooth eye movements that match the velocity of a moving visual stimulus and requires use of prediction and adjustment processes to stabilize the visual target. The goal of both pursuit and fixation is to retain a visual image on the fovea and hence these are often considered to be supported by the same system (Leigh and Zee, 1999). Each of these types of eye movements can be generated exogenously, in response to a compelling visual stimulus, or endogenously, guided by a voluntary plan. We will first describe the development of the basic aspects of each of these systems and subsequently, age-related improvements in their voluntary control. We argue that the development of controlled eye movements provides evidence that higher-level control functions show a protracted developmental trajectory. We end by presenting what is known about brain maturational processes that occur in parallel to improvements in voluntary eye movement control and conclude with a description of neurobehavioural processes that show a protracted developmental trajectory and which support the transition to mature, adult-level eye-movement control.

Development of reflexive/automatic eye movements

Fixation: development of the ability to retain gaze and suppress saccades

Visual fixation is an *active* process that permits retention of a stationary visual stimulus in the fovea such as when threading a needle which requires actively suppressing saccades. Visual fixation requires both maintenance of focused attention and inhibition of inappropriate eye movements. Visual fixation however does not exclude microsaccades around the target visual stimulus (Engbert, 2006). Subsequent saccades to new visual targets require that visual fixation be actively inhibited (Leigh and Zee, 1991). The visual fixation system is often considered part of the pursuit system (see below) because of the need to detect and correct drifts in fixation (Leigh and Zee, 1999). However, there is also evidence to support separation of the visual fixation system (Leigh and Zee, 1999). For example, single-cell studies in non-human primates demonstrate that active visual fixation recruits an adjacent but distinct brain circuitry including FEF (Goldberg et al., 1986), PPC (Mountcastle et al., 1981; Shibutani et al., 1984), and unique brain stem regions (Munoz and Wurtz, 1992).

While visual fixation is evident early in life, the stability and control of fixation continues to improve through adolescence. In particular, the distance of fixations around their 'centre of gravity' and numbers of intruding saccades decrease, while the duration of fixation increases from 4 to 15 years of age, indicating developmental improvement in the stability of fixation (Aring et al., 2007; Ygge et al., 2005). Important to the ability to retain fixation is engagement in the fixated target. For example, children between the ages of 8 and 10 years show a decrease in number of breaks of fixation towards distracting stimuli when the central stimulus is engaging (e.g. an animal to be named; Paus, 1989; Paus et al., 1990). This result suggests that the motoric ability to retain fixation is available early in development but that the top-down control continues to improve through adolescence as inhibitory function is enhanced.

Pursuit system: development of the ability to track a moving object

The ability to catch a ball or avoid being hit by a moving car requires that we monitor moving stimuli and is afforded by the smooth pursuit system. Similar to fixation, the pursuit system allows one to retain a visual image in the fovea. In order to approximate the velocity of a moving target and keep a visual stimulus foveated, the pursuit system generates slow eye movements that predict the trajectory of movement, together with small compensatory saccades that allow for adjustments. Pursuit eye movements are supported by a distributed brain circuitry that engages regions adjacent to the saccade system (Berman et al., 1999; MacAvoy et al., 1991) and overlaps with regions supporting the vestibular system (Fukushima et al., 2006). Cortical regions including motion processing regions in visual cortex (MT/V5), medial superior temporal cortex, caudal FEF and SEF have been found to support pursuit eye movements (Berman et al., 1999; MacAvoy et al., 1991; Newsome et al., 1988). These regions interact with subcortical regions including the cerebellar floccular region, dorsal vermis, caudal fastigial nucleus, dorsolateral pontine nucleus, and nucleus reticularis tegmenti pontis (for a review see Fukushima et al., 2006).

The pursuit system undergoes significant development in the first year of life. In the first two weeks of life, infants can track a moving object using optokinetic nystagmus, which invokes some smooth pursuit, but it is neither persistent or continuous (Haishi and Kokubun, 1998; Rosander, 2007; Shea and Aslin, 1990). In the next few months, saccadic eye movements are used to track moving objects (Roucoux et al., 1983; Shea and Aslin, 1990; Rosander and von Hofsten, 2002). Continuous smooth pursuit emerges around six months of age, but is initially slow and inaccurate (Gredebäck et al., 2005; Rosander and von Hofsten, 2002; Shea and Aslin, 1990). The velocity of smooth pursuit increases with development allowing faster moving stimuli to be tracked (Roucoux et al., 1983). The ability to coordinate head movements with gaze-shifts matures by approximately seven months improving pursuit accuracy (Daniel and Lee, 1990). However, consistent predictive gaze tracking is not present until 8 months (Gredebäck et al., 2005) and continues to improve through childhood (Salman et al., 2006).

With development, predictive gaze tracking, coupled with small corrective 'catch-up' saccades, continues to improve and enhances pursuit accuracy by more tightly matching pursuit eye movements with moving stimuli (Grönqvist et al., 2006; Jacobs et al., 1997; von Hofsten and Rosander, 1997; Shea and Aslin, 1990). Pursuit gain refers to the ratio of eye movement velocity to stimulus velocity, that is, how well moving fixation matches the moving target. Gain is used to assess accuracy independent of catch-up saccades and thus reflects the integrity of the pursuit system independent of the saccade system (Leigh and Zee, 1999). While saccadic mechanisms are present in infancy, pursuit gain continues to improve through childhood into adolescence, especially at higher speeds of pursuit tracking (Haishi and Kokubun, 1995; Katsanis et al., 1998; Ross et al., 1993; Rütsche et al., 2006) and some studies show continued improvement into mid-adolescence (Salman et al., 2006).

Throughout childhood the integration of cortical and cerebellar circuitries supporting the predictive processes underlying pursuit accuracy continues to mature (Rosander, 2007). Persistent asymmetries in upward pursuit eye movements during childhood indicate both immaturities in the organization of the floccular-vestibular system supporting accuracy, and immaturities in SEF which support cancellation of the downward vestibular ocular reflex (Fukushima et al., 2003; Takeichi et al., 2003). The integration of distributed cortical and cerebellar systems is critical to pursuit eye movements as well as cognitive control. Pursuit abnormalities in psychopathologies such as schizophrenia (Sweeney et al., 1998), which begin to emerge in adolescence, may reflect an underlying impairment in the maturation of the integration of cortical and subcortical circuits.

Visually-guided saccades: development of reflexive saccade responses

Saccadic eye movements are the fastest movements that the human body can make. They are essential to our moment to moment interaction with the environment, allowing us to attend to stimuli of interest in a dynamic fashion. Saccades are produced continuously from reading text to walking. The saccade system is supported by a widely distributed circuitry including regions in the cerebellum, brain stem, and cortical eye fields (Bruce and Goldberg, 1985; Goldberg and Bruce, 1990; Keating and Gooley, 1988; Leigh and Zee, 1999; Schlag and Schlag-Rey, 1987). Given the role of eye movements in guiding our behaviour it is not surprising that the saccade system shows substantial overlap with attentional systems (Corbetta et al., 1998). Reflexive saccades are generated automatically in response to exogenous stimuli. Saccades can also be generated voluntarily in accord with an endogenous purposive plan. In this section we describe the development of reflexive saccade performance.

The visually-guided saccade task, also referred to as the prosaccade task, requires that individuals look at a visual target that appears at an unpredictable location in the periphery. Saccade performance is assessed by measuring peak velocity, accuracy of end-point location (relative to the target), and the speed of saccade initiation (expressed in terms of latency). Saccade *velocity* is determined by burst neurons and omni-pause neurons in the brainstem (Leigh and Zee, 1999). In infancy, saccade velocity is slower than in adulthood (Hainline et al., 1984). While some studies have found that saccade velocity is comparable in children between the ages of 5–12 years and adults (Luna et al., 2004; Munoz et al., 1998), others have reported differences between these age groups (Fioravanti et al., 1995; Funk and Anderson, 1977; Irving et al., 2006). Among studies showing developmental differences, saccade velocity has generally been found to increase through childhood peaking at 10–15 years, and then to decrease with age (Irving et al., 2006). Across studies however, age ranges vary and, given the typically modest differences found between age groups (<100°/s), differences in results may reflect subtle methodological differences that impact sensitivity. To the extent that it is observed, a peak in saccade velocity in adolescence may reflect the peak in overall physical health that occurs during this developmental period.

Saccade *accuracy* or the precision with which a saccade terminates in a designated location for optimal foveation of a visual stimulus, is primarily determined by cerebellar circuits. Infants and children tend to make saccades that undershoot the target (hypometria) (Aslin and Salapatek, 1975; Fioravanti et al., 1995; Harris et al., 1993; Munoz et al., 1998; Regal et al., 1983). Accuracy is mature in adolescence (Irving et al., 2006) however there may be some speed-accuracy trade off reflected in slower saccades in adulthood that result in improved accuracy.

Saccade *latency* (or reaction time) refers to the time required to initiate an eye-movement following presentation of an eliciting stimulus. Saccade latencies for reflexive saccades decrease with age into mid-adolescence (Fischer et al., 1997; Fukushima et al., 2000; Klein and Foerster, 2001; Irving et al., 2006; Luna et al., 2004; Munoz et al., 1998) (see Fig. 35.1). The latency to initiate voluntary saccades, which is longer than for reflexive saccades because of the additional cognitive processes involved, shows a similar developmental trajectory. This developmental decrease in reaction time is similar to that found for manual reaction times (Kail and Park, 1992; Hale, 1990) suggesting that from birth to mid-adolescence there is general improvement in the speed of information processing. Increased myelination through this age period may underlie this general developmental speeding of responses. Enhanced functional integration of frontostriatal circuits through development (Olesen et al., 2003; Liston et al., 2006) may have a particular impact on the ability to initiate quick responses including saccadic responses.

Express saccades refer to saccades with very short latencies (from 80 to approximately 140 ms) (Fischer and Ramsperger, 1984). The speed with which these saccades are generated suggests that they do not depend on cortical systems and rather, that they are primarily supported by subcortical

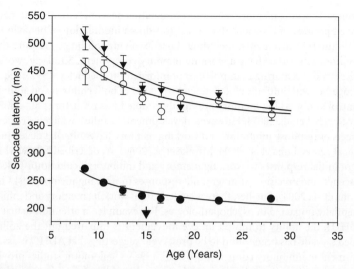

Fig. 35.1 Mean latency (+/ 1 standard error of the mean) to initiate a saccade during visually guided saccades (solid circles), antisaccades (open circles), and memory-guided saccades (solid triangles). Lines represent the inverse curve fit on the mean latencies by age in years. The arrow depicts the age at which changepoint analyses indicate adult levels of performance were reached. Reprinted from Luna, B., Garver, K.E., Urban, T.A., Lazar, N.A., Sweeney, J.A. Maturation of cognitive processes from late childhood to adulthood. *Child Development*, **75**(5), 1357–1372, with permission from John Wiley and Sons © 2004.

systems (Dorris and Munoz, 1995; Dorris et al., 1997; Guitton et al., 1985; Klein et al., 2005). Express saccades are considered to be the most reflexive type of eye movement toward a visual stimulus. Only modest developmental decreases in the number of express saccades have been found through childhood into adulthood (Fischer et al., 1997; Klein et al., 2005). The lack of developmental change in express saccades suggests that the subcortical fixation system matures earlier than the cortical systems supporting visually guided and voluntary eye movements.

To summarize, pursuit, fixation, and reflexive saccades appear by infancy or early childhood, but show continued refinement into adolescence as controlled processing matures. While subcortical systems are mostly in place by early childhood, there is evidence for some continued refinement through adolescence as reflected by improvements in saccade velocity and accuracy in childhood. Continued improvements in speed to initiate reflexive and voluntary saccades may reflect continued myelination, particularly in fronto-subcortical systems. The ability to effectively engage a widely distributed circuitry may underlie continued improvements in pursuit accuracy, prediction and in the ability to maintain fixation in the presence of salient distractors.

Voluntary control of eye movements

In addition to saccades being generated reflexively in response to a sensory stimulus, they can also be voluntarily generated in a goal-directed manner. Voluntary responses necessitate both inhibitory control and use of working memory. Inhibitory control permits the suppression of reflexive responses to distractors in favour of a planned response. Working memory refers to the sketch pad where responses are planned and retained on-line to guide behaviour in a voluntary fashion (Baddeley, 1986). Response inhibition and working memory operate in unison to support voluntary control (Asato et al., 2006; Miyake et al., 2000) and are sometimes considered a unitary process (Miller and Cohen, 2001). However, while the circuits that support inhibitory control and working memory overlap, the neuronal computations underlying each are distinct. Response inhibition depends on top-down modulation of behaviour as cortical regions operate to suppress subcortically-generated reflexive responses. Working memory relies on reverberating neuronal circuits that maintain activity across prolonged periods of time and that direct top-down modulation of behaviour (Funahashi et al., 1989). Voluntary movements, including those involving inhibition, require that a planned response be online, hence they have a working memory component. Similarly, working memory tasks, particularly those requiring manipulation of information (Baddeley, 1992), require retention of a task goal together with inhibition of distractors. Studies of both children and adults indicate that inhibitory control and working memory are tightly coupled (Eenshuistra et al., 2007; Kane et al., 2001; Van der Stigchel et al., 2007). However, developmental studies, which we review below, also show that aspects of response inhibition and working memory have differing developmental trajectories (Asato et al., 2006; Luna et al., 2004; Miyake et al., 2000). As described below, while the latency and accuracy of initial responses to working memory and inhibitory oculomotor tasks both mature in mid-adolescence, the precision of mnemonic responses in working memory tasks improves into adulthood (Luna et al., 2004). Further, there is evidence that working memory and inhibitory control may be differentially impacted in psychopathologies. For example, in attention deficit hyperactivity disorder (ADHD), the ability to inhibit an eye movement is impaired but the ability to make a memory-guided saccade has been found to be preserved, suggesting that ADHD is associated with a specific impairment in inhibitory control (Ross et al., 1994). Oculomotor studies provide an opportunity to better characterize the individual developmental profiles of specific control processes. For example, the antisaccade task emphasizes inhibitory control by having minimal working memory demands. In contrast, the oculomotor delayed response task emphasizes working memory in the absence of distractors or manipulation demands. Developmental findings from each of these paradigms offer unique insight into the nature of cognitive control.

Antisaccades: development of the ability to suppress a prepotent saccade

Reflexive saccades are automatic and generated throughout our daily lives in response to external sensory stimuli. Their suppression requires significant cognitive control. The antisaccade task requires active suppression of an impending reflexive saccade toward a visual stimulus. Specifically, subjects are instructed to suppress looking toward a peripherally-presented visual stimulus and to instead make a voluntary saccade to its mirror location (Hallett, 1978). Antisaccade errors occur when subjects are unable to suppress reflexive eye movements. Such errors are usually followed by a saccade to the correct mirror location indicating that the instruction was understood but that the reflexive saccade was not appropriately inhibited. A number of developmental studies have examined antisaccade performance in large samples of children as young as 4 years and adults and have found evidence for continued improvements in the ability to suppress reflexive saccades as well as in the time taken to initiate a voluntary response (Fischer et al., 1997; Fukushima et al., 2000; Klein and Foerster, 2001; Luna et al., 2004; Munoz et al., 1998; Nelson et al., 2000; Mayfrank et al., 1986).

Across studies, steep reductions in rates of inhibitory errors from childhood to adolescence have also been found (Fischer et al., 1997; Fukushima et al., 2000; Klein and Foerster, 2001; Luna et al., 2004; Mayfrank et al., 1986; Munoz et al., 1998; Nelson et al., 2000). Early studies found that from childhood to adolescence antisaccade errors decreased from 60% to 22% and continued to decrease at a slower rate until 25 years of age (Fischer et al., 1997; Fukushima et al., 2000). The high rate of antisaccade errors occurring at ages where prosaccade errors are few indicates that this developmental change in antisaccade performance is attributable to improvements in inhibition of reflexive saccades rather than to changes in saccade dynamics per se.

Subsequent research has shown that developmental improvement in voluntary saccade inhibition follows a curvilinear trajectory (Klein, 2001; Luna et al., 2004). For example, in our study of 245 8- to 30-year-olds, we found that an inverse regression $[Y = b0 + (b1/t)]$ best represented age-related changes in saccade latency and proportions of inhibitory errors (see Fig. 35.2) in comparison to linear, logarithmic, or cubic regressions (Luna et al., 2004). These results indicate that from childhood to adolescence there is a steep improvement in performance which then stabilizes through adulthood. Using change-point analyses, which determine the point when a function significantly changes its trajectory, we were able to specify that at 14–15 years of age antisaccade performance

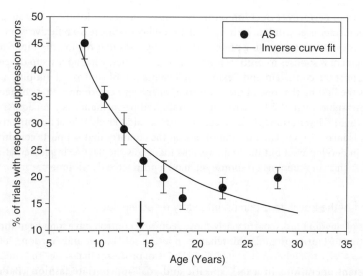

Fig. 35.2 Mean rate (+/ 1 standard error of the mean) of antisaccade errors by age. Line represents an inverse curve fit on antisaccade errors by age in years. The arrow indicates the age when adult level performance was reached as determined by changepoint analyses. Reprinted from Luna, B., Garver, K.E., Urban, T.A., Lazar, N.A., Sweeney, J.A. Maturation of cognitive processes from late childhood to adulthood. *Child Development*, **75**(5), 1357–1372, with permission from John Wiley and Sons © 2004.

becomes similar to that of adults. However, the exact age of maturity varies from study to study depending on sample size and context (Klein et al., 2005; Munoz et al., 1998). In a recent fMRI study we found that when performing the antisaccade task in an MRI scanner, adolescents committed significantly more errors than adults (Velanova et al., 2008). Further, when the difficulty of inhibiting a saccade is increased by adding a period with no fixation (a 'gap'), antisaccade errors are increased in children relative to adults, indicating that children rely more on the protective effects of fixation than mature individuals (Klein, 2001; Klein and Foerster, 2001; Klein et al., 2005). That is, children's performance is disproportionately impaired, relative to adults, when no stimulus is present to assist with maintenance of control. These results suggest that younger subjects can perform at adult levels but may have difficulty with sustained inhibitory processing in contexts that place greater demands on cognitive control.

As mentioned above, the latency to initiate an antisaccade also decreases with age (see Fig. 35.1) (Fischer et al., 1997; Fukushima et al., 2000; Klein and Foerster, 2001; Luna et al., 2004; Mayfrank et al., 1986; Munoz et al., 1998; Nelson et al., 2000). Specifically, studies have found continued decreases in latencies to initiate correct antisaccades (requiring inhibition of reflexive saccades), to initiate corrections to errors, and to make erroneous prosaccades (inhibition failures) (Fischer et al., 1997). These decreases are most pronounced from 9–15 years of age but continue up to 25 years of age. In addition to decreases in latency, there is a decrease in the variance of latency measures with age (Munoz et al., 1998). This may result from heterogeneity in maturational rates or suggest that the ability to perform at adult levels is present but inconsistent in adolescence. Some studies have found that antisaccade latencies have a more protracted development through adolescence in comparison to latencies for reflexive saccades (Fukushima et al., 2000). Our studies, described above, showed that despite there being longer latencies for antisaccades compared to prosaccades, latencies for both followed a similar developmental progression (Luna et al., 2004). This in turn suggests that latency to initiate responses may be determined by factors contributing to more general aspects of cognitive control such as continued myelination.

In summary, studies show that while children can perform an antisaccade trial correctly, the rate of correct responses significantly increases into adolescence and possibly into young adulthood.

Since children can perform correct inhibitory responses, albeit at a low rate, this suggests that the ability to inhibit responses is online early. Indeed, the ability to suppress a reflexive response has been documented as early as infancy using preferential looking tasks that require the suppression of head and eye-movement responses to probes (Johnson, 1995). Rather, what appears to develop are processes that support the consistent and flexible implementation of controlled inhibition. Supporting this notion is the finding that one of the main components of performance that changes with age is inter- and intrasubject variability such that by adulthood performance is even across participants (Klein et al., 2005). That is, some children can perform at adult levels at least on some trials but their performance is inconsistent. The implication is that the circuitry that supports cognitive control is on line early in development but the brain systems that allow the flexible implementation of executive abilities, such as in retaining a response set, have a protracted development.

Development of the ability to retain an inhibitory response set

Performance of ongoing tasks, particularly those requiring control, have long been thought to rely on the effective instantiation and maintenance of a task set (Logan and Gordon, 2001; Monsell, 1996). Task sets refer to higher-order supervisory control processes that select and modulate downstream transient operations in a task-specific and goal-appropriate fashion (Baddeley, 1996; Desimone and Duncan, 1995; Logan and Gordon, 2001; Norman and Shallice, 1986; Schneider and Shiffrin, 1977; Shiffrin and Schneider, 1977). For example, antisaccade performance requires the initiation and maintenance of top-down signals which modulate reflexive or prepotent responses in addition to operations executed on a trial-by-trial basis.

We have noted that children can perform at least some correct antisaccade trials, but that the rate of correct responses improves with age (Bedard et al., 2002; Brocki and Bohlin, 2004; Levin et al., 1991; Luciana and Nelson, 1998; Paus et al., 1990; Ridderinkhof et al., 1997, 1999; Tipper et al., 1989; Van den Wildenberg and van der Molen, 2004; Williams et al., 1999; Wise et al., 1975). Similar age-related improvements have been found in performance of dual-task and task-switching paradigms, which are thought to provide indirect measures of the integrity of task sets required for the coordination of multiple tasks (Dosenbach et al., 2006; Logan and Gordon, 2001; Monsell and Mizon, 2006; Schneider and Logan, 2006). Further, as with antisaccades, age-related variance in task-switching performance can be independent of that associated with task subprocesses such as perceptual speed and working memory (Cepeda and Kramer, 2001). Together, these findings suggest that task-set related (rather than trial-specific) processes may play an important role in development and more specifically, that task-set-related processes that enable consistent inhibitory control may be crucial for understanding the development of antisaccade performance and inhibitory control (see Velanova et al., 2009).

Development of brain function underlying response inhibition

Functional neuroimaging work in adult humans, consistent with extensive neurophysiological work in monkeys (Bruce and Goldberg, 1985; Robinson and Goldberg, 1978), demonstrates that antisaccade performance produces robust activation in a network of regions including DLPFC, SEF, FEF, lateral PPC, basal ganglia, SC, and cerebellum (Brown et al., 2006; Connolly et al., 2000; Miller et al., 2005; Matsuda et al., 2004; Muri et al., 1996). Further, single-cell studies demonstrate that crucial to the ability to perform an antisaccade trial is engagement of primary components of this circuitry during response preparation—before an antisaccade response is initiated (Amador et al., 2004; Everling and Munoz, 2000). Specifically, correct antisaccade responses occur when activity in saccade-related neurons in subcortical structures (SC) and in cortical regions (notably, FEF, and PPC) is dampened, and activity in fixation-related neurons is increased during presentation of preparatory cues (and prior to presentation of peripheral stimuli) (Munoz and Everling, 2004). fMRI studies indicate that DLPFC may play a central role in biasing the oculomotor network in anticipation of reflexive saccade suppression. DLPFC is active during antisaccade response preparation, but unlike SC, FEF, and PPC, which are active throughout antisaccade trials, DLPFC shows only minimal activity during saccade responses (Brown et al., 2007). Further, DLPFC has extensive projections to both cortical and subcortical regions (Fuster, 1997), which show increased activity in preparation for antisaccade versus prosaccade trials (Everling and Munoz, 2000; Everling et al., 1999). These results indicate that the ability to inhibit an impending saccade requires the concerted activity of prefrontal, premotor, and subcortical regions. The ability to make correct antisaccades in childhood implies that this circuitry is capable of functioning in a mature manner early on, albeit inconsistently. However, little data has been gathered to date documenting developmental change in antisaccade-related brain activity.

In the first study to investigate developmental changes in antisaccade performance using fMRI, we compared activity during blocks of antisaccade performance with activity during blocks of prosaccade performance in children aged 8–13 years, adolescents aged 14–17 years, and adults aged 18–30 years (Luna et al., 2001). Oculomotor control regions (FEF, PPC, SC) were more active in adults than in adolescents or children (see Fig. 35.3). Performance was worse in children, who showed increased activity in parietal regions, possibly reflecting a compensatory reliance on visuospatial processing. While adolescents performed similarly to adults, they showed increased activity in DLPFC, as do adults with increased cognitive load (Carpenter et al., 1999), suggesting that maintenance of performance at mature levels was more *effortful* for adolescents. Adults showed robust activity in oculomotor regions and less reliance on prefrontal systems, as well as recruitment of additional regions such as the lateral cerebellum suggesting engagement of a more highly integrated distributed circuitry that is less dependent on prefrontal systems. These results are supported by a recent topographical ERP study using the antisaccade task which shows that children rely on parietal regions, but by late adolescence a frontal predominance is evident (Klein and Feige, 2005).

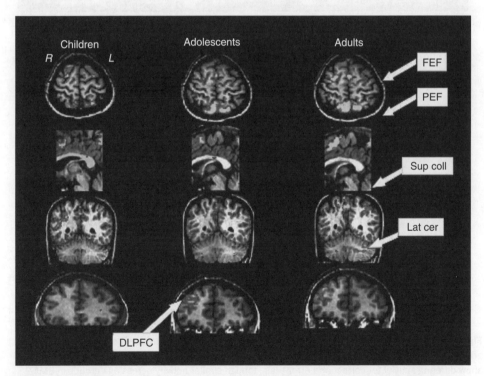

Fig. 35.3 Mean group activation during a block antisaccade task compared to prosaccade blocks for a group of children, adolescents, and adults overlaid on the structural anatomic image of a representative subject. Reprinted from *NeuroImage* **13**(5), B. Luna, K.R. Thulborn, D.P. Munoz, E.P. Merriam, K.E. Garver, N.J. Minshew, et al. Maturation of widely distributed brain function subserves cognitive development, pp. 786–793, (c) 2001, with permission from Elsevier.

We note, however, that in block fMRI designs of the sort we have described both error and correct trials contribute to measures of activity. More recently, event-related studies in our laboratory have allowed us to characterize age-related changes in brain function during correct and error trials separately (Velanova et al., 2008). We found that for correct trials, FEF, supplementary motor area/ presupplementary motor area (SMA/preSMA), PPC, and putamen showed increased activity relative to baseline but no age-group-related effects (see Fig. 35.4). We did, however, find age-related decreases in prefrontal activity, again likely reflecting less effortful processing with age.

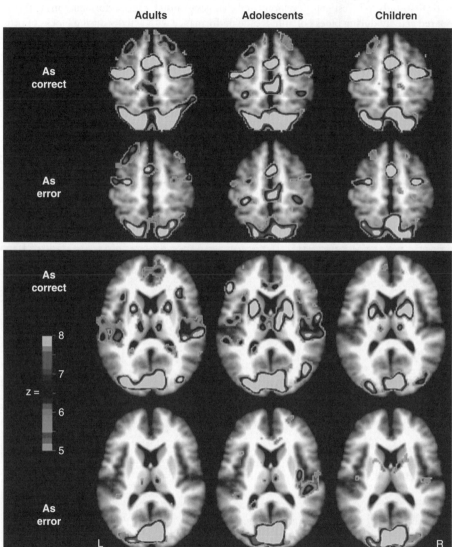

Fig. 35.4 (Also see Plate 18.) Mean group activation for a group of children, adolescents, and adults during correct and incorrect antisaccade task trials. Top panel) Horizontal sections at z = 54 show differing activity for correct and error trials, though similar activity across age groups in SMA/ preSMA, FEF and PPC. Bottom panel) Horizontal sections at z = 12 show increased activity in putamen for correct versus error trials in all age groups. Reproduced from *Cerebral Cortex*, **18**, Katerina Velanova, Mark E. Wheeler, and Beatriz Luna, Maturational Changes in Anterior Cingulate and Frontoparietal Recruitment Support the Development of Error Processing and Inhibitory Control, 2008, with permission from Oxford University Press.

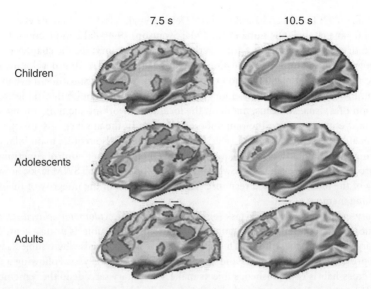

Fig. 35.5 (Also see Plate 19.) Mean group activation for antisaccade error trials in a group of children, adolescents, and adults overlaid on the partially inflated medial cortical surface of the right hemisphere. Activation is shown at two time points following trial onset—an 'early' time point at 7.5 s, and a 'late' time point at 10 s. The approximate location of rostral ACC is circled in green and dorsal ACC in blue. Reproduced from *Cerebral Cortex*, **18**, Katerina Velanova, Mark E. Wheeler, and Beatriz Luna, Maturational Changes in Anterior Cingulate and Frontoparietal Recruitment Support the Development of Error Processing and Inhibitory Control, 2008, with permission from Oxford University Press.

Brain activity underlying saccade inhibition *errors* was also investigated and showed significant developmental change, particularly in anterior cingulate cortex (ACC). Similar to findings from other adult studies (Polli et al., 2005), we found that dorsal anterior cingulate (dACC) showed increased modulation for error versus correct trials. In adults, peak activity in dACC occurred after antisaccade responses were made (Velanova et al., 2008). Children aged 8–12 years failed to show this late activity in dACC while adolescents aged 13–17 years showed an intermediate level of late recruitment (see Fig. 35.5). Importantly, in adults, dACC has been shown to provide signals that inform subsequent task performance (Kerns et al., 2004). Together, these results suggest that while the ability to recognize that an antisaccade error has occurred matures early, feedback signalling from dACC may have a protracted development.

Overall, imaging research using the antisaccade task demonstrates that systems implicated in successful eye-movement control are available early in development but that there is continued maturation of activity in regions that support accessing oculomotor systems in an efficient manner. Additionally, activation of regions implicated in error-detection, error-regulation and performance monitoring shows age-related modulation from childhood to adulthood, suggesting that maturation of these functions contributes to improvements in performance.

Memory guided saccades: development of the ability to direct eye movements with spatial working memory

Voluntary eye movements can also be directed in the absence of a visual stimulus, guided only by the representation of a goal maintained in working memory. Working memory (WM), the ability to maintain and manipulate information 'on-line' to guide responses in a voluntary manner (Baddeley, 1986), also demonstrates a protracted developmental trajectory (Demetriou et al., 2002;

Beveridge et al., 2002; Brocki and Bohlin, 2004; DeLuca et al., 2003; Gathercole et al., 2004; Hitch et al., 1989; Luciana et al., 2005; Luna et al., 2004; Swanson, 1999; Zald and Iacono, 1998). Spatial working memory (SWM) (as distinct from verbal working memory; see the chapter by Blythe and Joseph, Chapter 36, this volume for discussion of eye movements and reading development) supports the ability to maintain the spatial location of a target so as to guide a subsequent eye movement to that location. Prototypical working memory eye movement tasks require that subjects encode the spatial location of a visual stimulus, maintain the location in working memory during a delay, and then make an eye movement to the remembered location in the absence of sensory information (Funahashi et al., 1989; Hikosaka et al., 1989). Some SWM tasks also require manipulation of information during the delay period thus requiring engagement of other control functions including inhibitory processes (Kwon et al., 2002; Swanson, 1999). Common to all SWM tasks, however, is that the accuracy of the memory-guided response serves as an index of the integrity of the information held in working memory.

The *memory-guided saccade* (MGS) task (also referred to as the *oculomotor delayed response* task) is a sensitive measure of developmental change in WM. In this task, subjects fixate a central cross-hair as a visual target is briefly presented at an unpredictable location. Trials where subjects look toward the target represent inhibitory failures and are not considered in analyses. Following a delay, when the fixation cross-hair is extinguished, subjects make a voluntary saccade to the remembered target location. Subjects typically make several saccades, one initial long saccade that approximates gaze to the target location and then, one or more smaller corrective saccades that enhance precision of the final end fixation. When there are no manipulation requirements, the MGS task provides an optimal measure of WM encoding and maintenance.

Most studies examining MGS performance in children have done so with psychiatric populations (Fukushima et al., 2005; Goto et al., 2005). In one of the few studies examining normative *development,* Hikosaka (1997) examined MGS performance in 5- to 76-year-old subjects. Results indicated that young (<12 years of age) and elderly subjects (>50 years of age) showed increased inhibitory failures during the encoding phase of the task and overall longer latencies to initiate memory-guided saccades. Hikosaka (1997), however, did not examine age-related changes in the accuracy of MGS responses. In contrast, in our study of 245 8- to 30-year-olds we characterized the accuracy of memory-guided responses, in addition to examining latency and error rates (Luna et al., 2004). Similar to Hikosaka (1997), latencies to initiate correct memory-guided saccades decreased with age until 14–15 years of age (see Fig. 35.1), mirroring improvements in speed of processing found with the antisaccade and prosaccade tasks. Inhibitory errors during encoding also decreased with age, similar to antisaccade performance. We examined the accuracy of saccadic responses by measuring the distance between each saccade end point and the true location of the to-be-remembered stimulus. Results indicated that the accuracy of the first saccade was mature at approximately 15 years of age (see Fig. 35.6), again similar to antisaccade performance, suggesting that general processes supporting voluntary control mature in adolescence. The accuracy of the final saccade, however, continued to improve into the second decade of life, indicating that WM and performance monitoring are still immature in adolescence. These results provide further support for our interpretation of findings related to the protracted development of error processing in the antisaccade task (Velanova et al., 2008). We also found that age effects were present regardless of the duration of the delay period (1–8 s), indicating that encoding as well as mnemonic processes are implicated in the development of WM. These effects contrast with effects observed in aging populations. In another study using the MGS task in aging, we found that older subjects showed decreased accuracy of the initial saccade, but that accuracy of the final saccade was commensurate with young adults suggesting a sluggish response but preserved performance monitoring and WM (Sweeney et al., 2001) in older adults.

In summary, the ability to generate memory guided saccades improves with age and is supported by improvements in speed of processing and response inhibition, as well as by processes more directly related to the ability to guide behaviour based on a WM representation.

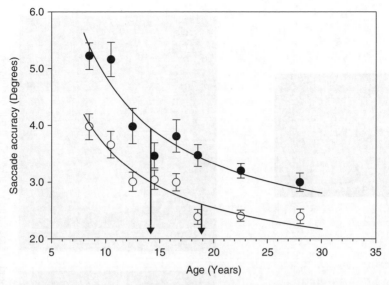

Fig. 35.6 Mean accuracy (+/ 1 standard error of the mean) of the initial (solid circles) and final gaze location (open circles) in the memory-guided saccade task for each age group. Lines represent the inverse curve fit on accuracy by age in years. Arrows depict the ages at which changepoint analyses indicate that adult levels of performance were reached. Luna, B., Garver, K.E., Urban, T.A., Lazar, N.A., Sweeney, J.A. Maturation of cognitive processes from late childhood to adulthood. *Child Development*, **75**(5), 1357–1372, with permission from John Wiley and Sons © 2004.

Development of brain function underlying working memory

A widely distributed brain circuitry, including DLPFC, FEF, ACC, insula, basal ganglia, thalamus, and lateral cerebellum (Hikosaka and Wurtz, 1983; Sweeney et al., 1996) underlies spatial working memory in the adult (Brown et al., 2004; Curtis et al., 2004; Geier et al., 2007; Postle et al., 2000; Sweeney et al., 1995). Working memory studies using neuroimaging have typically used memory-guided button press responses instead of saccades and have focused on the role of prefrontal cortex. These studies have generally found that with development there is decreased participation of prefrontal regions reflecting age-related decreases in effort required to perform the task (Crone et al., 2006; Klingberg et al., 2002; Olesen et al., 2007; Scherf et al., 2006).

We performed a blocked design fMRI study on 30 8 to 47-year-olds comparing activity during MGS performance and prosaccade performance in children, adults, and adolescents (Scherf et al., 2006). Results showed that children relied primarily on basal ganglia and insula. Adolescents showed increased recruitment of DLPFC, similar to findings from the antisaccade task (see Fig. 35.7). Adults recruited regions similar to adolescents but activity in prefrontal cortex was attenuated. Further, adults engaged additional areas including temporal cortex. When considering the distribution of activation across each group, results indicated a progression to more distributed activity with age, concurrent with decreasing recruitment of prefrontal regions. These results further support our proposal that there is a transition to reliance on prefrontal systems from childhood to adolescence while from adolescence to adulthood there is a shift to more evenly distributed function. Moreover, these studies suggest that SWM precision, which continues to improve into adulthood, may be supported by the recruitment of additional regions such as temporal areas (Maguire, 2001) implicated in navigation, and long term memory (Squire et al., 2004) that may provide better spatial resolution.

Thus, the ability to perform memory-guided saccades is present early in development. What continues to improve through adolescence is the precision of responses supported by enhanced

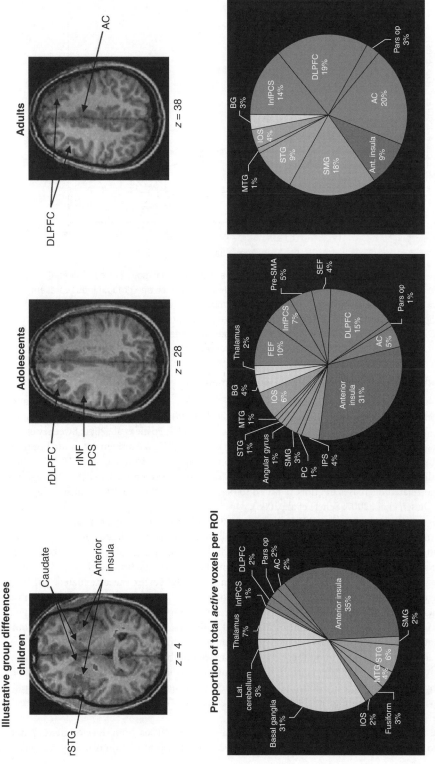

Fig. 35.7 (Also see Plate 20.) Mean group activation during a block memory-guided saccade task compared to prosaccade blocks for a group of children, adolescents, and adults overlaid on top of the structure of a representative subject. Each slice represents the location of primary activity for each group. Pie charts represent the proportion of total active voxels in each region of interest for each age group. From K.S. Scherf, J.A. Sweeney, B. Luna, Brain basis of developmental change in visuospatial working memory, *Journal of Cognitive Neuroscience*, **18**(7) (July, 2006), pp. 1045–1058. ©2006 by the Massachusetts Institute of Technology.

encoding and performance monitoring processes which in turn are subserved by a functionally integrated brain circuitry including prefrontal and posterior systems.

Brain maturation

The oculomotor system is subserved by a widely distributed neural circuitry, including frontal, parietal, and cerebellar regions as well as subcortical structures including the basal ganglia and thalamus. Interactions between these visual-sensory, attention, executive, motor planning, and motor execution regions are crucial to reflexive and controlled eye movements. In particular, this circuitry allows cortical regions to efficiently modulate subcortical signals to elicit or suppress eye movements. The neural processes underlying the function of these regions and their interconnectivity continue to mature into adolescence. Characterizing brain maturation allows us to better understand age-related changes in the execution of eye movements, particularly the ability to enact voluntarily controlled responses.

In particular, two maturational processes, synaptic pruning and myelination, continue from childhood through adulthood. Synaptic pruning refers to the programmed regulatory process by which the neural structure of the brain is refined via reduction of overproduced synapses. While the number of neurons is largely determined by birth, number of synaptic connections and dendritic arborization are known to have a protracted maturation through adolescence (Huttenlocher, 1990; Huttenlocher and Dabholkar, 1997). Specifically, in the first 2 years of life there is an increase in synaptic connections between neurons. After this initial synaptogenesis there is a loss of synaptic connections (i.e. synaptic pruning), that is believed to be determined by relative use: 'weak' connections are terminated, thus sculpting the brain to fit its particular environment (Rauschecker and Marler, 1987). Early morphological studies indicated that compared to area 17 of visual cortex, which showed mature synaptic density by 7 years of age, and Heschl's gyrus, which matured by 12 years of age, the middle frontal gyrus showed continued pruning up to 16 years of age. As a corollary, magnetic resonance imaging (MRI) studies have shown that there is protracted thinning of cortical grey matter in cortical association areas, notably in frontal and temporal regions (Gogtay et al., 2004; Giedd et al., 1999; Paus et al., 1999; Toga et al., 2006), as well as in basal ganglia (Sowell et al., 1999). Further, the pruning of unnecessary synaptic connections results not only in grey-matter thinning but also in more efficient and quick neuronal computations that support the complex processing needed for controlled behaviours including voluntary eye movements.

Another brain maturational process that is known to persist through childhood and adolescence is myelination. Myelination refers to the insulation of nerve tracts by fatty material thus providing a conduit for electrical transmission. As the myelin sheath thickens, neuronal transmission speeds (Drobyshevsky et al., 2005), supporting the efficient integration of widely distributed circuits. Morphometric studies indicate that myelination matures first in visual sensory regions while continuing through adolescence in frontal, parietal, and temporal regions. MRI studies measuring white matter volume and diffusion tensor imaging (DTI) studies measuring white matter integrity, indicate that there is continued white matter development in neocortical and subcortical regions throughout childhood, providing evidence for continued myelination with age (Ben Bashat et al., 2005; Klingberg et al., 1999; Li and Noseworthy, 2002; Mukherjee and McKinstry, 2006). The speeding of neuronal transmission associated with increased myelination allows for the functional integration of a widely-distributed circuitry via cortico-cortico connections needed for the integration of sensory, attentional, and executive processes together with cortico-subcortico connections needed for top-down modulation of behaviour, both necessary for the control of eye movements. Supporting the hypothesis that a shift toward reliance on more distributed brain systems underlies the transition from adolescence to adulthood are recent findings of a developmental shift from childhood to adolescence to adulthood in the establishment of long-range functional connections (Fair et al., 2007). Resting state activity results indicated that a frontoparietal network, known to support inhibitory control and working memory (Dosenbach et al., 2006) and a cingulo-opercular network, known to support the ability to retain a response state, continue to reorganize through adolescence by becoming distinct and segregated from one another and by integrating long distance connections.

Age related improvements in eye movement control thus can be viewed in the context of brain maturation. Basic aspects of neuronal processing that are present early in development support the large range of eye movement control evident at younger ages. The refinements afforded by continued maturation via processes such as synaptic pruning and myelination, allow for enhanced performance, particularly of more complex controlled eye movements. Synaptic pruning at the regional level may enhance the complex computations that support working memory and inhibition increasing the effectiveness of these processes. Increased myelination may support the consistent finding of decreases in the latency to initiate both reflexive and voluntary eye movements and may reflect a general speeding of information processing. Myelination may also support efficient top-down modulation of behaviour needed to support inhibitory processes in the antisaccade task as well as the ability to affect subcortically driven responses by working memory.

Summary and conclusions

The literature describing the development of oculomotor control indicates that basic aspects of sensorimotor function are, for the most part, mature by childhood. However, processes that support the cognitive control of eye movements have a protracted development into adolescence. While basic saccade metrics are mature early in development, the time to initiate an eye movement, be it reflexive or voluntary, continues to decrease into mid-adolescence, suggesting that processes underlying speed of information processing also have a protracted maturation. The accuracy of voluntary eye movements also shows continued refinement into adolescence as evidenced by developmental improvements in the performance of antisaccades and memory-guided saccades. While the ability to make such complex voluntary eye movements exists early in development, the ability to use executive systems in a consistent and flexible manner continues to mature through adolescence suggesting that brain systems supporting performance monitoring and retention of a task set are immature until adulthood. These developmental improvements in the ability to retain a task set and to monitor performance may underlie improvements in the cognitive control of behaviour.

The distinct developmental trajectories of different eye movement responses may parallel the maturational schedules of different brain systems. The early maturation of basic saccade metrics may be supported by the integrity of basic aspects of neuronal computations throughout cortex and subcortical regions. The more protracted development of the voluntary control of eye movements parallels the continuation of synaptic pruning and myelination into adolescence. Increased efficiency of brain regional processes afforded by synaptic pruning, which reaches adult levels in adolescence, would support the complicated computations necessary to perform voluntary saccades. Myelination, which continues through adolescence and enhances functional connectivity, may enhance top-down control and the functional integration of a widely distributed circuitry that supports voluntary control of eye movements and speed of information processing. In this manner, the development of the cognitive control of eye movements can be viewed as reflecting the development of a more widely distributed circuitry that entails less reliance on prefrontal systems as brain processes become better specialized and efficient. Importantly, developmental studies can inform us regarding basic systems by providing a unique window to identify what processes support the specific improvements that are seen in adulthood including appropriate error processing, the maintenance of a task set, and precision.

References

Amador, N., Schlag-Rey, M., and Schlag, J. (2004). Primate antisaccade. II. Supplementary eye field neuronal activity predicts correct performance. *Journal of Neurophysiology*, **91**, 1672–1689.

Aring, E., Grönlund, M.A., Hellström, A., and Ygge, J. (2007). Visual fixation development in children. *Graefe's Archive for Clinical and Experimental Ophthalmology*, **245**, 1659–1665.

Asato, M.R., Sweeney, J.A., and Luna, B. (2006). Cognitive processes in the development of TOL performance. *Neuropsychologia*, **44**, 2259–2269.

Aslin, R.N. and Salapatek, P. (1975). Saccadic localization of visual targets by the very young human infant. *Perception and Psychophysics*, **7**, 293–302.

Baddeley, A. (1986). *Working memory*. New York: Oxford University Press.

Baddeley, A. (1992). Working memory. *Science*, 255, 556–559.

Baddeley, A. (1996). Exploring the central executive. *Quarterly Journal of Experimental Psychology*, 494, 5–28.

Bedard, A.C., Nichols, S., Barbosa, J.A., Schachar, R., Logan, G.D., and Tannock, R. (2002). The development of selective inhibitory control across the life span. *Developmental Neuropsychology*, 21, 93–111.

Ben Bashat, D., Ben Sira, L., Graif, M., Pianka, P., Hendler, T., Cohen, Y., and Assaf, Y. (2005). Normal white matter development from infancy to adulthood: comparing diffusion tensor and high b value diffusion weighted MR images. *Journal of Magnetic Resonance Imaging*, 21, 503–511.

Berman, R.A., Colby, C.L., Genovese, C.R., Voyvodic, J.T., Luna, B., Thulborn, K.R., *et al.* (1999). Cortical networks subserving pursuit and saccadic eye movements in humans: an fMRI study. *Human Brain Mapping*, 8, 209–225.

Beveridge, M., Jarrold, C., and Pettit, E. (2002). An experimental approach to executive fingerprinting in young children. *Infant and Child Development*, 11, 107–123.

Bon, L. and Lucchetti, C. (1990). Neurons signalling the maintenance of attentive fixation in frontal area 6a beta of macaque monkey. *Experimental Brain Research*, 82, 231–233.

Brocki, K.C. and Bohlin, G. (2004). Executive functions in children aged 6 to 13: A dimensional and developmental study. *Developmental Neuropsychology*, 26, 571–593.

Brown, M.R., Vilis, T., and Everling, S. (2007). Frontoparietal activation with preparation for antisaccades. *Journal of Neurophysiology*, 98, 1751–1762.

Brown, M.R., Goltz, H.C., Vilis, T., Ford, K.A., and Everling, S. (2006). Inhibition and generation of saccades: rapid event-related fMRI of prosaccades, antisaccades, and nogo trials. *NeuroImage*, 33, 644–659.

Brown, M.R., Desouza, J.F., Goltz, H.C., Ford, K., Menon, R.S., Goodale, M.A., and Everling, S. (2004). Comparison of memory- and visually guided saccades using event-related fMRI. *Journal of Neurophysiology*, 91, 873–889.

Bruce, C.J. and Goldberg, M.E. (1985). Primate frontal eye fields. I. Single neurons discharging before saccades. *Journal of Neurophysiology*, 53, 603–635.

Carpenter, P.A., Just, M.A., Keller, T.A., and Eddy, W. (1999). Graded functional activation in the visuospatial system with the amount of task demand. *Journal of Cognitive Neuroscience*, 11, 9–24.

Cepeda, N.J. and Kramer, A.F. (2001). Changes in executive control across the life span: Examination of task-switching performance. *Developmental Psychology*, 37, 715–730.

Cohen, M.E. and Ross, L.E. (1978). Latency and accuracy characteristics of saccades and corrective saccades in children and adults. *Journal of Experimental Child Psychology*, 26, 517–527.

Connolly, J.D., Goodale, M.A., DeSouza, J.F.X., Menon, R.S., and Vilis, T. (2000). A comparison of frontoparietal fMRI activation during anti-saccades and anti-pointing. *Journal of Neurophysiology*, 84, 1645–1655.

Corbetta, M., Akbudak, E., Conturo, T.E., Snyder, A.Z., Ollinger, J.M., Drury, H.A., *et al.* (1998). A common network of functional areas for attention and eye movements. *Neuron*, 21, 761–773.

Crone, E.A., Wendelken, C., Donohue, S., van Leijenhorst, L., and Bunge, S.A. (2006). Neurocognitive development of the ability to manipulate information in working memory. *Proceedings of the National Academy of Sciences of the United States of America*, 103, 9315–9320.

Curtis, C.E., Rao, V.Y., and D'Esposito, M. (2004). Maintenance of spatial and motor codes during oculomotor delayed response tasks. *Journal of Neuroscience*, 24, 3944–3952.

Daniel, B.M. and Lee, D.N. (1990). Development of looking with head and eyes. *Journal of Experimental Child Psychology*, 50, 200–216.

DeLuca, C.R., Wood, S.J., Anderson, V., Bucanan, J., Proffitt, T.M., and Mahony, K. (2003). Normative data from the CANTAB: I. Development of executive function over the lifespan. *Journal of Clinical and Experimental Neuropsychology*, 25, 242–254.

Demetriou, A., Christou, C., Spanoudis, G., and Platsidou, M. (2002). The development of mental processing: efficiency, working memory, and thinking. *Monographs of the Society for Research in Child Development*, 67, 1–155; discussion 156.

Desimone, R. and Duncan, J. (1995). Neural mechanisms of selective visual attention. *Annual Reviews in Neuroscience*, 18, 193–222.

Dorris, M.C. and Munoz, D.P. (1995). A neural correlate for the gap effect on saccadic reaction times in monkey. *Journal of Neurophysiology*, 73, 2558–2562.

Dorris, M.C., Martin, P., and Munoz, D.P. (1997). Neuronal Activity in Monkey Superior Colliculus Related to the Initiation of Saccadic Eye Movements. *Journal of Neuroscience*, 17, 8566–8579.

Dosenbach, N.U., Visscher, K.M., Palmer, E.D., Miezin, F.M., Wenger, K.K., Kang, H.C., *et al.* (2006). A core system for the implementation of task sets. *Neuron*, 50, 799–812.

Drobyshevsky, A., Song, S.K., Gamkrelidze, G., Wyrwicz, A.M., Meng, F., Li, L., *et al.* (2005). Developmental changes in diffusion anisotropy coincide with immature oligodendrocyte progression and maturation of compound action potential. *Journal of Neuroscience*, 25, 5988–5997.

Eenshuistra, R.M., Ridderinkhof, K.R., Weidema, M.A., and van der Molen, M.W. (2007). Developmental changes in oculomotor control and working-memory efficiency. *Acta Psychologica*, 124, 139–158.

Engbert, R. (2006). Microsaccades: A microcosm for research on oculomotor control, attention, and visual perception. *Progress in Brain Research*, 154, 177–192.

Everling, S. and Munoz, D.P. (2000). Neuronal correlates for preparatory set associated with pro-saccades and anti-saccades in the primate frontal eye field. *Journal of Neuroscience*, **20**, 387–400.

Everling, S., Dorris, M.C., Klein, R.M., and Munoz, D.P. (1999). Role of primate superior colliculus in preparation and execution of anti-saccades and pro-saccades. *Journal of Neuroscience*, **19**, 2740–2754.

Fair, D.A., Dosenbach, N.U., Church, J.A., Cohen, A.L., Brahmbhatt, S., Miezin, F.M., *et al.* (2007) Development of distinct control networks through segregation and integration. *Proceedings of the National Academy of Sciences, U S A*, **104**, 13507–13512.

Fioravanti, F., Inchingolo, P., Pensiero, S., and Spanio, M. (1995). Saccadic eye movement conjugation in children. *Vision Research*, **35**, 3217–3228.

Fischer, B. and Ramsperger, E. (1984) Human express saccades: extremely short reaction times of goal directed eye movements. *Experimental Brain Research*, **57**, 191–195.

Fischer, B., Biscaldi, M., and Gezeck, S. (1997). On the development of voluntary and reflexive components in human saccade generation. *Brain Research*, **754**, 285–297.

Fukushima, J., Hatta, T., and Fukushima, K. (2000). Development of voluntary control of saccadic eye movements. I. Age-related changes in normal children. *Brain and Development*, **22**, 173–180.

Fukushima, J., Tanaka, S., Williams, J.D., and Fukushima, K. (2005). Voluntary control of saccadic and smooth-pursuit eye movements in children with learning disorders. *Brain and Development*, **27**, 579–588.

Fukushima, J., Akao, T., Takeichi, N., Kaneko, C.R.S., and Fukushima, K. (2003). Involvement of the frontal oculomotor areas in developmental compensation for the directional asymmetry in smooth-pursuit eye movements in young primates. *Annals of the New York Academy of Sciences*, **1004**, 451–456.

Fukushima, J., Akao, T., Kurkin, S., Kaneko, C.R., and Fukushima, K. (2006). The vestibular-related frontal cortex and its role in smooth-pursuit eye movements and vestibular-pursuit interactions. *Journal of Vestibular Research*, **16**, 1–22.

Funahashi, S., Bruce, C.J., and Goldman-Rakic, P.S. (1989). Mnemonic coding of visual space in the monkey's dorsolateral prefrontal cortex. *Journal of Neurophysiology*, **61**, 331–349.

Funk, C.J. and Anderson, M.E. (1977). Saccadic eye movements and eye-head coordination in children. *Perceptual and Motor Skills*, **44**, 599–610.

Fuster, J.M. (1997). *The Prefrontal Cortex* (3rd edn.) New York: Raven Press.

Gathercole, S.E., Pickering, S.J., Ambridge, B., and Wearing, H. (2004). The structure of working memory from 4 to 15 years of age. *Developmental Psychology*, **40**, 177–190.

Geier, C.F., Garver, K.E., and Luna, B. (2007). Circuitry underlying temporally extended spatial working memory. *Neuroimage*, **35**, 904–915.

Giedd, J.N., Blumenthal, J., Jeffries, N.O., Castellanos, F.X., Liu, H., Zijdenbos, A., *et al.* (1999). Brain development during childhood and adolescence: A longitudinal MRI study. *Nature Neuroscience*, **2**, 861–863.

Gogtay, N., Giedd, J.N., Lusk, L., Hayashi, K.M., Greenstein, D., Vaituzis, A.C., *et al.* (2004). Dynamic mapping of human cortical development during childhood through early adulthood. *Proceedings of the National Academy of Sciences of the U S A*, **101**, 8174–8179.

Goldberg, M.E. and Bruce, C.J. (1990). Primate frontal eye fields. III. Maintenance of a spatially accurate saccade signal. *Journal of Neurophysiology*, **64**, 489–508.

Goldberg, M.E., Bushnell, M.C., and Bruce, C.J. (1986). The effect of attentive fixation on eye movements evoked by electrical stimulation of the frontal eye fields. *Experimental Brain Research*, **61**, 579–584.

Goto, Y., Aihara, M., Hatakeyama, K., Kitama, T., Sato, Y., and Nakazawa, S. (2005). Study of saccadic eye movement in children with attention deficit/hyperactivity disorder. *No To Hattatsu*, **37**, 10–14.

Gredebäck, G., von Hofsten, C., Karlsson, J., and Aus, K. (2005). The development of two-dimensional tracking: a longitudinal study of circular pursuit. *Experimental Brain Research*, **163**, 204–213.

Grönqvist, H., Gredebäck, G., and Hofsten, C. (2006). Developmental asymmetries between horizontal and vertical tracking. *Vision Research*, **46**, 1754–1761.

Guitton, D., Buchtel, H.A., and Douglas, R.M. (1985). Frontal lobe lesions in man cause difficulties in suppressing reflexive glances and in generating goal-directed saccades. *Experimental Brain Research*, **58**, 455–472.

Hainline, L., Turkel, J., Abramov, I., Lemerise, E., and Harris, C.M. (1984). Characteristics of saccades in human infants. *Vision Research*, **24**, 1771–1780.

Haishi, K. and Kokubun, M. (1995). Developmental trends in pursuit eye movements among preschool children. *Perceptual and Motor Skills*, **81**, 1131–1137.

Haishi, K. and Kokubun, M. (1998). Development of psychological aspect in pursuit eye movements among preschoolers. *Perceptual and Motor Skills*, **86**, 146.

Hale, S. (1990). A global developmental trend in cognitive processing speed. *Child Development*, **61**, 653–663.

Hallett, P.E. (1978). Primary and secondary saccades to goals defined by instructions. *Vision Research*, **18**, 1279–1296.

Harris, C.M., Jacobs, M., Shawkat, F., and Taylor, D. (1993). The development of saccadic accuracy in the first seven months. *Clinical Vision Sciences*, **8**, 85–96.

Hikosaka, O. (1997) [Changes and disorders in voluntary saccades during development and aging]. *No To Hattatsu*, **29**, 213–219.

Hikosaka, O. and Wurtz, R.H. (1983). Visual and oculomotor functions of monkey substantia nigra pars reticulata. III. Memory-contingent visual and saccade responses. *Journal of Neurophysiology*, **49**, 1268–1284.

Hikosaka, O., Sakamoto, M., and Usui, S. (1989). Functional properties of monkey caudate neurons. I. Activities related to saccadic eye movement. *Journal of Neurophysiology*, **61**, 780–798.

Hitch, G.J., Halliday, M.S., Dodd, A., and Littler, J.E. (1989). Development of rehearsal in short-term memory: Differences between pictorial and spoken stimuli. *British Journal of Developmental Psychology*, **7**, 347–362.

Huttenlocher, P.R. (1990). Morphometric study of human cerebral cortex development. *Neuropsychologia*, **28**, 517–527.

Huttenlocher, P.R. and Dabholkar, A.S. (1997). Regional differences in synaptogenesis in human cerebral cortex. *Journal of Comparative Neurology*, **387**, 167–178.

Irving, E.L., Steinbach, M.J., Lillakas, L., Babu, R.J., and Hutchings, N. (2006). Horizontal saccade dynamics across the human life span. *Investigative Ophthalmology and Visual Science*, **47**, 2478–2484.

Jacobs, M., Harris, C.M., Shawkat, F., and Taylor, D. (1997). Smooth pursuit development in infants. *Australian and New Zealand Journal of Ophthalmology*, **25**, 199–206.

Johnson, M.H. (1995). The inhibition of automatic saccades in early infancy. *Developmental Psychobiology*, **28**, 281–291.

Kail, R. and Park, Y. (1992). Global developmental change in processing time. *Merrill-Palmer Quarterly*, **38**, 525–541.

Kane, M.J., Bleckley, M.K., Conway, A.R., and Engle, R.W. (2001). A controlled-attention view of working-memory capacity. *Journal of Experimental Psychology: General*, **130**, 169–183.

Katsanis, J., Iacono, W.G., and Harris, M. (1998). Development of oculomotor functioning in preadolescence, adolescence, and adulthood. *Psychophysiology*, **35**, 64–72.

Keating, E.G. and Gooley, S.G. (1988). Disconnection of parietal and occipital access to the saccadic oculomotor system. *Experimental Brain Research*, **70**, 385–398.

Kerns J.G., Cohen, J.D., McDonald A.W., Cho R.Y., Stenger V.A., and Carter C.S. (2004). Anterior cingulate conflict monitoring and adjustments in control. *Science*, **303**, 1023–1026.

Klein, C. (2001). Developmental functions for saccadic eye movement parameters derived from pro- and antisaccade tasks. *Experimental Brain Research*, **139**, 1–17.

Klein, C. and Feige, B. (2005). An independent components analysis (ICA) approach to the study of developmental differences in the saccadic contingent negative variation. *Biological Psychology*, **70**, 105–114.

Klein, C. and Foerster, F. (2001). Development of prosaccade and antisaccade task performance in participants aged 6 to 26 years. *Psychophysiology*, **38**, 179–189.

Klein, C., Foerster, F., Hartnegg, K., and Fischer, B. (2005). Lifespan development of pro- and anti-saccades: multiple regression models for point estimates. *Brain Research: Developmental Brain Research*, **160**, 113–123.

Klingberg, T., Forssberg, H., and Westerberg, H. (2002). Increased brain activity in frontal and parietal cortex underlies the development of visuospatial working memory capacity during childhood. *Journal of Cognitive Neuroscience*, **14**, 1–10.

Klingberg, T., Vaidya, C.J., Gabrieli, J.D.E., Moseley, M.E., and Hedehus, M. (1999). Myelination and organization of the frontal white matter in children: a diffusion tensor MRI study. *Neuroreport*, **10**, 2817–2821.

Kwon, H., Reiss, R.L., and Menon, V. (2002). Neural basis of protracted developmental changes in visuo-spatial working memory. *Proceedings of the National Academy of Sciences of the United States of America*, **99**, 13336–13341.

Leigh, R.J. and Zee, D.S. (1991). *The Neurology of Eye Movements* (2nd edN.) Philadelphia: F. A. Davis.

Leigh, R.J. and Zee, D.S. (1999). *The Neurology of Eye Movements* (3rd edN.) New York: Oxford University Press.

Levin, H.S., Culhane, K.A., Hartmann, J., Evankovich, K., and Mattson, A.J. (1991). Developmental changes in performance on tests of purported frontal lobe functioning. *Developmental Neuropsychology*, **7**, 377–395.

Li, T.Q. and Noseworthy, M.D. (2002). Mapping the development of white matter tracts with diffusion tensor imaging. *Developmental Science*, **5**, 293–300.

Liston, C., Watts, R., Tottenham, N., Davidson, M.C., Niogi, S., Ulug, A.M., and Casey, B.J. (2006). Frontostriatal microstructure modulates efficient recruitment of cognitive control. *Cerebral Cortex*, **16**, 553–560.

Logan, G.D. and Gordon, S.E. (2001). Executive control of visual attention in dual-task situations. *Psychological Review*, **108**, 393–434.

Luciana, M. and Nelson, C. (1998). The functional emergence of prefrontally-guided working memory systems in four- to eight-year-old children. *Neuropsychologia*, **36**, 273–293.

Luciana, M., Conklin, H.M., Hooper, C.J., and Yarger, R.S. (2005). The development of nonverbal working memory and executive control processes in adolescents. *Child Development*, **76**, 697–712.

Luna, B., Garver, K.E., Urban, T.A., Lazar, N.A., and Sweeney, J.A. (2004). Maturation of cognitive processes from late childhood to adulthood. *Child Development*, **75**, 1357–1372.

Luna, B., Thulborn, K.R., Munoz, D.P., Merriam, E.P., Garver, K.E., Minshew, N.J., *et al.* (2001). Maturation of widely distributed brain function subserves cognitive development. *NeuroImage*, **13**, 786–793.

Luna, B., Thulborn, K.R., Strojwas, M.H., McCurtain, B.J., Berman, R.A., Genovese, C.R., *et al.* (1998). Dorsal cortical regions subserving visually-guided saccades in humans: an fMRI study. *Cerebral Cortex*, **8**, 40–47.

MacAvoy, M.G., Gottlieb, J.P., and Bruce, C.J. (1991). Smooth pursuit eye movement representation in the primate frontal eye field. *Cerebral Cortex*, **1**, 95–102.

Maguire, E.A. (2001). The retrosplenial contribution to human navigation: a review of lesion and neuroimaging findings. *Scandinavian Journal of Psychology*, **42**, 225–238.

Matsuda, T., Matsuura, M., Ohkubo, T., Ohkubo, H., Matsushima, E., Inoue, K., *et al.* (2004). Functional MRI mapping of brain activation during visually guided saccades and antisaccades: cortical and subcortical networks. *Psychiatry Research*, **131**, 147–155.

Mayfrank, L., Mobashery, M., Kimmig, H., and Fischer, B. (1986). The role of fixation and visual attention in the occurrence of express saccades in man. *European Archives of Psychiatry and Neurological Sciences,* **235,** 269–275.

Miller, E.K. and Cohen, J.D. (2001). An integrative theory of prefrontal cortex function. *Annual Reviews in Neuroscience,* **24,** 167–202.

Miller, L.M., Sun, F.T., Curtis, C.E., and D'Esposito, M. (2005). Functional interactions between oculomotor regions during prosaccades and antisaccades. *Human Brain Mapping,* **26,** 119–127.

Miyake, A., Friedman, N.P., Emerson, M.J., Witzki, A.H., Howerter, A., and Wager, T.D. (2000). The unity and diversity of executive functions and their contributions to complex 'Frontal Lobe' tasks: a latent variable analysis. *Cognitive Psychology,* **41,** 49–100.

Monsell, S. (1996). Control of mental processes. In V.Bruce (ed.) *Unsolved mysteries of the mind: Tutorial essays in cognition* (pp. 93–148). London: Taylor and Francis.

Monsell, S. and Mizon, G.A. (2006). Can the task-cuing paradigm measure an endogenous task-set reconfiguration process? *Journal of Experimental Psychology: Human Perception and Performance,* **32,** 493–516.

Mountcastle, V.B., Andersen, R.A., and Motter, B.C. (1981). The influence of attentive fixation upon the excitability of the light-sensitive neurons of the posterior parietal cortex. *Journal of Neuroscience,* **1,** 1218–1225.

Mukherjee, P. and McKinstry, R.C. (2006). Diffusion tensor imaging and tractography of human brain development. *Neuroimaging Clinics of North America,* **16,** 19–43.

Munoz, D.P. and Everling, S. (2004). Look away: the anti-saccade task and the voluntary control of eye movement. *Nature Reviews Neuroscience,* **5,** 218–228.

Munoz, D.P. and Wurtz, R.H. (1992). Role of the rostral superior colliculus in active visual fixation and execution of express saccades. *Journal of Neurophysiology,* **67,** 1000–1002.

Munoz, D.P., Broughton, J.R., Goldring, J.E., and Armstrong, I.T. (1998). Age-related performance of human subjects on saccadic eye movement tasks. *Experimental Brain Research,* **121,** 391–400.

Muri, R.M., Nirkko, A.C., Ozdoba, C., Felblinger, J., Heid, O., Schroth, G., and Hess, C.W. (1996). Functional organization of cortical control of prosaccades and antisaccades in the frontal lobes. A functional magnetic resonance imaging (fMRI) study. *NeuroImage,* **3,** 352.

Nelson, C.A., Monk, C.S., Lin, J., Carver, L.J., Thomas, K.M., and Truwitt, C.L. (2000). Functional neuroanatomy of spatial working memory in children. *Developmental Psychology,* **36,** 109–116.

Newsome, W.T., Wurtz, R.H., and Komatsu, H. (1988). Relation of cortical areas MT and MST to pursuit eye movement. II. Differentiation of retinal from extraretinal inputs. *Journal of Neurophysiology,* **60,** 604–620.

Norman, D.A. and Shallice, T. (1986). Attention to action: Will and automatic control of behavior. In R.J. Davidson, G.E. Schwartz, and E. Shapiro (eds.) *Consciousness and self-regulation* (pp. 1–18). New York: Plenum Press.

Olesen, P.J., Macoveanu, J., Tegner, J., and Klingberg, T. (2007). Brain activity related to working memory and distraction in children and adults. *Cerebral Cortex,* **17,** 1047–1054.

Olesen, P.J., Nagy, Z., Westerberg, H., and Klingberg, T. (2003). Combined analysis of DTI and fMRI data reveals a joint maturation of white and grey matter in a fronto-parietal network. *Cognitive Brain Research,* **18,** 48–57.

Paus, T. (1989). The development of sustained attention in children might be related to the maturation of frontal cortical functions. *Acta Neurobiologiae Experimentalis,* **49,** 51–55.

Paus, T., Babenko, V., and Radil, T. (1990). Development of an ability to maintain verbally instructed central gaze fixation studied in 8- to 10-year-old children. *International Journal of Psychophysiology,* **10,** 53–61.

Paus, T., Zijdenbos, A., Worsley, K., Collins, D.L., Blumenthal, J., Giedd, J.N., *et al.* (1999). Structural maturation of neural pathways in children and adolescents: *in vivo* study. *Science,* **283,** 1908–1911.

Petit, L., Clark, V.P., Ingeholm, J., and Haxby, J.V. (1997). Dissociation of saccade-related and pursuit-related activation in human frontal eye fields as revealed by fMRI. *Journal of Neurophysiology,* **77,** 3386–3390.

Polli, F.E., Barton, J.J., Cain, M.S., Thakkar, K.N., Rauch, S.L., and Manoach, D.S. (2005). Rostral and dorsal anterior cingulate cortex make dissociable contributions during antisaccade error commission. *Proceedings of the National Academy of Sciences of the U S A,* **102,** 15700–15705.

Postle, B.R., Berger, J.S., Taich, A.M., and D'Esposito, M. (2000). Activity in human frontal cortex associated with spatial working memory and saccadic behavior. *Journal of Cognitive Neuroscience,* **12,** 2–14.

Rauschecker, J.P. and Marler, P. (1987). What signals are responsible for synaptic changes in visual cortical plasticity? In J.P. Rauschecker and P. Marler (eds.) *Imprinting and Cortical Plasticity* (pp. 193–200). New York: Wiley.

Regal, D., Ashmead, D., and Salapatek, P. (1983). The coordination of eye and head movements during early infancy: a selective review. *Behavioural Brain Research,* **10,** 125–132.

Ridderinkhof, K.R., Band, G.P.H., and Logan, G.D. (1999). A study of adaptive behavior: effects of age and irrelevant information on the ability to inhibit one's actions. *Acta Psychologica,* **101,** 315–337.

Ridderinkhof, K.R., van der Molen, M.W., Band, G.P., and Bashore, T.R. (1997). Sources of interference from irrelevant information: a developmental study. *Journal of Experimental Child Psychology,* **65,** 315–341.

Robinson, D.L. and Goldberg, M.E. (1978). Sensory and behavioral properties of neurons in posterior parietal cortex of the awake, trained monkey. *Federation Proceedings,* **37,** 2258–2261.

Robinson, D.L., Goldberg, M.E., and Stanton, G.B. (1978). Parietal association cortex in the primate: sensory mechanisms and behavioral modulations. *Journal of Neurophysiology*, **41**, 910–932.

Rosander, K. (2007). Visual tracking and its relationship to cortical development. *Progress in Brain Research*, **164**, 105–122.

Rosander, K. and von Hofsten, C. (2002). Development of gaze tracking of small and large objects. *Experimental Brain Research*, **146**, 257–264.

Ross, R.G., Radant, A.D., and Hommer, D.W. (1993). A developmental study of smooth pursuit eye movements in normal children from 7 to 15 years of age. *Journal of the American Academy of Child and Adolescent Psychiatry*, **32**, 783–791.

Ross, R.G., Hommer, D., Breiger, D., Varley, C., and Radant, A. (1994). Eye movement task related to frontal lobe functioning in children with attention deficit disorder. *Journal of the American Academy of Child and Adolescent Psychiatry*, **33**, 869–874.

Roucoux, A., Culee, C., and Roucoux, M. (1983). Development of fixation and pursuit eye movements in human infants. *Behavioural Brain Research*, **10**, 133–139.

Rütsche, A., Baumann, A., Jiang, X., and Mojon, D.S. (2006). Development of visual pursuit in the first 6 years of life. *Graefe's Archive for Clinical and Experimental Ophthalmology*, **244**, 1406–1411.

Salman, M.S., Sharpe, J.A., Lillakas, L., Dennis, M., and Steinbach, M.J. (2006). Smooth pursuit eye movements in children. *Experimental Brain Research*, **169**, 139–143.

Scherf, K.S., Sweeney, J.A., and Luna, B. (2006). Brain basis of developmental change in visuospatial working memory. *Journal of Cognitive Neuroscience*, **18**, 1045–1058.

Schlag, J. and Schlag-Rey, M. (1987). Evidence for a supplementary eye field. *Journal of Neurophysiology*, **57**, 179–200.

Schneider, D.W. and Logan, G.D. (2006). Hierarchical control of cognitive processes: switching tasks in sequences. *Journal of Experimental Psychology: General*, **135**, 623–640.

Schneider, W. and Shiffrin, R.M. (1977). Controlled and automatic human information processing: I. Detection, search, and attention. *Psychological Review*, **84**, 1–53.

Shea, S.L. and Aslin, R.N. (1990). Oculomotor responses to step-ramp targets by young human infants. *Vision Research*, **30**, 1077–1092.

Shibutani, H., Sakata, H., and Hyvarinen, J. (1984). Saccade and blinking evoked by microstimulation of the posterior parietal association cortex of the monkey. *Experimental Brain Research*, **55**, 1–8.

Shiffrin, R.M. and Schneider, W. (1977). Controlled and automatic human information processing: II. Perceptual learning, automatic attending and general theory. *Psychological Review*, **84**, 127–190.

Sowell, E.R., Thompson, P.M., Holmes, C.J., Jernigan, T.L., and Toga, A.W. (1999). In vivo evidence for post-adolescent brain maturation in frontal and striatal regions. *Nature Neuroscience*, **2**, 859–861.

Squire, L.R., Stark, C.E., and Clark, R.E. (2004). The medial temporal lobe. *Annual Review of Neuroscience*, **27**, 279–306.

Swanson, H.L. (1999). What develops in working memory? A life span perspective. *Developmental Psychology*, **35**, 986–1000.

Sweeney, J.A., Rosano, C., Berman, R.A., and Luna, B. (2001). Inhibitory control of attention declines more than working memory during normal aging. *Neurobiology of Aging*, **22**, 39–47.

Sweeney, J.A., Luna, B., Srinivasagam, N.M., Keshavan, M.S., Schooler, N.R., Haas, G.L., *et al.* (1998). Eye tracking abnormalities in schizophrenia: evidence for dysfunction in the frontal eye fields. *Biological Psychiatry*, **44**, 698–708.

Sweeney, J.A., Mintun, M.A., Kwee, S., Wiseman, M.B., Brown, D.L., Rosenberg, D.R., *et al.* (1995) PET studies of voluntary saccadic eye movements and spatial working memory. *Schizophrenia Research*, **15**, 100.

Sweeney, J.A., Mintun, M.A., Kwee, S., Wiseman, M.B., Brown, D.L., Rosenberg, D.R., *et al.* (1996). Positron emission tomography study of voluntary saccadic eye movements and spatial working memory. *Journal of Neurophysiology*, **75**, 454–468.

Takeichi, N., Fukushima, J., Kurkin, S., Yamanobe, T., Shinmei, Y., and Fukushima, K. (2003). Directional asymmetry in smooth ocular tracking in the presence of visual background in young and adult primates. *Experimental Brain Research*, **149**, 380–390.

Tipper, S.P., Bourque, T.A., Anderson, S.H., and Brehaut, J.C. (1989). Mechanisms of attention: a developmental study. *Journal of Experimental Child Psychology*, **48**, 353–378.

Toga, A.W., Thompson, P.M., and Sowell, E.R. (2006). Mapping brain maturation. *Trends in Neurosciences*, **29**, 148–159.

Van den Wildenberg, W.P.M. and van der Molen, M.W. (2004). Developmental trends in simple and selective inhibition of compatible and incompatible responses. *Journal of Experimental Child Psychology*, **87**, 201–220.

Van der Stigchel, S., Merten, H., Meeter, M., and Theeuwes, J. (2007). The effects of a task-irrelevant visual event on spatial working memory. *Psychonomic Bulletin and Review*, **14**, 1066–1071.

Velanova, K., Wheeler, M.E., and Luna, B. (2008). Maturational changes in anterior cingulate and frontoparietal recruitment support the development of error processing and inhibitory control. *Cerebral Cortex*, **18**, 2505–2522.

Velanova, K., Wheeler, M.E. and Luna, B. (2009). The maturation of task set-related activation supports late developmental improvements in inhibitory control. *Journal of Neuroscience*, **29**, 12558–12567.

von Hofsten, C. and Rosander, K. (1997). Development of smooth pursuit tracking in young infants. *Vision Research*, **37**, 1799–1810.

Williams, B.R., Ponesse, J.S., Schachar, R.J., Logan, G.D., and Tannock, R. (1999). Development of inhibitory control across the life span. *Developmental Psychology*, **35**, 205–213.

Wise, L.A., Sutton, J.A., and Gibbons, P.D. (1975). Decrement in Stroop interference time with age. *Perceptual and Motor Skills*, **41**, 149–150.

Ygge, J., Aring, E., Han Y., Bolzani R., and Hellström, A. (2005). Fixation stability in normal children. *Annals of the New York Academy of Sciences*, **1039**, 480–483.

Zald, D.H. and Iacono, W.G. (1998). The development of spatial working memory abilities. *Developmental Neuropsychology*, **14**, 563–578.

CHAPTER 36

Children's eye movements during reading

Hazel I. Blythe and Holly S.S.L. Joseph

Abstract

In this chapter, we evaluate the literature to date on children's eye movements during reading. We describe the basic developmental changes that occur in eye movement behaviour during reading, discuss age-related changes in the extent and time-course of information extraction during fixations in reading, and compare the effects of visual and linguistic manipulations in the text on children's eye movement behaviour in relation to skilled adult readers. We argue that future research will benefit from examining how eye movement behaviour during reading develops in relation to language and literacy skills, and use of computational modelling with children's eye movement data may improve our understanding of the mechanisms that underlie the progression from beginning to skilled reader.

Introduction

There has been a great deal of research that has used eye movement recordings to examine the psychological processes underlying skilled adult reading (see Rayner, 1998, 2009 for reviews). This line of research has grown to the point where there are several well-developed computational models that can account for many of the phenomena associated with eye movement behaviour during reading (e.g. the SWIFT model: Engbert et al., 2002, 2005; the E-Z Reader model: Pollatsek et al., 2006; Reichle et al., 1998, 1999, 2003, 2006; see also Reichle, Chapter 42, and Engbert and Kliegl, Chapter 43, this volume). These models are, however, currently limited to explaining the end point of development: the skilled adult reader. This is largely a consequence of there having been very few studies that have examined children's eye movements during reading in proportion to the vast body of research that has studied adults.

It is unsurprising that there has been little research in this area with children. Taking accurate eye movement recordings is a process that requires the participant to sit very still and follow instructions from the researcher, often for prolonged periods of time, requiring a lot of patience. This is difficult with adults and, understandably, even more so with children as participants. Finding young children who are willing and able to cooperate for the duration of an experiment can be extremely challenging and this has been a constraining factor in the sample size of some studies (depending on the particular equipment used and, consequently, the spatial and temporal accuracy of the data). As eye tracking technology improves, however, it is increasingly possible to take accurate eye movement recordings from larger samples of children across a broader range of ages.

In order to fully understand the cognitive processes underlying reading it is necessary to study the trajectory of reading development through online research methods such as eye movement recordings. In this chapter, we review the small, existing literature on children's eye movements during reading both to assess the current state of knowledge in this field, and also in an effort to highlight areas where future eye movement research might be effective in improving understanding of the cognitive changes underlying children's reading development. We do not discuss in detail the body of literature that exists on the eye movements during reading of children with dyslexia, as it is beyond the scope of this chapter. In experiments investigating the relationship between dyslexia and eye movements, typically develop- ing children are frequently used for both reading age and chronological age control groups; however, the data analyses are strongly focused upon comparisons of the different groups and the experiments are not designed to examine the characteristics of typically developing children's oculomotor control during reading. For a review of the literature on eye movements and dyslexia, see Kirkby et al. (2008).

In this chapter, we first comment on some theoretical and methodological issues which are partic- ularly relevant to conducting eye movement research with children. Second, we discuss several stud- ies which were largely exploratory and which examined the basic characteristics of children's eye movements during reading at different ages. The third section considers developmental changes in the encoding of visual information during fixations in reading. The latter half of the chapter then focuses on the influences of specific manipulations within text upon children's cognitive processing, as indexed by their eye movement behaviour. We give a review of studies which have manipulated lexical characteristics in text and then, following on from this, the influence of higher-level process- ing manipulations are considered. The chapter concludes with a discussion of how future research into children's eye movements during reading may inform our understanding of the cognitive devel- opmental changes underlying the progression from beginning to skilled reader.

Conducting eye movement research to investigate children's reading

Theoretical issues

First, it is vital to consider the possible contributions of chronological age and reading skill in relation to each other, and how they might impact on eye movement behaviour. As age increases, reading ability also improves as the child progresses from a beginning to a skilled reader. Thus, any changes in eye movement behaviour that are observed between different age groups may be attribut- able to the difference in chronological age, or they may be attributable to a difference in reading skill. When a skilled adult reads a line of text, their eyes make a sequence of extremely quick saccades that accurately position the eyes such that new information falls on the fovea. As with many different motor skills, it is possible that control of these eye movements improves with age in terms of speed and accuracy. Indeed, previous research using non-reading tasks has demonstrated developmental decreases in saccadic latency (e.g. Cohen and Ross, 1978; Groll and Ross, 1982; Huestegge et al., 2009) although saccadic accuracy, peak saccadic velocity, and saccadic overshoot have all been observed to be the same in children as in adults (e.g. Cohen and Ross, 1978; Fukushima et al., 2000; Salman et al., 2006). Thus, one possibility is that on a task such as reading, where optimal perform- ance depends on the execution of small but fast and accurate eye movements, improvements in motor control associated with increasing chronological age may be one factor underlying the observed developmental changes in eye movement behaviour.

On the other hand, and perhaps more obviously, developmental changes in eye movement control are also a behavioural consequence of increasing reading skill. As reading skill increases, changes in eye movements will reflect the decrease in cognitive processing difficulty associated with text compre- hension. In this case, we might expect to see differences between children of the same chronological age who vary significantly in reading skill. While several of the studies reviewed in this chapter have been careful to exclude children who were not within the normal range of reading ability for their age, to our knowledge no study has explicitly addressed this potential dichotomy. The possibility that differences in eye movement behaviour during reading between children and adults may be a combination of both age-related changes in motor skill and differences in reading proficiency should also be considered. The relative contributions of these two factors are not yet well understood in the eye movement literature; however, future research may allow separate examination of the causes underlying age-related change by including multiple child participant groups and matching both for chronological age and reading age, as well as making systematic manipulations of text difficulty in relation to reading skill (see discussion in the section 'Methodological issues').

Second, a critical issue with respect to age-related changes in eye movement behaviour during reading is that of cause and effect. Does increased processing difficulty cause readers to make more, longer fixations, etc., or is it the case that poor control of eye movements leads to difficulty in reading? The results of two eye movement studies with children have indicated that processing difficulty during reading causes changes in eye movement behaviour. Rayner (1986) found that, within a group of 9- to 10-year-old children, reading rates were slower, more fixations were made, fixation durations were longer, and the perceptual span was smaller when they read more difficult sentences compared to when they read relatively easy sentences. Thus, for an individual reader, the difficulty of the reading material impacts upon eye movement behaviour. Häikiö et al. (2009) found that less able readers (aged 8, 10, and 12 years as well as adults) have slower reading speeds and a smaller perceptual span than more able readers (see section 'Spatial limitations on information extraction' for an explanation of the perceptual span). Thus, processing difficulty is reflected in the reader's eye movement behaviour. It is less clear whether poor eye movement control can cause reading difficulty. Compared to their typically developing peers, children with dyslexia have been reported to have unstable fixation, increased numbers of express saccades, poor visual attention span, and limited perceptual span (see Kirkby et al., 2008 for a review). Most researchers agree, however, that differences in eye movement behaviour are either correlates or consequences of the reading difficulties experienced by children with dyslexia (e.g. Rayner, 1985). There are no published data, to date, which provide compelling evidence for a causal role of poor eye movement control in dyslexia.

Third, to reiterate, there are several well-developed computational models of eye movements during reading but they are based solely on data from skilled adult readers, (Engbert et al., 2002, 2005; Pollatsek et al., 2006; Reichle et al., 1998, 1999, 2003; Reilly and Radach, 2006). Recent work using artificial learning agents has shown how eye movements resembling those of a skilled adult reader can emerge as a consequence of reinforcement learning (Liu and Reichle, 2010; Reichle and Laurent, 2006). No a priori assumptions were made about the mechanisms underlying eye movement control; the agents were simply limited by constraints relating to factors known to impact on eye movements during reading (time taken to program saccades, word length as an index of processing difficulty associated with lexical identification, visual acuity limitations on lexical identification, and distribution of attention across words in a sentence). The agent was rewarded for each word that was identified, and was punished for time spent on word identification—the goal was that all the words in the sentence should be identified as quickly as possible. The behaviours that emerged were similar to those observed in skilled adult reading. The agent learned to target saccades toward the centres of words, and decisions about when (reading times) and where (refixation and word skipping probabilities) to move the eyes were affected by the processing difficulty associated with a word. In the future, modelling eye movement data collected from children as they read will provide the opportunity to understand the mechanisms underlying developmental changes in eye movement behaviour during reading, such as vision, language, attention, and basic oculomotor control, and interactions between such mechanisms during the progression from beginning to skilled reader.

Methodological issues

There are several methodological issues that should be considered in relation to developmental studies of eye movements during reading. The first issue is that of control groups, and this relates to the theoretical issue outlined above of how both chronological age and reading skill might contribute to the development of eye movement behaviour during reading. In the small number of studies which have used different groups of children in order to examine age-related changes in reading performance, groups have generally been split by chronological age. While this has certainly proven fruitful, it is worth noting that in other areas of developmental research (such as investigation of the language and literacy difficulties associated with developmental disorders), comparison groups are often controlled both for chronological age and for cognitive ability or mental age (e.g. Bishop and Snowling, 2004; Laing et al., 2001; Leonard, 1998; Snowling, 2000). It is important that research is undertaken to directly address the relative contributions of age and reading skill to the development of eye movement behaviour during reading. Until this is better understood, the inclusion of control groups for both chronological age and reading age would be helpful to avoid inadvertent confounding of one with the other.

A second methodological issue worth noting is the importance of the use of age-appropriate linguistic stimuli. One factor distinguishing between the studies reviewed in this chapter is their selection of stimuli for readers of different ages. Some studies have presented each group with age-appropriate stimuli. In this case, processing difficulty associated with reading can be equated across the groups (assuming careful stimulus selection), but the analysis of age group effects will necessarily be between-items; differences between groups may be attributable to their age, or may be attributable to the particular set of sentences that was read by each group. In other studies, participants of all ages read the same stimuli. In this latter case, analyses of age group effects are within-items, thus eliminating the concern that any effects observed are related to differences in materials rather than reflecting genuine effects of age group. There is, however, the concern that any set of reading materials will be inherently more difficult for younger readers compared to older readers. It is well documented that for skilled adult readers, increased processing difficulty impacts on eye movement behaviour. For example, word reading times are longer on low-frequency words than high-frequency words (e.g. Henderson and Ferreira, 1990), and reading times are longer and more regressions are made for sentences that are syntactically complex compared to those that are simple (Warren et al., 2009); for a summary see Rayner (1998, pp. 389–392). Clearly, having participants of different ages read the same materials will lead to differences in eye movement behaviour that are, at least partially, attributable to the processing difficulty associated with the text for readers of different ages.

A related point is that manipulations of text difficulty may affect readers differentially depending upon their reading skill and experience of processing printed text. Factors known to have a robust effect on adults' eye movements during reading, such as the length or frequency of a word, need to be carefully considered before being incorporated into experimental designs with children. For example, there are many words which are low frequency for adult readers but high frequency for children (e.g. *dragon*) and frequency of encounter, together with cumulative frequency (the total number of times a word is encountered over time) and age-of-acquisition (the age at which a word was acquired), may impact differently on lexical retrieval processes in adults and children. Ideally, future research would control for age-appropriateness by constructing multiple sets of experimental sentences, each designed for a different age group (e.g. Häikiö et al., 2009) and, if possible, by using extensive prescreening in order to compose sentences that are roughly equivalent in processing difficulty for all participant groups.

While creating stimuli that include linguistic processing manipulations but are also comparable in terms of processing difficulty across different age groups is extremely challenging, in certain circumstances it may be possible. For example, it is possible to set up a frequency manipulation in which items are high frequency for both adults and children of different ages. In addition, context can be made particularly relevant to children (e.g. sentences refer to well-known children's characters, school, etc.), thereby reducing (although not eliminating) the gap between how easy adults and children will find sentences to process. In addition, stimuli can prescreened for variables such as comprehension, plausibility, and predictability. Experimenters can attempt to equate these across age groups by prescreening more items than are needed and selecting a subset for the main experiment that are matched on these variables between adults and children.

Third, there is a methodological issue which inevitably arises when conducting research with children—increased variability in data. This usually exists not only in eye movement measures, but also in related measures such as reading ability, and can lead to problems with statistical analyses (e.g. violating the assumption of equal variance across groups for ANOVAs) as well as making it difficult to obtain reliable effects. One possible solution is to use large sample sizes. Alternatively, child participants may be grouped more closely with respect to either chronological age or reading skill. Both solutions are increasingly possible as new eye tracking devices make it far easier to test large numbers of children. Finally the increasing use of linear mixed effects (LME) analyses in eye movement research, in which both fixed and random effects are accounted for, may reduce the problems caused by this increased variance in child data. It may, however, also be the case that it is not realistic to expect reliable differences when experimental manipulations which generate only small effects are employed. Certainly, eye movement research into children's reading is at an early stage compared to the advanced literature on skilled adult readers where increasingly complex manipulations are employed to investigate relatively small effects. Currently, the basic questions that need addressing with respect to children's eye movements during reading allow studies to employ strong manipulations that generate large differences between groups of children. In the future, however, the issue of increased variability in children's data may be addressed by more sensitive approaches to the selective recruitment and screening of child participants, together with careful design and screening of experimental stimuli.

Basic characteristics of children's eye movements during reading

For comparative purposes, means for different eye movement measures at different ages from all of the published studies to date of typically developing children's eye movements during reading are shown in Table 36.1. The age-related changes are quite clear; as chronological age increases, sentence reading times and fixation durations decrease, saccade amplitudes increase, fewer fixations and regressions are made, refixation probability decreases, and word skipping probability increases (Blythe et al., 2006, 2009, 2011; Buswell, 1922; Häikiö et al., 2009; Huestegge et al., 2009; Joseph et al., 2009; McConkie et al., 1991; Rayner, 1986; Taylor, 1965; Taylor et al., 1960). While all studies show these same developmental changes in eye movement behaviour, they vary in their selection of stimuli for readers of different ages. Some studies have used different materials for readers of different ages in an effort to match reading difficulty across groups (Blythe et al., 2006; McConkie et al., 1991; Taylor, 1965). In contrast, other studies have presented readers of all ages with the same sentences in order to avoid differences in material as a confounding variable between groups (Blythe et al., 2009, 2011; Buswell, 1922; Häikiö et al., 2009; Huestegge et al., 2009; Joseph et al., 2008, 2009; Rayner, 1986). In this second group of studies, the stimuli were typically aimed at the level of the youngest readers tested and, as a consequence, were very easy to read for the adult participants.

Given their differences in age groupings of participants and the manner in which certain measures are reported (e.g. the number of regressions being reported either as the number made per sentence or as a percentage of all movements made), it is not possible to make meaningful comparisons between the magnitude of effects observed in studies that have used the same stimuli for readers of all ages and the magnitude of effects observed in studies that have used different stimuli for each age group. Importantly, though, all studies show the same basic developmental trends–it does not seem to be the case that the selection of more or less difficult materials for any given age group will differentially reflect age-related changes in eye movement behaviour to a substantive degree. Further, the results of these studies broadly agree that developmental changes in eye movement behaviour reach adult levels around the age of 11 years (see Table 36.1).

One interesting point to note is that, in studies where different sentences were written for each age group in order to try and control processing difficulty, age-related changes in eye movement behaviour may be a consequence of age-related changes in identification of the individual words in

Table 36.1 Developmental changes in eye movements during reading. Measures marked * are estimated from a graph. The data reported in Blythe et al. (2006, 2009) and Joseph et al. (2009) are from children in the UK, where most children begin formal education at the age of 3–4 years. The data reported in Blythe et al. (2011) and Häikiö et al. (2009) are from children in Finland, where most children begin formal education at the age of 6–7 years. Finally, the data reported in Buswell (1922), McConkie et al. (1991), Rayner (1986), and Taylor (1965) are from children in the US, where most children begin formal education at the age of 4–5 years

		Chronological age in years (US grade)		
Blythe et al. (2006)		7–11 (2–5)	Adult	
	Mean fixation duration (ms)	279	240	
	Mean saccade amplitude (characters)	7.1	8.2	
	Regression probability	0.28	0.21	
Blythe et al. (2009)		7–9 (2–3)	9–10 (3–4)	Adult
	Mean sentence reading time (ms)	5473	4666	2965
	Mean fixation duration (ms)	285	256	249
	Mean number of fixations per sentence	16.8	15.6	10.3
	Mean number of regressions per sentence	5.2	5.1	2.4
	Refixation probability	0.15	0.11	0.05
	Word skipping probability	0.39	0.44	0.44
Blythe et al. (2011)		8–9 (3)	10–11 (5)	Adult
	Mean sentence reading time (ms)	4563	3213	2092
	Mean fixation duration (ms)	253	232	206
	Mean number of fixations per sentence	18.0	13.9	10.1
	Mean number of regressions per sentence	3.1	2.9	1.5
	Refixation probability	0.45	0.30	0.19
	Word skipping probability	0.09	0.16	0.20

Buswell (1922)

	6–7 (1)	7–8 (2)	8–9 (3)	9–10 (4)	10–11 (5)	11–12 (6)	Adult
Mean fixation duration (ms)	432	364	316	268	252	263	252
Median number of fixations per line of text	15.5	10.7	8.9	7.3	6.9	7.3	5.9
Median number of regressions per line of text	4.0	2.3	1.8	1.4	1.3	1.6	0.5

Häikiö et al. (2009)

	8–9 (3)	10–11 (5)	12–13 (7)	Adult
Mean reading rate (words per minute)*	90	145	190	245
Mean fixation duration (ms)*	260	235	210	205
Mean saccade amplitude (characters)*	3.2	5.3	5.8	6.8
Word skipping probability*	0.05	0.08	0.11	0.15

Huestegge et al. (2009)

	8 (2)	10 (4)
Mean reading rate (words per minute)	66	103
Mean fixation duration (ms)	358	297
Mean saccade length (characters)	5.3	6.3
Mean number of fixations per sentence	35.9	27.2
Mean regression probability	0.36	0.42

Joseph et al. (2009)

	7–11 (2–5)	Adult
Mean sentence reading time (ms)	5381	2932
Mean fixation duration (ms)	283	235
Mean saccade amplitude (characters)	7.6	8.2
Regression probability	0.29	0.22

(continued)

Table 36.1 (continued) Developmental changes in eye movements during reading. Measures marked * are estimated from a graph. The data reported in Blythe et al. (2006, 2009) and Joseph et al. (2009) are from children in the UK, where formal education begins at the age of 5 years. The data reported in Blythe et al. (2011) and Häikiö et al. (2009) are from children in Finland, where formal education begins at the age of 7 years. Finally, the data reported in Buswell (1922), McConkie et al. (1991), Rayner (1986), and Taylor (1965) are from children in the US, where formal education begins at the age of 6-years

	Chronological age in years (US grade)						
McConkie et al. (1991)	6–7 (1)	7–8 (2)	8–9 (3)	9–10 (4)	10–11 (5)		Adult
Mean fixation duration (ms)	432	268	262	248	243		200
Mean saccade amplitude (characters)*	3.6	4.9	5.7	6.6	6.3		
Number of fixations per 100 words	168	138	125	132	135		118
Regression probability	0.34	0.33	0.34	0.36	0.36		0.21
Rayner (1986)	7–8 (2)	9–10 (4)	11–12 (6)	Adult			
Mean reading rate (words per minute)*	95	160	210	290			
Mean fixation duration (ms)*	280	275	240	235			
Mean saccade length (characters)*	2.8	6.0	6.4	6.6			
Mean number of fixations per sentence*	15	9	8	6			
Mean number of regressions per sentence*	4.0	2.3	2.5	0.6			
Taylor (1965)	6–7 (1)	7–8 (2)	8–9 (3)	9–10 (4)	10–11 (5)	11–12 (6)	Adult
Mean fixation duration (ms)	330	300	280	270	270	270	240
Mean number of fixations per 100 words	224	174	155	139	129	120	90
Regression probability	0.23	0.23	0.23	0.22	0.22	0.21	0.17

the sentences. Specifically, these differences in eye movement behaviour may reflect slower or less efficient lexical identification in children compared to adults, despite the sentences being age-appropriate. This suggestion is supported by more recent data showing that linguistic skills (word/picture naming speed) but not oculomotor skills (saccade latency on pro- and antisaccade tasks) at the age of 8 years predict sentence reading times at the age of 10 years (Huestegge et al., 2009). To be clear, these data indicate that a child's lexical processing ability can predict some aspects of their eye movement behaviour across sentences as wholes. The most important point to note, however, is that basic developmental changes in eye movement behaviour when reading sentences (as shown in Table 36.1) have been observed very consistently in all the studies published to date.

Saccadic targeting to words

An important aspect of eye movement behaviour during reading is where a reader locates their initial fixation (or subsequent refixation) on a word, and the consequences that landing positions on words have for ongoing language processing. This is important because we know that in adult readers, initial fixation location influences how quickly a word is processed (Vitu et al., 2001), and also how likely it is that the word will be refixated (McConkie et al., 1988, 1989). Three studies have examined landing position effects in children during normal text reading (Joseph et al., 2009; McConkie et al., 1991; Vitu et al., 2001).

McConkie et al. (1991) reported data from Grimes (1989), which showed that during their first year of reading instruction, children exhibited the same pattern of landing positions as adults, although full analyses were not reported. Furthermore, McConkie et al. found that, like adults, children were more likely to refixate a (five-letter) word following an initial fixation on the space before the word or on the first letter, than if the first fixation was close to the word centre (although these inferences were made from observing trends in the data rather than from conducting formal statistical analyses).

Vitu et al. (2001) conducted extensive analyses on three data sets, one of which used data from children who were approximately 12 years old. Although the aim of the study was not to compare children and adults, the data from the Vitu et al. study showed that children did not appear to differ from adults in the locations of their first or second fixations. Like adults, children targeted their saccades towards the word centre and landing position distributions shifted with word length (that is, the longer the word, the further into the word children's fixations were located). Also, like adults, and similar to the data reported by McConkie et al., children were more likely to refixate a word following an initial fixation away from the word centre (i.e. at the beginning or end of a word) than following a fixation close to the word centre.

Finally, Joseph et al. (2009) used tightly controlled experimental materials to make direct comparisons of landing positions between adults and children aged 7–11 years, as they read sentences containing target words which were four, six or eight letters long. They found no reliable differences in the location of initial fixations between adults and children for any word length. They also found, in line with previous studies, that both adults and children were more likely to refixate a word following an initial fixation away from the word centre. In addition, they found that children's refixation saccades were smaller than those of adults, and tended to be regressive more often than adults', although this trend was not significant.

Taken together, the data from these three studies show that very early in reading development (as young as 7 years), children target their saccades towards the word centre (McConkie et al., 1991; Vitu et al., 2001), and they do not differ reliably from adults in their initial landing positions (Joseph et al., 2009). Furthermore, children (like adults) are more likely to refixate a word following an initial fixation away from the word centre (that is at the beginning or end of a word) than following a fixation close to the word centre (Joseph et al., 2009; McConkie et al., 1991; Vitu et al., 2001), presumably because their initial fixation location does not allow them to extract the visual information necessary to complete lexical identification of the word. However, children appear to be less efficient than adults in targeting their refixation saccades (Joseph et al., 2009).

It seems, then, that although children are limited in the amount of parafoveal information availa-ble to them during reading compared to adults (i.e. they have smaller perceptual spans: see later section 'Spatial limitations on information extraction'), the parafoveal information that is available to them during normal text reading is used effectively to guide their oculomotor behaviour in order to maximize reading efficiency (although they appear to lag behind adult efficiency when more than one fixation on a word is required). It is worth noting that some aspects of eye movement behaviour during reading may arise due to basic oculomotor phenomena, independent of learning to read. While reading development might be linked to deciding which word to fixate, the actual saccade targeting and preview mechanisms may simply be a basic characteristic of the eye movement control; for example, the finding that both adults and children both tend to target saccades to the middle of words may be characterized as a global effect (Findlay, 1982), a phenomenon not necessarily associ-ated with reading. Nevertheless, research to date shows that children target their saccades to word centres, and this ability develops either before reading instruction begins or else within the first year of reading instruction.

Extent and time course of information extraction during fixations in reading

There have been several strands of research that have employed innovative methodologies to exam-ine in detail how visual characteristics of text affect children's ongoing language processing. This section reviews studies that have used the moving window technique, the boundary paradigm, and the disappearing text paradigm in order to investigate changes in both the spatial extent and the time course of information extraction during fixations with respect to development. We will consider each of these lines of research in turn.

Spatial limitations on information extraction

Two studies have examined developmental changes in the perceptual span, the area of text around the point of fixation from which useful information can be extracted (Häikiö et al., 2009; Rayner, 1986). Each of these will be discussed in turn, in some detail, as the ability to pre-process information from words to the right of fixation is a hallmark component of skilled adult reading, and being deprived of the opportunity to pre-process information from the right of fixation is extremely detri-mental to adults' reading (Rayner, 1975; Rayner et al., 1980, 1981, 1982, 2006).

The perceptual span has been measured using the moving window paradigm, in which there is an area of text around the point of fixation which is presented normally, and this window of text moves with the eyes as the reader progresses through the sentence (McConkie and Rayner, 1975). Outside the window, the text is mutilated in some way—typically replacing the letters with xs, or other, visually-similar letters. The size of the window of unmutilated text that is available to the reader is manipulated, and reading behaviour for different window sizes is compared to reading behaviour for text which is presented normally in its entirety. Small windows typically reduce reading speed, as the reader is unable to preprocess information outside the window. The window size at which reading speed becomes equal to that for normal text shows the perceptual span. As the reader can read at their full speed with a window of a particular size, it is inferred that they do not make use of informa-tion further from the point of fixation than is available to them in that window. The perceptual span for adults is asymmetric about the point of fixation, extending from the beginning of the fixated word to around 14 or 15 characters to the right (see Rayner, 1998 for a summary).

In 1986, Rayner published a paper on the development of the perceptual span during reading. Four experiments were conducted that examined the size and asymmetry of the perceptual span in children of different ages compared to skilled adult readers, as well as the influence of text difficulty upon the perceptual span. The first experiment used windows that were symmetrical about the point of fixation; the perceptual span was shown to extend 23 characters around the point of fixation

(11 characters to either side of fixation) for the two youngest groups of readers (7 and 9 years). In contrast, for 11-year-old children and the adults the perceptual span was larger, extending 29 characters around the point of fixation (or, 14 characters either side of fixation). When the window size was determined in terms of words rather than characters, and word spaces outside the window were preserved so that the reader had parafoveal access to upcoming word length information, both reading rate and eye movement data again showed that younger readers have a smaller perceptual span than older readers, with a span of one word to the right of fixation for 7-year-olds but a span of two words to the right of fixation for 9-year-olds, 11-year-olds, and adults. Comparisons across word- and character-defined window conditions also showed that, consistent with previous adult studies, readers as young as 7 years pre-process word-length information at a greater eccentricity from fixation than they preprocess letter-specific information.

With respect to the symmetry of the perceptual span, reading was equally disrupted for participants of all ages when the availability of information to the left of fixation was restricted; the characteristic asymmetrical span for adults is present in children by the age of 7 years. Finally, the data showed very clearly that the window size which allowed maximum reading speed was smaller for more difficult sentences—the perceptual span was reduced when the reader experienced greater processing difficulty. Thus, these experiments showed that several different aspects that characterize the perceptual span in skilled adult readers are established in readers as young as 7 years old (the acquisition of gross properties of the upcoming text at a greater eccentricity than more specific letter information, and the asymmetry of the perceptual span). Alongside these similarities, some differences were also found. Compared to adults, younger readers have a reduced perceptual span and proportionally more of their processing capacity is devoted to the fixated word. Manipulations of text difficulty with the children supported the argument that, when comparing adults and children, age-related changes in the overall size of the perceptual span were, at least partially, attributable to differences in processing difficulty. Note that increased processing difficulty has also been shown to reduce parafoveal pre-processing in skilled adult readers (Henderson and Ferreira, 1990; White et al., 2005).

Surprisingly, no research was conducted to extend or challenge these findings for 20 years. A recent study has, however, looked in detail at the development of the letter identity span—the eccentricity from fixation at which readers of different ages can access letter-specific information (Häikiö et al., 2009). Rayner showed that access to some degree of word-specific information was limited to either one or two words to the right of fixation depending on the reader's age, while word length information was processed at greater eccentricities. Häikiö et al. designed their experiment to examine more closely the level of detail associated with individual letters that readers can access during reading at varying eccentricities.

Letters outside the window were replaced by visually similar characters (i.e. replacing an *o* with a *c*), with word boundaries preserved. In this way, readers were able to preprocess both word length and letter feature information outside the moving window, but it was only inside the window that correct letter identities were available. First, the data clearly showed developmental change in the letter identity span. At 8 years, the letter identity span extends five characters to the right of fixation, at 10 years it extends seven characters, and at 12 years and for adults it extends nine characters to the right of fixation. These data were compared to those from Rayner's experiments and showed that, for all age groups, letter identity span was smallest, with letter feature information available relatively further to the right, and with word length information available further still from fixation. Interestingly, they also compared the letter identity spans of fast and slow readers of the same age. Clear differences were found at all ages, with slower readers having a smaller span than faster readers. These data again suggest that reading skill, rather than chronological age, is responsible for developmental differences in the perceptual span.

Some recent work, also investigating children's preprocessing of upcoming information in a sentence, has specifically examined whether pre-processing is different between words compared to within words (Häikiö et al., 2010). Häikiö et al. compared adults' and 8-, 10-, and 12-year-old children's preprocessing of the second constituent of compound words (e.g. of 'boy' in 'cowboy') to their preprocessing of the second word in adjective–noun pairs (e.g. of 'bad boy') using the boundary paradigm (Rayner, 1975). In this paradigm an invisible boundary was placed before the target word/s. Prior to the reader making a saccade that crossed the boundary, a preview letter string was presented in the target location; in this experiment, the letters of the target word/s were replaced with visually similar letters. When a saccade crossed the invisible boundary, the preview string changed to the target word. Since this change occurred during a saccade, when visual input is suppressed, the change was not noticed by the reader. In all age groups, preprocessing was greater within a compound word than between the words in an adjective-noun pair (see also Juhasz et al., 2009). They also found a significant parafoveal-on-foveal effect within the compound words, but not in the adjective-noun pairs, in both adults and children (for a full explanation and discussion of parafoveal-on-foveal effects, see Drieghe, Chapter 46, this volume). These data show that from as young as 8 years, the allocation of attention during reading and, thus, preprocessing of upcoming information is determined to a significant degree by the visual cues corresponding to word boundaries (rather than simply extending certain number of character spaces ahead, irrespective of whether this includes one or multiple words).

To summarize, developmental changes have been shown to occur in the preprocessing of three different aspects of text within the perceptual span (word length, letter feature, and letter identity) such that this information can be acquired further to the right from the point of fixation as age increases. Furthermore, these age-related increases in the perceptual span are driven by the underlying improvement in reading skill, reinforcing understanding of the perceptual span as an index of the allocation of attention and processing resources during reading rather than simply being a low-level perceptual restriction on eye movement behaviour. That said, the left–right asymmetry of the perceptual span is established by the age of 7 years; clearly, relatively little experience of processing printed text is necessary to develop one of the key characteristics of visual information processing during skilled adult reading. This asymmetry reflects the allocation of attention to upcoming words for parafoveal pre-processing. In our view, the development of parafoveal pre-processing during sentence reading is an integral aspect of the progression from beginning to skilled reader. The finding that the perceptual span is asymmetric in 7-year-olds is remarkable, given that reading skills at this age are still relatively basic and measures of eye movement behaviour during reading (such as fixation durations and sentence reading times) continue to show developmental change for a further 4 years, on average, before reaching adult levels of performance. To our knowledge, no research has been conducted to examine developmental changes in sensitivity to specific characteristics of upcoming words in parafoveal pre-processing, despite the large body of literature on this topic for adults (for a review, see Rayner, 1998, 2009). Future research must address how parafoveal pre-processing continues to develop with age and reading skill, as 7-year-olds are still a long way from being skilled readers.

Given that the perceptual span is related to the reader's cognitive processing of the text, we anticipate that as reading skills improve with age: 1) a beginning reader will become sensitive to increasingly detailed information from the word to the right of fixation; 2) the extent to which they preprocess information from the upcoming word will increase; 3) reading times on directly fixated words will decrease as a consequence of greater parafoveal preprocessing of those words. Through such mechanisms we believe that the process of lexical identification will become quicker and more efficient with age, not only due to more efficient linguistic processing during direct fixation but also, at least partially, due to developmental changes in parafoveal preprocessing. Increased parafoveal preprocessing of upcoming words in sentences will decrease the demand on processing resources necessary to identify that word during direct fixation; this in turn will facilitate parafoveal preprocessing of the next word. This cycle of preprocessing a word and subsequent facilitation of lexical identification during direct fixation will develop with reading skill, and it seems likely that this will be reflected in shorter fixation durations, fewer refixations, and increased word skipping probabilities—an increasingly mature pattern of eye movement behaviour during reading.

Temporal limitations on visual information extraction

Recent research has compared children of different ages with adults using the disappearing text paradigm (Liversedge et al., 2004; Rayner et al., 2003). This is a gaze-contingent change method, where there are invisible boundaries placed between all the words within the sentence. Each time the reader's eye crosses a boundary, the newly fixated word disappears after a specified delay while the previously fixated word reappears; there is only one word missing from the sentence at any one moment, but it is the word being fixated by the reader. Critically, a prespecified delay can be manipulated between the reader's eye crossing the boundary and the word disappearing, thus restricting the reader's opportunity to visually encode the word to the initial period (typically 60 ms) of the first fixation on the word. Work with skilled adult readers has demonstrated that they are able to read and understand sentences normally when presented as disappearing text with the word being presented for 60 ms from fixation onset (Liversedge et al., 2004; Rayner et al., 2003). Interestingly, word frequency effects were found upon fixation durations in the disappearing text condition; even when the word was no longer visible, the reader's cognitive processing determined when they would move their eyes onto the next word in the sentence.

An interesting question that arose from the disappearing text studies was whether children are able to encode visual information during fixations in reading as quickly and efficiently as adults. Beginning readers are, by nature, less familiar with the written forms of words than skilled adult readers. It may, therefore, be the case that they require longer presentation durations than adults to allow successful visual encoding and, consequently, the initiation of normal linguistic processing. Blythe and colleagues compared younger children (7–9 years), older children (10–11 years), and adults as they read sentences presented as disappearing text (Blythe et al., 2009). The sentences contained a target word that was manipulated for word frequency. In two experiments, four different presentation durations were used—40, 60, 80, and 120 ms disappearing text compared to normally-presented sentences. The results showed that even by the age of 7 years, there was a minimal impact of the disappearing text manipulation upon children's eye movement behaviour with all presentation durations tested. Effects of word frequency were found upon single and first fixation durations in the disappearing text conditions, providing strong evidence that even with very short periods of visual input, children aged 7 years are able to initiate normal lexical identification processes. These results are comparable to those obtained for adults.

In summary, the data from studies which have investigated visual information extraction during reading shows that: 1) the perceptual span for reading increases in size with chronological age, up to 11 years and is related to reading skill/processing difficulty; 2) the characteristic left–right asymmetry of the perceptual span associated with skilled adult reading of English has developed by the age of 7 years; 3) by the age of 7 years, children accurately target their saccades close to the word centre, as adults do; and 4) the speed of visual information encoding during reading does not increase significantly after the age of 7 years. Thus, while spatial aspects of information encoding continue to develop up to 11 years, where a child initially fixates a word and the speed with which a word is visually encoded are in place just a few years after beginning formal reading instruction, or perhaps even before (see 'Saccadic targeting to words' section).

In the latter half of this review, we will consider how various characteristics of the material being read can impact upon the eye movements of children compared to adults. Studies in this area have used eye movements as an index of the moment-to-moment psychological processing that underlies reading, to examine the process of development from beginning to skilled reader.

Word-based effects in children

Two of the most robust effects in the adult eye movement literature are those of word length and word frequency; that is, adults look longer at long than short words (Just and Carpenter, 1980; Rayner et al., 1996); and at low-frequency than high-frequency words (e.g. Henderson and Ferreira, 1990; Inhoff, 1984; Inhoff and Rayner, 1986; Just and Carpenter, 1980; Rayner, 1977; Rayner and Duffy, 1986; Rayner and Raney, 1996; Rayner et al., 2003). Perhaps for this reason, the majority of studies which have manipulated an aspect of text to examine its effect on children's eye movements during reading have focussed on precisely these two characteristics.

Word length

Four studies have manipulated word length to investigate whether these robust effects (whereby long words are fixated more often and for longer than short words) observed in adult readers are also present in children. Hyönä and Olson (1995) recorded the eye movements of both dyslexic children (mean age = 14.4 years) and reading-age-matched controls (mean age = 10.5 years) as they read aloud texts which contained words that were, subsequent to data collection, categorized as short (5–6 letters), medium (7–8 letters), or long (9–11 letters), resulting in a very high number of target words and, hence, a very rich data set. The reading material was set at a higher difficulty level than most participants' level of word recognition in order that some reading errors would be generated. Hyönä and Olson found a strong effect of word length in both groups which was apparent in gaze durations (the sum of all fixations made on a word before the eyes leave the word either to the right or to the left), number of first-pass fixations (the number of fixations made on a word before leaving that word to the right or left), second-pass reading time (the sum of all fixations made on a word after having left the word for at least one fixation); and number of second-pass fixations (the sum of all fixations associated with second-pass reading).

In a silent reading experiment, Joseph et al. (2009) took a different approach to that of Hyönä and Olson, and manipulated word length prior to data collection, which meant that they were able to control for word frequency and predictability in their target words (one per sentence). This allowed them to ensure that any effects observed were due to word length alone rather than being modulated by other linguistic variables. Furthermore, the experimental sentences were designed to be age-appropriate for the youngest of the children (aged 7 years), which meant that they were relatively easy for the older children (aged 11 years) and adults.

Like Hyönä and Olson, they found reliably longer gaze durations, more refixations, and longer total reading times on long than short words. They also found that both adults and children skipped short words more often than long words. Importantly, most of these effects were larger in children than adult readers, suggesting that not only do children experience an increased processing load when reading long as compared to short words, but the increase in word length has a more substantial effect on children's ongoing lexical processing as compared to that of adult readers. Furthermore, due to careful control of word frequency and predictability, it is likely that this difference between adults and children was due to the demands of visually encoding long as compared to short words, suggesting that children require more and/or longer visual samples of long words in order to reach the point at which lexical identification can proceed.

Similarly, Huestegge et al. (2009) found that children aged 8 and 10 years exhibited longer gaze durations and total fixation times on long (6–9-letter) compared to short (4–5-letter) words and, like the previous two studies, did not observe an effect of word length on children's first fixation durations. They also found an interaction between age group and word length on refixation time (gaze duration minus first fixation duration) showing that the word length effect was greater in younger compared to older children. These data from silent reading experiments suggest, therefore, that younger readers need additional processing time on long words compared to older readers, and that this need decreases with age.

A more recent experiment has directly investigated the question of why children make multiple fixations on long words (Blythe et al., 2011). Children aged 8–9 years, 10–11 years, and adults read sentences containing long (8-letter) or short (4-letter) words, that were presented either normally or as disappearing text (for an explanation of the disappearing text paradigm, see the section entitled 'Temporal limitations on visual information extraction'). The 8–9-year-old children made fewer refixations on long target words when they were presented under disappearing text conditions compared to normal conditions (resulting in shorter gaze durations). However, they subsequently made more regressions back to long words in the disappearing text condition, leading to no overall difference in total fixation times on those long words between the normal and disappearing text conditions. Thus, these younger children adopted an eye movement strategy by which they obtained a second visual sample on the long words without incurring any cost to overall processing time on this word. Such effects were reduced in the older children, and were minimal in the adults, indicating that while younger children do require a second visual sample on 8-letter words, by the age of 10 years one visual sample is usually sufficient.

Together, these studies provide compelling evidence that children (up to the age of around 9 years) are slower and less efficient at processing words, evidenced by their need for multiple and longer visual samples when reading long compared to short words; this applies in the domains of both silent and oral reading. Moreover, word length effects are found in text that is relatively difficult (Hyönä and Olson, 1995) or easy (Blythe et al., 2011; Joseph et al., 2009) for those children reading it, and the effects observed are more pronounced in younger readers compared to older readers (Huestegge et al., 2009).

Word frequency

Of the relatively small number of studies that have investigated word-based effects in children, several have specifically manipulated word frequency (Blythe et al., 2006, 2009; Huestegge et al., 2009; Hyönä and Olson, 1995). Word frequency refers to how often a word is encountered, as indexed by corpora such as CELEX (Baayan et al., 1995) and Kučera et al., 1967), which document how frequently a given word appears in a range of written texts. It is likely that this particular variable was chosen in all of the four studies because the word frequency effect is so robust in adult readers (e.g. Henderson and Ferreira, 1990; Inhoff, 1984; Just and Carpenter, 1980; Rayner and Duffy, 1986; Rayner and Raney, 1996). It was, therefore, important to establish whether children's eye movements were influenced as immediately and reliably as those of adults by the frequency with which a word is encountered.

In the same study outlined in the previous section, Hyönä and Olson (1995) also investigated word frequency effects. Words of each length were categorized into three frequency groups: low, medium, and high. They found a strong effect of word frequency in oral reading which could be seen in first fixation durations, showing that the frequency of a word has a very immediate effect on processing in children, as it is known to do in adults. Importantly, the word frequency counts of the target words were drawn from age-appropriate texts so that the high- and low-frequency words were high or low frequency for children, rather than for adults. While this study suggests that the frequency of occurrence of a word has an immediate effect on the reading behaviour of children as well as adults, a more recent study by Blythe et al. (2006) failed to find a frequency effect in children aged 7–11 years, despite finding a strong frequency effect in their adult participants in the same study. Importantly, this study used adult corpus data to index word frequency.

The discrepancy between these two studies suggests that adult frequency counts may be unsuitable for creating an effective manipulation with children. Blythe et al. (2009), however, did find robust frequency effects in children aged 7–9 years and 10–11 years across two separate experiments that used adult frequency counts in the target word manipulation (the disappearing text study outlined in section 'Temporal limitations on visual information extraction'). These effects occurred in very early measures of lexical identification, single and first fixation durations, in both children and adults. A third study that used adult frequency counts also found effects on 8–10-year-old children's eye movements, but only in gaze durations and total reading times (Huestegge et al., 2009). There was a numerical trend for longer first fixations on low frequency words compared to high frequency words, but this was not statistically significant. Unfortunately this study did not include a control group of adults, and so it is not possible to gauge how effective this manipulation of frequency was for skilled adult readers in comparison to children.

Overall, word frequency appears to exert a strong influence on the ease of lexical identification, as indexed by eye movement measures, from 7 years of age. It may, however, be the case that while it is possible for adult counts of frequency to generate effects in children (many words are, of course, high or low in frequency for adults and children alike), using frequency counts from age-appropriate texts is a more reliable means of obtaining robust effects. There is a clear need for a study to manipulate both adult and child frequencies and to examine whether they differentially affect eye movement behaviour in readers of different ages. Future research will also benefit from the careful control of potentially confounding linguistic variables such as age-of-acquisition and predictability, as well as the age-appropriateness of the texts used to index frequency, in order to establish more firmly how word frequency affects children's ongoing lexical processing. Finally, it should be noted that these data provide extremely strong evidence for cognitive control of eye movements during reading in children as young as 7 years. That is to say, by the age of 7 years, children's reading has developed to a level where their linguistic processing of the fixated word determines when they move their eyes on through the text.

Post-lexical processing

Only one study, to our knowledge, has used eye-movements during reading to examine children's processing during reading at a post-lexical level. Joseph et al. (2008) investigated how children (aged 7–11 years) and adults processed implausible and anomalous thematic relations during reading (see also Warren, Chapter 50, this volume). In their experiment, participants read sentences such as (1a–c), below. The sentences described events in which an individual performed an action with an instrument. In each case, the verb had three thematic roles (see sentences (1a–c)): an agent (*Robert*), an instrument (*trap*, *hook* or *radio*) and a patient/theme (*mouse*).

1a. Robert used a trap to catch the horrible mouse that was very scared.

1b. Robert used a hook to catch the horrible mouse that was very scared.

1c. Robert used a radio to play the horrible mouse that was very scared.

In all three sentences the instrument (*trap*, *hook*, or *radio*) could be plausibly used in conjunction with the main verb (*catch* or *play*). In the implausible condition (1b), however, the patient (*mouse*) was incongruous as the object of the verb (*catch*) given the particular instrument used (*hook*). That is, although hooks are often used to catch things (e.g. fish), and mice are often caught, a hook is not often used to catch a mouse. By contrast, in the anomalous condition (1c), the patient (*mouse*) could not be used in conjunction with the verb (in this case *play*).

Joseph et al. found that while children did not differ from adults in their anomaly detection (both groups exhibited longer gaze durations on the critical word in the anomalous than control conditions), they were delayed relative to adults in their implausibility detection. Adults showed disruption in go-past time (the sum of all the temporally contiguous fixations from the first fixation in a region until a fixation to the right of the region) in the post-target region, while children only showed disruption in total time in the post-target region. Thus, there was a difference in the time course of the disruption. The authors interpreted the data as showing that children and adults were similar in terms of basic thematic assignment processes that occur during reading, but that they differed in the efficiency with which they were able to integrate pragmatic and real world knowledge into their discourse representation.

While it is difficult to make any firm conclusions based on data from a single study, the results from Joseph et al. (2008) suggest that in some respects children may be adult-like in their post-lexical written language comprehension, although they appear to be slower than adults to incorporate real world knowledge information into their representation of sentence meaning. Clearly, much more research is needed before this claim can be more than speculative. If correct, however, this would suggest that early in reading development, children are very similar to adults in terms of the oculomotor mechanisms they have in place in order to make the eye movements necessary for written language comprehension, but that the efficiency and speed with this these mechanisms and processes function is reduced relative to adult reading performance. It may also be the case that there are developmental differences in how post-lexical processing influences eye movement control.

Future directions

Overall, despite the small number of studies that have investigated children's eye movements during reading, we believe great progress has been made towards understanding oculomotor control and online written language comprehension in children. This is an exciting time in the field of developmental eye movement research into reading, as technological improvements rapidly open up more possibilities for conducting well-controlled and innovative experiments with children. There are several directions in which we anticipate the field will head in the future.

First, we believe that it will be both timely and informative for new studies to examine the relative contributions of variables such as chronological age, reading age, and IQ to the development of oculomotor control during reading. From the existing literature on eye movements during reading, the large variance in children's data suggests that such factors are influential. By recording the broader cognitive profiles of children with respect to their language and literacy development, and analysing such information in relation to their eye movement data, we hope that research will allow a more detailed understanding of the relationships between development with age, reading skill and the moment-to-moment cognitive processing of text as indexed by eye movements.

Second, we hope that the use of portable, highly-accurate eye tracking equipment will enable well-controlled, longitudinal studies to be carried out. All of the research conducted in the field thus far has been cross-sectional in design. While this work has proved extremely informative, longitudinal studies will allow a more detailed examination of the developmental trajectory of reading behaviour in relation to different aspects of linguistic processing. This approach is already common in studies using offline measures of reading comprehension (e.g. Muter et al., 2004; Nation and Snowling, 2004). By adopting similar experimental designs and using an online measure of cognitive processing as it occurs during reading, researchers will be able to advance current understanding of literacy development by taking a range of variables into account that differ within typically developing children.

Third, there has only been one published study which has examined linguistic effects beyond the lexical level in children (Joseph et al., 2008). Further studies are needed to investigate aspects of higher order linguistic processing (e.g. syntactic and semantic processing, and even discourse processing) in children during sentence reading. While research thus far has shown that adults and children from the age of 7 years are very similar in their processing of visual linguistic stimuli at a lexical level, we consider it entirely possible that research examining post-lexical processing will reveal developmental changes that continue beyond the age of 7 years. One issue that may arise in relation to manipulations of higher order linguistic processing in children is that of stimulus selection. It is not yet clear whether the use of higher-level linguistic manipulations which have generated robust processing preferences in adult readers will produce reliable effects in children. For example, given the increased variability introduced by including children as participants, it may be that manipulations which result in small effect sizes in adult readers (e.g. lexical ambiguity effects) will not produce detectable effects in children.

Fourth, one very informative development in the field would be for eye movement studies with children to narrow the gap with the literature on literacy development based on studies that have used offline methods. There are many theoretical models of reading development that have resulted from offline research (see Ehri, 2005 for a review). We believe that, compared to offline studies, eye movement data will offer a more detailed understanding of the changes in cognitive processing that underlie the progression from beginning to skilled reader and such data will be extremely informative with respect to models of reading development. For example, there are developmental changes in the extent to which children use letter, syllable, and word representations as the access units in lexical identification; this varies across languages, and is thought to reflect fundamental characteristics of the structure of the adult mental lexicon—psycholinguistic grain size theory (Ziegler and Goswami, 2005). The sensitivity of eye movement behaviour to cognitive processing during reading would make eye movement recordings an ideal method with which to investigate such issues.

Finally, as discussed in the section 'Theoretical issues', recent work has shown that artificial learning agents can, with relatively few and simple constraints, develop eye movement behaviour resembling that of skilled adult readers. In our view, the next step will be for the increasingly large body of children's data to be incorporated into the existing computational models of eye movements during reading (e.g. the SWIFT model: Engbert et al., 2002, 2005; the E-Z Reader model: Pollatsek et al., 2006; Reichle et al., 1998, 1999, 2003, 2006; see Reichle, Chapter 42, and Engbert and Kliegl,

Chapter 43, this volume). To reiterate, modelling children's data in this way will facilitate our understanding of change in the mechanisms (visual, attentional, linguistic, oculomotor control) underlying reading.

In summary, an increasing body of literature now exists which provides important, preliminary data that document children's basic oculomotor behaviour, lexical processing, and, to a limited extent, post-lexical processing during sentence reading. It is hoped that future research will use these data as a benchmark to examine other populations such as younger children just beginning the process of learning to read and children with developmental disorders, in particular those with reading disabilities (e.g. dyslexia) or with more general language impairments (e.g. children with specific language impairment or comprehension problems). In the long term, research in this area might go some way towards informing the design of interventions for individuals who have difficulty learning to read. This may seem ambitious, but we believe that there is every reason to be optimistic that eye movement research investigating children's reading will continue to flourish as it has started to over the last few years.

Acknowledgements

Both H.I. Blythe and H.S.S.L. Joseph were supported by ESRC Postdoctoral Fellowships. We would like to thank Simon Liversedge and two anonymous reviewers for their helpful comments on an earlier version of this chapter.

References

Baayan, H., Piepenbrock, R., and Gulikers, L. (1995). *The CELEX lexical database* (CD-ROM). University of Pennsylvania, PA: Linguistic Data Consortium.

Bishop, D.V.M. and Snowling, M.J. (2004). Developmental dyslexia and specific language impairment: Same or different? *Psychological Bulletin*, **130**, 858–886.

Blythe, H.I., Liversedge, S.P., Joseph, H.S.S.L., White, S.J., and Rayner, K. (2009). The uptake of visual information during fixations in reading in children and adults. *Vision Research*, **49**, 1583–1591.

Blythe, H.I., Häikiö, T., Bertam, R., Liversedge, S.P., and Hyönä, J. (2011). Reading disappearing text: Why do children refixate words? *Vision Research*, **51**, 84–92.

Blythe, H.I., Liversedge, S.P., Joseph, H.S.S.L., White, S.J., Findlay, J.M., and Rayner, K. (2006). The binocular co-ordination of eye movements during reading in children and adults. *Vision Research*, **46**, 3898–3908.

Buswell, G.T. (1922). *Fundamental reading habits: A study of their development*. Chicago, IL: University of Chicago Press.

Cohen, M.E. and Ross, L.E. (1978). Latency and accuracy characteristics of saccades and corrective saccades in children and adults. *Journal of Experimental Child Psychology*, **26**, 517–527.

Ehri, L.C. (2005). Development of sight word reading: Phases and findings. In M.J. Snowling and C. Hulme (eds.) *The science of reading: A handbook* (pp. 135–154). Oxford: Blackwell.

Engbert, R., Longtin, A., and Kliegl, R. (2002). A dynamical model of saccade generation in reading based on spatially distributed lexical processing. *Vision Research*, **42**, 621–636.

Engbert, R., Nuthmann, A., Richter, E., and Kliegl, R. (2005). SWIFT: A dynamical model of saccade generation during reading. *Psychological Review*, **112**, 777–813.

Findlay, J.M. (1982). Global visual processing for saccadic eye movements. *Vision Research*, **22**, 1033–1045.

Fukushima, J., Hatta, T., and Fukushima, K. (2000). Development of voluntary control of saccadic eye movements: I. Age-related changes in normal children. *Brain and Development*, **22**, 173–180.

Grimes, J. (1989). Where first grade children look in words during reading. (Unpublished master's thesis). University of Illinois.

Groll, S.L. and Ross, L.E. (1982). Saccadic eye movements of children and adults to double-step stimuli. *Developmental Psychology*, **18**, 108–123.

Häikiö, T., Bertram, R., and Hyönä, J. (2010). Development of parafoveal processing within and across words in reading: Evidence from the boundary paradigm. *Quarterly Journal of Experimental Psychology*, **63**, 1982–1998.

Häikiö, T., Bertram, R., Hyönä, J., and Niemi, P. (2009). Development of the letter identity span in reading: Evidence from the eye movement moving window paradigm. *Journal of Experimental Child Psychology*, **102**, 167–181.

Henderson, J.M. and Ferreira, F. (1990). Effects of foveal processing difficulty on the perceptual span in reading: Implications for attention and eye movement control. *Journal of Experimental Psychology: Learning, Memory, and Cognition*, **16**, 417–429.

Huestegge, L., Radach, R., Corbic, D., and Huestegge, S.M. (2009). Oculomotor and linguistic determinants of reading development: A longitudinal study. *Vision Research*, **49**, 2948–2959.

Hyönä, J. and Olson, R.K. (1995). Eye fixation patterns among dyslexic and normal readers: effects of word-length and word-frequency. *Journal of Experimental Psychology: Learning Memory and Cognition*, **21**, 1430–1440.

Inhoff, A.W. (1984). Two stages of word processing during eye fixations in the reading of prose. *Journal of Verbal Learning and Verbal Behavior*, **23**, 612–624.

Inhoff, A.W. and Rayner, K. (1986). Parafoveal word processing during eye fixations in reading: effects of word frequency. *Perception and Psychophysics*, **40**, 431–439.

Joseph, H.S.S.L., Liversedge, S.P., Blythe, H.I., White, S.J., and Rayner, K. (2009). Word length and landing position effects during reading in children and adults. *Vision Research*, **49**, 2078–2086.

Joseph, H.S.S.L., Liversedge, S.P., Blythe, H.I., White, S.J., Gathercole, S.E., and Rayner, K. (2008). Children's and adults' processing of anomaly and implausibility during reading: Evidence from eye movements. *The Quarterly Journal of Experimental Psychology*, **61**, 708–723.

Juhasz, B.J., Pollatsek, A., Hyönä, J., Drieghe, D., and Rayner, K. (2009). Parafoveal processing within and between words. *Quarterly Journal of Experimental Psychology*, **62**, 1356–1376.

Just, M. and Carpenter, P. (1980). A theory of reading: from eye fixations to comprehension. *Psychological Review*, **87**, 329–354.

Kirby, J.A., Webster, L.A.D., Blythe, H.I., and Liversedge, S.P. (2008). Binocular coordination during reading and non-reading tasks. *Psychological Bulletin*, **134**, 742–763.

Kučera, H. and Francis, W.H. (1967). *Computational analysis of present-day American English*. Providence, RI: Brown University Press.

Laing, E., Hulme, C., Grant, J., and Karmiloff-Smith, A. (2001). Learning to read in Williams Syndrome: Looking beneath the surface of atypical reading development. *Journal of Child Psychology and Psychiatry*, **42**, 729–739.

Leonard, L.B. (1998). *Children with Specific language Impairment*. Cambridge, MA: MIT Press.

Liu, Y.-P. and Reichle, E.D. (2010). The emergence of adaptive eye movements in reading. In S. Ohlsson and R. Catrabone (Eds.), *Proceedings of the 32nd Annual Conference of the Cognitive Science Society* (pp. 1136–1141). Austin, TX: Cognitive Science Society.

Liversedge, S.P., Rayner, K., White, S.J., Vergilino-Perez, D., Findlay, J.M., and Kentridge, R.W. (2004). Eye movements when reading disappearing text: is there a gap effect in reading? *Vision Research*, **44**, 1013–1024.

McConkie, G.W. and Rayner, K. (1975). The span of effective stimulus during a fixation in reading. *Perception and Psychophysics*, **17**, 578–586.

McConkie, G.W., Kerr, P.W., Reddix, M.D., and Zola, D. (1988). Eye-movement control during reading: I. The location of initial eye fixations on words. *Vision Research*, **28**, 1107–1118.

McConkie, G.W., Kerr, P.W., Reddix, M.D., Zola, D., and Jacobs, A.M. (1989). Eye movement control during reading: II. Frequency of refixating a word. *Perception and Psychophysics*, **46**, 245–253.

McConkie, G.W., Zola, D., Grimes, J., Kerr, P.W., Bryant, N.R., and Wolff, P.M. (1991). Children's eye movements during reading. In J.F. Stein (Ed.), *Vision and visual dyslexia* (pp. 251–262). Boston: CRC Press.

Muter, V., Hulme, C., Snowling, M.J., and Stevenson, J. (2004). Phonemes, rimes, vocabulary and grammatical skills as foundations of early reading development: Evidence from a longitudinal study. *Developmental Psychology*, **40**, 665–681.

Nation, K. and Snowling, M.J. (2004). Beyond phonological skills: broader language skills contribute to the development of visual word recognition. *Journal of Research in Reading*, **27**, 342–356.

Pollatsek, A., Reichle, E.D., and Rayner, K. (2006). Tests of the E–Z Reader model: Exploring the interface between cognition and eye-movement control. *Cognitive Psychology*, **52**, 1–56.

Rayner, K. (1975). The perceptual span and peripheral cues in reading. *Cognitive Psychology*, **7**, 65–81.

Rayner, K. (1977). Visual attention in reading: Eye movements reflect cognitive processes. *Memory and Cognition*, **4**, 443–448.

Rayner, K. (1985). Do faulty eye movements cause dyslexia? *Developmental Neuropsychology*, **1**, 3–15.

Rayner, K. (1986). Eye movements and the perceptual span in beginning and skilled readers. *Journal of Experimental Child Psychology*, **41**, 211–236.

Rayner, K. (1998). Eye movements in reading and information processing: 20 years of research. *Psychological Bulletin*, **124**, 372–422.

Rayner, K. (2009). Eye movements and attention in reading, scene perception, and visual search. *The Quarterly Journal of Experimental Psychology*, **62**, 1457–1506.

Rayner, K. and Duffy, S.A. (1986). Lexical complexity and fixation times in reading: effects of word frequency, verb complexity, and lexical ambiguity. *Memory and Cognition*, **14**, 191–201.

Rayner, K. and Raney, G.E. (1996). Eye movement control in reading and visual search: Effects of word frequency. *Psychonomic Bulletin and Review*, **3**, 245–248.

Rayner, K., McConkie, G.W., and Zola, D. (1980). Integrating information across eye movements. *Cognitive Psychology*, **12**, 206–226.

Rayner, K., Sereno, S.C., and Raney, G.E. (1996). Eye movement control in reading: A comparison of two types of models. *Journal of Experimental Psychology-Human Perception and Performance*, **22**, 1188–1200.

Rayner, K., Well, A.D., Pollatsek, A., and Bertera, J.H. (1982). The availability of useful information to the right of fixation in reading. *Perception and Psychophysics,* **31**, 537–550.

Rayner, K., Liversedge, S.P., and White, S.J. (2006). Eye movements when reading disappearing text: The importance of the word to the right of fixation. *Vision Research,* **46**, 310–323.

Rayner, K., Liversedge, S.P., White, S.J., and Vergilino-Perez, D. (2003). Reading disappearing text: Cognitive control of eye movements. *Psychological Science,* **14**, 385–388.

Rayner, K., Inhoff, A.W., Morrison, R.E., Slowiaczek, M.L., and Bertera, J.H. (1981). Masking of foveal and parafoveal vision during eye fixations in reading. *Journal of Experimental Psychology: Human Perception and Performance,* **7**, 167–179.

Reichle, E.D., and Laurent, P.A. (2006). Using reinforcement learning to understand the emergence of 'intelligent' eye-movement behavior during reading. *Psychological Review,* **113**, 390–408.

Reichle, E.D., Rayner, K., and Pollatsek, A. (1999). Eye movement control in reading: accounting for initial fixation locations and refixations within the E-Z Reader model. *Vision Research,* **39**, 4403–4411.

Reichle, E.D., Rayner, K., and Pollatsek, A. (2003). The E-Z Reader model of eye-movement control in reading: Comparisons to other models. *Behavioral and Brain Sciences,* **26**, 445–476.

Reichle, E.D., Pollatsek, A., and Rayner, K. (2006). E-Z Reader: A cognitive-control, serial-attention model of eye-movement behavior during reading. *Cognitive Systems Research,* **7**, 4–22.

Reichle, E.D., Pollatsek, A., Fisher, D.L., and Rayner, K. (1998). Toward a model of eye movement control in reading. *Psychological Review,* **105**, 125–157.

Reilly, R.G. and Radach, R. (2006). Some empirical tests of an interactive activation model of eye movement control in reading. *Cognitive Systems Research,* **7**, 34–55.

Salman, M.S., Sharpe, J.A., Eizenman, M., Lillakas, L., Westall, C., To, T., *et al.* (2006). Saccades in children. *Vision Research,* **46**, 1432–1439.

Snowling, M.J. (2000). *Dyslexia.* Oxford: Blackwell.

Taylor, S.E. (1965). Eye movements while reading: Facts and fallacies. *American Educational Research Journal,* **2**, 187–202.

Taylor, S.E., Frackenpohl, H., and Pettee, J.L. (1960). Grade level norms for the components of fundamental reading skill. *EDL Research and Information Bulletin (Vol. 3).* Huntington, NY: Educational Development Laboratories.

Vitu, F., McConkie, G.W., Kerr, P., and O'Regan, J.K. (2001). Fixation location effects on fixation durations during reading: an inverted optimal viewing position effect. *Vision Research,* **41**, 3513–3533.

Warren, T., White, S.J., and Reichle, E.D. (2009). Investigating the causes of wrap-up effects: Evidence from eye movements and E-Z Reader. *Cognition,* **111**, 132–137.

White, S.J., Rayner, K., and Liversedge, S.P. (2005). Eye movements and the modulation of parafoveal processing by foveal processing difficulty: A reexamination. *Psychonomic Bulletin and Review,* **12**, 891–896.

Ziegler, J.C. and Goswami, U. (2005). Reading acquisition, developmental dyslexia, and skilled reading across languages: a psycholinguistic grain size theory. *Psychological Bulletin,* **131**, 3–29.

CHAPTER 37

Oculomotor developmental pathology: an 'evo-devo' perspective

Chris Harris

'All science is either physics or stamp collecting'.

Ernest Rutherford

Abstract

Human oculomotor developmental anomalies are difficult to explain in terms of causal events (such as lesions). Here we use ideas from evolutionary developmental biology (evo-devo) such as developmental plasticity and modularity to propose a framework for understanding early visuomotor development and sensitive periods in terms of the cost of phenotypic plasticity, using an optimality approach. With this framework, we explore two developmental disorders: infantile nystagmus syndrome (congenital nystagmus) and saccade initiation failure (ocular motor apraxia) as two examples of adaptive developmental plasticity in gaze maintenance and gaze shifting, with and without sensitive periods. We propose that early oculomotor developmental disorders can be understood as products of developmental plasticity in extreme environments constrained by modularity.

Introduction

Almost every paediatric ophthalmologist has been faced with a distraught and questioning parent asking *why* their child has incurable nystagmus for life, or has strange head movements and learning difficulties, or *why* patching the 'good' eye may improve vision in the 'poor' eye. When answering these awkward 'why' questions we tend to look for causal explanations, but in developmental disorders causality is elusive, and it is difficult to know even at what level to explain these developmental phenomena.

In acquired disorders we are often satisfied if we can find a lesion to explain the oculomotor dysfunction. The continuing editions of Leigh and Zee's, *The Neurology of Eye Movements* (Leigh and Zee, 2006) are testament to our impressive knowledge relating neurophysiology and behaviour. But, this approach is less satisfying for developmental disorders. Not only is our knowledge of the developing brain poor, but the neurophysiology is changing in time—there is a 'developmental trajectory'. Indeed, there may be no 'lesion' but the child may have a constellation of apparently disconnected abnormalities. Therefore, as clinicians, we tend to look at the whole patient to consult a public catalogue (or our personal stamp-album of experience) for the 'diagnosis'. A known label may provide reassurance, but a stamp is only phenomenological—not an explanation.

Increasingly we look for a mutation, which for many is where it all begins, and there is some comfort in having a starting point in the causal chain. Disconcertingly, we now find that there are networks of not-so-selfish genes signalling each other and collaborating to build different modular structures (e.g. the Pax/Six/Eya/Dach network). Microarray techniques have now revealed cascades of developmental genes involved in primate cortical development, whose expression may be modified by early visual experience (Lachance and Chaudhuri, 2004). McMullen et al. (2004) have shown changes in expression of a daunting array of genes in the mouse oculomotor system after dark rearing. Gene networks, like most other networks, have emergent properties, and it is hopelessly naïve to think of a single gene being responsible for any particular trait. It seems that each clinical condition is a complex product of genetic mutations, polymorphisms, pleitropy, a myriad of plasticity genes and neural growth factors—all directing an infant's developmental trajectory. Are we in danger of creating another stamp album full of disconnected phenomenology, or is there a science to this plethora?

I believe there is a framework to understand development, and especially oculomotor development. It is not to be found at the levels of genetics or physiology, but at the systems level of evolution, plasticity, and modularity. The recent explosion of the field of evolutionary developmental biology ('evo-devo') provides us with important insights, particularly into phenotypic plasticity (Pigliucci, 2001; West-Eberhard, 2003) and modularity (Sclosser and Wagner, 2004). It is surprising that eye movements are barely mentioned in this literature. The oculomotor system provides an extraordinary natural laboratory for understanding developmental plasticity. Oculomotor behaviour undergoes pre- and postnatal development, it is mostly canalized but can exhibit novel phenotypes (as I shall explore), and it is often conserved phylogenetically. Eye movements are clearly modularized and can be measured with some precision. The physiology is well understood, and progress is being made in oculomotor genetics. Moreover, an important component of the 'environment' for eye movements is afferent vision, which can also be measured.

Equally, though, oculomotorists can learn from the field of developmental plasticity, and take on board that development is not simply a sequence of behavioural phenomena, but organized (or perhaps orchestrated) by the logic of plasticity with its own genetic substrate. First and fundamental is the notion that the phenotype is not pre-ordained by the genotype, but it emerges as an interaction between genotype and environment. Second, developmental plasticity can be an *adaptive* evolutionary strategy that permits the developing phenotype to modify itself according to the local environment experienced by the individual phenotype. Whilst this may leave the developing phenotype vulnerable to abnormal environments, it provides the genotype with a means of fine-tuning individual phenotypes to improve their fitnesses for their particular environments. Although there are many examples of adaptive developmental plasticity, the unique case of the two-legged goat remains iconic. This animal was born with congenitally malformed forelimbs but survived by developing a bipedal hopping gait. This was made possible by remarkable postnatal adaptive changes in the development of bone structure and musculature—not seen in the normal quadrupedal goat (Slijpers, 1942). This goat was a 'one-off', it could not have been selected for. Instead, developmental plasticity was sufficiently flexible to allow this individual goat to modify its physical structure and behaviour beneficially. Clearly studying normal goats would give no inkling to the extent of caprine plasticity.

Developmental plasticity is often canalized, where most individuals of a species learn similar behaviours in similar environments—oculomotor behaviour is a case in point. This obscures the underlying plasticity at work. If we only study normal oculomotor development, it is easy to fall into the belief that the oculomotor systems are pre-programmed. By studying the 'abnormal' and 'exotic' we can observe plasticity outside this funnel of canalization. The purpose of this chapter is to examine oculomotor developmental pathologies, not from the traditional clinical perspective, or by proximal neuromimetic 'how' models, but as examples of phenotypic plasticity driven by extreme environments. The boundaries of 'environment' are inevitably ill-defined but we take a broad genocentric view, which includes (but is not limited to) effects from other genes (e.g. those that lead to fovea dysplasia), developmental noise (irreducible random fluctuations in development), influences that are external to the whole organism (e.g. nutrition, visual experience), as well as interactions among these.

My premise is that oculomotor control has evolved, either directly or indirectly via development, solely to support vision. For frontal and foveate eyes, there are three fundamental primate oculomotor behaviours: 1) yoking of the eyes which is important for the development of binocular visuomotor functions (manifested as fusion, stereopsis, vergence, accommodation, tracking in depth); 2) gaze maintenance which is important for maximizing visual contrast (vestibulo-ocular reflex (VOR), optokinetic nystagmus (OKN), fixation, smooth pursuit); 3) gaze shifting which is important for re-directing line of sight (saccades, head movements, scanning). All of these undergo post-natal development and are vulnerable to developmental redirection from extreme environments. In this chapter we will focus on the latter two for two reasons: first, gaze-maintenance and gaze-shifting have two well demarcated and dramatic developmental clinical ('novel') phenotypes: infantile nystagmus syndrome (INS) and saccade initiation failure (SIF). INS (formerly known as congenital nystagmus) is a type of spontaneous eye oscillation that starts only in the first few weeks of life, often secondary to an afferent deficit. INS is lifelong and incurable. SIF is abnormality of saccade triggering in which a young child refixates visual targets by making strange head-thrusts and blinks, which are clearly adaptive but unlike any normal behaviour. Second, we have fitness/cost models of saccades and fixations, which I will argue is central for understanding their development. There is no principled reason why we will not be able to apply our framework to yoking, but we do not yet have a fitness/cost model.

Before describing these two novel phenotypes, I will outline a framework for oculomotor developmental plasticity, where I introduce the concept of a developmental trajectory and the cost of plasticity to explain INS and SIF. I emphasize that this framework is based on a mathematical approach of optimality, and provide an appendix to demonstrate this grounding.

An 'evo-devo' perspective

The developmental fitness surface

I begin by introducing the idea of developmental fitness surfaces or 'landscapes'. Although the fitness landscape metaphor is familiar to most, here it means strictly a *phenotypic* fitness landscape. The height of the landscape is fitness, and the other dimensions are phenotype parameter values, and it is assumed that fitness is a smooth function of the parameter values. This description should not be confused with *genotypic* fitness landscapes, as modelled by population geneticists, where the dimensions are fitness and genotype (allelic) space. Genotype landscapes may be very rugged with inaccessible peaks. For further discussions of landscapes and smoothness, see Gavrilets (2004), McGhee (2007), and Godfrey-Smith (2009). Landscapes are typically high-dimensional, but to portray them on two-dimensional paper, I will collapse them into two dimensions labelled 'parameter x' and 'parameter y' (Fig. 37.1A).

In the phenotypic fitness landscape, the parameters may be structural (e.g. photoreceptor density, axial eye length, etc.) or behavioural (e.g. eye position, velocity, vergence angle, etc.). The topography of this landscape depends on the interaction of the phenotype (organism) with its environment. For a fixed environment (and identical organisms), we expect natural selection to maximize fitness by producing phenotypes with the optimal parameters that place them on or around a local fitness peak. Fitness is usually measured in terms of survival and viable progeny, which is virtually impossible to measure in mammals. Instead, it is usual to consider surrogate variables, which are expected to be monotonic functions of true fitness. For example, speed, accuracy, and energy efficiency are plausible surrogates, and much of the biological optimality literature has focused on how these surrogates are optimized (and traded-off against each other) in different behavioural tasks (e.g. foraging, locomotion, orienting).

However, when we consider development and plasticity, the phenotype and the environment are changing in time following some developmental trajectory through parameter space (arrowed line in

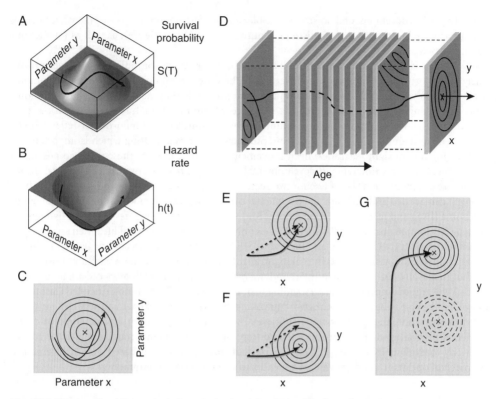

Fig. 37.1 Schematic of the cost of phenotypic plasticity shown for a two-dimensional parameter space (parameter x and parameter y). A) Local maximum of a fitness surface modelled as probability of survival until age T assuming constant x and y. Note that a developmental trajectory (solid line) involves changing x and y. B) Hazard surface at some time *t*. If surface is constant, cumulative hazard is given by the line integral along the developmental trajectory (see appendix). C) Contour map of (B) showing minimum at 'x' and the developmental trajectory (solid line). High fitness development would keep the trajectory short and near to the minimum. D) The hazard rate surface changes with age as the phenotype develops along the trajectory (arrow) until the adult optimum is reached. Note that the trajectory may pass through sub-optimal regions during development. E) Different trajectories have different overall fitnesses. The dashed line depicts the path of a fixed (non-plastic) phenotype and the solid line for a plastic phenotype. Both reach the adult optimum, but the fixed phenotype has higher fitness. F) The same phenotypes as in (E) but in a different environment (i.e. different hazard rate surface) with a different adult optimal phenotype. Now the plastic phenotype has more fitness. G) Illustration of how plasticity can be steered by sensitive periods, with parameter y developing before parameter x allowing the phenotype to avoid a region of the fitness surface with a local hazard minimum (dashed contour lines).

Fig. 37.1A), and the notion of a static phenotypic fitness landscape is too simple. Fitness depends on the developmental trajectory as well as the fitness of the adult product, and maximizing overall fitness will include development as well. Developing phenotypes also influence their own environments. For example, taking afferent vision as the environment for oculomotor development, early onset disorders (e.g. strabismus) can permanently affect sensory development (e.g. lack of stereopsis, amblyopia). To handle this kind of problem, we introduce the hazard surface (hazard landscape) (Fig. 37.1B), which nicely encapsulate the idea of fitness per unit time. From the theory of survival analysis, the hazard function (mortality rate) is the probability of dying (or becoming non-reproductive) in the infinitesimal time interval $(t, t+dt)$ given that the phenotype was alive (potentially reproductive) at time t (see 'Appendix'). Thus each point on the hazard surface is the mortality *rate* for the parameter values at some instant in time. One can view the hazard surface as a cost surface, since decreasing hazard is beneficial and increasing it is costly. Hence the surface appears inverted when compared to fitness landscapes, and the minimum has the same coordinates as the maximum survival probability in Fig. 37.1A. One can also plot the hazard surface as a contour map (Fig. 37.1C), where the minimum is shown by the cross.

When the phenotype changes in time (development, plasticity), it follows a trajectory on the hazard surface (arrowed line in Fig. 37.1B and C), and the probability of becoming non-reproductive (not surviving) is the total hazard accumulated along this trajectory (the line integral), called the 'cumulative hazard' (see 'Appendix'). For a fixed hazard surface, maximizing survival is equivalent to finding the trajectory that minimizes the cumulative hazard. Clearly, trajectories that are long and far from the hazard minimum have low fitness, whereas trajectories that are short and near the minimum would have high fitness. Fitness would be maximized by staying at the minimum as long as possible; that is, it would pay to reach this minimum as soon as possible, and stay there.

However, it is extremely unlikely that hazard landscapes remain fixed in early life. The background of physical (maturational) growth (e.g. changing head and eyeball size, height from ground, etc.), as well as postnatal development (macular and cortical development) imposes a milieu of ever-changing environments, which will continuously modify oculomotor hazard landscapes as the phenotype develops. As illustrated in Fig. 37.1D, there will be a changing hazard landscape during development, so that development becomes a trajectory in this space (arrowed line). The hazard landscape at any point in time will depend on previous developmental choices—it is as if the landscape changes on every step taken. For simplicity (although not necessary), assume that the hazard landscape changes minimally during adulthood and has a local minimum, marked by the cross in Fig. 37.1D. Development must reach this optimum, but there are many trajectories. Each will accumulate its own hazard as the young phenotype takes a different developmental path towards adulthood. The cost will be given by the hazard accumulated *along* the trajectory, so there is no straightforward way of determining the optimal trajectory ahead of time, other than generally being short and far away from high hazards. Tracking the minimum at each point in time is *not* necessarily the most successful strategy, as this could be a long tortuous route, and a short high-hazard route may actually have less *cumulative* hazard. So how could natural selection minimize this cost?

From the genotype stance, we can consider two extreme developmental strategies. One is to programme development to take a fixed trajectory to the adult optimum, so that all phenotypes arrive at the same point in phenotypic parameter space at the same time. Because this strategy is applied over and over again across individuals and down generations, it could be become highly optimized by natural selection. We will call this the 'fixed' genotypic strategy or phenotype. At the other extreme, development could be programmed to be entirely plastic and sensitive to the environment, so that each individual develops differently—tuned to its particular hazard topography. In this case, development must *search* for the trajectory in real time. Natural selection still acts, but it now favours a plasticity strategy to control development, rather than controlling development directly. We call this the 'plastic' genotypic strategy or phenotype. The two strategies will fare differentially. In a fixed environment, the fixed phenotype will be highly optimized and hence have high fitness (Fig. 37.1E, dashed arrow line). The plastic phenotype will still find the adult optimum, but will in general follow a less fit trajectory depending on the search algorithm (Fig. 37.1E, solid arrowed line). In a variable environment, however, the fixed phenotype will fair less well, as it may produce phenotypes that are not optimized for their environments (Fig. 37.1F, dashed arrowed line). In this case, the plastic phenotype will fare better as it can adjust each phenotype to its respective environment (Fig. 37.1F, solid arrowed line).

Modularity and sensitive periods

The plastic phenotype may be advantageous in variable environments, but it is no panacea. Searching phenotypic space can consume developmental time thereby increasing cumulative hazard, or it could become trapped in a local suboptimal minimum leaving the adult to a lifetime of increased hazard.

Phenotypic parameter spaces have very high dimensions, and to search the entire hypervolume for the optimal control of eye movements would be prohibitive. Modularity and sensitive periods permit steerage of development through this volume to reduce developmental time. As an illustration, consider a fully connected network in which any node can have two-way connections with any other node (Fig. 37.2A). These nodes could be genes, neurons, or subsystems, but for concreteness consider each to be an oculomotor nucleus containing homogenously functioning neurons. For N nodes there are N^2 possible connections (including recurrent connections; not shown). These connections can have different strengths or 'synaptic weights' (parameter values). The real-time behaviour of the entire network depends on the function of each node and the connection weights, but overall there are M^{N^2} different possible circuits. Except for trivial networks, this number is vast and virtually impossible to search in finite time. For example, a network of 10 nodes with binary synaptic weights will have 100 dimensions with a hypervolume of $\sim 10^{30}$ different circuits to search through (this is larger than the number of grains of sand in all of the world's beaches!). If the synaptic weights are trinary (e.g. inhibitory, off, excitatory) the hypervolume increases to $\sim 10^{47}$, and so on.

This search space needs to be reduced drastically by pruning connections. One way is to create clusters of weakly connected subnetworks or 'modules', where each module has functional significance (sometimes called a 'small world network'). Thus, in our toy example, if we divide the 10 nodes into two groups of 5 (Fig. 37.2B), then each has 25 dimensions, but we could optimize each in parallel. Afterwards we then optimize the link connecting the two groups (dashed line in Fig. 37.2B). This is equivalent to optimizing 27 dimensions, which is an enormous reduction in the search hypervolume, now $\sim 10^8$. If the modules have different sizes, then the smaller will be optimized before the larger, but the larger will determine the overall search time. The price to pay for this 'divide and conquer' strategy is that the two modules are only weakly connected and the total phenotypic space explored is reduced. Hierarchical nesting is another strategy (Fig. 37.2C). Here one module is optimized first, and becomes a node in the other module. The search explores more phenotypic space than the parallel subdivision, but will take longer and is equivalent to 61 dimensions or a hypervolume of $\sim 10^{18}$. It is important to recognize that when a module has been optimized, its internal connections must remain fixed when it is incorporated into a larger network, otherwise the search space will explode again. Modules can be further subdivided, and subdivided again, with parallel or hierarchal subdivisions. Clearly there are many ways to carve up the original network. Each is a compromise between search speed (developmental time) and explored space (plasticity) and their consequential hazards. Thus, we will see the plasticity of modules being switched on and off in time as the whole cluster is optimized, which to an observer would appear as cascades of 'sensitive periods'.

One advantage of this approach is that it is possible to steer plasticity to a region of the phenotypic space with potential value, or around unwanted local minima by temporally modulating plasticity in different dimensions (Fig. 37.1G). Another advantage is that a network of many weakly connected modules is more stable than a large highly connected network (see Wuensche 2004). This may be significant for the genotype. In large highly connected networks, small variations in connectivity ('developmental noise') could lead to wildly unpredictable phenotypes. Modularity reduces this susceptibility and hence draws a balance between novelty and canalization.

It is crucial to recognize that each module is optimized independently of the others. Thus each module is only locally adaptive—in both time and space—without feedback from its effect on other modules or the global network behaviour. This can have a serious downside when we consider extreme environments ('pathology'). Modifying an early module that is used by later modules could lead to an extreme environment for later modules with a suboptimal phenotype. Thus, what was locally adaptive in a primitive module could turn out to be maladaptive globally. For example, it has been proposed that pre- and postnatal infant growth is affected by maternal under-nutrition, and becomes adapted to an anticipated environment of poor nutrition. However, as an adult the phenotype may be more susceptible to disease (type 2 diabetes, coronary disease) if it encounters an affluent environment, rather than the poor one cued by the mother's nutrition (Bateson et al., 2004). Below we will look at INS from this viewpoint.

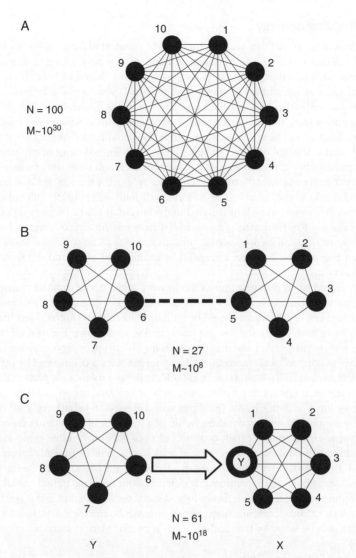

Fig. 37.2 Illustration of the benefit of modularity for network with 10 nodes (filled circles) with two-way interconnections (lines). A) Full network: a fully connected network with 100 connections (including self-recurrent connections not shown). If each connection can take on two values (binary) there are M~10^{30} different network circuits. Searching this volume is prohibitive. B) Parallel modularity: two self-contained modules, nodes 1–5, and nodes 6–10 (each having 25 connections) are optimized in parallel before the interconnection (dashed line) is optimized. This is equivalent to 27 connections with M~10^8. Note that each module must be frozen before the interconnection is optimized, thus exhibiting sensitive periods. C) Hierarchical modularity: nodes 6–10 form a self-contained module, Y, with 25 connections. This is optimized first and becomes a single node in the rest of the network with 36 connections, leading to a reduction in volume M~10^{18}. This hierarchical division requires sequential development with Y being searched first. Note that the connections within Y must be frozen to avoid the whole network from being searched later. Thus Y has a sensitive period.

The house-building analogy

I summarize these concepts with an analogy. Imagine the problem of building houses in a competitive market, given that you have a team of master builders who have a long tradition in building houses and know what constitutes a 'good' house. Such a house should be habitable to some minimum standard and stay upright for some minimum time. It also needs to be built as quickly as possible to compete with other builders. Each house will occupy a different plot of land with its own peculiar environment (soil, slope, climate, etc.) and materials will in general be variable. Building *exactly* the same house could be very fast (e.g. a completely prefabricated house), but it will result in failure in most cases as it could only ever be suitable for a very limited range of environments (fixed phenotype). An alternative approach would be to have a very rough blueprint of a house and let the builders construct each component (carving each stone, cutting the timbers, making cement manually, etc.). Such bespoke houses would all be different, well-built, and perfectly tailored to almost any environment, but they would take a long time to build (completely plastic phenotype). Now consider the modular approach. Pre-fabricated components (such as cement, bricks, window frames) can be reproduced very precisely and incorporated as primitive modules. Construction is now much faster. Modularity is a compromise between a very fast inflexible fixed build and the slow fully plastic bespoke construction.

This analogy runs deeper. Building houses has its own 'logic' which imposes constraints on the sequence of construction and hence the hierarchy of modules. For example, the plot must be cleared before construction can begin. A roof cannot be built until its supports are in place. If a foundation is needed, it must be built before the roof supports, and so on. Leaving the roof till last, however, exposes earlier work to the weather and may prevent some tasks from being completed (e.g. electrical wiring). In other words, the local environment for some modules is determined by other modules. There may be different overall solutions (such as building temporary roof supports and then removing them) but early decisions constrain later ones, and our builders' strong traditions (evolutionary constraints) may limit later flexibility. Buildings will still need to be tailored to their particular environment by the master builders, but there would be a strong similarity among the houses (canalization). A drawback is the need for high-quality control of the prefabricated components. A small error in a primitive (substandard cement, shape of bricks, etc.) could be potentially catastrophic. On the other hand, these errors may be overcome depending on the ingenuity of the master builders, who might produce a house that is considerably different from the usual mould (novel phenotype).

There is an optimal tradeoff between flexibility and speed of construction, but it will be a complex function of the logic of house building, materials, environments, and the master builders' traditions. In general, it can only be found by trial-and-error in the market place (natural selection).

Application to oculomotor development

So how could we build an oculomotor system? Clearly, the final product is a highly complex neural network of semi-autonomous subnetworks controlling various aspects of oculomotor control. These modules can also be hierarchical. For example, gaze holding (the eye position neural integrator) is a basic function that is nested within all the versional subsystems. Saccades are used in many different contexts for gaze-shifting (voluntary, reflexive, quick-phases, etc.), yet it is the same function that is repeatedly used. For most phenotypes, we label these stereotyped modules (VOR, saccades, smooth pursuit, etc.) as if they were independent systems. Modules are interconnected, but relatively weakly when compared to the intra-connectivity of individual modules. Indeed, it is their separate function and anatomy that has led to their identification. However, they all cooperate together to generate a remarkably sophisticated oculomotor behaviour. To appreciate the complexity, one only needs to consider the problem of aligning two two-dimensional retinas mounted on gimbals inside a bobbing head that is flexibly coupled to a body that is itself moving, while tracking a distant object that is moving independently of the body in three dimensions against a visual background. It is my contention that this level of sophistication could *only* be achieved by plastic modular development, as learning such behaviour *de novo* by a single fully connected large plastic network would take at least a life-time and would have zero fitness. Nevertheless, modularity in adulthood does not necessarily equate to modularity in development or developmental plasticity.

It seems likely that development follows some degree of modularity (although this could be self-fulfilling when experiments are designed to study the development of a specific module). The foundation of oculomotor control is the extraocular muscles, cranial nerves and brainstem nuclei. These develop very early during brainstem development (7–9 weeks' gestation; see Joseph, 2000). In vivo fetal eye movements have been detected via ultrasonography by 14 weeks (Horimoto et al., 1993). At birth spontaneous saccades, VOR, and monocular OKN (i.e. with nasotemporal asymmetry) can be elicited. Yoking of the eyes is present but alignment is variable. Smooth pursuit is rudimentary and difficult to distinguish from OKN (i.e. present to large stimuli) and develops post-natally (Aslin, 1981; Bloch and Carchon 1992; Dayton and Jones, 1964; Jacobs et al., 1997; Kremnitzer et al., 1979; Lengyel et al., 1998; Roucoux et al., 1983; Rütsche et al., 2006; Shea and Aslin 1990; von Hoftsen and Rosander 1996). Vergence and accommodation also develop post-natally (Banks, 1980; Thorn et al., 1994; Tondel and Candy, 2007; Weinacht et al., 1999).

However, normal oculomotor control reveals little, if any, evidence of developmental plasticity. Indeed, Weinacht et al. (1999) report that early visuomotor development is not advanced by early visual experience due to prematurity, but follows a gestational clock. However, as early sensory development is also gestational (excluding pathologies) moderate prematurity (>33 weeks' gestation) may not provide a sufficiently altered environment to drive postnatal oculomotor plasticity beyond the funnel of canalization. We need to examine more extreme environments (i.e. clinical conditions) for possible two-legged goats.

Saccade initiation failure (ocular motor apraxia)

Saccade initiation failure (SIF) is an abnormality of gaze-shifting, where the young affected child has a failure of saccade triggering (usually intermittent). Although unusual and seldom seen outside clinical circles, the condition has drawn much attention because of the extraordinary compensatory behaviour of head-thrusting and synkinetic blinking, which may even be seen in infants. Indeed the clinical literature is replete with cases, as most clinicians cannot resist adding another stamp to the album. In this section I will explore this condition as a novel phenotype in the framework of developmental plasticity, but first I briefly review the SIF phenotype.

The SIF phenotype

SIF was first described by David Cogan in 1952, who labelled it 'a type of congenital ocular motor apraxia presenting jerky head movements' because of its superficial similarity to adult-onset ocular motor apraxia (Cogan, 1952). The terms 'congenital ocular motor apraxia' (COMA) or 'Cogan's apraxia' have since become embedded in the literature. The term 'supranuclear gaze palsy' has also emerged in a largely separate neurometabolic literature. We introduced the term SIF to avoid the confusing term 'apraxia', which implies a deficit in voluntary or wilful movement in the presence of intact motor pathways (Harris et al., 1996). True acquired ocular motor apraxia is usually seen in adults with cortical lesions, who have difficulty in shifting attention and in generating voluntary saccades. The underlying brainstem saccadic machinery appears intact as deduced by the presence of normal optokinetic or vestibular nystagmus quick phases (Rambold et al., 2006). In contrast, children with SIF usually have no problems in shifting attention, as witnessed by their compensatory head movements, but invariably have abnormalities in quick phase triggering (Harris et al., 1996; Zee et al., 1977). Thus SIF is not an apraxia. This labelling issue is particularly problematic in older children who can acquire SIF (with quick phase failure), usually through cerebellar or brainstem disease, but to call this 'ocular motor apraxia' is clearly inappropriate.

SIF is primarily a disorder affecting the triggering (initiation) of saccades. Usually only horizontal saccades are affected, but vertical saccades may also be involved in midbrain and some neurometabolic disorders (Garbutt and Harris, 2000). The key feature of SIF is that the pathology is supranuclear with intact nuclear and infra-nuclear pathways, so that a full range of eye movements can be elicited with the VOR. Thus SIF is not a gaze palsy.

Without the normal saccadic mechanism, many children spontaneously learn to shift gaze with a characteristic head-thrusting strategy (provided head movement control is itself sufficiently developed), and affected infants may even develop headthrusting by a few months of age (Rosenberg and Wilson, 1987).

In the absence of any eye movements (total external ophthalmoplegia), gaze can be controlled purely by moving the head. This occurs in rare cases, and the trajectory of head movements are similar to saccades (Gilchrist et al., 1997). In SIF, however, the VOR is preserved, so that moving the head induces a VOR in the opposite direction to, and hence nullifying the effect of the head movement. To overcome the VOR, the head is moved rapidly beyond the target so that the eyes are 'locked-up' at the extreme limit of gaze and dragged over to align with the peripheral target. The head is then moved back towards the new target with the VOR maintaining gaze on the target. This procedure occurs in one movement and appears as a hypermetric head movement or 'head-thrust'. For a schematic, see Cassidy et al. (2000), and see Win and Laws (2006) for an illustrative video.

SIF also leads to a failure of quick-phases (saccades that reset eye position), which causes the eyes to deviate intermittently to the limit of gaze during optokinetic or induced vestibular nystagmus ('locking-up'). The degree of intermittency is variable both across and within patients (Harris et al., 1996). Because the lack of quick-phases can occur in complete darkness, it seems unlikely that SIF reflects an inability to break fixation (although gap/overlap studies have not been carried out in SIF). Some children will also adopt a compensatory strategy of synkinetic blinks. These blinks are synchronous with saccades and appear to help trigger a saccade (Lambert et al., 1989). They also speed up saccades in patients with slow saccades (Zee et al., 1983).

Recording of eye and head movements is challenging in these children, but it has revealed a range of strategies with some preserved saccadic component. Saccades may be delayed with the head being initiated first and leading to an initial VOR response in the opposite (and counterproductive) direction, taking gaze to an intermediate direction before long latency and hypometric saccades take gaze to the final position (Lambert et al., 1989). In milder cases, head and eye movements may be initiated synchronously. Although the eyes do not lock-up in extreme version, head movements may still overshoot possibly reflecting a phylogenetically earlier gaze-shifting mechanism (Zee et al., 1977). Thus there is probably a range of deficits in saccadic triggering involving different head movement compensation, but much of the 'compensation' is to counteract the intact VOR.

Causes and associations

There is no single pathophysiology. SIF can occur in infancy (congenital) or later in childhood (acquired). SIF can be associated with very many conditions including idiopaths, congenital malformations of the brain, a variety of developmental syndromes, peri- and postnatal disorders, early-onset neurometabolic diseases, and later-onset neurodegenerative conditions (reviewed by Cassidy et al., 2000).

In a large study, Shawkat et al. (1995) found delayed myelination, abnormalities of the cerebellum, brainstem, basal ganglia and cerebral cortex. Cerebellar abnormalities (especially the vermis) are a common finding in SIF, either as a midline malformation (e.g. the Joubert related syndromes), or as an acquired degeneration (e.g. ataxia telangiectasia). Recently the ataxin gene (APTX; MIM 606350) has been identified in the degenerative ataxia-oculomotor apraxia type 1 condition (Date et al., 2001), with typical onset at about 6–7 years of age (this should not be considered the 'SIF gene' as there many other associations). In non-syndromic children, SIF is usually sporadic but occasionally inherited with variable vermis involvement (MIM 257550; Harris et al., 1998). The role of the vermis in SIF is unclear, and although the possibility that the saccadic omnipause neurons (OPNs) may be disinhibited by the fastigial nucleus due to vermian Purkinje cell damage seems tantalizing, it is difficult to explain why the SIF is so often restricted to the horizontal meridian. In neurometabolic disease, direct involvement of the brainstem saccade generator seems most likely, as saccades (when they occur) are slow, falling far off the main sequence (Garbutt et al., 2001).

A variety of other oculomotor deficits are typically associated with SIF, including saccade dysmetria, and low gain smooth pursuit and OKN, regardless of underlying clinical diagnosis (Shawkat et al., 1995). Neurological nystagmus may also occur depending on the diagnosis. Neurodevelopmental delay is common (Marr et al., 2005) including fine and gross motor delay, and speech and language delays, but it is not clear to what extent SIF per se, or other structural abnormalities contribute. Jan et al. (1998) reported that even children without speech difficulties had reduced visual-perceptual IQ scores, presumably as a direct result of slow gaze-shifting.

In summary, the neural circuitry for triggering saccades is particularly vulnerable in young children to damage from many causes, some genetic, some sporadic with onset in infancy or later in childhood. The behavioural consequence of this disorder (however it originated) is a difficulty in gaze-shifting leading to reduced performance in visuospatial tasks. Most children spontaneously develop/learn compensatory strategies, headthrusting and/or synkinetic blinking. These behaviours are not adopted by the healthy infant or adult. Indeed, they are probably physiologically impossible unless there is a failure of saccades in the first place. Moreover, they are not the product of a genetic mutation, as these behaviours emerge as a response to a wide group of heterogeneous antecedent events. Nor are these delayed early neonatal reflexes or phylogenetic recapitulations (except possibly for the vestigial response described above). Finally, they are not learnt by imitation. There appears to be no sensitive period, as older children with acquired disorders also adopt these strategies.

SIF in an evo-devo context

Gaze shifting is a fundamental behaviour in all mammals as it allows reorientation relative to the visual field. In many afoveate species shifting gaze consists of closely coupled movements of the eyes and head, but in mammals with foveas (or similar specialized retinal regions) there is a considerable degree of eye–head decoupling so that eye saccades can be made without moving the head. This evolutionary bifurcation is probably also related to head size (brain size) as a fovea requires continual refixation to scan visual scenes, but moving a large head quickly is energetic and probably needs to be slower than eye saccades for a given accuracy (see below). The normal human newborn phenotype is endowed with a saccadic mechanism but head control is immature, so that gaze shifting is reliant on eye saccades. In this respect, ontogeny does not recapitulate phylogeny, and this decoupling is at the heart of SIF.

Adult optimum

Gaze shifting inevitably necessitates creating retinal image motion. One option is to move very slowly so as to maintain good visual contrast during the gaze-shift. However, this would require velocities below ~3°/s for an adult foveate visual system (Westheimer and McKee, 1975), so that a 10° 'saccade' would take more than 3 s to complete! This strategy is too costly. The alternative is to temporarily forego high-spatial frequency vision and move as quickly as possible to minimize the visual 'down-time' (Harris and Wolpert, 2006). Very rapid movements incur other crucial costs, however, which manifest as two sources of error in saccade accuracy: dynamic noise and targeting noise (van Beers, 2007).

For fast brief movements, the phasic motor control signal becomes intense (i.e. burst unit firing) and it appears that this drive becomes dominated by signal-dependent noise (Harris and Wolpert, 1998) in which noise standard deviation on the motor command increases with its mean level (proportional noise). The faster or larger the movement, the more noise is generated, thus causing a speed-accuracy tradeoff. Hence moving very quickly incurs more error, or equivalently, reducing error requires a slower movement. There is an optimal velocity profile that minimizes end-point variance, the minimum variance model (MV), which provides a good fit to observed adult saccade trajectories, as well as multi-joint arm movements (Harris and Wolpert, 1998). For arm movements, this noise seems to be intrinsic to the motor control machinery, probably motor unit recruitment (Jones et al., 2001), although this has not yet been firmly established for the oculomotor system.

From this model, the saccadic main sequence can also be explained as a fixed tradeoff between speed and accuracy (Harris and Wolpert 2006).

The above model would also be expected to hold for pure head movements. Because of the large mechanical inertia of the head, the MV model predicts that head movements would need to be slower than eye movements for a given end-point variance. There is surprisingly little data on head movement trajectories, but they do follow a slower 'main sequence' in normal subjects (Evinger et al., 1994; Liao et al., 2005; Stark et al., 1980).

Another price to pay for rapid saccades is the preclusion of visual feedback to guide the eye to its target. Hence the eyes are driven feedforward using local feedback (internal model). For visually guided saccades, this leads to localization errors, as accuracy cannot be greater than the spatial resolution of the peripheral retina that triggered the saccade, which increases with foveal eccentricity and hence saccade amplitude (van Beers, 2007). Although localization error seems irreducible, there is evidence that saccade accuracy may improve with latency (McSorley and Findlay, 2003; and others). Express saccades tend to be less accurate (Delinte et al., 2002), and multiple saccades made by school-age children have shorter latencies than single saccades (van Donkelaar et al., 2007). It is possible, therefore, that saccade latency is involved in a tradeoff between fast reaction time and accuracy. Recently, it has been proposed that latency is actually dependent on the attentional scale of the target (i.e. size/eccentricity), so that latency becomes large when the saccade amplitude is lower than the size of the attentional focus (Harwood et al., 2008).

So what do we expect from infants? What is the most cost-effective developmental path? Although the infant retina is immature with low resolution and low contrast sensitivity, it is still spatially inhomogeneous with peripheral resolution being about half of central resolution (Allen et al., 1995). Thus, as in adults, there is a fundamental need to re-orient the retinas, which is reflected by the powerful orienting reflex in infants (Fantz et al., 1962). Spatial frequency resolution is lower in the infant, and the 3°/s Westheimer-McKee maximum should be higher. Even with a tenfold increase, however, a 10° saccade would need 300 ms to complete, and presumably it would still pay to move as quickly as possible.

According to the MV theory, the low resolution of the neonatal vision places *less* demands on saccade accuracy than for adults, and perhaps contrary to intuition, there should be nothing to gain by making saccades slower than adults. Indeed, according to the speed–accuracy tradeoff, it would pay to make infant saccades even faster than for adults. Assuming there are no other physiological constraints, the optimal developmental strategy would be to make saccades from birth with speeds greater than adults. Empirically, full-term neonates generate conjugate-appearing saccades (Farroni et al., 1999). They also generate quick-phases during vestibular nystagmus induced by rotation, which can also be seen in premature infants (Cordero et al., 1983). The infant main sequence is similar to adults (Garbutt et al., 2006; Richards and Hunter, 1997). The velocity profiles of infant saccades have not been measured, but they also appear very similar to adult saccades (personal observation).

Infant saccade localization error is very high. It increases with target eccentricity and decreases with age (Harris et al., 1993; Richards and Hunter 1997), but how peripheral retinal maturation and internal model training contribute is unknown. Although localization error is substantial in infants, it cannot be reduced by slowing saccades and requires corrective saccades (in participants motivated to precisely fixate a single small target in the laboratory). As in adults, infant saccades show a strong undershoot bias in spite of the large errors, and it has been proposed that this is also an adaptive strategy to reduce the cost of localization error by minimizing total saccade flight-time (Harris 1995). Saccade latency is much longer in infants, whether for visually guided primary saccades (Matsuzawa and Shimojo, 1997), secondary saccades (Harris et al., 1993), or nystagmus quick phases (Cordero et al., 1983). It is interesting to note that infants and even newborns show a strong gap/overlap effect. This may reflect cortical/cognitive maturation of decision making, but it may reflect subcortical processing (Farroni et al., 1999). Whether it is also related to the immature *central* retina behaving as a large default region of attention (extrapolating from Harwood et al., 2008) remains unexplored.

The early development of fast saccades has implications for SIF. SIF from birth or in the first month or so will prevent gaze shifting until a compensatory strategy (head movement, synkinetic blinks) can be learnt, and it is not surprising that the condition can be misdiagnosed as an afferent problem (i.e. blindness). Head thrusting can begin by about 3 months (Rosenberg and Wilson, 1987), but if there is more generalized motor delay or an abnormality in head control, as in some cases of cerebral palsy, then head thrusting occurs later (if at all) and SIF may never be correctly diagnosed. When SIF is acquired later, the loss of saccades can be taken up by already developed head movements. Thus, if head control is present and plastically adaptable to compensate for the lack of saccades, we would *not* expect a sensitive period to modulate the plasticity, but allow it to act at all times.

An intriguing counterfactual question is why is VOR not suppressed during gaze-shifting in SIF? Eliminating VOR totally is probably too costly, as the gain in fitness in keeping the VOR for steady gaze maintenance outweighs the gain in suppressing the VOR during gaze shifts. But why not adaptively suppress the VOR during gaze shifts? Some degree of VOR attenuation can occur during gaze shifts in adults, but it is incomplete and highly variable across participants (and studies) (Cullen et al., 2004). It has been proposed that the VOR attenuation may be driven by saccade burst units inhibiting position-vestibular-pause neurons (Cullen et al., 2004). In which case, the failure to trigger a saccade would prevent any attenuation. Thus the VOR module may be 'disconnected' during head-only gaze shifts in SIF. Of course, one could ask why plasticity of VOR attenuation is not mediated by other means (e.g. via efference copy of higher collicular or frontal commands). In the normal phenotype, VOR and saccades are present from birth, but shifting gaze with the head does not develop until later and presumably is always accompanied by a saccade. Thus there is no selective pressure to evolve a different pathway, and it appears that new connections cannot be made after birth.

Thus, we can see how the strange 'novel' behaviour of headthrusting in SIF is both facilitated and constrained by plasticity. In the typical phenotype, the optimal developmental path is to endow the neonate with fast saccades, as this allows rapid redirection of the retina even at the price of inaccuracy (the alternative of moving slowly is worse). Head movements can help in large gaze-shifts, once their control is sufficiently mature. Plasticity allows head control to take over the gaze shift in the rare event of saccade failure, but modularity prevents the VOR from being suppressed during the shift, and hence prolongs the shift. This slow gaze-shifting then leads to visuospatial problems later in life (Jan et al., 1998).

Synkinetic blinking

The compensatory strategy of synkinetic blinking seems to take advantage of pre-existing connectivity between saccades and blinks. Spontaneous blinks are a physiological necessity for replenishing the evaporating tear film to prevent drying and damage to the cornea. The rate of spontaneous blink production varies widely across individuals but is typically 10–20 blinks per minute. Blinks are also periods of temporarily reduced vision, and it would seem an optimal strategy to time-lock blinks to saccades (Fogarty and Stern, 1989). The physiological link between saccades and blinks in healthy individuals is complex. During fixation a blink causes the eye to adduct and move downward, probably through co-contraction of all muscles except the superior oblique (Evinger et al., 1994). Omnipause neurons cease firing during blinks and microstimulation of pause neurons inhibits blinks (Mays and Morrisse, 1995). Blinks also reduce the firing rate of medium lead burst units and collicular saccade related burst units (Goosens and van Opstal, 2000b). Thus, blinks modulate saccade kinematics by slowing saccades in healthy adults (Goosens and van Opstal, 2000a; Rambold et al., 2002). This central connectivity may provide a way of compensating for mechanical interference. However, according to the MV model, it would pay to slow saccades to reduce dynamic noise by taking advantage of the slower blink. There would be no advantage in completing a saccade whilst the blink continues. This appears to be in agreement with experimental observations showing that saccade durations are extended to match the blink duration (based on data in Goosens and van Opstal (2000a) and Rambold et al. (2002)).

Although there has been no quantitative study, it is observed clinically that very young infants with SIF do not adopt the synkinetic blinking strategy. This may be due to the time needed to learn it, but it may also reflect the very low spontaneous blink rates in neonates—about 1–2 blinks per minute. The reason for this low rate is unclear but it is probably linked to the low rate of tear-film evaporation in infants, which in turn may be due to the relatively small palpebral fissures and/or the thickness of lipid layer in infants (Lawrenson et al., 2005).

Thus, it seems that the saccade and the spontaneous blink 'modules' are connected behaviourally and physiologically, but the connection is limited and their developments are separate. The young infant with SIF must wait until the blink system comes on-line before plasticity can exploit it to help initiate gaze shifts. Without blinks or head movements, the young infant with SIF has no other means to shift gaze. It is not surprising therefore that the SIF infant may appear to be behaviourally blind leading to fraught diagnostic issues.

Infantile nystagmus syndrome

INS (formerly known as 'congenital nystagmus') is an abnormality of gaze maintenance in which the eyes spontaneously oscillate. INS has an onset in the first few weeks of life, or occasionally at birth. Unlike many other types of nystagmus, INS cannot be acquired—it is a developmental condition. INS has a critical period, and from an evo-devo viewpoint it is considerably more complex than SIF. I will first review the phenotype before discussing INS in an evo-devo context.

The INS phenotype

INS is one specific type of nystagmus that can have an onset in infancy. Another common type is fusion maldevelopment nystagmus syndrome (FMNS) (formerly known as manifest latent nystagmus, see CEMAS (2000)), which tends to be associated with uniocular deficits (e.g. unilateral cataract) and/or early-onset strabismus. Other types are rare and similar to the adult-onset nystagmuses that occur secondary to neurological disorders (e.g. Arnold Chiari malformation, dysmyelinating disease), which we group under the umbrella term 'neurological nystagmus' (NN) (Casteels et al., 1992). (To add to the confusion, the term 'infantile nystagmus' is still used as an umbrella term for any nystagmus in infancy (Abadi and Bjerre, 2002), but I will always refer to the specific type.) Expertise and eye movement recording are needed to differentiate these types of nystagmus; the published literature, old and new, needs scrutiny and careful interpretation.

INS is typically horizontal and conjugate, but occasionally it can be vertical or asymmetric (more pronounced in one eye) (Shawkat et al., 2001). In their seminal work Dell'Osso and Daroff (1975) recorded eye movements and showed that INS typically can have 12 waveforms. Of particular importance was the discovery that horizontal INS jerk nystagmus frequently has accelerating (increasing velocity) slow phases, not seen in FMNS or NN, and virtually pathognomonic of INS (exceptions are extraordinarily rare). This has become the most definitive (sufficient but not necessary) diagnostic feature of INS.

Sensory defect versus idiopathic INS

Patients with INS can be divided into two groups, those with an underlying congenital visual sensory defect (SD-INS) and those with no detectable sensory defect, called idiopathic INS (I-INS). It is widely accepted that the nystagmus waveforms cannot reliably distinguish between them, although fine pendular waveforms may be more associated with congenital stationary night-blindness (CSNB) and cone dysfunctions. Essentially, SD-INS and I-INS are the same type of nystagmus, and only differ on aetiological grounds. However, the distinction between them is potentially very important, as it implies that there may be different underlying causes. There are, however, issues about identifying I-INS and about whether it really exists separate from SD-INS, which need clarifying.

SD-INS can be associated with a wide range of apparently unrelated sensory abnormalities including (but not limited to) achromatopsia, albinism (oculocutaneous and ocular), aniridia, cataract, retinal coloboma, corneal opacities, optic nerve hypoplasia, optic atrophy, CSNB, cone dysfunction, foveal hypoplasia (isolated), Leber's congenital amaurosis, retinopathy of prematurity (Casteels et al., 1992). INS can also be associated with Down's syndrome (even in the absence of strabismus or cataract), and remains unexplained (Lawson et al., 1996).

I-INS cannot be identified positively, but only diagnosed by exclusion (i.e. ruling out any known sensory defect), which depends on the resources used to search for any underlying sensory defect (and varies widely across clinical centres). Some sensory defects such as ocular albinism (OA), CSNB, and cone dysfunction can be subtle and missed by standard ophthalmoscopy. Electrophysiological investigations using the electroretinogram (ERGs) to detect subtle retinal disorders, and visual evoked potentials (VEPs) for detecting optic nerve abnormalities and chiasmal misrouting have long been recommended for more precise phenotyping and recently re-emphasized (Dorey et al., 2003). Even so, today many patients are not tested this way, and considerable caution is advised in interpreting studies that claim 'idiopathic' status without using electrophysiology. For example, two novel mutations of the ocular albino gene (OA1; GPR143; MIM 300500) in Chinese pedigrees have recently been claimed to be idiopathic (Liu et al., 2007; Zhou et al., 2008). However, the cardinal signs of albinism (iris transillumination, foveal hypoplasia, nystagmus, and excessive decussation at the chiasm), are notoriously variable. These studies did not employ electrophysiology in their phenotyping, so abnormal decussation cannot be excluded, and the status of idiopath is unproven. Apparent lack of foveal hypoplasia in idiopaths and some albinos is also problematic due to examiner subjectivity. The new technique of optical coherence tomography (OCT) is currently under development in various centres for use with nystagmats. It promises to become the standard objective technique for measuring foveal dysplasia (Cronin et al., 2009; Seo et al., 2007), and the longstanding question of the foveal status in idiopaths may be resolved.

The possibility that the underlying sensory defects may provide a clue to the pathophysiology and mechanism of INS has a long contentious history. Early studies tended to focus mostly on albinos that led to the hypothesis that INS may arise from excessive decussation at the chiasm and led to models based on anomalous positive feedback (Optican and Zee, 1984; Tusa et al., 1992; Zee et al., 1980). A similar argument has been proposed to account for the eye movements of a mutant zebrafish (Huang et al., 2006). However, the wide range of clinically unrelated sensory defects associated with INS implies that INS is a plasticity response to a congenital visual defect. Indeed Ohm (1958) presented a case of INS following corneal opacities acquired at birth by infection. The finding that prolonged bilateral dark rearing can induce INS in monkey is yet further support for the developmental plasticity argument (Tusa et al., 2001). Nevertheless, the diagnosis of I-INS implies that INS might emerge for some other reason, but does I-INS really exist? Genes may provide an answer.

Genetics

INS is often familial, but there is no single gene for INS. Inheritance for SD-INS is syndromic. The focus of geneticists is naturally on genotyping, but the problems of phenotyping are often overlooked (as described above). With this caveat, some idiopathic INS genes have been identified: X-linked NYS1 (Xq26.2 MIM 310700), autosomal dominant NYS2 (6p12 MIM 164100), autosomal dominant NYS3 (7p11.2 MIM 608345) and a rare autosomal recessive gene (MIM 257400) (see Self and Lotery, 2007 for a review) (another gene, NYS4, is not INS). These genes do not coincide with any known syndromic gene, so the claim of idiopathic status seems reasonable.

The recent identification of the NYS1 gene (FERM domain-containing 7, FRMD7 MIM 300628) by Tarpey et al. (2006) has provided new impetus to the molecular biology of I-INS, with a flurry of studies reporting novel FRMD7 mutations (He et al., 2008; Kaplan et al., 2008; Li et al., 2008; Schordert et al., 2007; Self et al., 2007; Shiels et al., 2007; B. Zhang et al., 2007; Q. Zhang et al., 2007). It is not clear how many idiopathic pedigrees can be accounted for by the FRMD7 gene, but it is low in sporadic cases, and there may be other I-INS genes (Self et al., 2007). The true significance of the discovery of FRMD7 is that it opens up the possibility for understanding the mechanism by which I-INS develops. FRMD7 is expressed in the retina and in the cerebellum (Tarpey et al., 2006), but little else is known at present. Whether it is involved in the timing of afferent and motor development is not known. However, this is currently a very active area of research.

Sensory defect or sensory delay?

As congenital sensory defects are sufficient to cause INS, it is puzzling why nystagmus does not develop in all infants—given the immaturity of neonatal macular vision. What cues development down the nystagmus route? Weiss and Kelly (2007) tracked the development of acuity in four groups of infants with INS: idiopath, albinism, aniridia, binocular optic nerve hypoplasia. Using Teller acuity cards presented vertically (horizontal grating bars), they found that acuity continued to improve after nystagmus onset in all conditions, and that it followed a developmental curve similar to controls, but slower (when plotted against linear rather than log age). Thus, nystagmus is not caused by the arrest of visual development. Instead, the most likely explanation is that the cue is age-specific visual function. One intriguing possibility is that INS results from *delayed* visual development (as indexed by acuity)—it may be a question of timing. Substantial delays between SD-INS infants and normal controls can be seen in the Weiss and Kelly data, but surprisingly even the idiopathic group exhibited delay. Of course, by adulthood there would be no evidence of this delay. Thus it is possible that even though vision may be poor in normal early infancy, provided it develops 'on time' normal oculomotor control will develop, but if it is late then nystagmus will develop. This is also consistent with INS emerging in monkeys after dark rearing (Tusa et al., 2001), as dark rearing commonly delays development. It may also explain why INS appears apparently idiopathically in some Down's infants (Lawson et al., 1996), who as a group also demonstrate delayed acuity development (John et al., 2004). Thus, sensory delay may be the common antecedent event to INS development, although the cause of delay in idiopaths remains a mystery.

However, the fundamental questions still remain as to why nystagmus develops when there is delay, and why specific waveforms occur that are not seen in acquired nystagmus. If we accept that INS results from plasticity, then we need to understand what drives plasticity and what the objective of plasticity is.

INS from an evo-devo viewpoint

The developmental strategy for maintaining gaze is complex. Clearly for the adult phenotype with a fully mature fovea, developmental plasticity must steer the phenotype towards maximizing visual function including contrast sensitivity at high spatial frequencies. This is achieved by near-zero retinal slip during foveal fixation, high gain smooth pursuit, and high gain VOR/OKN, which we call 'normal' eye movements. However, it is not so clear how to reach this point given the considerable development in spatial vision during the first few months of life. Near-zero retinal slip does not maximize contrast for low spatial frequencies which dominate early infant vision. To put this in perspective, the adult contrast sensitivity to a drifting grating with a spatial frequency of 0.75 cyc/° is maximized by an image speed approaching 10°/s in primary position or 20°/s at an eccentricity of 7.5° (Virsu et al., 1982). Similarly, the sensitivity to a bar of width 3° is maximized when it moves at 10°/s (Burr and Ross, 1982). Spatial contrast sensitivity in a young infant (<2 months) peaks below 0.5 cyc/° and falls off rapidly above 1 cyc/° (Banks and Salapatek, 1978), whereas temporal contrast sensitivity to luminance has a similar shape to adults (Dobkins et al., 1999). Thus, steady fixation is *not* the optimal strategy for a young infant—maximizing visual contrast of a stationary object would need to invoke some kind of retinal slip. However, retinal slip would move the image away from the incipient fovea and would reduce contrast. Therefore, we asked the mathematical question of what would be the optimal way to move the image (Harris and Berry, 2006a). Making some simplifying assumptions, we found that the optimal solution is to oscillate the eyes back-and-forth with alternating slow and quick phases. The shape of the optimal slow phase depends on the relative importance of maintaining foveation and matching the ideal image velocity. When the importance of foveation is relatively low, the optimal slow phase is linear (constant velocity), as seen in some young infants with INS (Reinecke et al., 1988) (Fig. 37.3A). As foveation becomes more important, the optimal slow phases become more curvilinear with increasing velocity profile. There are a variety of optimal solutions which bear a remarkably close resemblance to observed waveforms.

The implication is that nystagmus is beneficial for visual contrast in early infancy, but should be replaced by steady fixation once the fovea is fully developed. Transient nystagmus can occur in human infants (Good et al., 2003), but it is rare and not the typical developmental strategy. Why do not all infants develop nystagmus? Again we need to look at potential interactions between oculomotor control and afferent vision.

Whilst image motion enhances visual contrast of low spatial frequencies, it also deprives the system of high spatial frequency information (in the meridian of motion). Thus nystagmus occurring during the early sensitive period of afferent visual development may be amblyogenic (Abadi and King-Smith, 1979) and prevent or delay the optimal adult phenotype from developing. Nystagmus also raises thresholds for motion (Abadi et al., 1999) and stereovision (Ukwade and Bedell, 1999), and given that both functions may have their own early sensitive periods (Lewis and Maurer, 2005), it seems likely that INS may also interfere with their developments. Nystagmus also interferes with the acquisition of peripheral visual targets in adults (Wang and Dell'Osso, 2007). It seems most likely, therefore, that a strategy of maximizing contrast via transient nystagmus in infancy would eventually be counterproductive.

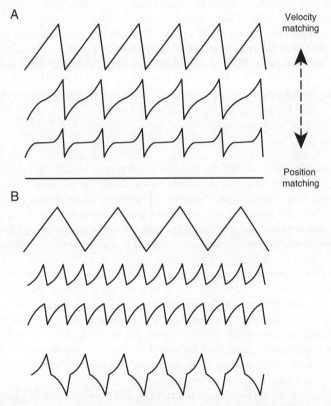

Fig. 37.3 Theoretical waveforms of optimal eye oscillations based on Harris and Berry (2006a) (ordinate is eye position, abscissa is time). A) Optimal waveform depends on relative importance of velocity and position matching, ranging from perfect velocity matching to perfect position matching. Note curvilinear waveforms for intermediate matching similar to some observed INS waveforms. B) Alternative optimal waveforms, which are also observed empirically. For more details and other waveforms see Harris and Berry (2006a, 2006b).

Natural selection would need to drive oculomotor plasticity genes to steer development around a local hazard minimum (i.e. nystagmus) by holding off maximizing visual contrast until foveal vision is sufficiently developed to avoid nystagmus (see Fig. 37.1G). Modularizing is necessary to achieve this, and it is plausible that one reason for the relatively late development of smooth pursuit is to avoid nystagmus. There must be a fine line between developing normal eye movements and INS. If there is a delay in the development of foveal vision (or possibly precocious oculomotor development) then INS will occur. Subsequent reduction in oculomotor plasticity will tend to fix the nystagmus permanently.

An important question is whether INS has a true critical period—can it be reversed? The disappearance of transient nystagmus by the end of the first year (Good et al., 2003) suggests some residual plasticity. In adults, there may be some residual plasticity as foveation periods can be extended by increasing visual demand (Wiggins et al., 2007), but the effect is small. Thus there may be an early window of opportunity for intervention in the first year or so.

Does reversing a sensory defect affect INS? Most congenital sensory defects that induce INS are not reversible with current technology. The obvious exception is congenital cataracts which are frequently removed in early infancy, but the effect on nystagmus is sadly unclear. Some large studies report that nystagmus usually remains, but less than 100%, and so by inference there are cases in which the nystagmus has presumably changed (Ondraek and Lokaj 2003). However, without recording waveforms pre- and post-surgery, it is impossible to distinguish INS from FMNS. Interestingly, Abadi et al. (2006) did record eye movements and found one case where INS converted to FMNS after surgery at 8 weeks of age, implying some degree of reversibility at this young age.

In a tantalizing experiment with gene therapy on dogs with the Leber's congenital amaurosis gene (*RPE65*) and pendular nystagmus, Jacobs et al. (2006) have not only restored retinal function but also eliminated the nystagmus. These are specially bred dogs, however, and it remains to be seen whether it is possible in 'wild type' primates with INS. If it turns out that *FRMD7* genes steer development, then it may be possible to extend the sensitive period, or even re-programme development—if we dare!

Discussion

Ernest Rutherford famously said 'All science is either physics or stamp collecting'. This may seem arrogant today, but evolution was not a consideration and deeply unpopular in his time. Nevertheless, his point is still pertinent today. Is development, whether normal or abnormal, a stamp album of genetic, physiological, and behavioural phenomenology, or is there an underlying 'physics' or logic to it—as in building houses? Surely, we should be able to answer the parent and the child as to why she has developed atypically, not by labelling her with a disorder, but by explaining the logic of development.

Developmental plasticity allows genotypes to cope with variable environments, but it must be under natural selection itself. The fitness (or cost) of plasticity is much debated, but the optimality approach provides a straightforward framework (see 'An 'evo-devo' perspective' and 'Appendix'). To develop a complex stable system in a short time, such as visuomotor control, requires modularity with sensitive periods where necessary. However, it also entails limited connectivity between modules, which reduces the total search space and implies that certain phenotypes cannot develop. I propose that SIF and INS are not only examples of developmental plasticity, but cannot be understood without this type of framework.

Gaze-shifting in afoveate lateral eyed mammals is usually accomplished by tightly coupled head and eye movements, so that saccades seldom occur without a head movement. A prerequisite for the evolution of frontal foveae in large heads (big brains) is the ability to re-orient the foveae frequently and rapidly. Optimizing speed probably favoured the fast saccadic system over the sluggish head movement system, weakening their coupling. The human neonate has poor control over its large head so is especially reliant on the saccadic system. Coupling between eye and head during gaze shifts is still needed, however. Maintaining eccentric gaze with only the eyes is noisy, unstable, and fatiguing

(Abel et al., 1978; Stahl 2001; Whyte et al., 2010), presumably from countering the strong centripetal elastic forces of the extraocular muscles. It pays therefore to use the head for large and/or sustained gaze-shifting (Oomen et al., 2004). This coupling is complex and not fully understood, but presumably requires some transient reduction in VOR gain driven by saccadic signals (discussed earlier). For the infant with SIF, the developing head control is exploited to generate the novel phenotype with head-thrusts. Blinks would seem, at first sight, to be unrelated to horizontal gaze shifting, but there is ample evidence of physiological and behavioural connectivity between these two systems. During blinks, the globe is retracted by co-contraction of recti muscles (or the retractor bulbi). Blinking is also time-locked to horizontal gaze shifts (eye and/or head saccades), presumably to optimize visual down-time (see earlier). These links are seen in other species (rabbit, birds) and are not a recent evolution. Developmental plasticity in SIF modifies this pre-existing connection to facilitate saccades by blinks. Overall, SIF is a condition that exists because of modularity in the first place, but plasticity can overcome the 'dysfunction' to some extent by developing novel head-thrusts and synkinetic blinks. The precise physiological mechanisms for these compensations remain unknown, but it appears that plasticity exploits existing rather than developing new connectivity.

The evolution of foveae also requires exceptional control of eye position to keep images registered on the foveae, which is mediated by the high gain fixation and smooth pursuit systems. Little is known about infant fixation accuracy, but the considerable postnatal development of smooth pursuit is well-documented. We propose that in the infant phenotype, delicate coordination of sensory and motor development is needed to avoid the long-term consequences (high hazards) of nystagmus and amblyopia. Maximizing visual contrast in a visual system dominated by low spatial frequencies will result in oscillatory eye movements that are locally adaptive, but are maladaptive in the long run. Not developing oculomotor strategies to maximize contrast will produce a suboptimal adult phenotype that under-utilizes the foveae. The optimal adult phenotype will be produced by staggering oculomotor development commensurate with sensory development, to avoid INS—an example of steerage around unwanted local hazard minima.

This chapter is an outline, and we are a long way from a complete theory of oculomotor development. There are many gaps to be filled. At the phenomenological level, our stamp album has many sketchy entries including how the timing of head movements and saccades develop both typically and in SIF. Little is known about oculomotor development prior to INS onset (Gottlob, 1997). At the theoretical level, the minimum variance model needs elaborating to include blinks and head movements for typical and atypical gaze shifting, and in the presence of INS. I have not discussed the development of yoking of the eyes because we do not yet have a fitness model for binocularity. Such a model would incorporate the fitness of a variety of phenotypic traits including fusion and Panum's area, accommodation and vergence, stereopsis, tracking of objects that are moving in depth, and the (apparent) advantage of monocular suppression of rivalrous static and moving images. By building such a model into the framework of adaptive developmental plasticity, we should be able to account for a wide variety of normal and abnormal phenomena such as the postnatal development of vergence and accommodation, single vision and stereopsis, strabismus and amblyopia, and monocular asymmetries of OKN and smooth pursuit. This is undoubtedly challenging, but in principle, it should be possible.

I have argued that modularity provides a tradeoff between plasticity and speed of development. Under pressure of natural selection and vulnerability of young phenotypes, one would expect modularity itself to be optimized. However, this is a complex problem (see the house building analogy in the earlier section). Moreover, how evolutionary history constrains development is a fundamental unresolved issue in the evo-devo field. The ideas outlined here have some resonance with the connectionist views of Elman et al. (1996) who proposed that development is constrained by the dynamics of learning in networks. More recent advances in network neuroscience have shown that clustered networks ('small world networks') tend to optimize information transmission and connection distances, but there is little work on learning times/rates (for a recent review, see Bullimore and Sporns, 2009). However, comparisons are typically made between regular lattice, small world and random networks, rather than fully connected networks. It remains to be seen whether this growing field can encompass ontogenetic and plasticity costs.

Finally, I stress the need to step outside our stereotyped 'boxes'. Understanding two-legged goats is as important as understanding the four-legged varieties because it tell us what developmental plasticity can achieve. Unfortunately, the normal–abnormal dichotomy is perpetuated by our organizational structures, with one group of investigators ('basic' scientists in universities) that studies the 'normal' system and screens out abnormal children, and another group ('clinical' scientists in hospitals) that screens out the normal. It is the same developmental system that is being studied. Without understanding the effects of extreme environments, we can never understand developmental plasticity in the typical environment.

Appendix: the cost of plasticity

Fitness is the number of progeny produced down the generations (Dewitt and Langerhans, 2004), or sometimes approximated by the expected number of offspring produced by an individual. For the infant, we consider the main component of fitness to be the probability of survival, which is captured by the survivor function, $S(t)$, defined as the probability of surviving at least until time t. Fitness is then $S(T)$, where T is an age of maturity where reproduction can occur. Following standard survival analysis (Cox and Oakes, 1984), we denote the probability of not surviving (i.e. dying or becoming infertile) in the time interval $(t,t+dt)$ given that the individual was alive at t by the hazard function, $h(t)$. Fitness is then given by $S(T)=\exp(-H(T))$, where $H(T)$ is the cumulative (integrated) hazard: $H(T)=\int_0^T h(t)dt$. Maximizing fitness is the same as maximizing the log survivor function $(S(T))=-H(T)$ or minimizing the cumulative hazard. This simple result provides a framework for the cost of plasticity.

The phenotype is defined by an N dimensional parameter vector $\mathbf{p}=(p_1,\cdots p_N)$ in phenotypic space, where we assume that each parameter can be manipulated independently of the others. In the context of plasticity, the phenotype may be changing in time given by $\mathbf{p}(t)$ which describes the developmental trajectory P. In a specified environment, E, the hazard function is a scalar function of the trait $h_E(t)=h_E(\mathbf{p}(t))$. The cumulative hazard for this path in this environment is given by the line integral along the trajectory P: $H_{P,E}(T)=\int_P h_E(p)ds$ where ds is the infinitesimal line segment, and fitness is $S_{P,E}(T)=\exp(-H_{P,E}(T))$. The average fitness of the genotype is the expected survival probability weighted by the frequency of different environments encountered by its phenotypes.

Acknowledgements

This work was supported by the charity Cerebra. I would like to thank Faith Budge and Jonathan Waddington for their help in writing this chapter. I would also like to thank the anonymous reviewers for their insightful comments.

References

Abadi, R.V. and Bjerre, A. (2002). Motor and sensory characteristics of infantile nystagmus *British Journal of Ophthalmology*, **86**, 1152–1160.

Abadi, R.V. and King-Smith, P.E. (1979). Congenital nystagmus modifies orientational detection. *Vision Research*, **19**, 1409–1411.

Abadi, R.V., Whittle, J.P., and Worfolk, R. (1999). Oscillopsia and tolerance for retinal image movement in congenital nystagmus. *Investigative Ophthalmology and Visual Science*, **40**, 339–345.

Abadi, R.V., Forster, J.E., and Lloyd, C. (2006). Ocular outcomes after bilateral and unilateral infantile cataracts. *Vision Research*, **46**, 940–952.

Abel, L.A., Parker, L., Daroff, R.B., Dell'Osso, L.F. (1978). End-point nystagmus. *Investigative Ophthalmology and Visual Science*, **17**, 539–544.

Allen D., Tyler, C.W., and Norcia, A.M. (1995). Development of grating acuity and contrast sensitivity in the central and peripheral visual field of the human infant. *Vision Research*, **36**, 1945–1953.

Aslin, R. (1981). Development of smooth pursuit in human infants. In D.F. Fischer, R.A. Monty, and E.J. Senders (eds.) *Eye movements: cognition and vision perception* (pp. 31–51). Hillsdale, NJ: Erlbaum.

Banks, M.S. (1980). The development of visual accommodation during early infancy. *Child Development*, **51**, 646–666.

Banks, M.S. and Salapatek, P. (1978). Acuity and contrast sensitivity in 1-, 2-, and 3-month-old human infants. *Investigative Ophthalmology and Visual Science*, **17**, 361–365.

Bateson, P., Barker, D., Clutton-Brock, T., Deb, D., D'Udine, B., Foley, R.A., *et al.* (2004). Developmental plasticity and human health. *Nature*, **430**, 419–421.

van Beers., R.J. (2007). The sources of variability in saccadic eye movements. *Journal of Neuroscience*, **27**, 8757–8770.

Bloch, H., and Carchon, I. (1992). On the onset of eye-head coordination in infants. *Behavioural Brain Research*, **49**, 85–90.

Bullimore, E., and Sporns, O. (2009). Complex brain networks: graph theoretical analysis of structural and functional systems. *Nature Reviews Neuroscience*, **10**, 186–198

Burr, D.C. and Ross, J. (1982). Contrast sensitivity at high velocities. *Vision Research*, **22**, 479–484.

Cassidy, L., Taylor, D., and Harris, C.M. (2000). Abnormal supranuclear eye movements in the child – a practical guide to examination and interpretation. *Survey of Ophthalmology*, **44**, 479–506.

Casteels. I, Harris, C.M., Shawkat, F., and Taylor, D. (1992). Nystagmus in infancy. *British Journal of Ophthalmology*, **76**, 434–437

CEMAS Working Group (2000). *A National Eye Institute Sponsored Workshop and Publication on The Classification of Eye Movement Abnormalities and Strabismus* (CEMAS). Bethesda, MD: National Institutes of Health, National Eye Institute. Available at: http://www.nei.nih.gov.

Cogan, D.G. (1952). A type of ocular motor apraxia presenting jerky head movements. *Transactions of the American Journal of Ophthalmology and Otolaryngology*, **56**, 853–862.

Cordero, L., Clark, D.L., and Urrutia, J.G. (1983). Postrotatory nystagmus in the full-term and premature infant. *International Journal of Pediatric Otorhinolaryngology*, **5**, 47–57.

Cox, D.R. and Oakes, D. (1984). *Analysis of survival data*. London: Chapman and Hall.

Cronin, T.H., Hertle, R.W., Ishikawa, H., Schuman, J.S. (2009). Spectral domain optical coherence tomography for detection of foveal morphology in patients with nystagmus. *Journal of the Association for Pediatric Ophthalmology and Strabismus*, **13**, 563–566.

Cullen, K.E., Huterer, M., Braidwood, D.A., Sylvestre, P.AA. (2004). Time course of vestibuloocular reflex suppression during gaze shifts. *Journal of Neurophysiology*, **92**, 3408–3422.

Date, H., Onoder, O., Tanaka, H., Iwabuchi, K., Uekawa, K., Igarashi, S., *et al.* (2001). Early-onset ataxia with ocular motor apraxia and hypoalbuminemia is caused by mutations in a new HIT superfamily gene. *Nature Genetics*, **29**, 184–188.

Dayton, G.O. and Jones, M.H. (1964). Analysis of characteristics of fixation reflex in infants by use of direct current electro-oculography. *Neurology*, **14**, 1152–1156.

Delinte, A., Gomez, C.M., Decostre, M.F., Crommelink, M., and Roucoux, A. (2002). Amplitude transition function of human express saccades. *Neuroscience Research*, **42**, 21–34.

Dell'Osso, L.F. and Daroff, R.B. (1975). Congenital nystagmus waveforms and foveation strategy. *Documenta Ophthalmologica*, **39**, 155–182.

Dewitt, T.J. and Langerhans, R.B. (2004). Integrated solutions to environmental heterogeneity. Theory of multimoment reaction norms. In T.J. Dewitt and S.M. Scheiner (eds.) *Phenotypic plasticity. Functional and conceptual approaches* (pp. 98–111). Oxford: Oxford University Press.

Dobkins. K.R., Anderson, C.M., and Lia, B. (1999). Infant temporal contrast sensitivity functions (tCSFs) mature earlier for luminance than for chromatic stimuli: evidence for precocious magnocellular development? *Vision Research*, **39**, 3223–3239

Dorey, S.E., Neveu, M.M., Burton, L.C., Sloper, J.J., and Holder, G.E. (2003). The clinical features of albinism and their correlation with visual evoked potentials. *British Journal of Ophthalmology*, **87**, 767–772.

Elman, J.L., Bates, E.A., Johnson, M.H., Karmiloff-Smith, A., Parisi, D., and Plunkett, K. (1996). *Rethinking innateness: A connectionist perspective on development*. Cambridge, MA: MIT Press.

Evinger, C., Manning, K.A., Pellegrini, J.J., Basso, M.A., Powers, A.S., and Sibony. P.A. (1994). Not looking while leaping: the linkage of blinking and saccadic gaze shifts. *Experimental Brain Research*, **100**, 337–344.

Fantz, R.L., Ordy, J.M., and Udelf, M.S. (1962). Maturation of pattern vision in infants during the first six months. *Journal of Comparative and Physiological Psychology*. **55**, 907–917

Farroni, T., Simion, F., Umiltà, C. and Barba, B.D. (1999). The gap effect in newborns. *Developmental Science*, **2**, 174–196.

Fogarty, C. and Stern, J.A. (1989). Eye movements and blinks: their relationship to higher cognitive processes. *International Journal of Psychophysiology*, **8**, 35–42.

Garbutt, S. and Harris, C.M. (2000). Abnormal vertical optokinetic nystagmus in infants and children. *British Journal of Ophthalmology*, **84**, 451–455.

Garbutt, S., Harwood, M.R., and Harris, C.M. (2001). A comparison of the main sequence of reflexive saccades and the quick phases of optokinetic nystagmus. *British Journal of Ophthalmology*, **85**, 1477–1483.

Garbutt, S., Harwood, M., and Harris, C.M. (2006). Infant saccades are not slow. *Developmental Medicine and Child Neurology*, **48**, 662–667.

Gavrilets, S. (2004). *Fitness landscapes and the origin of species*. Princeton, New Jersey: Princeton University Press.

Gilchrist, I.D., Brown, V., and Findlay, J.M. (1997). Saccades without eye movements. *Nature*, **390**, 130–131.

Godfrey-Smith, P. (2009). *Darwinian populations and natural selection*. Oxford: Oxford University Press.

Good, W.V., Hou, C., and Carden, S.M. (2003). Transient, idiopathic nystagmus in infants. *Developmental Medicine and Child Neurology*, **45**, 304–307.

Goosens, H.H. and van Opstal, A.J. (2000a). Blink-perturbed saccades in monkey. I. Behavioral analysis. *Journal of Neurophysiology*, **83**, 3411–3429.

Goosens, H.H. and van Opstal, A.J. (2000b). Blink-perturbed saccades in monkey. II. Superior colliculus activity. *Journal of Neurophysiology*, **83**, 3430–3452.

Gottlob, I. (1997). Infantile nystagmus. Development documented eye movement recording. *Investigative Ophthalmology and Visual Science*, **38**,767–773.

Harris, C.M. (1995). Does saccadic under-shoot minimize saccadic flight-time? A monte-carlo study. *Vision Research*, **35**, 691–701.

Harris, C.M. and Berry, D. (2006a). A distal model of congenital nystagmus as non-linear adaptive oscillations. *Nonlinear Dynamics*, **44**, 1–4.

Harris, C.M. and Berry, D. (2006b). A developmental model of infantile nystagmus. *Seminars in Ophthalmology*, **21**, 63–69.

Harris, C.M. and Wolpert, D.M. (1998). Signal-dependent noise determines motor planning. *Nature*, **394**, 780–784.

Harris, C.M. and Wolpert, D.M. (2006). The main sequence of saccades optimizes speed-accuracy trade-off. *Biological Cybernetics*, **95**, 21–29.

Harris, C.M., Jacobs, M., Shawkat, F., and Taylor, D. (1993). The development of saccadic accuracy in the first 7 months. *Clinical Visual Sciences*, **8**, 85–96.

Harris, C.M., Shawkat, F., Russell-Eggitt, I., Wilson, J., and Taylor, D. (1996). Intermittent horizontal saccade failure ('ocular motor apraxia') in children. *British Journal of Ophthalmology*, **80**, 151–158.

Harris, C.M., Hodgkins, P.R., Kriss, A., Chong, W.K., Thompson, D.S., Mezey, L.E., Shawkat, F.S., Taylor, D.S.I. and Wilson, J. (1998). Familial congenital saccade initiation failure and isolated cerebellar vermis hypoplasia. *Developmental Medicine and Child Neurology*, **40**, 775–779.

Harwood, M.R., Madelain, L., Krauzlis, R.J., Wallman, J. (2008). Spatial scale of attention strongly modulates saccade latencies. *Journal of Neurophysiology*, **99**, 1743–1757.

He, X., Gu, F., Wang, Y., Yan, J., Zhang, M., Huang, S., *et al.* (2008). A novel mutation in FRMD7 causing X-linked idiopathic congenital nystagmus in a large family. *Molecular Vision*, **14**, 56–60.

von Hofsten, VC. and Rosander, K. (1996). The development of gaze control and predictive tracking in young infants. *Vision Research*, **36**, 81–96.

Horimoto, N., Hepper, P.G., Shahidullah, S., and Koyanagi, T. (1993). Fetal eye movements. *Ultrasound in Obstetrics and Gynecology*, **3**, 362–369.

Huang, Y-Y., Rinner, O., Hedinger, P., Liu, S-C., and Neuhauss, C.F. (2006). Oculomotor instabilities in zebrafish mutant belladonna: a behavioral model for congenital nystagmus caused by axonal misrouting. *Journal of Neuroscience*, **26**, 9873–9880.

Jacobs, J.B., DellOsso, L.F., Hertle, R.W., Acland, G.M., and Bennett, J. (2006). Eye movement recordings as an effectiveness indicator of gene therapy in RPE65-deficient canines: implications for the ocular motor system. *Investigative Ophthalmology and Visual Science*, **47**, 2865–2875.

Jacobs M, Harris CM, Shawkat F, Taylor D (1997) Smooth pursuit development in infants. *Australian and New Zealand Journal of Ophthalmology* **25**, 199–206.

Jan, J.E., Kearney, S., Groenveld, M., Sargent, M.A., and Poskitt, K.J. (1998). Speech, cognition, and imaging studies in congenital ocular motor apraxia. *Developmental Medicine and Child Neurology*, **40**, 95–99.

John, F.M., Bromham, N.R., Woodhouse, J.M., and Candy, T.R. (2004). Spatial vision deficits in infants and children with Down syndrome. *Investigative Ophthalmology and Visual Science*, **45**, 1566–1572.

Jones, K.E., Hamilton. A.F., and Wolpert, D.M. (2001). Sources of signal-dependent noise during isometric force production. *Journal of Neurophysiology*, **88**, 1533–1544.

Joseph, R. (2000). Fetal brain behaviour and cognitive development. *Developmental Review*, **20**, 81–98.

Kaplan, Y., Vargel, I., Kansu, T., Akin, B., Rohmann, E., Kamaci, S., *et al.* (2008). Skewed X inactivation in an X linked nystagmus family resulted from a novel, p.R229G, missensense mutation in the FRMD7 gene. *British Journal of Ophthalmology*, **92**, 135–141.

Kelly, D.H. (1985). Visual processing of moving stimuli. *Journal of the Optical Society of America A*, **2**, 215–225.

Kremenitzer, J.P., Vaughan, H.G., Kurtzberg, D. and Dowling, K. (1979). Smooth-pursuit eye movements in the newborn infant. *Child Development*, **50**, 442–448.

Lachance, P.E.D., Chaudhuri, A. (2004). Microarray analysis of developmental plasticity in monkey primary visual cortex. *Journal of Neurochemistry*, **88**, 1455–1469.

Lambert, S.R., Kriss, A., Gresty, M., Benton, S., and Taylor, D. (1989). Joubert syndrome. *Archives of Ophthalmology*, **107**, 709–713.

Lawrenson, J.G., Birhah, R. and Murphy, P.J. (2005). Tear-film lipid layer morphology and corneal sensation in the development of blinking in neonates and infants. *Journal of Anatomy*, **206**, 265–270.

Lawson, J., Shawkat, F., Timms, C., Thompson, D., Kriss, A., Russell-Eggitt, I., *et al.* (1996). Eye movements in children with Down's syndrome. *Investigative Ophthalmology and Visual Science (Supplement)*, **37**, 278.

Leigh, R.J. and Zee, D.S. (2006). *The Neurology of Eye Movements* (4th ed).New York: Oxford University Press.

Lengyel, D., Weinacht, S., Charlier, J., and Gottlob, I. (1998). The development of visual pursuit during the first months of life. *Graefe's Archive for Clinical and Experimental Ophthalmology*, **236**, 440–444.

Lewis, T.L. and Maurer, D. (2005). Multiple sensitive periods in human visual development: evidence from visually deprived children. *Developmental Psychobiology*, **46**, 163–183.

Li, N., Wang, L., Cui, L., Zhang, Li., Dai, S., Li, H., *et al.* (2008). Five novel mutations of the FRMD7 gene in Chinese families with X-linked infantile nystagmus. *Molecular Vision*, **14**, 733–738.

Liao, K., Kumar, A.N., Han, Y.N.H., Grammer, V.A., Gedeon, B.T., and Leigh, R.J. (2005). Comparison of velocity waveforms of eye and head saccades. In S. Ramat and D. Straumann (eds.) *Clinical and Basic Oculomotor Research: in Honor of David S. Zee, Volume 1039* (pp. 477–479). New York: New York Academy of Sciences.

Liu, J.Y., Ren, X., Yang, X., Guo, T., Yao, Q., Li, L., Dai, X., Zhang, M., Wang, L., Liu, M., and Wang, Q.K. (2007). Identification of a novel GPR143 mutation in a large Chinese family with congenital nystagmus as the most prominent and consistent manifestation. *Journal of Human Genetics*, **52**, 565–570.

Marr, J.E., Green, S.H., and Willshaw, H.E. (2005). Neurodevelopmental implications of ocular motor apraxia. *Developmental Medicine and Child Neurology*, **47**, 815–819.

Mays, L.E. and Morisse, D.W. (1995). Electrical stimulation of the pontine omnipause area inhibits eye blink. *Journal of the American Optometric Association*, **66**, 419–422.

Matsuzawa, M. and Shimojo, S. (1997). Infants' fast saccades in the gap paradigm and development of visual attention. *Infant Behavior and Development*, **20**, 449–455.

McGhee, G. (2007). *The geometry of evolution*. Cambridge: Cambridge University Press.

McMullen, C.A., Andrade, F.H., and Stahl, J.S. (2004). Functional and genomic changes in the mouse ocular motor system in response to light deprivation from birth. *Journal of Neuroscience*, **24**,161–169.

McSorley, E. and Findlay, J.M. (2003). Saccade target selection in visual search: accuracy improves when more distracters are present. *Journal of Vision*, **11**, 877–892.

Ohm, J. (1958). *Nystagmus und Schielen bei Sehschwachen und Blinden*. Stuttgart: Enke.

Optican, L.M. and Zee, D.S. (1984). A hypothetical explanation of congenital nystagmus. *Biological Cybernetics*, **50**, 119–134.

Ondraek, O. and Lokaj, M. (2003). Visual outcome after congenital cataract surgery. Long term clinical results. *Scripta Medica (Brno)*, **76**, 95–102.

Oomen, B.S., Smith, R.M., Stahl, J.S. (2004). The influence of future gaze orientation upon eye-head coupling during saccades. *Experimental Brain Research*, **155**, 9–18.

Pigliucci, M. (2001). *Phenotypic plasticity; beyond nature and nurture*. Baltimore, MD: John Hopkins University Press.

Rambold, H., Sprenger, A., Helmchen, C. (2002). Effects of voluntary blinks on saccades, vergence eye movements, and saccade-vergence interactions in humans. *Journal of Neurophysiology*, **88**, 1220–1233.

Rambold, H., Moser, A., Zurowski, B., Gbadamosi, J., Kompf, D., Sprenger, A., *et al.* (2006). Saccade initiation in ocular motor apraxia. *Journal of Neurology*, **253**, 950–952.

Reinecke, R.D., Guo, S., and Goldstein, H.P. (1988). Waveform evolution in infantile nystagmus: an electro-oculographic study of 35 cases. *Binocular Vision*, **3**, 191–202.

Richards, J.E. and Hunter, S.K. (1997). Peripheral stimulus localization by infants with eye and head movements during visual attention. *Vision Research*, **37**, 3021–3035.

Rosenberg, M.L. and Wilson, E. (1987). Congenital ocular motor apraxia without head thrusts. *Journal of Clinical Neuro-Ophthalmology*, **7**, 26–28

Roucoux, A., Culee, C. and Roucoux, M. (1983). Development of fixation and pursuit eye movements in human infants. *Behavioural Brain Research*, **10**, 133–139.

Rütsche, A., Baumann, A., Jiang, X., and Mojon, D.S. (2006). Development of visual pursuit in the first 6 years of life. *Graefe's Archive for Clinical and Experimental Ophthalmology*, **244**, 1406–1411.

Schlosser, G., and Wagner, G.P. (2004). *Modularity in development and evolution*. Chicago, IL: University of Chicago Press.

Schorderet, D.F., Tiab, L., Gaillard, M., Lorenz, B., Klainguti, G., Kerrison, J.B., *et al.* (2007). Novel mutation in FRMD7 in X-linked congenital nystagmus. *Mutation in Brief #963 Online. Human Mutation*, **28**, 525.

Self, J. and Lotery, A. (2007). A review of the molecular genetics of congenital idiopathic nystagmus (CIN). *Ophthalmic Genetics*, **28**, 187–191.

Self, J.E., Shawkat, F., Malpas, C.T., Thomas, N.S., Harris, C.M., Hodgkins, P.R., *et al.* (2007). Allelic variation of the FRMD7 gene in congenital nystagmus. *Archives of Ophthalmology*, **125**, 1255–1263.

Seo, J.H., Yu, Y.S., Kim, J.H., Choung, H.K., Heo, J.W., Kim, and S-J. (2007). Correlation of visual acuity with foveal hypoplasia grading by optical coherence tomography in albinism. *Ophthalmology*, **114**, 1547–1551.

Shawkat, F.S., Kingsley, D., Kendall, B., Russell-Eggitt, I., Taylor, D.S.I, and Harris, C.M. (1995). Neuro-radiological and eye movement correlates in children with intermittent saccade failure: "ocular motor apraxia". *Neuropediatrics*, **26**, 298–305.

Shawkat, F., Kriss, A., Thompson, D., Russell-Eggitt, I., Taylor, D., and Harris, C.M. (2001). Outcome of children presenting with asymmetric pendular nystagmus. *Developmental Medicine and Child Neurology*, **43**, 622–627.

Shea, S.L. and Aslin, R.N. (1990). Oculomotor responses to step-ramp targets by young human infants. *Vision Research*, **30**, 1077–1092.

Shiels, A., Bennett, T.M., Prince, J.B., and Tychsen, L. (2007). X-linked idiopathic infantile nystagmus associated with a missense mutation in FRMD7. *Molecular Vision*, **13**, 22333–22241.

Slijper, E.J. (1942). Biologic-anatomical investigations on the bipepdal gait and upright posture in mammals, with special reference to a little goat, born without forelegs 1. *Proceedings of the Koninklijke Nederlandse Akadamie Wetenschappen*, **45**, 288–295.

Stahl, J.S. (2001). Eye-head coordination and the variation of eye-movement accuracy with orbial eccentricity. *Experimental Brain Research*, **136**, 200–210

Stark, L., Zangemesiter, W.H., Edwards, J., Grinberg, J., Jones, A., Lehman, S., *et al.* (1980). Head rotation trajectories compared with eye saccades by main sequence relationships. *Investigative Ophthalmology and Visual Science*, **19**, 986–988

Tarpey, P., Thomas, S., Sarvananthan, N., Mallya, U., Lisgo, S., Talbot, C.J., *et al.* (2006). Mutations in FRMD7, a newly identified member of the FERM family, cause X-linked idiopathic congenital nystagmus. *Nature Genetics*, **38**, 1242–1244.

Thorn, F. Gwiazda, J., Cruz, A.V., Bauer, J.A., and Held, R. (1994). The development of eye alignment, convergence, and sensory binocularity in young infants. *Investigative Ophthalmology and Visual Science*, **25**, 544–553.

Tondel, G.M. and Candy, T.R. (2007). Human infants' accommodation responses to dynamic stimui. *Investigative Ophthalmology and Visual Science*, **48**, 949–956.

Tusa, R.J., Zee, D.S., Hain, T.C., and Simonsz, H.J. (1992). Voluntary control of congenital nystagmus. *Clinical Visual Sciences*, **7**, 195–210.

Tusa, R.J., Mustari, M.J., Burrows, A.F., and Fuchs, A.F. (2001). Gaze-stabilizing deficits and latent nystagmus in monkeys with brief, early-onset visual deprivation: eye movement recordings. *Journal of Neurophysiology*, **86**, 651–661.

Ukwade, M.T. and Bedell, H.E. (1999). Stereothresholds in persons with congenital nystagmus and in normal observers during comparable retinal image motion. *Vision Research*, **39**, 2963–2973.

van Donkelaar, P., Saavedra, S., and Woollacott, M. (2007). Multiple saccades are more automatic than single saccades. *Journal of Neurophysiology*, **97**, 3148–3151.

Virsu, V., Rovamo, J., Laurinen, P. and Näsänen, R. (1982). Temporal contrast sensitivity and cortical magnification. *Vision Research*, **22**, 1211–1217.

Wang, Z.I. and Dell'Osso, L.F. (2007). Being "slow to see" is a dynamic visual function consequence of infantile nystagmus syndrome: Model predictions and patient data identify stimulus timing as its cause. *Vision Research*, **47**, 1550–1560.

Weinacht, S., Kind, C., Mönting, J.S., and Gottlob, I. (1999). Visual development in preterm and full-term infants: a prospective masked study. *Investigative Ophthalmology and Visual Science*, **40**, 346–353.

Weiss, A.H., and Kelly, J.P. (2007). Acuity development in infantile nystagmus. *Investigative Ophthalmology and Visual Science*, **48**, 4093–4099.

West-Eberhard, M.J. (2003). *Developmental plasticity and evolution*. Oxford: Oxford University Press.

Whyte, C.A., Petrock, A.M., and Rosenberg, M. (2010). Occurrence of physiologic gaze-evoked nystagmus at small angles of gaze. *Investigative Ophthalmology and Visual Science*, **51**, 2476–2478.

Wiggins, D., Woodhouse, M., Margrain, T.H., Harris, C.M., and Erichsen. J.T. (2007). Infantile nystagmus adapts to visual demand. *Investigative Ophthalmology and Visual Science*, **48**, 2089–2094.

Win, T.H. and Laws, D.E. (2006). Ocular motor apraxia. *British Journal of Ophthalmology*, **90**, 1045

Westheimer, G., and McKee, S.P. (1975). Visual acuity in the presence of retinal-image motion. *Journal of the Optical Society of America A*, **65**,847–850.

Wuensche, A. (2004). Basins of attraction in network dynamics: A conceptual framework for biomolecular networks, chapter 13. In G. Schlosser and G.P. Wagner (eds.) *Modularity in development and evolution* (pp. 288–311). Chicago: Chicago University Press.

Zee, D.S., Yee, R.D., Singer, and H.S. (1977). Congenital ocular motor apraxia. *Brain*, **100**, 581–599.

Zee, D.S., Leigh, R.J., and Mathieu-Millaire, F. (1980). Cerebellar control of ocular gaze stability. *Annals of Neurology*, **7**, 37–40.

Zee, D.S., Chu, F.C., Leigh, J., Savino, P.J., Schatz, N.J., Reingold, D.B., and *et al.* (1983). Blink-saccade synkinesis. *Neurology*, **33**, 1233–1236.

Zhang, B., Liu, Z., Zhao, G., Xie, X., Yin, X., Hu, Z., *et al.* (2007). Novel mutations of the FRMD7 gene in X-linked congenital motor nystagmus. *Molecular Vision*, **13**, 1674–1679.

Zhang, Q., Xiao, X., Li, S., and Guo, X. (2007). FRMD7 mutations in Chinese families with X-linked congenital motor nystagmus. *Molecular Vision*, **13**, 1375–1378.

Zhou, P., Wang, Z., Zhang, J., Hu Landian, and Kong, X. (2008). Identification of a novel GPR143 deletion in a Chinese family with X-linked congenital nystagmus. *Molecular Vision*, **14**, 1015–1019.

CHAPTER 38

Eye movements in psychiatric patients

Jennifer E. McDowell, Brett A. Clementz, and John A. Sweeney

Abstract

The study of eye movements in psychiatric disorders reflects two primary avenues of scientific investigation: 1) a search for valid markers that could identify risk for developing an illness, and 2) investigation into the neurobiological correlates of serious mental illness. The two types of eye movements most frequently studied for these purposes are smooth pursuit and saccades. The following summary provides information on deficits commonly reported in people with severe psychiatric conditions, along with any putative effects of psychiatric medications. When available, information about eye movement performance in the biological relatives of people with psychiatric illness also is reviewed. Finally, a brief synopsis of the neural substrates of eye movement abnormalities in psychiatric disorders is presented.

Introduction

Use of eye movement measures to assess neurological functioning has a long history (Diefendorf and Dodge, 1908). In patients with head injury, stroke, and movement disorders, a bedside evaluation of eye movements can efficiently yield useful information about the presence or absence of lateralized cortical and subcortical abnormalities (Leigh and Zee, 2006). Deviation from normal patterns of eye movements can include difficulty maintaining gaze, slow and/or poorly synchronized reaction times (how long it takes the eyes to initiate a movement), reduced movement accuracy (how well the eye movement locates and/or acquires the target), and/or directional errors.

In one of the first studies to use laboratory procedures to measure eye movements in any clinical population, Diefendorf and Dodge (1908) reported that 'the most marked variations are found in the pendulum pursuit-movements in dementia praecox [i.e. schizophrenia], where a marked hesitation to fall into the swing of the pendulum was found even in the mildest cases' (p. 468). They also noted that 'this peculiarity . . . was found in other patients [without dementia praecox] only where the disease process has produced marked deterioration' (p. 468). Despite Emil Kraepelin (1919/1971, p. 6) noting the potential significance of Diefendorf and Dodge's (1908) report for understanding the neuropathology of psychotic illness, this interesting area of investigation was rarely revisited (Couch and Fox, 1934) until the 1970s when Holzman and colleagues (1973) published a report of pursuit tracking impairment in schizophrenia patients and their relatives.

Since then, studies of eye movement abnormalities have been an active area in psychiatric research (Calkins et al., 2008; Clementz and Sweeney, 1990; Hutton and Ettinger, 2006; Levy et al., 2000; McDowell et al., 2008; Sweeney et al., 2007). Sustained efforts in this field reflect two primary avenues of scientific investigation. First, of greatest interest historically, have been attempts to develop valid 'intermediate phenotypes' (or 'endophenotypes'). These terms are applied to anatomical, physiological, or behavioural measures that can be quantified in the laboratory, are associated with the disorder of interest and are more closely associated with the predisposing genotype than clinical symptoms, such as psychosis (Gottesman and Gould, 2003). Ideally, endophenotypes are supported with established animal model analogues and rooted in modern cognitive or molecular neuroscience, and have the potential to resolve heritability and genetic heterogeneity of complex psychiatric diagnostic phenotypes (Braff et al., 2007; Iacono and Clementz, 1993). Second, of more recent and yet extensive interest, has been the use of specific eye movement abnormalities to investigate the neuropathological correlates of serious mental illness.

Numerous characteristics make eye movement performance particularly useful for investigating the neuropathological correlates of psychiatric disorders. First, eye movement tasks are easy to understand and require fairly simple behavioural responses, making them adaptable across a wide range of ages and illness severities. Second, eye movements can be elicited and measured precisely using a number of reliable methods (e.g. Smyrnis, 2008). Stimuli can be presented easily on computer screens or similar media, and are recorded using a number of available methods, including electro-oculography (EOG), infra-red oculography, or magnetic search coil (Young and Sheena, 1975). These methods use different technologies to provide a record of eye position over time, and changes in eye position relative to relevant stimuli to allow for later quantification of eye movement characteristics. Third, the neural circuitry supporting eye movements is particularly well understood based on an extensive literature that ranges from single unit recordings in primates (Johnston and Everling, 2008) to lesion (Pierrot-Deseilligny et al., 2004) and neuroimaging studies (McDowell et al., 2008; Sweeney et al., 2007) in humans. As such, eye movements have been extensively studied with great success in investigations of behavioural and brain alterations in psychiatric conditions, including schizophrenia, affective disorders, anxiety disorders (such as obsessive–compulsive disorder, OCD) and developmental disorders (such as attention deficit hyperactivity disorder (ADHD) and autism).

In navigating the environment, primates rely on various types of eye movements including: 1) smooth pursuit to follow a moving object's trajectory and 2) saccades to shift gaze between objects of interest in the visual field. Smooth pursuit occurs in response to a stimulus moving at a relatively slow rate (i.e. watching a train move across a distant horizon). Saccades rapidly redirect gaze from one location of interest to another (i.e. moving from one word to another on a page of text, or from one face to another in a crowded room).

Smooth pursuit and saccades are the two types of eye movements most commonly studied in psychiatric subjects. Despite the different characteristics and historical separation of these two types of motor output, there is increasing evidence for partial overlap of the supporting neural circuitry such that within a number of cortical and subcortical regions identified as common to both types, there appear to be subregions specialized for support of each type of response (Krauzlis, 2005; Liston and Krauzlis, 2005; Rosano et al., 2002). Indeed, this may explain some of the abnormalities observed in both smooth pursuit and saccadic systems seen in some neurological and psychiatric conditions.

The following review provides information on smooth pursuit and saccadic deficits commonly reported in people with various psychiatric conditions, as well as any putative effects of psychiatric medications. When available, information about eye movement performance in the biological relatives of people with psychiatric illness also is presented. Finally, a brief synopsis of the neural substrates of eye movement abnormalities in psychiatric disorders is offered.

General description of smooth pursuit

Smooth pursuit eye movements are evoked by moving visual stimuli and serve to maintain the image of the moving object on the fovea (the most sensitive part of the retina). In the laboratory, a stimulus (e.g. a small dot) is typically presented moving across a computer-controlled display screen. Different types of moving stimuli are optimal for evaluation of various components of smooth pursuit, including: pendular or sinusoid motion (a target that slides repeatedly and predictably across the screen from one side to the other with slower motion at the extremes and faster motion at the midpoint), ramp stimuli (a target that moves at a constant velocity from one location to another), and step-ramp or Rashbass (1961) stimuli (in which a target starts at a fixation point then jumps some distance in one direction before moving at a constant velocity in the opposite direction). These tasks are differentially sensitive to problems perceiving and using visual motion information, problems predicting target motion or problems making sensorimotor transformations (Chen et al., 2002; Sweeney et al., 1999; Thaker et al., 1996).

On pursuit tasks, subjects are instructed to follow the target as closely and accurately as possible. The periods of pursuit can be quantified, as can the frequency and characteristics of accompanying saccades that are sometimes generated. Indices of performance derived from smooth pursuit recordings are characterized as either global or specific measures (see Fig. 38.1, from Lencer et al., 2008).

Global measures

Global assessments capture the general, overall impression or 'fit' of eye-to-target synchrony using qualitative or quantitative measures. Early studies used primarily qualitative measures that consisted

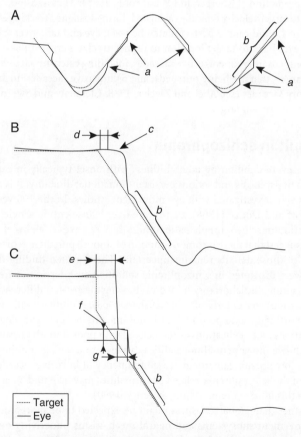

Fig. 38.1 Smooth pursuit paradigms showing target and eye position data for the A) oscillating, B) ramp, and C) step ramp tasks. *a* indicates corrective catch-up saccades; *b*, period when pursuit maintenance is assessed; *c*, pursuit initiation in the pure ramp task; *d*, pursuit initiation latency; *e*, latency of the initial catch-up saccade; *f*, saccade error of the initial catch-up saccade; and *g*, pursuit initiation in the step ramp task. From Lencer et al., (2008), Copyright © 2008 American Medical Association. All rights reserved.

of an observer's visual assessment of the recording as 'normal' or 'abnormal' (Holzman et al., 1973). Global quantitative measures include measures of 'root mean square error' (RMSE of the eye position relative to the target position such that greater values indicate greater disparity between the two (Iacono and Lykken, 1979)) and the total number of saccades generated during smooth pursuit (Calkins et al., 2008; Cegalis and Sweeney 1979; O'Driscoll et al., 2008).

Specific measures

In contrast to global measures, specific measures of smooth pursuit performance are more informative for discerning whether poor pursuit reflects a primary problem in the pursuit system, a primary problem in the saccadic system as indicated by the disruption of tracking by intrusive, extraneous saccades, or the disruption of both of these components of eye movement control. The following specific measures have been frequently quantified in studies of smooth pursuit control among psychiatric patients: 1) pursuit initiation is the time (in milliseconds) it takes to begin to pursue a moving target; 2) 'open loop' pursuit is evaluated by examining eye acceleration during the first 100 ms of target movement, with 'open loop' referring to the fact that movements during this period are driven solely by sensory input on the retina, as it is too early for any contribution from visual feedback or target prediction (Lisberger and Westbrook, 1985); 3) closed-loop pursuit gain is the ratio of eye velocity to target velocity typically calculated during sustained tracking after the first 100 ms of pursuit (a value of 1.0 indicates a perfect match between eye and target velocities); 4) 'catch-up' saccades bring the eyes back to target location to reduce tracking error if pursuit gain is too slow (more generally, compensatory, or corrective saccades, including catch-up saccades, re-align the eyes to slowly moving targets that are being pursued); and 5) intrusive saccades, including square wave jerks and anticipatory saccades (see Abel and Ziegler, 1988; Clementz and Sweeney, 1990), increase position error between eye and target.

Smooth pursuit in schizophrenia

Schizophrenia is a severe debilitating mental illness with onset typically in early adulthood and marked by episodes of psychosis and serious persistent functional disability. It is also the psychiatric illness most extensively investigated with eye movement studies. In the 100 years after the initial report by Diefendorf and Dodge (1908), there were over 900 scientific articles published on eye movement dysfunction in schizophrenia patients and their relatives (Calkins et al, 2008). The vast majority of studies suggest that there is some disruption of smooth pursuit in schizophrenia, although the precise nature of those deficits remains uncertain. The repeated finding that global smooth pursuit measures were disrupted in schizophrenia solidified an interest this field (see Levy et al., 1993); they are still among the laboratory measures showing the greatest differences between healthy and schizophrenia groups (see O'Driscoll and Callahan, 2008). A problem with the global measures, however, is that reporting general poor pursuit is not informative in a neurological sense because: 1) numerous conditions and medications are associated with poor smooth pursuit performance and 2) multiple types of eye movement abnormalities can lead to a deficient ability to track a slowly moving object (e.g. low pursuit gain, an increased frequency of intrusive saccades). Differentiating the precise nature of the schizophrenia-related abnormalities may help understand changes in brain function specific to this illness (Clementz and Sweeney, 1990).

Using specific rather than global measures might be expected to be more informative for determining the eye movement subsystems and neural mechanisms underlying overall poor pursuit observed in schizophrenia (Abel and Ziegler, 1988; Clementz and Sweeney, 1990; Sweeney et al., 1999). Among specific pursuit measures, reduced closed loop gain is commonly identified in schizophrenia (Hutton et al., 1998; Grove et al., 1994; Levy et al., 1994; Sweeney et al., 1994a) and was among the most informative specific measures in a recent meta-analysis (O'Driscoll and Callahan, 2008). Abnormalities among people with schizophrenia on this measure, however, are related to target characteristics such as predictability (Farber et al., 1997; Lencer et al., 2008). Open loop eye acceleration is also disrupted in schizophrenia (Clementz and McDowell, 1994; Lencer et al., 2008; Sweeney et al., 1998; Thaker et al., 1996), an abnormality which may be more prominent in deficit syndrome patients (Ross et al., 1996). Finally, a large proportion of the variance in smooth pursuit error among people with schizophrenia may be associated with an inability to properly predict the subsequent motion of slowly moving targets, maintain eye velocity at the predicted target velocity, and/or adjust eye movement velocity during less predictable tracking tasks (e.g. Chen et al., 1999; Lencer et al., 2008; Thaker et al., 1998, 1999).

The nature of the impairment can be examined further by quantifying the type and rate of saccades made during smooth pursuit. Several groups have demonstrated an increased frequency of saccades in people with schizophrenia compared with both normal and psychiatric comparison subjects (Hutton et al., 2001; Lencer et al., 2008; Sweeney et al., 1994a; for review, see Levy et al., 1994). Some groups have reported increased anticipatory saccades, in which the eyes seem to move ahead of the target apparently anticipating its trajectory (Abel et al., 1991; Clementz et al., 1994; Friedman et al., 1995; Sweeney et al., 1994a). Other reports document increased corrective saccades in schizophrenia, which presumably serve to compensate for lower gain pursuit (Fletchner et al., 1997; Levy et al., 1994; Lencer et al., 2008). Overall, people with schizophrenia appear to have reduced pursuit gain (an inability to match eye velocity to target velocity) and an increased rate of corrective saccades, findings consistent with dysfunction in some aspect of smooth pursuit control. It is uncertain from these results, however, whether deficient processing of visual motion information, a problem translating that information into a motor command, or an abnormality the motor output command itself accounts for the smooth pursuit findings.

Impact of antipsychotic medication on smooth pursuit

Smooth pursuit studies in schizophrenia most frequently include participants treated with various antipsychotic medications (with a few notable exceptions; e.g. Hutton et al., 1998, 2001a; Sweeney et al., 1999; Thaker et al., 1999). In general, studies of chronic patients who discontinued medications and those studied shortly after withdrawal from first-generation (or 'typical') antipsychotics indicate mostly the same smooth pursuit abnormalities as those observed among medicated patients (Gooding et al., 1994; Litman et al., 1994; Sweeney et al., 1999; Thaker et al., 1999; see review by Ettinger and Kumari, 2003). Further, first-episode schizophrenia patients with no or limited previous treatment have pursuit impairments indicating that eye tracking deficits are not a consequence of chronic drug therapy and that they are present at the time of illness onset (Friedman et al., 1992; Hutton et al., 1998 and 2001a; Sweeney et al., 1999). Longitudinal studies also typically indicate pursuit performance is relatively unaffected by first-generation antipsychotic medication (Muir et al., 1992; Schlenker and Cohen, 1995; Sweeney et al., 1998), although some studies showed greater deficits in treated than untreated chronically ill patients (Hutton et al., 1998 and 2001a; Sweeney et al., 1994b), perhaps an indication that greater illness severity is associated with more severe neurobehavioural deficits.

Contrary to the findings with first-generation medications, second-generation (or 'atypical') antipsychotics may deleteriously impact pursuit performance. For instance, decreased pursuit gain was reported in subjects with schizophrenia taking second-generation antipsychotic medications as compared to those taking first-generation medications or placebo (Litman et al., 1994). Additionally, a longitudinal study of medication effects on antipsychotic-naïve subjects indicated that pursuit gain was significantly reduced after treatment with second-generation medications (Lencer et al., 2008). After subjects had been on second-generation medications for 6 weeks, closed and open loop gain were reduced, and that effect persisted when patients were tested again at 6 months (with possible normalization by 1 year). Lencer et al. (2008) theorized that the persistent smooth pursuit abnormalities might be associated with antagonism at serotonergic 2A receptors, as that is a key difference between second and first-generation antipsychotics. In sum, while first-generation antipsychotics probably have negligible effects on smooth pursuit at least in lower doses (Reilly et al., 2008), second-generation antipsychotic medication appears more likely to impair pursuit, particularly in the initial months after treatment initiation.

Smooth pursuit in schizophrenia relatives

Clinically unaffected biological relatives of people with schizophrenia do not manifest the confound of treatment with antipsychotic medication or the deleterious effects of having a chronic disease, but still possess genetic risk for illness. Typically these relatives show deficits similar in form but, on average, with less severity compared with those observed among schizophrenia probands (a term referring to participants recruited into a study because they have the illness) (Clementz et al., 1995; Holzman et al., 1974; Iacono et al., 1992; Thaker et al., 1998). In a pair of studies, Ross and colleagues (Ross, 2003; Ross et al., 2002) reported that schizophrenia probands and their biological relatives showed reduced pursuit gain, an increased proportion of catch-up saccades, and a higher frequency of intrusive saccades (see also Clementz et al., 1990). When patients, relatives, and healthy comparison subjects were compared using a sinusoidal task (i.e. the target motion follows a predictable path which allows for extraretinal control of eye movements), both patients and their relatives showed reduced pursuit gain compared to controls (Iacono et al., 1992; Thaker et al., 2003), and the pattern of this abnormality among schizophrenia families is mathematically consistent with genetic transmission (Grove et al., 1992; see also Calkins et al., 2008). First-degree relatives also have disrupted predictive pursuit that, instead of being intermediate between normal and schizophrenia subjects, was similar to the schizophrenia group itself (Hong et al., 2008). These data support the notion that predictive pursuit may have the highest heritability of eye movement measures. In sum, the long history of smooth pursuit impairment in schizophrenia and the evidence for abnormalities in (unmedicated) biological relatives has made smooth pursuit one of the most investigated putative intermediate phenotypes for schizophrenia (Calkins et al., 2008; Clementz and Sweeney, 1990; Hutton and Kennard, 1998; Iacono and Clementz, 1993; Levy et al., 1993, O'Driscoll and Callahan, 2008).

Neural substrates of smooth pursuit and functional changes in schizophrenia

Successful performance of smooth pursuit tasks requires: 1) sufficient visual perception: a function of striate and extrastriate cortex (Zee et al., 1987), 2) adequate motion processing (Lisberger et al. 1987; Stanton et al. 2005): an extrastriate cortex function (Newsome and Paré 1988; Pasternak and Merigan 1994), and 3) integration of this perceptual motion information for generation of the correct motor response, which is primarily a frontal, parietal and cerebellar function (Lencer and Trillenberg, 2008). Functional neuroimaging studies indicate that the neural substrates of smooth pursuit include these and related regions: occipital visual areas, thalamus, basal ganglia, cuneus, frontal (FEF) and supplementary (SEF) eye fields and extrastriate cortical area V5 (Berman et al., 1999; Keedy et al., 2006; Kimming et al., 2008; O'Driscoll et al., 1998 and 2000). Researchers have attempted to determine, therefore, if dysfunction in brain regions supporting perceptual motion processing and/or motor output account for schizophrenia subjects' smooth pursuit abnormalities.

Some (Chen et al. 2003; Chen et al. 2004, 2005; Clementz et al. 2007; Kim et al. 2006; O'Donnell et al. 2006; Slaghuis et al. 2005; Stuve et al. 1997), but not all (Clementz 1996; Kim et al., 1997), behavioural research is consistent in reporting a motion perception deficit among people with schizophrenia. The behavioural research can be supported by blood flow-based functional neuroimaging techniques, such as functional magnetic resonance imaging (fMRI), which measures local haemodynamic changes via 'blood oxygen level dependent' (BOLD) signal that is associated with changes in neural activity. Generally, findings from these studies are consistent with the conclusion of a motion processing problem because schizophrenia patients have lower activity in cortical area V5 that is associated with poor smooth pursuit performance (Hong et al., 2005; Lencer et al., 2005). Cortical area V5 (also called area MT/MST) is an extrastriate cortical area specialized for processing of motion information (e.g. Dursteler and Wurtz 1988; Newsome et al. 1985).

Although consistent with a perceptual motion processing problem, the above results did not clarify the neurophysiological *stage* at which this abnormality is manifest. Some researchers posit that schizophrenia-related motion processing abnormalities are related to deficient early sensory input (e.g. Butler and Javitt 2005; Butler et al., 2005; Kim et al., 2005, 2006; Schechter et al., 2003), since this pathway provides the majority input to motion area V5 (Maunsell et al., 1990), although there are data inconsistent with this conclusion (e.g. Chen et al., 2003; Clementz 1996; Kim et al., 1997). Other researchers posit that motion processing deficits in schizophrenia are accounted for by dysfunction no earlier than V5 in the motion processing stream (Chen et al., 2003; Chen et al., 2004). Some fMRI studies, however, have shown reduced activation among people with schizophrenia compared to healthy individuals in brain areas more closely associated with motor output, like frontal, supplementary, and parietal eye fields, and anterior cingulate cortex (Keedy et al., 2006; Tregellas et al., 2004; Hong et al., 2005). The only study using measurements of brain activity (dense-array EEG) on a time scale that allows for differentiating between early perceptual and later decision-making stages of neural processing (Wang et al., 2010) found that early perceptual processing of motion information did not account for motion processing abnormalities among people with schizophrenia. Schulze et al. (2006) also found no evidence of structural abnormalities in extrastriate motion processing regions among people with schizophrenia. Determining the extent to which neurophysiological dysfunction at the levels of perceptual input, motion processing computations, or motor output cause schizophrenia subjects' smooth pursuit abnormalities, therefore, will require considerable additional investigation.

Smooth pursuit in affective disorders and their biological relatives

Affective disorders are characterized by episodes of extreme moods, such as desperate sadness (in major depression), or euphoria (during mania associated with bipolar disorder). Studies of smooth pursuit in affective disorder are less frequent, and often are reported as a psychiatric comparison sample in schizophrenia studies. Early evidence suggested that it was difficult to distinguish between schizophrenia and affective disorder groups (Abel et al., 1991; Amador et al., 1995; Friedman et al., 1992; Sweeney et al., 1994a), including in a study of groups who were currently off any medication (Sweeney et al., 1999). A report by Iacono et al. (1992), however, showed that overall smooth pursuit performance was specific to schizophrenia or schizophrenia-like disorders (psychotic depression without history of mania) among psychotic patients.

Findings among the biological family members of people with affective disorders have been inconclusive. Iacono et al. (1992) found that smooth pursuit eye tracking accuracy was fairly specific to schizophrenia families when compared to affective psychosis families. Kathmann and colleagues (2003) reported that groups of both schizophrenia and affective disorder subjects showed reduced pursuit gain. The biological relatives of those subjects also showed decreased pursuit gain, suggesting to the authors that these similarities point to a shared non-necessary genetic factor in schizophrenia and affective disorders. Studies of the offspring of subjects with affective disorder showed that, somewhat consistent with Iacono et al. (1992), those with depressed parents had similar gain problems as those with parents with schizophrenia, although the latter showed unique disruption of anticipatory saccades (Rosenberg et al., 1997).

Impact of affective disorder medication on smooth pursuit

Medications commonly used for affective disorders include antidepressants, lithium and anticonvulsants. Data on effects of antidepressant and anticonvulsant medication on smooth pursuit are rare, while more information is available for lithium (Reilly et al., 2008). Some studies suggest that lithium may be associated with deficits in smooth pursuit sometimes reported in affective disorder patients (Holzman et al., 1991; Iacono et al., 1982; Levy et al., 1985) while others have not. Gooding et al. (1993) showed no differences in smooth pursuit measures between mood disorder patients taking lithium and those who did not. In addition, she conducted a test re-test session that demonstrated no changes in smooth pursuit measures for subjects with bipolar illness whose medication status had changed between their first testing session and a second session 10 months later. Another study showed no impact of lithium on smooth pursuit after 2 weeks of clinically relevant doses in healthy subjects (Fletchner et al., 1992).

General description of saccades

Purposeful exploration of the visual environment relies primarily on two types of saccadic control. First, visually-guided (also known as 'pro-' or 'reflexive') saccades are generated to external cues and require simple and direct sensorimotor transformations for their successful implementation. Second, volitional saccades are controlled by internally generated cognitive plans that involve higher order control processes such as inhibition, spatial memory, and/or decisions based on an analysis of contextual cues. The same basic neural circuitry supporting the sensorimotor transformation aspect of saccade generation is utilized for reflexive and cognitively controlled saccadic responses (Leigh and Zee, 2006). As the factors determining saccadic response requirements get more complex, however, additional brain regions are recruited to support the requisite higher level processes (e.g. McDowell et al., 2001; Munoz and Everling, 2004; Pierrot-Deseilligny et al., 2005; Sweeney et al., 2007). These characteristics make the saccadic system extremely useful for investigating models of cognitive control that have applications across a diverse range of research literatures, extending from studies of basic motor function to normal cognitive neuroscience studies of executive control to investigations of behavioural and brain activity correlates of psychiatric conditions.

A prosaccade is a response that involves the simple redirection of gaze to a stimulus and typically is generated to align the fovea with visual targets. Prosaccade task performance measures include: 1) latency (time in ms from the appearance of the peripheral cue to the start of the saccade) and 2) accuracy (eye position/target position in degrees of visual angle). Prosaccade paradigms can be modified to increase the probability of eliciting fast latency saccades known as 'express saccades' (Fischer and Ramsperger, 1984). Insertion of a 'gap' (optimally 200 ms; Clementz, 1996a; Fischer and Weber, 1997; Weber and Fischer, 1995) between fixation point extinction and peripheral stimulus illumination facilitates this effect (Fischer et al., 1993) and produces a robust reduction of mean latency (Reuter-Lorenz et al., 1991; Saslow, 1967) that has been related to the release of fixation mechanisms (Munoz and Wurtz, 1992).

Saccades intended to foveate a target of interest are one component of the human ability to explore, and respond to, the visual environment. Such simple response capabilities, however, are not the only method for monitoring the visual environment. In order to visually attend to one aspect of the environment, automatic responses to other parts of the visual world that are not contextually relevant often need to be suppressed. Tasks requiring inhibition, working memory and/or other processes that require attendance to contextual cues are considered volitional saccades in that they are endogenously driven. In studies of people with psychiatric illness, the most frequently used volitional saccade paradigms are antisaccade and ocular motor delayed response (ODR or 'memory saccade') tasks. Below, the task parameters and response requirements are summarized by paradigm.

Antisaccade tasks

Antisaccades (Hallett, 1978) are volitional saccades during which participants must inhibit the prepotent response towards a peripheral (usually visual) cue in order to direct their gaze in the opposite (anti) direction. During typical antisaccade trials, subjects fixate on a central target and then the fixation point is extinguished and a peripheral cue is presented. Subjects are instructed to generate a saccade to the mirror image location (same amplitude, opposite direction) of the peripheral cue as quickly and accurately as possible without looking at the cue itself. An initial glance towards the cue is an error and may be conceptualized as a failure of inhibition. Latencies for correct antisaccade responses are usually about 50–100 ms longer (Evdokimidis et al., 1996; McDowell et al., 1999) than prosaccades, which represent in part the additional computations necessary for the co-ordinate transformation process. Standard measures of antisaccade performance include: 1) error rate (number of trials on which the first saccade is generated *towards* the cue/total number of trials), 2) latency (time in milliseconds from the appearance of the peripheral cue to the start of the saccade) for correct (volitionally-guided) and error (visually-driven) responses, and 3) accuracy (eye position/target position) for correct and error responses; see Fig. 38.2.

A

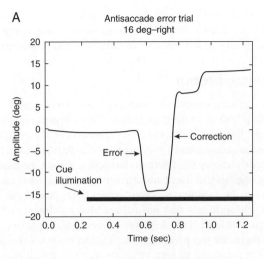

B

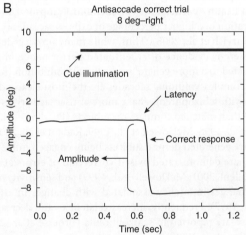

Fig. 38.2 Eye tracking data for A) incorrect and B) correct antisaccade trials. On both graphs, amplitude (degrees of visual angle) is shown on the y-axis (negative numbers indicating left and positive numbers indicating right), and time (seconds) is shown on the x-axis. On both graphs the eye position is shown fixated on the central target (indicated at 0°) during the start of the trial and the time and position of the cue onset is illustrated as a bold line. A) In the incorrect trial, the eyes move down (left) towards the cue illuminated at 16° left before an error correction is generated towards the correct location at 16° (right). B) In the correct trial, the response to an 8° right cue is correctly generated towards 8° left. Latency and amplitude of the saccade is indicated. Brett A. Clementz, Psychophysiological measures of (dis)inhibition as liability indicators for schizophrenia, *Psychophysiology*, **35**(6), pp. 648–668, figure 7 © 1998, Cambridge University Press.

Ocular motor delayed response (ODR) or memory saccade tasks

ODR paradigms are volitional saccade tasks that require both inhibitory and spatial working memory processes (e.g. Funahashi et al., 1989, 1993; Inoue et al., 2004; Sweeney et al., 1996; Walker et al., 1998). During ODR tasks, participants are instructed to remember the location of a briefly presented visual target in the periphery through a delay period (spatial working memory component) without making anticipatory saccades (inhibition component), and then to generate a 'memory' saccade (volitionally-guided) to that (unmarked) location after the delay period. Standard measures of ODR task performance include 1) error rate (frequency of saccades generated in response to the target presentation or during the following delay), 2) reaction time for memory saccades (generated to the remembered cue location), and 3) accuracy of memory saccades (eye position/target position).

Saccades in schizophrenia

Prosaccade performance based on standard paradigms (concurrent extinction of the fixation point and illumination of the peripheral target) in people with schizophrenia is mostly preserved, as demonstrated by normal latencies and accuracies (Clementz et al., 1994; Crawford et al., 1998; Ettinger et al., 2006; Hutton and Kennard 1998; Iacono et al., 1981; Smyrnis et al., 2004; Thaker et al., 1989). Normal prosaccade accuracy (and perhaps latency) is among the most frequently replicated behavioural results, and suggests that the neural circuitry supporting basic saccade performance may be intact in schizophrenia. Two studies, however, report faster prosaccade latencies in untreated, acutely ill people with schizophrenia that normalized after treatment with a second-generation antipsychotic (Reilly et al., 2005 and 2007). Faster responses in schizophrenia also are associated with the presentation of a prosaccade gap paradigm (the fixation point is extinguished roughly 200 ms before illumination of the peripheral target). While the gap prosaccade paradigm is well known to elicit express saccades in healthy participants (Fischer and Rampsberger, 1984), schizophrenia is associated with the generation of a higher percentage of express saccades (Clementz, 1996b; Matsue et al., 1994; Winograd-Gurvich et al., 2008). Thus, while many prosaccade paradigms elicit normal prosaccade dynamics, there is evidence of accentuated performance in specific visually-guided responses that may be related to a more general problem with inhibition (see below).

The more cognitively complex volitional saccades are the most clearly disrupted among schizophrenia subjects. People with schizophrenia make more antisaccade errors (glances *towards*, rather than away from, the cue) than matched comparison subjects (Everling et al., 1996; Fukushima et al., 1988 and 1990; Hutton et al., 1998; McDowell et al., 1999; Radant et al., 2007; Sereno and Holzman, 1995). Increased errors are generated despite subjects being engaged in the task and understanding the task demands, which are demonstrated by self-correction of errors at the same rate as normal subjects (Gooding and Tallent, 2001; McDowell et al., 1999) and sensitivity to changes in task parameters (i.e. appropriate changes in latency associated with changes in attentional manipulation; McDowell and Clementz, 1997). Frequently, increased latencies and decreased accuracies of correct antisaccade responses also are reported in schizophrenia (Broerse et al., 2001; Harris et al., 2006; Hutton et al., 1998; Everling et al., 1996).

Studies of ODR performance in schizophrenia show similar types of disruption as those observed in antisaccade tasks. Generally, the pattern of performance differences consists of memory saccades characterized by increased latencies and decreased accuracies (Everling et al., 1996; McDowell and Clementz, 1996; McDowell et al., 2001; Park et al., 1995, Reilly et al., 2007; Ross et al., 1998). An increased number of error (or anticipatory) saccades generated during cue presentation or the delay period also is reported in schizophrenia (Broerse et al., 2001; McDowell and Clementz, 1996; McDowell et al., 2001).

Similar patterns in deficits across antisaccade and ODR tasks may be due to their similarities in task demands. Correct responses on both paradigms require visual spatial attention, inhibition, spatial working memory, and generation of a (volitional) saccade to an unmarked location. More specifically, the patterns of saccadic abnormalities among people with schizophrenia may be consistent with a general problem with inhibitory abilities. Indeed, speeded prosaccade responding has been shown to predict increased antisaccade error rates among schizophrenia patients (Harris et al., 2006; Reilly et al., 2008). The combination of increased antisaccade and ODR errors and increased express saccades (during gap prosaccade paradigms) suggest a schizophrenia-related inability to inhibit context-inappropriate responses. The increased express saccade result is informative because *longer* reaction times are characteristic of schizophrenia, with speeded responses being infrequently observed among such patients. There are a number of regions in neural circuitry that have been identified as mediating regions for saccadic inhibition, including DLPFC, FEF, and SEF cortically, and BG and thalamus subcortically (see Munoz and Everling, 2004). While inhibition problems are apparent, there may also be difficulties generating volitional saccades to a correct location, particularly when it requires movement to a region that is not marked with a visual stimulus.

Impact of antipsychotic medication on saccades

As with smooth pursuit, the putative role of antipsychotics as a confounding factor must be considered with respect to interpreting reports of saccadic performance in schizophrenia. While some studies reported no evidence of medication associated prosaccade changes in people with schizophrenia (Broerse et al., 2001; Hommer et al., 1991; Hutton et al., 1998 and 2001b), reports to the contrary exist for both first- and second-generation medications. First-generation antipsychotics have been reported to reduce prosaccade gain (Crawford et al., 1995). A marked decrease in saccade gain also was observed for predictable prosaccades after treatment with a second-generation antipsychotic (despite normal gain before treatment; Harris et al., 2009). With regard to latencies, Reilly et al. (2005) reported that a group of acutely ill first-episode schizophrenia patients showed faster prosaccade reaction times than the control group. Prosaccade latencies stayed faster in the following months for the group treated with first-generation antipsychotics, while the group treated with second-generation antipsychotics got slower and longer than those of normal control subjects (see also Sweeney et al., 1997). In sum, recent studies suggest that prosaccade performance may be impacted particularly by second-generation antipsychotic medications.

For more complex saccades, there is no evidence that antisaccade error rate is *increased* by antipsychotic medication (either first- or second-generation). More antisaccade errors have been reported at all stages of schizophrenia illness: first-episode, chronic, remitted and even amidst changing clinical states (Broerse et al, 2002; Crawford et al., 1995; Curtis et al., 2001; Ettinger et al., 2004; Gooding et al., 2004; Hutton et al., 1998). Most studies show no relationships between antisaccade error rate and dose of antipsychotic medication (Curtis et al., 2001; Fukushima et al., 1990; Gooding and Tallent, 2001; McDowell et al., 1999; Müller et al., 1999), and similar error rates among treated, untreated, antipsychotic-naive, and chronically medicated patients (Crawford et al., 1995; Hutton et al. 1998; McDowell et al., 1999; Straube et al., 1999). There are indications that second-generation antipsychotics *decrease* antisaccade error rates and reduce antisaccade latencies among people with schizophrenia (Burke and Reveley, 2002; Ettinger and Kumari, 2003; Harris et al., 2006). Second-generation medications may help to *normalize* antisaccade performance, although it is noteworthy that even after one year of treatment, those antisaccade variables are improved but still are not at the levels observed among healthy comparison subjects (Harris et al., 2006).

One saccadic variable which antipsychotics may be more likely to disrupt is accuracy measures of volitional saccades. An initial study suggested that volitional saccade amplitude was impacted by first-generation antipsychotic medication, regardless of diagnosis (Crawford et al., 1995). Subsequent studies suggest a particular impact of second-generation medications on volitional saccade accuracy, but no difference between two of the commonly used second-generation drugs (Broerse et al., 2002). Specifically, people with first episode schizophrenia show initial decreased accuracy on memory saccades generated during an ODR task. Treatment with second-generation antipsychotics resulted in even worse accuracy performance, a pattern which did not recover over a year's time (Reilly et al., 2006 and 2007). As summarized by Reilly et al., (2007, p. 820):

> Although the mechanisms contributing to this adverse effect are not yet certain, neurophysiologic and neuro-chemical studies with nonhuman primates and imaging studies with patients treated with antipsychotic drugs suggest that altered dopaminergic function in dorsolateral prefrontal cortex or reduced thalamocortical drive are candidate mechanisms (Abi-Dargham et al. 2002; Camchong et al. 2006; Castner et al. 2000; Hirvonen et al. 2006; Lidow et al. 1997; Von Huben et al. 2006). Serotonin-2A receptor antagonism associated with antipsychotic treatment might also contribute to the worsening of ODR performance (Williams et al. 2002).

Saccades in schizophrenia relatives

Biological relatives show saccadic performance disruptions that are similar in kind to their schizophrenia probands, but intermediate in frequency/severity between the probands and healthy comparison subjects. For instance, most studies of antisaccade performance show increased errors among the biological relatives of schizophrenia subjects (Crawford et al., 1998; Curtis et al., 2001; Fukushima et al., 1988; Karoumi et al., 2001; Katsanis et al., 1997; McDowell et al., 1999), with few exceptions (Brownstein et al., 2003). Data from one of the largest existing family studies of antisaccade performance (N=365 subjects recruited from three diverse geographical locations) show that the probands had the highest error rate, followed by the first-degree biological relatives, who were followed by the second-degree relatives, who still made more errors than comparison subjects (McDowell et al., 1999). A similar pattern was observed in another large family study showing increased error rates in the first-degree relatives and grouping of poor performing family members with poor performing probands (Curtis et al., 2001). In contrast, a meta-analysis conducted by Levy and colleagues (2004) suggested that relatives of schizophrenia participants show similar volitional saccade performance to normal participants if similar criteria are used when recruiting participants from both groups. Calkins and colleagues (2004) addressed this hypothesis, however, and reported that relatives of schizophrenia participants recruited with the same selection criteria as the normal participants did show increased error rates. The latter group (Calkins et al., 2004) also reported that relatives of schizophrenia participants excluded from the analyses (who did not meet inclusion criteria used for the control groups) did not differ significantly in error rates from the relatives of people with schizophrenia included in the analyses. This is an important piece of biological evidence associated with heritable traits that indicate genetic vulnerability to the disease (Hutton and Ettinger, 2006). As a result, antisaccade performance specifically is generating interest as a possible endophenotype for schizophrenia (Calkins et al., 2008).

The first-degree relatives of patients with schizophrenia also have abnormalities on ODR tasks, including memory saccades characterized by increased latencies (McDowell and Clementz, 1996; Park et al., 1995) and decreased accuracy (Everling et al., 1996; Park et al.; 1995; Ross et al., 1998), and an increased frequency of delay period errors (Crawford et al., 1995; Landgraf et al., 2008). There is evidence that memory saccade accuracy or delay period errors may best distinguish between ill or at-risk group and control groups (Calkins et al., 2008; McDowell and Clementz, 1996; McDowell et al., 2001).

Neural substrates of saccades and functional changes in schizophrenia

Human brain imaging studies show that saccade generation is supported by fronto-basal ganglia-thalamocortical circuitry (O'Driscoll et al., 1995; Sweeney et al., 2007). Regions included in this saccadic circuitry are (Fig. 38.3): cerebellum, basal ganglia, thalamus, posterior eye fields (Simo et al., 2005) and supplementary and frontal eye fields (Rosano et al., 2002). With respect to the frontal eye fields, there is increasing evidence for two foci of activation within frontal eye fields: medial (inferior) and lateral (superior; Berman et al., 1999; Dyckman et al., 2007; Lobel et al., 2001; Luna et al. 1998; McDowell et al., 2005; Mort et al., 2003; Paus, 1996; Petit et al., 1997, Simo et al., 2005). The functional roles of these regions have yet to be fully delimited, although medial FEF may be associated with more complex tasks and the lateral FEF more associated with reflexive type movements. Typically in direct comparisons between prosaccades and volitional saccades, cortical brain regions are more active during volitional tasks (Connolly et al., 2000; Mort et al., 2003). More specifically, when cognitive control of the system is required for responses based on internal plans such as in antisaccade or ODR paradigms, changes of activation are observed in caudate nucleus, thalamus and prefrontal cortex (Camchong et al., 2006; Dyckman et al., 2007; Ford et al., 2005; Keedy et al., 2006; McDowell et al., 2002).

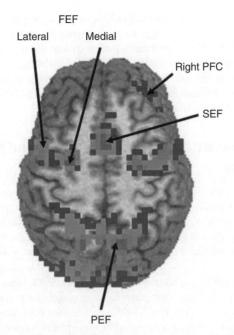

FEF

Lateral   Medial

Right PFC

SEF

PEF

Fig. 38.3 Cortical neural circuitry supporting antisaccade generation. This axial view displays percent blood oxygenation level-dependent signal change associated with antisaccade performance from 36 people (12 people at each of three time points). Colours from blue to pink to red indicate increasing percent signal change. FEF, frontal eye field; PEF is parietal eye fields; PFC, prefrontal cortex; SEF, supplementary eye field. Reprinted from *Neuroimage*, **36**(3), Kara A. Dyckman, Jazmin Camchong, Brett A. Clementz, Jennifer E. McDowell, An effect of context on saccade-related behaviour and brain activity, 774–784, © 2007 with permission from Elsevier.

People with schizophrenia show differences from normal individuals in BOLD response suggestive of reduced neural activation patterns in regions involved in saccadic control. People with schizophrenia have demonstrated antisaccade-related decreased activation in striatal (Raemaekers et al., 2006) and prefrontal (Ford et al., 2005; McDowell et al., 2002) regions. Additionally, groups of both medicated (Camchong et al., 2006) and unmedicated (Keedy et al., 2006) people with schizophrenia showed broadly reduced BOLD response in saccade structures including prefrontal cortex during volitional saccade tasks. More specific information is provided by a study on first-episode patients before and after the first month of treatment (Keedy et al., 2009). Initially, patients had less activation in frontal and parietal eye fields and cerebellum. After treatment, these disturbances were not present, suggesting improved function in attentional and sensorimotor systems. In contrast, while activity in striatum, thalamus and prefrontal cortex was not reduced at baseline, it was significantly reduced after treatment. These findings provide evidence for a complex impact of antipsychotic medication on functional brain systems in schizophrenia and illustrate the potential of neuroimaging biomarkers for both adverse and beneficial drug effects on functional brain systems (Keedy et al., 2009).

Similar patterns of abnormalities of brain activation also are reported in first-degree biological relatives of people with schizophrenia during antisaccade (Raemaekers et al., 2006) and ODR (Keshavan et al., 2002) tasks. As observed in the behavioural data, the abnormalities in relatives are generally attenuated compared to findings in patients. As an example, a study of volitional saccade control was conducted to investigate brain activity associated with volitional saccade generation in people with schizophrenia and their siblings (Camchong et al., 2008) by using a combination of antisaccade and ODR tasks. The data demonstrated that within the context of preserved activity in some neural regions in patients and relatives, there were two distinct patterns of disruptions in other regions. First, there were deficits observed only in the schizophrenia group (decreased activity in lateral FEF and SEF), suggesting a change associated with disease manifestation. Second, there were deficits observed in both the schizophrenia probands and the relatives (decreased activity in middle occipital gyrus, insula, cuneus, anterior cingulate and BA10 in prefrontal cortex), indicating a potential association with disease risk. Brain activation in regions involved in managing and evaluating early sensory and attention processing may be associated with poor volitional saccade control and a risk for developing schizophrenia.

Saccades in people with affective disorders and their biological relatives

Studies of saccade performance among people with affective disorders are less common. Generally, with respect to major depression, a variety of minor abnormalities are reported in some (Mahlberg et al., 2001; Sweeney et al., 1998; Winograd-Gurvich et al., 2006) but not all studies (Done and Frith, 1989). In bipolar disorder, studies generally show preserved prosaccade performance (Crawford et al., 1995; Sereno and Holzman, 1995; Tien et al., 1996). Studies of volitional saccades in major depressed subjects also show evidence of sporadic and mild differences in volitional saccade performance, such as no increase in antisaccades errors (Katsanis et al., 1997), or increased antisaccade errors for some, but not all, target conditions (for example when targets are presented further from rather than closer to central fixation; Sweeney et al., 1998). People with depression show normal accuracy of initial memory saccade but decreased accuracy of final eye position (Sweeney et al., 1998). A recent study suggests the melancholic subtype may be more prone to disruptions in saccadic variables (Winograd-Gurvich et al., 2006).

Studies of volitional saccades in people with bipolar disorder are divided in terms of antisaccade tasks. Some studies show no changes in error rates or intermediate error rates (Curtis et al., 2001; Clementz et al., 1994; Crawford et al., 1995) and others show increased errors (Gooding and Tallent, 2001; Katsanis et al., 1997; Sereno and Holzman, 1995; Tien et al., 1996). A possible explanation for these discrepancies is that antisaccade performance may be related to state factors in bipolar disorder (Gooding et al., 2004), rather than trait factors, as in schizophrenia. Another suggestion in the literature is that affective disorder with psychosis may be associated with increased antisaccade errors (Curtis et al. 2004; Sweeney et al., 1998), which is indirectly supported by a study showing that in borderline personality disorder subjects' antisaccade performance is only impaired when psychosis is present (Grootens et al., 2008). Performance on ODR in bipolar groups generally show preserved latency and accuracy of memory saccades (Crawford et al., 1995; Park and Holzman, 1992 and 1993).

In sum, it appears as if some prosaccade variables may show mild, if any, disruption in major depression or bipolar disorder. There also is evidence that volitional saccades of people with depression are not remarkably different from comparison subjects. In people with bipolar disorder, ODR seems preserved, while antisaccade error rate may vary with state factors such as episode severity or history of psychosis. As such, it is apparent that the volitional saccade abnormalities observed in schizophrenia are most frequently differentiated from psychiatric comparison groups in their severity and extent.

Impact of affective disorder medication on saccades

One study of two groups of people with bipolar affective disorder who were either treated with antipsychotics or antipsychotic-free, suggested that antipsychotic treatment (in bipolar disorder *and* schizophrenia) was associated with undershoot of memory saccades (Crawford et al., 1995). In another study of people with bipolar disorder, major depression, and schizophrenia, subjects were treated with varying doses of antipsychotics, lithium, anticholinergics, antidepressants, and benzodiazepines (Katsanis et al., 1997). The association between medication status (i.e. those patients who were or were not taking a particular agent) and antisaccade variables showed only a relationship between anticholinergic medications and longer correct antisaccade latencies. Although to date, the data are not consistent with the conjecture that results on saccadic tasks are due entirely to medication effects, it is clear that more needs to be known about the effects of medications commonly prescribed for mood disorders—and their potential interactions. For studies of neuropathology or marking genetic risk, drug effects can be a troubling confound. From a different perspective, however, eye movement measures may prove to be a useful biomarker for dose-dependent drug effects on different functional brain systems.

Summary

The use of eye movement measures to assess neurological status has a long and productive history. The use of eye movements to learn about underlying impairments in psychiatric conditions, and particularly schizophrenia, has been pursued vigorously over the past three decades and has been informative on three fronts. First, evidence from people with schizophrenia and their biological relatives demonstrates that some eye movement measures may be promising endo- or intermediate phenotypes useful for resolving the genetic transmission of brain abnormalities placing persons at risk for developing this illness (Calkins et al., 2008). Second, evidence from behavioural and brain imaging studies shows great promise that eye movement measures may assist understanding of the neuropathological underpinnings of serious mental illnesses, particularly psychotic disorders. Third, data on the impact of antipsychotic medications on behaviour and brain function have been particularly illuminating. Medication effects appear to change across the course of treatment, and may have differential short- and long-term implications for remediation of psychotic symptoms. There is evidence for both improvements in some, and deterioration in other brain-related behavioural functions (see Keedy et al., 2009). The extent to which eye movement measures are useful for research on the aetiology, genetics, and treatment of psychiatric disorders is impressive. The research reviewed here indicates that there may be patterns of eye movement disruption specific to particular diagnoses; this is a possibility that should be actively evaluated in future, large-scale studies.

Acknowledgements

The authors thank Cynthia Krafft, Qingyang Li, and Michael Amlung for their contributions. This work was supposed by USPHS with the following grants: MH001852 and MH076998 (JEM), MH51129 and MH57886 (BAC) and MH080066, MH077862 and MH62134 (JAS).

References

Abel, L.A. and Ziegler, A.S. (1988). Smooth pursuit eye movements in schizophrenics—what constitutes quantitative assessment? *Biological Psychiatry*, **24**(7), 747–761.

Abel, L.A., Friedman, L., Jesberger, J., Malki, A., and Meltzer, H.Y. (1991). Quantitative assessment of smooth pursuit gain and catch-up saccades in schizophrenia and affective disorders. *Biological Psychiatry*, **29**(11), 1063–1072.

Abi-Dargham, A., Mawlawi, O., Lombardo, I., Gil, R., Martinez, D., Huang, Y., *et al.* (2002). Prefrontal dopamine D1 receptors and working memory in schizophrenia. *Journal of Neuroscience*, **22**, 3708–3719.

Amador, X.F., Malaspina, D., Sackeim, H.A., Coleman, E.A., Kaufmann, C.A., Hasan, A., *et al.* (1995). Visual fixation and smooth pursuit eye movement abnormalities in patients with schizophrenia and their relatives. *Journal of Neuropsychiatry and Clinical Neuroscience*, **7**(2), 197–206.

Berman, R.A., Colby, C.L., Genovese, C.R., Voyvodic, J.T., Luna, B., Thulborn, K.R., *et al.* (1999). Cortical networks subserving pursuit and saccadic eye movements in humans: an FMRI study. *Human Brain Mapping*, **8**(4), 209–225.

Braff, D.L., Freedman, R., Schork, N.J., and Gottesman, I.I. (2007). Deconstructing schizophrenia: an overview of the use of endophenotypes in order to understand a complex disorder. *Schizophrenia Bulletin*, **33**(1), 21–32.

Broerse, A., Crawford, T.J., and den Boer, J.A. (2002). Differential effects of olanzapine and risperidone on cognition in schizophrenia? A saccadic eye movement study. *Journal of Neuropsychiatry and Clinical Neuroscience*, **14**(4), 454–460.

Broerse, A., Holthausen, E.A., van den Bosch, R.J., and den Boer, J.A. (2001). Does frontal normality exist in schizophrenia? A saccadic eye movement study. *Psychiatry Research*, **103**(2–3), 167–178.

Brownstein, J., Krastoshevsky, O., McCollum, C., Kundamal, S., Matthysse, S., Holzman, P.S., *et al.* (2003). Antisaccade performance is abnormal in schizophrenia patients but not in their biological relatives. *Schizophrenia Research*, **63**(1–2), 13–25.

Burke, J.G. and Reveley, M.A. (2002). Improved antisaccade performance with risperidone in schizophrenia. *Journal of Neurology, Neurosurgery and Psychiatry*, **72**(4), 449–454.

Butler, P.D., and Javitt, D.C. (2005). Early-stage visual processing deficits in schizophrenia. *Current Opinion in Psychiatry*, **18**(2), 151–157.

Butler, P.D., Zemon, V., Schechter, I., Saperstein, A.M., Hoptman, M.J., Lim, K.O., *et al.* (2005). Early-stage visual processing and cortical amplification deficits in schizophrenia. *Archives of General Psychiatry*, **62**(5), 495–504.

Calkins, M.E., Iacono, W.G., and Ones, D.S. (2008). Eye movement dysfunction in first-degree relatives of patients with schizophrenia: a meta-analytic evaluation of candidate endophenotypes. *Brain and Cognition*, **68**(3), 436–461.

Calkins, M.E., Curtis, C.E., Iacono, W.G., and Grove, W.M. (2004). Antisaccade performance is impaired in medically and psychiatrically healthy biological relatives of schizophrenia patients. *Schizophrenia Research*, **71**(1), 167–178.

Camchong, J., Dyckman, K.A., Austin, B.P., Clementz, B.A., and McDowell, J.E. (2008). Common neural circuitry supporting volitional saccades and its disruption in schizophrenia patients and relatives. *Biological Psychiatry*, **64**(12), 1042–1050.

Camchong, J., Dyckman, K.A., Chapman, C.E., Yanasak, N.E., and McDowell, J.E. (2006). Basal ganglia-thalamocortical circuitry disruptions in schizophrenia during delayed response tasks. *Biological Psychiatry*, **60**(3), 235–241.

Castner, S.A., Williams, G.V., and Goldman-Rakic, P.S. (2000). Reversal of antipsychotic induced working memory deficits by short-term dopamine D1 receptor stimulation. *Science*, **287**, 2020–2022.

Cegalis, J.A., and Sweeney, J.A. (1979). Eye movements in schizophrenia: a quantitative analysis. *Biological Psychiatry*, **14**(1), 13–26.

Chen, Y., Holzman, P.S., and Nakayama, K. (2002). Visual and cognitive control of attention in smooth pursuit. *Progress in Brain Research*, **140**, 255–265.

Chen, Y., Bidwell, L.C., and Holzman, P.S. (2005). Visual motion integration in schizophrenia patients, their first-degree relatives, and patients with bipolar disorder. *Schizophrenia Research*, **74**(2–3), 271–281.

Chen, Y., Levy, D.L., Sheremata, S., and Holzman, P.S. (2004). Compromised late-stage motion processing in schizophrenia. *Biological Psychiatry*, **55**(8), 834–841.

Chen, Y., Nakayama, K., Levy, D., Matthysse, S., and Holzman, P. (2003). Processing of global, but not local, motion direction is deficient in schizophrenia. *Schizophrenia Research*, **61**(2–3), 215–227.

Chen, Y., Palafox, G.P., Nakayama, K., Levy, D.L., Matthysse, S., and Holzman, P.S. (1999). Motion perception in schizophrenia. *Archives of General Psychiatry*, **56**(2), 149–154.

Clementz, B.A. (1996a). The ability to produce express saccades as a function of gap interval among schizophrenia patients. *Experimental Brain Research*, **111**(1), 121–130.

Clementz, B.A. (1996b). Saccades to moving targets in schizophrenia: evidence for normal posterior cortex functioning. *Psychophysiology*, **33**(6), 650–654.

Clementz, B.A. and McDowell, J.E. (1994). Smooth pursuit in schizophrenia: abnormalities of open- and closed-loop responses. *Psychophysiology*, **31**(1), 79–86.

Clementz, B.A. and Sweeney, J.A. (1990). Is eye movement dysfunction a biological marker for schizophrenia? A methodological review. *Psychological Bulletin*, **108**(1), 77–92.

Clementz, B.A., McDowell, J.E., and Zisook, S. (1994). Saccadic system functioning among schizophrenia patients and their first-degree biological relatives. *Journal of Abnormal Psychology*, **103**(2), 277–287.

Clementz, B.A., McDowell, J.E., and Dobkins, K.R. (2007). Compromised speed discrimination among schizophrenia patients when viewing smooth pursuit targets. *Schizophrenia Research*, **95**(1–3), 61–64.

Clementz, B.A., Reid, S.A., McDowell, J.E., and Cadenhead, K.S. (1995). Abnormality of smooth pursuit eye movement initiation: specificity to the schizophrenia spectrum? *Psychophysiology*, **32**(2), 130–134.

Connolly, J.D., Goodale, M.A., Desouza, J.F., Menon, R.S., and Vilis, T. (2000). A comparison of frontoparietal fMRI activation during anti-saccades and anti-pointing. *Journal of Neurophysiology*, **84**(3), 1645–1655.

Couch, F.H. and Fox, J.C. (1934). Photographic study of ocular movements in mental disease. *Archives of Neurology and Psychiatry*, **34**, 556–578.

Crawford, T.J., Haeger, B., Kennard, C., Reveley, M.A., and Henderson, L. (1995). Saccadic abnormalities in psychotic patients. II. The role of neuroleptic treatment. *Psychological Medicine*, **25**(3), 473–483.

Crawford, T.J., Sharma, T., Puri, B.K., Murray, R.M., Berridge, D.M., and Lewis, S.W. (1998). Saccadic eye movements in families multiply affected with schizophrenia: the Maudsley Family Study. *American Journal of Psychiatry*, **155**(12), 1703–1710.

Curtis, C.E., Rao, V.Y., and D'Esposito, M. (2004). Maintenance of spatial and motor codes during oculomotor delayed response tasks. *Journal of Neuroscience*, **24**(16), 3944–3952.

Curtis, C.E., Calkins, M.E., Grove, W.M., Feil, K.J., and Iacono, W.G. (2001). Saccadic disinhibition in patients with acute and remitted schizophrenia and their first-degree biological relatives. *American Journal of Psychiatry*, **158**(1), 100–106.

Diefendorf, A.R. and Dodge, R. (1908). An experimental study of the ocular reactions of the insane from photographic records. *Brain*, **31**(3), 451–489.

Done, D.J. and Frith, C.D. (1989). Automatic and strategic volitional saccadic eye movements in psychotic patients. *European Archives of Psychiatry and Neurological Sciences*, 239(1), 27–32.

Dursteler, M.R. and Wurtz, R.H. (1988). Pursuit and optokinetic deficits following chemical lesions of cortical areas MT and MST. *Journal of Neurophysiology*, 60(3), 940–965.

Dyckman, K.A., Camchong, J., Clementz, B.A., and McDowell, J.E. (2007). An effect of context on saccade-related behavior and brain activity. *Neuroimage*, 36(3), 774–784.

Ettinger, U. and V. Kumari (2003). Pharmacological studies of smooth pursuit and antisaccade eye movements in schizophrenia: current status and directions for future research. *Current Neuropharmacology*, 1(4), 285–300.

Ettinger, U., Kumari, V., Chitnis, X.A., Corr, P.J., Crawford, T.J., Fannon, D.G., *et al.* (2004). Volumetric neural correlates of antisaccade eye movements in first-episode psychosis. *American Journal of Psychiatry*, 161(10), 1918–1921.

Ettinger, U., Picchioni, M., Hall, M.H., Schulze, K., Toulopoulou, T., Landau, S., *et al.* (2006). Antisaccade performance in monozygotic twins discordant for schizophrenia: the Maudsley twin study. *American Journal of Psychiatry*, 163(3), 543–545.

Evdokimidis, I., Constantinidis, T.S., Liakopoulos, D., and Papageorgiou, C. (1996). The increased reaction time of antisaccades. What makes the difference? *International Journal of Psychophysiology*, 22(1–2), 61–65.

Everling, S., Krappmann, P., Preuss, S., Brand, A., and Flohr, H. (1996). Hypometric primary saccades of schizophrenics in a delayed-response task. *Experimental Brain Research*, 111(2), 289–295.

Farber, R.H., Clementz, B.A., and Swerdlow, N.R. (1997). Characteristics of open—and closed-loop smooth pursuit responses among obsessive-compulsive disorder, schizophrenia, and nonpsychiatric individuals. *Psychophysiology*, 34(2), 157–162.

Fischer, B. and Ramsperger, E. (1984). Human express saccades: extremely short reaction times of goal directed eye movements. *Experimental Brain Research*, 57(1), 191–195.

Fischer, B. and Weber, H. (1997). Effects of stimulus conditions on the performance of antisaccades in man. *Experimental Brain Research*, 116(2), 191–200.

Fischer, B., Weber, H., Biscaldi, M., Aiple, F., Otto, P., and Stuhr, V. (1993). Separate populations of visually guided saccades in humans: reaction times and amplitudes. *Experimental Brain Research*, 92(3), 528–541.

Flechtner, K.M., Steinacher, B., Sauer, R., and Mackert, A. (1997). Smooth pursuit eye movements in schizophrenia and affective disorder. *Psychological Medicine*, 27(6), 1411–1419.

Flechtner, K.M., Mackert, A., Thies, K., Frick, K., and Muller-Oerlinghausen, B. (1992). Lithium effect on smooth pursuit eye movements of healthy volunteers. *Biological Psychiatry*, 32(10), 932–938.

Ford, K.A., Goltz, H.C., Brown, M.R., and Everling, S. (2005). Neural processes associated with antisaccade task performance investigated with event-related FMRI. *Journal of Neurophysiology*, 94(1), 429–440.

Friedman, L., Jesberger, J.A., and Meltzer, H.Y. (1992). Effect of typical antipsychotic medications and clozapine on smooth pursuit performance in patients with schizophrenia. *Psychiatry Research*, 41(1), 25–36.

Friedman, L., Kenny, J.T., Jesberger, J.A., Choy, M.M., and Meltzer, H.Y. (1995). Relationship between smooth pursuit eye-tracking and cognitive performance in schizophrenia. *Biological Psychiatry*, 37(4), 265–272.

Fukushima, J., Fukushima, K., Chiba, T., Tanaka, S., Yamashita, I., and Kato, M. (1988). Disturbances of voluntary control of saccadic eye movements in schizophrenic patients. *Biological Psychiatry*, 23(7), 670–677.

Fukushima, J., Morita, N., Fukushima, K., Chiba, T., Tanaka, S., and Yamashita, I. (1990). Voluntary control of saccadic eye movements in patients with schizophrenic and affective disorders. *Journal of Psychiatric Research*, 24(1), 9–24.

Funahashi, S., Bruce, C.J., and Goldman-Rakic, P.S. (1989). Mnemonic coding of visual space in the monkey's dorsolateral prefrontal cortex. *Journal of Neurophysiology*, 61(2), 331–349.

Funahashi, S., Chafee, M.V., and Goldman-Rakic, P.S. (1993). Prefrontal neuronal activity in rhesus monkeys performing a delayed anti-saccade task. *Nature*, 365(6448), 753–756.

Gooding, D.C. and Tallent, K.A. (2001). The association between antisaccade task and working memory task performance in schizophrenia and bipolar disorder. *Journal of Nervous and Mental Disease*, 189(1), 8–16.

Gooding, D.C., Iacono, W.G., and Beiser, M. (1994). Temporal stability of smooth-pursuit eye tracking in first-episode psychosis. *Psychophysiology*, 31(1), 62–67.

Gooding, D.C., Mohapatra, L., and Shea, H.B. (2004). Temporal stability of saccadic task performance in schizophrenia and bipolar patients. *Psychological Medicine*, 34(5), 921–932.

Gooding, D.C., Iacono, W.G., Katsanis, J., Beiser, M., and Grove, W.M. (1993). The association between lithium carbonate and smooth pursuit eye tracking among first-episode patients with psychotic affective disorders. *Psychophysiology*, 30(1), 3–9.

Gottesman, I.I. and Gould, T.D. (2003). The endophenotype concept in psychiatry: etymology and strategic intentions. *American Journal of Psychiatry*, 160(4), 636–645.

Grootens, K.P., van Luijtelaar, G., Buitelaar, J.K., van der Laan, A., Hummelen, J.W., and Verkes, R.J. (2008). Inhibition errors in borderline personality disorder with psychotic-like symptoms. *Progress in Neuropsychopharmacology and Biological Psychiatry*, 32(1), 267–273.

Grove, W.M. and Iacono, W.G. (1994). Comment on Levy et al. "Eye tracking dysfunction and schizophrenia". *Schizophrenia Bulletin*, 20(4), 781–786.

Grove, W.M., Clementz, B.A., Iacono, W.G., and Katsanis, J. (1992). Smooth pursuit ocular motor dysfunction in schizophrenia: evidence for a major gene. *American Journal of Psychiatry*, 149(10), 1362–1368.

Hallett, P.E. (1978). Primary and secondary saccades to goals defined by instructions. *Vision Res*, 18(10), 1279–1296.

Harris, M.S., Reilly, J.L., Keshavan, M.S., and Sweeney, J.A. (2006). Longitudinal studies of antisaccades in antipsychotic-naive first-episode schizophrenia. *Psychological Medicine*, **36**(4), 485–494.

Harris, M.S., Wiseman, C.L., Reilly, J.L., Keshavan, M.S., and Sweeney, J.A. (2009). Effects of risperidone on procedural learning in antipsychotic-naive first-episode schizophrenia. *Neuropsychopharmacology*, **34**(2), 468–476.

Holzman, P.S., Proctor, L.R., and Hughes, D.W. (1973). Eye-tracking patterns in schizophrenia. *Science*, **181**(95), 179–181.

Holzman, P.S., O'Brian, C., and Waternaux, C. (1991). Effects of lithium treatment on eye movements. *Biological Psychiatry*, **29**(10), 1001–1015.

Holzman, P.S., Proctor, L.R., Levy, D.L., Yasillo, N.J., Meltzer, H.Y., and Hurt, S.W. (1974). Eye-tracking dysfunctions in schizophrenic patients and their relatives. *Archives of General Psychiatry*, **31**(2), 143–151.

Hommer, D.W., Clem, T., Litman, R., and Pickar, D. (1991). Maladaptive anticipatory saccades in schizophrenia. *Biological Psychiatry*, **30**(8), 779–794.

Hong, L.E., Tagamets, M., Avila, M., Wonodi, I., Holcomb, H., and Thaker, G.K. (2005). Specific motion processing pathway deficit during eye tracking in schizophrenia: a performance-matched functional magnetic resonance imaging study. *Biological Psychiatry*, **57**(7), 726–732.

Hong, L.E., Turano, K.A., O'Neill, H., Hao, L., Wonodi, I., McMahon, R.P., et al. (2008). Refining the predictive pursuit endophenotype in schizophrenia. *Biological Psychiatry*, **63**(5), 458–464.

Hutton, S.B. and Ettinger, U. (2006). The antisaccade task as a research tool in psychopathology: a critical review. *Psychophysiology*, **43**(3), 302–313.

Hutton, S. and Kennard, C. (1998). Oculomotor abnormalities in schizophrenia: a critical review. *Neurology*, **50**(3), 604–609.

Hutton, S.B., Crawford, T.J., Puri, B.K., Duncan, L.J., Chapman, M., Kennard, C., et al. (1998). Smooth pursuit and saccadic abnormalities in first-episode schizophrenia. *Psychological Medicine*, **28**(3), 685–692.

Hutton, S.B., Crawford, T.J., Gibbins, H., Cuthbert, I., Barnes, T.R., Kennard, C., and Joyce, E.M. (2001). Short and long term effects of antipsychotic medication on smooth pursuit eye tracking in schizophrenia. *Psychopharmacology (Berl)*, **157**(3), 284–291.

Hutton, S.B., Cuthbert, I., Crawford, T.J., Kennard, C., Barnes, T.R., and Joyce, E.M. (2001). Saccadic hypometria in drug-naive and drug-treated schizophrenic patients: a working memory deficit? *Psychophysiology*, **38**(1), 125–132.

Iacono, W.G. and Clementz, B.A. (1993). A strategy for elucidating genetic influences on complex psychopathological syndromes (with special reference to ocular motor functioning and schizophrenia). *Progress in Experimental Personality and Psychopathology Research*, **16**, 11–65.

Iacono, W.G. and Lykken, D.T. (1979). Electro-oculographic recording and scoring of smooth pursuit and saccadic eye tracking: a parametric study using monozygotic twins. *Psychophysiology*, **16**(2), 94–107.

Iacono, W.G., Tuason, V.B., and Johnson, R.A. (1981). Dissociation of smooth-pursuit and saccadic eye tracking in remitted schizophrenics. An ocular reaction time task that schizophrenic perform well. *Archives of General Psychiatry*, **38**(9), 991–996.

Iacono, W.G., Peloquin, L.J., Lumry, A.E., Valentine, R.H., and Tuason, V.B. (1982). Eye tracking in patients with unipolar and bipolar affective disorders in remission. *Journal of Abnormal Psychology*, **91**(1), 35–44.

Iacono, W.G., Moreau, M., Beiser, M., Fleming, J.A., and Lin, T.Y. (1992). Smooth-pursuit eye tracking in first-episode psychotic patients and their relatives. *Journal of Abnormal Psychology*, **101**(1), 104–116.

Inoue, M., Mikami, A., Ando, I., and Tsukada, H. (2004). Functional brain mapping of the macaque related to spatial working memory as revealed by PET. *Cerebral Cortex*, **14**(1), 106–119.

Johnston, K., and Everling, S. (2008). Neurophysiology and neuroanatomy of reflexive and voluntary saccades in non-human primates. *Brain and Cognition*, **68**(3), 271–283.

Karoumi, B., Saoud, M., d'Amato, T., Rosenfeld, F., Denise, P., Gutknecht, C., et al. (2001). Poor performance in smooth pursuit and antisaccadic eye-movement tasks in healthy siblings of patients with schizophrenia. *Psychiatry Research*, **101**(3), 209–219.

Kathmann, N., Hochrein, A., Uwer, R., and Bondy, B. (2003). Deficits in gain of smooth pursuit eye movements in schizophrenia and affective disorder patients and their unaffected relatives. *American Journal of Psychiatry*, **160**(4), 696–702.

Katsanis, J., Kortenkamp, S., Iacono, W.G., and Grove, W.M. (1997). Antisaccade performance in patients with schizophrenia and affective disorder. *Journal of Abnormal Psychology*, **106**(3), 468–472.

Keedy, S.K., Ebens, C.L., Keshavan, M.S., and Sweeney, J.A. (2006). Functional magnetic resonance imaging studies of eye movements in first episode schizophrenia: smooth pursuit, visually guided saccades and the oculomotor delayed response task. *Psychiatry Research*, **146**(3), 199–211.

Keedy, S.K., Rosen, C., Khine, T., Rajarethinam, R., Janicak, P.G., and Sweeney, J.A. (2009). An fMRI study of visual attention and sensorimotor function before and after antipsychotic treatment in first-episode schizophrenia. *Psychiatry Research*, **172**(1), 16–23.

Keshavan, M.S., Diwadkar, V.A., Spencer, S.M., Harenski, K.A., Luna, B., and Sweeney, J.A. (2002). A preliminary functional magnetic resonance imaging study in offspring of schizophrenic parents. *Progress in Neuropsychopharmacology and Biological Psychiatry*, **26**(6), 1143–1149.

Kim, C.E., Thaker, G.K., Ross, D.E., and Medoff, D. (1997). Accuracies of saccades to moving targets during pursuit initiation and maintenance. *Experimental Brain Research*, **113**(2), 371–377.

Kim, D., Zemon, V., Saperstein, A., Butler, P.D., and Javitt, D.C. (2005). Dysfunction of early-stage visual processing in schizophrenia: harmonic analysis. *Schizophrenia Research*, **76**(1), 55–65.

Kim, D., Wylie, G., Pasternak, R., Butler, P.D., and Javitt, D.C. (2006). Magnocellular contributions to impaired motion processing in schizophrenia. *Schizophrenia Research*, **82**(1), 1–8.

Kimmig, H., Ohlendorf, S., Speck, O., Sprenger, A., Rutschmann, R.M., Haller, S., *et al.* (2008). fMRI evidence for sensorimotor transformations in human cortex during smooth pursuit eye movements. *Neuropsychologia*, **46**(8), 2203–2213.

Krauzlis, R. J. (2005). The control of voluntary eye movements: new perspectives. *Neuroscientist*, **11**(2), 124–137.

Landgraf, S., Amado, I., Bourdel, M.C., Leonardi, S., and Krebs, M.O. (2008). Memory-guided saccade abnormalities in schizophrenic patients and their healthy, full biological siblings. *Psychological Medicine*, **38**(6), 861–870.

Leigh, R.J and Zee, D.S. (2006). *The Neurology of Eye movements*. Oxford University Press.

Lencer, R. and Trillenberg, P. (2008). Neurophysiology and neuroanatomy of smooth pursuit in humans. *Brain and Cognition*, **68**(3), 219–228.

Lencer, R., Nagel, M., Sprenger, A., Heide, W., and Binkofski, F. (2005). Reduced neuronal activity in the V5 complex underlies smooth-pursuit deficit in schizophrenia: evidence from an fMRI study. *Neuroimage*, **24**(4), 1256–1259.

Lencer, R., Sprenger, A., Harris, M.S., Reilly, J.L., Keshavan, M.S., and Sweeney, J.A. (2008). Effects of second-generation antipsychotic medication on smooth pursuit performance in antipsychotic-naive schizophrenia. *Archives of General Psychiatry*, **65**(10), 1146–1154.

Levy, D.L., Holzman, P.S., Matthysse, S., and Mendell, N.R. (1993). Eye tracking dysfunction and schizophrenia: a critical perspective. *Schizophrenia Bulletin*, **19**(3), 461–536.

Levy, D.L., Holzman, P.S., Matthysse, S., and Mendell, N.R. (1994). Eye tracking and schizophrenia: a selective review. *Schizophrenia Bulletin*, **20**(1), 47–62.

Levy, D.L., Dorus, E., Shaughnessy, R., Yasillo, N.J., Pandey, G.N., Janicak, P.G., *et al.* (1985). Pharmacologic evidence for specificity of pursuit dysfunction to schizophrenia. Lithium carbonate associated with abnormal pursuit. *Archives of General Psychiatry*, **42**(4), 335–341.

Levy, D.L., Lajonchere, C.M., Dorogusker, B., Min, D., Lee, S., Tartaglini, A., *et al.* (2000). Quantitative characterization of eye tracking dysfunction in schizophrenia. *Schizophrenia Research*, **42**(3), 171–185.

Levy, D.L., O'Driscoll, G., Matthysse, S., Cook, S.R., Holzman, P.S., and Mendell, N.R. (2004). Antisaccade performance in biological relatives of schizophrenia patients: a meta-analysis. *Schizophrenia Research*, **71**(1), 113–125.

Lidow, M.S., Elsworth, J.D., and Goldman-Rakic, P.S. (1997). Down-regulation of the D1 and D5 dopamine receptors in the primate prefrontal cortex by chronic treatment with antipsychotic drugs. *Journal of Pharmacology and Experimental Therapeutics*, **281**, 597–603.

Lisberger, S.G. and Westbrook, L.E. (1985). Properties of visual inputs that initiate horizontal smooth pursuit eye movements in monkeys. *Journal of Neuroscience*, **5**(6), 1662–1673.

Lisberger, S.G., Morris, E.J., and Tychsen, L. (1987). Visual motion processing and sensory-motor integration for smooth pursuit eye movements. *Annual Review of Neuroscience*, **10**, 97–129.

Liston, D. and Krauzlis, R.J. (2005). Shared decision signal explains performance and timing of pursuit and saccadic eye movements. *Journal of Vision*, **5**(9), 678–689.

Litman, R.E., Hommer, D.W., Radant, A., Clem, T., and Pickar, D. (1994). Quantitative effects of typical and atypical neuroleptics on smooth pursuit eye tracking in schizophrenia. *Schizophrenia Research*, **12**(2), 107–120.

Lobel, E., Kahane, P., Leonards, U., Grosbras, M., Lehericy, S., Le Bihan, D., and Berthoz, A. (2001). Localization of human frontal eye fields: anatomical and functional findings of functional magnetic resonance imaging and intracerebral electrical stimulation. *Journal of Neurosurgery*, **95**(5), 804–815.

Luna, B., Thulborn, K.R., Strojwas, M.H., McCurtain, B.J., Berman, R.A., Genovese, C.R., and Sweeney, J.A. (1998). Dorsal cortical regions subserving visually guided saccades in humans: an fMRI study. *Cerebral Cortex*, **8**(1), 40–47.

Mahlberg, R., Steinacher, B., Mackert, A., and Flechtner, K.M. (2001). Basic parameters of saccadic eye movements— differences between unmedicated schizophrenia and affective disorder patients. *European Archives of Psychiatry and Clinical Neuroscience*, **251**(5), 205–210.

Matsue, Y., Osakabe, K., Saito, H., Goto, Y., Ueno, T., Matsuoka, H., *et al.* (1994). Smooth pursuit eye movements and express saccades in schizophrenic patients. *Schizophrenia Research*, **12**(2), 121–130.

Maunsell, J.H., Nealey, T.A., and DePriest, D.D. (1990). Magnocellular and parvocellular contributions to responses in the middle temporal visual area (MT) of the macaque monkey. *Journal of Neuroscience*, **10**(10), 3323–3334.

McDowell, J.E. and Clementz, B.A. (1996). Ocular-motor delayed-response task performance among schizophrenia patients. *Neuropsychobiology*, **34**(2), 67–71.

McDowell, J.E., and Clementz, B.A. (1997). The effect of fixation condition manipulations on antisaccade performance in schizophrenia: studies of diagnostic specificity. *Experimental Brain Research*, **115**(2), 333–344.

McDowell, J.E., Dyckman, K.A., Austin, B.P., and Clementz, B.A. (2008). Neurophysiology and neuroanatomy of reflexive and volitional saccades: evidence from studies of humans. *Brain and Cognition*, **68**(3), 255–270.

McDowell, J.E., Myles-Worsley, M., Coon, H., Byerley, W., and Clementz, B.A. (1999). Measuring liability for schizophrenia using optimized antisaccade stimulus parameters. *Psychophysiology*, **36**(1), 138–141.

McDowell, J.E., Brenner, C.A., Myles-Worsley, M., Coon, H., Byerley, W., and Clementz, B.A. (2001). Ocular motor delayed-response task performance among patients with schizophrenia and their biological relatives. *Psychophysiology*, **38**(1), 153–156.

McDowell, J.E., Brown, G.G., Paulus, M., Martinez, A., Stewart, S.E., Dubowitz, D.J., and Braff, D.L. (2002). Neural correlates of refixation saccades and antisaccades in normal and schizophrenia subjects. *Biological Psychiatry*, **51**(3), 216–223.

McDowell, J.E., Kissler, J.M., Berg, P., Dyckman, K.A., Gao, Y., Rockstroh, B., and Clementz, B.A. (2005). Electroencephalography/magnetoencephalography study of cortical activities preceding prosaccades and antisaccades. *Neuroreport*, **16**(7), 663–668.

Mort, D.J., Perry, R.J., Mannan, S.K., Hodgson, T.L., Anderson, E., Quest, R., et al. (2003). Differential cortical activation during voluntary and reflexive saccades in man. *Neuroimage*, **18**(2), 231–246.

Muir, W.J., St Clair, D.M., Blackwood, D.H., Roxburgh, H.M., and Marshall, I. (1992). Eye-tracking dysfunction in the affective psychoses and schizophrenia. *Psychological Medicine*, **22**(3), 573–580.

Muller, N., Riedel, M., Eggert, T., and Straube, A. (1999). Internally and externally guided voluntary saccades in unmedicated and medicated schizophrenic patients. Part II. Saccadic latency, gain, and fixation suppression errors. *European Archives of Psychiatry and Clinical Neuroscience*, **249**(1), 7–14.

Munoz, D.P. and Everling, S. (2004). Look away: the anti-saccade task and the voluntary control of eye movement. *Nat Rev Neurosci*, **5**(3), 218–228.

Munoz, D.P. and Wurtz, R.H. (1992). Role of the rostral superior colliculus in active visual fixation and execution of express saccades. *Journal of Neurophysiology*, **67**(4), 1000–1002.

Newsome, W.T. and Paré, E.B. (1988). A selective impairment of motion perception following lesions of the middle temporal visual area (MT). *Journal of Neuroscience*, **8**(6), 2201–2211.

Newsome, W.T., Wurtz, R.H., Dursteler, M.R., and Mikami, A. (1985). Deficits in visual motion processing following ibotenic acid lesions of the middle temporal visual area of the macaque monkey. *J Neurosci*, **5**(3), 825–840.

O'Driscoll, G.A., and Callahan, B.L. (2008). Smooth pursuit in schizophrenia: a meta-analytic review of research since 1993. *Brain and Cognition*, **68**(3), 359–370.

O'Donnell, B.F., Bismark, A., Hetrick, W.P., Bodkins, M., Vohs, J.L., and Shekhar, A. (2006). Early stage vision in schizophrenia and schizotypal personality disorder. *Schizophrenia Research*, **86**(1–3), 89–98.

O'Driscoll, G.A., Alpert, N.M., Matthysse, S.W., Levy, D. L., Rauch, S.L., and Holzman, P.S. (1995). Functional neuroanatomy of antisaccade eye movements investigated with positron emission tomography. *Proceedings of the National Academy of Sciences U S A*, **92**(3), 925–929.

O'Driscoll, G.A., Strakowski, S.M., Alpert, N.M., Matthysse, S.W., Rauch, S.L., Levy, D.L., et al. (1998). Differences in cerebral activation during smooth pursuit and saccadic eye movements using positron-emission tomography. *Biological Psychiatry*, **44**(8), 685–689.

O'Driscoll, G.A., Wolff, A.L., Benkelfat, C., Florencio, P.S., Lal, S., and Evans, A.C. (2000). Functional neuroanatomy of smooth pursuit and predictive saccades. *Neuroreport*, **11**(6), 1335–1340.

Park, S. and Holzman, P.S. (1992). Schizophrenics show spatial working memory deficits. *Archives of General Psychiatry*, **49**(12), 975–982.

Park, S. and Holzman, P.S. (1993). Association of working memory deficit and eye tracking dysfunction in schizophrenia. *Schizophrenia Research*, **11**(1), 55–61.

Park, S., Holzman, P.S., and Goldman-Rakic, P.S. (1995). Spatial working memory deficits in the relatives of schizophrenic patients. *Archives of General Psychiatry*, **52**(10), 821–828.

Pasternak, T., and Merigan, W.H. (1994). Motion perception following lesions of the superior temporal sulcus in the monkey. *Cerebral Cortex*, **4**(3), 247–259.

Paus, T. (1996). Location and function of the human frontal eye-field: a selective review. *Neuropsychologia*, **34**(6), 475–483.

Petit, L., Clark, V.P., Ingeholm, J., and Haxby, J.V. (1997). Dissociation of saccade-related and pursuit-related activation in human frontal eye fields as revealed by fMRI. *Journal of Neurophysiology*, **77**(6), 3386–3390.

Pierrot-Deseilligny, C., Milea, D., and Muri, R.M. (2004). Eye movement control by the cerebral cortex. *Current Opinion in Neurology*, **17**(1), 17–25.

Pierrot-Deseilligny, Ch., Muri, R.M., Nyffeler, T., and Milea, D. (2005). The role of the human dorsolateral prefrontal cortex in ocular motor behavior. *Annals of the New York Academy of Sciences*, **1039**, 239–251.

Radant, A.D., Dobie, D.J., Calkins, M.E., Olincy, A., Braff, D.L., Cadenhead, K.S., et al. (2007). Successful multi-site measurement of antisaccade performance deficits in schizophrenia. *Schizophrenia Research*, **89**(1–3), 320–329.

Raemaekers, M., Ramsey, N.F., Vink, M., van den Heuvel, M.P., and Kahn, R.S. (2006). Brain activation during antisaccades in unaffected relatives of schizophrenic patients. *Biological Psychiatry*, **59**(6), 530–535.

Rashbass, C. (1961). The relationship between saccadic and smooth tracking eye movements. *Journal of Physiology*, **159**, 326–338.

Reilly, J.L., Harris, M.S., Keshavan, M.S., and Sweeney, J.A. (2005). Abnormalities in visually guided saccades suggest corticofugal dysregulation in never-treated schizophrenia. *Biological Psychiatry*, **57**(2), 145–154.

Reilly, J.L., Harris, M.S., Keshavan, M.S., and Sweeney, J.A. (2006). Adverse effects of risperidone on spatial working memory in first-episode schizophrenia. *Archives of General Psychiatry*, **63**(11), 1189–1197.

Reilly, J.L., Harris, M.S., Khine, T.T., Keshavan, M.S., and Sweeney, J.A. (2007). Antipsychotic drugs exacerbate impairment on a working memory task in first-episode schizophrenia. *Biological Psychiatry*, **62**(7), 818–821.

Reilly, J.L., Lencer, R., Bishop, J.R., Keedy, S., and Sweeney, J.A. (2008). Pharmacological treatment effects on eye movement control. *Brain and Cognition*, **68**(3), 415–435.

Reuter-Lorenz, P.A., Hughes, H.C., and Fendrich, R. (1991). The reduction of saccadic latency by prior offset of the fixation point: an analysis of the gap effect. *Perception and Psychophysics*, **49**(2), 167–175.

Rosano, C., Krisky, C.M., Welling, J.S., Eddy, W.F., Luna, B., Thulborn, K.R., *et al.* (2002). Pursuit and saccadic eye movement subregions in human frontal eye field: a high-resolution fMRI investigation. *Cerebral Cortex*, **12**(2), 107–115.

Rosenberg, D.R., Sweeney, J.A., Squires-Wheeler, E., Keshavan, M.S., Cornblatt, B.A., and Erlenmeyer-Kimling, L. (1997). Eye-tracking dysfunction in offspring from the New York High-Risk Project: diagnostic specificity and the role of attention. *Psychiatry Research*, **66**(2–3), 121–130.

Ross, R.G. (2003). Early expression of a pathophysiological feature of schizophrenia: saccadic intrusions into smooth-pursuit eye movements in school-age children vulnerable to schizophrenia. *Journal of the American Academy of Child and Adolescent Psychiatry*, **42**(4), 468–476.

Ross, R.G., Hommer, D., Radant, A., Roath, M., and Freedman, R. (1996). Early expression of smooth-pursuit eye movement abnormalities in children of schizophrenic parents. *Journal of the American Academy of Child and Adolescent Psychiatry*, **35**(7), 941–949.

Ross, R.G., Harris, J.G., Olincy, A., Radant, A., Adler, L.E., and Freedman, R. (1998). Familial transmission of two independent saccadic abnormalities in schizophrenia. *Schizophrenia Research*, **30**(1), 59–70.

Ross, R.G., Olincy, A., Mikulich, S.K., Radant, A.D., Harris, J.G., Waldo, M., *et al.* (2002). Admixture analysis of smooth pursuit eye movements in probands with schizophrenia and their relatives suggests gain and leading saccades are potential endophenotypes. *Psychophysiology*, **39**(6), 809–819.

Saslow, M.G. (1967). Latency for saccadic eye movement. *Journal of the Optical Society of America*, **57**(8), 1030–1033.

Schechter, I., Butler, P.D., Silipo, G., Zemon, V., and Javitt, D.C. (2003). Magnocellular and parvocellular contributions to backward masking dysfunction in schizophrenia. *Schizophrenia Research*, **64**(2–3), 91–101.

Schlenker, R., and Cohen, R. (1995). Smooth-pursuit eye-movement dysfunction and motor control in schizophrenia: a follow-up study. *European Archives of Psychiatry and Clinical Neuroscience*, **245**(2), 125–126.

Schulze, K., MacCabe, J.H., Rabe-Hesketh, S., Crawford, T., Marshall, N., Zanelli, J., *et al.* (2006). The relationship between eye movement and brain structural abnormalities in patients with schizophrenia and their unaffected relatives. *Journal of Psychiatric Research*, **40**(7), 589–598.

Sereno, A.B. and Holzman, P.S. (1995). Antisaccades and smooth pursuit eye movements in schizophrenia. *Biological Psychiatry*, **37**(6), 394–401.

Simo, L.S., Krisky, C.M., and Sweeney, J.A. (2005). Functional neuroanatomy of anticipatory behavior: dissociation between sensory-driven and memory-driven systems. *Cerebral Cortex*, **15**(12), 1982–1991.

Slaghuis, W.L., Bowling, A.C., and French, R.V. (2005). Smooth-pursuit eye movement and directional motion-contrast sensitivity in schizophrenia. *Experimental Brain Research*, **166**(1), 89–101.

Smyrnis, N. (2008). Metric issues in the study of eye movements in psychiatry. *Brain and Cognition*, **68**(3), 341–358.

Smyrnis, N., Malogiannis, I.A., Evdokimidis, I., Stefanis, N.C., Theleritis, C., Vaidakis, A., *et al.* (2004). Attentional facilitation of response is impaired for antisaccades but not for saccades in patients with schizophrenia: implications for cortical dysfunction. *Experimental Brain Research*, **159**(1), 47–54.

Stanton, G.B., Friedman, H.R., Dias, E.C., and Bruce, C.J. (2005). Cortical afferents to the smooth-pursuit region of the macaque monkey's frontal eye field. *Experimental Brain Research*, **165**(2), 179–192.

Straube, A., Riedel, M., Eggert, T., and Muller, N. (1999). Internally and externally guided voluntary saccades in unmedicated and medicated schizophrenic patients. Part I. Saccadic velocity. *European Archives of Psychiatry and Clinical Neuroscience*, **249**(1), 1–6.

Stuve, T.A., Friedman, L., Jesberger, J.A., Gilmore, G.C., Strauss, M.E., and Meltzer, H.Y. (1997). The relationship between smooth pursuit performance, motion perception and sustained visual attention in patients with schizophrenia and normal controls. *Psychological Medicine*, **27**(1), 143–152.

Sweeney, J.A., Haas, G.L., Li, S., and Weiden, P.J. (1994b). Selective effects of antipsychotic medications on eye-tracking performance in schizophrenia. *Psychiatry Research*, **54**(2), 185–198.

Sweeney, J.A., Luna, B., Keedy, S.K., McDowell, J.E., and Clementz, B.A. (2007). fMRI studies of eye movement control: investigating the interaction of cognitive and sensorimotor brain systems. *Neuroimage*, **36 Suppl 2**, T54–60.

Sweeney, J.A., Clementz, B.A., Haas, G.L., Escobar, M.D., Drake, K., and Frances, A.J. (1994a). Eye tracking dysfunction in schizophrenia: characterization of component eye movement abnormalities, diagnostic specificity, and the role of attention. *Journal of Abnormal Psychology*, **103**(2), 222–230.

Sweeney, J.A., Bauer, K.S., Keshavan, M.S., Haas, G.L., Schooler, N.R., and Kroboth, P.D. (1997). Adverse effects of risperidone on eye movement activity: a comparison of risperidone and haloperidol in antipsychotic-naive schizophrenic patients. *Neuropsychopharmacology*, **16**(3), 217–228.

Sweeney, J.A., Luna, B., Haas, G.L., Keshavan, M.S., Mann, J.J., and Thase, M.E. (1999). Pursuit tracking impairments in schizophrenia and mood disorders: step-ramp studies with unmedicated patients. *Biological Psychiatry*, **46**(5), 671–680.

Sweeney, J.A., Mintun, M.A., Kwee, S., Wiseman, M.B., Brown, D.L., Rosenberg, D.R., and Carl, J.R. (1996). Positron emission tomography study of voluntary saccadic eye movements and spatial working memory. *Journal of Neurophysiology*, **75**(1), 454–468.

Sweeney, J.A., Luna, B., Srinivasagam, N.M., Keshavan, M.S., Schooler, N.R., Haas, G.L., and Carl, J.R. (1998). Eye tracking abnormalities in schizophrenia: evidence for dysfunction in the frontal eye fields. *Biological Psychiatry*, **44**(8), 698–708.

Thaker, G.K. and Avila, M. (2003). Schizophrenia, V: risk markers. *American Journal of Psychiatry*, **160**(9), 1578.

Thaker, G.K., Nguyen, J.A., and Tamminga, C.A. (1989). Increased saccadic distractibility in tardive dyskinesia: functional evidence for subcortical GABA dysfunction. *Biological Psychiatry*, **25**(1), 49–59.

Thaker, G.K., Nguyen, J.A., and Tamminga, C.A. (1989). Saccadic distractibility in schizophrenic patients with tardive dyskinesia. *Archives of General Psychiatry*, **46**(8), 755–756.

Thaker, G.K., Ross, D.E., Buchanan, R.W., Adami, H.M., and Medoff, D.R. (1999). Smooth pursuit eye movements to extra-retinal motion signals: deficits in patients with schizophrenia. *Psychiatry Research*, **88**(3), 209–219.

Thaker, G.K., Ross, D.E., Buchanan, R.W., Moran, M.J., Lahti, A., Kim, C., and Medoff, D. (1996). Does pursuit abnormality in schizophrenia represent a deficit in the predictive mechanism? *Psychiatry Research*, **59**(3), 221–237.

Thaker, G.K., Ross, D.E., Cassady, S.L., Adami, H.M., LaPorte, D., Medoff, D.R., and Lahti, A. (1998). Smooth pursuit eye movements to extraretinal motion signals: deficits in relatives of patients with schizophrenia. *Archives of General Psychiatry*, **55**(9), 830–836.

Tien, A.Y., Ross, D.E., Pearlson, G., and Strauss, M.E. (1996). Eye movements and psychopathology in schizophrenia and bipolar disorder. *Journal of Nervous and Mental Disease*, **184**(6), 331–338.

Tregellas, J.R., Tanabe, J.L., Miller, D.E., Ross, R.G., Olincy, A., and Freedman, R. (2004). Neurobiology of smooth pursuit eye movement deficits in schizophrenia: an fMRI study. *American Journal of Psychiatry*, **161**(2), 315–321.

Von Huben, S.N., Davis, S.A., Lay, C.C., Katner, S.N., Crean, R.D., Taffe, M.A. (2006). Differential contributions of dopaminergic D(1)- and D(2)-like receptors to cognitive function in rhesus monkeys. *Psychopharmacology (Berl)* **188**, 586–596.

Walker, R., Husain, M., Hodgson, T.L., Harrison, J., and Kennard, C. (1998). Saccadic eye movement and working memory deficits following damage to human prefrontal cortex. *Neuropsychologia*, **36**(11), 1141–1159.

Wang, J., Brown, R., Dobkins, K.R., McDowell, J.E., and Clementz, B.A. (2010). Diminished parietal cortex activity associated with poor motion direction discrimination performance in schizophrenia. *Cerebral Cortex*, **20**(7), 1749–1755.

Weber, H. and Fischer, B. (1995). Gap duration and location of attention focus modulate the occurrence of left/right asymmetries in the saccadic reaction times of human subjects. *Vision Research*, **35**(7), 987–998.

Williams, G.V., Rao, S.G., and Goldman-Rakic, P.S. (2002). The physiological role of 5-HT2A receptors in working memory. *Journal of Neuroscience*, **22**, 2843–2854.

Winograd-Gurvich, C., Georgiou-Karistianis, N., Fitzgerald, P.B., Millist, L., and White, O.B. (2006). Self-paced and reprogrammed saccades: differences between melancholic and non-melancholic depression. *Neuroscience Research*, **56**(3), 253–260.

Winograd-Gurvich, C., Fitzgerald, P.B., Georgiou-Karistianis, N., Millist, L., and White, O. (2008). Inhibitory control and spatial working memory: a saccadic eye movement study of negative symptoms in schizophrenia. *Psychiatry Research*, **157**(1–3), 9–19.

Young, L.R. and Sheena, D. (1975). Eye-movement measurement techniques. *American Psychologist*, **30**(3), 315–330.

Zee, D.S., Tusa, R.J., Herdman, S.J., Butler, P.H., and Gucer, G. (1987). Effects of occipital lobectomy upon eye movements in primate. *Journal of Neurophysiology*, **58**(4), 883–907.

CHAPTER 39

Eye movements in autism spectrum disorder

Valerie Benson and Sue Fletcher-Watson

Abstract

Autism spectrum disorder (ASD) is a term encompassing a range of developmental conditions principally characterized by impairments in social interaction and communication. It is unclear to what extent the social difficulties experienced by people with ASD result from differences in sampling the social environment, or differences in interpreting the information sampled, or both. In addition, perceptual and attentional atypicalities are common in the disorder. This chapter reviews how eye tracking has been used to explore all of these issues. We organize the literature into sections covering low-level eye-movement characteristics; perception of complex stimuli; and processing of, and attention to social information. The heterogeneity of the disorder, changes across development, and the effect of general ability and linguistic level all impact upon findings. We interpret the studies reviewed in terms of these effects and link findings to theoretical accounts of autism, as well as considering the future of eye-movement research in ASD.

Introduction

Autism spectrum disorders (ASDs) are lifelong neurodevelopmental conditions, including autism, pervasive developmental disorder (PDD) and Asperger's syndrome (AS). These disorders are united by impairments in three diagnostic domains: social interaction, communication, and flexibility/imagination (APA, 1994; Wing and Gould, 1979). Autism may also entail deficits in cognitive processing such as poor executive function (Russell, 1997) and atypical attention and perception have also been highlighted (Ames and Fletcher-Watson, 2010; Behrmann et al., 2006; Burack et al., 1997; Dakin and Frith, 2005; Happé and Frith, 2006; Mottron et al., 2005). Recently, eye movement recording techniques have begun to be used to explore cognitive and perceptual processes in autism. One of the reasons for this is that there is a very tight link between eye movements and cognitive processing for many tasks (Liversedge and Findlay, 2000; Rayner, 2009). This means that measuring eye movements can be informative in relation to sampling and processing differences that might exist in autism.

This chapter seeks to consolidate and present evidence to date concerning eye movement research in this clinical population. The many theories as to the possible causes of autism (which remain unknown) are not presented in detail, but these will be referred to as they are addressed by the eye movement studies reported here.

A note on terminology: throughout this chapter participants with a clinical diagnosis of an ASD will be referred to as 'people with ASD' or similar, regardless of their specific diagnosis. This is because many studies combine, for example, people with high-functioning autism and Asperger's syndrome into a single sample. The exception will be when two different groups of people with ASD are compared with each other, or when a specific diagnostic category is otherwise relevant. When referring to ASDs in the abstract, the term 'autism' will be used for brevity, again referring to the whole spectrum of disorders. As is standard in reports of research with people with ASD, comparison participants will be referred by the acronym TD, meaning typically-developed or typically-developing (in the case of children).

Why investigate eye movements in autism?

Unusual visual orienting patterns in people with ASD are potentially of major clinical relevance, not least because such individuals often interact socially in ways that are inappropriate and/or ineffective, frequently failing to read the social cues of others. Is this because they simply do not look at the appropriate visual information source, or could it be that relevant information is visually sampled but not processed in the 'normal' way? An advantage of measuring eye movements as opposed to just reaction times or using self-report measures is that they can give an online measure of cognitive processing as it occurs during particular tasks. Patterns of saccades and fixations can inform us not only whether participants have an intact saccadic orienting system, but also what features in a display are being attended to and for how long, and thus we can make inferences about what is of significance in terms of capturing, driving, and holding attention in autism.

Eye movement recordings have, to date, been used to explore three major aspects of autism. Firstly, basic oculomotor characteristics have been investigated using low-level eye movement control paradigms. Such paradigms are used to explore the typical functioning of the oculomotor system, and assessment of any possible neurological atypicalities in people with ASD. These experiments are important since atypical eye movements may be indicative of central processing problems per se, irrespective of social function, and there is some evidence to suggest that this may be the case (e.g. Brenner et al., 2006). Some higher-level paradigms have also provided insight into the atypical attention processes apparent in autism, which may include difficulties shifting between two items, and broadening the focus of attention. Records of eye movements during tasks such as the gap-overlap paradigm (Saslow, 1967), and the antisaccade task (Hallet, 1978) produce online measures of voluntary and reflexive attentional control in autism, and are explained in more detail below. Secondly, attentional processes that operate for more complex tasks, or tasks that use more complex stimuli, have been explored using eye movement recordings. Studies have investigated whether there are perceptual processing advantages in ASD for various tasks, including visual search. Finally, and most prolifically, eye tracking has been deployed to provide insight into the social impairments which are so characteristic of autism. A large number of studies exploring scan paths for faces, and a smaller number of more recent studies examining complex social scenes have been reported, often combined with measures such as emotion recognition and social competence scores.

Observed processing differences in autism could plausibly be related to problems with basic oculomotor control, problems with higher-level cortical control, or cognitive or social processing problems that impact upon eye movement sampling, or a combination of these. Currently there are about 60 papers published on eye movements in autism that have attempted to address these possibilities.

What have eye movement studies revealed about basic oculomotor control in autism?

In the field of eye movement research there are several very well established experimental paradigms assessing low-level oculomotor function in which performance is highly predictable, and where deviations from such performance are indicative of dysfunction in either specific brain regions, or the connectivity between those regions (Pierrot-Deseillingny et al., 2004). Measures such as the time to initiate a saccade (latency), the speed of the saccade (velocity), the size of the saccade (amplitude) and the accuracy of the landing position of eye movements executed to simple targets can inform as to whether participants have an intact saccadic orienting system and whether observed deficits are a result of abnormalities in brainstem, cerebellar, or cerebral cortex anatomy or functioning (Leigh and Kennard, 2004).

One of the first studies to examine oculomotor control in autism measured saccade amplitude, velocity and latency to non-predictive, peripherally presented saccade targets (Rosenhall et al., 1988). Most participants with ASD showed reduced maximum velocity, and saccadic landing positions that fell short of the target location (hypometria) in this visually-guided saccade task. Whilst these findings may be indicative of brainstem dysfunction, unfortunately no firm conclusions concerning atypical autistic behaviour can be drawn from the study since the ASD group differed from the TD comparison group on a number of variables that could also have affected oculomotor control.

The next study (Kemner et al., 1998) used a variation of the visual odd ball paradigm (where participants are presented with rare or novel target stimuli embedded in a sequential stream of frequently appearing stimuli). Children aged between 6–12 years with ASD (n = 10) compared to TD (n = 10) and other clinical control groups were presented with novel (an ampersand on zig-zag background), rare or frequent non-social (abstract figures) stimuli, and frequency of eye movements was recorded during inspection of these and also for two intertrial interval presentations of a blank screen. Previous work had shown that individuals with ASD make more eye movements in between (visual) stimulus presentations (Roelofs, 1987) and have shorter fixation durations for task irrelevant (frequently presented) stimuli. The clearest finding from the Kemner et al. study was that participants with ASD compared to all control groups, showed increased numbers of fixations made to the blank screen presented between stimulus presentation trials. The authors suggest that this provides evidence for the involvement of higher brain structures during this task in autism. However, since the ASD group had a lower mean IQ (by 20 points) than the TD group, again caution must be used in interpreting these findings.

A more informative investigation with a larger sample (n = 26) of age and IQ matched ASD and TD groups (Minshew et al., 1999), employed three oculomotor tasks to investigate the functional integrity of the frontal and cerebellar systems in autism. In a visually guided saccade task, performance for the ASD group did not differ from the TD group on all measures including latency, accuracy, duration, and peak velocity. This is interesting since it implies that oculomotor control is normal in autism for this task. It is known that cerebellar vermal lobules VI and VII play a key role in guiding eye movements (e.g. Keller, 1989). The cerebellar model of autism (Courchesne et al., 1993) argues that cognitive deficits in shifts of attention, for example, result from dysfunction of the cerebellar vermal lobules. Deficits should therefore result in dysmetric (inaccurate) saccades. The findings from this study provide evidence for an absence of disturbance in VI and VII lobules, and in automatic shifts of visual attention for the ASD group.

The neocortical model of autism (e.g. Bennetto et al., 1996; Ozonoff et al., 1991) predicts intact saccade metrics, such as those seen in the visually-guided saccade task, but impairment on tasks that require higher-level voluntary control of saccades. This was tested in a second oculomotor delayed response task (Minshew et al., 1999). Here participants had to maintain central fixation during a 1s presentation of a peripheral target. Following a variable delay period after the target had been extinguished, participants had to make an eye movement to the 'remembered' target location. These memory-guided saccades are thought to be a standard test of spatial working memory: deficits are indicative of reduced prefrontal cortex capacity, and also indicate dysfunction of the functional connectivity between prefrontal and parietal cortex (Funahashi et al., 1993). In this task, compared to the TD group, participants with ASD showed a greater proportion of response suppression errors, i.e. an inability to suppress the execution of a reflexive saccade toward the target, and less accuracy in terms of landing position in relation to target presentation location. Latency to initiate the saccade was equivalent between groups.

In a third task participants had to make an eye movement in the opposite direction to a target onset (the antisaccade paradigm) (Minshew et al., 1999). Whether saccades can be made in this task provides a clear indication as to how effective individuals are at imposing voluntary control over their eye movements (Hallett, 1978). Erroneous saccades made toward the target are indicative of executive function abnormalities that are directly related to frontal lobe processing problems (Munoz and Everling, 2004). The ASD group produced a greater proportion of errors, but there were no other group differences for latency, accuracy, or velocity of correctly initiated saccades.

The data from the memory guided saccade task, and the antisaccade task strongly support the cortical systems model of autism, since the deficits observed on these tasks were restricted to deficits in cognitive processing such as spatial working memory deficits and deficits in inhibiting context inappropriate responses, rather than in basic saccade metrics. Minshew and colleagues concluded that autism reflects neocortical dysfunction, not cerebellar, and that in parallel with this, the elementary attentional and sensorimotor system in autism is intact and the observed deficits are in higher-order cognitive mechanisms. The obvious conclusion from these findings is that the reflexive saccadic orienting system is intact in autism, whereas the voluntary orienting system is impaired for tasks that require higher cognitive control.

Visual fixation stability has been measured as a means of further investigating cerebellar dysfunction in autism (Nowinski et al., 2005). The large (n = 52) sample in this study ranged in age from 8–46 years and were matched on IQ. Suppression of intrusive saccades (small eye movements made whilst fixating a target) and the ability to maintain eccentric gaze (keep looking at a peripheral position) were compared and were found not to be increased in the ASD group. The authors interpret these findings as indicating the functional integrity of the cerebellar brainstem networks involved in oculomotor control in autism. However, between the two participant groups there were subtle differences that showed increased amplitude of intrusive saccades, and increased latency of target re-fixation following these, for the ASD group, especially in a task where fixation had to be maintained to remembered target locations. Furthermore, these findings correlated with age in the ASD group. Atypical metrics of intrusive saccades may be attributable to faulty functional connectivity in corticocerebellar networks—so there may be subtle abnormality of the cerebellar vermis function, possibly involving reduced inhibitory input from the cerebellar to the brainstem. However, the findings of disturbances when fixating target locations in the dark without sensory guidance, are more consistent with reduced capacity for integration in sensorimotor systems that alters vermal modulation of brainstem function, and the data here suggest that dysfunction in the circuitry may increase with age at an accelerated rate in autism.

Minshew et al.'s (1999) findings have been supported by Goldberg et al. (2002) who found no group differences in basic measures such as accuracy, latency, amplitude, or peak velocity for a predictive saccade task (where participants had to look back and forth between two alternating illuminated LEDs), an antisaccade task and a memory guided saccade task. There were group differences in proportion of errors in the antisaccade task and in proportion of response suppression errors in the memory guided saccade task, similar to the findings reported in the Minshew et al., study. This confirmation of the deficits affecting inhibition of reflexive responses in the ASD group provides further support for cortical models of autism.

One difference between the Minshew and the Goldberg studies was that the ASD group were slower, compared to the TD group, to initiate saccades in the memory-guided saccade task and there was evidence for greater latency variability in the predictive saccade task. The ASD group were also slower overall to move their eye to the target in a gap-overlap task (where the central fixation was removed prior to, at the same time as, or after, the target was presented) in the Goldberg study. However there was no actual difference in the gap effect (gap minus overlap latencies) between the two groups, and this essentially means that there was no evidence for attentional disengagement differences between the two groups.

This finding contrasts with earlier reports from Landry and Bryson (2004) and van der Geest et al. (2001). The former reported a large gap effect for children with ASD compared to a TD group, while the latter found a smaller gap effect in their ASD sample. One methodological difference is that Landry and Bryson monitored eye movements using video-recording only, and analysed these frame by frame at a rate of 30 frames per second. However, the most important distinction between these studies is likely to be the choice of stimuli, which were particularly appealing to the children with ASD in the Landry and Bryson study: they used abstract images of colourful shapes falling across the screen. Marshall et al. (2009) have convincingly demonstrated that the apparent impairment in disengagement demonstrated by the children with ASD was likely due to their greater interest in the stimuli, which made it harder for them to shift attention to the periphery. Likewise, Chawarska et al. (2010) have demonstrated faster disengagement from a central stimulus when that stimulus is a face (and therefore of less interest to children with ASD), whereas disengagement is slower for TD children for face stimuli.

Van der Geest et al. predicted a smaller gap effect because they believed that the ASD group had attentional *engagement* deficits, as opposed to attentional *disengagement* deficits (Goldberg et al., 2002). Their findings and interpretation are in line with Kemner et al., (1998), and they suggest that the reduced gap effect could reflect lower activity in the fixation cells in the superior solliculus, a mid brain region thought to be involved in the integration of incoming sensory information (Stein and Meredith, 1993), and in the generation of saccades (Schiller et al., 1987). Since the frontal eye fields project directly to the superior colliculus, then in the future, the hypothesis that weaker attentional engagement in autism results in higher saccadic frequency may be found to be supported.

The examples above serve to illustrate that there is still debate as to whether differences exist in basic oculomotor control in autism for simple stimuli that require voluntary control. As we have seen, stimulus design may be an important factor affecting the pattern of results (e.g. Speer et al., 2007; see the 'What have eye movement studies revealed about social processing in autism?' section). Another factor affecting outcome may be the ages or developmental stages of the participants including the degree or severity of autism that participants' exhibit.

For example, language development in childhood is used to distinguish between high-functioning autism and AS, and it appears that this difference can affect oculomotor control (Takarae et al., 2004a). The ASD sample in their study was divided into participants with high-functioning autism who did (n = 28) or did not (n = 18) exhibit delayed language development in childhood and a large group (n = 104) of age and IQ-matched TD children, all at least 8 years old. A visually-guided saccade task using peripheral targets was used to investigate cerebellar function. Participants with ASD and language delay showed increased variability in hypometric (short) and hypermetric (long) saccade accuracy, but there were no differences in peak velocity and latency. Because these accuracy differences were observed with normal latency Takrae et al. proposed the deficit to be motor rather than attentional. The findings challenge Minshew et al's. earlier conclusion that cerebellar function is intact in autism and highlight the importance of within autism differences that may be related to language development. Figure 39.1 shows the variability in saccade landing position.

An important message from this study is that, rather than relying on the mean as the definitive measurement (for any metric), the distribution of saccades should be examined at an individual level. It is not known at present whether the pathophysiology at the level of the cerebellum differs depending on language development in high functioning autism. The current move towards eliminating the diagnostic category of AS (essentially defined as a high-functioning form of autism without developmental language delay) from the DSM-V (Frith, 2004; Ghaziuddin, 2010) will only serve to further complicate such issues.

In addition to investigating how the saccadic system operates for simple target presentation, some research has also been conducted on the ability to track moving objects in autism. It has been shown that visual motion processing is abnormal in autism (Bertone et al., 2003; Milne et al., 2005) but there is limited investigation of eye movement control for moving stimuli. Kemner et al. (2004) examined both smooth pursuit eye movements and visually guided saccades in 16 high-functioning school-aged children with ASD, and found both systems to be intact and suggested that earlier reported abnormalities in visual motion processing may need to be reinterpreted in light of their findings.

However, a more detailed study (Takarae et al., 2004b) compared pursuit eye movements in adults with ASD (n = 60 mean age 20 years) for three different tasks. Their findings pointed to some abnormalities in the smooth pursuit system in autism, but once again participant variables, in this case age, were shown to affect performance in this study. Given that autism is a developmental disorder then

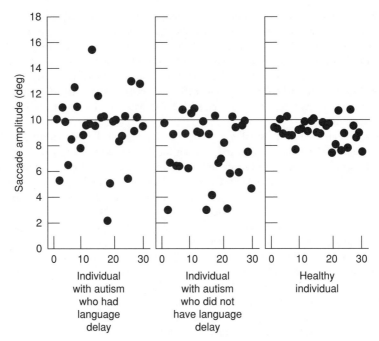

Fig. 39.1 Variability in saccade landing positions. Illustrative examples of the increased 'within-individual' variability in saccade landing positions seen in an individual with autism who had language delay, an individual without early language delay and a healthy individual. Each point in the figure represents the landing position of one saccade. The x-axis in the graph is organized from first (leftmost) to last (rightmost) eccentric saccade for each of the three subjects. The solid line indicates the 10° target step amplitude. Reproduced from *Journal of Neurology, Neurosurgery and Psychiatry*, Takarae, Y., Minshew, N., Luna, B., and Sweeney, J.A. (2004). Oculomotor abnormalities parallel cerebellar histopathology in autism, **75**(9), 1359–1361, 2004 with permission from BMJ Publishing Group Ltd.

it is not surprising that some differences manifest only at particular stages of development, and it is likely that these may either result in, and/or reflect, anatomical reorganization and functional adaptivity in different brain structures involved in both the saccadic and the smooth pursuit systems.

In summary, the work on basic oculomotor control in autism has shown that there are some subtle differences that affect performance on low-level eye movement tasks using simple stimuli, and higher-level attentional control and memory-guided saccade tasks. However, the evidence is not conclusive and basic eye movement characteristics may be affected by symptom severity, stimulus type, task demand, and developmental effects upon the neurophysiology of the brain, at various levels. Language development in autism may be a particular modulating factor of oculomotor control. Although the evidence to date suggests normal reflexive orienting with impaired voluntary orienting at the level of the cortex in autism, one must still be cautious in accepting this conclusion if group differences have not been accounted for. Studies using eye tracking to explore higher-level atypicalities in autism should not assume an absence of group differences at the level of individual eye movement control.

What have eye movement studies revealed about perceptual processing of more complex stimuli in autism?

Individuals with ASD have shown processing advantages for some complex tasks such as visual search tasks (e.g. O'Riordan et al., 2001) and the embedded figures test (EFT), in which a simple geometric shape must be found, hiding inside a more complex line-drawing, (e.g. Shah and Frith, 1983). Although there have been reaction time studies for both tasks, and functional magnetic resonance imaging (fMRI) recordings during the EFT (Manjaly et al., 2007), there is limited work on eye movement control in these tasks. One recent study by Kemner et al. (2008), recorded eye movements for a group of participants with ASD (n = 8, mean age 22 years), and a TD group (n = 8, mean age 21 years), matched on IQ, for an easy visual search task—'look for the upright bar amongst tilted bars', and a hard task—'look for the tilted bar amongst the upright bars', manipulating set size. The goal was to see whether the reason that people with ASD are better at visual search was a result of enhanced stimulus discrimination abilities, or whether they simply used a more effective search strategy. Fewer, shorter fixations to identify the target would support the former, whereas fewer, longer fixations would provide evidence for the latter hypothesis. For all set sizes participants with ASD were faster to respond, and made fewer eye movements compared to the TD group supporting the view that enhanced stimulus discrimination exists in autism. The authors have suggested that the advantage may be due to differences in basic perceptual processes.

How this activation is related to eye movement parameters is unclear, but it is known that stimulus discriminability affects the number of fixations and fixation duration (Hooge and Erkelens, 1999). However, and in contrast to the Kemner findings, data from a different visual search task has shown slower target-identification by people with ASD compared to a TD comparison group (Kourkoulou et al., 2008). This slower response was reflected by longer fixations as they scanned the display, though once they identified the target the ASD group were as quick to respond as the TD group.

The findings from the Kemner study do concur with fMRI findings for the EFT (Manjaly et al., 2007) showing evidence of enhanced local processing in early visual areas, as opposed to impaired processing of global context. This finding supports a recent reconceptualization of the weak central coherence (WCC) model of ASD (Happé and Frith, 2006). While the original model posited both enhanced local and impaired global processing (Frith and Happé, 1994), the emphasis has lately switched to focus on a processing style in autism which favours local elements, but allows for intact global processing. Further support for the updated WCC model of autism comes from a recent study, which examined fixation duration and frequency during the EFT (Keehn et al., 2009). The authors found similar first fixation durations for baseline and test conditions in the ASD group as well as shorter fixations for correct responses, indicating low-level perceptual enhancement in autism. It is inferred from the Kemner and Manjaly studies that local processing advantages observed in autism result from an amplification of early perceptual processes, which boosts the processing of local stimulus properties, but does not affect processing of global context.

A diagnostic characteristic of autism is the observation of restricted imagination/flexibility. This manifests itself in repetitive behaviours and rigid activities (in younger or low-functioning individuals) or circumscribed, intense interests (in more able individuals). In an attempt to quantify circumscribed attention, Sasson and Turner-Brown, (2008) employed eye movement recording to measure active exploration of picture arrays that included objects that were categorized as being of high or low interest to the ASD group. Arrays were also matched for social or non-social content. It was hypothesized that the severity of repetitive behaviour in the ASD group would be related to the amount of exploration of the picture arrays. Participants with ASD explored fewer images (as measured by the number of fixations to images), had longer fixation times on the images they looked at, and also showed a greater number of discrete fixations on the images that they explored. A subsequent study found the same pattern of results in a sample of young children with ASD (Sasson et al., 2010).

The authors of these studies conclude that visual attention in autism is more detail oriented, more circumscribed, and more perseverative, and that eye movements as discrete measures of visual attention may be a valid way to quantify aspects of the repetitive behaviour phenotype in autism. Although a similar eye movement pattern for arrays of social and non-social objects was seen in the ASD group as a whole, the severity of repetitive behaviour symptoms in the ASD group correlated positively with exploration of non-social arrays, and negatively with perseveration on social arrays. An interesting interaction also revealed that individuals with ASD explored fewer social images when the alternative array contained high-interest objects: arrays featuring low-interest objects and arrays featuring social information were explored equally, implying that social objects are low interest to people with ASD. This study has shown that measuring eye movements can reveal differences in attentional distribution in autism for objects that have high salience for those individuals. Whilst it is known that measures of saccadic landing positions and the duration of fixations on a visual stimulus are informative regarding the visual salience of items to particular individuals (Klin et al., 2002) this study provides compelling evidence that eye movement behaviour is related to the severity of repetitive behaviour symptoms in autism.

Complex stimuli have also been used to examine attentional cueing effects in autism (Kuhn et al., 2010). This study permitted an examination of both voluntary and involuntary orienting. Participants had to saccade to a simple peripheral target and ignore centrally presented eye gaze or arrow pointing distractors, that were either congruent (pointing in the same direction of the target) or incongruent (pointing in the opposite direction to the target). See Fig. 39.2 for an example of the stimuli and a summary of the eye movement results for correct latencies and directional errors. Both groups made more errors, and had longer latencies, for incongruent versus congruent distractor cues (showing a typical cueing effect). Both cue types elicited reflexive (involuntary) saccades in the cued but unintended direction and both groups also made faster (voluntary) saccades when distractors were eyes rather than arrows. Importantly, there was no interaction with group on any of the measures. Essentially this means that both distractor cues impact upon performance in the same way for both ASD and TD groups. Since it is known that face processing, and in particular eye gaze following (see next section) is impaired in autism then this implies that this particular paradigm reflects attentional cueing per se, exclusive of any social processing demands.

In summary, a small set of studies has investigated eye movements and perceptual processing in ASD for more complex stimuli with higher-level task demands. The finding of a perceptual processing advantage is present in the eye movement measures, and although this is not entirely consistent across the visual search studies, local processing advantages fit well with contemporary theoretical models of the spectrum such as WCC (Frith and Happe, 1994; Happe and Frith, 2006). The discovery of a possible link between eye movement patterns and the flexibility/imagination element of the autistic triad of impairments (Wing and Gould, 1979) is encouraging as this validates the utility of eye movements as a means of exploring in much more detail the attentional processing differences in those that score high on this element. Finally, the Kuhn and colleagues (2010) study shows that there are sometimes more similarities than there are differences between ASD and TD individuals for simple attentional orienting tasks with complex stimuli.

What have eye movement studies revealed about social processing in autism?

The principal area in which eye movement studies have been employed to explore social impairments in autism is the specific topic of face processing. People with ASD have long been known to process faces atypically (Langdell, 1978; Sasson, 2006) though there remains some debate about the exact nature and extent of this abnormality (Jemel et al., 2006). Eye tracking is an obvious way to provide new insight into this debate and the first study on this topic was by Pelphrey and colleagues (Pelphrey et al., 2002) who presented just five male adults with ASD with a selection of Ekman and Friesen emotional faces which they were asked to view with no special instructions. Participants with ASD showed reduced fixation on 'core features' of the faces, especially eyes, regardless of emotional expression, compared with a group of non-matched TD participants.

Subsequent studies of face perception with matched comparison participants have largely reinforced the conclusions from Pelphrey et al. (2002), in particular reporting reduced fixation on the eye-region in people with ASD (Boraston et al., 2008; Corden et al., 2008; Dalton et al., 2007; Klin et al., 2002b; Sterling et al., 2008). Unfortunately, the agreement between research studies on abnormal face processing in autism ends there. Some studies of face scanning do not find differences between people with and without ASD for 'looking to the eyes' (de Wit et al., 2008; Falck-Ytter et al., 2010; Rutherford and Towns, 2008; van der Geest et al., 2002).

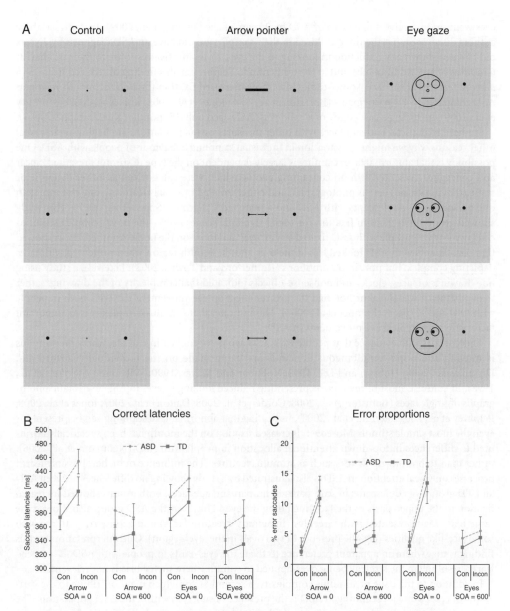

Fig. 39.2 A) Stimuli and sequence of presentation for each condition. B) Saccade latencies for correct saccades for congruent (Con) and incongruent (Incon) trials, for each distractor type, SOA and group. C) Percentage of error saccades made on congruent (Con) and incongruent (Incon) trials, for each distractor type, SOA and group. With kind permission from Springer Science+Business Media: *Experimental Brain Research*, Eye movements affirm: automatic overt gaze and arrow cueing for typical adults and adults with autism spectrum disorder. **201**(2) 2010, 155–165, Gustav Kuhn et al.

In other areas, there is also inconsistency between the outcomes of apparently very similar studies. For example, diagnosed toddlers have been found to show reduced percentages of total fixation time on the eyes from 2 years old (Jones et al., 2008) while another study found no autistic reduction in fixation on core features until 4 years old (Chawarska and Shic, 2009). Early data indicated that younger siblings of children with autism, who are 'at risk' to develop an ASD but have no diagnosis, look less at eyes than TD counterparts (Dalton et al., 2007; Merin et al., 2006). However, a recent follow-up study finds that none of those children identified at 6 months old who looked less at the eyes went on to receive a diagnosis of ASD by 2 years of age (Young et al., 2009). In contrast, these authors discovered that the three children in their sample who did have an ASD diagnosis by 2 years old had not shown any reduction in looking to the eyes, or in affective response to their mother, at 6 months of age. Additionally, and in contradiction to Pelphrey et al.'s finding of reduced fixation to *all* core features of the face, some studies also show increased fixation time on the mouth region in ASD compared to TD participants (Boraston et al., 2008; Jones et al., 2008; Klin et al., 2002b; Norbury et al., 2009), including a case-study of a child with ASD aged only 15 months (Klin and Jones, 2008).

Studies linking scan paths to faces with other measures or manipulations are beginning to reveal other reasons why we might see variation in the visual sampling behaviour of people with ASD. One possibility is that abnormal face scanning is largely dependent on the type of stimuli presented. Speer and colleagues presented stimuli containing people which were categorized as either dynamic or static (moving images versus photographs) and either isolated or social (featuring one or more than one person) to 12 adolescents with ASD and a matched TD group (Speer et al., 2007). This study showed group differences in fixation for social-dynamic scenes only—the most complex stimulus category—where people with ASD fixated less on eyes and more on the body. Another report showed that participants with ASD looked less at the eyes and the mouth region when presented with faces depicting complex, but not simple emotions (Rutherford and Towns, 2008). Likewise, a study using line drawings of faces, clocks and nonsense-objects indicated that complexity of the drawing, rather than whether it was social or not, had the greater effect on eye-movement patterns, both in people with ASD and TD peers (Kemner et al., 2007). This indicates that stimulus complexity is an important factor affecting atypical eye movements in ASD.

This concurs with evidence that people with ASD avoid eye contact in real life, where the stimulus is moving and other simultaneous demands are being made on the individual (Clifford and Dissanayake, 2008; Hobson and Lee, 1998; Volkmar and Mayes, 1990; Willemsen-Swinkels et al., 1998). In contrast, most of the reports presenting reduced looking to eyes in ASD used static photographs of single faces (Boraston et al., 2008; Corden et al., 2008; Dalton et al., 2007; Jones et al., 2008; Pelphrey et al., 2002; Sterling et al., 2008), indicating that abnormal face scanning can be present for even the most simple stimuli. Moreover, increased fixation on the mouth has been specifically attributed to differences in top-down attentional allocation in people with ASD (Neumann et al., 2006), rather than to bottom-up factors such as stimulus features. The influence of higher, possibly learnt processes on visual attention in ASD is also illustrated by a study showing no differences between ASD and TD groups of adolescents in scan paths to human and ape faces: both groups showed increased fixation to the upper-parts of the face, including the eyes. However, the ASD group also showed the same bias when presented with Greebles (imaginary-creature faces) and geometric patterns with some face-like qualities (e.g. the presence of two ovals in the 'eye' region). One interpretation for this finding is that where an apparent preference to fixate the eyes exists in people with ASD, it has been learnt, resulting in the strategy being over-applied to stimuli where such a bias is not relevant.

In addition to the issue of stimulus complexity, a second factor which may contribute to the variability of results on face scanning in ASD is the presence of subtypes within the ASD population. The studies reviewed in this chapter represent work with a range of ages and specific diagnostic groups, and these and other relevant variations in the ASD population, especially those that are not readily observable, may impact upon atypical sampling strategies. One specific possibility is that atypical looking to the eye region is underpinned by individual differences in amygdala function. A pair of studies combining eye tracking and MRI revealed that reduced fixation on eyes in people with ASD was predicted by having a small amygdala (Nacewicz et al., 2006). Small amygdalas were also related to slower emotion identification and degree of social impairment. Finally, an interaction with age suggested a complex developmental relationship between social skills, eye-region fixation and amygdala size which needs further exploration. Another study using eye-tracking and fMRI reported a relationship between eye-fixation and amygdala activation in participants with ASD exclusively (Dalton et al., 2007). These findings are supported by a number of theoretical accounts which place abnormalities in amygdala development and function at the root of autism (Baron-Cohen et al., 2000; Dawson et al., 2002; Howard et al., 2000; Kleinhans et al., 2008; Schultz, 2005).

The amygdala theory of autism could also explain the particular deficit people with ASD have in fear recognition, which is also related to eye-fixation (Corden et al., 2008; Pelphrey et al., 2002). Poor fear recognition in people with ASD correlates with low eye-region fixation (Corden et al., 2008), demonstrating how unusual facial fixation patterns could underlie some of the wider behavioural problems exhibited by people with ASD. A large number of face-scanning studies have related fixation patterns to either symptom profiles or behavioural measures and these are revealing of the role of eye-movements for successful social interaction. For example, Boraston et al. (2008), found that their participants with ASD looked less at the eyes and more at the mouth when presented with a series of photos depicting real or faked smiles (Boraston et al., 2008). Likewise, people with ASD were worse at correctly identifying faked smiles, though accuracy was not directly correlated with fixation location. People with ASD who fixate less on eyes are also slower and less accurate to identify emotions (Ba et al., 2010; Kirchner et al., 2011; Nacewicz et al., 2006; Pelphrey et al., 2002) and less accurate at familiar face recognition (Dalton et al., 2007) though others report differences in fixation but not in face recognition (Sterling et al., 2008). These contradictory findings are replicated in behavioural paradigms which have produced similarly conflicting results on the use of eyes as a source of information by people with ASD in emotion recognition tasks (Back et al., 2007; Hobson et al., 1988).

One study to explore the role of fixation-location in social proficiency in detail was an emotion-recognition task combined with so-called 'Bubbles' masking (Spezio et al., 2007). This technique presents a large number of stimuli which have been partially masked, with isolated 'bubbles' allowing a glimpse of the image underneath. By relating the bubble locations to task accuracy, one can discover what information from the underlying stimulus is most valuable to the task at hand. Participants with ASD and a TD comparison group showed no gross differences in accuracy, response time or overall fixation to the eye-regions of the emotional faces presented. However, people with ASD did exhibit less reliance on the eye region, and more reliance on the mouth to make emotional judgements. They were also more likely to look at the mouth in trials where information was also available from the eye-region. A similar pattern of looking for the same task was found in parents of people with ASD who were categorized as having traits of the Broader Autistic Phenotype (Adolphs et al., 2008) indicating a continuous relationship between looking-behaviour and autistic traits in the general population.

To date, the majority of the research on face-scanning in autism has focused on fixation on the eye region in particular. For some time, degree of eye gaze exhibited in real-life has been considered an implicit measure of social insight in people with ASD (Clements and Perner, 1994; Ruffman et al., 2001). Eye movement recordings reinforce this contention, by demonstrating that degree of fixation on the eyes is often related to social disability (Corden et al., 2008; Jones et al., 2008; Nacewicz et al., 2006; Speer et al., 2007). Conversely, it must be acknowledged that the eye region is not the only social region of the face: looking at the mouth is a valid attentional priority when engaged in conversation, for example. In fact, three studies have found relationships between looking to the mouth region and social and communicative ability in people with ASD (de Wit et al., 2008; Klin et al., 2002b; Norbury et al. 2009). A more detailed exploration of this issue indicated that looking at the mouth is associated with communicative competence, while looking at the eyes is an indicator of social ability, in people with ASD only (Falck-Ytter et al., 2010). To extend this argument, studies that present images of faces in isolation, as in most of those cited above, are limited in their relevance to the daily social difficulties experienced by people with ASD. Increasingly, eye tracking work in the autism research field has presented realistic scenes or moving images to participants, to explore eye movements across a wider range of social and non-social information.

The first of these studies by Klin and colleagues, presented participants with clips from the film 'Who's afraid of Virginia Woolf?' (Klin et al., 2002b). They divided the image into regions of interest: mouths, eyes, bodies, and objects, and painstakingly coded the location of fixation for every frame of the 2-minute, 42-second clip. Frames in which the regions of interest were too small for fixation location to be accurately identified were excluded. Group differences were found for the proportion of fixations in each region, such that the participants with ASD fixated less on the eyes and more on every other region presented. There was also a relationship between social competence and fixation time on the mouth and on objects, such that increased fixation on the mouth region was associated with greater social competence, whilst the opposite pattern was found for fixation time on objects.

Although it is not entirely clear why, this paper has frequently been cited in support of theories of autism which propose that a deficit in attention to social information in infancy is at the root of the disorder (Klin et al., 2003; Schultz, 2005). However, it is rarely noted that as well as showing diminished fixation on eyes, the (adult) participants with ASD in this study also made a much larger proportion of fixations on both the mouth region of the face and on bodies: items which are also social in nature and convey social information. The paper has also been criticized for showing participants a very extreme social scenario—the film depicts the surreal relationship of a couple who have gone to the lengths of inventing an imaginary son—which presents a real challenge to the comprehension of even the most socially able viewer. Furthermore, it has been pointed out that the stimulus properties such as concurrent multimodal information (image and soundtrack), moving images, and film-cuts (Kemner and van Engeland, 2003) might have been particularly difficult for the autistic viewer to interpret. We have already noted that complex stimulus properties may play a significant role in producing the atypical eye movements often observed in autism (Kemner et al., 2007; Rutherford and Towns, 2008; Speer et al., 2007). In this light, we might reinterpret the increased fixation time on mouth regions in the participants with ASD as evidence of effortful processing of information from both visual and aural modalities.

This account, while it clearly cannot explain atypical scanning of static photos, can be applied to some intriguing findings from biological motion paradigms. Here, it has been found that TD children show a preference to look at point-light displays which depict upright biological motion (e.g. a person dancing) more than inverted images, which appear as nonsense movements (Klin and Jones, 2008; Klin et al., 2003). Children with ASD do not show this preference, with one exception: one particular display which showed an adult person playing a clapping game was preferentially-fixated by children with ASD. This was the only stimulus presented which featured an aural-visual contingency. Again, this may be due to effortful processing of the simultaneously presented aural and visual signals. Further research is needed to tease apart the extent to which atypical patterns of fixation in autism can be attributed to aspects of the task or stimulus, as opposed to abnormal attention in the participants.

The evidence from eye movement patterns made to realistic social scenes closely reflects that found for face perception. First of all, many studies find reductions in fixation on the eyes in their participants with ASD, relative to TD peers (Klin et al., 2002a, 2002b; Riby and Hancock, 2008a, 2008b). These complex scenes also offer the opportunity for participants to look less at faces as a whole, and it is found that this is often the case for people with ASD (Benson et al., 2009; Riby and Doherty, 2010; Riby and Hancock, 2008, 2009a, 2009b; Stagg et al., 2008). However, there is also evidence of normal looking to faces and to the eye-region specifically in people with ASD (Fletcher-Watson et al., 2009; Freeth et al., 2010a, 2010b; van der Geest et al., 2002). Fletcher-Watson and Freeth and their colleagues both found that although people with ASD looked equally at the face, compared with their TD peers, they were slower to look at people and were less likely to follow the gaze of the person depicted in the scene. Figure 39.3 shows an example of the stimuli used in Fletcher-Watson et al. (2009), and a summary of the viewing time and first fixation results. These findings have been replicated in a study with children with ASD which also found reduced accuracy for the ASD group when they were required to identify which of a number of potential targets was being fixated by the person depicted (Riby and Doherty, 2010) . The '. . . Virginia Woolf?' study also showed that people with ASD were less likely than TD counterparts to follow the point of a person depicted on film (Klin et al., 2002a). These results indicate a subtle but important atypicality in initial orienting to social information and joint attention in autism and emphasize the importance of using measures such as the first eye fixation (duration or landing position) to look for sampling and processing differences between groups.

In agreement with findings from studies of processing of isolated faces, there is evidence of a relationship between looking preferences for social information and symptom profiles in autism, such that looking to faces is associated with higher social functioning (Riby and Hancock, 2008a; 2008b). In an imaginative study, Stagg and colleagues presented stimuli which showed two cartoon people

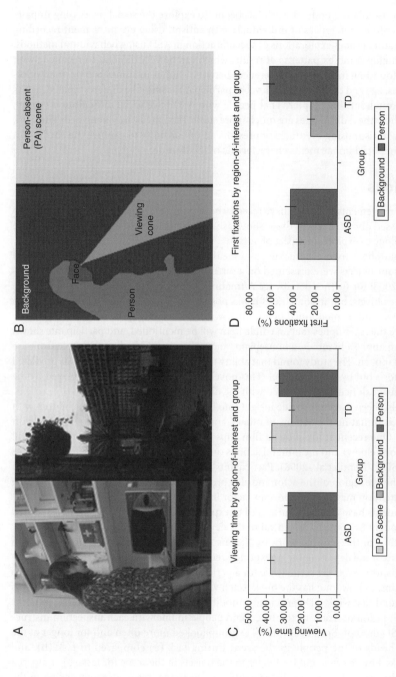

Fig. 39.3 A) Example of stimuli. B) Regions of interest demarcated by grey shading. The 'viewing cone' shows the region being fixated by the person in the scene. Items in this region were fixated at a rate no more than chance by people with ASD, whereas TD participants showed a level of interest in these objects significantly above chance. C) Viewing time results. D) First fixation results. From Fletcher-Watson, S., Leekam, S. R., Benson, V., Frank, M. C. and Findlay, J. M. (2009). First fixations reveal attention to social information in autism spectrum disorder. *Neuropsychologia* **47**, 248–257.

either facing each other or back-to-back (Stagg et al., 2008). Participants with high-functioning autism, but not AS, looked less at the facing pair than TD participants. For participants with AS, degree of preference for the interacting pair was correlated with a measure of their social ability in the real world.

In summary, an accumulating body of work has begun to explore the social processing impairments and social attention preferences of individuals with autism, using eye movement recording techniques. This literature echoes explorations of social function in ASD using behavioural methods, in producing some highly complex patterns of results which can be very difficult to reconcile with each other. The confounding influence of differences between studies in stimulus type, methodology, specific diagnosis, age and developmental level of participants cannot be underestimated, as has been emphasized throughout this chapter. That people with ASD have social difficulties is typical, but these data show how these difficulties are much more subtle than previously imagined. The work on social function in autism using eye tracking presents an opportunity to capture the elusive but significant roots of the social impairments characteristic of the disorder.

Future directions

Three studies on eye movements in autism have recently been published which do not fall neatly into the categories discussed above. Each of these showcases a promising new way of harnessing eye movement methodology to explore an aspect of autism.

Brock and colleagues have used eye tracking as a measure of linguistic ability, in a visual world paradigm in which four objects were presented on a screen, while a sentence was played to participants (Brock et al., 2008; for further details, see Altmann, Chapter 54, this volume). The sentence referred to one of the objects, but in some cases it was possible to use the context of the sentence to predict which object would be mentioned before that word was actually spoken. For example, the sentence 'The boy ate the . . .' implies that an edible item will be mentioned, and participants shown a display depicting an apple, a hammer, a houseplant, and a chair would look at the apple from the point that the verb is spoken. The study found that ability to fixate on target items early was predicted not by autism diagnosis but by language level. This novel finding highlights the role played by the often-neglected language difficulties associated with the disorder.

Eye tracking has also been used to provide insight into imitation abilities in autism: children with ASD are often poor at imitating the actions of others, and may not do so spontaneously (Meltzoff and Gopnik, 1993). One recent study showed film clips of someone performing non-meaningful gestures (e.g. lifting one elbow) and meaningful actions on objects (e.g. opening a jar) to adolescents with and without ASD (Vivanti et al., 2008). Participants' eye movements indicated that those with ASD looked less at the eye region of the actor and also produced less accurate imitations, indicating that interpersonal attention may be an important factor in imitation.

Finally, eye movements have also been measured to explore the executive dysfunctions associated with autism, and thought by some to be central to the development of the disorder (Russell, 1997). In a partial replication of the seminal work by Yarbus (1967) participants were presented with a picture of a complex scene depicting the unexpected return home of a father from a war (Benson et al., 2009). Participants viewed the scene twice for a period of 20 s, each time following one of two inspection instructions: a) how long has the unexpected visitor been absent? And, b) how wealthy is the family? It was found that while TD participants modified their eye movement patterns, in terms of proportion and duration of fixations to objects and people in line with each inspection instruction, people with ASD did not. Specifically, the TD group looked more often and for longer at the people, and to the heads of the people in the scene during task (a) compared to task (b), and conversely, they looked more often and for longer to the objects in the scene for task (b) compared to task (a). This indicates that they sampled the different elements in the scene according to the top-down instructions given prior to each inspection. These online sampling differences for the two complex task instructions were absent for the ASD group. See Fig. 39.4 for a summary of the findings and a description of how the stimulus picture was divided into interest areas.

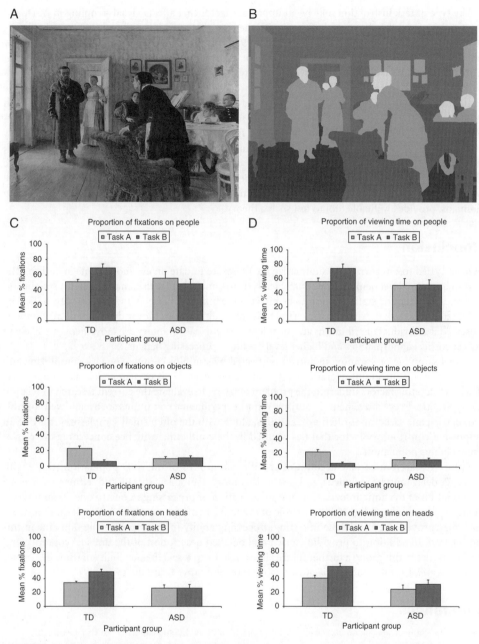

Fig. 39.4 Stimuli. A) The 'Repin' picture and (B) regions of interest, which were categorized as people (heads and bodies), objects (on the floor and wall) and background items (doors and windows, walls and ceiling, floor, window panes). Results: C) proportion of fixations directed to the people domain (top), the object domain (middle), and the heads only domain (bottom). D) Proportion of viewing time spent in the people domain (top), the object domain (middle), and the heads only domain (bottom). Error bars denote ±1 S.E.M. Reprinted from *Neuropsychologia*, **47**(4), Valerie Benson, Jenna Piper and Sue Fletcher-Watson, Atypical saccadic scanning in autistic spectrum disorder, pp. 1178–1182, © 2009, with permission from Elsevier.

The type of task instruction may be an important factor that affects visual sampling in ASD, and the findings from the above study fit well with the view that autism is a disorder of complex information processing (Minshew and Goldstein, 1998) with an intact visuospatial system. This view implies that the problem is not with acquisition of information, but with the processing of information. Minshew and Goldstein argue that for many cognitive domains processing demands that are simple or mechanical are intact in ASD, whereas processing of more complex information within the same domain may be impaired. The earlier reported finding which showed that participants with ASD increase the number of fixations to people in a simple gender discrimination task (Fletcher-Watson et al., 2009), coupled with the finding from the partial replication of the Yarbus study (Benson et al., 2009) which showed a lack of modulation on eye movement patterns for complex task instructions (i.e. those that demand a high-level value judgement to be made in order to complete the task) support this theory. What they also show is that the recording and examination of eye movements for simple and complex task instructions, for cognitive, and perhaps other processing domains, provide a valuable tool to test such a theory.

Conclusion

We have tried to categorize and summarize the literature to date on eye movements in autism. The research on low-level oculomotor control leads us to conclude that the smooth pursuit system and the saccadic orienting system appear to be intact at the brainstem level in individuals with ASD. Any subtle differences that exist in basic characteristics resulting from motor dysfunction may only be observed if individual distributions are considered. Abnormal voluntary eye movements are likely to reflect cortical abnormalities and higher level cognitive processing deficits.

Visual sampling or scanning in autism is affected by stimulus complexity, task complexity, and symptom profile, including age, severity, whether language delay is present and social competence. These moderating factors underpin the problem of trying to evaluate the current research in relation to atypicalities in eye movements in autism. Whilst experimental conditions are usually well controlled, participant variation is often not, and this, along with the often small sample sizes, may be an important contributory factor that has resulted in the conflicting evidence concerning eye movements in this population.

Future research must take account of specific sub groups of the ASD population (those with language delay must be included), and also employ more naturalistic stimuli and settings, such as the presentation of dynamic information and investigation of processing in one to one social interactions (as suggested by Klin, 2008). The role of eye movements for simple and complex task instruction may prove to be invaluable in testing processing ability in many processing domains in this population. In addition to providing a rich and detailed description of the unusual cognitive and social profiles in this group a further future aim should be to assess the possibility of using eye movement research to contribute to diagnostic tools or rehabilitative techniques.

References

APA (1994). *Diagnostic and Statistical Manual of Mental Disorders* (4th edn.).Washington, DC: American Psychiatric Association.

Adolphs, R., Spezio, M.L., Parlier, M., and Piven, J. (2008). Distinct face processing strategies in parents of autistic children. *Current Biology*, **18**(14), 1090–1093.

Ames, C. and Fletcher-Watson, S. (2010). A review of methods in the study of attention in autism. *Developmental Review*, **30**(1), 52–73.

Back, E., Ropar, D., and Mitchell, P. (2007). Do the eyes have it? Inferring mental states from animated faces in autism. *Child Development*, **78**(2), 397–411.

Bal, E., Harden, E., Lamb, D., Van Hecke, A., Denver, J., and Porges, S. (2010). Emotion recognition in children with autism spectrum disorders: relations to eye gaze and autonomic state. *Journal of Autism and Developmental Disorders*, **40**(3), 358–370.

Baron-Cohen, S., Ring, H.A., Bullmore, E.T., Wheelwright, S., Ashwin, C., and Williams, S.C.R. (2000). The amygdala theory of autism. *Neuroscience and Biobehavioral Reviews*, **24**(3), 355–364.

Behrmann, M., Thomas, C., and Humphreys, K. (2006). Seeing it differently: Visual processing in autism. *Trends in Cognitive Sciences*, **10**(6), 258–264.

Bennetto, L., Pennington, B.F., and Rogers, S.J. (1996). Intact and impaired memory functions in autism. *Child Development*; **67**, 1816–1835.

Benson, V., Piper, J., and Fletcher-Watson, S. (2009). Atypical saccadic sampling in autistic spectrum disorder. *Neuropsychologia*, **47**(4), 1178–1182.

Bertone, A., Mottron, L., Jelenic, P., and Faubert, J. (2003). Motion perception in autism: A complex issue. *Journal of Cognitive Neuroscience*, **15**, 218–225.

Boraston, Z.L., Corden, B., Miles, L.K., Skuse, D., and Blakemore, S.J. (2008). Brief report: Perception of genuine and posed smiles by individuals with autism. *Journal of Autism and Developmental Disorders*, **38**, 574–580.

Brenner, L.A., Turner, K.C., and Muller, R.-A. (2006). Eye movement and visual search: Are there elementary abnormalities in autism? *Journal Autism and Developmental Disorders*, **37** (7), 1289–1309.

Brock, J., Norbury, C., Einav, S., and Nation, K. (2008). Do individuals with autism process words in context? Evidence from language-mediated eye-movements. *Cognition*, **108**(3), 896–904.

Burack, J.A., Enns, J.T., Stauder, J.E.A., Mottron, L., and Randolph, B. (1997). Attention and autism: Behavioural and electrophysiological evidence. In D.J. Cohen and F.R. Volkmar (eds.) *Handbook of autism and pervasive developmental disorders* (pp. 226–247). New York: Wiley.

Chawarska, K. and Shic, F. (2009). Looking but not seeing: Atypical visual scanning and recognition of faces in 2 and 4-year-old children with autism spectrum disorder. *Journal of Autism and Developmental Disorders*, **39**(12), 1663–1672.

Chawarska, K., Volkmar, F., and Klin, A. (2010). Limited attentional bias for faces in toddlers with autism spectrum disorders. *Archives of General Psychiatry*, **67**(2), 178–185.

Clements, A. and Perner, J. (1994). Implicit understanding of belief. *Cognitive Development* **9**, 377–395.

Clifford, S. and Dissanayake, C. (2008). The early development of joint attention in infants with autistic disorder using home video observations and parental interview. *Journal of Autism and Developmental Disorders*, **38**(5), 791–805.

Corden, B., Chilvers, R., and Skuse, D. (2008). Avoidance of emotionally arousing stimuli predicts social–perceptual impairment in asperger's syndrome. *Neuropsychologia*, **46**, 137–147.

Courchesne, E., Townsend, J.P., Akshoomoff, N.A., Yeung-Courchesne, R., Press, G.A., Murakmi, J.W., *et al.* (1993). A new finding: Impairment in shifting of attention in autistic and cerebellar patients. In S.H. Broman, and J. Grafman (eds.) *Atypical deficits in developmental disorders: Implications for brain function* (pp. 101–137). Hillsdale, NJ: Erlbaum.

Dakin, S. and Frith, U. (2005). Vagaries of visual perception in autism. *Neuron* **48**(3), 497–507.

Dalton, K.M., Nacewicz, B.M., Alexander, A.L. and Davidson, R.J. (2007). Gaze-fixation, brain activation and amygdala volume in unaffected siblings of individuals with autism. *Biological Psychiatry*, **61**(4), 512–520.

Dawson, G., Carver, L., Meltzoff, A.M., Pagagiotides, H., McPartland, J., and Webb, S.J. (2002). Neural correlates of face and object recognition in young children with autism spectrum disorder, developmental delay and typical development. *Child Development*, **73**, 700–717.

de Wit, T.C.J., Falck-Ytter, T., and von Hofsten, C. (2008). Young children with autism spectrum disorder look differently at positive versus negative emotional faces. *Research in Autism Spectrum Disorders*, **2**(4), 651–659.

Falck-Ytter, T., Fernell, E., Gillberg, C. and von Hofsten, C. (2010). Face scanning distinguishes social from communication impairments in autism. *Developmental Science*, **13**(6), 864–875.

Fletcher-Watson, S., Leekam, S.R., Benson, V., Frank, M.C., and Findlay, J.M. (2009). Eye-movements reveal attention to social information in autism spectrum disorder. *Neuropsychologia*, **47**, 248–257.

Freeth, M., Ropar, D., Mitchell, P., Chapman, P. and Loher, S. (2010a). Brief report: How adolescents with ASD process social information in complex scenes: Combining evidence from eye movements and verbal descriptions. *Journal of Autism and Developmental Disorders*, **41**(3), 364–371.

Freeth, M.M., Chapman, P., Ropar, D. and Mitchell, P. (2010b). Do gaze cues in complex scenes capture and direct the attention of high functioning adolescents with ASD? Evidence from eye-tracking. *Journal of Autism and Developmental Disorders*, **40**(5), 534–547.

Frith, U. (2004). Emmanuel Miller Lecture: Confusions and controversies about Asperger syndrome. *Journal of Child Psychology and Psychiatry*, **45**(4), 672–686.

Frith, U. and Happé, F. (1994). Autism: Beyond 'theory of mind'. *Cognition*, **50**, 115–132.

Funahashi, S., Bruce, C.J., Goldman–Rakic, P.S. (1993). Dorsolateral prefrontal lesions and oculomotor delayed-response performance: evidence for mnemonic scotomas. *Journal of Neuroscience*, **13**, 1479–1497.

Ghaziuddin, M. (2010). Brief Report: Should the DSM-V drop Asperger syndrome? *Journal of Autism and Developmental Disorders*, **40**(9), 1146–1148.

Goldberg, M.C., Zee, D.S., Lasker, A.G., Garth, E., Tien, A., and Landa, R.J. (2002). Deficits in the initiation of eye movements in the absence of visual targets in adolescents with high functioning autism. *Neuropsychologia*, **1426**, 1–11.

Hooge, I.T. and Erkelens, C.J. (1999). Peripheral vision and oculomotor control during visual search. *Vision Research*, **39**, 1557–1575.

Hallett, P.E. (1978). Primary and secondary saccades to goals defined by instructions. *Vision Research*, **18**, 1279–1296.

Happé, F. and Frith, U. (2006). The weak coherence account: Detail-focused cognitive style in autism spectrum disorders. *Journal of Autism and Developmental Disorders*, **36**(1), 5–25.

Hobson, P. and Lee, A. (1998). Hello and goodbye: A study of social engagement in autism. *Journal of Autism and Developmental Disorders*, **28**, 117–127.

Hobson, P., Ouston, J., and Lee, A. (1988). Emotion recognition in autism: Co-ordinating faces and voices. *Psychological Medicine*, **18**, 911–923.

Howard, M.A., Cowell, P.E., Boucher, J., Broks, P., Mayes, A., Farrant, A. *et al.* (2000). Convergent neuroanatomical and behavioural evidence of an amygdala hypothesis of autism. *Neuroreport*, **11**, 2931–2935.

Jemel, B., Mottron, L., and Dawson, M. (2006). Impaired face processing in autism: Fact or artefact? *Journal of Autism and Developmental Disorders*, **36**, 91–106.

Jones, W., Carr, K., and Klin, A. (2008). Absence of preferential looking to the eyes of approaching adults predicts level of social disability in 2-year-old toddlers with autism spectrum disorder. *Archives of General Psychiatry*, **65**(8), 946–954.

Keehn, B., Brenner, L A., Ramos, A.I., Lincoln, A.J., Marshall, S.P., and Müller, R.-A. (2009). Eye movement patterns during an embedded figures test in children with ASD. *Journal of Autism and Developmental Disorders*, **3**(2), 383–387.

Keller E.L. (1989). The cerebellum. In: R.H. Wurtz and M.E. Goldberg (eds.) *The neurobiology of saccadic eye movements* (pp. 391–411). Amsterdam: Elsevier.

Kemner, C. and van Engeland, H. (2003). Autism and visual fixation. *American Journal of Psychiatry*, **160**(7), 1358–1359.

Kemner C, van der Geest J.N., Verbaten M.N., van Engeland H. (2004). In search of neurophysiological markers of pervasive developmental disorders: smooth pursuit eye movements? *Journal of Neural Transmission*, **111**(12), 1617–1626.

Kemner, C., van der Geest, J.N., Verbaten, M.N., and van Engeland, H. (2007). Effects of object complexity and type on the gaze behavior of children with pervasive developmental disorder. *Brain and Cognition*, **65**, 107–111.

Kemner, C., van Ewijk, L., van Engeland, H., and Hooge, I.T.C. (2008). Brief report: Eye movements during visual search tasks indicate enhanced stimulus discriminability in subjects with PDD. *Journal of Autism and Developmental Disorders*, **38**(3), 553–557.

Kemner, C., Verbaten, M.N., Cuperus, J.M., Camfferman, G., and van Engeland, H. (1998). Abnormal saccadic eye movements in autistic children. *Journal of Autism and Developmental Disorders*, **28**(1), 61–67.

Kirchner, J.C., Hatri, A., Heekeren, H.R., and Dziobek, I. (2011). Autistic symptomatology, face processing abilities and eye fixation patterns. *Journal of Autism and Developmental Disorders*, **41**, 158–167

Kleinhans, N.M., Richards, T., Sterling, L., Stegbauer, K.C., Mahurin, R., Johnson, L.C., *et al.* (2008). Abnormal functional connectivity in autism spectrum disorders during face processing. *Brain*, **131**, 1000–1012.

Klin A. (2008). In the eye of the beholden: tracking developmental psychopathology. *Journal of the American Academy of Child and Adolescent Psychiatry*, **47** (4), 362–3.

Klin, A. and Jones, W. (2008). Altered face scanning and impaired recognition of biological motion in a 15-month-old infant with autism. *Developmental Science*, **11**(1), 40–46.

Klin, A., Jones, W., Schultz, R., Volkmar, F., and Cohen, D. (2002a). Defining and quantifying the social phenotype in autism. *American Journal of Psychiatry*, **159**(6), 895–908.

Klin, A., Jones, W., Schultz, R. and Volkmar, F. (2003). The enactive mind or from actions to cognition: Lessons from autism. *Philosophical Transactions of the Royal Society*, B, **358**, 345–360.

Klin, A., Jones, W., Schultz, R., Volkmar, F. and Cohen, D. (2002b). Visual fixation patterns during viewing of naturalistic social situations as predictors of social competence in individuals with autism. *Archives of General Psychiatry*, **59**, 809–815.

Kourkoulou, A., Findlay, J.M. and Leekam, S.R. (2008). Implicit memory of visual context is intact in autism spectrum disorders. Paper presented at the Applied Vision Association Annual Meeting, University of Manchester, Manchester, UK.

Kuhn, G., Benson, V., Fletcher-Watson, S., Kovshoff, H., McCormick, C., Kirkby, J., *et al.* (2010). Eye movements affirm: automatic overt gaze and arrow cueing for typical adults and adults with autism spectrum disorder. *Experimental Brain Research*, **201**(2), 155–165.

Landry, R. and Bryson, S.E. (2004). Impaired disengagement of attention in young children with autism. *Journal of Child Psychology and Psychiatry and Allied Disciplines*, **45**(6), 1115–1122.

Langdell, T. (1978). Recognition of faces: An approach to the study of autism. *Journal of Child Psychology and Psychiatry and Allied Disciplines*, **19**, 255–268.

Leigh R.J. and Kennard C. (2004). Using saccades as a research tool in the clinical neurosciences. *Brain*, **127**, 460–77.

Liversedge, S.P. and Findlay, J.M. (2000). Eye movements reflect cognitive processes. *Trends in Cognitive Sciences*, **4**, 6–14.

Manjaly Z.M., Bruning N., Neufang S., Stephan K.E., Brieber S., Marshall J.C., *et al.*(2007) Neuro-physiological correlates of relatively enhanced local visual search in autistic adolescents. *NeuroImage*, **35**, 283–291.

Marshall, D., Findlay, J.M. and Leekam, S.R. (2009). Stimulus Interest, Disengagement of Attention and Children with ASD. Paper presented at the British Psychological Society, Developmental Psychology Section.

Meltzoff, A.M. and Gopnik, A. (1993). The role of imitation in understanding persons and developing a theory of mind. In S. Baron-Cohen, H. Tager-Flusberg, and D. Cohen (eds.) *Understanding other minds: Perspectives from autism* (pp. 335–366). New York: Oxford University Press.

Merin, N., Young, G.S., Ozonoff, S., and Rogers, S. (2006). Visual fixation patterns during reciprocal social interaction distinguish a sub-group of 6-month-old infants at risk for autism from comparison infants. *Journal of Autism and Developmental Disorders*, **37**, 108–121.

Milne, E., Swettenham, J., and Campbell, R. (2005). Motion perception and autistic spectrum disorder: A review. *Current Psychology of Cognition*, **23**(1), 3–36.

Minshew, N.J. and Goldstein, G. (1998). Autism as a disorder of complex information processing. *Mental Retardation and Developmental Disabilities Research Reviews*, **4**, 129–136.

Minshew, N.A., Luna, B., and Sweeney, J.A. (1999). Oculomotor evidence for neocortical systems but not cerebellar dysfunction in autism. *Neurology*, **52**, 917–922.

Mottron, L., Dawson, M., Soulieres, I., Hubert, B., and Burack, J. (2005). Enhanced perceptual functioning in autism: An update and eight principles of autistic perception. *Journal of Autism and Developmental Disorders*, **36**(1), 27–43.

Munoz, D.P. and Everling, S. (2004). Look away: The anti-saccade task and the voluntary control of eye movement. *Nature Reviews Neuroscience*, **5**, 218–228.

Nacewicz, B.M., Dalton, K.M., Johnstone, T., Long, M.T., McAuliff, E.M., Oakes, T.R., *et al.* (2006). Amygdala volume and nonverbal social impairment in adolescent and adult males with autism. *Archives of General Psychiatry*, **63**, 1417–1428.

Neumann, D., Spezio, M.L., Piven, J., and Adolphs, R. (2006). Looking you in the mouth: Abnormal gaze in autism resulting from impaired top-down modulation of visual attention. *Social Cognition and Affective Neuroscience*, **1**(3), 194–202.

Norbury, C., Brock, J., Cragg, L., Einav, S., Griffiths, H., and Nation, K. (2009). Eye-movement patterns are associated with communicative competence in autistic spectrum disorders. *Journal of Child Psychology and Psychiatry*, **50**(7), 834–842.

Nowinski, C.V., Minshew, N.J., Luna, B., Takarae, Y., and Sweeney, J.A. (2005). Oculomotor studies of cerebellar function in autism. *Psychiatry Research*, **137** (1–2), 11–19.

O'Riordan, M.A., Plaisted, K.C., Driver, J., and Baron-Cohen, S. (2001). Superior visual search in autism. *Journal of Experimental Psychology. Human Perception and Performance*, **27**(3), 719–730.

Ozonoff, S., Pennington, B.F., and Rogers S.J. (1991). Executive function deficits in high-functioning autistic individuals: relationship to theory of mind. *Journal of Child Psychology and Psychiatry*, **32**, 1081–1103.

Pelphrey, K.A., Sasson, N., Reznick, J. S., Paul, G., Goldman, B., and Piven, J. (2002). Visual scanning of faces in autism. *Journal of Autism and Developmental Disorders*, **32**, 249–261.

Pierrot-Deseilligny, C., Milea, D., and Muri, R.M. (2004). Eye movement control by the cerebral cortex. *Current Opinion Neurology*, **17**, 17–25.

Rayner, K. (2009). The 35th Sir Frederick Bartlett lecture: Eye movements and attention in reading, scene perception, and visual search. *Quarterly Journal of Experimental Psychology*, **62**(8), 1457–1506.

Riby, D. and Doherty, M.J. (2010). Tracking eye movements proves informative for the study of gaze direction detection in autism. *Research in Autism Spectrum Disorders*, **3**(3), 723–733.

Riby, D. and Hancock, P.J.B. (2008a). Research note: Viewing it differently: Social scene perception in Williams syndrome and autism *Neuropsychologia*, **46**(11), 2855–2860.

Riby, D. and Hancock, P.J.B. (2008b). Looking at movies and cartoons: Eye-tracking evidence from wiliam's syndrome and autism. *Journal of Intellectual Disability Research*, **53**, 169–18.

Riby, D. and Hancock, P.J.B. (2009a). Do faces capture the attention of children with Williams syndrome or autism? Evidence from tracking eye-movements. *Journal of Autism and Developmental Disorders*, **39**(3), 421–431.

Riby, D. and Hancock, P.J.B. (2009b). Looking at movies and cartoons: Eye-tracking evidence from wiliam's syndrome and autism. *Journal of Intellectual Disability Research*, **53**(2), 169–181.

Roelofs, J.W. (1987). Processing of information in autistic children. Unpublished doctoral dissertation, Utrecht University, The Netherlands.

Rosenhall, U., Johansson, E., and Gillberg, C. (1988). Oculomotor findings in autistic children. *Journal of Laryngology and Otology*, **102**(5), 435–439.

Ruffman, T., Garnham, W., and Rideout, P. (2001). Social understanding in autism: Eye gaze as a measure of core insights. *Journal of Child Psychology and Psychiatry and Allied Disciplines*, **42**(8), 1083–1094.

Russell, J. (1997). *Autism as an executive disorder*. Oxford: Oxford University Press.

Rutherford, M. and Towns, A. (2008). Scan path differences and similarities during emotion perception in those with and without autism spectrum disorders. *Journal of Autism and Developmental Disorders*, **38**(7), 1371–1381.

Saslow, M.G. (1967). Effects of components of displacement-step stimuli upon latency for saccadic eye movement. *Journal of the Optical Society of America*, **57**, 1030–1033.

Sasson, N. (2006). The development of face processing in autism. *Journal of Autism and Developmental Disorders*, **36**(3), 381–394.

Sasson, N., Turner-Brown, L., Holtzclaw, T.N., Lam, K.S.L., and Bodfish, J. (2008). Children with autism demonstrate circumscribed attention during passive viewing of complex social and nonsocial picture arrays. *Autism Research*, **1**(1), 31–42.

Sasson, N., Elison, J.T., Turner-Brown, L.M., Dichter, G., and Bodfish, J. (2010). Brief report: Circumscribed attention in young children with autism. *Journal of Autism and Developmental Disorders*, **41**(2), 242–247.

Schiller, P.H., Sandell, J.H. and Maunsell, J.H.R. (1987). The effect of frontal eye field and superior colliculus lesions on saccadic latencies in the rhesus monkeys. *Journal of Neurophysiology*, **57**, 1033–1049.

Schultz, R.T. (2005). Developmental deficits in social perception in autism: The role of the amygdala and fusiform face area. *International Journal of Developmental Neuroscience*, **23**, 125–141.

Shah, A. and Frith, U. (1983). An islet of ability in autistic children: A research note. *Journal of Child Psychology and Psychiatry and Allied Disciplines*, **24**, 613–620.

Speer, L.L., Cook, A.E., McMahon, W.N., and Clark, E. (2007). Face processing in children with autism: Effects of stimulus contents and type. *Autism*, **11**(3), 265–277.

Spezio, M.L., Adolphs, R., Hurley, R.S.E., and Piven, J. (2007). Analysis of face gaze in autism using 'Bubbles'. *Neuropsychologia* **45**: 144–151.

Stagg, S., Heaton, P., Linnell, K., and Valentine, T. (2008). Social perception in children with high functioning autism and Asperger syndrome. British Psychological Society, Annual Conference. Dublin, Ireland.

Stein, B.E. and Meredith, M.A. (1993). *The Merging of the Senses*. Cambridge, MA: A Bradford Book, MIT Press.

Sterling, L., Dawson, G., Webb, S., Murias, M., Munson, J., Panagiotides, H. *et al.* (2008). The role of face familiarity in eye tracking of faces by individuals with autism spectrum disorders. *Journal of Autism and Developmental Disorders*, **38**(9), 1666–1675.

Takarae, Y., Minshew, N., Luna, B., and Sweeney, J.A. (2004a). Oculomotor abnormalities parallel cerebellar histopathology in autism. *Journal of Neurology, Neurosurgery and Psychiatry*, **75**(9), 1359–1361.

Takarae, Y., Minshew, N., Luna, B., Krisky, C.M., and Sweeney, J.A. (2004b). Pursuit eye-movement deficits in autism. *Brain*, **127**(Pt 12), 2584–2594.

van der Geest, J.N., Kemner, C., Verbaten, M.N., and van Engeland, H. (2002). Gaze behaviour of children with pervasive developmental disorder towards human faces: A fixation time study. *Journal of Child Psychology and Psychiatry and Allied Disciplines*, **43**(5), 669–678.

van der Geest, J.N., Kemner, C., Camfferman, G., Verbaten, M.N., and van Engeland, H. (2002). Looking at images with human figures: Comparison between autistic and normal children. *Journal of Autism and Developmental Disorders*, **32**(2), 69–75.

van der Geest, J.N., Kemner, C., Camfferman, G., Verbaten, M.N., and van Engeland, H. (2001). Eye movements, visual attention and autism: a saccadic reaction time study using the gap and overlap paradigm. *Biological Psychiatry*, **50**, 614–619.

Vivanti, G., Nadig, A., Ozonoff, S., and Rogers, S.J. (2008). What do children with autism attend to during imitation tasks? *Journal of Experimental Child Psychology*, **101**(3), 186–205.

Volkmar, F.R. and Mayes, L.C. (1990). Gaze behaviour in autism. *Development and Psychopathology* **2**, 61–69.

Willemsen-Swinkels, S.H., Buitelaar, J.K., Weijenen, F.G., and van Engeland, H. (1998). Timing of social gaze behaviour in children with a pervasive developmental disorder. *Journal of Autism and Developmental Disorders*, **28**, 199–210.

Wing, L. and Gould, J. (1979). Severe impairments of social interaction and associated abnormalities in children: epidemiology and classification. *Journal of Autism and Developmental Disorders*, **9**(1), 11–12.

Yarbus, A.L. (1967). *Eye movements and vision*. New York: Plenum Press.

Young, G.S., Merin, N., Rogers, S.J., and Ozonoff, S. (2009). Gaze behaviour and affect at 6 months: predicting clinical outcomes and language development in typically developing infants and infants at risk for autism. *Developmental Science*, **12**(5), 798–814.

PART 6

Eye movement control during reading

CHAPTER 40

On the role of visual and oculomotor processes in reading

Françoise Vitu

Abstract

In the present chapter, I provide an analysis of the last 40 years of research on eye movements in reading, but from visual and oculomotor points of view. I first report rather robust and universal eye movement patterns that arise from the effects of two main variables, word length and fixation position, on where and when the eyes move. I then show that such regularities of eye behaviour cannot be solely explained by the strong visual constraints that apply to letter extraction and word identification during a fixation. These more likely reflect low-level visuomotor mechanisms associated with the computation of saccade metrics and adaptive visuomotor strategies that aim at maximizing visual-information intake by regulating when the eyes move. I conclude in favour of a rather low-level view of eye guidance in reading, where visual attention and spatial-selection processes play only a minor, delayed role.

Introduction

Saccades are brief movements of our eyes which bring poorly-resolved peripheral input onto the central, foveal part of our retinas. They are a major component of reading since they form the basis of early visual letter-extraction processes and higher-level lexical, syntactic, and semantic processes. One may intuitively think that saccades are driven step-by-step by the language processes they enable. However, if language processes certainly contribute to determine when and where the eyes move, lower-level visuomotor processes associated with saccade planning also play an important, if not greater, role. The aim of the present chapter is not to estimate the relative contribution of high- versus low-level, language-related versus visuomotor processes, but rather to clearly establish that there is a default visuomotor reading mode. This depends entirely on the basic properties of visual and oculomotor systems and the readers' perceptual experience with word identification.

In the first part, I describe rather universal reading eye movement patterns, the ones that arise from the effects of two main visual variables, word length and fixation location.[1] In the next two parts,

---

[1] Note that the effects on eye behaviour of several other visual variables were tested, but these are either less documented (e.g. the position of the word on the screen or the line of text; Vitu and McConkie, 2003; Vitu et al. 2004a) or less stable than the effects of word length and fixation location, and their origin is not as clear. These findings are not discussed here.

I explore the origin of these phenomena. I first consider the strong visual constraints that apply to letter extraction and word identification as a potential explanation. I then specify the visuomotor mechanisms and scanning strategies which more likely account for the regularities of eye behaviour. In the last, concluding part, I present my own conception of eye guidance in reading, and to clarify my point, I discuss the role of visual attention in relation with saccadic eye movements during reading.

Universal eye movement patterns: a main role of word length and fixation location

During reading, our eyes move along the lines of text with saccades of variable sizes and directions, interspaced with fixations of variable durations. Typically, the eyes move forward from one word to an upcoming word, but they sometimes make an additional fixation on the currently fixated word (a case which is referred to as within-word refixation) or they move back towards one of the previous words (inter-word regression), before progression starts again. Nearly two-thirds of the words are fixated, some words being skipped in the first eye pass on the line of text; only a few skipped words are subsequently fixated following an inter-word regression. Despite the apparent chaos and the great variability of saccade parameters, eye behaviour shows a number of regularities when two major variables, word length and fixation location (or the distance of the eyes with respect to word boundaries), are taken into account. The role of these variables is described below for inter- and intra-word eye behaviour.

Word skipping and initial landing sites in words

As just mentioned, some words are skipped during the first eye pass. These are mainly the shortest words. The likelihood of word skipping dramatically decreases with word length, dropping from about 0.76 for 1- and 2-letter words to about 0.42 for 4-letter words and 0.05 for words of 9–10 letters (Vitu et al., 1995; see also Rayner and McConkie, 1976). Word skipping also depends strongly on the location of the prior eye fixation on the line of text, that is, the eyes' launch-site distance to the beginning of a word; for launch sites of 1 letter, the probability of skipping a 5-letter word is near 0.65, but this decreases to about 0.30 for launch sites of 7–8 letters, and gets near zero for launch sites of 10 letters and more (Kerr, 1992; see also Brysbaert and Vitu, 1998).

In a manner similar to word-skipping behaviour, the eyes' landing sites in words greatly vary with word length and launch site. The effect of word length exemplifies in the well-known *preferred viewing(/landing) position effect* (or PVP/PLP effect; Rayner, 1979). This shows, in languages read from left to right that the eyes' landing position in words is most frequently towards the centre of short words (5 letters) and slightly to the left of the centre of long words (see also Coëffé, 1985; Dunn-Rankin, 1978; Hyönä, 1995; Nuthmann et al., 2005; Radach and Kempe, 1993; Radach and McConkie, 1998; Vitu et al., 1990). As shown in Fig. 40.1, there is still some variability in where the eyes land on words (see also Erdmann and Dodge, 1898), the typical Gaussian-shape distribution of landing sites extending from the very-beginning to the end of words.

The PVP effect is already present in young English-speaking children (1st grade or 6–7 years old; Grimes, 1989; for older children see Joseph et al., 2009) and it generalizes to languages read from right to left, with a maximum near the centre of short words, but slightly right of the centre of long words (Deutsch and Rayner, 1999). The effect is also present in Asian languages, though being sometimes weaker, and/or with a maximum at the very beginning of words (Kajii et al., 2001; Sainio et al., 2007; Yan et al., 2007; Yang and McConkie, 1999a; but see Tsai and McConkie, 2003). Note that these differences could arise, at least partly, from the lack of inter-word spacing in some Asian languages. Several studies indeed revealed that during the reading of English texts deprived of spaces, the distribution of landing sites in words tends to slightly shift towards the beginning of words (Morris et al., 1990; Rayner et al., 1998; see also Epelboim et al., 1997). However, the visual complexity and density of logographic characters could also contribute (Tsai and McConkie, 2003).

As originally revealed by McConkie et al. (1988), the PVP effect is the resultant of a more basic effect, the effect of launch site. The typical PVP distribution of all eye fixation positions in words is a

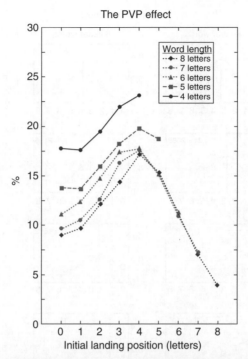

Fig. 40.1 The preferred viewing position effect as shown by the distribution of the eyes' initial landing sites in words for the case of adult readers; re-plotted from Vitu et al. (2001) in a replication of Rayner's (1979) original findings. Note that in contradiction with the classical description of the effect, the eyes did not preferentially land at the centre of short words (4–5 letters in length), but most frequently overshot the centre of these words. Reprinted from *Vision Research* **41**(25–26), F. Vitu, G.W. McConkie, P. Kerr, and J.K. O'Regan, Fixation location effects on fixation durations during reading: an inverted optimal viewing position effect, pp. 3513–3533, © 2001, with permission from Elsevier.

composite distribution, which is a summation of many landing-site distributions, each contingent on where the eyes come from on the line (see also Nuthmann et al., 2005; Radach and McConkie, 1998; for children see Huestegge et al., 2009; McConkie et al., 1991; but for Chinese see Tsai and McConkie, 2003). When the eyes come from close to the beginning of a word the landing site distribution is deviated towards the word's end, illustrating the fact that the eyes most often overshoot the centre of the word; as the eyes are launched from further away, the landing-site distribution gradually shifts towards the beginning of the word, meaning that the eyes undershoot and no longer overshoot the centre of the word (see Fig. 40.2). Interestingly, the relationship between launch site and mean landing site is linear and independent of word length; its estimated slope is on average about 0.5 character positions for 4- to 8-letter words, which indicates that for every one-letter increment of the launch-site distance, the landing position shifts on average by only half a letter (see also Nuthmann et al., 2005; but see Krügel and Engbert, 2010). More importantly, when the launch-site distance to the centre of words is held constant, the eyes land on average with about the same variability in words of different lengths, thus suggesting that launch site, more than word length, determines where the eyes land in words.

Within-word eye behaviour and fixation times

The eyes' initial landing position in a word strongly constrains the subsequent eye behaviour, affecting both the likelihood of within-word refixations and the durations of individual fixations.

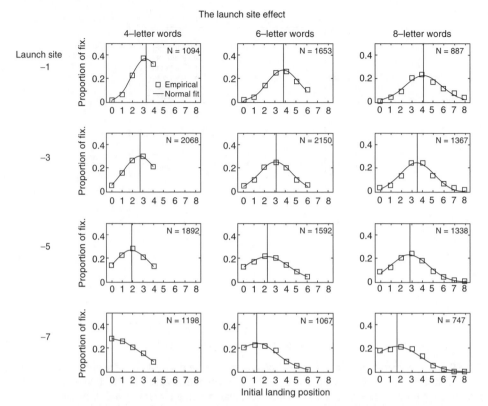

Fig. 40.2 Distributions of the eyes' initial landing sites in words of 4, 6, and 8 letters (for adult readers) as a function of the saccade's launch site measured from the space in front of the word (for the case of adult readers). A normal distribution was fitted to each of the distributions; vertical lines represent the mean of the estimated curves. From Nuthmann et al. (2005) in a replication of McConkie et al.'s (1988) original findings. Reprinted from *Vision Research* 45(17), A. Nuthmann, R. Engbert, and R. Kliegl, Mislocated fixations during reading and the inverted optimal viewing position effect, pp. 2201–2217, © 2005, with permission from Elsevier.

As shown in Fig. 40.3A, the probability of refixating a word is lower when the eyes initially land in the central region of the word than when they first fixate the beginning or end of the word. This first phenomenon has a typical U shape, with a minimum at the centre of short words and to the left of the centre of long words; it is referred to as *the refixation-optimal viewing position effect* (or *refixation-OVP effect*). It is related to another phenomenon, the OVP effect, showing that a word presented in isolation is more easily and more quickly identified when the eyes first fixate near the word's centre (O'Regan, 1990; O'Regan, et al., 1984). The refixation-OVP effect was originally shown during the recognition of isolated words presented at variable locations relative to a previously displayed fixation point (O'Regan and Lévy-Schoen, 1987). It was later found to generalize to natural reading in many different languages for the case of adults (McConkie et al., 1989; see also Hyönä, 2003; Kajii et al., 2001; Nuthmann et al., 2005; Radach and McConkie, 1998; Rayner et al., 1996; Yang and McConkie, 1999b), as well as children (McConkie et al., 1991; see also Joseph et al., 2009). The effect is weaker for words in texts than for isolated words (Vitu et al., 1990), but the likelihood of refixating a long word (6–8 letters) in reading still increases by about 50% as the initial fixation location shifts from the central region of the word to one of its ends (Vitu et al., 2001).

Fixation durations present a reverse pattern as a function of fixation location in both adults and children (Huestegge et al., 2009; McDonald et al., 2005; Nuthmann et al., 2005; Vitu et al., 2001).

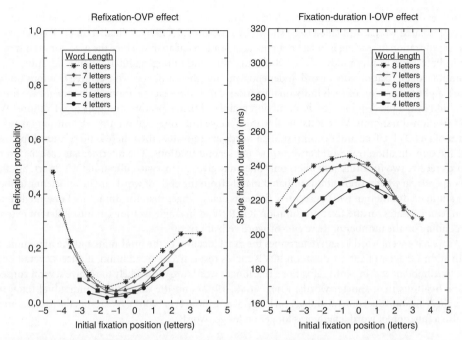

Fig. 40.3 The refixation-OVP and the fixation-duration IOVP effects in adult readers. A) The likelihood of refixating words of 4 to 8 letters as a function of the eyes' initial fixation location in words, and (B) the mean duration of single fixations on 4- to 8-letter words as a function of fixation location. Re-plotted from *Vision Research* **41**(25–26), F. Vitu, G.W. McConkie, P. Kerr, and J.K. O'Regan, Fixation location effects on fixation durations during reading: an inverted optimal viewing position effect, pp. 3513–3533, © 2001, with permission from Elsevier.

As shown in Fig. 40.3B, for the case of adults, fixation durations are longest when the eyes are near the centre of short words and to the left of the centre of long words. This inverted-U shape effect, is referred to as the *fixation-duration inverted OVP (IOVP) effect* because it is exactly opposite to the prediction one would make if fixation durations were, as suggested by previous research, uniquely determined by the difficulties of ongoing word identification processing (for a review see Rayner, 1998); since a word is most easily and most quickly identified when the eyes fall near the centre of the word (i.e. the OVP effect; see above), fixation durations should be shortest and not longest near the centre of words. This very robust phenomenon applies to first fixation durations, whether or not they are followed by an additional fixation. The durations of second fixations in two-fixation cases also tend to be longest when the eyes are near the centre of words, but these are additionally affected by the eyes' initial fixation position. Actually, there is a *fixation-duration trade-off* between the first and the second of two fixations; the first tends to be longest, and the second tends to be shortest when the eyes initially fall near the centre of a word (O'Regan and Lévy-Schoen, 1987; Vitu et al., 2001). As described by Vitu et al. (2001), the critical variable in accounting for the duration of second fixations in two-fixation cases, is more likely the distance between the first and the second fixation location; as the distance becomes greater, the duration of the second fixation becomes longer. Note that within-word refixation saccades bring the eyes preferentially towards the end of a word when they are launched from the middle of the word; otherwise, they move the eyes to the part of the word that is opposite to where they initially landed, though sometimes landing at the centre of the word (O'Regan and Lévy-Schoen, 1987; Vitu and O'Regan, 1989; see also Joseph et al., 2009).

Following O'Regan et al.'s (1984) original findings, Vitu et al. (1990) reported a *gaze-duration-OVP effect* in text reading; they found that the time the eyes remain on a word during a first eye pass is shorter when the initial fixation falls near the centre of the word than when it is towards one of the word's ends (see also Nuthmann et al., 2005). However, the effect was somewhat weaker than in the case of isolated words, and failed to be shown by Rayner et al. (1996). Whether an OVP effect exists for gaze duration in reading is in fact not crucial at our level of analysis since the gaze duration is only an indirect, composite, index of eye behaviour (Vitu and O'Regan, 2004).[2] Being the sum of the durations of all fixations on a word, it depends on both the number of consecutive fixations on the word and the duration of each individual fixation. Thus, the exact relationship between gaze duration and initial fixation location is a function mainly of the respective strengths of refixation-OVP and fixation-duration IOVP effects. If all words receive only one fixation, the relationship takes the form of an IOVP effect, and in contrast, if all words are refixated, then there is no relationship given the fixation-duration trade-off between first and second fixations. The intermediate case, i.e. some words receive two fixations and others only one, may give rise to a gaze-duration OVP effect, but this all depends on whether refixations initiated mainly from the ends of words are in sufficient number; the summed duration of two consecutive fixations being longer than the duration of one single fixation, compensates for the fixation-duration IOVP trend in single fixations, but to different extents depending on the number of these end-of-word refixations.

As we have seen, word length determines the exact location of the minimum and the maximum of refixation-OVP and fixation-duration IOVP curves respectively. In addition, it affects overall both the likelihood of within-word refixations (i.e. longer words are more likely to receive several consecutive fixations than shorter words; Kliegl et al., 1982) and the duration of individual fixations (i.e. single fixation durations are longer on longer words; Vitu et al., 2001). As a result, the gaze duration is also a function of word length; it is longer on longer words.

Inter-word regressions

The eyes mainly move forward along the lines of text, but they sometimes return to previous regions of text (in about 21% of the cases in adult readers and 34% in 1st-grade children according to McConkie et al., 1991). About 70% of the regressive saccades made by adults are inter-word regressions. They are mainly small-amplitude saccades, which bring the eyes to the immediately prior word, but in some instances, particularly when a text or a sentence comprehension difficulty is experienced they are longer saccades (e.g. Frazier and Rayner, 1982). Only a few studies have investigated systematically the determinants of inter-word regressions. However, it seems that visuomotor variables again play a critical role. As originally shown by Andriessen and de Voogd (1973), the likelihood of making a regressive saccade is primarily a function of the length of the prior, progressive, saccade; the longer the prior saccade, the more likely a regression occurs. Regressions are also a function of whether or not a word was skipped with the prior saccade. They are more likely in word-skip than in non-word-skip cases, and in word-skip cases, they are more frequent following the skipping of longer words, and when the prior saccade was launched from a far distance from the beginning of the skipped word (Vitu and McConkie, 2000; Vitu et al., 1998). Still, regressions seem to differ fundamentally from progressive saccades. They almost invariably send the eyes to the centre of the prior word, irrespective of their launch-site distance to the end of the prior word (Radach and McConkie, 1998; Vitu, 2005; Vitu et al., 1998).

Visual information processing and the limited role of parafoveal preview

Because of the many limiting factors in the extraction of visual information during a fixation, word length and fixation location are two critical variables which greatly affect both letter extraction and

---

[2] This view was developed in collaboration with G.W. McConkie, but was never published.

word-identification processes. Here, I consider the possibility that these early perceptual processes,[3] combined with higher-level language processes, are responsible for the rather universal eye-movement patterns described above. As we will see after a short description of visual-information processing in reading, perceptual processes in the time course of an eye fixation may contribute to the regularities of inter- and intra-word eye behaviour, but they cannot be the sole explanation.

The notions of visual and perceptual span

Due to the much greater density of photoreceptors in the central part of the retina than in the periphery, *visual acuity* is maximal at the centre of the fovea and decreases as retinal eccentricity increases. Thus, when a single letter is presented at a variable eccentricity from an initial fixation point, the likelihood it is identified decreases as the letter is presented more peripherally. In reading, letters are not presented in isolation, but they are surrounded by other letters, and as suggested by Bouma's (1970) original findings, this adds more constraints to letter extraction processes. The likelihood of correctly identifying a letter is lower when the letter is flanked by other characters than when it is presented in isolation. This effect, referred to as *lateral masking* or crowding, is particularly critical since it becomes greater as letter eccentricity increases (Pelli et al., 2007). It suggests that a small number of letters only may be extracted from a given eye fixation in reading.

Several authors measured the *visual span*, or the number of letters that can be extracted in a single eye fixation, when both visual acuity and lateral masking are taken into account (for reviews see O'Regan, 1989, 1990). Their findings suggest that the visual span, as defined by the number of letters that can be identified with a performance greater than 90% correct at a viewing distance of 60 cm, is of about 10 letters or 5 letters on each side of the fixation point (O'Regan et al., 1983). However, these estimations may not completely reflect the limitations associated with letter extraction in natural reading. In that case, the letters are embedded in words, and words are embedded in sentences. As known since the work of Cattell (1886), a letter is more easily identified when it is presented in a word than in a pseudoword (a non-word constructed by replacing one letter of a word with the resulting string remaining orthographically legal), or an illegal string of consonants (see also Reicher, 1969). This effect, known as the word superiority effect, suggests top-down influences on letter identification. It may be further reinforced in normal reading where most words can be predicted from the sentence context.

The *perceptual span*, measured in the time course of natural reading, takes these additional variables into account. Its first estimations were given in the mid-seventies, by two American researchers, G.W. McConkie and K. Rayner, who developed a very neat technique, referred to as the moving window technique (McConkie and Rayner, 1975; for a review see Rayner, 1998). This consists of moving a window of visible text with the reader's eyes, with all letters outside of the foveal window being replaced by irrelevant material such as xs. The perceptual span corresponds to the maximal window size below which reading speed and eye-movement characteristics remain unaffected by the manipulation. By using different window sizes and symmetrical versus asymmetrical windows, as well as different variants of the original paradigm (e.g. the foveal mask technique; Rayner and Bertera, 1979), the authors found, in the reading of English, that letter identity is extracted up to 6–8 letters to the right of fixation, and only up to 4 letters to the left; coarse information about inter-word spacing and hence word length is extracted further to the right (up to about 12 letters). O'Regan (1990) discussed these findings and techniques. He raised the possibility that the moving window technique measures perturbations of the eye movement pattern, but not the limitations of letter extraction processes. The dispute was never resolved (but see Rayner, 1998), but the fact is that estimates of both the visual and the perceptual span clearly emphasize the strong limitations that apply to letter extraction in reading.

---

[3] Note that other authors may refer to these as language processes. I prefer to speak in terms of perceptual processes because these are low-level non-language-specific processes reflecting visual-information intake, though being modulated by top-down language-related influences.

Many studies investigated whether readers benefit from words being displayed in parafoveal vision before being fixated (for a review see Rayner, 1998; see also Drieghe, Chapter 46, and Hyönä, Chapter 45, this volume). They came to about the same conclusion. Using the boundary technique, a variant of the moving window, these studies revealed that word identification was facilitated and the time spent fixating a word was shortened (as indexed by refixation probability, individual fixation duration and gaze duration) when the word was visible on a previous eye fixation (thus, while being in parafoveal vision) compared to when it was masked. However, *parafoveal preview benefit* was found to result on average from extraction of the first three letters of the words only (e.g. Lima and Inhoff, 1985).

Visual and perceptual span theories of eye guidance

In 1979, McConkie proposed a perceptual span theory of eye guidance in reading. This relied on two main principles: 1) the durations of individual fixations reflect the time required to process letters and words in the perceptual span, and 2) the length of saccades is adjusted such that the set of letters extracted from a new eye fixation juxtaposes the perceptual span of the previous fixation. This hypothesis was rapidly abandoned, based on the simple fact that the average length of forward saccades in reading (about 8 letters) is of about the same size as the perceptual span (6–8 letters to the right of fixation); this suggested that the perceptual spans from consecutive fixations in reading do not juxtapose, but overlap. Another argument came from O'Regan et al.'s (1983) study. The authors measured both the size of the visual span (as defined above) and the characteristics of eye movements in reading as a function of viewing distance (or angular character size). Results showed that the visual span comprised a smaller number of letters as the viewing distance increased from 60 to 120 cm, while the mean length of progressive saccades (measured in number of letters traversed) remained unchanged for the same viewing distances. Thus, how far the eyes moved forward was relatively independent of letter visibility. At the same time, the lack of an effect of viewing distance (or angular character size) on saccade amplitude (Morrison and Rayner, 1981) comforted the already well-established tradition of using letters and not degrees of visual angle for measuring saccade lengths in reading.

Mr Chips, an ideal-observer model for the case of reading with macular scotomas (Legge et al., 1997), relies on a set of assumptions that are quite similar to McConkie's (1979) original principles. This integrates three sources of information, visual, lexical, and oculomotor, in order to read a text in a minimal number of fixations. It relies on the notion of visual, and not perceptual span, but since the length and direction of each saccade is computed based on available visual information combined with lexical information (i.e. words are derived from the set of available letters), it is more or less the same as assuming that eye guidance is under perceptual-span control. Mr Chips seems to be a very good candidate to account for the scanning strategies developed by patients suffering from age-related macular degeneration (for a more recent two-dimensional model see Bernard et al., 2009)). It also successfully predicts some eye-movement patterns of normally-sighted readers (e.g. the relationship between the likelihood of word skipping and word length; see section 'Universal eye-movement patterns'). However, as will be further developed below, other, more basic, interpretations of these phenomena are more likely.

Inter-word eye behaviour and parafoveal preview

We have seen that the eyes tend to undershoot the centre of long and eccentric words, while they tend to skip or at least overshoot the centre of short and near words. A very simple explanation of this effect is suggested by perceptual-span views of eye guidance in reading. As words get longer and they are presented more peripherally, their letters are less likely to fall within the perceptual span. This reduces the likelihood of parafoveal word identification and may in turn increase the necessity of a fixation on the word and at a location in the word which allows all previously non-extracted letters to become available. Furthermore, if due to oculomotor aiming errors, several letters of a word fail to fall in the perceptual span on two consecutive eye fixations, as for instance when a word is skipped, the lexical ambiguity associated with the word may not be resolved. This increases in turn the likelihood of a regressive saccade as suggested by previous studies showing that inter-word regressions are more likely following the skipping of longer and initially more distant words (see 'Universal eye-movement patterns' section).

In line with this explanation, we found that the likelihood of an inter-word regression to a previously skipped word is further increased when the word has a low frequency of occurrence in the language as compared to when it is very frequent (Vitu et al., 1998; Vitu and McConkie, 2000). This suggests that online word identification contributes to determine the probability of moving the eyes backward through the line of text (see also Rayner and Liversedge, Chapter 41, this volume). However, note that the effect may purely result from the information which was extracted on the prior eye fixation and not the fixation just preceding the regressive saccade (see Vitu, 2005); thus a perceptual-span account of regression patterns cannot be asserted unambiguously.

Forward saccades are simpler to investigate and their study reveals with less ambiguity that they cannot be accounted for by a perceptual-span explanation. As pointed out by McConkie et al. (1988), if the effect of launch site on initial landing sites resulted from the amount of word information extracted in parafoveal vision, it should asymptote at launch sites above the limits of the perceptual span. As the perceptual span extends to about 6–8 letters to the right of fixation (McConkie and Rayner, 1975), the relationship between launch site and landing site should break up at launch sites of about 6 letters or even less if the visual span was taken as a reference for the number of letters extracted on a given eye fixation. However, the relationship between launch site and landing site is linear over a larger range. In addition, as shown in several other studies, the eyes' initial landing position in words is only slightly influenced by the processing of parafoveal word information. First, it varies quite systematically, but only slightly, with the orthography of parafoveal words (White and Liversedge, 2004, 2006). Second, it does not unambiguously vary with the location in the word of the most informative sequence of letters (for a review see Rayner, 1998). Third, there are some effects of the semantic predictability of words on initial landing sites; the eyes tend to land slightly further into predictable compared to unpredictable words (Lavigne-Tomps et al., 2000; but see Rayner et al., 2001). However, again, the effects are small and hard to find; they actually occur mainly when visual and lexical evidence about the upcoming word is relatively high (e.g. the word is of high frequency and it is close enough to fixation to benefit from parafoveal preview).

The probability of word skipping depends on the ease of processing associated with the words. It is greater for high- compared to low-frequency words; it is also greater for words which are predictable from the sentence context and words which are visible (as opposed to being masked) in parafoveal vision (Brysbaert and Vitu, 1998; Brysbaert et al., 2005; O'Regan, 1990). However, as noted by Brysbaert and colleagues, these effects are relatively unstable, and their magnitude is rather small, exceeding no more than about 10% on average across a large set of studies; this is actually much smaller than the effects of word length and launch site. Thus, ongoing letter extraction and word identification processes cannot be the sole explanation of the effects of word length and launch site on inter-word eye behaviour. The recent finding that the effects of word length and word predictability on the likelihood of word skipping are independent from one another (Rayner et al., 2011) is consistent with this view.

OVP, IOVP effects, and letter visibility

Several authors considered the possibility that letter visibility and hence ongoing word identification processes are responsible for the refixation-OVP effect (McConkie et al., 1989; see also Engbert et al., 2005; Reilly and Radach, 2003). As the eyes' initial fixation position in a word moves away from the centre of the word, the number of letters from the word that fall within the perceptual span decreases, which reduces the likelihood of word identification (Nazir et al., 1991), and in turn increases the probability of a refixation saccade. Although quite nice and intuitive, this assumption wrongly predicts that the strength of the refixation-OVP effect should vary with word-related variables.

While both the frequency of occurrence of a word in the language and its predictability from the prior sentence context overall influence the likelihood of within-word refixations, neither of them affect the refixation-OVP effect (McConkie et al., 1989; Vitu, 1991b).

The fixation-duration IOVP effect is also clearly not a result of ongoing letter extraction and word identification processes. The first argument comes from the many studies which tested the effects of word-related variables (e.g. word frequency, word predictability) on fixation durations and unambiguously showed that longer fixations are indicative of processing difficulties (for a review see Rayner, 1998). Since a word is more rapidly recognized when the initial fixation falls near the centre of the word than towards one of the word's ends, initial fixations, at least, should be shortest, but not longest near the centre of words. Furthermore, if by any means, the Fixation-Duration IOVP effect was related to online letter extraction and word identification, then it should vary with the linguistic properties of the words. However, as for the refixation-OVP effect, the IOVP effect remains unaffected by word frequency (Nuthmann et al., 2005; Vitu et al., 2001).

Further elements from 'z-reading' studies

Probably the strongest and most obvious argument against an account of universal eye-movement patterns in terms of online letter extraction and word identification is the fact that the same phenomena can be found in the absence of linguistic and meaningful material. Several years ago, we conducted an experiment where we compared participants' eye movements, while they were viewing either normal texts or non-texts that preserved the visual, spatial layout of words in a text, but carried no meaningful, word-related information (Vitu et al., 1995). There were four conditions; a normal reading condition with a normal text, a condition with z-texts where all letters of the original texts had been replaced by the letter 'z' and participants were asked to move their eyes as if they were reading (i.e. z-reading), and two visual search conditions in which participants were asked to search for the letter 'c' in normal texts and in z-texts where all letters except the letter 'c' had been replaced by the letter 'z'. Results first revealed a great similarity in the overall distributions of saccade lengths, and to a lesser extent in the distributions of fixation durations, fixation durations being overall longer in z-texts than in normal texts (Nuthmann et al., 2007; Rayner and Fischer, 1996).

More critically, the regularities of eye behaviour described above were all observed in z-text conditions. First, the likelihood of skipping z-letter strings was a function of string length and launch site in a manner quite similar to the probability of word skipping being a function of word length and launch site (see also Rayner and Fischer, 1996). Second, the typical PVP distribution of landing sites in words replicated almost perfectly for the case of z-strings (see also Nuthmann et al., 2007). Third, both the refixation-OVP effect and the fixation-duration IOVP effect were present, although the IOVP effect in z-reading was exaggerated as noted by Nuthmann et al. (2007). Rayner and Fischer (1996) rightly noted that there were differences between normal reading and z-reading. For instance, the likelihood of skipping short words was slightly higher (by about 10%) than the likelihood of skipping short strings. However, these small differences most likely came from the effect of ongoing parafoveal word identification processes adding up on top of the more basic, language-unrelated, word/string length effect.

Low-level visuomotor processes and strategies

We have seen that the regularities of inter- and intra-word eye behaviour as a function of word length and fixation location cannot entirely result from online letter-extraction and word-identification processes. In the present section, I present the basic, low-level, visuomotor processes and strategies, which more likely account for these regularities.

PVP and launch-site effects

Since its discovery, the PVP effect, or preference for the central region of words, was taken as evidence for the assumption that the eyes, while proceeding forward along the lines of text, aim for the centre of words, and that the variability of initial landing sites around this location results from oculomotor aiming errors (Rayner, 1979). The effect of word length on landing sites in words attested for the role of word-boundary information, and suggested that extraction of this information serves the preparation of goal-directed movements towards the centre of words. Later discovery of OVP-related phenomena provided the functional explanation of the word-centre targeting strategy by showing that a word is indeed best identified when the eyes initially fixate the centre of the word or slightly left of it (O'Regan and Lévy-Schoen, 1987). However, it was the finding of a more fundamental phenomenon, the launch-site effect, which provided the strongest arguments for this already general assumption, while defining more clearly the oculomotor constraints that may sometimes deviate the eyes away from the centre of words (McConkie et al., 1988).

As we saw in the first section in this chapter, the launch-site effect, the fact that the eyes land further into a word as their initial launch-site distance to the beginning of the word decreases, forms the basis of the typical PVP distribution of all landing sites in words. Its original account was in terms of saccadic range error (SRE), a tendency to move the eyes always the same distance forward, despite the underlying strategy of aiming at the centre of peripherally-selected target words (McConkie et al., 1988). It suggested that the eyes' effective landing position in a given word results from a compromise between an intended, goal-directed movement and an average saccade length. This interpretation was proposed on the basis of two main properties of the launch site effect. The first is the slope of the linear relationship between launch site and mean landing site (0.5); this is exactly intermediate between the slope value one would expect if the eyes always moved to the centre of words (0) and the slope value if the eyes systematically made movements of the same length (slope of 1). The second is the finding that the eyes land on average at the same distance from the centre of words of differing lengths when the eyes' initial launch-site distance to the centre of words is held constant, and quite importantly, that the eyes attain the aimed-for location mainly when executing saccades of an average length in the reading task (about 7 letters).

Further support for the SRE assumption came from another similar but more basic phenomenon, the *range effect*. Originally shown for a wide range of motor tasks (Poulton, 1981), the range effect was also found in simple oculomotor tasks (Kapoula, 1985; Kapoula and Robinson, 1986; but see Findlay, 1982). It shows that saccades bring the eyes accurately on a peripheral singleton target-object mainly when the eccentricity of the target corresponds to the middle of the range of possible target eccentricities in the block of trials; when the target is presented at smaller or greater eccentricities, the eyes respectively overshoot and undershoot the target locations. The effect suggests that saccades are subject to a systematic bias, that of moving the eyes always an average, optimal, distance in the task (Engbert and Krügel, 2010). This bias, likely at work in reading, would thus account for the variability of landing sites around the centre of words.

The SRE account of the launch site effect is nowadays well accepted. It has been implemented in different models of eye-movement control in reading, and it predicts quite well the distributions of initial landing sites in words (Engbert et al., 2005; McDonald et al., 2005; Reichle et al., 2003; see also Engbert and Kliegl, Chapter 43, and Reichle, Chapter 42, this volume); it also predicts, but to a lesser extent, an effect of launch site on the likelihood of word skipping. However, it was recently challenged based on the simple fact that the strength of the launch-site effect varies depending on whether or not the incoming saccade skips an intervening word; this finding contradicts the assumption that all saccades in a given reading task are biased towards the same length (Krügel and Engbert, 2010). As I noted 20 years ago, these are two other arguments against the SRE assumption. The first is the possibility that there is no systematic range error in saccadic eye movements; several studies indeed failed to replicate the oculomotor range effect with singleton stimuli (Coëffé and O'Regan, 1987; Findlay, 1982) and words (Vitu, 1991c). The second is the simple fact that another, more robust, oculomotor phenomenon known as the global effect could be found with isolated words (Vitu, 1991a).

The *global effect*, originally discovered by Findlay (1982), shows the general tendency to move the eyes towards the centre of gravity of the peripheral configuration formed by the presented stimuli. When, for instance, two singleton stimuli are presented simultaneously in peripheral vision, the eyes quite systematically move to an intermediate location between the two; this is true whether both stimuli are targets to be fixated in a sequence or one is a target and the other is a distractor. In contrast, when a target is presented in isolation, the eyes land relatively accurately on the target, and the landing position error, if any, is much reduced relative to that observed in two-stimulus visual displays (see also Coren and Hoenig, 1972). The global effect is, today, well documented; it was found to generalize to a large range of perceptual and oculomotor tasks, from simple saccade target tasks and visual search to reading and the free viewing of visual displays (for a review see Vitu, 2008). Present in humans as well as monkeys, it is assumed to operate at the level of the superior colliculus, a structure involved in the generation of saccadic eye movements; it reflects spatial integration processes in the motor map. When two neighbouring sites in the map are simultaneously active, the two corresponding peaks merge into a single, intermediate, peak, which in turns favours the execution of a saccade towards an intermediate location between the stimuli.

Importantly, the global effect was observed when participants were presented with pairs of words in an orthographic comparison task (Vitu, 1991a). In one of our original experiments, the two words were displayed in peripheral vision either simultaneously or sequentially, the second word appearing only when a saccade towards the first word was detected. Results showed that the distribution of initial landing sites was shifted towards the end of the first word in the simultaneous as compared to the consecutive condition, with the effect being greater when the first word was short (5 letters). Thus, letters from the two words were spatially integrated, but as suggested by further analyses and preliminary modelling, all letters did not contribute to the same extent to computation of saccade amplitude. While letters too close to fixation had no influence, more eccentric letters had less and less influence as their eccentricity increased, as predicted by the cortical magnification factor (see also Findlay, 1982). This, as well as other findings obtained in different variants of the original paradigm, led us to propose that the eyes move towards a cortically-weighted centre of gravity of the configuration formed by a subset of the letters in the periphery, irrespective of the word they belong to (see also Vitu, 2008). The critical peripheral window over which spatial integration operates excludes the letters that fall in a central foveal dead-zone of about 1° radius (Vitu et al., 2006), and may extend to a few degrees in the periphery, although the exact size of the critical peripheral window as well as the properties of the filtering mechanism remain to be determined.

Our centre-of-gravity assumption provides a nice framework to account for the launch site effect (Vitu, 1991a, 2003, 2008). As the eyes are launched from closer to the beginning of a given word, more letters from the following words fall in the critical peripheral window where spatial-integration processes operate. This shifts the weighted centre of gravity towards more peripheral locations, and in turn increases the likelihood the eyes overshoot the centre of the word or even skip the word. In a reverse manner, the eyes undershoot the centre of distant words because the letters of intervening words prevent the eyes from moving too far. Further research is certainly needed to disentangle range-error and centre-of-gravity assumptions. The possibility remains that both systematic oculomotor range error and spatial-integration processes contribute to determine the launch site effect and hence the PVP phenomenon. However, our recent investigations quite clearly argue for a spatial-integration account of the launch-site effect, with no recourse to SRE (Vitu and Blanes, 2009).

In any case, it seems quite clear that the regularities of inter-word eye behaviour depend mainly on low-level visuomotor processes associated with saccade programming. As proposed by several authors, readers' expectations of the ease of processing words of different lengths in parafoveal and peripheral vision may also contribute to determine inter-word eye behaviour (Brysbaert and Vitu, 1998; Kerr, 1992; McDonald et al., 2005). A simple strategy of skipping short and near words, which often do not require to be fixated for being identified, could potentially account for the effects of word length and launch site on word skipping probability (see also Reilly and O'Regan, 1998). However, this hypothesis was never tested experimentally.

Refixation-OVP and fixation-duration IOVP effects

The observation that refixations are less likely when the eyes initially fixate the centre of a word (i.e. the refixation-OVP effect) was made before observation of a fixation-duration IOVP effect.

In O'Regan and Lévy-Schoen's (1987) original work, only the duration of first fixations in two-fixation cases showed an inverted-U shape as a function of initial fixation location; the likelihood of single fixations being relatively low, the authors assumed, based on a few data points only, that single-fixation durations were independent of the eyes' initial fixation position. Thus, they focused mainly on the origin of the refixation-OVP effect, and actually their hypothesis cannot account for the IOVP phenomenon observed in single fixation durations. However, the authors' assumption remains interesting as it formed the basis of another, more appropriate, assumption.

O'Regan and Lévy-Schoen's (1987) rationale was based on two main, apparently contradicting, results. The first was the fact that the refixation-OVP effect could be predicted based on the likelihood of correctly identifying a word presented at variable locations with respect to initial fixation location (the basic perceptual OVP phenomenon; O'Regan, 1990; see also Brysbaert et al., 1996). The second was the finding that the refixation-OVP effect is independent of word frequency and hence unlikely the result of ongoing word identification processes (see 'Visual information processing and the limited role of parafoveal preview' section); this was later confirmed by observation of a refixation-OVP effect in z-letter strings (Vitu et al., 1995). To get around what seemed to be a contradiction, the authors assumed that the effect results from predetermined visuomotor scanning routines (or within-word tactics). These, elaborated on the basis of readers' perceptual experience that a word is more easily identified when their eyes are near its centre, are based on early localization of fixation location. They automatically trigger a refixation to the part of the word that is opposite to where the eyes initially landed, when the eyes are estimated to be far from the centre of the word (see also Reilly and Radach, 2003). In contrast, when the eyes are estimated to be near the centre of the word, the main strategy of moving the eyes to the centre of the next word takes over.

To account for fixation durations, O'Regan and Lévy-Schoen (1987) made two additional assumptions. First, every last fixation on a word terminates when the word is identified, and all words take about the same time to be identified. Second, the localization process, which relies on extraction of word-boundary information, is realized quicker when the eyes are near one of the word's ends than when they are near the middle of the word. This additional set of assumptions rightly predicts that the duration of first fixations in two-fixation cases should increase as the eyes get closer to the centre of words. It also correctly predicts that the durations of second fixations should present a reverse pattern as a function of initial fixation location (i.e. the fixation-duration trade-off); the longer the time spent during the first fixation, the quicker the word can be accessed during the second fixation. However, when a single fixation is made, both localization and word identification processes presumably happen during the same time interval; this wrongly predicts that fixation duration should remain unaffected by fixation location.

In more recent work, we preserved O'Regan and Lévy-Schoen's (1987) original assumption that readers' perceptual experience affects eye behaviour, but proposed that this primarily determines when, and not where the eyes move. In that framework, where the eyes move, and hence the refixation-OVP effect is mainly a consequence of the fixation-duration IOVP effect or how long the eyes remain at a given location. Our assumption, referred to as the *perceptual-economy* hypothesis, is that fixation durations are prolonged when the eyes are estimated to be at an optimal location for letter extraction and word identification processes (Vitu et al., 2001, 2007). When the eyes land on a word, a localization process estimates how far the eyes are from the word boundaries and how long the word is; supposedly, this is done relatively quickly based on extraction of word-boundary information. If the eyes are estimated to be near the centre of a short word or left of the centre of a long word, saccade onset is delayed. In contrast, when the eyes are estimated to be near one of a word's ends, fixation duration is determined based on default low-level visuomotor processes associated with saccade generation.

In a recent series of experiments, we provided evidence for the perceptual-economy hypothesis (Vitu et al., 2007). First, we confirmed that the fixation-duration IOVP effect generalizes to meaningless material (see 'Visual information processing and the limited role of parafoveal preview' section). Second, we showed that this effect is not obligatory given that its strength is a function of the expected amount of information in the fixation area; the effect was strongly reduced when the fixated stimulus (e.g. a string of numbers) was irrelevant for the task (i.e. an animal name search task), and this irrelevant stimulus appeared at a location where a word was never displayed. Third, we found that for the particular case of short 5-letter words inserted at variable locations in longer strings of symbols (e.g. 'xvoilexxxxx', 'xxxvoilexxx' or 'xxxxxvoilex'), fixation durations were first defined with respect to the string boundaries and hence with respect to inter-stimulus spaces as in normal reading. In all presentation conditions, short fixation durations (less than about 325–400 ms depending on the conditions) were longest when the eyes were located to the left of the string's centre, or at the optimal location for identifying words of a similar length (see O'Regan, 1990). In contrast, when fixations lasted for more than 325–400 ms, thus when there was enough time for detailed visual information to arrive and word boundaries to be distinguished from irrelevant embedded symbols, prolonged fixations were observed at the centre of the short 5-letter words in all cases. These findings clearly demonstrate in accordance with our perceptual-economy hypothesis, that fixation durations are prolonged when fixations fall at locations in words/stimuli which are usually optimal for letter extraction and word identification, and that in natural reading this operates quickly based on extraction of inter-word spaces.

An alternative to the perceptual-economy hypothesis was proposed by Nuthmann et al. (2005, 2007); they considered that mechanisms associated with the detection of oculomotor aiming errors contribute to the effect. Their assumption, referred to as the *mislocated fixation* hypothesis, directly follows the explanation of the relationship between launch site and landing site in reading. It assumes that due to systematic oculomotor range error (see above), the eyes sometimes fail to land on the intended word; a word may be unexpectedly skipped or alternatively, a word may be unexpectedly refixated. These instances which most likely correspond to fixations near the ends of words, trigger the execution of early saccade programs, and hence decrease the mean duration of the corresponding fixations. The authors implemented this assumption in the framework of the SWIFT model of eye movement control in reading, and succeeded in simulating an IOVP effect with longer fixations near the centre of words than towards the words' ends (see also Engbert et al., 2005). However, there are two main reasons why the assumption proposed by the authors cannot be the sole explanation of the IOVP effect. First, unlike the observed data, simulated IOVP curves were relatively flat in the central region of words. Second, in our experiments, an IOVP effect was found when the word was experimentally displayed at variable locations relative to the reader's previously defined fixation position, thus in the absence of oculomotor aiming errors resulting from the execution of a saccade to a given word (Vitu et al., 2007).

The remaining question concerns the origin of the refixation-OVP effect. I mentioned above that this may simply be a consequence of the fixation-duration IOVP effect. How might this be? Actually, this may come about from a simple rule, that small-amplitude and/or refixation saccades become less likely as time goes by. Since fixation durations are longer when the eyes are near the centre of a word, more information accumulates than when the eyes quickly fixate less optimal locations such as the beginning or end of a word. This reduces, in turn, the need to refixate the word in the former case, at least under the assumption that within-word refixations depend to some extent on ongoing word identification processes (Engbert et al., 2005; Vitu et al., 2007). Lower-level processes may also contribute to reduce the likelihood of small-amplitude saccades as time goes by. In recent studies, we showed that the presentation of an irrelevant distractor string of letters in the foveal region either favours the execution of short-latency small-amplitude saccades within the distractor string or delays the onset of saccades made to more peripheral locations (Vitu et al., 2006). These results suggest that small-amplitude saccades occur early on, and that they are suppressed at longer time intervals. Small-amplitude, within-word-refixation saccades are thus quite unlikely to occur when the eyes fall near the centre of a word in reading since in that case, fixation duration is prolonged.

On the role of visual attention

So far, I did not discuss the role of visual attention in reading. One first, main issue is whether visual attention intervenes in the process of driving the eyes along the lines of text. In most models of eye-movement control in reading, it implicitly plays a major role. Indeed, the common assumption that the eyes aim for the centre of peripherally selected target words necessarily implies attention-based spatial selection processes (Engbert et al., 2005; McDonald et al., 2005; Reilly and O'Regan, 1998;

Reilly and Radach, 2003; but see Reichle et al., 2003). There is evidence in the literature for a coupling between saccadic eye movements and attention shifts; in simple letter-identification tasks for instance, it was shown that perceptual performance is enhanced at the saccade-target location (e.g. Deubel and Schneider, 1996). However, the role of attention-based, selective eye guidance in reading remains debated. As recently proposed, it may well be that the eyes move forward along the lines of text without aiming for a specific location.

One such view is that developed by Yang and McConkie (2001, 2004) in their competition-interaction model of eye-movement control in reading. The authors propose that the default is to move the eyes forward with saccades of constant length, thus irrespective of word boundaries and that selective eye guidance intervenes quite late, that is, after rather long fixation durations. As their findings suggest, the extraction of visual and word-related information takes too long to determine within an average fixation interval where to move the eyes next. Thus, it is only when saccade onset is delayed that the extracted information can modulate the default move-forward strategy. An alternative is to consider that undetailed low-level visual information determines where the eyes move. As I proposed several years ago, eye movements may be determined online by low-level visuomotor processes, such as those processes which are responsible for the global effect (Vitu, 2003, 2008). By default, the eyes would move forward towards a weighted centre of gravity of the visual configuration formed by all or a subset of the letters and words in the periphery. We have seen in an earlier section ('Low-level visuomotor processes and strategies') that several reading findings are consistent with this centre-of-gravity assumption. However, the main argument comes from basic oculomotor research.

As we have seen, there is a general tendency, irrespective of the perceptual task, for our eyes to move towards the centre of gravity of the peripheral configuration. This general trend, interpreted in terms of spatial-integration processes, reflects a default saccade-programming mode, which takes place until descending influences from various visual-cortical areas arrive at the superior colliculus and visual information becomes more detailed (e.g. Findlay & Walker, 1999). It suggests that early on, the oculomotor system simply cannot isolate a visual target within a set of other visual elements, and hence that spatial selection, which in the case of reading means eye guidance towards the centre of peripherally-selected target words, cannot be the default. Now, the fact is that the global effect attenuates only for saccade latencies greater than about 260–300 ms when distractor and target stimuli are singletons separated by 3° (e.g. McSorley and Findlay, 2003), and latencies as long as 400–600 ms when the target (a letter) is embedded in a homogenous string of characters (Coëffé and O'Regan, 1987; Jacobs, 1987; Vitu et al., 2006). This indicates that spatial selection takes rather long delays to exert an influence. Since these delays are longer than average fixation intervals (225–250 ms) in reading, it seems quite obvious that spatial selection can only play a minor role, and hence that the majority of our saccades along the lines of text are simply determined by low-level spatial integration processes. In fact, the effect of launch site on initial landing sites in words, which can be interpreted in terms of spatial-integration processes (see 'Low-level visuomotor processes and strategies' section), is maintained up to fixation durations of at least 300 ms (Yang and Vitu, 2007); this further confirms that spatial selection comes in late, too late to have a major impact. Thus, to conclude, the role of attention in driving the eyes along the lines of text is not impossible, but quite implausible to us. Future studies will probably help us clarify this issue.

Whether attention intervenes in the processing of adjacent words and allows words to be processed one at a time (as proposed for instance in the E-Z reader model, e.g., Reichle et al., 2003), is another issue. As we previously argued, instead, adjacent words may be processed in parallel (Vitu et al., 2004b). The strong decrease of visual acuity with retinal eccentricity would naturally ensure that once a word is fixated this word is accessed first, without suffering too much from other words being processed more slowly in the parafovea. Note that our perceptual-economy assumption is not inconsistent with this view; it does not require selective attentional word processing.

Conclusion

To sum up, inter- and intra-word eye behaviour during reading varies greatly with visual variables such as word length and fixation location. The rather universal eye-movement patterns that these effects generate cannot be purely explained by online letter extraction and word identification processes. They more likely reflect the fact that *where* eye-movement decisions primarily depend on low-level visuomotor mechanisms, and *when* decisions result first from adaptive visuomotor strategies associated with readers' perceptual experience. These phenomena and their interpretation suggest that online language processes may only intervene as modulators of default visuomotor mechanisms and strategies.

References

Andriessen, J.J. and De Voogd, A.H. (1973). Analysis of eye movement patterns in silent reading. *IPO Annual Progress Report*, **8**, 29–34.

Bernard, J.-B., Moscoso Del Prado, F., Montagnini, A., and Castet, E. (2009). A model of optimal oculomotor strategies in reading for normal and damaged visual fields [abstract]. *Journal of Vision*, **9**(8), 824, 824a.

Bouma, H. (1970). Interaction effects in parafoveal letter recognition. *Nature*, **226**, 177–178.

Brysbaert, M. and Vitu, F. (1998). Word skipping: Implications for theories of eye movement control in reading. In G. Underwood (ed.) *Eye guidance in reading and scene perception* (pp. 125–147). Oxford: Elsevier.

Brysbaert, M., Drieghe, D., and Vitu, F. (2005). Word skipping: Implications for theories of eye movement control in reading. In G. Underwood (ed.) *Cognitive processes in eye guidance.* (pp. 53–77). Oxford: Oxford University Press.

Brysbaert, M., Vitu, F., and Schroyens, W. (1996). The right visual field advantage and the optimal viewing position effect: On the relation between foveal and parafoveal word recognition. *Neuropsychologia*, **10**, 385–395.

Cattell, J. (1886). The time it takes to see and name objects. *Mind*, **11**(41), 63–65.

Coëffé, C. (1985). La visée du regard sur un mot isolé. *L'Année Psychologique*, **85**, 169–184.

Coëffé, C. and O'Regan, J.K. (1987). Reducing the influence of non-target stimuli on saccade accuracy: Predictability and latency effects. *Vision Research*, **27**, 227–240.

Coren, S. and Hoenig, P. (1972). Effects of non-target stimuli upon length of voluntary saccades. *Perceptual and Motor Skills*, **34**, 499–508.

Deubel, H. and Schneider, W.X. (1996). Saccade target selection and object recognition: Evidence for a common attentional mechanism. *Vision Research*, **36**(12), 1827–1837.

Deutsch, A. and Rayner, K. (1999). Initial fixation location effects in reading Hebrew words. *Language and Cognitive Processes*, **14**, 393–421.

Dunn-Rankin, P. (1978). The visual characteristics of words. *Scientific American*, **238**, 122–130.

Engbert, R. and Krügel, A. (2010). Readers use Bayesian estimation for eye movement control. *Psychological Science*, **21**(3), 366–371.

Engbert, R., Nuthmann, A., Richter, E., and Kliegl, R. (2005). Swift: A dynamical model of saccade generation during reading. *Psychological Review*, **112**(4), 777–813.

Epelboim, J., Booth, J.R., Ashkenazy, R., Taleghani, A., and Steinman, R.M. (1997). Fillers and spaces in text: The importance of word recognition during reading. *Vision Research*, **37**, 2899–2914.

Erdmann, B., and Dodge, R. (1898). *Psychologische untersuchungenuber das lesen auf experimenteller grundlage*. Halle: Niemeyer.

Findlay, J.M. (1982). Global visual processing for saccadic eye movements. *Vision Research*, **22**, 1033–1045.

Findlay, J.M. and Walker, R. (1999). A model of saccade generation based on parallel processing and competitive inhibition. *Behavioral and Brain Sciences*, **22**(4), 661–720.

Frazier, L. and Rayner, K. (1982). Making and correcting errors during sentence comprehension: Eye movements in the analysis of structurally ambiguous sentences. *Cognitive Psychology*, **14**, 178–210.

Grimes, J. (1989). Where first grade children look in words during reading. Unpublished Doctoral Dissertation, University of Illinois at Urbana-Champaign, Champaign, IL, USA.

Huestegge, L., Radach, R., Corbic, D., and Huestegge, S.M. (2009). Oculomotor and linguistic determinants of reading development: A longitudinal study. *Vision Research*, **49**, 2948–2959.

Hyönä, J. (1995). Do irregular letter combinations attract readers' attention? Evidence from fixation locations in words. *Journal of Experimental Psychology: Human Perception and Performance*, **21**, 68–81.

Hyönä, J. (2003). Initial fixation position in words affects fixation durations. Paper presented at the ECEM 12 (European Conference on Eye Movements), August 20–24, Dundee.

Jacobs, A. (1987). On localization and saccade programming. *Vision Research*, **27**(11), 1953–1966.

Joseph, H.S.S.L., Liversedge, S.P., Blythe, H.I., White, S.J., and Rayner, K. (2009). Word length and landing position effects during reading in children and adults. *Vision Research*, **49**, 2078–2086.

Kajii, N., Nazir, T.A., and Osaka, N. (2001). Eye movement control in reading unspaced text: The case of the Japanese script. *Vision Research*, **41**, 2503–2510.

Kapoula, Z. (1985). Evidence for a range effect in the saccadic system. *Vision Research*, **25**(8), 1155–1157.

Kapoula, Z. and Robinson, D.A. (1986). Saccadic undershoot is not inevitable: Saccades can be accurate. *Vision Research*, **26**(5), 735–743.

Kerr, P.W. (1992). Eye movement control during reading: The selection of where to send the eyes. Unpublished Doctoral Dissertation, University of Illinois at Urbana-Champaign.

Kliegl, R., Olson, R.K., and Davidson, B.J. (1982). Regression analysis as a tool for studying reading processes: Comments on just and carpenter's eye fixation theory. *Memory and Cognition*, **8**, 336–344.

Krügel, A., and Engbert, R. (2010). On the launch-site effect for skipped words during reading. *Vision Research*, **50**, 1532–1539.

Lavigne-Tomps, F., Vitu, F., and d'Ydewalle, G. (2000). The influence of semantic context on initial landing sites in words. *Acta Psychologica*, **104**, 191–214.

Legge, G.E., Klitz, T.S., and Tjan, B.S. (1997). Mr Chips: An ideal-observer model of reading. *Psychological Review*, **104**, 524–553.

Lima, S.D. and Inhoff, A.W. (1985). Lexical access during eye fixations in reading: Effects of word-initial letter sequence. *Journal of Experimental Psychology: Human Perception and Performance*, **11**, 272–285.

McConkie, G.W., and Rayner, K. (1975). The span of the effective stimulus during a fixation in reading. *Perception and Psychophysics*, **17**, 578–586.

McConkie, G.W., Kerr, P.W., Reddix, M.D., and Zola, D. (1988). Eye movement control during reading: I. The location of initial eye fixations on words. *Vision Research*, **28**(10), 1107–1118.

McConkie, G.W., Kerr, P.W., Reddix, M.D., Zola, D., and Jacobs, A.M. (1989). Eye movement control during reading: Ii. Frequency of refixating a word. *Perception and Psychophysics*, **46**, 245–253.

McConkie, G.W., Zola, D., Grimes, J., Kerr, P.W., Bryant, N.R., and Wolff, P.M. (1991). Children's eye movement during reading. In J.F. Stein (ed.), *Vision and visual dyslexia* (pp. 251–262). London: Macmillan Press.

McDonald, S.A., Carpenter, R.H.S., and Shillcock, R.C. (2005). An anatomically constrained, stochastic model of eye movement control in reading. *Psychological Review*, **112**, 814–840.

McSorley, E. and Findlay, J.M. (2003). Saccade target selection in visual search: Accuracy improves when more distractors are present. *Journal of Vision*, **3**, 877–892.

Morris, R.K., Rayner, K., and Pollatsek, A. (1990). Eye movement guidance in reading: The role of parafoveal letter and space information. *Journal of Experimental Psychology: Human Perception and Performance*, **16**, 268–281.

Morrison, R.E., and Rayner, K. (1981). Saccade size in reading depends upon character spaces and not visual angle. *Perception and Psychophysics*, **30**, 395–396.

Nazir, T., O'Regan, J.K., and Jacobs, A.M. (1991). On words and their letters. *Bulletin of the Psychonomic Society*, **29**, 171–174.

Nuthmann, A., Engbert, R., and Kliegl, R. (2005). Mislocated fixations during reading and the inverted optimal viewing position effect. *Vision Research*, **45**, 2201–2217.

Nuthmann, A., Engbert, R., and Kliegl, R. (2007). The iovp effect in mindless reading: Experiment and modeling. *Vision Research*, **47**, 990–1002.

O'Regan, J.K. (1989). Visual acuity, lexical structure and eye movements in word recognition. In B. Elsendoorn and H. Bouma (eds.) *Working models of human perception*. (pp. 261–292). London: Academic Press.

O'Regan, J.K. (1990). Eye movements and reading. In E. Kowler (ed.) *Eye movements and their role in visual and cognitive processes* (pp. 395–453). Amsterdam: Elsevier.

O'Regan, J.K. and Lévy-Schoen, A. (1987). Eye movement strategy and tactics in word recognition and reading. In M. Coltheart (ed.) *Attention and performance xii: The psychology of reading* (pp. 363–383). Hillsdale, NJ: Erlbaum.

O'Regan, J.K., Lévy-Schoen, A., and Jacobs, A. (1983). The effect of visibility on eye movement parameters in reading. *Perception and Psychophysics*, **34**, 457–464.

O'Regan, J.K., Levy-Schoen, A., Pynte, J., and Brugaillère, B. (1984). Convenient fixation location within isolated words of different lengths and structures. *Journal of Experimental Psychology: Human Perception and Performance*, **10**, 250–257.

Pelli, D.G., Tillman, K.A., Freeman, J., Su, M., Berger, T.D., and Majaj, N.J. (2007). Crowding and eccentricity determine reading rate. *Journal of Vision*, **7**(2), 1–36.

Poulton, E.C. (1981). Human manual control. In V.B. Brooks (ed.), *Handbook of physiology. Section 1: The nervous system. Volume ii: Motor control. Part 2* (pp. 1337–1389). Bethesda, MD: American Physiological Society.

Radach, R. and Kempe, V. (1993). An individual analysis of initial fixation positions in reading. In G. d'Ydewalle and J. Van Rensbergen (eds.) *Perception and cognition: Advances in eye movement research* (pp. 213–225). Amsterdam: North-Holland/Elsevier Science Publishers.

Radach, R. and McConkie, G.W. (1998). Determinants of fixation positions in words during reading. In G. Underwood (ed.), *Eye guidance in reading and scene perception* (pp. 77–100). Oxford: Elsevier.

Rayner, K. (1979). Eye guidance in reading: Fixation location within words. *Perception*, **8**, 21–30.

Rayner, K. (1998). Eye movements in reading and information processing: 20 years of research. *Psychological Bulletin*, **124**(3), 372–422.

Rayner, K., and Bertera, J.H. (1979). Reading without a fovea. *Science*, **206**, 468–469.

Rayner, K. and Fischer, M.H. (1996). Mindless reading revisited: Eye movements during reading and scanning are different. *Perception and Psychophysics*, **58**(5), 734–747.

Rayner, K. and McConkie, G.W. (1976). What guides a reader's eye movements? *Vision Research*, **16**, 829–837.

Rayner, K., Sereno, S.C., and Raney, G.E. (1996). Eye movement control in reading: A comparison of two types of models. *Journal of Experimental Psychology: Human Perception and Performance*, **22**(5), 1188–1200.

Rayner, K., Fischer, M.H., and Pollatsek, A. (1998). Unspaced text interferes with both word identification and eye movement control. *Vision Research*, **38**, 1129–1144.

Rayner, K., Binder, K.S., Ashby, J., and Pollatsek, A. (2001). Eye movement control in reading: Word predictability has little influence on initial landing positions in words. *Vision Research*, **41**(7), 943–954.

Rayner, K., Slattery, T.J., Drieghe, D., and Liversedge, S.P. (2011). Eye movements and word skipping during reading: Effects of word length and predictability. *Journal of Experimental Psychology: Human Perception and Performance*, **37**(2), 514–528.

Reicher, G.M. (1969). Perceptual recognition as a function of meaningfulness of stimulus material. *Journal of Experimental Psychology*, **81**, 275–280.

Reichle, E.D., Rayner, K., and Pollatsek, A. (2003). The e-z reader model of eye movement control in reading: Comparisons to other models. *Behavioral and Brain Sciences*, **26**, 445–526.

Reilly, R. and O'Regan, J.K. (1998). Eye movement control during reading: A simulation of some word-targeting strategies. *Vision Research*, **38**(2), 303–317.

Reilly, R. and Radach, R. (2003). Foundations of an interactive model of eye movement control in reading. In J. Hyönä, R. Radach and H.H. Deubel (eds.) *Cognitive and applied aspects of eye movement research* (pp. 429–455). Amsterdam: Elsevier.

Sainio, M., Hyönä, Y., Bingushi, K., and Bertram, R. (2007). The role of interword spacing in reading japanese: An eye movement study. *Vision Research*, **47**, 2575–2584.

Tsai, J.L., and McConkie, G.W. (2003). Where do chinese readers send their eyes? In J. Hyönä, R. Radach and H. Deubel (eds.) *The mind's eye: Cognitive and applied aspects of eye movement research* (pp. 159–176). Oxford: Elsevier.

Vitu, F. (1991a). The existence of a center of gravity effect during reading. *Vision Research*, **31**(7/8), 1289–1313.

Vitu, F. (1991b). The influence of parafoveal preprocessing and linguistic context on the optimal landing position effect. *Perception and Psychophysics*, **50**, 58–75.

Vitu, F. (1991c). Research note: Against the existence of a range effect during reading. *Vision Research*, **31**(11), 2009–2015.

Vitu, F. (2003). The basic assumptions of e-z reader are not well-founded. *Behavioral and Brain Sciences*, **26**(4), 506–507.

Vitu, F. (2005). Visual extraction processes and regressive saccades in reading. In G. Underwood (Ed.), *Cognitive processes in eye guidance.* (pp. 1–32). Oxford, NY: Oxford University Press.

Vitu, F. (2008). About the global effect and the critical role of retinal eccentricity: Implications for eye movements in reading. *Journal of Eye Movement Research*, **2**(3): **6**, 1–18.

Vitu, F. and Blanes, C. (2009). From the global effect to eye movements in reading: The missing link. *15th European Conference on Eye Movements (ECEM)*.

Vitu, F. and McConkie, G.W. (2000). Regressive saccades and word perception in adult reading. In A. Kennedy, R. Radach, D. Heller and J. Pynte (eds.) *Reading as a perceptual process* (pp. 301–326). Oxford: Elsevier.

Vitu, F. and McConkie, G.W. (2003). *Visuo-motor influences on eye movements in reading: How word position on line affects landing positions in words.* Paper presented at the ECEM12 (12th European Conference on Eye Movements), Dundee.

Vitu, F. and O'Regan, J.K. (1989). Le rôle du prétraitement périphérique dans la lecture de textes. *Journal de Médecine Nucléaire et Biophysique*, **13**(5), 359–366.

Vitu, F. and O'Regan, J.K. (2004). Les mouvements oculaires comme indice on-line des processus cognitifs: Rêve ou réalité? In L. Ferrand and L. Grainger (eds.) *Psycholinguistique cognitive: Essai en l'honneur de Juan Segui* (pp. 189–214). Bruxelles: De Boeck Université, Collection Neurosciences et Cognition.

Vitu, F., O'Regan, J.K., and Mittau, M. (1990). Optimal landing position in reading isolated words and continuous text. *Perception and Psychophysics*, **47**(6), 583–600.

Vitu, F., McConkie, G.W., and Zola, D. (1998). About regressive saccades in reading and their relation to word identification. In G. Underwood (ed.) *Eye guidance in reading and scene perception* (pp. 101–124). Oxford: Elsevier Science Ltd.

Vitu, F., Brysbaert, M., and Lancelin, D. (2004b). A test of parafoveal-on-foveal effects with pairs of orthographically related words. *European Journal of Cognitive Psychology*, **16**(1/2), 154–177.

Vitu, F., O'Regan, J.K., Inhoff, A.W., and Topolski, R. (1995). Mindless reading: Eye-movement characteristics are similar in scanning letter strings and reading texts. *Perception and Psychophysics*, **57**, 352–364.

Vitu, F., McConkie, G.W., Kerr, P., and O'Regan, J.K. (2001). Fixation location effects on fixation durations during reading: An inverted optimal viewing position effect. *Vision Research*, **41**, 3513–3533.

Vitu, F., Lancelin, D., Jean, A., and Farioli, F. (2006). Influence of foveal distractors on saccadic eye movements: A dead zone for the global effect. *Vision Research*, **46**, 4684–4708.

Vitu, F., Lancelin, D., and Marrier d'Unienville, V. (2007). A perceptual-economy account for the inverted-optimal viewing position effect. *Journal of Experimental Psychology: Human Perception and Performance*, **33**(5), 1220–1249.

Vitu, F., Kapoula, Z., Lancelin, D., and Lavigne, F. (2004a). Eye movements in reading isolated words: Evidence for strong biases towards the center of the screen. *Vision Research*, **44**(3), 321–338.

White, S.J. and Liversedge, S.P. (2004). Orthographic familiarity influences initial eye fixation positions in reading. *European Journal of Cognitive Psychology*, **16**, 52–78.

White, S.J. and Liversedge, S.P. (2006). Foveal processing difficulty does not modulate non-foveal orthographic influences on fixation positions. *Vision Research*, **46**, 426–437.

Yan, M., Kliegl, R., Richter, H., Nuthmann, A., and Shu, H. (2007). Flexible saccade-target selection in Chinese reading. *Quarterly Journal of Experimental Psychology*, **63**(4), 705–725.

Yang, H.-M., and McConkie, G.W. (1999a). Reading chinese: Some basic eye-movement characteristics. In J. Wang, A.W. Inhoff and *et al.* (eds.) *Reading Chinese script: A cognitive analysis* (pp. 207–222). Mahwah, NJ: Lawrence Erlbaum Associates.

Yang, S.-N., and McConkie, G.W. (1999b). Reading chinese: Some basic eye- movement characteristics. In J. Wang and A.W. Inhoff (eds.) *Reading Chinese script: A cognitive analysis.* (pp. 207–222). Mahwah, NJ: Lawrence Erlbaum Associates.

Yang, S.-N. and McConkie, G.W. (2001). Eye movements during reading: A theory of saccade initiation times. *Vision Research*, **41**, 3567–3585.

Yang, S.-N., and McConkie, G.W. (2004). Saccade generation during reading: Are words necessary? *European Journal of Cognitive Psychology*, **16**, 226–261.

Yang, S.-N., and Vitu, F. (2007). Dynamic coding of saccade length in reading. In R.P.G. van Gompel, M.H. Fischer, W.S. Murray, and R.L. Hill (eds.) *Eye movements: A window on mind and brain* (pp. 293–318). Oxford: Elsevier Science.

CHAPTER 41

Linguistic and cognitive influences on eye movements during reading

Keith Rayner and Simon P. Liversedge

Abstract

In this chapter we consider the extent to which eye movements are influenced by linguistic processing during reading. We contrast the linguistic/cognitive position, according to which eye movements are influenced to a significant degree by language processing with the oculomotor view, according to which fixation durations are largely independent of linguistic processing. We then briefly discuss eye movement measures in relation to language processing, before turning to four topics associated with lexical processing during reading (frequency effects, predictability effects, disappearing text, and distributional analyses of word frequency effects). We conclude this section by considering how processing associated with lexical identification is distributed across fixations during reading. In the next section we discuss higher order linguistic influences on reading. In particular, we examine plausibility effects, referential effects, and focus operator effects. We then describe some recent findings from studies investigating mindless reading. Finally, we conclude that any comprehensive account of eye movements during reading must specify the nature of linguistic processes associated with comprehension in relation to the oculomotor decisions of where and when to move the eyes.

There have been many debates over the years about the nature of eye movement control during reading. For example, one current debate revolves around the extent to which reading involves serial versus parallel lexical processing as exemplified in differences that exist between the E-Z Reader model of eye movement control (Pollatsek et al., 2006; Rayner et al., 2007; Reichle et al., 1998, 2003, 2009) and the SWIFT model (Engbert et al., 2005; Kliegl et al., 2006). Is lexical processing of the currently fixated word completed before lexical processing begins for the next word (see Reichle, Chapter 42, and Engbert and Kliegl, Chapter 43, volume)? Another current debate, which is very much related to the prior one, concerns the exact nature of parafoveal-on-foveal effects (see Rayner, 2009 and Drieghe, Chapter 46, this volume for discussion). Do properties of the word to the right of fixation influence how long readers look at the currently fixated word, and to what extent do readers preprocess the word to the right of fixation (see the chapter by Hyönä, Chapter 45, this volume)? In this chapter, we take a step back from these immediate and ongoing discussions and review the literature in relation to a more general question, namely, the extent to which eye movements (and, predominantly, eye fixation times) are influenced on a moment-to-moment basis by linguistic and cognitive variables. According to this view (which we'll call the linguistic/cognitive view), how long readers look at a given word is largely driven by inherent or contextual properties of that word. The time spent processing a word reflects the ease with which its meaning can be accessed and readily incorporated into the semantic representation of the sentence or text that has been developed up to that point. It is also assumed that the online development of a meaningful interpretation of the text necessarily entails the evaluation of the word under fixation in relation to existing interpretation on the basis of real world knowledge. Consequently, according to the linguistic/cognitive view, the formation of a fully specified meaningful interpretation of text involves exchange and interaction between core language processing systems and other, more generic higher order cognitive processes (e.g. memory or even, ultimately, problem solving). To the extent that such effects occur during reading and are observable in the eye movement record, they too may be cognitive determinants of oculomotor behaviour during reading.

The linguistic/cognitive position can be contrasted with an alternative view (often termed the oculomotor view; see Vitu, Chapter 40, this volume) in which eye fixation times are assumed to be relatively independent of moment-to-moment cognitive processing. According to this view, eye movement behaviour during reading is largely pre-determined, reflecting strategies or heuristics that lead to the visual material being sampled in a way that is most often optimal for subsequent language processing. Implicit here is the idea that there is a stage of visual processing during reading that precedes any language processing, with eye movements being central to the former, but not to the latter. From an experimentalist's point of view, if this latter position is correct, then eye movements are far more limited as a methodological tool for the investigation of psychological processes under-lying reading, than is the case if the linguistic/cognitive position is correct.

At one time, the view that eye movements are unrelated to ongoing cognitive processes was widely accepted (e.g. see Bouma and deVoogd, 1974; Kolers, 1976; Viviani, 1990). The general nature of the argument was that the eyes largely served the function of 'scooping up' the printed information, with lexical and semantic processing necessarily lagging behind perceptual processing of the stimulus material; the so-called 'cognitive lag' position. Inherent in this argument was the view that because saccade latency in a simple oculomotor task is on the order of 175–200 ms, and given that the average fixation duration in reading is on the order of 200–250 ms, there wouldn't be enough time in any given eye fixation to program an eye movement based on the nature of the linguistic information associated with the word under fixation. Saccade latency, the time to initiate a saccade, is typically determined in tasks in which participants are initially required to look at a fixation point and when a new fixation point appears elsewhere in the visual field, they must make a saccade to fixate the new location (see Rayner et al., 1983a for an example of such a study). Thus, the actual saccade latency is the period from when the new fixation point appears until the point at which the eyes start moving. Logically then, the latency includes both the time: 1) to perceive the new saccade target location and 2) to program and execute the saccade. Given that the time it takes to carry out oculomotor processes required to move the eyes from one location to another is close to the amount of time that readers typically fixate during reading, proponents of the cognitive lag position argued that there would be little opportunity for linguistic processing associated with the fixated word to actually influence when a saccade is initiated.

Research over the past 30 years, however, has made it abundantly clear that fixation time on a word and saccade length, are both strongly influenced by aspects of the word currently being processed (Liversedge and Findlay, 2000; Rayner, 1979, 1998, 2009). Implicit in the cognitive lag position was the assumption that a serial processing relationship existed between saccade programming and language processing. However, it has become quite clear that saccade programming occurs in parallel with linguistic processing, as exemplified in the E-Z Reader model (Reichle et al., 1998; see also Reichle, Chapter 42, this volume) and other models that followed it, most notably, the Glenmore model (Reilly and Radach, 2006) and the SWIFT model (Engbert et al., 2005; see also Engbert and Kliegl, Chapter 43, this volume). More critically, there have now been numerous demonstrations that linguistic properties of the fixated word strongly influence how long readers look at that word. Some of this evidence is reviewed in chapters elsewhere in this volume (see Juhasz and Pollatsek, Chapter 48, and Clifton and Staub, Chapter 49). Here, we will further review the evidence and discuss how far one can push the view that linguistic/cognitive factors are the primary determinants of when, and (to a much lesser extent), where to move the eyes in reading.

The linguistic/cognitive position versus the oculomotor position

Elsewhere, we (Rayner, 1995, 1998; Rayner and Liversedge, 2004) have pointed out that there are two research groups at opposite extremes of a continuum, each comprised of researchers who use eye movement data during reading, and each of which has a set of goals that are somewhat different. We hasten to note that our distinction is really a characterization, and like most characterizations it probably oversimplifies the situation somewhat. Nevertheless, we'd suggest that one group is primarily concerned with understanding the nature of oculomotor behaviour in its own right and particularly interested in how relatively low-level visual factors influence eye movements. It is probably fair to say that those in this research group appear to be more interested in eye movements per se than in reading. For them, reading is simply a convenient way to study oculomotor control since the visual stimuli are very structured and constrained, and eye movement behaviour during reading is relatively easy to characterize. The other group is primarily interested in language processing (such as, lexical processing, ambiguity resolution, syntactic parsing, discourse processing and the like). Those in this group largely appear to have little interest in eye movements per se, and simply use eye movements as a convenient (and very good) online measure of linguistic processing. Unfortunately, these two groups often do not communicate with each other as well as perhaps they should; they tend to publish in different journals and go to different conferences resulting in a failure to share ideas and findings.

However, there is also a third group of researchers who are interested both in the oculomotor aspects of eye movements during reading, as well as lexical and higher order linguistic influences on eye movements. We consider ourselves to be part of this group, and in our own work, have engaged in both types of research. We have done this in a very considered way since our goal is to understand the relationship between eye movements and the psychological processes that occur during reading (whether they be visual or linguistic). Furthermore, this reflects a very core belief that the two aspects of reading are tightly bound together, though we also hold a very strong bias that eye movements during reading are largely driven by linguistic/cognitive processing. We recognize that there are clearly occasions when visual/oculomotor processes have strong effects. For example, consider the important distinction between the decision of when to move the eyes (the *when* decision) and the decision of where to move (the *where* decision). Our view of the evidence is that the when decision is primarily driven by linguistic/cognitive processing (though there are cases where low-level visual characteristics of words can have an effect, e.g. long words that are comprised of more letters are fixated for longer than short words comprised of fewer letters), while the decision of where to move the eyes is largely driven by low-level visual processes (though, similarly, there are also instances in which linguistic processing has an impact, e.g. predictable words are skipped more often than unpredictable words).[1] Very consistent with this distinction is the finding that linguistic variables such as

---

[1] The topic of where readers target their initial saccades to words has received considerable attention within the literature (e.g. Hyona, 1995; Pollatsek et al., 2006; Rayner, 1979; White and Liversedge, 2004), and as we have described, the visual characteristics of words have been shown to be the primary determinant of where fixations are made. However, a different aspect of saccadic targeting that has received far less attention within the literature concerns targeting of regressive saccades. Early studies such as Frazier and Rayner (1982) and Rayner et al. (1983b) were the first to consider where, within a sentence, participants fixated after experiencing disruption to processing. Similarly, Kennedy (1992; see also Baccino and Pynte, 1994; Murray and Kennedy, 1988) advocated the Spatial Coding Hypothesis as a preliminary, working account of how spatial coordinates

word frequency, word predictability, and age-of-acquisition have major influences on when readers move their eyes, while word length information has a major influence on where readers move their eyes (see Rayner, 1998, 2009 for summaries). Of course, we recognize that word length also very much influences gaze duration (see below) on a word since readers make more refixations on long words than short words.

We (Rayner and Liversedge, 2004) have previously reviewed a number of low-level visual/oculomotor factors that have been studied in the context of reading. But, given that our central thesis in this chapter is that linguistic/cognitive factors primarily influence when to move the eyes, we will focus the remainder of our discussion on these factors and try to provide evidence to substantiate our claim.

Eye movement measures

Before moving to a discussion of lexical influences on fixation times, we need to briefly note the different processing time measures typically used in the research we discuss. They are: 1) first fixation duration (the duration of the first fixation on a word independent of the total number of fixations), 2) single fixation duration (cases when only a single fixation is made on a word), 3) gaze duration (the sum of all fixations on a word prior to moving to another word), and 4) go-past time (the time from when a word is first fixated until the reader moves forward in the text; this measure includes regressions back to earlier words as well as the time on the word itself). All of these measures are contingent on there being a first-pass fixation on the target word in the first place. There are obviously a number of other time-based measures, such as total time on a word (which includes first past fixations and all rereading of a word) and second pass time that researchers use to deal with the large and complex data sets that eye movement experiments yield. Other variables such as word skipping rates and regressions are obviously also important. Regressions can be a particularly useful measure when investigating higher-order cognitive processing in reading (e.g. pronoun resolution or other aspects of semantic processing), since such eye movements are often made in order for readers to undertake processing associated with the computation of a coherent representation of the discourse (though see Footnote 1). Generally, first fixation duration, single fixation duration, and gaze duration typically (though not invariably) yield similar patterns of effects, with effects typically larger (numerically speaking) in gaze duration than the other two measures (which follows because first and single fixations are subsumed in the gaze duration measure, and gaze duration is very much increased when readers make more than one fixation on a word). Go-past time (like total time) is generally assumed to reflect later processing than the other three measures, which are typically assumed to be fairly good indices of initial lexical processing.

Before leaving this discussion of eye movement measures, it is perhaps worth saying something about how the different types of measures are related to different types of linguistic processing. It can be appealing to think that there is a direct correspondence between particular reading time measures and specific types of processing (e.g. gaze duration might be assumed to exclusively reflect

---

may be associated with particular portions of text, or sentential constituents and this information could be used to guide targeting of regressive saccades. More recently, Mitchell and colleagues (Mitchell et al., 2008) have put forward a more radical suggestion, namely, that regressive eye movements are (at least to some extent) decoupled from ongoing cognitive processing. According to this position, regressive saccades are targeted on the basis of low level visual characteristics of text (e.g. spatial layout), as well as, on some occasions, higher order linguistic information and processing. In our view, it seems quite likely that linguistic processing does affect such saccadic targeting, and that regressive saccades reflect important aspects of processing associated with recovery from disruption, or the processing of referring expressions. However, the formalization of theoretical accounts of such processing is still in its infancy, and will need to occur in relation to better specification of the role of memory (spatial and linguistic) in ongoing language processing. It seems likely that this topic will receive considerable interest in the future.

lexical identification). However, it is not the case that there is an unambiguous and transparent link between different stages of language processing and particular reading time measures. Different types of linguistic manipulations (e.g. a lexical manipulation compared with a syntactic manipulation) can produce effects in the same eye movement measure (e.g. first fixation duration, or gaze duration). Also, although effects due to a particular type of linguistic manipulation might appear in early measures in some studies, effects due to other similar manipulations might not appear quite so immediately in other studies (see Clifton et al., 2007 for a review). This is particularly true of manipulations that involve higher-order linguistic processing. For example, disruption to processing due to detection of a syntactic misanalysis, known as a garden path effect, has been shown to occur in the earliest of eye movement measures, such as the duration of the first fixation on the syntactically disambiguating word, or in much later measures such as go past time, or even on the region of the sentence downstream from the critical word or phrase (see Clifton et al. 2007). At present it is not fully understood why there are such differences in the immediacy of effects across experimental studies. Suffice it to say that there is variability in this respect, and this leads us to conclude that the relationship between eye movement measures and linguistic processes is not always unambiguous and entirely transparent.

A related point concerns the interpretations that it is possible to make regarding the time course of different stages of linguistic processing. Implicit in most eye movement research investigating reading is the idea of different levels or stages of processing, each of increasing complexity. And from some perspectives at least, there is often assumed to be sequentiality to the separate stages of processing, and that dependency relations between the stages of processing exist. For example, most researchers would probably agree that, under normal circumstances, lexical identification occurs very early after a word has been initially fixated (and sometimes before it is fixated, as when a word is skipped). Furthermore, only when the word has been lexically identified, does information about its syntactic category become available in order that it can be incorporated into the syntactic structure that is currently being developed for the sentence. Also, when a word has been lexically identified, information about its meaning becomes available such that the representation of the overall meaning of the sentence can be developed based on the individual word meanings and the syntactic structure of the sentence. What should be apparent from this example is that syntactic and semantic processing *necessarily* follow lexical processing sequentially, and are dependent on successful lexical identification for them to occur (at least if we assume that syntactic and semantic processing occur non-predictively, based on information associated with the word itself, rather than based on preceding sentential context and partial information about the word).

As mentioned above, adopting this theoretical approach allows researchers to consider the time-course of different linguistic processes in relation to each other. In line with this, most researchers broadly assume that effects associated with early stages of language processing (e.g. lexical processing) will appear in earlier reading time measures (first and single fixation durations, gaze durations), while effects associated with later stages of processing (e.g. semantic and discourse processing) will affect later reading time measures (go past and total reading times).

In most psycholinguistic experiments the researchers are principally interested in when a variable that they have manipulated first has a discernible influence in the eye movement record. Arguably, however, eye movements are not always as effective in providing insight into when a stage of linguistic processing has been fully completed. One of the best ways to determine that a particular process must have been carried out successfully (and therefore completed) is to establish that another, different, effect has occurred that reflects processing dependent on the completion of the former process. The main points to note here are that eye movements provide a very good indication of the time course of processing, and in particular, when a linguistic variable first shows an influence. Such information can be extremely useful in distinguishing between different theoretical accounts. Establishing when a stage of processing has been completed can be trickier, however, though there are ways in which this can be established, and in principle, there is no reason to assume that the eye movement record is not transparent in this respect. We will now turn our attention to a discussion of lexical influences on eye movements.

Lexical influences on fixation times on words

Frequency effects

As noted above, there is now a great deal of evidence to indicate that lexical properties of the fixated word influence how long readers' eyes remain on a word during first-pass processing. Specifically, there have been numerous demonstrations, starting with Rayner and Duffy (1986) and Inhoff and Rayner (1986), that when word length is controlled readers look at low frequency words longer than high frequency words. Likewise, numerous experiments starting with Ehrlich and Rayner (1981) and Rayner and Well (1996) have demonstrated that when word length is controlled, readers look at low predictable words longer than high predictable words (see Rayner, 1998, 2009 for other references for frequency and predictability effects). Interestingly, Chinese readers show frequency effects (Yan et al., 2006, see also Zang et al., Chapter 53, this volume) and predictability effects (Rayner et al., 2005) that are comparable to readers of English.

Predictability effects

In addition to frequency and predictability effects (which have been referred to, along with word length, as the 'big three' variables influencing fixation times on words, see Kliegl et al., 2006), age-of-acquisition (Juhasz and Rayner, 2003, 2006), word familiarity (Williams and Morris, 2004), and number of meanings of a word (Duffy et al., 1988; Rayner et al., 2006; Sereno et al., 2006) also have influences on how long readers look at a word; the effects of age-of-acquisition and familiarity are generally independent of word frequency. Some advocates of a largely oculomotor view of eye movement influences on reading (see, for example, Yang and McConkie, 2003) have argued that lexical variables, like word frequency, have an inhibitory role, only influencing long fixations (and therefore resulting in a skew to the rightward tail of the frequency distribution). However, we believe that this position is now largely untenable given two recent findings. First, the *disappearing text* paradigm clearly shows that eye fixations are under cognitive control. Second, recent analyses show very clearly that there is a distribution shift associated with word frequency effects. We consider each of these in turn.

Disappearing text

In the disappearing text paradigm (Blythe et al., 2009; Ishida and Ikeda, 1989; Liversedge et al., 2004; Rayner et al., 1981, 2003a, 2006, 2011), the text that is being read either disappears after a fixed interval (50–60 ms) after the fixation begins or is replaced by a pattern mask for the remainder of the fixation; the results are pretty much the same whether the fixated word disappears or is masked. A very interesting finding in these experiments is that, when the word that is fixated disappears (or is masked), there is little or no effect on overall reading. In other words, reading proceeds rather smoothly and naturally despite the fact that the text (or fixated words) disappears quite early in a fixation. This does not mean that the words are fully processed in 50–60 ms, but rather that the visual information needed for reading gets into the processing system within that time frame and reading proceeds quite normally. Another, perhaps more dramatic finding, is that when specific target words are examined, the word frequency effect on the word is unaffected (Blythe et al., 2009; Liversedge et al., 2004; Rayner et al., 2003, 2006, 2011). Even though the word is no longer there, its frequency determines how long the eyes remain in place. We take this as rather strong evidence that linguistic/cognitive processes are the engine driving eye movements in reading.

Distributional analyses

As we noted above, it has sometimes been argued (see Yang and McConkie, 2003 for such an argument) that the frequency effect is due to some very long fixations on low frequency words, and hence it is only the right tail of the distribution (or the skew of the distribution) that is affected when frequency effects emerge in any given data set. Rayner (1995; see also Rayner et al., 2003) presented frequency distributions for high and low frequency words and argued that the distribution for low frequency words shifted to the right in comparison to the distribution of high frequency words. More recently, Staub et al. (2010) presented formal analyses of frequency distributions and demonstrated quite conclusively that with low frequency words there is both a distribution shift and more long fixations on the right tail of the distribution.

Lexical identification: a broader context

Before moving from lexical influences on eye movements, we would like to briefly consider them in the broader context of models of lexical processing, and specifically in relation to research investigating isolated word recognition. Most research examining lexical processing uses an alternative methodology to eye movement recordings, such as word naming, semantic categorization, or most often, a lexical decision task. All of these methodologies involve the presentation of quite long lists of words, each word being presented one at a time in isolation, and each requiring some form of behavioural response. The behavioural response usually involves the participant making a decision (e.g. is the string a word or nonword). Advocates of these methodologies argue that one of their significant advantages is that they allow for very precise control of the visual stimulus on which word identification processes operate. The visual stimulus often has an abrupt onset (though they can be forward and backward masked) and is presented central to fixation. It is also often argued that the use of these approaches allows for the study of lexical identification processes in isolation, that is, in the absence of other linguistic processing that occurs when we read normally. To this extent, advocates of these methodologies argue that isolated word recognition allows an investigation of 'pure' lexical processing, and we recognize and acknowledge that this may be the case (though we note that decision processes are not usually associated with word identification).

In our view, however, this approach is fundamentally limited in relation to what it can tell us about the process of word identification as it happens when we read normally. In normal reading situations word recognition occurs in the context of many other types of ongoing language processing, and given this, the study of isolated word identification represents an oversimplification of the situation that exists when we read normally. Consider a simple question for a moment: When was the last time that you read a list of 50 or so words and nonwords one by one, each having no relation to its predecessor? In all probability, if the reader is an experimental psychologist, then the response will be 'The last time I was a participant in a lexical decision experiment'. The point here is that we carry out this type of processing *very* infrequently.

A different and more serious concern with isolated word recognition methodologies, however, is that they do not accurately or adequately approximate the manner in which visual information about words is delivered to the lexical processing system by the visual system. Given this, it is our view that lexical identification processes will not be initiated, nor proceed in the way that they would normally during reading. We view this as a fundamental shortcoming of the isolated word identification approach, if the experimenter's objective is to understand written language comprehension as it occurs when we read normally.

During normal reading, visual and orthographic information first becomes available in the parafovea and is processed to a comparatively shallow level prior to direct inspection. Thus, words are processed to differing degrees over time and across fixations. The precise pattern of fixations in relation to the visual stimulus fundamentally determines the quality of and the rate at which orthographic information enters and is processed by the word identification system. Implicit in this statement is the important idea that the precise mechanics of eye movement behaviour and the time course of linguistic processing are fundamentally related and inextricably bound together. If this suggestion is correct (and we believe it is), then it further reinforces our primary claim in this chapter, namely, that eye movements provide an accurate online index of the cognitive processing that occurs during normal reading. Furthermore, given the dependency relation that exists between oculomotor behaviour and the delivery of abstract representations of the linguistic information on the page or screen to the lexical processor, it appears to us that methodologies in which, single, isolated words that are presented centrally at fixation are fundamentally constrained in the extent to which they can elucidate core linguistic processes that occur during normal reading. A criticism often levelled at eye movement researchers by those adopting isolated word methodologies is that lexical decision methodology is the benchmark method for the investigation of word identification. Our view is the precise opposite to this, namely, that if one is interested in the nature of word identification that occurs during normal reading, rather than that which occurs under unnatural reading conditions, then isolated word methodologies are limited, whilst eye movement methodology is far more advantageous. Given these views, it is perhaps unsurprising that we believe a central research issue in forthcoming years will be to develop models of lexical processing that are ecologically valid in relation to how visual information about words becomes available for processing across fixations in reading.

Beyond lexical influences on fixation times

The discussion above makes it very clear that there are immediate lexical effects on eye fixation times in reading (see also Juhasz and Pollatsek, Chapter 48, this volume). But, how far do cognitive/linguistic effects extend in terms of their influence on eye fixations? Do other higher order linguistic variables have an influence? In fact, it is very clear that variables like plausibility, syntactic ambiguity and disambiguation, and higher-order discourse factors such as clause and sentence wrap up, anaphora, elaborative inferences, and so on can influence how long the eyes remain in place (Liversedge and Findlay, 2000; Rayner, 1998, 2009). In the next section, we do not provide a comprehensive review of this literature (indeed, we could not do it justice in the space available). Instead, we have selected several relevant lines of recent research, some of which we have been involved in, that fall in this category of work. We have chosen to focus on those areas that we consider have produced, and will continue to produce, results that are interesting and challenging to current theoretical accounts of eye movements in reading.

Plausibility

Rayner et al. (2004) examined the time course of plausibility/anomaly effects on eye movements during reading. In this experiment, we presented readers with normal sentences, sentences that were possible but somewhat implausible, or sentences that were anomalous (see (1)–(3)):

1. John used a knife to chop the large carrots for dinner. (Normal control)
2. John used an axe to chop the large carrots for dinner. (Implausible)
3. John used a pump to inflate the large carrots for dinner. (Anomalous)

The first of these sentences was designed to describe an everyday event. The second was designed to be minimally different from the first, but to describe a situation that was unlikely, but still possible. Thus, whilst it is reasonable to chop logs with an axe, it would be quite unusual (though still possible) to chop carrots with an axe. Finally, the third type of sentence was created to describe a situation that was very strange, and almost could not happen within a 'normal' context. Thus, while it is possible to use a pump to inflate something like a tyre, or a balloon, it would be very strange to use one to inflate a carrot that does not have the properties required to allow it to be inflated. Note that all of the sentences make perfect sense up until the critical word *carrot*, and only upon reading this word can any oddity with sentences (2) and (3) be detected. Thus, these stimuli were useful to examine the immediacy and magnitude of disruption to processing associated with implausibility and anomaly effects by identifying both the fixations made during the initial encounter with the critical word, and later fixations made during revisits to that word (for further details see Warren, Chapter 50, this volume). Basically, we found that the anomalous condition had a fairly immediate effect on eye movement measures. The anomalous nature of the sentence more or less hit the reader 'between the eyes' and there was an effect on gaze duration for the critical word (though there was no effect on first fixation duration). However, in the implausible condition, the effect was much delayed and first started to appear in the go-past measure (though it was only marginally significant). In addition, the amount of disruption that was observed was greater in the anomalous relative to the implausible condition, indicating that the nature of the linguistic violation was related to the severity of disruption observed in the eye movement record.

This experiment led to a number of follow-up studies (see Joseph et al., 2008; Patson and Warren, 2010; Warren and McConnell, 2007; Warren et al., 2008) that have replicated the original findings, though some of the studies found somewhat earlier effects than the original (for both implausible and anomalous sentences), but with the same general pattern. In addition, Warren et al. (2008) demonstrated that if the anomalous sentences were embedded in a cartoon-like context (e.g. where John is using a pump to inflate a large carrot for a parade), there is only a brief initial boggle on *carrot* (see Filik, 2008 for a similar, but slightly delayed effect).

We took the results of the original study to suggest that whereas gross anomaly can immediately override lexical processes and cause disruption to the system, plausibility effects only appear in later measures and don't influence immediate decisions about when to move the eyes. In the context of the current discussion, these findings are a good example of how eye movements during reading are differentially sensitive to linguistic manipulations both in relation to immediacy and magnitude of disruption—the greater the degree of semantic violation in relation to what we know about the world, then the faster and larger the effects. We also argued that the effect of anomaly that we observed in this study is very much like a strong garden-path effect wherein readers are initially led to adopt one syntactic parse of the sentence but then detect an initial misanalysis and have to revise their initial analysis (Frazier and Rayner, 1982). For example, in sentence (4):

4. While Mary was mending the sock fell off her lap

readers typically take *the sock* to be the object of *was mending* and have to reanalyse when they realize that it is actually the beginning of a new constituent. In many ways this is like encountering anomalous material and fixations will be lengthened (as a number of experiments starting with Frazier and Rayner, 1982 and Rayner et al., 1983b demonstrated).

Referential discourse effects

The next topic we will consider is that of referential effects. We have chosen this topic for two reasons. First, a clear and strong theoretical line has developed over a significant period of time, from the earliest studies that were carried out quite a number of years ago (e.g. Altmann and Steedman, 1988; Crain and Steedman, 1985). These studies did not use eye movement methodology, though a number of later studies did (e.g. see Clifton and Ferrreira, 1989; Clifton et al., 2003; Ferreira and Clifton, 1986; Murray and Liversedge, 1994; Rayner et al., 1992; Trueswell et al., 1994). In these experiments, the nature of the preceding referential context was explicitly manipulated. In more recent eye movement experiments, focus operators have been used to manipulate the referential properties of the discourse representation, thereby avoiding the need for explicit preceding context (e.g. Ni et al., 1996; Clifton et al., 2000; Filik et al., 2005, 2009; Liversedge et al., 2002; Paterson et al., 1999, 2007; for a detailed discussion of this work see Filik et al., Chapter 51, this volume). The second reason that we feel these studies are relevant to this chapter is that they provide another good example of work in which the nature of higher order linguistic processing, namely, the online construction of a discourse representation, affects eye movement behaviour during reading. The underlying theoretical commonality between these studies is that characteristics of the text are manipulated in order to cause readers to instantiate a discourse representation with particular referential properties. When a subsequent sentence is read, it can be shown that it is interpreted fairly rapidly in relation to that discourse representation. That is to say, the current sentence is semantically (referentially) evaluated in relation to the understanding of the preceding text that has been developed up to that point. Specifically, this work has shown that the particular referential properties of the discourse representation cause the reader to adopt one particular interpretation of an ambiguous sentence rather than another, and that this is evident from the eye movement record. In other words, the work again demonstrates very clearly that higher order linguistic and cognitive processes directly influence eye movements during reading.

As noted above, the earliest experiments investigating referential context effects did not actually use eye movement methodology (e.g. Altmann and Steedman, 1988; Crain and Steedman, 1985). Instead, self paced reading or grammaticality decision methodologies were employed. The basic manipulation, however, was to set up a brief context that either mentioned two similar but distinct entities (e.g. a safe and a strongbox), or two entities that were the same (e.g. two safes). These contexts were then followed by a syntactically ambiguous target sentence that referred to one of the entities in the preceding context (e.g. (5) and (6)).

5. The burglar blew open the safe with the diamonds.

6. The burglar blew open the safe with the dynamite.

One version of the target sentence was referentially restrictive, that is, providing further information about which safe was being referred to (e.g. (5)), and in the other it was not (e.g. (6)). The aim was to assess whether readers would be more likely to initially interpret the ambiguous target sentence as restrictive (i.e. specifying the entity to which the sentence referred) when they had just read a context that mentioned two entities that were the same compared to when they had just read a context that mentioned two entities that were different. By making the target sentences either congruous or incongruous with the context sentences, it was possible to assess the influence of context on the interpretation of the target sentence. Thus, these early experiments, along with those that followed, were designed in part to demonstrate a direct influence of the nature of the discourse representation (i.e. a high order cognitive representation of the meaning of the text) on eye movements during reading.

Focus operator effects

The early experiments investigating referential processing were presented in the context of the modularity debate in relation to syntactic parsing, specifically, whether semantic information was used to guide initial syntactic commitments. However, to a significant degree, this debate has moved on, and more recent studies have used the ideas behind the referential theory to consider more generally the function of focus operators, their referential properties, and how these shape the nature of the discourse representation and influence sentence interpretation.

Focus operators are words like *only* and *even* and they serve the linguistic purpose of indicating that a contrast should be made between an entity that is mentioned in the sentence and some set of alternatives (again, see Filik et al., Chapter 51, this volume). For example, in the sentence fragment *Only actresses who were sent flowers . . .* the focus operator *only* indicates that a contrast should be made between two sets of individuals. One of these groups is referred to in the sentence (*actresses*), whilst the other is not explicitly specified in the text, and must be inferred by the reader prior to its instantiation in the developing discourse representation. However, there is ambiguity as to how this process might proceed. For instance, the reader might instantiate a representation in which a set of actresses might be contrasted with an alternative such as, say, a group of non-actresses. Alternatively, contrasting groups of actresses who were, and were not sent flowers may be instantiated. The point is that if the reader commits to an interpretation of the sentence in relation to contrast sets in the discourse representation, then they have to make higher-order inferences about the nature of those contrasting sets. The information is not explicitly provided in the sentence. The relationship between these experiments investigating focus operator effects and the earlier work investigating the effects of an explicit preceding referential context effects should be apparent. Effectively the later studies used the focus operators to cause the reader to instantiate discourse representations with contrasting sets in a similar way to the manner in which the preceding referential contexts were used explicitly to cause the reader to set up discourse representations (that, for example, explicitly contained contrasting entities like safes and strongboxes).

One of the earliest eye movement experiments to investigate focus operator effects was carried out by Paterson et al. (1999), who used sentences like (7):

7. Only teenagers allowed a party invited a juggler straightaway

They were interested to investigate whether the presence of *only* at the beginning of the sentence would prevent readers from an initial syntactic misanalysis. Their rationale was that if *only* caused readers to initially instantiate contrasting sets of teenagers in their discourse representation, then they would treat *allowed a party* as the information specifying the nature of the distinction between the two sets (i.e. two groups of teenagers, one of whom was allowed a party, and the other not). If readers did this, then they would not experience an initial syntactic misanalysis. In fact, Paterson et al. showed garden path effects in gaze durations on the disambiguating region of the sentence regardless of whether *only* did or did not appear at the beginning of the sentence, suggesting that the focus operator did not prevent a misanalysis. However, there were differences in later measures indicating less disruption to processing when the focus operator was present than when it was not. Paterson et al. concluded that the focus operator did cause readers to instantiate contrasting sets in the discourse representation, but the influence of the discourse representation was not sufficient to prevent a garden path, though it did facilitate recovery from the initial syntactic misanalysis.

In a follow up experiment, Liversedge et al. (2002) adopted a very similar approach, but in this experiment they used slightly different sentences like (8):

8. Only motorists stopped in the car park received a warning about their outdated permits.

For such sentences, the bias to initially process them syntactically one way rather than another is much weaker, and consequently, Liversedge et al. anticipated that the focus operator might be much more influential in relation to the interpretation of the sentence that the reader initially formed. In fact, there were no first pass reading time effects (suggesting a lack of a garden path). However, there were fewer regressions and shorter re-reading times for sentences with *only* than for sentences without. Liversedge et al. again concluded that the focus operator did cause readers to instantiate contrasting sets in the discourse representation and that these did affect the ease with which readers formed a meaningful interpretation of the ambiguous sentence.

More recently, we have extended this work to examine whether manipulating where a focus operator appears in a sentence affects the nature of the interpretation that the reader forms. Paterson et al. (2007) carried out an experiment using sentences like (9)–(12):

9. At dinner Jane passed only the salt to her mother, but not the pepper as well . . .

10. At dinner Jane passed only the salt to her mother, but not her father as well . . .

11. At dinner Jane passed the salt to only her mother, but not the pepper as well . . .

12. At dinner Jane passed the salt to only her mother, but not her father as well . . .

Here the focus operator *only* appeared early or late in the sentence. Paterson et al. argued that when it appeared early in the sentence (i.e. preceding *the salt*), then it would cause readers to draw a contrast between what was, and was not, being passed from person to person. In this way, they argued that readers should form a discourse representation containing two contrasting sets of entities that would be likely candidates to be passed to someone at the dinner table (e.g. salt and pepper). In contrast, when *only* appeared late (i.e. preceding *her mother*), then it would cause readers to draw a contrast between two likely candidates that might be passed something at the dinner table (e.g. mother and father). Thus, Paterson et al. predicted that when the contrasting clause (*but not the pepper/her father*) was congruent with the discourse representation that the focus operator caused the reader to develop (as in sentences (9) and (12)), then processing difficulty would be minimal, whereas when it was incongruent (as in sentences (10) and (11)), disruption should occur.

In fact, as is often the case in eye movement experiments investigating the influence of the discourse representation, the effects emerged quite late, appearing in go-past reading times for the region downstream from the critical region. Nonetheless, the effects patterned in the way Paterson et al.

expected, with incongruent continuations producing more disruption to processing than congruent continuations. Taken together, these three studies investigating focus operator effects provide good examples of how it is possible to use eye movement methodology to examine higher order cognitive processes that occur during reading. Once again, these studies add to our argument that eye movements are sensitive to higher order linguistic processing.

Mindless reading

The final topic we will cover in this section concerns a phenomenon that might not, by some, actually be regarded as higher order processing at all. Indeed, according to Reichle et al. (2010) the phenomenon of mindless reading occurs when the reader disengages from processing the text even though they continue to move their eyes from word to word as if they were actually reading. There are very few readers who will not have experienced this; you reach the end of a paragraph in a book that you are reading and realize that you did not take in any of what you have just read.

We consider that mindless reading is relevant to the current discussion because studying it provides a very different way of assessing whether eye movements do reflect higher-order linguistic processing. If, as we have argued throughout this chapter, eye movements do reflect ongoing linguistic processing, then a very strong prediction is that during mindless reading linguistically mediated effects should be reduced or even might not occur. That is to say, if linguistic processing is disengaged such that no meaningful interpretation of the text is available to the reader, then effects associated with linguistic processing should be much reduced in the eye movement record. It was exactly this rationale adopted by Reichle et al. in their very recent experiment in which they required participants to read very long passages of text (*Sense and Sensibility* by Jane Austen) during a number of sessions over several days. During the time that participants were reading, it was assumed that they would periodically disengage and drop into a mindless reading state (perhaps as their minds wandered). Critical to this paradigm is being able to detect when participants have dropped into a mindless reading state, and Reichle et al. adopted two methods for such detection, namely, self-caught mind wandering and probe-caught mind wandering (see Rayner and Fischer, 1996 and Vitu et al., 1995, for earlier, but less elegant, attempts to study mindless reading). Self-caught mind wandering episodes were signalled by the reader themselves pressing a button to indicate that they had just realized that they had come out of a mindless reading episode. In addition to participants' mindless reading self-reports, participants were also periodically probed to respond *yes* or *no* to a question asking them whether they were in a mindless reading state. The two methods of detecting mindless reading were also useful to investigate whether there were any differences in eye movements immediately prior to probed and self-report responses. Presumably, fixations immediately prior to a self-report of mindless reading would reflect cognitive processing associated with a developing self-awareness of a failure to engage in proficient reading. In contrast, if the probe interrupted a mindless reading session, then it would be likely that eye movements immediately prior to the probe appearing would reflect 'pure' mindless reading without any processing related to meta-awareness of disengagement. Note also that when the reader made a negative response to a probe for mindless reading, then the fixations prior to such a response represent the perfect control data against which to compare those occasions when they responded positively (i.e. such periods would reflect normal reading). Finally, Reichle et al. reported a series of global measures offering broadly descriptive indices of general processing across the text as a whole, as well as a series of local measures related to the individual words that were read during the mindless reading episode. These measures were computed for several time windows prior to probed or self-reported responses (2.5, 5, 10, 30, 60, and 120 s).

For the global measures, the most important effects occurred for the smallest time windows and showed that there were fewer first-pass fixations, fewer words fixated, and fewer regressions during mindless reading than during normal reading. Furthermore, readers made more fixations away from the text immediately prior to self-caught mindless reading than probed mindless reading, which suggests that erratic reading behaviour, including failing to look at the text that is being read, seems to be associated with a self awareness of mindless reading.

For the local measures, the effects seemed strongest in the later time intervals (10 to 120 s), and showed consistently longer first fixations, gaze durations, and total times on words during self-reported mindless reading episodes than normal reading, and often during probe caught mindless reading episodes than during normal reading. Thus, not only does mindless reading result in longer fixations than normal reading, it is also the case that such episodes can last for considerable periods (up to 2 min). To assess whether linguistic processing was engaged during mindless reading, the local measures for each of the words that were processed during each time period were analysed in relation to several variables that are known to influence lexical and post-lexical processing (and therefore fixation durations). For our purposes, the most critical of these were word length and frequency, and the analyses clearly showed that fixations during mindless reading (both probed and self-caught) were far less influenced by length and frequency than they were during normal reading. Thus, Reichle et al. took these results to indicate that readers did indeed disengage from cognitive processing during mindless reading, and consequently, eye movements showed less systematic variability in relation to lexical and post-lexical variables than occurred when cognitive processing was fully engaged. Thus, the strong prediction that linguistic effects would be reduced was borne out in the data, and it is for this reason that we consider the Reichle et al. experiment to provide further evidence that eye movements during reading reflect higher-order linguistic processing. The results from Reichle et al. are also consistent with the results of Rayner and Fischer (1996) and Rayner and Raney (1996) who showed reliable frequency effects for a target word in a text during reading, but no such effects when participants were simply required to search for a word in the same text. Again, the idea in these earlier studies was to demonstrate that processing associated with language comprehension largely determines fixation durations during reading, and that when no such processing occurs, then the relationship between the linguistic properties of words and fixation durations is not apparent.

Summary

In this chapter we have tried to make the strong case that cognitive processes associated with lexical and higher-order linguistic processing affect eye movements during reading. We have not tried to provide a comprehensive review of all of the relevant literature, but instead have tried to focus on studies that we believe make our points effectively. In our view, the 'battle' over what influences eye movements appears to be largely resolved in favour of the view that whilst visual characteristics of text do affect where and when we fixate during reading, it is the case that cognitive and linguistic processing also have a very significant, if not predominant, influence. Indeed, if we go simply by popular vote, the cognitive/linguistic account maintains clear credibility given all the psycholinguists who use eye movement methodology to study language processing in reading; they implicitly, if not explicitly, maintain this view.

We conclude this chapter by making a key point that we believe may be of some importance. If the argument that we have developed seems be reasonable, and it apparently does to many, then a primary objective of those developing models or theories of eye movements and reading has to be to better specify how the nature of ongoing linguistic processing impacts on oculomotor control decisions. This issue simply cannot be sidestepped, if the goal is to develop comprehensive, psychologically valid theories and models of eye movements. The eye movements that we make when we read do not take place in a linguistic processing vacuum. To reiterate, our argument is simple: cognitive processes associated with linguistic processing affect when (and to a lesser extent where) we move our eyes during reading. Models of eye movement control attempt to explain in detail when (and where) we move our eyes during reading. Thus, to adequately account for eye movement control during reading, we necessarily must understand and specify the nature of cognitive processes associated with language comprehension in relation to oculomotor decisions. In essence, a more detailed understanding of the interface between the system responsible for language comprehension and the eye movement control system is needed.

Acknowledgements

During the preparation of this chapter, the first author was supported by grant HD26765 from the National Institute of Health. The second author was supported by UK Economic and Social Research Council Research Grants (RES-000-22-3398) and (RES-000-22-4218). The authors are grateful to Tian Jing for her assistance with the References section of the chapter and Denis Drieghe for his comments on an earlier version.

References

Altmann, G.T.M. and Steedman, M.J. (1988). Interaction with context during human sentence processing. *Cognition,* **30**, 191–238.

Baccino, T. and Pynte, J. (1994). Spatial coding and discourse models during text reading. *Language and Cognitive Processes,* **9**, 143–155.

Blythe, H.I., Liversedge, S.P., Joseph, H.S.S.L., White, S.J., and Rayner, K. (2009). Visual information capture during fixations in reading for children and adults. *Vision Research,* **49**, 1583–1591.

Bouma, H. and deVoogd, A.H. (1974). On the control of eye saccades in reading. *Vision Research,* **14**, 272–284.

Clifton, C. and Ferreira, F. (1989). Ambiguity in context . *Language and Cognitive Processes,* **4**, SI77–SI104.

Clifton, C., Jr, Bock, J., and Radó, J. (2000). Effects of the focus particle only and intrinsic contrast on comprehension of reduced relative clauses. In A. Kennedy, R. Radach, D. Heller, and J. Pynte (eds.) *Reading as a perceptual process* (pp. 591–619). Oxford: Elsevier.

Clifton, C., Staub, A., and Rayner, K. (2007). Eye movements in reading words and sentences. In R. van Gompel, M.H. Fischer, W.S. Murray, and R.L. Hill (eds.) *Eye movements: A window on mind and brain* (pp. 341–372). New York: Elsevier.

Clifton, C., Traxler, M.J., Mohamed, M.T., Williams, R.S., Morris, R.K. and Rayner, K. (2003). The use of thematic role information in parsing: Syntacic processing autonomy revisited. *Journal of Memory and Language,* **49**, 317–334.

Crain, S., and Steedman, M.J. (1985). On not being led up the garden path: the use of context by the psychological parser. In D. Dowty, L. Karttunen, and A. Zwicky (eds.) *Natural language parsing: Psychological, computational, and theoretical perspectives* (pp. 320–358). Cambridge: Cambridge University Press.

Duffy, S.A., Morris, R.K., and Rayner, K. (1988). Lexical ambiguity and fixation times in reading. *Journal of Memory and Language,* **27**, 429–446.

Ehrlich, S.F. and Rayner, K. (1981). Contextual effects on word perception and eye movements during reading. *Journal of Verbal Learning and Verbal Behavior,* **20**, 641–655.

Engbert, R., Nuthmann, A., Richter, E.M., and Kliegl, R. (2005). SWIFT: A dynamical model of saccade generation during reading. *Psychological Review,* **112**(4), 777–813.

Ferreira, F. and Clifton, C. (1986). The independence of syntactic processing. *Journal of Memory and Language,* **25**(3), 348–368.

Filik, R. (2008). Contextual override of pragmatic anomalies: Evidence from eye movements. *Cognition,* **106**, 1038–1046.

Filik, R., Paterson, K.B., and Liversedge, S.P. (2005). Parsing with focus particles in context: Evidence from eye movements in reading. *Journal of Memory and Language,* **53**, 473–495.

Filik, R., Paterson K.B., and Liversedge, S.P. (2009). The influence of only and even on online semantic interpretation. *Psychonomic Bulletin and Review,* **16**(4), 678–683.

Frazier, L. and Rayner, K. (1982). Making and correcting errors during sentence comprehension: Eye movements in the analysis of structurally ambiguous sentences. *Cognitive Psychology,* **14**, 178–210.

Hyönä, J. (1995). Do irregular letter combinations attract readers' attention? Evidence from fixation locations in words. *Journal of Experimental Psychology: Human Perception and Performance,* **21**(1), 68–81.

Ishida, T. and Ikeda, M. (1989). Temporal properties of information extraction in reading studied by a text-mask replacement technique. *Journal of the Optical Society A: Optics and Image Science,* **6**, 1624–1632.

Inhoff, A.W. and Rayner, K. (1986). Parafoveal word processing during eye fixations in reading. *Perception and Psychophysics,* **40**, 431–439.

Joseph, H.S.S.L., Liversedge, S.P., Blythe, H.I., White, S.J., Gathercole, S.E., and Rayner, K. (2008). Children's and adults' processing of anomaly and implausibility during reading: Evidence from eye movements. *Quarterly Journal of Experimental Psychology,* **61**, 708–723.

Juhasz, B.J. and Rayner, K. (2003). Investigating the effects of a set of intercorrelated variables on eye-fixation durations in reading. *Journal of Experimental Psychology: Learning, Memory, and Cognition,* **29**, 1312–1318.

Juhasz, B.J. and Rayner, K. (2006). The role of age-of-acquisition and word frequency in reading: Evidence from eye fixation durations. *Visual Cognition,* **13**, 846–863.

Kennedy, A. (1992). The spatial coding hypothesis. In K. Rayner (ed.) *Eye movements and visual cognition: Scene perception and reading* (pp. 379–396). New York: Springer-Verlag.

Kliegl, R., Nuthmann, A., and Engbert, R. (2006). Tracking the mind during reading: The influence of past, present, and future words on fixation durations. *Journal of Experimental Psychology: General,* **135**, 12–35.

Kolers, P.A. (1976). Buswell's discoveries. In R.A. Monty and J.W. Senders (eds.) *Eye movements and psychological processes* (pp. 373–395). Hillsdale, NJ: Erlbaum.

Liversedge, S.P. and Findlay, J.M. (2000). Saccadic eye movements and cognition. *Trends in Cognitive Sciences,* **4**, 6–14.

Liversedge, S.P., Paterson, K.B., and Clayes, E.L. (2002). The influence of 'only' on syntactic processing of 'long' relative clause sentences. *Quarterly Journal of Experimental Psychology,* **55A**, 225–240.

Liversedge, S.P., Rayner, K., White, S.J., Vergilino-Perez, D., Findlay, J.M., and Kentridge, R.W. (2004). Eye movements when reading disappearing text: Is there a gap e ect in reading? *Vision Research,* **44**, 1013–1024.

Mitchell, D., Shen, X., Green, M., and Hodgson, T. (2008). Accounting for regressive eye-movements in models of sentence processing: A reappraisal of the Selective Reanalysis hypothesis. *Journal of Memory and Language,* **59**, 266–293.

Murray, W.S. and Kennedy, A. (1988). Spatial coding in the processing of anaphor by good and poor readers: Evidence from eye movement analyses. *Quarterly Journal of Experimental Psychology,* **40A**, 693–718.

Murray, W.S. and Liversedge, S.P. (1994). Referential context effects on syntactic processing. In C. Clifton, L. Frazier, and K. Rayner (eds.) *Perspectives on sentence processing* (pp. 359–388). Hillsdale, NJ: Erlbaum.

Ni, W., Crain, S., and Shankweiler, D. (1996). Sidestepping garden paths: The contribution of syntax, semantics and plausibility in resolving ambiguities. *Language and Cognitive Processes,* **11**, 283–334.

Paterson, K.B., Liversedge, S.P., and Underwood, G. (1999). The influence of focus operators on syntactic processing of 'short' relative clause sentences. *Quarterly Journal of Experimental Psychology,* **52A**, 717–737.

Paterson, K.B., Liversedge, S.P., Filik, R., Juhasz, B.J., White, S.J., and Rayner, K. (2007). Processing contrastive focus during silent reading: Evidence from eye movements. *Quarterly Journal of Experimental Psychology,* **60**, 1423–1445.

Patson, N.D. and Warren, T. (2010). Eye movements when reading implausible sentences: Investigating potential structural influences on semantic integration. *Quarterly Journal of Experimental Psychology,* **63**(8), 1516–1532.

Pollatsek, A., Reichle, E.D., and Rayner, K. (2006). Tests of the E-Z Reader model: Exploring the interface between cognition and eye-movement control. *Cognitive Psychology,* **52**(1), 1–56.

Rayner, K. (1979). Eye guidance in reading: Fixation locations within words. *Perception,* **8**, 21–30.

Rayner, K. (1995). Eye movements and cognitive processes in reading, visual search, and scene perception. In J.M. Findlay, R. Walker, and R.W. Kentridge (eds.) *Eye movement research: Mechanisms, processes and applications* (pp. 3–22). North Holland.

Rayner, K. (1998). Eye movements in reading and information processing: 20 years of research. *Psychological Bulletin,* **124**(3), 372–422.

Rayner, K. (2009). The Thirty-Fifth Sir Frederick Bartlett Lecture: Eye movements and attention in reading, scene perception, and visual search. *Quarterly Journal of Experimental Psychology,* **62**, 1457–1506.

Rayner, K. and Duffy, S.A. (1986). Lexical ambiguity and fixation times in reading: Effects of word frequency, verb complexity, and lexical ambiguity. *Memory and Cognition,* **14**, 191–201.

Rayner, K. and Fischer, M.H. (1996). Mindless reading revisited: Eye movements during reading and scanning are different. *Perception and Psychophysics,* **58**, 734–747.

Rayner, K. and Liversedge, S.P. (2004). Visual and linguistic processing during eye fixations in reading. In F. Ferreira and J. Henderson (eds.) *The interface of language, vision and action: Eye movements and the visual world* (pp. 59–104). New York: Psychology Press.

Rayner, K. and Raney, G.E. (1996). Eye movement control in reading and visual search: Effects of word frequency. *Psychonomic Bulletin and Review,* **3**, 245–248.

Rayner, K. and Well, A.D. (1996). Effects of contextual constraint on eye movements in reading: A further examination. *Psychonomic Bulletin and Review,* **3**, 504–509.

Rayner, K., Carlson, M., and Frazier, L. (1983b). The interaction of syntax and semantics during sentence processing: Eye movements in the analysis of semantically biased sentences. *Journal of Verbal Learning and Verbal Behavior,* **22**, 358–374.

Rayner, K., Garrod, S., and Perfetti, C.A. (1992). Discourse influences during parsing are delayed. *Cognition,* **45**, 109–139.

Rayner, K., Liversedge, S.P., and White, S.J. (2006). Eye movements when reading disappearing text: The importance of the word to the right of fixation. *Vision Research,* **46**, 310–323.

Rayner, K., Li, X., and Pollatsek, A. (2007). Extending the E-Z Reader Model of eye movement control to Chinese readers. *Cognitive Science,* **31**, 1021–1033.

Rayner, K., Slowiaczek, M.L., Clifton, C., and Bertera, J.H. (1983a). Latency of sequential eye movements: Implications for reading. *Journal of Experimental Psychology: Human Perception and Performance,* **9**, 912–922.

Rayner, K., Liversedge, S.P., White, S.J., and Vergilino-Perez, D. (2003). Reading disappearing text: Cognitive control of eye movements. *Psychological Science,* **14**, 385–389.

Rayner, K., Warren, T., Juhasz, B.J., and Liversedge, S.P. (2004). The effect of plausibility on eye movements during reading. *Journal of Experimental Psychology: Learning, Memory, and Cognition,* **30**, 1290–1301.

Rayner, K., Li, X., Juhasz, B.J., and Yan, G. (2005). The effect of word predictability on the eye movements of Chinese readers. *Psychonomic Bulletin and Review,* **12**, 1089–1093.

Rayner, K., Cook, A.E., Juhasz, B.J., and Frazier, L. (2006). Immediate disambiguation of lexically ambiguous words during reading: Evidence from eye movements. *British Journal of Psychology,* **16**, 467–482.

Rayner, K., Yang, J., Castelhano, M.S., and Liversedge, S. (2011). Eye movements of older and younger readers when reading disappearing text. *Psychology and Aging,* **26**(1), 214–223.

Rayner, K., Inhoff, A.W., Morrison, R., Slowiczek, M.L., and Bertera, J.H. (1981). Masking of foveal and parafoveal vision during eye fixations in reading. *Journal of Experimental Psychology: Human Perception and Performance, 7*, 167–179.

Reichle, E.D., Rayner, K., and Pollatsek, A. (2003). The E-Z Reader model of eye movement control in reading: Comparison to other models. *Brain and Behavioral Sciences, 26*, 445–476.

Reichle, E.D., Warren, T., and McConnell, K. (2009). Using E-Z Reader to model the effects of higher level language processing on eye movements during reading. *Psychonomic Bulletin and Review, 16*(1), 1–21.

Reichle, E.D., Reineberg, A.E., and Schooler, J.W. (2010). Eye movements during mindless reading. *Psychological Science. 21*, 1300–1310.

Reichle, E.D., Pollatsek, A., Fisher, D.L., and Rayner, K. (1998). Toward a model of eye movement control in reading. *Psychological Review, 105*(1), 125–157.

Reilly, R.G. and Radach, R. (2006). Some empirical tests of an interactive activation model of eye movement control in reading. *Cognitive Systems Research, 7*, 34–55.

Sereno, S.C., O'Donnell, P., and Rayner, K. (2006). Eye movements and lexical ambiguity resolution: Investigating the subordinate bias effect. *Journal of Experimental Psychology: Human Perception and Performance, 32*(2), 335–350.

Staub, A., White, S.J., Drieghe, D., Hollway, E.C., and Rayner, K. (2010). Distributional effects of word frequency on eye fixation durations. *Journal of Experimental Psychology: Human Perception and Performance, 36*, 1280–1293.

Trueswell, J.C., Tanenhaus, M.K., and Garnsey, S.M. (1994). Semantic influence on parsing: Use of thematic role information in syntactic ambiguity resolution. *Journal of Memory and Language, 33*, 285–318.

Vitu, F., O'Regan, J.K., Inhoff, A.W. and Topolski, R. (1995). Mindless reading: eye-movement characteristics are similar in scanning letter strings and reading texts. *Perception and Psychophysics, 57*, 352–364.

Viviani, P. (1990). Eye movements in visual search: Cognitive, perceptual and motor control aspects. *Reviews in Oculomotor Research, 4*, 353–393.

Warren, T. and McConnell, K. (2007). Investigating effects of selectional restriction violations and plausibility violation severity on eye-movements in reading. *Psychonomic Bulletin and Review, 14*, 770–775.

Warren, T., McConnell, K., and Rayner, K. (2008). Effects of context on eye movements when reading about plausible and impossible events. *Journal of Experimental Psychology: Learning, Memory, and Cognition, 34*, 1001–1010.

White, S.J. and Liversedge, S.P. (2004). Orthographic familiarity influences initial eye fixation positions in reading. *European Journal of Cognitive Psychology, 16*(1and2), 52–78.

Williams, R.S. and Morris, R.K. (2004). Eye movements, word familiarity, and vocabulary acquisition. *European Journal of Cognitive Psychology, 16*, 312–339.

Yan. G., Tian, H., Bai, X., and Rayner, K. (2006). The effect of word and character frequency on the eye movements of Chinese readers. *British Journal of Psychology, 97*, 259–268.

Yang, S- N. and McConkie, G.W. (2003). Saccade generation during reading: Are words necessary? *European Journal of Cognitive Psychology, 16*(1–2), 226–261.

CHAPTER 42

Serial-attention models of reading

Erik D. Reichle

[W]e are limited, in the amount that we can read during a reading pause, by the inadequacy of the retinal structure, by our inability to attend to more than a few parts of the total picture presented, and by the necessity of our attention's concerning itself with interpretations.

Huey (1908, p. 70)

Abstract

This chapter will provide an overview of *serial-attention* models of eye-movement control in reading, which share the core assumptions that attention is allocated sequentially to support the lexical processing of only one word at a time, and that lexical processing normally causes the eyes to move from one word to the next. Two such models (Reader: Just and Carpenter, 1980; EMMA: Salvucci, 2001) are briefly described and a third (E-Z Reader: Reichle et al., 1998) is described in detail. The chapter then reviews simulations completed using the E-Z Reader model to evaluate the plausibility and generality of its assumptions, and to examine various reading phenomena. These simulations are consistent with the hypothesis that attention is allocated serially during reading.

The basic question of how attention is allocated during reading has a long history in psychology. A century of research has clearly demonstrated that limitations of visual acuity *and* the capacity to attend impose severe restrictions on the rate at which readers can process information on the printed page. Despite our progress in understanding the psychology of reading, however, there is still no consensus about how attention is allocated during reading (Rayner and Juhasz, 2004; Reichle et al., 2009a; Starr and Rayner, 2001). As a result, models of eye-movement control in reading make very different assumptions about how attention is allocated. For example, *serial-attention* models posit that attention is focused on one word at a time, in a strictly serial manner, with lexical processing only occurring on the word being attended (Reichle, 2006). In contrast, *attention-gradient* models (e.g. see Engbert et al., 2005; Reilly and Radach, 2006; see also Engbert and Kliegl, Chapter 43, this volume) posit that attention is distributed to support concurrent lexical processing of multiple words. This chapter provides an overview of the former class of models—those consistent with the hypothesis that attention is allocated in a strictly serial manner.

Although there are several theories consistent with serial-attention hypothesis (e.g. Morrison, 1984), only three have been implemented as computational models. In their chronological order of development, they are: 1) *Reader* (Just and Carpenter, 1980); 2) *E-Z Reader* (Reichle et al., 1998); and 3) *EMMA* (Salvucci, 2001). In addition to sharing the serial-attention assumption, these models share an assumption that lexical processing is the 'engine' that determines when the eyes will move from one word to the next during reading. The models are therefore *cognitive control* models, in contrast to models in which cognition plays a reduced (Engbert et al., 2005; McDonald et al., 2005; Reilly and Radach, 2006) or negligible (Feng, 2006; Yang, 2006) role in deciding when to move the eyes.

This chapter reviews all three serial-attention models of reading. However, because only E-Z Reader (Reichle et al., 2009b) is currently being used to guide reading research, the descriptions of Reader (Just and Carpenter, 1980) and EMMA (Salvucci, 2001) will be brief, with most of the discussion focused on E-Z Reader and its assumptions. This chapter then reviews the simulations completed using E-Z Reader to evaluate the plausibility and generality of its assumptions, as well as various reading phenomena. One goal in doing this is to show how the phenomena being simulated are consistent with (and in some cases depend upon) the assumption that attention is allocated in a serial manner during reading.

The Reader and EMMA models

Reader (Just and Carpenter, 1980, 1987; Thibadeau et al., 1982) and EMMA (Salvucci, 2001) are implemented within *cognitive architectures* (Anderson, 1983; Newell, 1973, 1990; Rumelhart, 1989) or general computational frameworks used to simulate and understand the perceptual, cognitive, and motor processes that mediate human performance in a variety of tasks (e.g. problem solving; Newell and Simon, 1972). Reader and EMMA are both implemented within a particular type of cognitive architecture called a *production system* (Newell, 1990). Production systems consist of (often very large) collections of *condition-action* or *if-then* pairs, called *productions*, which describe the elementary perceptual, cognitive, and/or motor processes that support human cognition and behaviour.

In the context of reading, for example, the following production might encode the orthographic features corresponding to three letters arranged in a particular spatial configuration, and upon detecting this configuration provide new information (to other productions) that a particular word has been perceived:

if⟨ letter$_1$ = "c" and letter$_2$ = "a" and letter$_3$ = "t" ⟩, *then* ⟨ word percept = "cat" ⟩

Another production might then test for the word percept 'cat' and, upon detecting it, make the word's meaning available for further linguistic processing. Productions thus consist of units of procedural knowledge that operate on declarative information (e.g. the forms and meaning of words), making this information available to working memory for further processing. Available information can trigger other productions that, when executed in sequence, support a variety of (often complex) cognitive activities. In Reader and EMMA, this activity is reading.

Reader

The Reader model (Just and Carpenter, 1980, 1987; Thibadeau et al., 1982) was implemented in the CAPS production system (Just and Varma, 2002). The model's productions perform a wide variety of different processes related to reading, including encoding word percepts, making their meanings available for syntactic and semantic processing, and using the results of this processing to build propositional representations of the text. Perhaps not too surprisingly, these activities require a large number of different productions; for example, a small-scale version of Reader capable of reading a short passage of text included 225 separate productions. Because of this, and because several productions are often concurrently active, the model has been criticized because its 'inner workings' are not as transparent as those of the other models (e.g. see Rayner et al., 2003a). Despite this limitation, however, the model has been influential because of its broad theoretical scope, and because its core assumptions can be described by two simple—even intuitive—principles.

The first is the *immediacy assumption*, or the hypothesis that readers always attempt to process each word to the fullest extent possible as soon as possible. In the model, this means that whenever the eyes move to a new word, whatever processing of that word can be completed is done as quickly as possible. As a result, most words are rapidly encoded and linguistically processed before the eyes leave the word—consistent with the model's second core assumption, the *eye-mind assumption*, or the hypothesis that readers' eyes remain on a word as long as it is being processed. In the model, this means that the time that is spent looking at a word is a direct indicator of the time required to process that word. It also means that, at any point in time, processing is completely restricted to the word being fixated, making Reader the strongest version of the serial-attention hypothesis. (As will be described below, in both the EMMA and E-Z Reader models, attention is not always coupled to the current fixation location, so that words are often processed prior to being fixated.)

Although one might argue that—on some coarse level—the immediacy and eye-mind assumptions are reasonable approximations, there is considerable evidence against strong versions of both hypotheses. For example, the processing of difficult words often 'spills over' onto subsequent words, increasing the fixation times on those words (Rayner and Duffy, 1986; Rayner et al., 1989). These *spillover effects* are inconsistent with the immediacy assumption. Similarly, words usually undergo some amount of parafoveal processing before they are fixated (Balota et al., 1985; Binder et al., 1999; Pollatsek et al., 1992; Rayner, 1975). These *parafoveal preview effects* are inconsistent with the eye-mind assumption.

Finally, the Reader model has been criticized because it includes implausible assumptions and lacks predictive precision (e.g. see Reichle et al., 2003). For example, the model assumes that the minimal time to programme a saccade is 30 ms, which is much shorter than current estimates (e.g. 125–150 ms; Becker and Jürgens, 1979; Rayner et al., 1983). The model also only predicts an indirect composite measure of looking time—one generated by converting the number of production processing cycles into units of time, and one that averages across skips, single fixations, and multiple fixations. Reader therefore predicts neither the durations nor the locations of individual fixations. Such limitations have resulted in the model being viewed more as a 'straw man' hypothesis than a serious model of reading.

EMMA

The EMMA model (i.e. *Eye Movements and Movements of Attention*; Salvucci, 2001) was implemented within the ACT-R production system (Anderson and Lebiere, 1998). The core assumptions of EMMA are that: 1) only one visual object can be attended (and thus encoded) at a time, and 2) the encoding of an object causes both attention and the eyes to shift to another object (so that it can be encoded). In the context of reading, the visual 'objects' are words, but in non-reading tasks (e.g. driving) can correspond to any number of different objects (e.g. vehicles). EMMA thus instantiates Morrison's (1984) verbal theory of eye-movement control because the identification of word n causes both attention *and* the eyes to be directed towards word $n+1$. The mean time to encode a visual object, T_{enc}, is given by:

$$T_{enc} = K\left[-\log(freq)\right]e^{k\varepsilon} \tag{1}$$

where *freq* is the frequency of the object (e.g. how often a word occurs in printed text) after it has been normalized to the range (0, 1), and ε is the angular distance between the centre of vision and the centre of the object being encoded. Frequently encountered objects thus require less time to encode than less frequent objects, and because visual acuity decreases from the centre of vision, objects close to fixation require less time to encode than objects in peripheral vision. The free parameter K (= 0.006) scales the base time to encode an object, and k (= 0.4) determines how much this time is modulated by visual acuity. Finally, Equation 1 gives the mean time to encode an object; the actual time to encode an object during any given Monte-Carlo simulation[1] is sampled from a γ distribution with $\mu = T_{enc}$ and $\sigma = 0.33\mu$.

---

[1] In this type of stochastic modeling, the durations of individual processes are often subject to random variability to simulate the 'noise' inherent to neural systems and factors that vary among individuals (e.g. reading skill).

All of the remaining assumptions of EMMA are related to saccadic programming. The first is that saccades are programmed in two stages: an initial *preparatory stage* that is cancelled by the initiation of another saccadic programme, followed by an *execution stage* that cannot be cancelled and that includes the actual saccade. This distinction was motivated by 'double-step' experiments (Becker and Jürgens, 1979) showing that, if a cue to move the eyes to a target location is rapidly followed by another such cue in a different location, then the eyes often move directly to the second location, presumably because the first saccadic programme was cancelled. However, if the second cue occurs later (i.e. after the initial programming stage has presumably been completed), then the first saccade is executed, resulting in a brief fixation on the first location followed by a saccade to the second location. Based on these results, the mean time to complete the preparatory stage of saccadic programming, T_{prep}, is set equal to 135 ms The mean time (in milliseconds) to complete the execution stage, T_{exec}, is given by:

$$T_{exec} = \beta_1 + \beta_2 + \beta_3 x° \tag{2}$$

where β_1 (= 50 ms) is the time to actually complete the second stage of programming, β_2 (= 20 ms) is the minimal saccade duration, and β_3 (= 2 ms) is the amount by which the saccade duration increases per degree of visual angle, x. As with object-encoding times, the actual times to complete the two stages of saccadic programming during any given simulation are sampled from γ distributions with means as specified and $\sigma = 0.33\mu$.

These assumptions allow EMMA to explain both skipping and refixations. If the eyes are on word n and it is encoded, then attention moves to word $n+1$ (so that it can be encoded) and a saccadic programme to move the eyes to word $n+1$ is initiated. However, if word $n+1$ happens to be encoded before the preparatory stage of programming is completed, then this initiates another programme to move the eyes to word $n+2$, cancelling the first programme that would have otherwise moved the eyes to word $n+1$ and thereby causing it to be skipped. However, if the eyes happen to move to word $n+1$ before it is encoded, then a saccadic programme to refixate word $n+1$ is initiated. Because the first situation is more likely to happen if word $n+1$ is encoded rapidly, and because the second situation is more likely to happen if word $n+1$ is encoded slowly, words that are easy to encode (e.g. short, frequent, and/or predictable words) are skipped more often and refixated less often than words that are difficult to encode, consistent with empirical results (see Rayner, 1998).

In contrast to Reader, EMMA makes realistic assumptions about the nature of saccadic programming and the time required to complete it (185 ms, on average). EMMA also generates direct predictions about the durations of individual fixations, distinguishing between skips, single fixations, and cases involving two or more fixations. The model's assumptions about word frequency and visual acuity (see Equation 1) also allow it account for two important 'benchmark' findings in reading: Readers tend to look at infrequent words longer and more often than frequent words (Schilling et al., 1998), and readers identify words in central vision more rapidly than in peripheral vision (Rayner and Morrison, 1981). And because EMMA allows for some 'slippage' between where attention and the eyes are located, it can account for both parafoveal preview and spillover effects (which are problematic for the Reader model).

Finally, although Reader provides a more comprehensive account of reading than EMMA does, the principles that allow EMMA to explain eye movements in reading are applicable to other domains, allowing the model to explain eye movements in other tasks (e.g. solving algebra problems; Salvucci, 2001). These simulations provide an existence proof that the serial encoding of visual objects is plausible, suggesting that the cognitive demands imposed by the encoding of (complex) visual stimuli may be similar across many tasks. For example, the serial allocation of attention may be necessary to 'bind' the features of complex visual stimuli into unitary representations that can be used for further

---

The amount of variability is often selected so that the distribution of whatever dependent measure is being simulated (e.g. fixation durations) approximates the observed variability.

cognitive processing (Reichle et al., 2009; Reichle et al., 2008; Treisman and Gelade, 1980; Treisman and Schmidt, 1982). This role of attention is one factor that motivated the development of the E-Z Reader model (Reichle et al., 1998).

The E-Z Reader model

The E-Z Reader model (Reichle et al., 1998) is actually a family of models developed over the past decade to provide increasingly sophisticated descriptions of how various perceptual, cognitive, and motor processes guide readers' eye movements. A minimalist strategy of model development has entailed adding assumptions only as necessary to account for phenomena that cannot be explained by simpler versions of the model (e.g. fixation landing-site distributions; Reichle et al., 1999), and to make the model consistent with known biological or psychological constraints (e.g. the eye-to-brain neural transmission time; Reichle et al., 2003). Although the critical benchmark phenomena used to evaluate eye-movement models have been simulated with successive versions of the model (see Table 42.1), the versions are not 'nested' in the strictest sense (Jacobs and Grainger, 1994) because a few of the simulations (see Table 42.2) have not been replicated using more recent versions of the model. (These latter simulations are discussed in the final section of this chapter.)

Table 42.1 The family of E-Z Reader models (listed in their chronological order of development), their theoretical assumptions, and the phenomena that they explain. (All of the listed assumptions and phenomena are nested; that is, the assumptions of early versions are true of subsequent versions, as are the phenomena that are explained.)

Version	Model assumptions	Benchmark phenomena explained by the model
1–5	• Core assumptions about L_1 and L_2 (using multiplicative versions of Equations 3 and 5) • Core assumptions about M_1 and M_2	• Word-frequency effects • Word-predictability effects • Word-length effects • Parafoveal preview • Preview foveal load • Spillover effects • Skipping 'costs' • Predicted spatial accuracy = words
6	• Saccade targeting assumptions (Equations 6–7)	• Predicted spatial accuracy = letters • Landing-site distributions • Range bias launch-site fixation duration • Refixation probabilities
7	• Pre-attentive vision stage (t = 90 ms; duration modulated by visual acuity) • Substages of labile saccade programming • Automatic refixations modulated by saccadic error (Equation 8)	• See Table 42.2
8	• (Current) additive version of Equations 3 and 5	• Frequency predictability
9	• Constant pre-attentive vision stage (t = 50 ms)	• See Table 42.2
10	• Explicit (t > 0 ms) attention shifts • Post-lexical integration stage • Proportionally smaller L_2 duration (Δ = 0.25)	• Pauses/inter-word regressions • Post-lexical processing effects

Note: The primary references for the different versions of E-Z Reader are: (1) E-Z Reader 1–5: Reichle et al. (1998); (2) E-Z Reader 6: Reichle et al. (1999); (3) E-Z Reader 7: Reichle et al. (2003); (4) E-Z Reader 8: Rayner et al. (2004b); (5) E-Z Reader 9: Pollatsek et al. (2006a); and (6) E-Z Reader 10: Reichle et al. (2009b).

Table 42.2 Reading-related phenomena that have been examined using the E-Z Reader model. (The version of the model used in each simulation is indicated, as are the primary references describing the simulations.)

Simulation	Manipulated variables	Theoretical questions	Versions
1	50-ms vs. 90-ms eye-to-brain lag	What is the precise nature of the vision–cognition interface?	
2	Continuous vs. discontinuous lexical processing during saccades		
3	Word n vs. word n+1 disappears 60 ms after fixating word n	How is attention allocated?	9
4	1 vs. 2 stage(s) of lexical processing	Is the L_1 vs. L_2 distinction necessary?	
5	Word n+1 appears vs. disappears 140 ms after word n is fixated	How is attention allocated?	
6	College-aged vs. elderly readers	Are the model's assumptions general across different populations, writing systems, and/or materials?	7
7	French language, short text passage		
8	Chinese (non-alphabetic) language		9
9	Advertisements (text and pictures)		
10	Various embedded assumptions about compositional morphology	How are compound words identified?	7
11	Various embedded assumptions about lexical ambiguity resolution	How are ambiguous words identified?	
12	Frequency/length of nouns in noun-adjective pairs	What causes the reverse word-length effect?	9

Note: The primary references for the listed simulations are: (1–4) Pollatsek et al. (2006a); (5) Pollatsek et al. (2006b, 2006c); (6) Rayner et al. (2006); (7) Miellet et al. (2007); (8) Rayner et al. (2007); (9) Reichle and Nelson (2003); (10) Pollatsek et al. (2003); (11) Reichle et al. (2007); and (12) Pollatsek et al. (2008).

Figure 42.1 is a schematic diagram of the E-Z Reader model. The boxes represent the perceptual, cognitive, and motor processes posited to guide readers' eye movements. The black arrows indicate how information and control passes between processes, and the dashed arrows indicate how difficulty with post-lexical processing can intermittently influence the eyes and attention, resulting in pauses and/or regressions. The following description is of the most recent version of E-Z Reader (i.e. version 10; Reichle et al., 2009), but Table 42.1 shows how the model has been developed to explain an increasing number of empirical results (for a review, see Reichle et al., 2006).

As with the other models reviewed in this chapter, E-Z Reader posits that attention is allocated to one word at a time, and that lexical processing is the 'engine' that moves the eyes forward during reading. However, in contrast to Reader and EMMA, the coupling between cognition and the eyes is much looser, with a preliminary stage of lexical processing providing the signal to start programming a saccade to move the eyes from one word to the next. Most of the model's other assumptions about saccadic programming are similar to those of EMMA[2], but with additional specification about saccade execution. The most recent version of E-Z Reader (Reichle et al., 2009) also includes a stage of higher-level language processing that, when it fails, can interrupt the progression of the eyes, resulting in pauses and/or regressions. The precise details of how all of this happens will now be described.

---

2 The EMMA and E-Z Reader models are similar because many assumptions of the former were borrowed from the latter (Salvucci, 2001, p. 202).

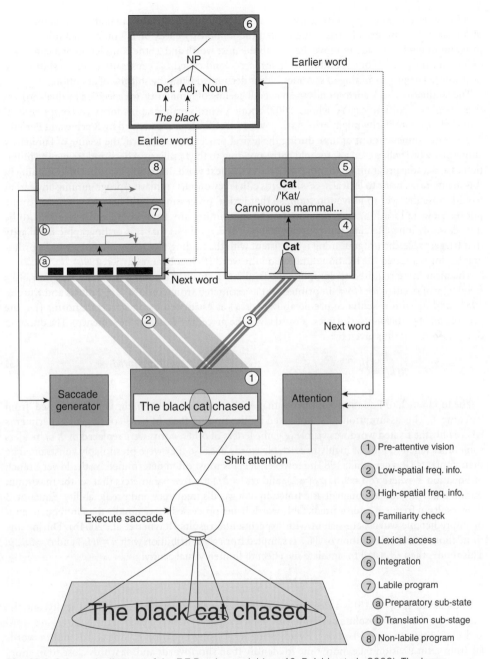

Fig. 42.1 Schematic diagram of the E-Z Reader model (ver. 10; Reichle et al., 2009). The boxes represent the perceptual, cognitive, and motor processes posited by the model. The thick arrows indicate the flow of information and control among the processes. The thin vertical line projecting from the 'c' in 'cat' to the eye indicates the current fixation location; visual acuity decreases symmetrically from either side of this location. The attention 'spotlight' is on the word 'cat,' and while that word is being identified, the previous word ('black') is being integrated into the sentence representation. (See the text for a complete description of the model's assumptions.)

With respect to lexical processing, the core assumptions of E-Z Reader are that: 1) the completion of an early stage of lexical processing (called the *familiarity check* or L_1) on a word initiates the programming of a saccade to move the eyes to the next word; and 2) the completion of a later stage of lexical processing (corresponding to *lexical access* and called L_2) causes attention to shift to the next word. The programming of saccades is thus decoupled from the shifting of attention.

The familiarity check corresponds to an overall 'feeling of familiarity' (as specified by dual-process theories of recognition; e.g. Yonelinas, 2002) about a word's orthographic form. (A computational model of how familiarity might arise during word identification is provided by Reichle and Perfetti, 2003.) After some amount of time during the lexical processing of a word, the feeling of familiarity about that word will exceed a threshold corresponding to the familiarity check and trigger the initiation of a saccadic programme to move the eyes to the next word. Initiating saccadic programming in this manner (i.e. prior to lexical access) affords efficiency because initiating programming any earlier would cause the eyes to move too soon, so that lexical processing would have to continue from a poorer viewing location, whereas initiating programming any later would cause fixations to be unnecessarily long (Reichle and Laurent, 2006). The hypothesis that it is orthographic familiarity that triggers saccadic programming is consistent with the finding that the quality of a word's orthographic form affected the fixation duration on the word (Reingold and Rayner, 1996).

The mean time required to complete the familiarity check, $t(L_1)$, on a word is a function of its frequency of occurrence (*freq*) in printed text as estimated from corpora (e.g. Francis and Kučera, 1982) and its within-sentence predictability (*pred*) as estimated using *cloze-task* norms (i.e. the proportion of participants who guess a word given the preceding words in the sentence). The duration of $t(L_1)$ (in ms) is thus given by:

$$t(L_1) = \begin{cases} 0 & \text{with } p = pred \\ \alpha_1 - \alpha_2 \ln(freq) - \alpha_3(pred) & \text{with } p = (1 - pred) \end{cases} \tag{3}$$

The top branch of Equation 3 stipulates that, with some probability p, the word is 'guessed' from its context. This assumption was motivated by the finding that, in gaze-contingent experiments where only the fixated word was visible (e.g. the letters of other words were replaced by X's), readers sometimes failed to look at highly predictable words because they were presumably constrained by their contexts (Rayner et al., 1982). However, $t(L_1)$ is most often determined by the lower branch of Equation 3, where α_1 (= 98), α_2 (= 2), and α_3 (= 27) are free parameters that set the maximum duration of $t(L_1)$ and attenuate it as a function of a word's frequency and predictability. Equation 3 thus results in frequent and/or predictable words being processed more rapidly than infrequent and/or unpredictable words, consistent with experimental results (Rayner et al., 2004b). During any simulation, the actual duration of $t(L_1)$ is sampled from a γ distribution with $\mu = t(L_1)$ and $\sigma = 0.22\mu$. This time is then adjusted to simulate the effect of limited visual acuity:

$$t(L_1) = t(L_1)\varepsilon^{\sum_i |letter_i - fixation|/N} \tag{4}$$

In Equation 4, ε (= 1.15) is a free parameter that scales the slowing effect of visual acuity, and the exponent is the mean absolute deviation (in character spaces) between each of the N letters in a word and the centre of vision (*fixation*). By adjusting $t(L_1)$ using Equation 4, long words and/or words far from central vision take more time to identify than short words and/or words close to fixation, consistent with empirical results (Lee et al., 2003; Rayner and Bertera, 1979; Rayner and Morrison, 1981).

In E-Z Reader, lexical access corresponds to the process of activating a word's meaning so that it can be used in further linguistic processing. The time to complete lexical access, $t(L_2)$, is always non-zero because even the meanings of 'guessed' words have to be activated. Furthermore, $t(L_2)$ is not affected by visual acuity because the information being accessed is semantic, not visual. The duration of $t(L_2)$ is specified by:

$$t(L_2) = \Delta(L_1) \tag{5}$$

where Δ (= 0.25) is a free parameter that sets $t(L_2)$ equal to some fixed proportion of $t(L_1)$, using the value of $t(L_1)$ given by the lower branch of Equation 3. As with $t(L_1)$, the actual duration of $t(L_2)$ during any simulation is sampled from a γ distribution with $\mu = t(L_2)$ and $\sigma = 0.22\mu$.

Because $t(L_2)$ is a fixed proportion of $t(L_1)$, and because the time to programme saccades is (on average) a constant (see below), the amount of time that is available for parafoveal processing (i.e. the time between when attention shifts from word n to word $n+1$ and when the eyes move from word n to word $n+1$) decreases as the foveal word (i.e. word n) becomes more difficult to process. This allows the model to explain the interaction between foveal processing difficulty and preview benefit: Because difficult-to-process words require more time to identify, less time is available for parafoveal processing of the next word, thereby increasing the fixation on that word (Henderson and Ferreira, 1990; Kennison and Clifton, 1995). This also allows the model to explain spillover effects: Because less parafoveal processing is carried out on difficult-to-process words, the next word receives less parafoveal processing, thereby increasing the fixation on that word (Rayner and Duffy, 1986; Rayner et al., 1989).

The remaining model assumptions are related to early visual processing, saccadic programming, the movement of attention, and post-lexical processing. As Fig. 42.1 illustrates, a preliminary stage of pre-attentive processing propagates visual information from the eye to the brain (t = 50 ms). This stage is 'pre-attentive' because all of the information on the page is processed in parallel and thus potentially available for further processing (subject to visual acuity limitations). Low-spatial frequency information (e.g. word boundaries) is used by the oculomotor system to select upcoming saccade targets, and some portion of the high-spatial frequency information is selectively attended for further lexical processing.

Figure 42.1 also indicates that that saccadic programming is completed in two stages (as in EMMA). This assumption was motivated by numerous results showing that the initiation of a saccadic programme can cancel an earlier programme, but that two programmes initiated far enough apart in time can be programmed in parallel (Becker and Jürgens, 1979; Leff et al., 2001; McPeek et al., 2000; Molker and Fischer, 1999; Vergilino and Beauvillain, 2000). Thus, an initial, *labile* stage of programming, M_1, can be cancelled by the initiation of a subsequent programme. The time required to complete this first stage, $t(M_1)$, is sampled from a γ distribution with $\mu = 125$ ms and $\sigma = 0.22\mu$. This stage can also be further divided into two sub-stages that require equal amounts of time to complete—a *preparatory* substage in which a saccade's spatial target (e.g. the centre of the next word) is identified, followed by a *translation* stage in which the spatial target is converted into a distance (i.e. muscle force) metric.

The second, *non-labile* stage of saccadic programming, M_2, cannot be cancelled by the initiation of a new saccadic programme under the assumption that a programme that has reached this 'point of no return' has been instantiated in the brainstem circuitry responsible for executing the saccade and will be obligatorily executed. Thus, initiating a saccadic programme after an earlier programme has reached the non-labile stage will result in two programmes being completed in parallel. The time required to complete the non-labile stage, $t(M_2)$, is sampled from a γ distribution with $\mu = 25$ ms and $\sigma = 0.22\mu$.

Finally, saccades require 25 ms to execute. During the saccades, lexical processing continues using information from the previous viewing location until the new fixation begins and enough time has passed (i.e. the 50-ms eye-to-brain lag) for processing to continue using information from the new location. In contrast to both Reader and EMMA, E-Z Reader specifies how saccades are actually executed: They are always directed towards the centres of words, with the actual saccade length (in character spaces) being the sum of the *intended saccade length* (ISL), a *range bias* (RB) that causes short/long saccades to over/undershoot their intended targets (McConkie et al., 1988, 1991; Rayner, 1979; Rayner et al., 1996), and *random motor error*.

The range bias (in character spaces) is modulated by the launch-site fixation duration (*fixation*) as specified by:

$$RB = (\psi - ISL)\{[\Omega_1 - \ln(fixation)]/\Omega_2\} \tag{6}$$

where $\Psi (= 7)$ is the saccade length (in English) that is unbiased, and Ω_1 $(= 7.3)$ and Ω_2 $(= 3)$ are free parameters that control the degree to which the launch-site fixation duration modulates the range bias. The second term of Equation 6 thus causes the range bias to decrease as saccadic programming time increases, consistent with empirical findings (McConkie et al., 1988, 1991; Rayner, 1979; Rayner et al., 1996).

Finally, the third component of saccades, the random motor error, is sampled from a Gaussian distribution with $\mu = 0$ and σ (in character spaces) given by Equation 7. The random error thus has a minimal value ($\eta_1 = 0.5$) that increases (by $\eta_2 = 0.15$ per character space) with the intended saccade length.

$$\sigma = \eta_1 - \eta_2 ISL \tag{7}$$

With these assumptions about saccade execution, the model accurately simulates fixation landing-site distributions that are centred on words and approximately Gaussian in shape, with missing tails due to saccades that occasionally miss their targets, and with variability that increases with saccade length and decreases with launch-site fixation duration (McConkie et al., 1988, 1991; O'Regan, 1981; O'Regan and Lévy-Schoen, 1987; Rayner, 1979; Rayner et al., 1996).

In addition to the primary saccades that move the eyes from one word to the next, there are also corrective saccades that can be initiated whenever a primary saccade deviates from its intended target. The probability of initiating a corrective saccade, p, is:

$$p = \lambda \,|\, \text{landing position} - \text{saccade target} \,| \tag{8}$$

where λ $(= 0.05)$ is a parameter that scales the absolute deviation (in character spaces) between the intended saccade target (i.e. the centre of the word being targeted) and the initial fixation location. The logic behind this assumption is that an *efference copy* or predicted trajectory of the primary saccade (Carpenter, 2000) provides immediate feedback about its accuracy and is used to move the eyes to a better viewing location with a probability that reflects saccadic error. The model thus explains why refixations are more likely following initial fixations near the ends of words (Rayner et al., 1996; Vitu et al., 2001). And because corrective saccades are initiated immediately after the eyes land on a word, first fixations near the edges of a word are shorter in duration (on average) than fixations near the centre (i.e. the *inverted optimal viewing position effect*; Vitu et al., 2001).

Finally, as Fig. 42.1 indicates, E-Z Reader includes assumptions about: 1) how word identification influences attention and post-lexical language processing (i.e. integration), and 2) how integration in turn influences lexical processing, attention, and eye movements. With respect to the former, the model assumes that the completion of lexical access causes attention to shift from the identified word to the next, allowing it to be processed. At the same time, post-lexical processing also begins on the word that was just identified. This integration corresponds to the minimal amount of processing that is necessary to continue moving attention and the eyes forward though the text. Thus, whereas lexical access is like a signal to 'step on the gas' (i.e. move attention to the next word), the completion of integration is like a signal to 'not step on the brakes' (i.e. allow lexical processing to continue). In most instances, integration completes without difficulty, so that both attention and the eyes continue their progression and post-lexical processing has only a minimal effect on readers' eye movements. However, in cases involving integration difficulty, the effects of post-lexical processing can rapidly manifest themselves as pauses and/or inter-word regressions back to previously read portions of the text.

Of course, it takes time to both shift attention and complete integration. The time to shift attention, $t(A)$, is sampled from a γ distribution with $\mu = 50$ ms and $\sigma = 0.22\mu$, giving values consistent with empirical estimates (e.g. Eriksen and Schultz, 1977; Jolicoeur et al., 1983; Posner, 1978; Shulman et al. 1979; Tsal, 1983). Similarly, the time to complete integration, $t(I)$, is also sampled from a γ distribution with $\mu = 25$ ms and $\sigma = 0.22\mu$. Although 25 ms may seem to be too little time to allow any reasonable amount of post-lexical processing to be completed, this processing is meant to be roughly consistent with the notion of 'good enough' processing (e.g. see Ferreira and Patson, 2007; Ferreira et al., 2002; Swets et al., 2008) in that it is the amount of processing that is needed to support minimal comprehension and thereby prevent a pause or regression.

As mentioned, the model also stipulates two ways that integration can influence lexical processing, attention, and eye movements. The first is that a word's meaning must be integrated before predictability information (which reflects the syntactic and/or semantic constraints of the sentence up through that word) can be used to help constrain the identity of the next word in the sentence. Thus, prior to integrating the meaning of word $n-1$, the predictability of word n (i.e. the value assigned to *pred* in Equations 3) is set equal to 0.

Second, on some occasions, integration fails, causing the eyes and attention to pause and/or move backwards. These integration failures happen by default whenever word $n+1$ is identified before the meaning of word n has been integrated, under the assumption that this situation is inherently problematic because the meaning of word $n+1$ has to be maintained in the face of having not yet integrated the meaning of word n. Integration failure can also happen rapidly, as might be expected if a reader mis-parses a syntactically ambiguous 'garden path' sentence (Frazier and Rayner, 1982) or encounters a word that violates semantic plausibility (Rayner et al., 2004b; Warren and McConnell, 2007). These rapid integration failures are assumed to occur with probability p_F that varies across situations. Both types of integration failure cause lexical processing of word $n+1$ to halt and the initiation of a regressive saccadic programme. This can result in a pause, however, if integration fails before the eyes have actually moved to word $n+1$; in such cases, the new saccadic programme that would have produced a regression cancels the labile programme that would have moved the eyes to word $n+1$, thereby prolonging the fixation on word n. Irrespective of what actually happens, however, both the eyes and attention are directed back to word n (i.e. where integration failed) with probability p_N, and to some earlier sentence location (e.g. word $n-1$) with probability $1.0-p_N$. This last assumption allows the model some flexibility because, without a detailed model of language processing and how such processing fails, all inter-word regressions would move the eyes back exactly one word. Finally, the labile stage of programming for regressions requires an additional 30 ms to complete, consistent with evidence that regressions to previously fixated locations take longer to programme than other saccades (Rayner et al., 2003b).

Each successive version of the E-Z Reader model (see Table 42.1) has been evaluated using the 48 sentences used by Schilling et al. (1998) to examine word-frequency effects using eye movements, lexical decision, and the naming task. To evaluate the model, all of the words except the first and last in each sentence are first grouped into five frequency classes. (The first and last words are excluded because the processing of these words starts and ends abruptly in both the experiment and the simulations.) Means are then calculated across participants and words within each frequency class for six dependent measures: first-fixation, single-fixation, and gaze duration, and the probabilities of skipping, making one fixation, or making two or more fixations. The model's parameter values are then selected by fitting the model to these means. Figure 42.2 shows the results of such a simulation (Reichle et al., 2009).

E-Z Reader simulations

This section will briefly review the E-Z Reader simulations that have been completed to: 1) develop and test the model's core assumptions; 2) evaluate how well those assumptions generalize to other populations and materials; and 3) examine various reading phenomena. This chapter will not review the phenomena that have been used to 'benchmark' the model against other models (see Table 42.1) because those simulations have been reviewed elsewhere (e.g. see Reichle et al., 2006). The simulations discussed below are listed in Table 42.2.

Testing model assumptions

Pollatsek et al. (2006a) completed several simulations to test core assumptions of the E-Z Reader model. The simulations were of *gaze-contingent paradigms* in which the information being displayed on the computer monitor was contingent upon where participants were looking (Rayner, 1975). The first simulation examined the hypothesized duration of the eye-to-brain lag, which was set equal to

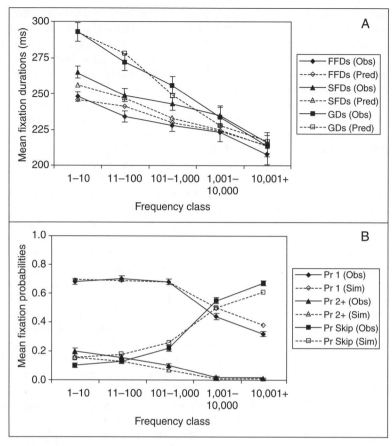

Fig. 42.2 Observed (*Obs*; Schilling et al., 1998) and simulated (*Sim*; Reichle et al., 2009) means for five frequency classes of words (bars indicate standard errors of observed means). A) First-fixation (*FFDs*), single-fixation (*SFDs*), and gaze durations (*GDs*). B) Probabilities of making one fixation (*Pr 1*), two or more fixations (*Pr 2+*), and skipping (*Pr Skip*).

either 90 ms (i.e. the value used in E-Z Reader 7; Reichle et al., 2003) or 50 ms (i.e. a value based on empirical estimates; Clark et al., 1995; Foxe and Simpson, 2002; Mouchetant-Rostaing et al., 2000; Van Rullen and Thorpe, 2001). These two variants of the model were then used to simulate the *boundary paradigm* (Rayner, 1975), where the parafoveal processing of a target word that normally occurs prior to it being fixated is prevented by replacing all of its letters with random letters until the reader's eyes move past the blank space to the left of the target. Gaze durations on target words typically increase by 40–50 ms when their preview is prevented (Hyönä et al., 2004). Consistent with this, the model with a 50-ms lag predicted a 46-ms preview effect, whereas the model with the 90-ms lag predicted a 59-ms effect. This suggests that 50 ms is a reasonable estimate of the eye-to-brain lag.

The second simulation examined the assumption that lexical processing continues during each saccade using visual information from the previous viewing location. Two versions of E-Z Reader were compared: 1) the standard model in which lexical processing continues during each saccade, and 2) a variant in which lexical processing halts with the onset of each saccade and then resumes only after the pre-attentive stage of visual processing has completed, providing visual information from the new fixation location. Although both models performed equally well simulating the measures shown in Fig. 42.2, the model with discontinuous lexical processing predicted a 20-ms preview effect—much smaller than the 40–50 ms effects that are typically observed (Hyönä et al., 2004). The discontinuous model also generated bi-modal fixation-duration distributions (i.e. very short or very long fixations) because words that were not completely identified in the parafovea could only undergo further lexical processing after the eyes had moved and enough time had passed (i.e. the duration of the eye-to-brain lag) to allow lexical processing to resume. This simulation suggests that the assumption that lexical processing continues during saccades is valid.

The third simulation examined the results of another gaze-contingent paradigm—one in which, whenever participants fixated on a high- or low-frequency target word, that word or the one immediately to its right disappeared after 60 ms (Rayner et al., 2005). Somewhat surprisingly, the former manipulation had little effect (e.g. a word-frequency effect was still evident), but the latter manipulation disrupted reading. The explanation for this paradoxical finding is that, while 60 ms is enough time for attended visual information to be converted into more stable lexical (e.g. orthographic) codes, any visual information that is not being attended during this time will be lost (because it will not have been converted into more stable codes). This explanation was tested with the model by assuming that whatever word was being attended when the fixated word (word n) or the one to its right (word $n+1$) disappeared was converted into more stable lexical codes and was thus resistant to loss. With these assumptions, the model predicted normal gaze durations and frequency effects on word n in both conditions, but inflated gaze durations on word $n+1$ in the condition where word $n+1$ disappeared. This simulation suggests that the model's assumption about serial attention allocation may be necessary to account for these key findings.

The last simulation examined the L_1 versus L_2 distinction in E-Z Reader by pitting the standard version of the model against a variant in which the completion of a single stage of lexical processing (i.e. lexical access) caused both the initiation of saccadic programming and the shifting of attention to the next word (in a manner similar to Morrison's, 1984 theory). To provide a fairer test of the one-stage model, the visual-acuity restriction was relaxed (i.e. the value of the ε parameter in Equation 4 was reduced) to allow more rapid parafoveal processing. (Without relaxing this constraint, it would have been necessary to posit unrealistically fast rates of lexical processing or unrealistically long fixations because more lexical processing would have to be completed from the fovea.) With these assumptions, the one-stage model simulated the measures shown in Fig. 42.2 as well as the standard model, but predicted an 87-ms preview effect, suggesting that the L_1 versus L_2 distinction is necessary.

Finally, in response to Inhoff et al. (2005), Pollatsek et al. (2006b, 2006c) completed simulations to show that E-Z Reader could account for experimental results that were touted as problematic for serial-attention models. In this experiment, specific target words either remained visible (full preview), remained masked until fixated (no preview), or appeared (late preview) or disappeared (early preview) 140 ms after the previous word had been fixated. Relative to the no-preview condition, the full-, late-, and early-preview conditions produced 99-ms, 40-ms, and 24-ms preview effects, respectively. Inhoff et al. argued that this pattern was incompatible with serial-attention models because attention would presumably be focused on either the pre-target or target word when the display changed, but not both. However, without any special assumptions, the E-Z Reader model predicted the correct qualitative pattern of results: In the late-preview condition, attention shifted to the target word prior to its appearance 46.2% of the time, while in the early-preview condition, attention shifted to the target word after its disappearance 36.9% of the time. If one assumes that only words that have been attended up to the time of the display change are converted into more stable lexical codes, then the predicted results are roughly consistent with the observed because both the late- and early-preview conditions produced less preview benefit than the full-preview condition. This simulation thus provides further support for the serial-attention hypothesis (cf. Inhoff et al., 2006).

Testing model generality

One limitation of using the Schilling et al. (1998) sentence corpus to evaluate E-Z Reader is that it does not indicate how well the model's assumptions generalize to other populations of readers and/or materials. The simulations reported in this section are important because they show that the model's assumptions are not specific to university students reading English sentences, but instead apply remarkably well across different populations of readers, different languages and writing systems, and different materials.

For example, Rayner et al. (2006) used E-Z Reader to simulate the eye movements of college-aged versus elderly readers. The key differences between these two populations were that the older readers made longer fixations and skipped words more often, but also made more regressions after skipping. To simulate older readers, it was only necessary to: 1) adjust the model's parameters to slow the rate of lexical processing; and 2) assume that older readers are more likely to use linguistic constraints to 'guess' the identity of (and skip) words, but that some of these 'guesses' are incorrect, making inter-word regressions to re-read the misidentified words more likely. With these assumptions, the model simulated the age-related differences in readers' eye movements, suggesting how age affects reading.

E-Z Reader has also been used to simulate the eye movements of readers of other, non-English languages. For example, Miellet et al. (2007) simulated the eye movements of native French speakers reading a short passage of text (see also Sparrow et al., 2003), and Rayner et al. (2007) simulated the eye movements of native Chinese speakers reading sentences. These simulations show that the model's assumptions—and the serial-attention hypothesis—are sufficient to simulate eye movements during the reading of both alphabetic and non-alphabetic languages, suggesting that many of the cognitive processes involved in reading are similar across languages and writing systems as different as English and Chinese.

Finally, Reichle and Nelson (2003) used E-Z Reader to simulate the eye movements of participants reading advertisements containing text and images (Liechty et al., 2003). To do this, it was necessary to convert the model's distance metric (e.g. see Equation 4) from character spaces to visual angle, and to adopt a few simple assumptions about the participants' goals in performing the task. With these modifications, the model simulated the observed number and length of saccades, again showing that its assumptions generalize across participants and materials.

Examining reading phenomena

E-Z Reader has also been used to examine various reading phenomena. For example, the model was used to evaluate various explanations of how Finnish compound words might be identified (Pollatsek et al., 2003). In the experiments that were simulated, the frequencies and lengths of both the compound words and their constituents were orthogonally varied to determine if and when these variables influenced readers' eye movements (Hyönä and Pollatsek, 1998; Pollatsek et al., 2000). The experiments revealed systematic effects of these variables, with the frequency and length of the first constituents influencing the durations and locations of the first fixations on the words, and the frequencies and lengths of both the second constituents and of the whole words influencing subsequent fixation durations and locations. The results thus suggest that both constituent and whole-word processing somehow affect the process of generating the overall meaning of the compound word.

E-Z Reader was used to test several possible accounts of how this might happen. The one that was successful implemented a composition model of word identification (Jarvella and Meijers, 1983; MacKay, 1978), with the individual constituents first being identified and then combined to generate the overall word meaning. The individual constituents were thus processed like small words (that happened to not be separated by blank spaces), with the completion of the familiarity check on the first constituent triggering a saccade to the second, the completion of the familiarity check on that constituent triggering a saccade to yet another viewing location on the word, and the completion of the compositional stage triggering a saccade to the next word. The time (in ms) required to complete the compositional stage, $t(C)$, was assumed to be a function of the compound word's overall frequency, as given by:

$$t(C) = \gamma_1 - \gamma_2 \ln(freq) \tag{9}$$

where the parameter γ_1 (= 115) is the maximum time to complete the compositional stage, and with γ_2 (= 70) attenuating this time as a function of the word's frequency. [The value of $t(C)$ was restricted so that it could not be less than 0 ms]

The above assumptions were sufficient to simulate the patterns of eye movements that were observed on the compound words, and the manner in which the fixation durations and locations were affected by the frequencies and lengths of both the whole words and their constituents. The fact that this simulation required the sequential processing of sub-word units suggests that, with long poly-morphemic words, attention may actually be focused on units that are smaller than individual words. This suggests that attention may occasionally be focused in a manner that is even more serial than the standard serial-attention models currently posit (e.g. on individual syllables or graphemes; see Ans et al., 1998).

E-Z Reader has also been used to test various explanations of *lexical ambiguity resolution*, or how words with multiple meanings are interpreted with and without prior disambiguating sentence contexts (Reichle et al., 2007). For example, how is the correct meaning of 'port' accessed when it occurs in the absence of biasing context versus a context that evokes either the *dominant* or common 'harbor' meaning or the *subordinate* or less common 'wine' meaning? In an experiment addressing this question (Duffy et al., 1988), ambiguous words having strongly biased (e.g. 'port') and more equi-biased (e.g. 'count') interpretations were embedded in sentences that were either neutral or that supported the subordinate meanings of the words. In the neutral contexts, the biased ambiguous words were read as rapidly as (frequency-matched) unambiguous control words, but the equi-biased words were read more slowly. But when the preceding sentence context supported the subordinate meanings of the words, the biased ambiguous words were read more slowly than the control words, and the equi-biased words were read as rapidly as the control words.

To simulate this pattern of results, it was necessary to assume that the time to complete the familiarity check (i.e. $t(L_1)$, as specified by Equation 3) included an additional fourth term, $t(D)$, reflecting the relative disparities between the dominant and subordinate meanings of the ambiguous words, and how these disparities are modulated by prior sentence context. The duration of this term (in ms) is given by:

$$t(D) = \alpha_4 / \left\{ z \left[p\left(meaning_{dom} + \phi \right) \right] - z \left[p\left(meaning_{sub} + \phi \right) \right] \right\} \qquad (10)$$

where $p(meaning_{dom})$ and $p(meaning_{sub})$ are the proportions of participants that gave the dominant versus subordinate meanings of a word when it was displayed in isolation, and ϕ is a parameter that attenuates any disparity between these values when the word appears in supporting context ($\phi = 0$ without context and $\phi = 0.36$ with context). The two probabilities are then z-transformed so that values close to 0 and 1 become very large, and the difference between the two resulting values is then scaled by a free parameter ($\alpha_4 = 7$) that modulates the overall size of the ambiguity effect.

These assumptions are consistent with the *re-ordered access model* (Duffy et al., 2001; Pacht and Rayner, 1993) of lexical ambiguity resolution in that the time needed to identify an ambiguous word is a function of its overall frequency and the relative disparities of its different meanings, with the contribution of the latter also being modulated by whether or not the word appears in a disambiguating context. And when implemented within E-Z Reader, these assumptions were sufficient to simulate the patterns of eye movements associated with ambiguity resolution (Dopkins et al., 1992; Duffy et al., 1988, 2001; Rayner and Duffy, 1986; Rayner and Frazier, 1989). This simulation thus lends additional support to the re-ordered access account and underscores the computational challenge that ambiguous words place on the word-identification system—one that seemingly demands the serial allocation of attention (e.g. see Reichle et al., 2009).

Pollatsek et al. (2008) have also used E-Z Reader to examine the *reverse word-length effect*—the paradoxical finding that the gaze durations on the nouns in adjective-noun pairs tended to be longer when the preceding adjective was short (e.g. 'bald merchant') rather than long (e.g. 'corrupt merchant'). The explanation of this finding included three assumptions: 1) that the adjectives had some probability of being misidentified because of their having higher-frequency orthographic neighbours (e.g. 'bold' is a high-frequency neighbour of 'bald'); 2) that the misidentification of the adjectives subsequently slowed lexical processing of the nouns; and 3) that shorter adjectives tended to be inadvertently skipped more often than the longer adjectives, necessitating their processing from the nouns and thereby inflating the gaze durations on the nouns. When implemented in E-Z Reader, these assumptions were sufficient to simulate the complex pattern of results that—without the model—seemed to defy explanation.

Finally, Reichle and Laurent (2006) used a machine-learning algorithm called *Reinforcement Learning* (Sutton and Barto, 1998) to examine how, given an initial set of biological (e.g. limited visual acuity) and psychological (e.g. minimal word-identification latencies) constraints, a virtual reading 'agent' might learn to move its eyes and attention to read as efficiently as possible. When constrained to allocate attention serially and to process one word at a time, these agents learned to direct their eyes towards the centres of words, where the words could be identified most rapidly. The agents also learned to skip the easy-to-identify short words and to refixate the difficult-to-identify long words, with refixations being more likely whenever initial fixations landed near the beginnings of words, on poor viewing locations. Finally, the agent learned the relationship between the lengths of the words and their identification times, and learned to initiate saccadic programming so that the eyes would leave the words just as they were identified. This strategy was optimal because initiating saccadic programming any earlier would cause the eyes to move prematurely, making it necessary to continue lexical processing from a poorer viewing location and thereby slowing the overall rate of reading, while initiating saccadic programming any later would cause the fixations to be unnecessarily long, also slowing the overall rate of reading. By learning to initiate saccadic programming in this manner, the reading agents learned something akin to the familiarity check that is posited in the E-Z Reader model. The simulations thus show how a familiarity check might be learned as a way of enhancing reading efficiency.

Conclusion

This chapter started with a review of those computational models of eye movement control in reading that share the assumptions that attention is allocated serially, to only one word at a time, and that lexical processing is the 'engine' that causes the eyes to move forward through the text. These models are important because they explain how cognition influences the readers' eye movements, and because they indicate the feasibility of the serial-attention hypothesis. And in terms of their theoretical scope, these models provide a standard against which other models should be evaluated.

The second half of this chapter reviewed the simulations that have been completed using the E-Z Reader model. These simulations show that the model can handle a range of gaze-contingent phenomena and that the basic model assumptions generalize across different reading populations, writing systems, and materials. These simulations also show how the model can be used to examine theoretical issues related to language processing during reading. Together, the simulations suggest that the serial-attention hypothesis provides a plausible and parsimonious description of how attention is allocated during reading (Reichle et al., 2009).

Acknowledgements

The writing of this chapter was supported by NIH grant RO1 HD053639. I would like to thank Denis Drieghe, Patryk Laurent, Simon Liversedge, Polina Vanyukov, and Tessa Warren for their helpful suggestions on earlier versions of this chapter.

References

Anderson, J.R. (1983). *The architecture of cognition*. Cambridge, MA: Harvard University Press.
Anderson, J.R. and Lebiere, C. (1998). *The atomic components of thought*. Hillsdale, NJ: Erlbaum.

Ans, B., Carbonnel, S., and Valdois, S. (1998). A connectionist multiple-trace memory model for polysyllabic word reading. *Psychological Review*, **105**, 678–723.

Balota, D.A., Pollatsek, A., and Rayner, K. (1985). The interaction of contextual constraints and parafoveal visual information in reading. *Cognitive Psychology*, **17**, 364–390.

Becker, W. and Jürgens, R. (1979). An analysis of the saccadic system by means of double step stimuli. *Vision Research*, **19**, 967–983.

Binder, K., Pollatsek, A., and Rayner, K. (1999). Extraction of information to the left of the fixated word in reading. *Journal of Experimental Psychology: Human Perception and Performance*, **25**, 1162–1172.

Carpenter, R.H.S. (2000). The neural coding of looking. *Current Biology*, **10**, R291–R293.

Clark, V.P., Fan, S., and Hillyard, S.A. (1995). Identification of early visual evoked potential generators by retinotopic and topographic analyses. *Human Brain Mapping*, **2**, 170–187.

Dopkins, S. Morris, R.K., and Rayner, K. (1992). Lexical ambiguity and eye fixations in reading: A test of competing models of lexical ambiguity resolution. *Journal of Memory and Language*, **31**, 461–476.

Duffy, S.A., Morris, R.K., and Rayner, K. (1988). Lexical ambiguity and fixation times in reading. *Journal of Memory and Language*, **27**, 429–446.

Duffy, S.A., Kambe, G., and Rayner, K. (2001). The effect of prior disambiguating context on the comprehension of ambiguous words: Evidence from eye movements. In D.S. Gorfein (ed.) *On the consequences of meaning selection* (pp. 27–43). Washington, DC: APA Books.

Engbert, R., Nuthmann, A., Richter, E., and Kliegl, R. (2005). SWIFT: A dynamical model of saccade generation during reading. *Psychological Review*, **112**, 777–813.

Eriksen, C.W. and Shultz, D.W. (1977). Retinal locus and acuity in visual information processing. *Bulletin of the Psychonomic Society*, **9**, 81–84.

Feng, G. (2006). Eye movements as time-series random variables: A stochastic model of eye movement control in reading. *Cognitive Systems Research*, **7**, 70–95.

Ferreira, F. and Patson, N.D. (2007). The 'good enough' approach to language comprehension. *Language and Linguistics Compass*, **1**, 71–83.

Ferreira, F., Bailey, K.G.D., and Ferraro, V. (2002). Good-enough representations in language comprehension. *Current Directions in Psychological Science*, **11**, 11–15.

Foxe, J.J. and Simpson, G.V. (2002). Flow of activation from V1 to frontal cortex in humans: A framework for defining 'early' visual processing. *Experimental Brain Research*, **142**, 139–150.

Francis, W.N. and Kučera, H. (1982). *Frequency analysis of English usage: Lexicon and grammar*. Boston, MA: Houghton Mifflin.

Frazier, L. and Rayner, K. (1982). Making and correcting errors during sentence comprehension: Eye movements in the analysis of structurally ambiguous sentences. *Cognitive Psychology*, **14**, 178–210.

Henderson, J.M. and Ferreira, F. (1990). Effects of foveal processing difficulty on the perceptual span in reading: Implications for attention and eye movement control. *Journal of Experimental Psychology: Learning, Memory, and Cognition*, **16**, 417–429.

Huey, E.B. (1908). *The psychology and pedagogy of reading*. New York: Macmillian.

Hyönä, J. and Pollatsek, A. (1998). Reading Finnish compound words: Eye fixations are affected by component morphemes. *Journal of Experimental Psychology: Human Perception and Performance*, **24**, 1612–1627.

Hyönä, J., Bertram, R., and Pollatsek, A. (2004). Are long compound words identified serially via their constituents? Evidence form an eye-movement contingent display change study. *Memory and Cognition*, **32**, 523–532.

Inhoff, A.W., Eiter, B.M., and Radach, R. (2005). The time course of linguistic information extraction from consecutive words during eye fixations in reading. *Journal of Experimental Psychology: Human Perception and Performance*, **31**, 979–995.

Inhoff, A.W., Radach, R., and Eiter, B.M. (2006). Temporal overlap in the linguistic processing of successive words in reading: Reply to Pollatsek, Reichle, and Rayner (2006). *Journal of Experimental Psychology: Human Perception and Performance*, **32**, 1490–1495.

Jacobs, A.M. and Grainger, J. (1994). Models of visual word recognition—Sampling the state of the art. *Journal of Experimental Psychology: Human Perception and Performance*, **20**, 1311–1334.

Jarvella, R. and Meijers, G. (1983). Recognizing morphemes in spoken words: Some evidence for a stem-organized mental lexicon. In G.B. Flores d'Arcaos and R. Jarvella (eds.) *The process of language understanding* (pp. 81–112). New York, NY: Wiley.

Jolicoeur, P., Ullman, S., and Mackay, M.F. (1983). Curve tracing: A possible basic operation in the perception of spatial relations. *Memory and Cognition*, **14**, 129–140.

Just, M.A. and Carpenter, P.A. (1980). A theory of reading: om eye fixations to comprehension. *Psychological Review*, **87**, 329–354.

Just, M.A. and Carpenter, P.A. (1987). *The psychology of reading and language comprehension*. Newton, MA: Allyn and Bacon.

Just, M.A. and Varma, S. (2002). A hybrid architecture for working memory: Reply to MacDonald and Christiansen (2002). *Psychological Review*, **109**, 55–65.

Kennison, S.M. and Clifton, C. (1995). Determinants of parafoveal preview benefit in high and low working memory capacity readers: Implications for eye movement control. *Journal of Experimental Psychology: Learning, Memory, and Cognition,* **21**, 68–81.

Lee, H.-W., Legge, G.E., and Ortiz, A. (2003). Is word recognition different in central and peripheral vision? *Vision Research,* **43**, 2837–2846.

Leff, A.P., Scott, S.K., Rothwell, J.C., and Wise, R.J.S. (2001). The planning and guiding of reading saccades: A repetitive transcranial magnetic stimulation study. *Cerebral Cortex,* **11**, 918–923.

MacKay, D.G. (1978). Derivational rules and the internal lexicon. *Journal of Verbal Learning and Verbal Behavior,* **17**, 61–71.

McConkie, G.W., Kerr, P.W., Reddix, M.D., and Zola, D. (1988). Eye movement control during reading: I. The location of initial eye fixations in words. *Vision Research,* **28**, 1107–1118.

McConkie, G.W., Zola, D., Grimes, J., Kerr, P.W., Bryant, N.R., and Wolff, P.M. (1991). Children's eye movements during reading. In J.F. Stein (ed.), *Vision and visual dyslexia 13.* London: MacMillan.

McDonald, S.A., Carpenter, R.H.S., and Shillcock, R.C. (2005). An anatomically constrained, stochastic model of eye movement control in reading. *Psychological Review,* **112**, 814–840.

McPeek, R.M., Skavenski, A.A., and Nakayama, K. (2000). Concurrent processing of saccades in visual search. *Vision Research,* **40**, 2499–2516.

Miellet, S., Sparrow, L., and Sereno, S.C. (2007). Word frequency and predictability effects in reading French: An evaluation of the E-Z Reader model. *Psychonomic Bulletin and Review,* **14**, 762–769.

Molker, A. and Fischer, B. (1999). The recognition and correction of involuntary prosaccades in an antisaccade task. *Experimental Brain Research,* **125**, 511–516.

Morrison, R.E. (1984). Manipulation of stimulus onset delay in reading: Evidence for parallel programming of saccades. *Journal of Experimental Psychology: Human Perception and Performance,* **10**, 667–682.

Mouchetant-Rostaing, Y., Giard, M.-H., Bentin, S., Aguera, P.-E., and Pernier, J. (2000). Neurophysiological correlates of face gender processing in humans. *European Journal of Neuroscience,* **12**, 303–310.

Newell, A. (1973). You can't play 20 questions with nature and win. In W.G. Chase (ed.), *Visual information processing* (pp. 283–308). New York: Academic Press.

Newell, A. (1990). *Unified theories of cognition.* Cambridge, MA: Harvard University Press.

Newell, A. and Simon, H.A. (1972). *Human problem solving.* Englewood Cliffs, NJ: Prentice-Hall.

O'Regan, J.K. (1981). The 'convenient viewing location' hypothesis. In D.F. Fisher, R.A. Monty, and J.W. Senders (eds.) *Eye movements: Cognition and visual perception* (pp. 289–298). Hillsdale, NJ: Erlbaum.

O'Regan, J.K. and Lévy-Schoen, A. (1987). Eye-movement strategy and tactics in word recognition and reading. In M. Coltheart (ed.), *Attention and performance, XII* (pp. 363–384). Hillsdale, NJ: Erlbaum.

Pacht, J.M. and Rayner, K. (1993). The processing of homophonic homographs during reading: Evidence from eye movement studies. *Journal of Psycholinguistic Research,* **22**, 251–271.

Pollatsek, A., Hyönä, J., and Bertram, R. (2000). The role of morphological constituents in reading Finnish compound words. *Journal of Experimental Psychology: Human Perception and Performance,* **26**, 820–833.

Pollatsek, A., Reichle, E.D., and Rayner, K. (2003). Modeling eye movements in reading: Extensions of the E-Z Reader model. In J. Hyönä, R. Radach and H. Deubel (eds.) *The mind's eyes: Cognitive and applied aspects of oculomotor research* (pp. 361–390). Oxford: Elsevier.

Pollatsek, A., Reichle, E.D., and Rayner, K. (2006a). Tests of the E-Z Reader model: Exploring the interface between cognition and eye-movement control. *Cognitive Psychology,* **52**, 1–56.

Pollatsek, A., Reichle, E.D., and Rayner, K. (2006b). Attention to one word at a time is still a viable hypothesis: Rejoinder to Inhoff, Eiter, and Radach. *Journal of Experiment Psychology: Human Perception and Performance,* **32**, 1496–1500.

Pollatsek, A., Reichle, E.D., and Rayner, K. (2006c). Serial processing is consistent with the time course of linguistic information extraction from consecutive words during eye fixations in reading: A response to Inhoff, Eiter, and Radach (2005). *Journal of Experiment Psychology: Human Perception and Performance,* **32**, 1485–1489.

Pollatsek, A., Lesch, M., Morris, R.K., and Rayner, K. (1992). Phonological codes are used in integrating information across saccades in word identification and reading. *Journal of Experimental Psychology: Human Perception and Performance,* **18**, 148–162.

Pollatsek, A., Juhasz, B.J., Reichle, E.D., Machacek, D., and Rayner, K. (2008). Immediate and delayed effects of word frequency and word length on eye movements in reading: A delayed effect of word length. *Journal of Experiment Psychology: Human Perception and Performance,* **34**, 726–750.

Posner, M.I. (1978). *Chronometric explorations of mind.* Hillsdale, NJ: Erlbaum.

Rayner, K. (1975). The perceptual span and peripheral cues in reading. *Cognitive Psychology,* **7**, 65–81.

Rayner, K. (1979). Eye guidance in reading: Fixation locations with words. *Perception,* **8**, 21–30.

Rayner, K. (1998). Eye movements in reading and information processing: 20 years of research. *Psychological Bulletin,* **124**, 372–422.

Rayner, K. and Bertera, J.J. (1979). Reading without a fovea. *Science,* **206**, 468–469.

Rayner, K. and Duffy, S.M. (1986). Lexical complexity and fixation times in reading: Effects of word frequency, verb complexity, and lexical ambiguity. *Memory and Cognition,* **14**, 191–201.

Rayner, K. and Juhasz, B. (2004). Eye movements in reading: Old questions and new directions. *European Journal of Cognitive Psychology*, **16**, 340–352.

Rayner, K. and Morrison, R.E. (1981). Eye movements and identifying words in parafoveal vision. *Bulletin of the Psychonomic Society*, **17**, 135–138.

Rayner, K., Sereno, S.C., and Raney, G.E. (1996). Eye movement control in reading: A comparison of two types of models. *Journal of Experimental Psychology: Human Perception and Performance*, **22**, 1188–1200.

Rayner, K., Pollatsek, A., and Reichle, E.D. (2003a). Eye movements in reading: Models and data. *Behavioral and Brain Sciences*, **26**, 507–518.

Rayner, K., Liversedge, S.P., and White, S.J. (2005). Eye movements when reading disappearing text: The importance of the word to the right of fixation. *Vision Research*, **46**, 310–323.

Rayner, K., Li, X., and Pollatsek, A. (2007). Extending the E-Z Reader model of eye movement control to Chinese readers. *Cognitive Science*, **31**, 1021–1033.

Rayner, K., Slowiaczek, M.L., Clifton, C., and Bertera, J.H. (1983). Latency of sequential eye movements: Implications for reading. *Journal of Experimental Psychology: Human Perception and Performance*, **9**, 912–922.

Rayner, K., Juhasz, B., Ashby, J., and Clifton, C. (2003b). Inhibition of saccade return in reading. *Vision Research*, **43**, 1027–1034.

Rayner, K., Ashby, J., Pollatsek, A., and Reichle, E.D. (2004a). The effects of frequency and predictability on eye fixations in reading: Implications for the E-Z Reader model. *Journal of Experimental Psychology: Human Perception and Performance*, **30**, 720–732.

Rayner, K., Warren, T., Juhasz, B.J., and Liversedge, S.P. (2004b). The effect of plausibility on eye movements in reading. *Journal of Experimental Psychology: Learning, Memory, and Cognition*, **30**, 1290–1301.

Rayner, K., Pollatsek, A., Liversedge, S.P., and Reichle, E.D. (2009). Eye movements and non-canonical reading: Comments on Kennedy and Pynte (2008). *Vision Research*, **49**, 2232–2236.

Rayner, K., Sereno, S.C., Morris, R.K., Schmauder, A.R., and Clifton, C. (1989). Eye movements and on-line language comprehension processes. *Language and Cognitive Processes*, **4**, 21–49.

Rayner, K., Reichle, E.D., Stroud, M.J., Williams, C.C., and Pollatsek, A. (2006). The effects of word frequency, word predictability, and font difficulty on the eye movements of young and elderly readers. *Psychology and Aging*, **21**, 448–465.

Reichle, E.D. and Laurent, P.A. (2006). Using reinforcement learning to understand the emergence of 'intelligent' eye-movement behavior during reading. *Psychological Review*, **113**, 390–408.

Reichle, E.D. and Nelson, J.R. (2003). Local vs. global attention: Are two states necessary? Comment on Liechty et al., 2003. *Psychometrika*, **68**, 543–549.

Reichle, E.D. and Perfetti, C.A. (2003). Morphology in word identification: A word experience model that accounts for morpheme frequency effects. *Scientific Studies of Reading*, **7**, 219–237.

Reichle, E.D., Rayner, K., and Pollatsek, A. (1999). Eye movement control in reading: Accounting for initial fixation locations and refixations within the E-Z Reader model. *Vision Research*, **39**, 4403–4411.

Reichle, E.D., Rayner, K., and Pollatsek, A. (2003). The E-Z Reader model of eye movement control in reading: Comparisons to other models. *Behavioral and Brain Sciences*, **26**, 445–476.

Reichle, E.D., Pollatsek, A., and Rayner, K. (2006). E-Z Reader: A cognitive-control, serial-attention model of eye-movement control during reading. *Cognitive Systems Research*, **7**, 4–22.

Reichle, E.D., Pollatsek, A., and Rayner, K. (2007). Modeling the effects of lexical ambiguity on eye movements during reading. In R.P.G. Van Gompel, M.F. Fischer, W.S. Murray, and R.L. Hill (eds.) *Eye movements: A window on mind and brain* (pp. 271–292). Oxford: Elsevier.

Reichle, E.D., Warren, T., and McConnell, K. (2009b). Using E-Z Reader to model the effects of higher-level language processing on eye movements during reading. *Psychonomic Bulletin and Review*, **16**, 1–21.

Reichle, E.D., Pollatsek, A., Fisher, D.L., and Rayner, K. (1998). Toward a model of eye movement control in reading. *Psychological Review*, **105**, 125–157.

Reichle, E.D., Vanyukov, P.M., Laurent, P.A., and Warren, T. (2008). Serial or parallel? Using depth-of-processing to examine attention allocation during reading. *Vision Research*, **48**, 1831–1836.

Reichle, E.D., Liversedge, S.P., Pollatsek, A., and Rayner, K. (2009a). Encoding multiple words simultaneously in reading is implausible. *Trends in Cognitive Sciences*, **13**, 115–119.

Reingold, E.M. and Rayner, K. (2006). Examining the word identification stages hypothesized by the E-Z Reader model. *Psychological Science*, **17**, 742–746.

Reilly, R. and Radach, R. (2006). Some empirical tests of an interactive activation model of eye movement control in reading. *Cognitive Systems Research*, **7**, 34–55.

Rumelhart, D.E. (1989). The architecture of mind: A connectionist approach. In M.I. Posner (ed.), *Foundations of cognitive science* (pp. 133–159). Cambridge, MA: MIT Press.

Salvucci, D.D. (2001). An integrated model of eye movements and visual encoding. *Cognitive Systems Research*, **1**, 201–220.

Schilling, H.E.H., Rayner, K., and Chumbley, J.I. (1998). Comparing naming, lexical decision, and eye fixation times: Word frequency effects and individual differences. *Memory and Cognition*, **26**, 1270–1281.

Shulman, G.L., Remington, R.W., and McLean, J.P. (1979). Moving attention through visual space. *Journal of Experimental Psychology: Human Perception and Performance*, **15**, 522–526.

Starr, M.S. and Rayner, K. (2001). Eye movements during reading: Some current controversies. *Trends in Cognitive Science*, **5**, 156–163.

Sutton, R.S. and Barto, A.G. (1998). *Reinforcement learning: An introduction*. Cambridge, MA: MIT Press.

Swets, B., Desmet, T., Clifton, C., and Ferreira, F. (2008). Underspecification of syntactic ambiguities: Evidence from self-paced reading. *Memory and Cognition*, **36**, 201–216.

Thibadeau, R., Just, M.A., and Carpenter, P.A. (1982). A model of the time course and content of reading. *Cognitive Science*, **6**, 157–203.

Treisman, A. and Gelade, G. (1980). A feature integration theory of attention. *Cognitive Psychology*, **12**, 97–136.

Treisman, A. and Schmidt, H. (1982). Illusory conjuctions in the perception of objects. *Cognitive Psychology*, **14**, 107–141.

Tsal, Y. (1983). Movements of attention across the visual field. *Journal of Experimental Psychology: Human Perception and Performance*, **9**, 523–530.

Van Rullen, R. and Thorpe, S. (2001). The time course of visual processing: From early perception to decision-making. *Journal of Cognitive Neuroscience*, **13**, 454–461.

Vergilino, D. and Beauvillain, C. (2000). The planning of refixation saccades in reading. *Vision Research*, **40**, 3527–3538.

Vitu, F., McConkie, G.W., Kerr, P., and O'Regan, J.K. (2001). Fixation location effects on fixation durations during reading: an inverted optimal viewing position effect. *Vision Research*, **41**, 3513–3533.

Warren, T. and McConnell, K. (2007). Disentangling the effects of selectional restriction violations and plausibility violation severity on eye-movements in reading. Psychonomic Bulletin and Review, **14**, 770–775.

Yang, S.-N. (2006). A oculomotor-based model of eye movements in reading: The competition/activation model. *Cognitive Systems Research*, **7**, 56–69.

Yonelinas, A.P. (2002). The nature of recollection and familiarity: A review of 30 years of research. *Journal of Memory and Language*, **46**, 441–517.

CHAPTER 43

Parallel graded attention models of reading

Ralf Engbert and Reinhold Kliegl

Abstract

Models of eye movement control based on parallel graded attention contribute theoretical solutions to various problems related to distributed processing, word skipping, and regressions. Here we give an overview of the key concepts of the theoretical framework, its plausibility, and its application and present the assumptions and simulation results for the SWIFT model (Engbert et al., 2005) as an example for a parallel graded attention model of reading.

Introduction

A key feature of language is its serial order. While the importance of word order varies between different languages, there is generally a strong need to keep track of serial order during word processing. As a consequence, the first models of eye movement control in reading (Reichle et al., 1998; see also Engbert and Kliegl, 2001) operated on the assumption of the two principles that: 1) attention is allocated to exactly one word at a time and that 2) attentional shifts mandatorily move from one word to the next, i.e. in strict serial order. Models based on these principles, summarized under the name *sequential attention shifts* (SAS), turned out to be extremely stimulating to the research on eye movements in reading (see Reichle, Chapter 42, this volume). Thus, the value of computational modelling of cognitive processes has been demonstrated in the study of eye movements in reading and is an active area of cognitive research (e.g. Reichle et al., 2003; again see Reichle, Chapter 42, this volume).

During reading, our eyes are actively scanning a well-structured visual environment using saccadic eye movements. Roughly 50% of all saccades move our eye's fixation point from word *n* to the next word *n*+1. The remaining 50% of cases is divided into three different categories of saccades (e.g. Rayner, 2009). First, we observe *word-skipping* saccades which contribute about 20% to all saccades. These are rapid eye movements from word *n* to word *n*+2 (note, however, that sometimes more than one word is skipped). Second, *refixations* represent another 20% of all saccades. Refixations are saccades which update the eye's fixation position within the same word. The third and last category is represented by *regressions*, which are saccades from word *n* to word *n-k* (*k*>0), i.e. to a word located in a previously fixated region of text. Regressions contribute roughly 10% to all saccades. As a consequence, the eye's scan path during reading is generally complex, even when reading simple texts, where difficulties in text comprehension are rather exceptional. The E-Z Reader model (Reichle et al., 1998) was able to explain some aspects of scanpath complexity (Engbert et al., 2004), namely word skipping and refixations, using the parsimonious SAS principle, while regressions were outside the focus of the E-Z Reader framework.[1]

In recent years, experimental evidence has been argued to demonstrate that SAS models might be too limited to account for a number of phenomena. Developed as a theoretical alternative to SAS models and, in particular, the E-Z Reader model, *processing gradient* (PG) models relax the assumption that attention is confined to exactly one word at a time by postulating spatially distributed processing according to an attentional gradient (Engbert et al., 2002; Reilly and Radach, 2003). As an example, in the SWIFT model (Engbert et al., 2002) spatially-distributed processing is used to build up activation fields for movement planning. We will review the key concepts of PG models in the following section ('Processing gradient models of reading') and discuss the SWIFT model as a particular example of a PG model in the section 'SWIFT as a processing gradient model of eye movement control'. Next, we discuss the experimental basis for moving from the SAS to PG framework. First, SAS models are incompatible with patterns of lag and successor effects (Kliegl et al., 2006). Second, fixation durations before skipped words (Kliegl and Engbert, 2005) are decreased for short and/or high frequency words, while SAS models always generate inflated fixation durations before skipped words due to their architecture. Third, PG models can explain key patterns of regressions observed in reading (Engbert et al., 2005). We will discuss each of these issues separately in later sections and demonstrate how PG models can solve these problems within a theoretically coherent framework.

Processing gradient models of reading

Why should the two categories of serial (SAS) and parallel (PG) models be distinguished? The problem of serial versus parallel processing is a natural research topic in psychology and cognitive science because of its relation to the capacity of our mind (Townsend, 1990). For example, it is well-established in eye movement research on reading that saccade preparation and word recognition do not compete for cognitive capacity, so that lexical processing continues during saccade programming (Morrisson, 1984). Thus, the notion of parallel processing of saccade preparation and lexical processing is well-accepted. However, the assumption of temporally overlapping lexical processing of multiple words at a time is controversial (Kliegl, 2007; Kliegl et al., 2006; Rayner et al., 2006; Reichle et al., 2009a).

The development of *processing gradient* models of eye movement control in reading was driven by the hypothesis that all types of saccades (i.e. forward, skipping, refixation saccades, and regressions) might emerge from a single underlying principle which is related to parallel processing of multiple words at a time. The theoretical background for PG models is the dynamic field theory of movement preparation (Erlhagen and Schöner, 2002), which might be looked upon as the most general cognitive framework to explain the control of motor systems. In the dynamic field theory, spatially-distributed activations (or an activation field) determine probabilities for target selection during movement planning. This approach guarantees the existence of a movement target at any point in time, even in the absence of a decision to command a new movement. Such a framework is necessary, if temporal decisions ('when' to move the eyes) are partially independent of spatial decisions ('where' to move the eyes). Interestingly, this property is an essential requirement derived from oculomotor physiology (Findlay and Walker, 1999).

The temporal evolution of the activation fields is related to both external (e.g. sensory) and internal (e.g. memory) influences, which is determined by an equation of motion. From a mathematical point of view, the most fundamental difference between SAS and PG models of eye movement control is that SAS models (e.g. Reichle et al., 1998) are *state-based, stochastic automata* with an explicit assumption for every single processing state, while PG models are *dynamical systems*, which focus on generalized equations of motion in *phase space* to capture the unfolding dynamics of cognitive

---

[1] The *E-Z Reader* model (Reichle et al., 1998) generates regressions in very special situation and with low probability. In the *E-Z Reader* framework, regressions were considered to represent a consequence of higher-level language processing (see Reichle et al., 2009).

processes shaped by internal and external constraints (Beer, 2000; Busemeyer and Townsend, 1993; van Gelder, 1998). One of the major advantages of dynamical models is their structural similarity to neural and physiological models. Fortunately, predictions of dynamical models of cognition are highly specific (Beer, 2000). For example, an attentional gradient produces preview effects almost naturally, since processing is not restricted to a single word at a time. However, it is a challenge to implement a PG model, which satisfies constraints for processing the currently fixated word and constraints from the previously fixated and the upcoming word (Engbert et al., 2005).

In the *Glenmore* PG model (Reilly and Radach, 2003, 2006), key elements are a visual input module, a competitive word processing module where several words can be simultaneously active, a fixate centre, and a saccade generator, which produces the actual saccadic movement. The input vector represents the current perceptual span and is used for coding of the visual configuration. During processing, information is transferred to the saliency map and to a linguistic processing module implementing processing on the letter and word level within an interactive activation framework. Activation values are calculated as an additive function of bottom-up visual activation from the input units and top-down letter and (indirectly) word activation. The time course of activation at the word level is a function of both competitive inhibition from neighbouring words and a word's frequency. Words feed back to the letter level with inhibitory links that serve to slow the decay of the letter units. Thus, the *Glenmore* model focuses explicitly on processing at the letter level and provides a coherent framework for parallel processing at both letter and word level.

Processing gradient models like SWIFT (Engbert et al., 2002, 2005) and Glenmore (Reilly and Radach, 2003, 2006) produce all saccade types experimentally found in reading from a single principle: Saccade targets are selected from an activation field which evolves over time contingent on cognitive and visuomotor processing. In this approach, words of a sentence serve as units of the activation field. The word-based activation field is a set of variables that changes continuously over time. This architecture can explain why eye movements in reading are similar across a wide range of other visuomotor behaviour like visual search (e.g. Trukenbrod and Engbert, 2007) and z-string scanning (e.g. Nuthmann and Engbert, 2009; though see Rayner et al., 2007a).

SWIFT as a processing gradient model of eye movement control

As noted in the previous section, two independent pathways for spatial ('where') and temporal ('when') control of saccades during reading have been identified (Findlay and Walker, 1999). The SWIFT model represents an example for the computational implementation of this principle (Fig. 43.1A). In the temporal pathway ('when'), a decision to initiate a new saccade programme is generated by a random timer. In the spatial pathway ('where'), the activation field determines the probability to select a word as the next saccade target (Fig. 43.1B). A general form of transforming activations into probabilities for action selection is given by the computation of relative activations, i.e. the proportion of the activation $a_n{}^\gamma(t)$ of the current word n divided by the sum of all activations,

$$\pi(n,t) = \frac{a_n^\gamma(t)}{\sum_{m=1}^{N} a_m^\gamma},$$

(1)

where N is the number of words in a sentence (or a given region of text) and γ is an exponent which controls the amount of stochasticity in target selection. Two limiting cases are: 1) random target selection, $\gamma \to 0$, which is equivalent to selecting targets with equal probability from the set of all words with non-vanishing activations, and 2) winner-takes-all selection (or deterministic selection), $\gamma \to \infty$, i.e. the word with highest activation is selected as the next saccade target with probability $\pi=1$. In previous studies of the SWIFT model, we fixed $\gamma=1$, i.e. the probability for target selection was equal to its relative activation (Luce's choice rule; Luce, 1959).

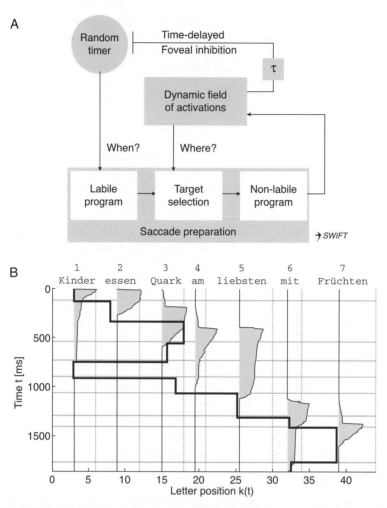

Fig. 43.1 The SWIFT model. A) A key feature of the SWIFT model is the separation into spatial ('where') and temporal ('when') pathways of saccade preparation. B) Activation-based target selection in SWIFT. Activations (plotted for each word to the right) evolve over time (ordinate) as a consequence of word processing. Saccades (time windows marked by bars) shift gaze to a new fixation position. The eye's scan path is indicated by the bold line (vertical parts are fixations, horizontal parts are saccades). Word skippings, refixations, and regressions are the outcome of the competition of words for saccade target selection.

How are temporal and spatial aspects synchronized in the SWIFT model? Here we implemented an inhibition of random saccade timing by the amount of activation of the currently fixated word. This process of *foveal inhibition* modulates fixation durations by processing difficulty. However, it can be shown mathematically and numerically (Richter et al., 2006) that the form of foveal inhibition implemented in the SWIFT model (Engbert et al., 2002, 2005) can add only relatively small amounts of additional fixation time. Thus, stochastic timing with a limited (local) adjustment to the current fixation duration might be a parsimonius account of the systematic and random variability observed in experimental distributions of fixation durations. As a result, the SWIFT model captures the experimental data on fixation durations as indicators of ongoing cognition, while at the same time it is compatible with the partial independence of spatial and temporal pathways of the oculomotor system.

It is important to note that the mechanism of foveal inhibition offers an interesting answer to the question of why additional fixation time during processing of difficult (e.g. low-frequency or

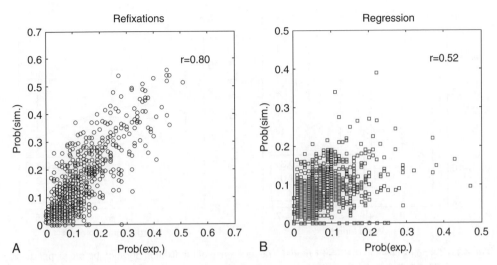

Fig. 43.2 Correlations of observed and simulated fixation probabilities in SWIFT. A) Refixations. B) Regressions.

unpredictable) words is mainly acquired by multiple fixations—and not by prolongation of individual fixation durations. First, foveal inhibition cannot delay a new saccade programme by arbitrarily long time intervals. Second, the activation-field dynamics keep track of the processing of all words, so that refixations emerge from the model's architecture without additional assumptions (Fig. 43.2A). Thus, the SWIFT model solves the problem of refixation by its dynamical principles (Beer, 2000; van Gelder, 1998), while additional assumptions for refixations are needed in state-based models (e.g. Engbert and Kliegl, 2001).

Not only refixations, however, but all types of saccades are explained by target selection from the dynamically evolving field of activation in SWIFT (e.g. regressions in Fig. 43.2B). A high activation of the currently fixated word n at the time of saccade target selection triggers the preparation of a *refixation* saccade to word n (Fig. 43.1B, word 3 at 550 ms), while high activations of the next two words, word $n+1$ and word $n+2$, induce *forward saccades* and *word skipping* (word 4 at 1100 ms) respectively. In the SWIFT model, a *regression* to a word $n-k$ ($k>0$) is the consequence of incomplete processing (word 1 at 700 ms). In general, the relative activations determine the probabilities for target selection. As a consequence of activation-field dynamics, PG models generate scan paths, which are indistinguishable from those produced by human readers. Compatible with experimental findings (Kennedy and Pynte, 2008), model simulations show that violations of the serial order of fixation do not necessarily slow down processing.

After we addressed the basic concepts of PG models, we will now discuss a set of experimentally observed phenomena which lend support to these models.

Word skipping and the need for parallel processing

The principles underlying the theoretical explanation of word skipping in computational models generate an interesting side effect, which can be exploited to construct a qualitative model test. As noted by Kliegl and Engbert (2005), fixation durations before long and/or low-frequency skipped words are on average increased (*skipping costs*) compared to when these words are fixated. Interestingly, however, before short and/or high-frequency words, decreased fixation durations were observed when they are skipped (*skipping benefits*).

In the SWIFT model, inflated fixation durations before skipped words are a cause of word skipping. If there is longer fixation time on word n than on average (i.e. by chance due to random timing), then there will be more parafoveal processing on both words $n+1$ and $n+2$ due to the

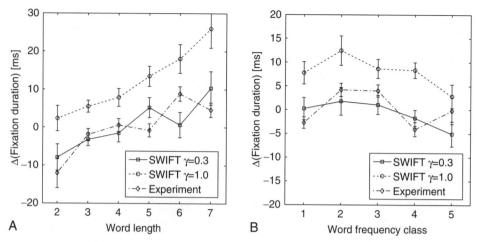

Fig. 43.3 Skipping costs in the SWIFT model. The difference of the fixation duration before skipped words and the fixation duration before fixated words is plotted as function of word length (A) and word frequency (B). A negative difference indicates skipping benefits for short and/or high-frequency words, while there are skipping costs (positive difference) for all other cases. In the SWIFT model, the target selection exponent γ determines the amount of skipping costs and benefits. For $\gamma=1$ (Engbert et al., 2005), we did not observe skipping benefits, while for $\gamma=0.3$, the approximately linear increase from skipping benefits to skipping costs in experimental data is reproduced by the model.

processing gradient. This generates increased activations of these two words (compared to the baseline). Because relative activations determine the probability for target selection, the increased activation of word $n+2$ implies an increase in the probability to select word $n+2$ as the next saccade target, that is, an increase in skipping probability. From this qualitative analysis, we can generate the prediction that there are always skipping costs in the SWIFT model, i.e. fixation durations are longer before skipped words than before fixated words. A numerical analysis (Fig. 43.3) shows that the SWIFT model ($\gamma=1$, see Engbert et al., 2005) produced a skipping cost for all word lengths (and all frequency classes), while experimental data indicated skipping benefits for short and/or high-frequency words. However, the model reproduces the linear increase of skipping costs, which was found in the data. According to the SWIFT model, the interpretation of this effect is that more fixation time is needed to skip a long (or low-frequency word) compared to the skipping of a short (or high-frequency) word. Therefore, the linear increase of skipping costs support the activation-field explanation of word skipping implemented in the SWIFT model.

Target words are selected with probabilities proportional to relative activations (see Eq. (1)). In earlier numerical simulation studies (Engbert et al., 2002, 2005), we fixed the target selection exponent at $\gamma=1$, however, different values for γ might explain the existence of skipping benefits, which we found in experimental data. In Fig. 43.3, we plotted the simulated data of the SWIFT model for a value of $\gamma=0.3$. Such a variation of the exponent γ favours words with low activations to be selected as a saccade target (compared to $\gamma=1$). The new simulations show that the model reproduces the linear increase from skipping benefits to skipping costs. Thus, the pattern of skipping benefits and costs are highly compatible with the dynamic field approach to saccade planning in reading, which is demonstrated by the numerical simulations of the SWIFT model.[2]

---

[2] Changing the value of the target selection exponent from $\gamma=1$ to $\gamma=0.3$, however, also affects skipping probabilities and measures of distributed processing. Therefore, a full solution of the problem of skipping benefits and costs needs to be addressed in a future version of the SWIFT model.

According to the SAS models, however, there is parafoveal processing of word $n+1$ while the saccadic eye movement to word $n+1$ is programmed. If recognition of word $n+1$ terminates earlier than the saccade programme, then the saccade programme is cancelled and restarted to word $n+2$ as a new saccade target (see Engbert and Kliegl, 2003, for a mathematical analysis of word skipping in the E-Z Reader model, where lexical processing stage L_1 triggers saccade programmes). As a consequence there is an inflated fixation duration before word skipping according to the SAS model.

Distributed processing: lag and successor effects

Properties of the fixated word (e.g. word frequency, word length) influence its fixation duration. Attempts to explain statistical properties of eye movements during reading from a cognitive perspective focused on these *immediacy effects*. However, Kliegl et al. (2006) identified five additional principles of the control of fixation duration during reading which represent important challenges to any theoretical model of saccade generation during reading. The first two of these principles are related to the concept of distributed processing.

Successor effects

Fixation duration is modulated by properties of the upcoming word (word $n+1$ during fixation of word n). The perceptual span determines the limits of information processing based on parafoveal information, which influences measures of fixation durations on the currently fixation word. The observation of these parafoveal-on-foveal effects can be interpreted as evidence for parallel processing on multiple words at a time (Kliegl et al., 2006; Kennedy and Pynte, 2005; see also Drieghe, Chapter 46, this volume).

Lag effects

Word recognition continues to have an impact on subsequent fixation durations after gaze position has moved forward to the next word (properties of word $n-1$ influence the fixation duration on word n). This lag effect is highly compatible with the time lines of word recognition obtained from research on event-related potentials (Dambacher and Kliegl, 2007). Based on numerical simulations of the SWIFT model (Engbert et al., 2005) we demonstrated that the lag and successor effects can be explained by the assumption of parallel lexical processing in PG models.

How does distributed processing in the SWIFT model capture lag and successor effects? While several words are processed simultaneously in the SWIFT model, it is not obvious how lag and successor effects are produced, because only properties of the fixated words can *directly* modulate fixation durations by *foveal* inhibition. Two different mechanisms generate the lag effect in SWIFT. First, the lag effect is produced by parafoveal processing of word n during fixation of word $n-1$. If word $n-1$ is a long (or low-frequency) word, then parafoveal preprocessing will be reduced, so that subsequent fixation durations are longer than on average for word n. Second, the time-delay in foveal inhibition can lead to inhibition of the current fixation duration by activation of the previous fixation. We assumed that word processing at time $t-\tau$ (delay of τ) might influence fixation times at a later time t due to the long feedback loops involved in word recognition.

Successor effects are due to the simultaneous activation of several words. Simultaneous activations can produce time-dependent selection effects for saccade targets. Let us consider a fixation on word n with a low- versus high-frequency word $n+1$. Because of parallel processing, activations on both word n and word $n+1$ will be non-zero in general.[3] The selection of the saccade target for the saccade terminating the fixation on word n will be based on the relative activations. If word $n+1$ is a high-frequency

---

[3] For simplicity, we focus on word n and word $n+1$ only.

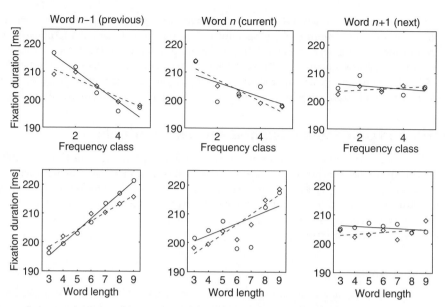

Fig. 43.4 Analysis of lag and successor effects. Bottom row: Average single fixation durations as a function of word length of the previous word (word *n*-1, left column), the current word (word *n*, middle column), and the next word (word *n*+1, right column). Top row: Corresponding plots as a function of word-frequency class. In each panel, we compare the experimental data (with solid line indicating the linear regression) with simulated data (with dashed line as linear fit).

word, then the activation is lower than in the case of a low-frequency word *n*+1, because the maximum activation is related to the word's processing difficulty. As a consequence, a forward saccade from word *n* to word *n*+1 is more likely for a low-frequency word *n*+1 than for a high-frequency word *n*+1, since the relative activation (or probability for target selection) is higher in the low-frequency case. The difference of target selection probabilities in the two conditions, however, is time-dependent. The longer the eye fixates word *n*, the more probable it will move forward to a low-frequency word *n*+1, whereas a refixation of word *n* will become more and more likely for longer fixations, if word *n*+1 is a high-frequency word. However, a refixation of word *n* will move the corresponding fixation duration to the category of first (of multiple) fixations, so that overall single-fixation durations will be shorter for high- than low-frequency words *n*+1. This qualitative explanation is based on the numerical simulations by Engbert et al. (2005), which demonstrated that the SWIFT model produces lag and successor effects compatible with experimental data (Fig. 43.4).

The interpretation that lag and successor effects are due to distributed processing has been criticized (Rayner et al., 2006; but see Kliegl, 2007). Among the most frequently discussed alternative explanations for lag and successor effects are processes related to mislocated fixations (Engbert and Nuthmann, 2008; Nuthmann et al., 2005, 2007). In a mislocated fixation, oculomotor errors induce a fixation on a word different from the selected saccade target (McConkie et al., 1988). In an SAS model, attention moves sequentially from word *n* to the next word *n*+1. A saccadic error with an overshoot to word *n*+2 would result in a mislocated fixation. Because attentional selection is more reliable than saccadic landing positions (Deubel and Schneider, 1996), it is compatible with the SAS assumption that the intended target word (i.e. word *n*+1) is processed during this mislocated fixations, while the eyes fixate a different word (word *n*+2 in the case considered here). As a consequence, the fixation duration observed for a mislocated fixation would be better correlated with properties of the intended word *n*+1 than with the properties of the fixated word *n*+2.

While an explanation of effects of distributed processing as artefacts generated by mislocated fixations seems attractive, it is incompatible with at least two findings on misguided saccades in reading.

First, Nuthmann et al. (2005, 2007; see also Engbert et al., 2005) suggested that mislocated fixations are related to the *inverted optimal viewing position* (IOVP) effect (Vitu et al., 2001), the phenomenon that fixation durations are decreased near word edges. According to this theory, a mislocated fixation triggers a new saccade programme immediately. Such a new saccade programme might be functional to correct a mislocated fixation. Due to the immediate triggering of the saccade programme, the average fixation duration of a mislocated fixation is decreased and, more importantly, it will be unrelated to ongoing processing during the mislocated fixation. Therefore, fixation durations of mislocated fixations should be modulated neither by properties of the current word nor by properties of the intended target word and should not mimic the specific pattern of distributed processing.

Second, the hypothesis that mislocated fixations can mimic distributed processing is incompatible with quantitative estimations of the prevalence of mislocated fixations. Using a self-consistent iterative method to estimate different types of mislocated fixations, Engbert and Nuthmann (2008) showed that there is a general tendency to produce undershoot errors during reading, while overshoot errors are negligible. Because the lag effect is the strongest linear frequency effect we observe in reading of isolated sentences (Kliegl et al., 2006), however, the frequency of overshoot errors is incompatible with the size of the lag effect.

In summary, the SWIFT model demonstrates that processing gradient models can explain the experimental findings on lag and successor effects based on the principle of distributed processing. Moreover, the hypothesis that lag and successor effects are related to parafoveal processing during mislocated fixations is incompatible with the observation that mislocated fixations induce rather short fixation durations not related to word recognition (i.e. the IOVP effect) and that overshoot errors necessary to explain the lag effect are quantitatively negligible.

Regressions: support for activation-based saccade planning

The activation field dynamics naturally generate regressions as a consequence of unfinished processing. If there is some activation of a word $n-k$ (with $k>0$) to the left of the currently fixated word n, then with probability $p>0$ word $n-k$ will be selected as the next saccade target. In the development of the SWIFT model (Engbert et al., 2002), we interpreted the increasing part of the activation as lexical preprocessing, while the decreasing part was interpreted as lexical completion process. According to this hypothesis, regressions are the result of incomplete processing: Whenever the eye moves forward to word n before activation of word $n-k$ was fully removed (i.e. lexical processing was completed), a regression is likely to occur. This mechanism can explain important statistical patterns in experimental data. Most importantly, we observed a high correlation ($r=0.52$, $p<0.01$) between observed and predicted regression probabilities (Fig. 43.2B). A comparison with the same plot for refixation probabilities (Fig. 43.2A) indicates that regressions are more difficult to predict. This observation is compatible with the assumption that regressions are triggered by post-lexical integration failures (e.g. Reichle et al., 2009). Nevertheless, the correlation between experimental and predicted data lends support to the mechanism of incomplete lexical processing for regression in the SWIFT model.

Recently findings on z-string scanning paradigm, however, suggest that regressions represent a very general phenomenon found in various visuomotor tasks (e.g. Trukenbrod and Engbert, 2007). In z-string scanning, all letters of a text are replaced by the letters 'z' and 'Z' (Vitu et al., 1995; Rayner and Fischer, 1996). Interestingly, regressions occur frequently in this task, although word processing is completely absent. This finding suggests that a certain proportion of regressions is unrelated to lexical processing. Additionally, there is theoretical support for this interpretation. Nuthmann and Engbert (2009) investigated SWIFT modelling for z-string scanning. Generally, the model was able to reproduce the statistical pattern of eye movements. For example, the model could reproduce the effects of string length on fixation duration. Furthermore, the SWIFT model reproduced the pattern of regressions in z-string scanning accurately. From these findings, we developed the hypothesis that some regressions were caused by the activation-field dynamics per se. After the build-up of the activation field necessary to form a dynamic saliency map for target selection, the decrease of activation might be an active (inhibitory or removal) and time-consuming process, that is, activation cannot simply be switched off. In reading, the removal process might occur simultaneously with post-lexical processing, so that post-lexical integration failures could modulate the decrease of activations. Such an interpretation is compatible with the observation of regressions across a wide range of visuomotor tasks.

Lines of research triggered by processing gradient models

Reading, one of the most complex processes the human brain is capable of, involves the coordinated timing of many psychologically distinguishable subprocesses, of which the two most basic ones are word recognition and oculomotor control. Much of the impact of the current generation of computational models of eye movement control is related to their success in recovering benchmark results relating to various eye movement measures as functions of length and frequency of words. In this final section, we sketch three lines of research along which PG models are currently generalized: 1) multivariate analyses of eye movement corpora, 2) perceptual span, and 3) attentional span.

Multivariate analyses

In the previous sections we illustrated how one PG model, SWIFT, copes with new lag and successor word-frequency effects reliably established in corpora of reading eye movements. Our expectation is that this line of research will lead to new challenges for computational models and help expose many of their theoretical infelicities. We have barely started to model any of the influences of well over 50 word properties with reliable influences on processing time in word recognition research (e.g. familiarity, lemma frequency, cumulative frequency of words starting with the same two letters, neighbourhood size). In addition, as illustrated for lag and successor word frequency in this chapter, the influence of these properties may also depend on whether they are associated with the fixated word n, the left word $n-1$, or the right word $n+1$. Actually, in ongoing research some of these effects span the words from $n-2$ to $n+2$ (Heister et al., 2011). In the end, to the degree that a computational model adequately captures the varying processing difficulties associated with them, all these effects should 'fall out' from the implementation of the theoretical principles.

Perceptual span

The corpus-analytic research, handicapped by substantial correlations between the variables carrying processing-relevant information, stands in a productive tension with eye movement research focusing on effects of one to three target words per sentence (see exchange by Kliegl, 2007, and Rayner et al., 2007). Indeed, some of the fundamental constraints guiding the design of computational models of eye movement control were established in such experiments, most notably with the moving-window paradigm (McConkie and Rayner, 1975) and the boundary paradigm (Rayner, 1975) that in one way or another change the display contingent on a subject's direction of gaze. Currently such experiments are often designed with the explicit purpose to decide between SAS and PG models. Therefore, we describe two controversial lines of research and discuss their implications for computational models of eye movement control.

The moving-window paradigm led to what is known now as the perceptual span during reading that is the rather narrow area from which information can be extracted during a fixation (i.e. about 3 letters to the left and 13–15 letters to the right of the point of fixation for alphabetic languages with left to right reading direction). The boundary paradigm has taught us much about what type information from word $n+1$ (visual, lexical, orthographic, phonological, semantic, etc.) becomes available during a fixation on word n. If visual or orthographic information of word $n+1$ was available during fixation on word n, shorter fixation durations result on the subsequent fixation on word $n+1$.

Such a preview benefit had not been obtained for semantic previews (e.g. synonyms) during fixations in alphabetic writing systems (Rayner et al., 2003; see also Drieghe, Chapter 46, this volume). Indeed, Rayner et al. (2003) concluded from their review that 'the basis for the robust parafoveal preview benefit obtained in numerous studies is not any type of semantic code', noting also that such effects would be problematic for serial attention shift models. Recently, however, such results have been reported for reading Chinese (e.g. Yan et al., 2009) and also German (e.g. Hohenstein et al., 2010). The generalizability of these effects still needs to be determined.

The second controversial question is whether we obtain useful linguistic information from the word beyond the next parafoveal word ($n+2$). Again, in principle, but not always, this should be the case according to PG models but not SAS models. Consistent with SAS conception, preview of word $n+2$ during word n viewing did not convey any benefit when the word was subsequently fixated (e.g. Angele et al., 2008; Rayner et al., 2007b). This null effect is not uncontested, however, as subtle $n+2$ effects are reported when word $n+1$ is a short word (e.g. Kliegl et al., 2007; Risse and Kliegl, in press).

As already indicated above, much of this research was inspired by the desire to provide critical experiments to decide between SAS and PG models. There is, however, a major problem with parafoveal effect sizes. With the exception of the largest preview benefit which is around 30 ms (i.e. the lengthening of fixation duration on a word if the word had been completely denied any preview during the fixation on the previous word), the PG models we are aware of may not reliably reproduce effects of this size even if they were found in experimental settings. Nevertheless, these controversies are very productive because they test the limits of what should be possible in principle. Indeed, some of the experimental results have been quite influential on how we conceptualize processing efficiency around the point of fixation.

Attentional span

The asymmetry of the perceptual span is parameterized in the SWIFT model as two Gaussian functions with different standard deviations for the left and right visual fields (see Fig. 43.1, Engbert et al., 2005). Although we did not elaborate on this aspect, we take the agreement of parameter estimates with expectations about the size of the perceptual span as further evidence for the model validity. The ordinate of this asymmetric Gaussian curve represents processing rate and, because of its asymmetry, may be better referred to as an attentional span (Henderson and Ferreira, 1990; Rayner and Pollatsek, 1987). There has always been the option of having the size of the attentional span be modulated by foveal processing difficulty (Henderson and Ferreira, 1990; Inhoff and Rayner, 1986). Engbert (2007) presented such an implementation with two distinctive features for a variant of the SWIFT model. First, the area under the curve was kept constant. Second, the curve was symmetric for maximum focusing (see Fig. 43.5A). Therefore, given maximum foveal load, a reduction of right parafoveal processing rate was traded off against an increase of foveal processing rate.

Links to earlier research in visual spatial attention

Graded attention has been a central concept in visual spatial attention for the last 30 years. Indeed, the hypothetical symmetric attentional span under maximum foveal load is similar to a number of classical conceptualizations. Figure 43.5B–E illustrate four of them (cited after Tsotsos, 2005, who calls them optical metaphors). The classic spotlight metaphor assumed that attention is moved through space with equal resolution within its beam (Fig. 43.5B) (e.g. Shulman et al., 1979). This notion was replaced or augmented by a zoom lens model allowing for a variable size of the spotlight with higher processing efficiency for narrow settings (Fig. 43.5C) (Eriksen and St James, 1986). The notion of attentional gradient was introduced by LaBerge and Brown (1989) (Fig. 43.5D). The first computational approach dates to the inhibitory beam model by Tsotsos (1990) (Fig. 43.5E). The relation between these classical models of spatial attention and PG attention models of reading needs to be explored in future research.

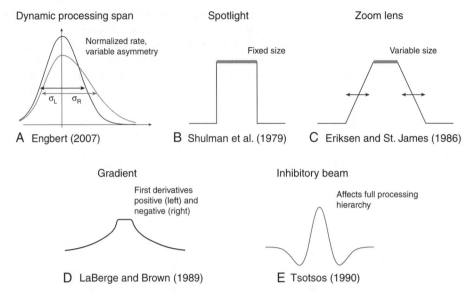

Fig. 43.5 Concepts of spatial selective attention. A) Dynamical processing spans for normal and maximum foveal load during reading (Engbert, 2007) and four optical metaphors of spatial attention (Tsotsos, 2005): B) spotlight (Shulman et al., 1979), C) zoom lens (Eriksen and St James, 1986), D) gradient (LaBerge and Brown, 1989), and E) inhibitory beam (Tsotsos, 1990). With kind permission from Springer Science+Business Media: *Attention, Perception, & Psychophysics*, Visual attention within and around the field of focal attention: A zoom lens model, **40**(4), 1986, 225-240, Charles W. Eriksen.

Conclusion

In this chapter we argue that oculomotor programming and lexical processing during reading can be conceptualized within the framework of a parallel graded attention model. We present in some detail how one of these models, SWIFT, generates a complex profile of relations to frequencies of three neighbouring words and associated skipping probabilities. In our view, SWIFT provides an excellent account for a large variety of effects relating to distributed processing in the perceptual or attentional span. There certainly are many empirical regularities of reading beyond SWIFT's current horizon, but we see no principled reason that the lines of evidence reviewed in the discussion cannot be assimilated within its general framework.

Acknowledgements

We would like to thank Denis Drieghe and Simon Liversedge for valuable comments on the manuscripts. This work was supported by Deutsche Forschungsgemeinschaft (FOR 868, project A1).

References

Angele, B., Slattery, T., Yang, J., Kliegl, R., and Rayner, K. (2008). Parafoveal processing in reading: Manipulating n+1 and n+2 previews simultaneously. *Visual Cognition*, 16, 697–707.

Beer, R.D. (2000). Dynamical approaches to cognitive science. *Trends in Cognitive Sciences*, 4, 91–99.

Busemeyer, J.R. and Townsend, J.T. (1993). Decision field theory: a dynamic–cognitive approach to decision making in an uncertain environment. *Psychological Review*, 100, 432–459.

Dambacher, M. and Kliegl, R. (2007). Synchronizing timelines: Relations between fixation durations and N400 amplitudes during sentence reading. *Brain Research*, 1155, 147–162.

Deubel, H. and Schneider, W.X. (1996). Saccade target selection and object recognition: Evidence for a common attentional mechanism. *Vision Research*, **36**, 1827–1837.

Engbert, R. (2007). *Reading with a dynamic processing span.* Presentation at 14th ECEM, Potsdam, Germany.

Engbert, R. and Kliegl, R. (2003). The game of word skipping: Who are the competitors? *Behavioral and Brain Sciences*, **26**, 481–482.

Engbert, R. and Nuthmann, A. (2008). Self-consistent estimation of mislocated fixations during reading. *PLoS ONE*, **3**, e1534: 1–6.

Engbert, R. and Kliegl, R. (2001). Mathematical models of eye movements in reading: A possible role for autonomous saccades. *Biological Cybernetics*, **85**, 77–87.

Engbert, R., Longtin, A. and Kliegl, R. (2002). A dynamical model of saccade generation in reading based on spatially distributed lexical processing. *Vision Research*, **42**, 621–636.

Engbert, R., Kliegl, R., and Longtin, A. (2004). Complexity of eye movements in reading. *International Journal of Bifurcation and Chaos*, **14**, 493–503.

Engbert, R., Nuthmann, A., Richter, E.M., and Kliegl, R. (2005). SWIFT: A dynamical model of saccade generation during reading. *Psychological Review*, **112**, 777–813.

Eriksen, C.W. and St James, J.D. (1986). Visual attention within and around the field of focal attention: A zoom lens model. *Perception & Psychophysics*, **40**, 225–240.

Erlhagen, W. and Schöner, G. (2002). Dynamic field theory of movements preparation. *Psychological Review*, **109**, 545–572.

Findlay, J.M. and Walker, R. (1999). A model of saccade generation based on parallel processing and competitive inhibition. *Behavioral and Brain Sciences*, **22**, 661–721.

Heister, J., Würzner, K.-M., Bubenzer, J., Pohl, E., Hanneforth, T., Geyken, A., *et al.* (2011). dlex—eine lexikalische Datenbank für die psychologische und linguistische Forschung *Psychologische Rundschau*, **61**, 10–20.

Henderson, J.M. and Ferreira, F. (1990). Effects of foveal processing difficulty on the perceptual span in reading: Implications for attention and eye movement control. *Journal of Experimental Psychology: Learning, Memory, and Cognition*, **16**, 417–429.

Hohenstein, S., Laubrock, J., and Kliegl, R. (2010). Semantic preview benefit in eye movements during reading: A parafoveal fast-priming study. *Journal of Experimental Psychology: Learning, Memory, and Cognition*, **36**, 1150–1170.

Inhoff, A.W. and Rayner, K. (1986). Parafoveal processing during eye fixations in reading: Effects of word frequency. *Perception and Psychophysics*, **40**, 431–439.

Kennedy, A. and Pynte, J. (2005). Parafoveal-on-foveal effects in normal reading. *Vision Research*, **45**, 153–168.

Kennedy, A. and Pynte, J. (2008). The consequences of violations to reading order: An eye movement analysis. *Vision Research*, **48**, 2309–2320.

Kliegl, R. (2007). Toward a perceptual-span theory of distributed processing in reading: A reply to Rayner, Pollatsek, Drieghe, Slattery, and Reichle (2007). *Journal of Experimental Psychology: General*, **136**, 530–537.

Kliegl, R. and Engbert, R. (2005). Fixation durations before word skippings in reading eye movements. *Psychonomic Bulletin and Review*, **12**, 132–138.

Kliegl, R., Nuthmann, A. and Engbert, R. (2006). Tracking the mind during reading: The influence of past, present, and future words on fixation durations. *Journal of Experimental Psychology: General*, **135**, 12–35.

Kliegl, R., Risse, S., and Laubrock, J. (2007). Preview benefit and parafoveal-on-foveal effects from word N+2. *Journal of Experimental Psychology: Human Perception and Performance*, **33**, 1250–1255.

LaBerge, D. and Brown, V. (1989). Theory of attentional operations in shape identification. *Psychological Review*, **96**, 101–124.

Luce, R.D. (1959). *Individual choice behavior: A theoretical analysis.* New York: Wiley.

McConkie. G.W., and Rayner, K. (1975). The span of the effective stimulus during a fixation in reading. *Perception and Psychophysics*, **17**, 578–586.

McConkie, G.W., Kerr, P.W., Reddix, M.D., and Zola, D. (1988). Eye movement control during reading: I. The location of initial fixations on words. *Vision Research*, **28**, 1107–1118.

Nuthmann, A. and Engbert, R. (2009). Mindless reading revisited: An analysis based on the SWIFT model of eye-movement control. *Vision Research*, **49**, 322–336.

Nuthmann, A., Engbert, R., and Kliegl, R. (2007). The IOVP effect in mindless reading: Experiment and modeling. *Vision Research*, **47**, 990–1002.

Nuthmann, A., Engbert, R., and Kliegl, R. (2005). Mislocated fixations during reading and the inverted optimal viewing position effect. *Vision Research*, **45**, 2201–2217.

Rayner, K. (1975). The perceptual span and peripheral cues during reading. *Cognitive Psychology*, **7**, 65–81.

Rayner, K. (2009). Eye movements and attention in reading, scene perception, and visual search. *Quarterly Journal of Experimental Psychology*, **62**, 1457–1506.

Rayner, K. and Fischer, M.H. (1996). Mindless reading revisited: Eye movements during reading and scanning are different. *Perception and Psychophysics*, **58**, 734–747.

Rayner, K. and Pollatsek, A. (1987). Eye movements in reading: A tutorial review. In M. Coltheart (ed.) *Attention and Performance 12*. New York: Academic Press.

Rayner, K., Juhasz, B.J., and Brown, S.J. (2007b). Do readers obtain preview benefit from word n+2? A test of serial attention shift versus distributed lexical processing models of eye movement control in reading. *Journal of Experimental Psychology: Human Perception and Performance*, **33**, 230–245.

Rayner, K., White, S.J., Kambe, G., Miller, B., and Liversedge, S.P. (2003). On the processing of meaning from parafoveal vision during eye fixation in reading. In J. Hyönä, R. Radach, and H. Deubel (eds.) *The mind's eye: Cognitive and applied aspects of eye movements* (pp. 213–234). Amsterdam: Elsevier Science.

Rayner, K., Pollatsek, A., Drieghe, D., Slattery, T.J., Reichle, E.D. (2006). Tracking the mind during reading via eye movements: Comments on Kliegl, Nuthmann, and Engbert (2006). *Journal of Experimental Psychology: General*, **136**, 520–529.

Rayner, K., Li, X., Williams, C.C., Cave, K.R., and Well, A.D. (2007a). Eye movements during information processing tasks: Individual differences and cultural effects. *Vision Research*, **47**, 2714–2726.

Reichle, E.D., Rayner, K., and Pollatsek, A. (2003). The E-Z Reader model of eye movement control in reading: Comparisons to other models. *Behavioral and Brain Sciences*, **26**, 446–526.

Reichle, E.D., Warren, T., and McConnel, K. (2009b). Using E-Z Reader to model the effects of higher level language processing on eye movements during reading. *Psychonomic Bulletin and Review*, **16**, 1–21.

Reichle, E.D., Pollatsek, A., Fisher, D.L., and Rayner, K. (1998). Toward a model of eye movement control in reading. *Psychological Review*, **105**, 125–157.

Reichle, E.D., Liversedge, S.P., Rayner, K., and Pollatsek, A. (2009a). Encoding multiple words simultaneously in reading is implausible. *Trends in Cognitive Sciences*, **13**, 115–119.

Reilly, R. and Radach, R. (2003). Glenmore: An interactive activation model of eye movement control in reading. In J. Hyönä, R. Radach, and H. Deubel (eds.) *The mind's eye: Cognition and applied aspects of eye movement research* (pp. 429–456). Oxford, England: Elsevier.

Reilly, R. and Radach, R. (2006). Some empirical tests of an interactive activation model of eye movement control in reading. *Cognitive Systems Research*, **7**, 34–55.

Richter, E.M., Engbert, R. and Kliegl, R. (2006). Current advances in SWIFT. *Cognitive Systems Research*, **7**, 23–33.

Risse, S. and Kliegl, R. (in press). Investigating age differences in the perceptual span with the N+2-boundary paradigm. *Psychology and Aging*.

Shulman, G., Remington, R., and McLean, J. (1979). Moving attention through visual space. *Journal of Experimental Psychology*, **92**, 428–431.

Townsend, J.T. (1990). Serial vs. parallel processing: Sometimes they look like tweedledum and tweedledee but they can (and should) be distinguished. *Psychological Science*, **1**, 46–54.

Tsotsos, J.K. (1990). A complexity level analysis of vision. *Behavioral and Brain Sciences*, **13**, 423–445.

Tsotsos, J.K. (2005). A brief and selective history of attention. In L. Itti, G. Rees, and J.K. Tsotsos (eds.) *Neurobiology of attention*. Amsterdam: Elsevier Press.

Trukenbrod, H.A. and Engbert, R. (2007). Oculomotor control in a sequential search task. *Vision Research*, **47**, 2426–2443.

van Gelder, T. (1998). The dynamical hypothesis in cognitive science. *Behavioral and Brain Sciences*, **21**, 615–628.

Vitu, F., O'Regan, J.K., Inhoff, A.W., and Topolski, R. (1995). Mindless reading: Eye movement characteristics are similar in scanning letter strings and reading texts. *Perception and Psychophysics*, **57**, 352–364.

Vitu, F., McConkie, G.W., Kerr, P., and O'Regan, J.K. (2001). Fixation location effects on fixation durations during reading: An inverted optimal viewing position effect. *Vision Research*, **41**, 3513–3533.

Yan, M., Richter, E.M., Shu, H., and Kliegl, R. (2009). Chinese readers extract semantic information from parafoveal words during reading. *Psychonomic Bulletin and Review*, **16**, 561–566.

CHAPTER 44

Binocular coordination during reading

Julie A. Kirkby, Sarah J. White, and Hazel I. Blythe

Abstract

The chapter reviews a range of evidence that suggests that the fixation positions of the two eyes are not perfectly coordinated during reading, such that fixation disparity is frequently observed. The chapter focuses on three critical issues. First, evidence is reviewed for whether the visual or linguistic characteristics of text can influence binocular coordination. Second, a possible link between developmental factors and binocular coordination is discussed (that is, whether children show different patterns of binocular coordination compared to adults). Third, evidence for and against the possibility that dyslexia might be associated with differences in binocular coordination is assessed. On the basis of the existing evidence we conclude that: fixation disparity is, at most, minimally affected by linguistic processing demands; that binocular coordination develops with age such that by the age of 12 children display patterns of binocular coordination equivalent to that of adults; and that the issue of a possible link between binocular coordination and dyslexia demands much further research. The conclusions also highlight the implications of these findings for our understanding of word processing mechanisms, eye movement control during reading, and research with dyslexic readers.

Binocular vision extends our visual field and allows us to perceive and interact with our environment with greater precision than monocular vision would permit (Jones and Lee, 1981). In reading, saccadic eye movements serve to bring new portions of the text onto the high-acuity region of the retina, the fovea, allowing successful lexical identification of words within the sentence (Liversedge and Findlay, 2000). Critically, reading is a unique visual task, which requires accurate encoding and complex processing of relatively small-sized visual stimuli (letters within words). Consequently, it might plausibly be assumed that, in order for reading to progress undisturbed, two precisely coupled retinal inputs must be necessary for visual encoding and lexical identification. Indeed, much research has been undertaken recording the position of just one of the eyes, on the implicit assumption that the position of one eye accurately represents the positions of both eyes. Throughout this chapter, however, we will review a range of evidence suggesting that the assumption of precise binocular coordination during reading is not, in fact, always correct and demonstrates that fixation disparity is frequently observed during reading.

The aim of this chapter is to provide a concise review of the influential and topical research in the area of binocular coordination during reading in order to address three critical questions: 1) do visual or linguistic characteristics of text influence binocular coordination?; 2) Do developmental factors influence binocular coordination? (see also Luna and Velanova, Chapter 35, this volume); (3) Is there a link between binocular coordination and dyslexia? We begin with a brief review of the literature describing the basic characteristics of binocular coordination during reading and the fusion of disparate retinal inputs during reading. For a broader review of binocular coordination during both reading and non-reading tasks, see Kirkby et al. (2008). Note that work in this area has, so far, largely focused on empirical studies and the content of the chapter reflects this. Nevertheless, the chapter will conclude by summarising some recent theoretical work, as well as noting the implications of fixation disparity for studies of eye movement control during reading in general.

Basic characteristics of binocular coordination during reading

Both the distance from and the direction of target locations must be accounted for in accurate saccade programming and, hence, in accurate binocular coordination. Three different types of eye movement have been studied in order to characterize the accuracy and binocular coordination of saccades: 1) pure version (also referred to as conjugate movements, a change in direction while maintaining a constant angle of sight between the two eyes); 2) pure vergence movements (a change in depth only, where the angle of sight between the two eyes changes but there is no directional change in the point of fixation); 3) combined eye movements (also referred to as disjunctive movements, movements with both version and vergence components, such that the point of fixation changes in both depth and direction).

Until recently, the majority of research examining binocular coordination had focused upon analyses of the two eyes' saccades. Among the handful of early studies examining binocular coordination during reading, researchers found that there was frequently disparity between saccades of the two eyes. There was, however, some disagreement regarding the source of binocular disparity. The results of Smith et al. (1971) indicated that subtle temporal differences in the timing of the two eyes' saccadic onsets were observed during reading, leading to disparity during saccades. Williams and Fender (1977) questioned these findings and measured the characteristics of binocular coordination when the eyes were saccading between LEDs rather than during reading. Williams and Fender demonstrated that differences in the two eyes' saccadic velocity occurred frequently; however, in contrast to the results of Smith et al., they did not find differences in the timing of the two eyes' saccadic onsets. Further research has established that there are differences between the abducting eye (the eye moving temporally) and the adducting eye (the eye moving nasally) with respect to the timing of saccade onset, peak saccadic velocity, saccade duration, skewness (the relative durations of the eyes' acceleration and deceleration periods during a saccade), and amplitude (Collewijn et al., 1988). As a consequence of the asymmetry of the abducting and adducting eyes' saccadic parameters, the two eyes typically become diverged during a saccade.

With respect to reading, however, it is important to consider binocular coordination during fixations, as it is while the eyes are relatively still that linguistic information is primarily encoded and subsequently processed (Liversedge and Findlay, 2000; but see Yatabe et al., 2009). In recent years there has been an upsurge of interest in binocular coordination during reading, resulting in a number of important empirical findings. Most notably, frequent disparity between the two eyes' points of fixation during reading has now been demonstrated to occur in both sentence reading studies (e.g. Blythe et al., 2006; Heller and Radach, 1999; Hendriks, 1996; Juhasz et al., 2006; Kliegl et al., 2006; Liversedge et al., 2006a) and in single word reading studies (Paterson et al., 2009; Bucci and Kapoula, 2006).

The article published by Liversedge et al. (2006a) provided one of the first demonstrations of the extent to which binocular disparity is found in skilled readers. They described both the magnitude and the direction of fixation disparity that occurred during a single line sentence reading experiment, with the magnitude of disparity measured as the absolute difference between the fixation positions of the two eyes at both fixation onset and offset. On average, fixation disparity at fixation offset was found to be 1.1 character spaces. For nearly half of all fixations the two eyes were more than one character space apart in either direction (categorized as non-aligned). For these non-aligned fixations, the magnitude of the fixation disparity was, on average, 1.9 character spaces. The direction of

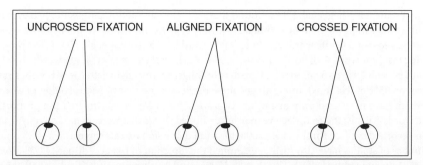

Fig. 44.1 Categories of fixation disparity: *Uncrossed*, fixation disparity greater than one character with the left eye to the left of the right eye; *Aligned*, fixation disparity less than one character; *Crossed*, fixation disparity greater than one character with the left eye to the right of the right eye.

non-aligned fixation disparity was classified as either crossed (where the left eye was fixated further to the right than the right eye), which accounted for 8% of all fixations, or uncrossed (where the right eye was fixated further to the right than the left eye), which accounted for 39% of fixations. The nature of uncrossed, aligned, and crossed fixations is illustrated in Fig. 44.1.

As noted above, Liversedge et al. (2006a) reported fixation disparity at both fixation onset and offset, enabling some estimate of the slow vergence movements (non-parallel movements of the two eyes) that occurred during fixations. Overall, the proportion of aligned fixations was greater at the end of fixations (53%) compared to the beginning of fixations (48%), which resulted from vergence movements during fixations. Liversedge, White et al. demonstrated that fixation vergence movements were more often convergent than divergent (i.e. moving the points of fixation closer together, thus being in a corrective direction for the uncrossed disparity that was prevalent during the majority of disparate fixations). Overall, their results were consistent with the data reported by Collewijn et al. (1988). Recall that in Collewijn's study the two eyes were shown to diverge during saccades, due to binocular asymmetries in saccadic onset timing, peak velocity, amplitude, duration, and skewness. Thus, the fact that the data from Collewijn's study showed a divergence between the two eyes during saccades complements Liversedge, et al.'s (2006a) finding that the two eyes are frequently uncrossed at the start of fixations. Interestingly, despite the observed corrective vergence movements during fixations, Liversedge, White et al. showed that at the end of 47% of fixations the two eyes remained unaligned, of which 39% were uncrossed, with an overall average disparity of 1.1 characters.

To summarize, the results reported by Liversedge et al. (2006a) revealed that: 1) fixation disparity frequently occurs during reading; 2) fixation disparity is regularly more than one character space; 3) fixation disparity is more often uncrossed than crossed; 4) vergence movements reduce disparity between the two eyes during fixations; 5) despite these vergence movements, at fixation offset some degree of disparity is still evident. While the data from both reading (Liversedge et al., 2006a) and non-reading studies (Collewijn et al., 1988) are complementary in describing the divergence that occurs during saccades, and the resulting disparity followed by slow convergence during fixations, the presence of fixation disparity during reading raised two critical issues that were investigated further in other studies. First, the observation of large fixation disparities during reading led researchers to consider whether the two eyes might, occasionally, be fixating different words in the sentence. Second, additional studies examined whether the predominant tendency is for unaligned fixations to be crossed or uncrossed in skilled adult readers. We will discuss each of these issues in turn.

The disparities observed during the majority of fixations in reading are not substantial (as noted above, on average, approximately one character space). On some occasions, however, the disparity is much greater than the average; for example, for the non-aligned fixations in the Liversedge, et al. (2006a) study, the average disparity was 1.9 characters. Consequently, particularly for cases in which fixation disparity is larger than normal, disparities may result in the two eyes fixating on adjacent words in a sentence. Kliegl et al. (2006) found that in 23% of all valid[1] fixations the two eyes fixated different words within the sentence. Similarly, Kirkby et al. examined the frequency with which the two eyes fixated two separate words as a function of word length (Kirkby et al., 2008). The probability of fixating the same word with both eyes was smaller for shorter words (four-letter words were fixated with both eyes on 79% of fixations) and greater for longer words (eight-letter words were fixated by both eyes on 95% of fixations). Interestingly, these results suggest that previous studies of word skipping, which have measured only one of the two eyes, may have over-estimated the proportion of skipped words. That is, the recorded eye may have skipped words that were, in fact, directly fixated by the non-recorded eye (see Kirkby et al., 2008, for a full discussion on this subject).

A number of studies have also further examined the direction of fixation disparity (i.e. crossed or uncrossed) during reading. Both Kliegl et al. (2006) and Nuthmann and Kliegl (2009) found the direction of binocular disparity to be predominantly crossed, whereas other studies have found it to be predominantly uncrossed for skilled adult readers (Blythe et al., 2006; Juhasz et al., 2006; Liversedge et al., 2006a). The differences in overall fixation alignment across different studies might be accounted for by differences in the physical experimental set-ups. Kliegl et al.'s and Nuthmann and Kliegl's data were recorded using an EyeLink eye tracker (SR Research Ltd), while the data reported by Blythe et al., Juhasz et al., and Liversedge et al. (2006a) were recorded using Dual Purkinje Image (DPI) eye trackers (Fourward Technologies). These eye tracking systems tend to be used in physical set-ups which differ in, for example, viewing distance, background lighting, and stimulus luminance (Kirkby et al., 2008; Nuthman and Kliegl, 2009, Shillcock et al., 2010).

Further research is needed in order to address which factors impact on the direction of binocular disparity, as no studies have directly examined this and suggestions for contributing factors are based on informal comparisons between papers. Recently, however, Shillcock and colleagues (2010) have developed a theory and computational model of binocular foveation in reading, in which it is argued that binocular disparity is a functional, adaptive response to the relative processing difficulty associated with reading under a range of viewing conditions (rather than being a simple, reflexive response to the visual environment). Shillock et al.'s model is discussed further at the end of this chapter, but critically they argue that uncrossed fixation disparities facilitate binocular fusion more than crossed fixation disparities and, hence, should occur more often under viewing conditions that make fusion difficult. Accordingly, in a review of the eye movement literature, they suggest that the different viewing conditions employed in each study are the reason why a predominance of either crossed or uncrossed fixations was observed. Clearly, further research is needed in order to experimentally determine which factors relating to the physical set-up might influence binocular coordination during reading.

The fusion of disparate retinal inputs and neural control of binocular saccades

Given the established finding of disparity during fixations in reading, several recent studies have examined how disparate retinal inputs might be processed during reading and how information from the two eyes impacts on programming of saccades. Importantly, despite the disparity that occurs during saccades and persists into fixations, readers experience a unified percept. That is, the two eyes frequently fixate different letters within a word, and so the letters of the word fall on slightly different locations on each of the two retinae. The reader is, however, able to fuse the two disparate retinal inputs, resulting in a single percept (as opposed to diplopia—double vision). There are limits to the magnitude of disparity that can be successfully fused, and the range of fuseable disparities (Panum's area) has been widely studied for simple stimuli such as lines and dots presented in an

---

[1] A fixation was considered valid if the duration was between 80 and 1200 ms and further, if the disparity between the points of fixation was within two standard deviations of the mean for that individual.

impoverished visual environment (e.g. Ogle, 1952; Fender and Julesz, 1967) (note that the visual characteristics of stimuli also affect the fusional range (Fender and Julesz, 1967)).

A recent study by Blythe et al. (2010) investigated the range of disparities that could be successfully fused for word stimuli in 7- to 11-year-old children compared to adults. Participants' binocular eye movements were recorded as they made lexical decisions for stereoscopically presented words (in a stereoscopic presentation, the same image is presented independently to each eye; see Fig. 44.2). In this experiment, the entire word/non-word was presented to both eyes, but on some trials a horizontal

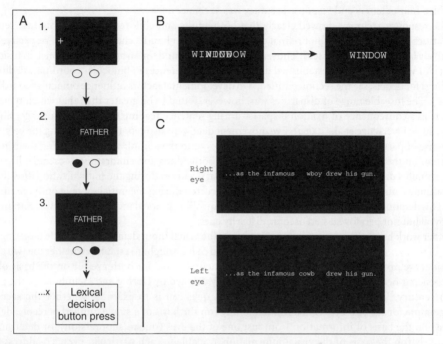

Fig. 44.2 Examples of the stereoscopic presentation used by Blythe et al. (2010), and the dichoptic presentation used by Liversedge et al. (2006b). Panel (A) shows the sequence of events during a trial in the experiment reported by Blythe et al. (2010). The black and white circles under each of the three displays represent the shutter glasses in front of each of the participant's eyes being either open (white) or closed (black), thus allowing stimuli to be presented independently to each eye. A fixation cross appeared on the left side of the screen for 1 s, before disappearing. When the cross disappeared, the target word was presented stereoscopically in the centre of the screen. This example shows a stimulus being presented with 2 character spaces of uncrossed disparity—the word presented to the right eye is 2 character spaces further to the right on the screen than the word presented to the left eye. The two images alternated on the screen every 8 ms, in synchrony with the opening and closing of the shutter glasses. This continued until the participant pressed a button to make their lexical decision. Panel (B) shows the typical perceptual experience for a participant in the experiment reported by Blythe et al. (2010). Again, this represents a trial where the stimulus was presented with 2 character spaces of stereoscopic disparity. The stimulus initially appeared as a jumbled blur of letters, and only when fused could the participant reliably decide whether or not the letter string was a correct word. Panel (C) shows an example of the dichoptic stimulus presentation used in the experiment reported by Liversedge et al. (2006b). Shutter glasses were used to present a different image uniquely to each eye. Here, the positions of these two images on the screen were the same—there was no stereoscopic disparity. This example shows a congruent display, where the initial portion of the target word was presented to the left eye and the end portion of the word was presented to the right eye.

offset (stereoscopic disparity) was manipulated between the two eyes' stimuli. The stereoscopic stimuli were, therefore, either presented aligned (thus appearing normally), or with a manipulated disparity of one or two character spaces in either a crossed or uncrossed direction. In addition to this stereoscopic manipulation, following data collection, the recorded fixation disparity for each participant was also taken into account on a fixation by fixation basis. This provided a measure of the total retinal disparity (summed stereoscopic disparity and fixation disparity) experienced during each fixation as participants looked at the letter strings and made a lexical decision. Accurate lexical decisions were only possible if the stimuli were successfully fused (otherwise, the stimuli appeared as a jumbled blur of letters and response accuracy was at chance).

The response accuracy showed clearly that both adults and children could reliably fuse retinal disparities of up to 0.37°, but not retinal disparities of 0.74° (1 and 2 character spaces, respectively; a relatively large font size was used). Thus, no evidence was found for an age-related change in fusional limits for words, despite the established developmental differences in binocular coordination during reading (for details, see the section entitled, 'Do developmental factors influence binocular coordination?'). The fuseable range of disparities was, however, found to be greater than that which typically occurs as a consequence of fixation disparity during sentence reading (0.2–0.3° on average; Blythe et al., 2006; Liversedge et al., 2006a). Eye movement data were also reported, comparing the vergence response of participants during their initial saccades onto the stimuli with that during their initial fixations on the stimuli. The data showed that, for both adults and children, stereoscopic disparity (e.g. stimulus disparity) determined the vergence that occurred during the initial fixation directly on the stimulus, but did not affect the vergence that occurred during the initial saccade onto the stimulus. This demonstrated that the vergence system, controlling binocular coordination, was responsive to foveal but not parafoveal stereoscopic disparity cues.

Other work has more specifically examined how the visual input determines saccade targeting for each of the eyes (Liversedge et al., 2006b). Such research has sought to establish whether the two eyes' saccades are programmed on the basis of a single neural signal for both eyes or on the basis of an independent neural signal for each eye, as originally debated by Hering and Helmholtz in the early 19th century. One way in which to address this question is to examine whether the saccade programme for the two eyes is determined jointly (on the basis of a single, unified percept), determined on the basis of information from just one of the eyes (due to suppression), or determined separately (on the basis of the visual information available to each particular eye). To address this issue, Liversedge et al. (2006b) presented participants with sentences containing a compound target word, such as 'cowboy', which were presented dichoptically (in a dichoptic presentation, a different image is presented uniquely to each eye, see Fig. 44.2). The first half of the word, 'cowb', was presented to one eye and the second half of the word, 'wboy', was presented to the other eye. The rationale was that if saccades were programmed to a single, unified percept based on the two fused retinal inputs, then the distribution of landing positions on the target word would be unaffected by the dichoptic manipulation. Alternatively, if saccades were programmed independently for each eye on the basis of their own perceptual input, then each eye should have been directed to the word portion that was presented independently to that eye.

In line with previous research, the mean initial landing positions on the critical words in Liversedge et al.'s (2006b) study were at, or just left of, the word centre, at the preferred viewing position (Rayner, 1979). Note that although most fixations land at the preferred viewing position, saccades tend to undershoot this location when launched from distant launch sites, and tend to overshoot when launched from near launch sites (known as the range effect) (McConkie et al. 1988). In line with previous research showing disparate fixations, and predominantly more uncrossed than crossed non-aligned fixations (Blythe et al., 2006; Juhasz et al., 2006; Liversedge et al., 2006a), mean fixation positions on the critical word in Liversedge et al.'s study (2006b) were disparate such that the fixation positions for the left eye were significantly to the left of those for the right eye. Crucially, though, Liversedge et al. (2006b) found no effect of dichoptic viewing condition on initial landing positions on the critical word. That is, regardless of whether the two halves of the target word (e.g. 'cowb' and 'wboy') were each presented independently to different eyes or were presented to both eyes, the landing positions on these target words were the same. These data are, therefore, strong evidence that readers programme their saccades towards a single percept resulting from combination of the information from both of the eyes. These data also indicate that the two eyes' saccades during reading are programmed as a single neural signal (Hering, 1868, as cited in Howard, 1999) rather than being programmed independently (Helmholz, 1910, as cited in Howard, 1999).

Note that the different presentation techniques employed by Blythe et al. (2010) and by Liversedge et al. (2006b) lead to complementary conclusions that might, at first, seem contradictory. Blythe et al. used a stereoscopic presentation, where the content of the two eyes' images were identical but with a horizontal disparity manipulated between the two images. On the basis of their data, they concluded that participants had not fused the images prior to direct fixation (i.e. in the parafovea), thus suggesting that the visual system is either not sensitive to or not responsive to parafoveal disparity cues. Liversedge et al. (2006b) used a dichoptic presentation, where there is no disparity manipulation in the stimuli but the content of the two eyes' images is different (e.g. 'cowb' to one eye and 'wboy' to the other eye). On the basis of their data, they concluded that participants were able to target saccades to the words as a whole, indicating that saccade programming was operating over a combined percept of the two eyes' inputs. Thus, parafoveal information from the two retinal signals seems to be integrated (but not necessarily fused) in order for saccades to be programmed to a single percept.

Supporting the argument for a single neural signal underlying saccades, other research has shown that the degree of synchronization between binocular saccades is independent of whether words are viewed monocularly or binocularly (e.g. Williams and Fender, 1977; Heller and Radach, 1999). Were it the case that saccades for the two eyes are programmed independently, then gross differences ought to be observed between normal, binocular viewing and monocular viewing (where one eye has no visual input by which to guide its saccades). In contrast though, these studies showed that when reading monocularly, saccades of the occluded eye are coordinated with the viewing eye in the same manner as when both eyes are viewing the text. Together with the data from Liversedge et al. (2006b) this work provides converging evidence that binocular saccades are generated on the basis of a single neural signal. Furthermore, these studies also indicate that the frequently observed disparity between the two eyes during reading is not a consequence of the eyes being driven by two independent neural signals. Instead, researchers have argued that differences in neural transmission or in the two eyes' musculature may underlie the characteristic binocular disparity that occurs during saccades (e.g. Bains et al., 1992; Collewijn et al., 1988).

In summary, it appears that the visual system computes saccades on the basis of a single percept of the upcoming word and, during direct fixation, can fuse relatively large retinal disparities for word stimuli (greater than those which naturally occur as a consequence of binocular disparity during reading). We now turn to the three critical questions outlined in the Introduction: 1) do visual or linguistic characteristics of text influence binocular coordination?; 2) Do developmental factors influence binocular coordination?; 3) Is there a link between binocular coordination and dyslexia?

Do visual or cognitive factors influence binocular coordination?

Several studies have investigated which aspects of text processing (if any) may influence binocular coordination (e.g. Blythe et al., 2006; Bucci and Kapoula, 2006; Heller and Radach, 1999; Hendriks, 1996; Juhasz et al., 2006; Liversedge et al., 2006b; Yang and Kapoula, 2003). These studies specifically manipulated linguistic and/or visual characteristics of text and examined whether they impacted on binocular coordination in skilled adult readers.

One of the first empirical studies to investigate the modulation of binocular coordination during reading was Hendriks (1996). Hendriks assessed the influence of linguistic factors on vergence velocity during fixations. Binocular coordination was compared when participants read prose passages or lists of unrelated words, and were instructed either to read for meaning or to 'sound out' the pronunciations of the words subvocally without reading for meaning. Reading prose passages requires syntactic and semantic processing in addition to the identification of individual words, and thus requires greater depth of processing than reading lists of unrelated words. Similarly, reading text for meaning requires greater depth of processing than simply sounding out words. Hendriks found that the velocity of vergence movements was higher when reading for meaning than when sounding out words, and when reading passages of text than when reading lists of words. Hendriks suggested that under conditions where reading is more dependent on the visual input, vergence velocities are slower, compared to conditions where more top-down information is available to the reader. Hendriks argued, therefore, that the nature of the text and the task demands associated with linguistic processing impact on binocular coordination, at least in terms of vergence velocities. Critically though, Hendriks' data also showed a relationship between processing difficulty and saccade amplitude, with smaller saccades made when 'sounding out' or reading unrelated words. Non-reading studies have established that there is a strong relationship between saccade amplitude and fixation disparity, whereby the greater the amplitude of the incoming saccade, the greater the disparity between the two eyes' positions during the subsequent fixation (Collewijn et al., 1988; Kirkby et al., 2010). Hendriks (1996) argued that linguistic processing difficulty affected the amplitude of saccades that were made as the reader progressed through the stimuli, and it was saccade amplitude (rather than processing difficulty per se) that determined the velocity of vergence movements during the subsequent fixation. Thus, although Hendriks' data showed a relationship between processing difficulty and vergence movements, this link may be at least partially attributable to preceding saccade amplitude.

Other studies have directly manipulated the characteristics of text in order to investigate whether binocular coordination is modulated by visual or cognitive processing. Heller and Radach (1999) examined the influence of visual task demands on binocular coordination during reading, by presenting readers with MiXeD cAsE text compared to normal text.[2] They found an increase in fixation durations and the number of fixations being made when reading mixed case text, indicating that mixed case text incurred more processing difficulty than normal text in their study. Heller and Radach also describe an increase in both the magnitude of disparity as well as the velocity of the vergence movements during fixations for normal text compared to that observed during the mixed case condition. However saccade amplitudes were also reduced for mixed case, compared to normally presented text. Similar to Hendriks' (1996) data, therefore, the modulation of binocular disparity shown in Heller and Radach's study may be explained either by an effect of processing difficulty or by differences in saccade amplitude.

Other studies have failed to find effects of processing difficulty on binocular coordination. Smith et al. (1971) measured the difference in saccade onset asymmetry as a method of assessing binocular coordination. They measured the movements of the two eyes while participants read text that was manipulated for difficulty (although the authors did not specify the nature of this manipulation), as well as for the orientation of the constituent letters (the text was either rotated along the horizontal axis or presented normally). Although saccades of the two eyes were asymmetric during all conditions, in contrast to Hendriks (1996) and Heller and Radach (1999), Smith et al. found no effects of text difficulty on binocular coordination during reading.

One study that has specifically measured the influence of processing difficulty upon binocular coordination in terms of the magnitude and direction of fixation disparity is that of Juhasz et al. (2006). Juhasz et al. aimed to further test Heller and Radach's (1999) suggestion that binocular coordination is modulated by difficulty as induced by MiXeD cAsE text presentation. In addition, to provide a test of whether binocular coordination is modulated by linguistic difficulty, Juhasz et al. also manipulated the frequency of target words within sentences. There were significant effects of both word frequency and case on fixation durations, clearly showing that the processing difficulty manipulations were effective (fixation durations reflect the ease with which words are identified; Liversedge and Findlay, 2000; Rayner, 1998). In contrast to the findings of Heller and Radach,

---

[2] Mixed case text is often used in reading research in order to preserve abstract orthographic and lexical information whilst disrupting the familiarity of the visual input (McConkie and Zola, 1979). Note that although mixed case text can be more difficult to read than normally presented text, such effects diminish with practice (Inhoff et al., 2005).

however, there was no evidence to suggest that processing difficulty influenced the direction or magnitude of fixation disparity. It is not clear, however, whether saccade amplitudes were also shorter during mixed case reading in Juhasz et al.'s study (hence the relationship between processing difficulty, saccade amplitude, and fixation disparity cannot be assessed for this data set).

Given that processing difficulty impacts on fixation durations, this raises the broader question of whether fixation duration in general is linked to the magnitude of fixation disparity and, in particular, whether vergence movements occur throughout the entire duration of a fixation. Liversedge et al. (2006a) showed that the duration of a fixation correlated with the magnitude of disparity reduction during the fixation. On this basis it might be predicted that end of fixation disparities should be smaller for more difficult text as fixation durations are generally longer on more difficult text (Rayner, 1998), thus allowing more time for the eyes to converge and reduce disparity. Two recent studies have examined the time course of vergence movements during fixations (Jainta et al., 2010; Vernet and Kapoula, 2009). Vernet and Kapoula (2009) examined binocular coordination over multiple time periods during reading, these periods were: just prior to a saccade, during a saccade, and at two time periods after a saccade. They found that at fixation onset (defined as the initial 48 ms after the end of the saccade) the disconjugacy between the two eyes' points of fixation was greatest. Over the subsequent 80 ms there was a reduction in disparity and by the end of the fixation the alignment of the eyes was quite stable (but still disparate). Jainta et al. found that the magnitude of fixation disparity at its minimum point in the fixation did not differ significantly from that at the end of fixations and, as such, fixation durations were not found to correlate with the magnitude of disparity. These data indicate that the relationship between fixation duration and vergence during the fixation is more complex than had been suggested by Liversedge et al. (2006a).

To summarize, only a few studies have specifically investigated the effect of linguistic processing difficulty on binocular coordination in skilled adult readers, and these studies have provided mixed evidence. One study (Hendriks, 1996) has shown significant effects of processing difficulty on binocular coordination (specifically, fixation vergence velocities); however, this effect could, at least partially, be attributable to a confounding variable (preceding saccade amplitude). Heller and Radach (1999) also argued that processing difficulty influenced binocular coordination. Similar to Hendriks' data, though, the effects reported by Heller and Radach may also be attributable to differences in saccade amplitudes. In contrast, a more recent investigation using several different manipulations of processing difficulty found no effects of these manipulations on binocular coordination (Juhasz et al., 2006). Finally, there is little evidence to suggest that fixation duration is related to the magnitude of fixation disparity (Jainta et al., 2010; Kliegl et al., 2006; Vernet and Kapoula, 2009). Given these mixed results in the literature, further research is needed to clarify whether or not visual/cognitive manipulations influence binocular coordination, as well as to determine the role of any mediating variables (e.g. saccade length, fixation duration).

Do developmental factors influence binocular coordination?

Research comparing the binocular coordination of children and adults has revealed differences in both the magnitude and the direction of fixation disparity. An important question to consider is whether these differences are a consequence of the increased processing difficulty experienced by child readers compared to skilled adult readers. The cognitive demands associated with processing linguistic stimuli are far greater for younger children (in particular those who have recently learnt to read), compared to older children and adult skilled readers who have years of reading experience (e.g. Rayner, 1986). Hence any differences in binocular coordination between beginning and skilled readers could be due to at least three possible factors: the development of binocular coordination control in general; the development of binocular coordination specifically in relation to reading; or greater language processing difficulties for beginning compared to skilled readers.

The data from several studies have shown that children tend to have a greater magnitude of disparity between the two points of fixation than adults; furthermore, where adults tend to show a predominance of uncrossed fixation disparities, children tend to show a higher proportion of crossed fixation disparities than adults. This pattern of differences between adults and children has been found on both reading (Blythe et al., 2006) and non-reading tasks (Bucci and Kapoula, 2006; Fioravanti et al., 1995; Yang and Kapoula, 2003). Given that children and adults show differences in binocular coordination for non-reading based tasks, the observed developmental changes in binocular coordination during reading cannot be attributed solely to high-level cognitive processing of linguistic stimuli. Rather, these differences between adults and children appear to be more low-level in nature and perhaps improvements in binocular coordination during reading reflect age-related improvements in oculomotor control more generally.

Overall, it is clear that developmental changes in binocular coordination during reading occur, but the differences between adults and children whilst reading cannot necessarily be attributed to children's increased processing difficulty as beginning readers as they also occur during non-reading tasks. What remains uncertain as yet is why these age-related changes in binocular coordination occur (see Kirkby et al., 2008 for a discussion of this issue). However several studies have described a general development of eye movement control maturing at around adolescence, perhaps linked to the maturation of the brain via synaptic pruning and myelination (see Luna and Velanova, Chapter 35, this volume).

Is there a link between binocular coordination and dyslexia?

The third of our three questions is currently something of a greater challenge to address, partly due to the lack of empirical studies specifically investigating which aspects of reading are affected by binocular coordination for those with dyslexia, and partly due to the conflicting evidence in the literature. We will, therefore, first provide an overview of the eye movement research associated with the argument that poor binocular coordination and reading difficulties may be causally related. Then, although there are only a few studies that have directly measured the binocular eye movements of individuals with reading difficulties, we will discuss the data (often based on non-reading tasks) supporting this claim.

The 1994 DSM-IV Criteria for Reading Disorder (dyslexia) are: a) reading achievement, as measured by an individually administered, standardized test of reading accuracy or comprehension, substantially below that expected given the person's chronological age, measured intelligence, and age-appropriate education; b) the disturbance interferes with academic achievement or activities of daily living that require reading skills; c) if a sensory deficit is present, the reading difficulties are in excess of those usually associated with the specific sensory deficit (APA, 1994). After several decades of research there is still considerable disagreement over the neurological and cognitive basis of dyslexia and this remains strongly debated. The most influential theory of dyslexia is the phonological-deficit hypothesis (Liberman, 1973; Snowling, 2000; Stanovich, 1988), where cognitive deficits in processing the relationships between printed letters and speech sounds cause the reading problems experienced by dyslexics (Ramus, 2003). A far more controversial approach to understanding the pattern of deficits associated with dyslexia is the magnocellular-deficit theory, where causation is attributed to sensory deficits as a result of impairments in the magnocellular pathway of the visual system (Stein, 2001). The magnocellular theory of dyslexia will be the main focus of this section, as the proponents of this theory have argued that poor binocular coordination can be causally linked to reading difficulty.

Stein (2001) suggests that visual deficits, such as unstable binocular coordination during fixation and poor vergence control, can lead to letter and word processing difficulties (Bigelow and McKenzie, 1985; Cornelissen et al., 1992, 1993; Eden et al., 1994; Evans and Drasdo, 1990; Kapoula et al., 2007; Stein and Fowler, 1993; Stein et al., 1986; 1988). Stein proposed that children with dyslexia make reading errors due to their inability to perform appropriate vergence movements during fixation (Kapoula et al., 2007; Stein et al., 1988). Recall that vergence movements (non-parallel movements of the two eyes) are made by adult and child readers during fixations, such that the residual disparity from the preceding saccade is reduced (Blythe et al., 2006; Liversedge et al., 2006a, 2006b). Stein argued that vergence movements are necessary in order to maintain a stable, fused visual percept of the words on a page, and that up to two thirds of the dyslexic population may be affected by the inability to perform appropriate vergence movements during fixations (Kapoula et al., 2007; Stein et al., 1988). Specifically, it was claimed that individuals with dyslexia fail to make appropriate vergence movements during fixations in reading and, thus, experience an unstable single percept from the two retinal inputs (there are often anecdotal reports that dyslexic readers experience blurring of letters, letters moving around in a word, and letters obscuring one another).

The magnocellular deficit theory postulates deficient functioning of the magnocellular stream of the visual system, and neurological problems are suggested to affect visual contrast sensitivity as well as reduced binocular stability (Stein and Fowler, 1993; Cornelissen et al., 1993; see Boden and Giaschi, 2007, for a review). Both these deficits in magnocellular function would obviously negatively impact on a child's ability to learn to read; however, deficits in binocular coordination in dyslexia remain inadequately investigated to date (Kirkby et al., 2008). In particular, some intervention programs already focus on improving binocular coordination in dyslexic children (Stein et al., 2000), even though there has been little empirical evaluation of the extent to which such a deficit exists. Importantly, the present chapter highlights that binocular disparity is commonplace during reading and non-reading tasks for both skilled adult and child readers, hence binocular disparity is not unique to dyslexic readers. In addition to examining whether dyslexic readers do show poorer binocular coordination we must also ask, therefore, whether fixation disparity in dyslexic readers impacts on their reading performance.

Interestingly, there are also some eye movement experiments indicating that dyslexic children's fixations are largely adequate in reading-like, visual scanning tasks (De Luca et al., 1999, 2002; Hutzler et al., 2006; Hutzler and Wimmer, 2004). However, these studies only recorded the movements of one eye during the task and, therefore, they provide no information in relation to binocular coordination during reading.

If dyslexia is caused by poor binocular control then dyslexic individuals should exhibit different binocular coordination behaviour compared to skilled readers in general, and not only during reading. In order to support the claim that poor binocular coordination is a cause of children's reading difficulties, it would be necessary to demonstrate poor binocular coordination in such children both during tasks that require linguistic processing and during tasks that do not, compared to typically developing children. A difference between typically developing and dyslexic children on a reading task alone would leave the researcher unable to distinguish between whether poor binocular coordination is a cause, consequence, or correlate of reading difficulty. In contrast, if poor binocular coordination was found to occur for dyslexic children during non-reading tasks in the absence of any linguistic processing demands, at least it would then be shown that reading difficulty is not the cause of poor binocular coordination in dyslexic children. We will now briefly outline research that has attempted to examine whether reading difficulty is associated with poor binocular coordination in reading and non-reading tasks (e.g. Bucci et al., 2008; Jaschinski et al., 2004; Kapoula et al., 2007; Kirkby et al., submitted; Stein et al., 1988).

Stein and colleagues examined children's vergence eye movements in response to simulated movements of small targets in depth. Using both subjective reports and more objective eye movement recordings, the findings led Stein and colleagues to suggest that a number of children with dyslexia are unable to maintain stable binocular fixation (Stein, 1989, 2001; Stein and Fowler, 1981, 1982, 1993; Stein et al., 1988). Other studies have investigated binocular coordination in individuals with dyslexia by using dichoptic methodologies in which different images are presented to each of the eyes using a synoptophore.[3] In these studies, the images presented to the two eyes were gradually drawn apart in either a convergent or a divergent direction. The children were asked to report the moment at which they experienced double vision (i.e. the moment at which the magnitude of disparity between the two retinal inputs became too great for them to be successfully fused). Several studies

---

[3] The Synoptophore is a haploscope that allows the experimenter to present separate slides to each eye in order to test various aspects of binocular vision.

were conducted using this method, reporting eye movement data in one instance whilst relying on the subjective self-report of children in other cases (Bigelow and McKenzie, 1985; Stein, 1989; Stein and Fowler, 1981, 1982, 1993). While typically developing children did make vergence movements up until the point at which fusion broke, Stein et al.'s (1988) data showed that children with dyslexia failed to make appropriate, stimulus-driven vergence movements (instead, they made parallel drift movements of the two eyes). Together, these results indicate that dyslexic children have poorer binocular coordination compared to non-dyslexic children, at least during certain non-reading tasks.

In addition to the studies by Stein and colleagues, two recent studies have demonstrated a reduced capacity to verge the eyes during fixation in children with dyslexia on both non-reading and single-word reading tasks (Bucci et al., 2008; Kapoula et al., 2007). Similarly, Jaschinski et al. (2004) used dichoptically presented nonius lines to determine a psychophysical measure of fixation disparity. In this test of disparity, the participant views dichoptically presented vertical lines, one above the other, and they are required to make small adjustments until the lines appear vertically aligned. The remaining disparity between the two lines following the participants' adjustment is taken as a measure of their fixation disparity. Jaschinski et al. found that the mean fixation disparity for dyslexic children was larger in magnitude than that of typically developing children. Thus, several studies examining fixation disparity on non-reading tasks have found evidence of relatively poor binocular coordination in dyslexic children compared to their typically developing peers. Note, however, that the non-reading tasks used in these studies have not required oculomotor behaviour analogous to that observed during reading. This raises the question of whether the results would generalize to reading or to scanning tasks that demand similar eye movement behaviour to reading.

There are, however, studies which have not found differences between groups of typically developing children and children with dyslexia in their capacity to verge the eyes. Lennerstrand and colleagues conducted a longitudinal study employing a number of different methods for examining binocular coordination (Lennerstrand et al., 1993, 1994). A synoptophore test was used to examine vergence capacity when viewing small, simple pictures. In addition, participants completed other orthoptic tests, and their binocular eye movements were recorded during a sentence reading task. Vergence control was found to be comparable for children with and without dyslexia during the synoptophore test. Interestingly, however, for the sentence reading task, the children with dyslexia were found to have greater binocular asymmetry during saccades compared to the typically developing children. Given that there were no differences in binocular coordination between the dyslexic and typically developing children in the non-reading task, but a difference in the reading task, these data indicate that a cognitive modulation of binocular coordination may be present for children with dyslexia.

Recently Kirkby et al. (submitted) conducted a study that measured binocular coordination in adults, typically developing children, and children with dyslexia during both a reading and a non-linguistic dot scanning task. Participants were required to either scan (from left to right) horizontal arrays of dot strings or to silently read sentences as their binocular eye movements were recorded. The dot stimuli were carefully designed to appear visually similar to horizontal arrays of words (sentences), without requiring any linguistic processing. The resulting oculomotor behaviour observed during the dot scanning task was similar to that observed during reading (highly stylized patterns of fixations and saccades). With respect to binocular coordination, Kirkby et al. found that fixation disparity was significantly greater for dyslexic children compared to both adults and typically developing children during reading, but not during the non-reading task. Kirkby et al. concluded that observation of poorer binocular coordination in dyslexic readers exclusively when reading (in both Kirkby et al. and Lennerstrand et al.'s studies) casts serious doubt on the claims of the magnocellular theory. Given the lack of a difference in binocular coordination between dyslexic and typically developing children on non-reading tasks, it seems highly unlikely that a low-level dysfunction in binocular coordination causes the reading difficulties associated with dyslexia. Rather, Kirkby et al. propose that increased fixation disparity during reading in children with dyslexia may result either from inadequate attentional or cognitive resource allocation in the reading process, or from suboptimal linguistic processing.

It could also be argued that the differences in binocular coordination during reading for dyslexic children might arise due to the greater linguistic processing difficulty that dyslexic children experience in the reading task compared to their typically developing peers. Such a suggestion contrasts, however, with the research with skilled adult readers, discussed above, showing little direct evidence for a link between processing difficulty and binocular coordination (e.g. Heller and Radach, 1999; Hendriks, 1996; Juhasz et al., 2006). We suggest that the manipulations of processing difficulty used with adults (such as word frequency) do not approximate the difference in cognitive effort required for reading in children with dyslexia compared to that in skilled (adult or child) readers.

In summary, a number of studies (Bigelow and McKenzie, 1985; Bucci et al., 2008; Cornelissen et al., 1992, 1993; Eden et al., 1994; Evans and Drasdo, 1990; Jaschinski et al., 2004; Kapoula et al., 2007; Stein and Fowler, 1993; Stein et al., 1986, 1988) have shown differences in binocular coordination between readers with dyslexia and matched controls. To date, however, only one study has recorded binocular eye movements from the same group of dyslexic children during both a reading and a non-reading task (Kirkby et al., submitted). Kirkby et al.'s results indicate that dyslexia is associated with increased fixation disparity exclusively during reading and, hence, poor binocular coordination is unlikely to cause reading difficulties. Overall, it is clear that there are conflicting findings in the literature on binocular coordination and dyslexia, and it is evident that much more research is needed. First, further studies must confirm whether or not poor binocular coordination occurs exclusively during reading for children with dyslexia. Second, if differences in binocular coordination are specific to reading, then further studies must be conducted to distinguish between two possible explanations: 1) poor binocular coordination is a consequence of severe processing difficulty and, hence, is seen in children with dyslexia but is not necessarily specific to that group (stronger manipulations with adults could result in an effect on their binocular coordination); 2) poor binocular coordination during reading is an inherent characteristic of dyslexia and reflects the particular attentional/linguistic abnormalities associated with that pheneotype.

Conclusions

The chapter has provided an overview of the current topical issues surrounding binocular coordination during reading. A number of studies now illustrate that precise coordination of the eyes is not necessary for fluent reading. In fact the two points of fixation are frequently disparate, with the two eyes often fixating different letters within a word (though disparity rarely exceeds two character spaces). Vergence movements occur during fixations and tend to be in a corrective direction for the residual binocular disparity from the preceding saccade. Nevertheless, disparity remains until the end of fixation albeit reduced in magnitude. Readers can fuse up to $0.37°$ of retinal disparity during reading, and no age-related changes for fusional limits have been found. Furthermore, evidence from a range of studies indicates that saccades are programmed on the basis of a single unified percept.

The chapter focused on three critical issues. Our review of whether visual/cognitive factors impact on binocular coordination in skilled readers concluded that disparity during reading is, at most, minimally affected by the processing demands of the task. Further research is necessary, though, to confirm whether processing difficulty, or mediating variables such as saccade amplitude or fixation duration can, in some circumstances, impact on binocular coordination. Second, our review indicated that binocular coordination develops with age; at around 12 years of age children display a pattern of binocular coordination similar to that for adults. Importantly, comparisons of reading and non-reading data indicate that these changes are not associated with changes in reading skill but rather reflect a low-level development in oculomotor control. Finally, we considered whether variability in binocular coordination is linked to dyslexia. Although there is some evidence that dyslexia in children is associated with poor binocular coordination, a recent direct comparison of binocular coordination in reading and a non-reading task indicates that increased fixation disparity for dyslexic children during reading may in fact be a consequence of reading difficulties. Further research is needed to clarify the extent to which increased fixation disparity in dyslexic readers might be attributable to reading material itself, or the cognitive/linguistic processing demands associated with reading and comprehending text.

The research outlined in this chapter not only has important implications for our understanding of binocular coordination in general, but is also critical for our understanding of eye movement control during reading. In terms of methodology, the finding of disparate fixations has implications for inferring the precise location of overt attention (as determined by where the eyes are fixating). That is, the two eyes are frequently disparate during fixations and yet the two retinal inputs are fused; even if the positions of both eyes are recorded, it is unclear where overt attention should be considered to be located (especially if the two eyes are fixating different letters). Research based on the recording of just one eye produces particular uncertainty about the precise location of overt attention in the text. In some cases, it may even be that the non-recorded eye is fixating a different word to the recorded eye.

The fixation disparities that occur during reading raise questions about the interpretation of some existing findings based on the recordings of just one eye. For example, some studies have shown that the characteristics of a word can influence eye movement behaviour on the prior word (parafoveal-on-foveal effects) (Kennedy, 2000). Such findings are central to determining whether attention can be allocated to more than one word at any one time. However, a contributing factor to such effects may be a subset of fixations in which the non-recorded eye is actually fixating the next word in the sentence (and affecting fixation durations which are associated with the prior word in the sentence that is being fixated by the recorded eye). Thus, it is possible that 'parafoveal-on-foveal' effects in such circumstances may not be driven by parafoveal processing (for a thorough discussion of parafoveal-on-foveal effects, see Drieghe, Chapter 46, this volume). Similarly, words that are thought to have been skipped might actually have been fixated by the non-recorded eye. Importantly, given that the two eyes occasionally fixate on different words, a fully comprehensive model of eye movement control in reading will need to account for the position of the two eyes separately, rather than assuming that the two eyes fixate in precisely the same location as is currently the case (e.g. Engbert et al., 2005; Reichle et al., 1998).

One recent model does take into account the relative positions of the two eyes (Shillcock et al., 2010). Shillcock et al. (2010) simulated the effect of a range of both crossed and uncrossed fixation disparities in their model. The results indicated that fixation disparity would impact on lexical identification, as disparity increases the width of the foveal window (thereby increasing the range of information that falls within high-acuity vision). The results also indicated that crossed disparities would facilitate lexical identification more than uncrossed fixation disparities. In addition to binocular disparity, their model also incorporates foveal splitting, whereby the left half of a fixated word is initially projected to the right hemisphere and the right half of a word is initially projected to the left hemisphere of the brain via contralateral projections (e.g. Lavidor et al., 2001). Model simulations indicated that the processing advantage associated with crossed fixation disparities was increased by precise foveal splitting, such that the greater the simulated overlap between hemifoveas the smaller the difference between crossed and uncrossed fixation disparities. Note, however, that the assumption of precise foveal splitting is controversial and strongly debated (see Jordan and Paterson, 2009, 2010).

Finally, the issues outlined here have particular implications for our understanding of the role of binocular coordination in dyslexia. As emphasized above, much more research is needed to clarify the nature of any difference in binocular coordination in dyslexic compared to typical populations, and to identify whether any differences are specific to reading. The issue is of particular importance due to the potential implications of this research for intervention programmes.

Acknowledgements

J.A. Kirkby was supported by the Leverhulme Trust. Portions of this work were completed while S.J. White was on Study Leave granted by the University of Leicester. H.I. Blythe was supported by an ESRC Postdoctoral Fellowship. We would like to thank Kevin Paterson and Denis Drieghe for their helpful comments on an earlier version of this chapter.

References

American Psychiatric Association (2001). *Diagnostic and Statistical Manual of Mental Disorders* (4th Ed.). Washington, DC: APA.

Bains, R.A., Crawford, J.D., Cadera, W., and Vilis, T. (1992). The conjugacy of human saccadic eye movements. *Vision Research*, 32, 1677–1684.

Bigelow, E.R., and McKenzie, B.E. (1985). Unstable ocular dominance and reading ability. *Perception*, 14, 329–335.

Blythe, H.I., Liversedge, S.P., and Findlay, J.M. (2010). The effective fusional range for words in a natural viewing situation. *Vision Research*, 50, 1559–1570.

Blythe, H.I., Liversedge, S.P., Joseph, H.S.S.L., White, S.J., Findlay, J.M., and Rayner, K. (2006). The binocular coordination of eye movements during reading in children and adults. *Vision Research*, 46, 3898–3908.

Boden, C. and Giaschi, D. (2007). M-stream deficits and reading-related visual processing in developmental dyslexia. *Psychological Bulletin*, 133, 346–366.

Bucci, M.P., Brémond-Gignac, D., and Kapoula, Z. (2008). Latency of saccades and vergence eye movements in dyslexic children. *Experimental Brain Research*, 188, 1–12.

Bucci, M.P. and Kapoula, Z. (2006). Binocular coordination of saccades in 7 years-old children in single word reading and target fixation. *Vision Research*, 46, 457–466.

Collewijn, H., Erkelens, C.J., and Steinman, R.M. (1988). Binocular co-ordination of human horizontal saccadic eye movements. *Journal of Physiology*, 404, 157–182.

Cornelissen, P., Bradley, L., Fowler, S., and Stein, J.F. (1992). Covering one eye affects how some children read. *Developmental Medicine and Child Neurology*, 34, 296–304.

Cornelissen, P., Munro, N., Fowler, S., and Stein, J.F. (1993). The stability of binocular fixation during reading in adults and children. *Developmental Medicine and Child Neurology*, 35, 777–787.

De Luca, M., Borrelli, M., Judica, A., Spinelli, D., and Zoccolotti, P. (2002). Reading words and pseudowords: An eye movement study of developmental dyslexia. *Brain and Language*, 80, 617–626.

De Luca, M., Di Pace, E., Judica, A., Spinelli, D., and Zoccolotti, P. (1999). Eye movement patterns in linguistic and non-linguistic tasks in developmental surface dyslexia. *Neuropsychologia*, 37, 1407–1420.

Eden, G.F., Stein, J.F., Wood, H.M., and Wood, F.B. (1994). Differences in eye movements and reading problems in dyslexic and normal children. *Vision Research*, 34, 1345–1358.

Engbert, R., Nuthmann, A., Richter, E.M., and Kliegl, R. (2005). SWIFT: A dynamical model of saccade generation during reading. *Psychological Review*, 112, 777–813.

Evans, B.J. and Drasdo, N. (1990). Review of ophthalmic factors in dyslexia. *Ophthalmic and Physiological Optics*, 10, 123–132.

Fender, D. and Julesz, B. (1967). Extension of Panum's fusional area in binocularly stabilized vision. *Journal of the Optical Society of America*, 57, 819–830.

Fioravanti, F., Inchingolo, P., Pensiero, S., and Spanios, M. (1995). Saccadic eye movement conjugation in children. *Vision Research*, 35, 3217–3228.

Heller, D. and Radach, R. (1999). Eye movements in reading: Are two eyes better than one? In W. Becker, H. Deubel, and T. Mergner (eds.) *Current oculomotor research: Physiological and psychological aspects.* (pp. 341–348). New York: Plenum Press.

Hendriks, A.W. (1996). Vergence eye movements during fixations in reading. *Acta Psychologica*, 92, 131–151.

Howard, I.P. (1999). The Helmholtz - Hering debate in retrospect. *Perception*, 28, 543–549.

Hutzler, F. & Wimmer, H. (2004). Eye movements of dyslexic children when reading in a regular orthography. *Brain and Language*, 89, 235–242.

Hutzler, F., Kronbichler, M., Jacobs, A.M., and Wimmer, H. (2006). Perhaps correlational but not causal: No effect of dyslexic readers' magnocellular system on their eye movements during reading. *Neuropsychologia*, 44, 637–648.

Inhoff, A.W., Eiter, B.M., and Radach, R. (2005). Time course of linguistic information extraction from consecutive words during eye fixations in reading. *Journal of Experimental Psychology: Human Perception and Performance*, 31, 979–995.

Jainta, S., Hoormann, J., Kloke, W.B., and Jaschinski, W. (2010). Binocularity during reading fixations: Properties of the minimum fixation disparity. *Vision Research*, 50, 1775–1785.

Jaschinski, W., König, M., Schmidt, R., and Methling, D. (2004). Vergence dynamics and variability of fixation disparity in dyslexic children. *Klin monatsbl augenheilkd*, 221, 854–861.

Jones, R.K. and Lee, D.N. (1981). Why two eyes are better than one: the two views of binocular vision. *Journal of Experimental Psychology: Human Perception and Performance*, 7, 30–40.

Jordan, T.R. and Paterson, K.B. (2009). Re-evaluating split-fovea processing in word recognition: A critical assessment of recent research. *Neuropsychologia*, 47, 2341–2353.

Jordan, T.R. and Paterson, K.B. (2010). Where is the evidence for split-fovea processing in word recognition? *Neuropsychologia*, 48, 2782–2783.

Juhasz, B.J., Liversedge, S.P., White, S.J., and Rayner, K. (2006). Binocular coordination of the eyes during reading: Word frequency and case alternation affect fixation duration but not fixation disparity. *Quarterly Journal of Experimental Psychology*, 59, 1614–1625.

Kapoula, Z., Bucci, M.P., Jurion, F., Ayoun, J., Afkhami, F., and Bre´mond-Gignac, D. (2007). Evidence for frequent divergence impairment in French dyslexic children: Deficit of convergence relaxation or of divergence per se? *Graefe's Archives for Clinical and Experimental Ophthalmology*, **245**, 931–936.

Kennedy, A. (2000). Parafoveal processing in word recognition. *Quarterly Journal of Experimental Psychology*, **53A**, 429–455.

Kirkby, J.A., Blythe, H.I., Benson, V., and Liversedge, S.P. (2010). Binocular coordination during the scanning of simple dot stimuli. *Vision Research*, **50**, 171–180.

Kirkby, J.A., Blythe, H.I., Drieghe, D., and Liversedge, S.P. Reading text increases binocular disparity in dyslexic children. (Manuscript submitted.)

Kirkby, J.A., Webster, L.A.D., Blythe, H.I., and Liversedge, S.P. (2008). Binocular coordination during reading and non-reading tasks. *Psychological Bulletin*, **134**, 742–763.

Kliegl, R., Nuthman, A., and Engbert, R. (2006). Tracking the mind during reading: The influence of past, present, and future words on fixation durations. *Journal of Experimental Psychology: General*, **135**, 12–35.

Lavidor, M., Ellis, A.W., Shillcock, R., and Bland, T. (2001). Evaluating a split processing model of visual word recognition: Effects of word length. *Cognitive Brain Research*, **12**, 265–272.

Lennerstrand, G., Ygge, J., and Jacobson. C. (1993). Control of binocular eye movements in normals and dyslexics. *Annals of New York Academy of Sciences*, **682**, 231–239.

Lennerstrand, G., Ygge, J., and Rydberg, A. (1994). Binocular control in normally reading children and dyslexics. In J. Ygge and G. Lennerstrand (eds.) *Eye movements in reading* (pp. 291–300). Oxford: Pergamon Press.

Liberman, I.Y. (1973). Segmentation of the spoken word and reading acquisition. *Bulletin of the Orton Society*, **23**, 65–76.

Liversedge, S.P. and Blythe, H.I. (2009). There is no such thing as a free trip across the corpus callosum. *Manuscript in preparation*.

Liversedge, S.P. and Findlay, J.M. (2000). Saccadic eye movements and cognition. *Trends in Cognitive Sciences*, **4**, 6–14.

Liversedge, S.P., Rayner, K., White, S.J., Findlay, J.M., and McSorley, E. (2006b). Binocular Coordination of the Eyes during Reading. *Current Biology*, **16**, 1726–1729.

Liversedge, S.P., White, S.J., Findlay, J.M., and Rayner, K. (2006a). Binocular coordination of eye movements during reading. *Vision Research*, **46**, 2363–2374.

McConkie, G.W., Kerr, P.W., Reddix, M.D., and Zola, D. (1988). Eye movement control during reading: I. The location of initial eye fixations on words. *Vision Research*, **28**, 1107–1118.

McConkie, G.W. and Zola, D. (1979). Is visual information integrated across successive fixations in reading? *Perception and Psychophysics*, **25**, 221–224.

Nuthmann, A. and Kliegl, R. (2009). An examination of binocular reading fixations based on sentence corpus data. *Journal of Vision*, **9**, 1–28.

Ogle, K.N. (1952). On the limits of stereoscopic vision. *Journal of Experimental Psychology*, **44**, 253–259.

Paterson, K.B., Jordan, T.R., and Kurtev, S. (2009). Binocular fixation disparity in single word displays. *Journal of Experimental Psychology: Human Perception and Performance*, **35**, 1961–1968.

Ramus, F. (2003). Developmental dyslexia: Specific phonological deficit or general sensorimotor dysfunction? *Current Opinion in Neurobiology*, **13**, 212–218.

Rayner, K. (1979). Eye guidance in reading: fixation locations within words. *Perception*, **8**, 21–30.

Rayner, K. (1986). Eye movements and the perceptual span in beginning and skilled readers. *Journal of Experimental Child Psychology*, **41**, 211–236.

Rayner, K. (1998). Eye movements in reading and information processing: 20 years of research. *Psychological Bulletin*, **124**, 372–422.

Reichle, E.D., Rayner, K., and Pollatsek, A. (2003). The E-Z Reader model of eye movement control in reading: Comparisons to other models. *Behavioral and Brain Sciences*, **26**, 445–526.

Shillcock, R.C., Roberts, M., Kreiner, H., and Obregón, M. (2010). Binocular foveation in reading. *Attention, Perception, and Psychophysics*, **72**, 2184–2203.

Smith, K.U., Schremser, R., and Putz, V. (1971). Binocular coordination in reading. *Journal of Applied Psychology*, **55**, 251–258.

Snowling, M.J. (2000). *Dyslexia* (2nd edn.). Oxford: Blackwell Publishers.

Stanovich, K.E. (1988). Explaining the differences between the dyslexic and the garden-variety poor reader: The phonological-core variable-difference model. *Journal of Experimental Child Psychology*, **38**, 175–190.

Stein, J.F. (1989). Visuospatial perception and reading problems. *Irish Journal of Pyschology*, **10**, 521–533.

Stein, J.F. (2001). The magnocellular theory of developmental dyslexia. *Dyslexia*, **7**, 12–36.

Stein, J.F. and Fowler, M.S. (1981). Visual dyslexia. *Trends in Neurosciences*, **4**, 77–80.

Stein, J.F. and Fowler, M.S. (1982). Diagnosis of dyslexia by means of a new indicator of eye dominance. *British Journal of Ophthalmology*, **66**, 332–336.

Stein, J.F. and Fowler, M.S. (1993). Unstable binocular control in children with specific reading retardation. *Journal of Research in Reading*, **16**, 30–45.

Stein, J.F., Riddell, P., and Fowler, M.S. (1986). The Dunlop Test and reading in primary school children. *British Journal of Ophthalmology*, **70**, 3–17.

Stein, J.F., Riddell, P. and Fowler, M.S. (1988). Disordered vergence control in dyslexic children. *British Journal of Ophthalmology*, **72**, 162–166.

Stein, J.F., Richardson, A.J., and Fowler, M.S. (2000). Monocular occlusion can improve binocular control and reading in dyslexics. *Brian*, **123**, 164–170.

Vernet, M. and Kapoula, Z. (2009). Binocular motor coordination during saccades and fixations while reading: A magnitude and time analysis. *Journal of Vision* **9**, 1–13.

Williams, R.A. and Fender, D.H. (1977). The synchrony of binocular saccadic eye movements. *Vision Research*, **17**, 303–306.

Yang, Q. and Kapoula, Z. (2003). Binocular coordination of saccades at far and at near in children and in adults. *Journal of Vision*, **3**, 554–561.

Yatabe, K., Pickering, M.J., and McDonald, S.A. (2009). Lexical processing during saccades in text comprehension. *Psychonomic Bulletin and Review*, **16**, 62–66.

CHAPTER 45

Foveal and parafoveal processing during reading

Jukka Hyönä

Abstract

Eye movement studies on foveal and parafoveal word processing in reading are reviewed. The studies show that when a word in a text is fixated, identities of letters and their corresponding phonemes are activated early during the fixation. Orthographic and phonological coding give rise to lexical and meaning activation, which is also reflected in fixation times on words. As regards parafoveal processing, the research shows that lower-level visual features, such as the length and the visual shape of words, are extracted during reading. Moreover, readers also gain orthographic and phonological information from the parafoveal word. On the other hand, the evidence for parafoveal processing of lexical and semantic information is equivocal and inconclusive. It seems lexical and semantic parafoveal processing is not standardly achieved during reading.

Introduction

Readers' eye behaviour consists of fixations during which the eyes remain relatively stable and saccades that move the eyes rapidly from one text region to another. Intake of textual information takes place during fixations, whereas during saccades readers are functionally blind (the so-called saccadic suppression). Two key objectives in the research on eye movements during reading have been to determine what factors govern when to terminate a fixation to move on in the text and where in the text to send the eyes next. It is widely agreed that the duration of fixations is controlled by the ongoing comprehension processes, while saccadic targeting is primarily determined by oculomotor constraints and lower-level visual features of the text.

As information intake takes place during fixations, one of the key questions is to examine how much textual information around the centre of the current fixation readers are able to extract. The area from which useful information can be gleaned is very significantly constrained by the physiology of the eyes. The cones that are responsible for detailed visual perception are heavily concentrated in the foveal area of the retina. In order to recognize the words in a text, readers need to locate the foveal area such that light from the word to be fixated falls directly on it. High visual acuity is needed in word recognition, as the identity of written words in alphabetic scripts is marked by letter codes, many of which closely resemble one another (e.g. *l* vs. *t*, or *k* vs. *h*). The visual acuity of the eyes is best around the fovea (it comprises about 2° of visual angle around the fovea centre), and it drops off quite steeply as a function of distance from the centre of the fovea. The area outside the fovea is further divided into two functionally distinct regions: parafovea and periphery. The parafoveal area extends up to 5° of visual angle to the right and left from the fixation point, while the visual periphery refers to the area beyond the parafovea. What is relevant for the present discussion, is that readers can extract useful information from the parafovea, whereas peripheral information is of very little use (with the exception of content structure signals, such as headings, that may be perceived in the periphery, see Cauchard et al., 2010).

The pertinence of foveal vision in reading was convincingly demonstrated by Rayner et al. (1981) by using the moving window paradigm introduced by McConkie and Rayner (1975). In one version of this paradigm (Experiment 2), a set of letters around the fixation point was visually masked (using an interlaced square wave grating), and the size of the mask was varied from 1 to 17 characters. The mask moved along with the eyes so that wherever the reader looked in the text, a set of letters around the fixation point was masked. When the size of the mask was 7 letters (average word length in English texts), the foveal region was completely masked, and reading was dramatically slowed down (from 295 words per minute, as observed in the normal, unmasked condition, to a mere 15 words per minute). With the 7-letter mask, readers were still able to correctly report 78% of the words; with the 15-letter mask the accuracy went down to 18% and the reading rate was less than 10 words per minute. Thus, reading becomes virtually impossible, or at least extremely cumbersome, when the use of foveal vision is prevented (Rayner and Bertera, 1979; see also studies of patients suffering a central scotoma, e.g. Legge et al. (1997)).

Although foveal vision is necessary for reading, only a limited foveal exposure time is required for the reading to proceed normally. In Experiment 3, Rayner et al. (1981) demonstrated that when the text was masked 50 ms after the fixation onset, readers' eye behaviour mirrored that of reading under normal conditions. Thus, visual information necessary for reading can be acquired within the fixation's first 50 ms. However, this does not mean that the processing of visual information is completed during this time. This was demonstrated by Liversedge et al. (2004) using a disappearing text paradigm, where the fixated word always disappeared 60 ms after the fixation onset (i.e. the word was replaced with a blank space). Even though the word was no longer visible, readers continued to fixate the blank space. Even more importantly, they fixated the blank space for longer time if the word that had disappeared was infrequent relative to a frequent word, which is a nice demonstration of the ongoing linguistic processing affecting fixation durations in reading. The only noticeable difference compared to normal reading was that, quite understandably, readers did not make a second fixation on the blank space, as they occasionally do when a word is difficult to process and the word stays available throughout the fixation.

In the present chapter, I review what is known of foveal and parafoveal processing in reading. Before going into details of individual studies, one important caveat related to the terminology needs to be discussed. In eye movement research on reading, it has become a standard to refer to the fixated word as the foveal word and the word(s) adjacent to the fixated word as the parafoveal word. Many times this usage is consistent with the physiologically based definition (see above) of the foveal and parafoveal area, but this is not always the case. For example, if 1° of visual angle corresponds to about five letters (as is the case when reading this text from a distance of 40 cm) and the fixated word and the adjacent word both comprise three letters, also the adjacent word falls onto the foveal region. However, the non-fixated word will be nevertheless called the parafoveal word. On the other hand, if the fixated word is long (e.g. *institutionalization*), the most exterior letters fall onto the parafoveal region. Nevertheless, the fixated word is called the foveal or foveated word.

The remainder of this chapter is organized as follows. I first discuss the foveal processing of words as revealed by readers' eye movement registration, followed by a discussion of parafoveal word processing. Only those studies are discussed where words are read in a sentence or discourse context (i.e. unless stated otherwise, studies using isolated word presentation are not included). I also limit the discussion to skilled reading, with sporadic observations related to less skilled readers.

Foveal processing

In this section, I go over the factors that are shown to affect fixation times on foveated words. The discussed word-level factors include oculomotor, orthographic, phonological, lexical, and semantic factors.

Effects related to syntactic processing are not covered here; the interested reader should consult a comprehensive review of Clifton et al. (2007; see also Clifton and Staub, Chapter 49, this volume).

Location of initial fixation position

When readers fixate a word in a text, they tend to position the point of fixation on a letter close to the word's centre (the preferred viewing location is established to be somewhat to the left of the word's centre, Rayner, 1979). This facilitates word identification, as the positioning of the eyes in the word centre makes all or most letters of the word (depending on word length) fall within the foveal reach. Studies (Nuthmann et al., 2005; O'Regan et al., 1984; Vitu et al., 1990) have shown that the time fixating a word before fixating away from it (i.e., so called gaze duration) increases linearly as a function of the distance of the initial fixation from the word centre. The further away the initial fixation is from the optimal location, the more likely it is that a refixation is made on a word (McConkie et al., 1989; Nuthmann et al., 2005; Rayner et al., 1996; Vitu et al., 1990, 2001). These optimal viewing position (OVP) effects were first established with isolated word presentation (O'Regan et al., 1984), but they have subsequently been extended to normal reading (see the above references). The OVP effects observed in gaze duration and refixation probability are readily explained by visual acuity constraints: when the initial fixation lands on the word beginning or ending, the letters at the other end of the word are less visible than when the eyes are positioned in the word centre. However, there is one OVP effect that is clearly at odds with this account. When a single fixation is made on the word, the duration of this single fixation is longest when positioned in the word centre and shortest when positioned furthest away from the centre (hence the name Inverted OVP effect; Vitu et al., 2001; though see Rayner et al., 1996, for findings that are inconsistent with this work). Although efforts have been made to account for this counterintuitive observation (Nuthmann et al., 2005, 2007; Vitu et al., 2001, 2007), it may be fair to say that it still remains somewhat controversial. However, at present there is quite general agreement that the Inverted OVP effect is at least partly explained by the single fixation positioned toward the word beginning and end being mislocated (e.g. a fixation landing in the word beginning is intended to land on the previous word; Nuthmann et al., 2005; 2007). According to another plausible account, called the perceptual-economy account (Vitu et al., 2007), a single fixation on the word centre is longer than a fixation on the word beginning or end simply because there is more visual information pertinent to word recognition to be processed around the centre than at the edges.

Word length

Given the pertinence of foveal vision in reading, it probably comes as no surprise that word length has a significant effect on foveal word processing. Gaze duration on long words is longer than that on short words (e.g. Calvo and Meseguer, 2002; Hyönä and Olson, 1995; Just and Carpenter, 1980; Kliegl et al., 2004). As visual acuity is not equally distributed across the whole of the fovea, the final letters of a long word are not as visible as those of a short word (assuming a fixation equally far into each word), which in turn gives rise to the need for a refixation, which in turn lengthens the time spent on a long word relative to a short one. However, the foveal constraint is not the only determinant of the word length effect. McDonald (2006) manipulated word length while keeping constant the horizontal extent; this was achieved by varying the width of letters. His main observation was that the more letters a word contains, the more and longer fixations are made on the word, despite the fact that the words subtend the same visual angle. McDonald concludes that the word length effect is likely due to longer words being subject to a greater degree to visual crowding than short words. To counteract the adverse crowding effect, more and longer fixations are needed.

Orthographic coding of letters, letter clusters, and letter position

As words are identified via the individual letters they contain, it is relevant to examine how letter information influences the foveal processing of words during reading. For example, it is possible that the frequency of letter clusters (e.g. bigrams or trigrams) influences the foveal processing time: words containing an infrequent letter cluster require longer fixation times than words comprising frequent letter clusters. White and Liversedge (2004) introduced misspellings in the word-initial trigram, while varying at the same time the trigram frequency (e.g. *laboratory/liboratory/luboratory/lyboratory/lwboratory*). They found that gaze duration on the target word increased as a function of word-initial trigram frequency: Gaze duration was shortest for a correctly spelled word and longest for illegally spelled, unpronounceable initial-trigram words (for an effect of misspelling on gaze duration, see also Inhoff and Topolski, 1994; Rayner et al., 1998a; Underwood et al., 1988). An effect of the familiarity of word-initial letter sequence was also obtained by Lima and Inhoff (1985) for correctly spelled words. Words containing an infrequent letter sequence (e.g. *dwarf*) received longer first fixations but not reliably longer gaze durations than words containing a frequent letter sequence (e.g. *clown*). However, Hand et al. (2008) obtained a reversed effect: longer first fixation and gaze durations on words containing a frequent than an infrequent word-initial trigram, which suggests an infrequent trigram helps constrain the set of possible lexical candidates (i.e. there exist fewer words starting with an infrequent trigram).

A second question related to orthographic coding that has attracted attention is to what extent readers code letter position information in words. Can letters swap positions within a word without lengthening the fixation time on the word? White et al. (2008a) demosntrated taht jubmling up lettres in wrods increases their foveal processing: gaze duration was longer for the transposed-letter words than for the correctly spelled words (see also Rayner et al., 2006). Moreover, this transposed letter effect was more pronounced when the external letters were transposed (e.g. *problme* or *rpoblem*) instead of the internal letters (e.g. *probelm*). Transposing the word-initial letters tended to produce the largest disruption in processing. Despite these significant effects, it is noteworthy that the overall reading speed was slowed down only by 11%, which suggests that 'word recognition processes must be quite flexible in the way letter position information is encoded' (White et al., 2008a, p. 1268).

Finally, Lee et al. (2001) demonstrated that consonants are processed faster than vowels during the early stages of foveal word processing. This became evident in two experiments that employed a version of the so-called fast priming paradigm (Sereno and Rayner, 1992). In their version of the paradigm, when the reader fixated the target word the presentation of one letter (either a consonant or vowel) was delayed for either 30 or 60 ms. Delaying a consonant for 30 ms after fixation onset caused significantly longer gaze durations on the target word than delaying a vowel. However, in the 60-ms delay condition, there was no difference between the consonant and vowel conditions. Thus, in the earliest stages of foveal processing, consonants play a more important role than vowels that appear to be of minimal significance (see also Lee et al., 2002, for a similar pattern of results using another version of the fast priming paradigm), as evidenced in Experiment 2 where delaying both a vowel and a consonant for 30 ms did not lengthen gaze duration more than simply delaying a consonant.

Phonological coding

When we read a text silently, most people 'hear' the text as if spoken by an inner voice. This type of subvocal speech may serve the purpose of temporarily retaining words and sentence fragments to be integrated to a coherent sentence meaning. A related, but different question is whether readers use phonological codes during lexical access. In English, one way to examine the activation of the word's phonological representation during foveal processing is to compare fixation times on words having a regular pronunciation (e.g. *mood*) to those having an irregular pronunciation (e.g. *weird*). Inhoff and Topolski (1994) obtained a regularity effect in the first fixation duration: it was significantly longer on irregular than regular words. The effect was short-lived as it no longer was significant in gaze duration. Sereno and Rayner (2000) extended and refined these results by showing a regularity effect in gaze duration for low-frequency but not for high-frequency words (the parafoveal processing aspect of the study is reported below). This suggests that phonological coding is more important in identifying infrequent than frequent words. Folk and Morris (1995) demonstrated longer gaze durations for words containing multiple phonological codes in comparison to words having a single phonological code.

Another way to examine the role of phonological representations in lexical access during reading is to compare the foveal processing of correct word forms (*bear*) to that of incorrect homophones (*bare*) and orthographic controls (*barn*), as was done in the study of Rayner et al. (1998a). Readers were told that some of the passages contained a misspelled word but they were to focus on comprehending the passage. Rayner et al. observed in Experiment 1 no difference in first fixation and single duration between the correct and incorrect homophones when they shared one or two letters in the word beginning (*break–brake*). This is taken as evidence for an early activation of phonological codes. On the other hand, incorrect homophones received longer gaze durations than correct homophones indicating a meaning activation a bit later in the processing time line. Experiment 2 and 3 demonstrated that the effect reflects phonological rather than orthographic similarity; evidence for early activation of phonology was obtained in the conditions where the target word was predictable from the prior sentence context. This pattern of results is inconsistent with that observed by Daneman and Reingold (1993) and Daneman et al. (1995) who failed to find evidence for activation of phonological codes during foveal processing, only at a later, postlexical stage, as evidenced by the number of regressions back to the target word (see Rayner et al., 1998, for a detailed discussion of the discrepancies between the Daneman et al. studies and that of Rayner et al., which all employed similar manipulations).

Sparrow and Miellet (2002) made use of homophones in French. They asked readers to proofread a text that contained different types of spelling errors. They observed equally long first fixation durations on correctly spelled words and homophonic non-words—a finding that was taken as evidence for early activation of phonological representations in reading French.

Evidence for an early activation of phonological codes during foveal processing is also obtained by the fast priming paradigm (Sereno and Rayner, 1992). The presentation of a visually similar homophone for 32–36 ms at the beginning of a fixation (after which it is replaced by the correct word) speeds up the gaze duration (a 30–40 ms difference between the homophone and the orthographically similar conditions) on the word (Lee et al., 1999; Rayner et al., 1995). In Experiment 2 of Lee et al., a phonological priming effect was obtained only for high-frequency prime words (not for pseudoword primes). This indicates that the phonological prime needs be to accessed fast for the priming effect to occur.

Yates et al. (2008) compared fixation times on words containing several phonological neighbours (*bait* and *get* are phonological neighbours of *gate*, as they sound similar when pronounced) to those on words having only a few phonological neighbours. They demonstrated phonological neighbourhood density to facilitate foveal processing of words. Again, the phonological effect was short-lived, as it showed up in first fixation and single fixation duration, but not in gaze duration, which indicates that phonological codes are used in the early stages of foveal processing (for negligible effects of orthographic neighbours, see Perea and Pollatsek, 1998; Pollatsek et al., 1999; Sears et al., 2006).

Finally, Ashby and Clifton (2005) examined whether prosodic information is activated during silent reading. More specifically, they studied whether the prosodic property of lexical stress is processed during reading. In order to do that, they compared the foveal processing of words containing either one or two stressed syllables (e.g. *significant* vs. *fundamental*). They observed that words with two stressed syllables were read with significantly longer gaze durations and a greater number of fixations. These effects are taken to suggest that readers obtain stress information during silent reading.

In sum, the majority of studies speak for an activation of phonological codes during the early stages of foveal processing. Moreover, the activation appears to be short-lived, as it is typically observed in first fixation duration but not usually in gaze duration.

Word frequency and age of acquisition

Probably the most well documented effect in foveal word processing is the word frequency effect (e.g. Henderson and Ferreira, 1990; Hyönä and Olson, 1995; Inhoff and Rayner, 1986; Rayner and Duffy, 1986; Raney and Rayner, 1995; Schilling et al., 1998; White, 2008). The higher the frequency, the shorter the gaze duration is on a word. In other words, the more frequently a reader has been exposed to a written word, the less time is needed to identify it during reading. Frequency is capable of influencing either individual fixation durations or the probability of making a refixation on a word, or both. As the effects of word frequency are robust, the simulation of the effect has become a part of the standard 'testbed' when assessing the goodness of fit of eye guidance models in reading (see Reichle, Chapter 42, this volume).

Novel words comprise an extreme group of words in the frequency continuum. Chaffin et al. (2001) examined how readers establish the meaning of novel words from the sentence context. Perhaps surprisingly, readers did not spend more time on novel than low-frequency words when they were first encountered. On the other hand, they regressed back to novel words more than to low-frequency words and read for longer time the informative context following the novel versus the familiar words, which effects were taken to suggest that the readers inferred on-line the meaning of the novel word on the basis of the informative context.

The age at which a word is acquired also influences the time it takes to fixate it during text reading. This was demonstrated by Juhasz and Rayner (2006), who orthogonally varied target words' age of acquisition and frequency. They reported significantly longer gaze durations for late- than early-acquired words (see also Juhasz and Rayner, 2003). As word frequency was equated, the effect does not reflect a more frequent exposure to early-acquired words, but it is likely to be semantic in nature.

Word meaning

Activation of word meaning during foveal processing has been studied by comparing the processing of words with multiple meanings (homonyms) to that of words with only a single meaning (Binder and Morris, 1995; Dopkins et al., 1992; Duffy et al., 1988; Folk and Morris, 1995; Rayner and Duffy, 1986; Rayner and Frazier, 1989; Rayner et al., 1994; Sereno, 1995; Sereno et al., 1992). The following picture emerges from these studies. When the two meanings of a word are equally frequent (in such a situation the homonym is called balanced) and the prior sentence context does not constrain either meaning, the homonym is fixated for longer time than a single-meaning word or a word that has one dominant and another less dominant meaning. This is taken as evidence to support the view that both meanings of a balanced homonym are activated during the word's foveal processing. On the other hand, when the preceding context instantiates the less likely meaning of an unbalanced homonym (one meaning is more frequent than the other), a word with one dominant and one less dominant meaning is fixated for longer time than a balanced homonym or a control word. This effect suggests that meaning dominance determines the order of accessing the multiple meanings (for a review, see Duffy et al., 2001). In other words, the most dominant is accessed first, but if it is not the meaning supported by prior context, a less dominant meaning needs to be activated, which is responsible for the extra fixation time.

Morphological structure of words

The meaning structure of words varies in that some words contain only one single meaning unit (e.g. *car*), while other words consist of multiple meaning units (e.g. *caring*, *caretaker*). These meaning units are called morphemes, which can be divided into free morphemes (*care* and *taker* in *caretaker*) or bound morphemes (*-ing* in *caring*). Most of the eye movement studies of morphological processing during reading have focused on the role of free morphemes in processing morphologically complex compound words.

A number of studies (e.g. Andrews et al., 2004; Bertram and Hyönä, 2003; Hyönä and Pollatsek, 1998; Juhasz et al., 2003; Pollatsek et al., 2000a) have shown that the foveal processing of long compounds consisting of two free morphemes is serial in the sense that these compounds are identified via their constituents (for a review, see Pollatsek and Hyönä, 2006). This is evidenced by a reliable effect of first constituent frequency in an early measure of foveal processing (first fixation duration) and a reliable effect of second constituent effect in a measure indexing later foveal processing (gaze duration).

These effects are more robust in Finnish than in English, probably due to the fact that Finnish is a morphologically much richer language than English (i.e. word compounding is much more productive in Finnish than in English).

On the other hand, Bertram and Hyönä (2003) demonstrated that short (7–9 letters) Finnish two-constituent compound words are processed holistically, as evidenced by a reliable word frequency effect combined with no effect of first-constituent frequency. According to the visual acuity principle put forth by Bertram and Hyönä, short compound words can be processed holistically, because the entire word is simultaneously available in the foveal vision when the word is fixated, while long compound words are processed via the morphological components, because a part of the word (the second constituent) falls outside the foveal area during the initial fixation on the word. However, these claims were not fully supported by the study of Juhasz (2008), who observed a reliable first-constituent frequency effect for short English compound words but not for long compound words (for which there was a non-significant reversed frequency effect).

A few studies have examined the foveal processing of affixed words (comprising a bound and a free morpheme, as in *remove*). Lima (1987) compared the processing of prefixed words (*remove*) to that of pseudoprefixed words (*relish*) and observed longer gaze durations (Experiment 2) for pseudopre-fixed than prefixed words. This finding was taken to suggest that readers automatically decompose the word into morphemes or morpheme-looking units. For pseudoprefixed words the unnecessary decomposition leads to a processing delay, as evidenced in longer gaze duration. Niswander-Klement and Pollatsek (2006) extended the visual acuity principle of Bertram and Hyönä (2003) to the processing of shorter and longer affixed words. Experiment 2 of Niswander-Klement and Pollatsek demonstrated a morphological effect (as indexed by a root frequency effect of similar magnitude as the frequency effect for free morphemes without an affix) in gaze durations for long words (>8 letters, such as *unfamiliar*) but not for short words (<7 letters, such as *unpack*).

Contextual predictability

As noted above, context has an influence on accessing the meaning of words. There is now ample evidence demonstrating that sentence-level or paragraph-level semantic predictability affects fixation times on words during reading (Ashby et al., 2005; Balota et al., 1985; Calvo and Meseguer, 2002; Calvo et al., 2001; Drieghe et al., 2004, 2005; Ehrlich and Rayner, 1981; Frisson et al., 2005; Hyönä, 1993; Kliegl et al., 2004; Morris, 1994; Rayner et al., 2004a; Rayner and Well, 1996; White et al., 2005a). Contextually predictable words are read with shorter fixation times than less predictable words. Also local, purely lexically based predictability effects have been observed. When a verb strongly constrains the identity of the following word (e.g. 'hunched his back'), gaze duration on the noun is shorter than when it is preceded by a non-constraining verb (Schustack et al., 1987; Vainio et al., 2009). There is also a large body of literature on the effects of syntactic prediction (for a comprehensive review, see Clifton et al., 2007; Clifton and Staub, Chapter 49, this volume). For example, readers expect to encounter a syntactic object after a transitive verb. However, if this expectation is violated, processing difficulty will ensue, which is reflected in the eye movement record.

Parafoveal processing

In this section, I review the research evidence on what features of the text are extracted from para-foveal vision during reading. Before doing that, a note on the use of terminology is in order. I follow the practice mentioned in the Introduction where the fixated word is called the foveal word and the word to the right (i.e. when reading from left to right) of the fixated word is called the parafoveal word, irrespective of whether or not it falls entirely outside foveal vision.

Two types of methodological tools have been used to examine what aspects of the parafoveal word are processed. In the moving window paradigm (McConkie and Rayner, 1975), the researcher varies the amount of parafoveal (or foveal) information available around the current fixation point. For example, using a symmetric 15-character moving window, 7 letters to the right and left of the fixated letter are visible, while all the remaining text is mutilated (e.g. replaced by x's or random letters). The window moves along with the eyes, so that wherever the reader looks in the text, (s)he sees 15 intact letters around the fixation point. By varying the size of the window and the type of changes made to the text outside the window, the researcher is in a position to determine what type of information is extracted from the parafovea and what the size of effective vision is for different types of textual information.

Another very popular paradigm is the so-called boundary paradigm (Rayner, 1975), also known as the eye-movement contingent display change method (Fig. 45.1). In this paradigm, only prespecified target words are initially mutilated. An invisible boundary is set to the left of the target word. During the saccade crossing the boundary, the target word is changed to its correct form (due to saccadic suppression the reader does not see the actual change). If the reader detects a discrepancy between the parafoveally available information and the foveated word, a processing cost will ensue when the target word is fixated (apparent in a longer fixation time on the target word), which is interpreted to indicate that information of the parafoveal word was processed prior to its fixation. By varying the type of parafoveal preview preceding the target, the researcher can determine the exact nature of the type of parafoveal processing that is carried out.

A third phenomenon related to parafoveal word processing is the so-called parafoveal-on-foveal effect (Kennedy, 1998; see Drieghe, Chapter 46, this volume, for a review). As the name indicates, such effects indicate that some aspect of the parafoveal word (or of the experimentally defined para-foveal preview) influences the processing of the fixated word. Investigation of parafoveal on foveal effects may be carried out with or without the display change paradigm. For example, if in the display change paradigm all the letters of the parafoveal word are initially replaced by random letters and this manipulation increases gaze duration on the foveal word (as a response to perceiving a strange letter cluster in the parafovea), we have detected a parafoveal-on-foveal effect.

In the following, I go over the effects related to the same word features that have been demonstrated to affect foveal word processing.

Distance to the parafoveal word (or preview)

A general finding is that the closer the reader is fixating to the parafoveal word (or preview), the more parafoveal processing is carried out (e.g. Kennison and Clifton, 1995). When the fixation is very close to the parafoveal word, it is likely that at least a part of the parafoveal word is within foveal vision, as determined strictly physiologically. Thus, a subset of the reported parafoveal effects reflect a mixture of foveal and parafoveal on foveal processing.

Word length

McConkie and Rayner (1975) employed the moving window paradigm to examine how far in the parafovea word length information is perceived. In order to do that they either preserved the spaces

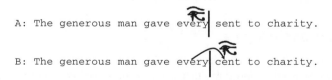

Fig. 45.1 A graphical depiction of the eye-contingent display change paradigm. During Phase A, a parafoveal preview (*sent*) is presented of the intended target word (*cent*); the eyes are located to the left of the invisible boundary (marked by a vertical bar). During a saccade crossing the invisible boundary (Phase B), the parafoveal preview is changed to the intended form. Due to vision being suppressed during saccades, readers do not see the actual change taking place. Thus, when the eyes fixate the target word, it always appears in the correct form. The sentences are adopted from the study of Pollatsek et al. (1992).

between words or filled them with extra letters. Their study showed that readers acquire word-length information up to 15 character positions to the right of fixation (see also Rayner, 1986) and that this information primarily affects saccade length (readers use parafoveal word length information to target a saccade to the centre of next unidentified word in the parafovea). Inhoff et al. (1998) demonstrated that correct length information provided for the parafoveal word (*barclohqo → movement*) speeds up the target word processing when it is fixated, compared to incorrect length information (*barc ohqo → movement*) (see also Inhoff et al., 2003; White et al., 2005a). Parafoveal word length information, in combination with sentence context, can also be used to narrow down the possible lexical candidates for the upcoming word (Juhasz et al., 2008).

Orthographic coding

Apart from word length information, readers also acquire information about the visual shape of letters comprising the parafoveal word. This has been demonstrated in studies using the boundary paradigm. Intact parafoveal previews have been compared to previews preserving the word's visual shape (letters are replaced with visually similar letters, e.g. *l* is replaced with *t*), or to previews dissimilar in shape with the intended word. When the parafoveal preview comprises letters visually dissimilar to those of the intended word, the word's subsequent foveal processing (it appears in the intended form when fixated) is delayed by about 40 ms (for a review, see Hyönä, et al., 2004; Rayner, 1998). On the other hand, when the letters are replaced with visually similar letters, the processing cost is reduced to 15 ms.

Also letter identity information is processed parafoveally. The seminal studies suggested that parafoveal letter identity processing is primarily limited to the beginning letters, as no processing cost was observed when the first two or three letters are kept intact and the remaining letters are replaced with visually similar letters (Henderson and Ferreira, 1990; Pollatsek et al., 1992; Rayner et al., 1982). More recently, there is accumulating evidence suggesting that parafoveal letter identity processing is not entirely limited to the initial letters. The discrepancy in results between the seminal and more recent studies may be due to improvements in the quality of cathode ray tube (CRT) screens used to present experimental texts (see also Drieghe et al., 2005). With greater precision of screens, the text appearing in the parafovea may be more recognizable in the modern screens.

Using the moving window technique, Häikiö et al. (2009) recently showed that the letter identity span extends up to 9 letters to the right of fixation. In a similar vein, Inhoff (1989a) showed that not only the parafoveal availability of word-initial letters but also that of word-final letters facilitates a word's subsequent foveal processing. The effect size was not modulated by the reading direction (left to right versus right to left)—a manipulation which was included to vary the relative distance of the critical parafoveal information from the current fixation location. On the other hand, the preview effect for word-final letters was eliminated when the remaining letters were replaced with dissimilar letters (rather than *x*'s) rendering the word-final letters less discriminable. Johnson et al. (2007) examined further the parafoveal processing of letter identity information for interior and final letters. In order to do that they provided parafoveal previews for which two interior or final letters of 5-letter words were either transposed (e.g. *clekr* instead of *clerk*) or substituted with other letters (e.g. *clefn* instead of *clerk*). In Experiment 1, they observed a 31-ms penalty in gaze duration when the first three letters were kept intact but the final two letters were initially changed (i.e. the mean of the transposition and substitution conditions; see also Hyönä and Häikiö, 2005). This is further evidence for the view that parafoveal letter processing is not limited to the first 2–3 word-initial letters. Experiments 2 and 3 provided evidence for a privileged role of word-final (and word-initial) letters over word-internal letters. In Experiment 3, changing the two final letters in 7-letter words led to significantly longer gaze durations in comparison to the no-change condition, whereas changing two word-internal letters (5th and 6th) did not significantly disrupt subsequent foveal processing. The results led Johnson et al. to the conclusion that 'readers are able to extract information from the first five letters of the word to the right of fixation plus the word-final letter' (p. 222). This conclusion compares favourably with the study of Briihl and Inhoff (1995) who observed a greater preview benefit from beginning (*thuxxxx → thunder*) and exterior letters (*thxxxxr → thunder*) than from the word-interior letters (*xxundxx → thunder*), which yielded no preview benefit when compared to no preview (*xxxxxx*). This is due to interior letters suffering more from visual crowding than exterior letters.

Johnson et al. (2007) also demonstrated that letter identity information can be obtained from the parafovea outside of absolute letter position. This became evident in the previews containing transposed letters producing generally less disruption in subsequent foveal processing than previews where the corresponding letters were substituted with other visually similar letters.

Evidence for the effect of the frequency of letter clusters constituting the parafoveal word has been mixed. Some studies have established a parafoveal-on-foveal effect of orthographic familiarity (Inhoff et al., 2000a; Pynte et al., 2004; Rayner, 1975; Starr and Inhoff, 2004; Underwood et al., 2000; White, 2008), while others have not (Rayner et al., 2007; White and Liversedge, 2004; 2006). An example of a positive effect is provided by a recent study by White (2008) that manipulated orthographic familiarity by the sum of the frequencies of the words that contain particular letter sequences (e.g. for a four-letter word, the letter sequences comprise two trigrams, three bigrams, and four monograms). White obtained a small effect of orthographic familiarity: the duration prior to fixating the target word was 6 ms longer in the orthographically familiar than unfamiliar condition.

Finally, Williams et al. (2006) demonstrated that parafoveal letter processing is modulated by the frequency of the parafoveal word. In Experiment 1, a low-frequency target word (e.g. *sleet*) was parafoveally previewed by a high-frequency orthographic neighbor (*sweet*), a non-word orthographic neighbour (*speet*), or an identical preview (*sleet*); two words are orthographic neighbours when they look similar visually (i.e. they share most of the same letters). Gaze duration on target revealed that a high-frequency orthographic neighbour was almost as good a preview as the target word itself and significantly better than the non-word orthographic preview. In Experiment 2, the situation was reversed in that a low-frequency orthographic neighbour served as a preview for a high-frequency target word. Now both orthographic previews were significantly poorer previews than the identical preview. Taken together, the two experiments indicate that there is no general advantage for having a word as a parafoveal preview over a non-word. Rather, there is a distinct advantage for a high-frequency orthographic neighbour. This pattern of results is interpreted to indicate that the parafoveal processing takes place at the level of activating letter identities, which process is boosted by the partial activation of lexical entries. The reason for why the preview effect for high-frequency orthographic neighbours is not interpreted to reflect lexical level activation is that full lexical activation should have inhibited (due to competition between two lexical candidates), not facilitated the foveal processing of target words (e.g. Carreiras, Perea, and Grainger, 1997).

Phonological coding

Several studies show that a word's phonological representation is activated parafoveally. Pollatsek et al. (1992) provided parafoveally either homophone previews (*cite → site*), visually matched control previews (*cake → sake*), or identical previews (*site → site*). When the previewed word was fixated (it always appeared in the correct from), the duration of first fixation (but not gaze duration) on the target word was significantly shorter when preceded by a homophone preview than a visually matched non-homophonic control. Similarly, Miellet and Sparrow (2004) found no difference in first fixation duration on the target word when it was preceded either by an identical preview or a homophonic pseudoword; the study was conducted in French. Henderson et al. (1995) observed that parafoveally presented words with phonologically regular initial trigrams (e.g. *but* in *button*) produced greater preview benefits than did words with phonologically irregular initial trigrams (e.g. *but* in *butane*). Pollatsek et al. (2000b), Liu et al. (2002) and Tsai et al. (2004) provided evidence for parafoveal phonological coding even in Chinese—a non-alphabetic language with a deep orthography. Liu et al. further observed that for the parafoveal phonological coding to occur, the preview and the target need to share the same phonological radical (see also Tsai et al. (2004) for further evidence). Chace et al. (2005) reported a parafoveal homophone effect for skilled readers but not for less skilled readers.

Finally Ashby et al. (2006) examined parafoveal phonological coding using non-word parafoveal previews in which the vowel phoneme was concordant (*cherg → chirp*) or discordant (*chorg → chirp*) with the vowel phoneme in the target word (note that in both preview conditions the identity of the critical letter was incorrect). In Experiment 1, they observed that gaze durations were 15 ms shorter for targets preceded by concordant previews than for those preceded by discordant previews. In Experiment 2, the vowel concordance effect was replicated by keeping the critical vowel constant (also its letter identity) but manipulating in non-word previews the following consonant that influences the preceding vowel sound (concordant: *raff → rack*; discordant: *rall → rack*).

In sum, the eye movement studies reviewed above provide evidence for an early involvement of phonological codes during reading. This conclusion compares favourably with theorizing based on visual word recognition studies (see Frost, 1998).

Lexical-semantic effects

The question of whether words are identified parafoveally has recently gained increased interest, as the answer to this question is highly pertinent to the competing eye guidance models of reading (see Reichle, Chapter 42, and Engbert and Kliegl, Chapter 43, this volume). Parafoveal word identification has been investigated by examining whether a manipulation of the frequency of the parafoveal word or its contextual predictability or plausibility leads to discernible effects in the eye movement record prior to its direct fixation. Word frequency effects index parafoveal lexical processing, while predictability effects reflect parafoveal semantic activation. As becomes evident from the following review, the evidence for parafoveal lexical and semantic processing is rather mixed.

Parafoveal lexical-semantic effects have been examined using several different experimental setups. Kennedy (1998) introduced a logic where effects of parafoveal word features on the foveal word processing are investigated (so-called parafoveal-on-foveal effects; for a more thorough review, see Drieghe, Chapter 46, this volume). The idea here is that if the parafoveal word is identified while fixating on a previous word, its lexical or semantic features should affect the processing of the fixated word. Kennedy (2000) and Kennedy et al. (2002) reported a parafoveal-on-foveal effect of frequency using a word search target (e.g. participants were asked to search for words referring to clothing among a set of unrelated words; for a criticism of the use of this task to study normal reading, see Rayner et al., 2003). An effect of parafoveal word frequency on gaze duration of the foveal word was also reported in a corpus study of Pynte and Kennedy (2006) for English but not for French and in another corpus study of Kennedy and Pynte (2005) for short foveal words but not for long foveal words (see also Kliegl et al., 2006). However, other studies on normal reading using experimentally manipulated variables have not been able to confirm this effect (see Calvo and Meseguer, 2002; Carpenter and Just, 1983; Henderson and Ferreira, 1993; Hyönä and Bertram, 2004; Inhoff et al., 2000b; Rayner et al., 1998b; White, 2008; White and Liversedge, 2004; see Schroyens et al., 1999, for a replication failure using a non-reading task). For example, in five experiments Hyönä and Bertram manipulated either the whole word frequency or the frequency of the first constituent of two-noun compounds. Of the five experiments, only one demonstrated longer gaze durations on the fixated word when the parafoveal word was of low- rather than of high-frequency.

Another way to study parafoveal word identification is to vary the semantic relatedness of the parafoveal word to the preceding context. This was done by Murray (1998) and Murray and Rowan (1998) in a study where participants were asked to judge whether two sentences were physically identical or not (when they differed, they differed only by one word). Murray found that when word *n* and *n*+1 resulted in a semantically implausible reading (*uranium smacked*), the fixation time on word *n* was increased, compared to a condition where the two words conformed to a semantically plausible reading (*savages smacked*). However, in a normal reading study this parafoveal implausibility effect was not replicated by Rayner et al. (2003) or Rayner et al. (2004b). Inhoff et al. (2000b) varied the semantic relatedness of two adjacent words with three conditions: identical (*mother's mother*), semantically associated (*mother's father*), and unassociated (*mother's garden*) condition. Gaze duration on the preceding word was significantly shorter when the following word was either identical or semantically related in comparison to the unassociated condition (for an effect of semantic relatedness in processing two-noun compound words, see White et al., 2008b). Finally, Kliegl et al. (2006) obtained a parafoveal predictability effect: when the parafoveal word was predictable from the previous sentence context; the duration of single fixation on the foveal word was longer than when the parafoveal word was unpredictable. This surprising finding is interpreted to suggest that the reader stays fixating the foveal word longer when (s)he cannot guess what the next word is.

Parafoveal lexical-semantic processing has also been investigated using the display change paradigm. In these studies, semantically related and unrelated parafoveal previews have not differed from each other (see Altarriba et al., 2001; Balota et al., 1985; Hyönä and Häikiö, 2005; Rayner et al., 1986). When the target word *song* was previewed either by *tune* (semantically related) or *door* (unrelated), Pollatsek et al. observed no difference in target word fixation time. Altarriba et al. tested Spanish-English bilinguals reading Spanish and English sentences, where a target word was parafoveally previewed by a translation equivalent (among other things) in the other language. No evidence was observed to support parafoveal semantic processing. Hyönä and Häikiö (2005) examined parafoveal lexical processing by presenting in the parafovea emotionally-laden words (many of them were obscene or curse words), emotionally neutral words, or identical words. Identical previews resulted in shorter gaze durations on the target word than the other two conditions when the target was subsequently foveated. More importantly, however, there was no effect of emotionality, which indicates that the preview word was not identified parafoveally.

There is yet another way to assess parafoveal lexical-semantic processing that makes use of the data on word skipping (i.e. reading a word without fixating on it). The underlying logic here is that when a word is skipped, it is identified parafoveally when their eyes are fixating a previous word. Brysbaert et al. (2005) have provided an informative review of the relevant studies. They identified eight studies where the frequency of the parafoveal word was manipulated. In all studies skipping rate was higher or equal for frequent than infrequent parafoveal words. However, the overall difference in skipping rate is rather small (5%), and it is slightly greater for short than long words (see also a recent study of White, 2008). As for contextual predictability, Brysbaert et al. identified 15 studies that all showed the skipping rate to be larger for predictable than less predictable words. The overall difference amounted to 8%. Thus, the studies examining word skipping provide clearer evidence for parafoveal lexical-semantic processing than the other studies cited above. Note that other phenomena related to word skipping (e.g. prolonged fixation times prior to skipping) is beyond the scope of the present chapter. An interested reader should consult the review of Brysbaert et. al. (2005), studies by Drieghe and colleagues (Drieghe, 2008; Drieghe et al., 2004, 2005, 2007) and that of White et al. (2005a) and Kliegl and Engbert (2005).

Morphological structure

The evidence to support the notion of parafoveal morphological processing in alphabetic languages is meagre; however, the notion has obtained support in non-alphabetic languages. Lima (1987) and Kambe (2004) failed to find evidence in English for parafoveal morphological processing of prefixed words (e.g. *revive*). The same was true for parafoveal morphological processing of two-noun compound words (e.g. *cowboy*) either in English (Inhoff, 1989b; Juhasz et al., 2008) or in Finnish (Bertram and Hyönä, 2007). For example, Juhasz et al. (2008, Experiment 4) did not observe a greater preview benefit for incorrectly previewed compounds (*pop corn*) than for incorrectly previewed (a space was inserted in the middle of the word) monomorphemic words containing a pseudo-lexeme in the beginning (*dip loma*). On the other hand, Deutsch et al. (2003) found evidence for parafoveal morphological processing in Hebrew. They studied the processing of Hebrew nouns that consist of the root morpheme carrying the core meaning of the word and the word pattern defining the grammatical features of the word. These two components are interwoven into each other so that the word's morphological structure is orthographically non-transparent. In the study, they provided three types of parafoveal previews for the target nouns: identical, morphological related (the preview and the target were derivations of the same root) and orthographic control (the preview and the target were derived from different roots). Both the identical and the morphological related preview yielded shorter gaze durations on the target than the orthographic control condition; moreover, the identical and the morphologically related previews did not differ significantly from each other. Thus, the data lend clear support for a morphological preview benefit in Hebrew.

Yen et al. (2008) investigated the processing of Chinese two-character compound words. In Experiment 2, they provided three types of previews of the second character (in relation to the target word): same-morpheme preview (the compound meaning was nevertheless different between the previewed and the target compound), different-morpheme preview, and pseudoword preview. The invisible boundary was set in the space to the left of the first character (which was always kept intact). Yen et al. obtained significantly shorter gaze durations on the second character for the same-morpheme previews than for the pseudoword previews, while the different-morpheme preview did not differ from the pseudoword preview. This finding is taken as evidence for parafoveal morphological processing in Chinese.

Effect of foveal load

Parafoveal word processing is also found to be affected by the relative difficulty of processing the foveal word. Henderson and Ferreira (1990) varied the foveal processing difficulty by manipulating the frequency (Experiment 1) and the syntactic complexity (Experiment 2) of the foveal word. The degree of parafoveal processing was assessed by the observed difference between the identical preview and two non-word previews (orthographically similar or dissimilar to the target). In both experiments, less parafoveal information was acquired when foveal processing was difficult. This finding suggests that the parafoveal attentional span is constrained by foveal processing difficulty. That is, when increased attentional resources are required for foveal processing, relatively less is left for parafoveal processing. Kennison and Clifton (1995) replicated this effect but only for trials for which the location of the final fixation was close to the parafoveal word. White et al. (2005b), on the other hand, observed the foveal difficulty effect for participants who did not become aware of the display change, but not for participants who noticed the change (these participants were excluded from the Henderson and Ferreira study). The source of these individual differences is still unknown.

Parafoveal processing within and across words

There is evidence to support the view that parafoveal processing is carried out to a greater extent within one long compound word than across two short words (Hyönä et al., 2004; Juhasz et al., 2009). The preview effect in gaze duration obtained by Juhasz et al. obtained in Experiment 1 for unspaced compound words (e.g. *basketball*) was about double the size than that for spaced compound words (e.g. *tennis ball*). Thus, it appears readers attend more 'strongly' to a spatially unified visual object (an unspaced compound) than to two spatially separate objects. This 'stronger attention' may either mean swift shifting of visual attention from the first compound word component to the second and/or attempt to process in parallel all letters within a spatially unified word object.

Parafoveal processing seems to be limited to the word to the right of fixation (when reading from left to right), and may extend to word $n+2$ when word $n+1$ is very short (2–3 letters; Kliegl et al., 2007; Risse et al., 2008) but not when word $n+1$ is 4 letters or longer (Angele et al., 2008). On the other hand, readers do not obtain useful visual information of the word to the left of fixation (Rayner et al., 1980) or the information intake is rather limited (Binder et al., 1999), which suggests that English readers' perceptual span is asymmetric to the right. When reading from right to left, the perceptual span is asymmetric to the left (Pollatsek et al., 1981); in vertical reading of Japanese, more information is gleaned from the text appearing below than above the current fixation (Osaka, 1993).

Summary of the observed effects

The present chapter has reviewed the eye movement literature on foveal and parafoveal word processing during reading. A number of features have been found to affect foveal and parafoveal word processing.

Table 45.1 Summary of evidence for foveal and parafoveal effects

	Foveal processing	Parafoveal processing
Location of initial fixation	Yes	N/a
Word length	Yes	Yes
Orthographic coding	Yes	Yes
Phonological coding	Yes	Yes
Word frequency	Yes	Mixed
Age of acquisition	Yes	?
Word meaning	Yes	Mixed
Morphological structure	Yes	Mixed (language-dependent?)
Contextual predictability	Yes	Mixed

These effects are summarized in Table 45.1.The following picture emerges from the reviewed studies. When a word in a text is fixated, identities of letters and their corresponding phonemes are activated early during the fixation. Word-external (particularly word-initial) letters are activated more strongly than word-internal letters. Moreover, consonants are activated earlier than vowels. If the word consists of several letters, the likelihood is increased that a refixation is made on the word (also fixation duration may be lengthened). Orthographic and phonological coding give rise to lexical and meaning activation, which is also reflected in fixation times on words: Words that the reader has seldom seen in print require more foveal fixation time than words (s)he is frequently exposed to. Moreover, meaning activation for words containing two meanings requires more fixation time than that for single-meaning words. When the word is morphologically complex, its identification takes place via the constituent morphemes, particularly when the word is long. Finally, words that are highly predictable from previous discourse context are fixated for less time than non-predictable words. This fixation time difference is likely to reflect both lexical access and meaning integration.

As regards parafoveal processing, the research shows that lower-level visual features, such as the length and the visual shape of words, are extracted during reading. Moreover, readers also gain orthographic and phonological information from the parafoveal word. Word-external (particularly word-initial) letters are perceived better than word-internal letters. Phonological coding is also carried out for parafoveal words. On the other hand, the evidence for parafoveal processing of lexical (including morphological) and semantic information is equivocal and inconclusive. It seems lexical and semantic parafoveal processing is not standardly achieved. It remains for the future studies to disentangle the conditions under which parafoveal lexical-semantic processing is possible. Greater care should also be taken to guarantee that the non-fixated word really lies outside the foveal boundaries. Finally, studies show that more parafoveal processing is done within a long word than across two short words and that parafoveal processing is limited to the word to the right of fixation (when reading from left to right) unless the parafoveal word is very short, in which case also features of word $n+2$ may be parafoveally processed.

References

Altarriba, J., Kambe, G., Pollatsek, A., and Rayner, K. (2001). Semantic codes are not used in integrating information across eye fixations in reading: Evidence from fluent Spanish- English bilinguals. *Perception and Psychophysics,* **63**, 875–890.

Andrews, S., Miller, B., and Rayner, K. (2004). Eye movements and morphological segmentation of compound words: There is a mouse in mousetrap. *European Journal of Cognitive Psychology,* **16**, 285–311.

Angele, B., Slattery, T.J., Yang, J., Kliegl, R., and Rayner, K. (2008). Parafoveal processing in reading: Manipulating n+1 and n+2 previews simultaneously. *Visual Cognition,* **16**, 697–707.

Ashby, J. and Clifton, C. Jr (2005). The prosodic property of lexical stress affects eye movements during silent reading. *Cognition,* **96**, B89–B100.

Ashby, J., Rayner, K., and Clifton, C. (2005). Eye movements of highly skilled and average readers: Differential effects of frequency and predictability. *Quarterly Journal of Experimental Psychology*, **58A**, 1065–1086.

Ashby, J., Treiman, R., Kessler, B., and Rayner, K. (2006). Vowel processing during silent reading: Evidence from eye movements. *Journal of Experimental Psychology: Learning, Memory, and Cognition*, **32**, 416–424.

Balota, D.A., Pollatsek, A., and Rayner, K. (1985). The interaction of contextual constraints and parafoveal visual information in reading. *Cognitive Psychology*, **17**, 364–390.

Bertram, R. and Hyönä, J. (2003). The length of a complex word modifies the role of morphological structure: Evidence from eye movements when reading short and long Finnish compounds. *Journal of Memory and Language*, **48**, 615–634.

Bertram, R. and Hyönä, J. (2007). The interplay between parafoveal preview and morphological processing in reading. In R.G. van Gompel, M.H. Fischer, W.S. Murray and R.L. Hill (eds.) *Eye movements: A window on mind and brain* (pp. 391–407). Oxford: Elsevier Science.

Binder, K.S. and Morris, R.K. (1995). Eye movements and lexical ambiguity resolution: Effects of prior encounter and discourse topic. *Journal of Experimental Psychology: Learning, Memory, and Cognition*, **21**, 1186–1196.

Binder, K.S., Pollatsek, A., and Rayner, K. (1999). Extraction of information to the left of the fixated word in reading. *Journal of Experimental Psychology: Human Perception and Performance*, **25**, 1162–1172.

Briihl, D. and Inhoff, A.W. (1995). Integrating information across fixations during reading: The use of orthographic bodies and exterior letters. *Journal of Experimental Psychology: Learning, Memory, and Cognition*, **21**, 55–67.

Brysbaert, M., Drieghe, D., and Vitu, F. (2005). Word skipping: Implications for theories of eye movement control in reading. In G. Underwood (ed.) *Cognitive processes in eye guidance* (pp. 53–77). Oxford, UK: Oxford University Press.

Calvo, M.G. and Meseguer, E. (2002). Eye movements and processing stages in reading: Relative contribution of visual, lexical and contextual factors. *Spanish Journal of Psychology*, **5**, 66–77.

Calvo, M.G., Meseguer, E., and Carreiras, M. (2001). Inferences about predictable events: Eye movements during reading. *Psychological Research*, **65**, 158–169.

Carpenter, P.A. and Just, M.A. (1983). What your eyes do while your mind is reading. In K. Rayner (ed.) *Eye movements in reading: Perceptual and language processes* (pp. 275–307). New York: Academic Press.

Carreiras, M., Perea, M., and Grainger, J. (1997). Effects of the orthographic neighborhood in visual word recognition: Cross-task comparisons. *Journal of Experimental Psychology: Learning, Memory, and Cognition*, **23**, 857–871.

Cauchard, F., Eyrolle, H., Cellier, J.M., and Hyönä, J. (2010). Visual signals vertically extend the perceptual span in searching a text: A gaze-contingent window study. *Discourse Processes*, **47**, 617–640.

Chace, K.H., Rayner, K., and Well, A.D. (2005). Eye movements and phonological parafoveal preview: Effects of reading skill. *Canadian Journal of Experimental Psychology*, **59**, 209–217.

Chaffin, R., Morris, R.K., and Seely, R.E. (2001). Learning new word meanings from context: A study of eye movements. *Journal of Experimental Psychology: Learning, Memory, and Cognition*, **27**, 225–235.

Clifton, C., Jr, Staub, A., and Rayner, K. (2007). Eye movements in reading words and sentences. In R.G. van Gompel, M.H. Fischer, W.S. Murray and R.L. Hill (eds.) *Eye movements: A window on mind and brain* (pp. 341–371). Oxford: Elsevier Science.

Daneman, M., and Reingold, E. (1993). What eye fixations tell us about phonological recoding during reading. *Canadian Journal of Experimental Psychology*, **47**, 153–178.

Daneman, M., Reingold, E., and Davidson, M. (1995). Time course of phonological activation during reading: Evidence from eye fixations. *Journal of Experimental Psychology: Learning, Memory, and Cognition*, **21**, 884–898.

Deutsch, A., Frost, R., Pelleg, S., Pollatsek, A., and Rayner, K. (2003). Early morphological effects in reading: Evidence from parafoveal preview benefit in Hebrew. *Psychonomic Bulletin and Review*, **10**, 415–422.

Dopkins, S., Morris, R.K., and Rayner, K. (1992). Lexical ambiguity and eye fixations in reading: A test of competing models of lexical ambiguity resolution. *Journal of Memory and Language*, **31**, 461–477.

Drieghe, D. (2008). Foveal processing and word skipping in reading. *Psychonomic Bulletin and Review*, **15**, 856–860.

Drieghe, D., Rayner, K., and Pollatsek, A. (2005). Eye movements and word skipping during reading revisited. *Journal of Experimental Psychology: Human Perception and Performance*, **31**, 954–969.

Drieghe, D., Desmet, T., and Brysbaert, M. (2007). How important and linguistic factors in word skipping during reading? *British Journal of Psychology*, **98**, 157–171.

Drieghe, D., Brysbaert, M., Desmet, T., and De Baecke, C. (2004). Word skipping in reading: On the interplay of linguistic and visual factors. *European Journal of Cognitive Psychology*, **16**, 79–103.

Duffy, S.A., Morris, R.K., and Rayner, K. (1988). Lexical ambiguity and fixation times in reading. *Journal of Memory and Language*, **27**, 429–446.

Duffy, S.A., Kambe, G., and Rayner, K. (2001). The effect of prior disambiguating context on the comprehension of ambiguous words: Evidence from eye movements. In D. S. Gorfein (ed.) *On the consequences of meaning selection: Perspectives on resolving lexical ambiguity* (pp. 27–43). Washington, DC: American Psychological Association.

Ehrlich, S.F. and Rayner, K. (1981). Contextual effects on word perception and eye movements during reading. *Journal of Verbal Learning and Verbal Behavior*, **20**, 641–655.

Folk, J.R. and Morris, R.K. (1995). Multiple lexical codes in reading: Evidence from eye movements, naming time, and oral reading. *Journal of Experimental Psychology: Learning, Memory, and Cognition*, **21**, 1412–1429.

Frisson, S., Rayner, K., and Pickering, M.J. (2005). Effects of contextual predictability and transitional probability on eye movements during reading. *Journal of Experimental Psychology: Learning, Memory, and Cognition*, 31, 862–877.

Frost, R. (1998). Toward a strong phonological theory of visual word recognition: True issues and false trails. *Psychological Bulletin*, 123, 71–99.

Häikiö, T., Bertram, R., Hyönä, J., and Niemi, P. (2009). Development of the letter identity span in reading: Evidence from the eye movement moving window paradigm. *Journal of Experimental Child Psychology*, 102, 167–181.

Hand, C., O'Donnell, P., and Sereno, S. (2008). Clown vs. dwarf: Every little bit helps. Poster presented at the 49th Annual Meeting of the Psychonomic Society, November 13–16, Chicago, IL.

Henderson, J.M. and Ferreira, F. (1990). Effects of foveal processing difficulty on the perceptual span in reading: Implications for attention and eye movement control. *Journal of Experimental Psychology: Learning, Memory, and Cognition*, 16, 417–429.

Henderson, J.M. and Ferreira, F. (1993). Eye movement control during reading: Fixation measures reflect foveal but not parafoveal processing difficulty. *Canadian Journal of Experimental Psychology*, 47, 201–221.

Henderson, J.M., Dixon, P., Petersen, A., Twilley, L.C., and Ferreira, F. (1995). Evidence for the use of phonological representations during transsaccadic word recognition. *Journal of Experimental Psychology: Human Perception and Performance*, 21, 82–97.

Hyönä, J. (1993). Effects of thematic and lexical priming on readers' eye movements. *Scandinavian Journal of Psychology*, 34, 293–304.

Hyönä, J. and Bertram, R. (2004). Do frequency characteristics of non-fixated words influence the processing of non-fixated words during reading? *European Journal of Cognitive Psychology*, 16, 104–127.

Hyönä, J. and Häikiö, T. (2005). Is emotional content obtained from parafoveal words during reading? An eye movement analysis. *Scandinavian Journal of Psychology*, 46, 475–483.

Hyönä, J. and Olson, R.K. (1995). Eye fixation patterns among dyslexic and normal readers: Effects of word length and word frequency. *Journal of Experimental Psychology: Learning, Memory, and Cognition*, 21, 1430–1440.

Hyönä, J. and Pollatsek, A. (1998). The role of component morphemes on eye fixations when reading Finnish compound words. *Journal of Experimental Psychology: Human Perception and Performance*, 24, 1612–1627.

Hyönä, J., Bertram, R., and Pollatsek, A. (2004). Are long compound words identified serially via their constituents? Evidence from an eye-movement contingent display change study. *Memory and Cognition*, 32, 523–532.

Inhoff, A.W. (1989a). Parafoveal processing of words and saccade computation during eye fixations in reading. *Journal of Experimental Psychology: Human Perception and Performance*, 15, 544–555.

Inhoff, A.W. (1989b). Lexical access during eye fixations in reading: Are word access codes used to integrate lexical information across interword fixations? *Journal of Memory and Language*, 28, 444–461.

Inhoff, A.W. and Rayner, K. (1986). Parafoveal word processing during eye fixations in reading: Effects of word frequency. *Perception and Psychophysics*, 40, 431–439.

Inhoff, A.W., Starr, M., and Shindler, K.L. (2000a). Is the processing of words during eye fixations in reading strictly serial? *Perception and Psychophysics*, 62, 1474–1484.

Inhoff, A.W., Starr, M., Liu, W., and Wang, J. (1998). Eye-movement-contingent display changes are not compromised by flicker and phosphor persistence. *Psychonomic Bulletin and Review*, 5, 101–106.

Inhoff, A.W., Radach, R., Starr, M., and Greenberg, S. (2000b). Allocation of visuo-spatial attention and saccade programming during reading. In A. Kennedy, R. Radach, D. Heller and J. Pynte (eds), *Reading as a perceptual process* (pp. 221–246). Oxford: Elsevier.

Inhoff, A.W., Radach, R., Eiter, B.M., and Juhasz, B. (2003). Distinct subsystems for the parafoveal processing of spatial and linguistic information during eye fixations in reading. *Quarterly Journal of Experimental Psychology*, 56A, 803–827.

Johnson, R.L., Perea, M., and Rayner, K. (2007) Transposed-letter effects in reading: Evidence from eye movements and parafoveal preview. *Journal of Experimental Psychology: Human Perception and Performance*, 33, 209–229.

Juhasz, B.J. (2008). The processing of compound words in English: Effects of word length on eye movements during reading. *Language and Cognitive Processes*, 23, 1057–1088.

Juhasz, B.J. and Rayner, K. (2003). Investigating the effects of a set of intercorrelated variables on eye fixation durations in reading. *Journal of Experimental Psychology: Learning, Memory, and Cognition*, 29, 1312–1318.

Juhasz, B.J. and Rayner, K. (2006). The role of age of acquisition and word frequency in reading: Evidence from eye fixation durations. *Visual Cognition*, 13, 846–863.

Juhasz, B.J., Starr, M., Inhoff, A.W., and Placke, L. (2003). The effects of morphology on the processing of compound words: Evidence from naming, lexical decisions, and eye fixations. *British Journal of Psychology*, 94, 223–244.

Juhasz, B.J., White, S.J., Liversedge, S.P., and Rayner, K. (2008) Eye movements and the use of parafoveal word length information in reading. *Journal of Experimental Psychology: Human Perception and Performance*, 34, 1560–1579.

Juhasz, B.J., Pollatsek, A., Hyönä, J., Drieghe, D., and Rayner, K. (2009). Parafoveal processing within and between words. *Quarterly Journal of Experimental Psychology*, 62, 1356–1376.

Just, M.A. and Carpenter, P.A. (1980). A theory of reading: From eye fixations to comprehension. *Psychological Review*, 87, 329–354.

Kambe, G. (2004). Parafoveal processing of prefixed words during eye fixations in reading: Evidence against morphological influences on parafoveal preprocessing. *Perception and Psychophysics*, 66, 279–292.

Kennedy, A. (1998). The influence of parafoveal words on foveal inspection time: Evidence for a processing trade off. In G. Underwood (ed.) *Eye guidance in reading and scene perception* (pp. 149–179). Oxford, England: Elsevier.

Kennedy, A. (2000). Attention allocation in reading: Sequential or parallel? In A. Kennedy, R. Radach, D. Heller and J. Pynte (eds.) *Reading as a perceptual process* (pp. 193–220). Oxford, UK: Elsevier.

Kennedy, A. and Pynte, J. (2005). Parafoveal-on-foveal effects in normal reading. *Vision Research*, **45**, 153–168.

Kennedy, A., Pynte, J., and Ducrot, S. (2002). Parafoveal-on-foveal interactions in word recognition. *Quarterly Journal of Experimental Psychology*, **55A**, 1307–1337.

Kennison, S.M. and Clifton. C. (1995). Determinants of parafoveal preview benefit in high and low working memory capacity readers: Implications for eye movement control. *Journal of Experimental Psychology: Learning, Memory, and Cognition*, **21**, 68–81.

Kliegl, R. and Engbert, R. (2005). Fixation durations before word skipping in reading. *Psychonomic Bulletin and Review*, **12**, 132–138.

Kliegl, R., Nuthmann, A., and Engbert, R. (2006). Tracking the mind during reading: The influence of past, present, and future words on fixation durations. *Journal of Experimental Psychology: General*, **135**, 12–35.

Kliegl, R., Risse, S., and Laubrock, J. (2007). Preview benefit and parafoveal-on-foveal effects from word n + 2. *Journal of Experimental Psychology: Human Perception and Performance*, **33**, 1250–1255.

Kliegl, R. Grabner, E., Rolfs, M., and Engbert, R. (2004). Length, frequency, and predictability effects of words on eye movements in reading. *European Journal of Cognitive Psychology*, **16**, 262–284.

Lee, H.W., Rayner, K., and Pollatsek, A. (2001). The relative contribution of consonants and vowels to word identification during silent reading. *Journal of Memory and Language*, **44**, 189–205.

Lee, H.W., Rayner, K., and Pollatsek, A. (2002). The processing of consonants and vowels in reading: Evidence from the fast-priming paradigm. *Psychonomic Bulletin and Review*, **9**, 766–772.

Lee, Y.-A., Binder, K.S., Kim, J.O., Pollatsek, A., and Rayner, K. (1999). Activation of phonological codes during eye fixations in reading. *Journal of Experimental Psychology: Human Perception and Performance*, **25**, 948–964.

Legge, G.E., Klitz, T.S., and Tjan, B.S. (1997). Mr Chips: An ideal-observer model of reading. *Psychological Review*, **104**, 524–553.

Lima, S.D. (1987). Morphological analysis in sentence reading. *Journal of Memory and Language*, **26**, 84–99.

Lima, S.D. and Inhoff, A.W. (1985). Lexical access during eye fixations in reading: Effects of word-initial letter sequences. *Journal of Experimental Psychology: Human Perception and Performance*, **11**, 272–285.

Liu, W., Inhoff, A.W., Ye, Y., and Wu, C. (2002). Use of parafoveally visible characters during the reading of Chinese sentences. *Journal of Experimental Psychology: Human Perception and Performance*, **28**, 1213–1227.

Liversedge, S.P., Rayner, K., White, S.J., Vergilino-Perez, D., Findlay, J.M., and Kentridge, R.W. (2004). Eye movements when reading disappearing text: Is there a gap effect in reading? *Vision Research*, **44**, 1013–1024.

McConkie, G.W. and Rayner, K. (1975). The span of effective stimulus during a fixation in reading. *Perception and Psychophysics*, **17**, 578–586.

McConkie, G.W., Kerr, P.W., Reddix, M.D., Zola, D., and Jacobs, A.M. (1989). Eye movement control during reading: II. Frequency of refixating a word. *Perception and Psychophysics*, **46**, 245–253.

McDonald, S.A. (2006). Effects of number-of-letters on eye movements during reading are independent from effects of spatial word length. *Visual Cognition*, **13**, 89–98.

Miellet, S. and Sparrow, L. (2004). Phonological codes are assembled before word fixation: Evidence from boundary paradigm in sentence reading. *Brain and Language*, **90**, 299–310.

Morris, R.K. (1994). Lexical and message-level sentence context effects on fixation times in reading. *Journal of Experimental Psychology: Learning, Memory, and Cognition*, **20**, 92–103.

Murray, W.S. (1998). Parafoveal pragmatics. In G. Underwood (ed.) *Eye guidance in reading and scene perception* (pp. 181–200). Oxford, England: Elsevier.

Murray, W. and Rowan, M. (1998). Early, mandatory, pragmatic processing. *Journal of Psycholinguistic Research*, **27**, 1–22.

Niswander-Klement, E. and Pollatsek, A. (2006). The effects of root frequency, word frequency, and length on the processing of prefixed English words during reading. *Memory and Cognition*, **34**, 685–702.

Nuthmann, A., Engbert, R., and Kliegl, R. (2005). Mislocated fixations during reading and the inverted optimal viewing position effect. *Vision Research*, **45**, 2201–2217.

Nuthmann, A., Engbert, R., and Kliegl, R. (2007). The IOVP effect in mindless reading: Experiment and modeling. *Vision Research*, **47**, 990–1002.

O'Regan, J.K., Lévy-Schoen, A., Pynte, J., and Brugaillere, B. (1984). Convenient fixation location within isolated words of different lengths and structure. *Journal of Experimental Psychology: Human Perception and Performance*, **10**, 250–257.

Osaka, N. (1993). Asymmetry of the effective visual field in vertical reading as measured with a moving window. In G. d'Ydewalle and J. Van Rensbergen (eds.) *Perception and cognition: Advances in eye movement research* (pp. 275–283). Amsterdam: North-Holland.

Perea, M. and Pollatsek, A. (1998). The effects of neighborhood frequency in reading and lexical decision. *Journal of Experimental Psychology: Human Perception and Performance*, **24**, 767–779.

Pollatsek, A. and Hyönä, J. (2006). Processing of morphologically complex words in context: What can be learned from eye movements. In S. Andrews (Ed.), *From inkmarks to ideas: Current issues in lexical processing* (pp. 275–298). Hove: Psychology Press.

Pollatsek, A., Perea, M., and Binder, K.S. (1999). The effects of 'neighborhood size' in reading and lexical decision. *Journal of Experimental Psychology: Human Perception and Performance*, 25, 1142–1158.

Pollatsek, A. Hyönä, J., and Bertram, R. (2000a). The role of morphological constituents in reading Finnish compound words. *Journal of Experimental Psychology: Human Perception and Performance*, 26, 820–833.

Pollatsek, A., Tan, L.H., and Rayner, K. (2000b). The role of phonological codes in integrating information across saccadic eye movements in Chinese character identification. *Journal of Experimental Psychology: Human Perception and Performance*, 26, 607–633.

Pollatsek, A., Bolozky, S., Well, A.D., and Rayner, K. (1981). Asymmetries in the perceptual span for Israeli readers. *Brain and Language*, 14, 174–180.

Pollatsek, A., Lesch, M., Morris, R.K., and Rayner, K. (1992). Phonological codes are used in integrating information across saccades in word identification and reading. *Journal of Experimental Psychology: Human Perception and Performance*, 18, 148–162.

Pynte, J. and Kennedy, A. (2006). An influence over eye movements in reading exerted from beyond the level of the word: Evidence from reading English and French. *Vision Research*, 46, 3786–3801.

Pynte, J., Kennedy, A., and Ducrot, S. (2004). The influence of parafoveal typographical errors in eye movements in reading. *European Journal of Cognitive Psychology*, 16, 178–202.

Raney, G.E., and Rayner, K. (1995). Word frequency effects and eye movements during two readings of a text. *Canadian Journal of Experimental Psychology*, 49, 151–173.

Rayner, K. (1975). The perceptual span and peripheral cues in reading. *Cognitive Psychology*, 7, 65–81.

Rayner, K. (1979). Eye guidance in reading: Fixation locations within words. *Perception*, 8, 21–30.

Rayner, K. (1986). Eye movements and the perceptual span in beginning and skilled readers. *Journal of Experimental Child Psychology*, 41, 211–236.

Rayner, K. (1998). Eye movements in reading and information processing: 20 years of research. *Psychological Bulletin*, 124, 372–422.

Rayner, K. and Bertera, J.H. (1979). Reading without a fovea. *Science*, 206, 468–469.

Rayner, K. and Duffy, S.A. (1986). Lexical complexity and fixation times in reading: Effects of word frequency, verb complexity, and lexical ambiguity. *Memory and Cognition*, 14, 191–201.

Rayner, K. and Frazier, L. (1989). Selection mechanisms in reading lexically ambiguous words. *Journal of Experimental Psychology: Learning, Memory, and Cognition*, 15, 779–790.

Rayner, K. and Raney, G.E. (1996). Eye movement control in reading and visual search: Effects of word frequency. *Psychonomic Bulletin and Review*, 3, 238–244.

Rayner, K. and Well, A.D. (1996). Effects of contextual constraint on eye movements in reading: A further examination. *Psychonomic Bulletin and Review*, 3, 504–509.

Rayner, K., Well, A.D., and Pollatsek, A. (1980). Asymmetry of the effective visual field in reading. *Perception and Psychophysics*, 27, 537–544.

Rayner, K., Balota, D.A., and Pollatsek, A. (1986). Against parafoveal semantic preprocessing during eye fixations in reading. *Canadian Journal of Psychology*, 40, 473–483.

Rayner, K., Pacht, J.M., and Duffy, S.A. (1994). Effects of prior encounter and global discourse bias on the processing of lexically ambiguous words: Evidence from eye fixations. *Journal of Memory and Language*, 33, 527–544.

Rayner, K., Sereno, S.C., and Raney, G.E. (1996). Eye movement control in reading: A comparison of two types of models. *Journal of Experimental Psychology: Human Perception and Performance*, 22, 1188–1200.

Rayner, K., Pollatsek, A., and Binder, K.S. (1998a). Phonological codes and eye movements in reading. *Journal of Experimental Psychology: Learning, Memory, and Cognition*, 24, 476–497.

Rayner, K., Fischer, M.H., and Pollatsek, A. (1998b). Unspaced text interferes with both word identification and eye movement control. *Vision Research*, 38, 1129–1144.

Rayner, K., Juhasz, B.J., and Brown, S.J. (2007). Do readers obtain preview benefit from word n + 2? A test of serial attention shift versus distributed lexical processing models of eye movement control in reading. *Journal of Experimental Psychology: Human Perception and Performance*, 33, 230–245.

Rayner, K., Well, A.D., Pollatsek, A., and Bertera, J.H. (1982). The availability of useful information to the right of fixation in reading. *Perception and Psychophysics*, 31, 537–550.

Rayner, K., Sereno, S.C., Lesch, M.F., and Pollatsek, A. (1995). Phonological codes are automatically activated during reading: Evidence from an eye movement priming paradigm. *Psychological Science*, 6, 26–32.

Rayner, K., Ashby, J., Pollatsek, A., and Reichle, E.D. (2004a). The effects of frequency and predictability on eye fixations in reading: Implications for the E-Z reader model. *Journal of Experimental Psychology: Human Perception and Performance*, 30, 720–732.

Rayner, K., Warren, T., Juhasz, B.J., and Liversedge, S.P. (2004b). The effect of plausibility on eye movements in reading. *Journal of Experimental Psychology: Learning, Memory, and Cognition*, 30, 1290–1301.

Rayner, K., Inhoff, A.W., Morrison, R., Slowiaczek, M.L., and Bertera, J.H. (1981). Masking of foveal and parafoveal vision during eye fixations in reading. *Journal of Experimental Psychology: Human Perception and Performance*, 7, 167–179.

Rayner, K., White, S.J., Kambe, G., Miller, B., and Liversedge, S.P. (2003). On the processing of meaning from parafoveal vision during eye fixations in reading. In J. Hyönä, R. Radach and H. Deubel (eds.) *The mind's eye: Cognitive and applied aspects of eye movement research* (pp. 213–234). Amsterdam: Elsevier.

Risse, S., Engbert, R., and Kliegl, R. (2008). Eye movement control in reading: Experimental and corpus-analysis challenges for a computational model. In K. Rayner, D. Shen, X. Bai and G. Yan (eds.) *Cognitive and cultural influences on eye movements* (pp. 65–91). Tianjin: Tianjin People's Publishing Company.

Schilling, H.E.H., Rayner, K., and Chumbley, J.I. (1998). Comparing naming, lexical decision, and eye fixation times: Word frequency effects and individual differences. *Memory and Cognition*, 26, 1270–1281.

Schroyens, W., Vitu, F., Brysbaert, M., and d'Ydewalle, G. (1999). Eye movement control during reading: Foveal load and parafoveal processing. *Quarterly Journal of Experimental Psychology*, 52(A), 1021–1046.

Schustack, M., Ehrlich, S.F., and Rayner, K. (1987). Local and global sources of contextual facilitation in reading. *Journal of Memory and Language*, 26, 322–340.

Sears, C.R., Campbell, C.R., and Lupker, S.J. (2006). Is there a neighborhood frequency effect in English? Evidence from reading and lexical decision. *Journal of Experimental Psychology: Human Perception and Performance*, 32, 1040–1062.

Sereno, S.C. (1995). Resolution of lexical ambiguity: Evidence from an eye movement priming paradigm. *Journal of Experimental Psychology: Learning, Memory, and Cognition*, 21, 582–595.

Sereno, S.C. and Rayner, K. (1992). Fast priming during eye fixations in reading. *Journal of Experimental Psychology: Human Perception and Performance*, 18, 173–184.

Sereno, S.C. and Rayner, K. (2000). Spelling-sound regularity effects on eye fixations in reading. *Perception and Psychophysics*, 62, 402–409.

Sereno, S.C., Pacht, J.M., and Rayner, K. (1992). The effect of meaning frequency on processing lexically ambiguous words: Evidence from eye fixations. *Psychological Science*, 3, 296–300.

Sparrow, L. and Miellet, S. (2002). Activation of phonological codes during reading: Evidence from errors detection and eye movements. *Brain and Language*, 81, 509–516.

Starr, M.S., and Inhoff, A.W. (2004). Attention allocation to the right and left of a fixated word: Use of orthographic information from multiple words during reading. *European Journal of Cognitive Psychology*, 16, 203–225.

Tsai, J., Lee, C., Tzeng, O.J.L., Hung, D.L., and Yen, N. (2004). Use of phonological codes for Chinese characters: Evidence from processing of parafoveal preview when reading sentences. *Brain and Language*, 91, 235–244.

Underwood, G., Bloomfield, R., and Clews, S. (1988). Information influences the pattern of eye fixations during sentence comprehension. *Perception*, 17, 267–278.

Underwood, G., Binns, A., and Walker, S. (2000). Attentional demands on the processing of neighbouring words. In A Kennedy, R. Radach and D. Heller (eds.) *Reading as a perceptual process* (pp. 247–268). Amsterdam: North-Holland.

Vainio, S., Hyönä, J., and Pajunen, A. (2009). Lexical predictability exerts robust effects on fixation duration, but not on initial landing position during reading. *Experimental Psychology*, 56, 66–74.

Vitu, F., O'Regan, J.K., and Mittau, M. (1990). Optimal landing position in reading isolated words and continuous text. *Perception and Psychophysics*, 47, 583–600.

Vitu, F., McConkie, G.W., Kerr, P., and O'Regan, J.K. (2001). Fixation location effects on fixation durations during reading: An inverted optimal viewing position effect. *Vision Research*, 41, 3513–3533.

Vitu, F., Lancelin, D., and Marrier d'Unienville, V. (2007). A perceptual-economy account for the inverted-optimal viewing position effect. *Journal of Experimental Psychology: Human Perception and Performance*, 33, 1220–1249.

White, S.J. (2008). Eye movement control during reading: Effects of word frequency and orthographic familiarity. *Journal of Experimental Psychology: Human Perception and Performance*, 34, 205–223.

White, S.J. and Liversedge, S.P. (2004). Orthographic familiarity influences initial eye fixation positions in reading. *European Journal of Cognitive Psychology*, 16, 52–78.

White, S.J. and Liversedge, S. (2006). Foveal processing difficulty does not modulate non-foveal orthographic influences on fixation positions. *Vision Research*, 46, 426–437.

White, S.J., Rayner, K., and Liversedge, S.P. (2005a). The influence of parafoveal word length and contextual constraints on fixation durations and word skipping in reading. *Psychonomic Bulletin and Review*, 12, 466–471.

White, S.J., Rayner, K., and Liversedge, S.P. (2005b). Eye movements and the modulation of parafoveal processing by foveal processing difficulty: A re-examination. *Psychonomic Bulletin and Review*, 12, 891–896.

White, S.J., Bertram, R., and Hyönä, J. (2008b). Semantic processing of previews within compound words. *Journal of Experimental Psychology: Learning, Memory and Cognition*, 34, 988–993.

White, S.J., Johnson, R.L., Liversedge, S.P., and Rayner, K. (2008a). Eye movements when reading transposed text: The importance of word beginning letters. *Journal of Experimental Psychology: Human Perception and Performance*, 34, 1261–1276.

Williams, C.C., Perea, M., Pollatsek, A., and Rayner, K. (2006). Previewing the neighborhood: The role of orthographic neighbors as parafoveal previews in reading. *Journal of Experimental Psychology: Human Perception and Performance*, **32**, 1072–1082.

Yates, M., Friend, J., and Ploetz, D. (2008). Phonological neighbors influence word naming through the least supported phoneme. *Journal of Experimental Psychology: Human Perception and Performance*, **34**, 1599–1608.

Yen, M.-H., Tsai, J.-L., Tzeng, O.J.-L., and Hung, D.L. (2008). Eye movements and parafoveal word processing in reading Chinese. *Memory and Cognition*, **36**, 1033–1045.

CHAPTER 46

Parafoveal-on-foveal effects on eye movements during reading

Denis Drieghe

Abstract

Parafoveal-on-foveal effects refer to the possibility that processing of the parafoveal word can influence the fixation durations on the foveal word during reading. In this chapter, I will review the literature of studies examining this issue. Effects observed in reading-like tasks have been questioned on methodological grounds with regards to the generalizability to normal reading. The clearest evidence for the existence of parafoveal-on-foveal effects comes from experiments allowing tight control over the stimuli but restricting the observations to fixation locations very close to the parafoveal word, and from corpus studies showing reliable but numerically small effects. I will make the claim that with regards to taking reported parafoveal-on-foveal effects as evidence for parallel lexical processing, the jury is still out. The argument is that as long as parafoveal-on-foveal effects are numerically small and difficult to replicate in a controlled experiment, they can be explained on the basis of mislocated fixations, machine error, and binocular disparity. These latter three influences can create apparent parafoveal-on-foveal effects without being linked to parallel lexical processing.

Introduction

This chapter deals with what is undoubtedly one of the most controversial issues in the research field of eye movements in reading during the past decade, namely the existence of so-called parafoveal-on-foveal effects. In this chapter I start by defining what these effects are and explaining the theoretical importance of the debate surrounding this topic. After this, I review the research pointing towards the existence of such parafoveal-on-foveal effects, and some of the studies that cast doubts on the validity of those findings. Several theoretical explanations for these effects or indeed the lack of them will be discussed and suggestions are made for future research to resolve the ongoing dispute with regards to this issue.

Eye movements in reading are characterized by a succession of periods of steadiness (fixations) and fast movements (saccades). The main purpose of saccades is to bring new information into foveal vision, which comprises the central 2° of the visual field. Acuity at this location is highest and readers need to get most of the words into foveal vision in order to proceed smoothly through the text. Research has shown that denying the reader access to useful foveal information and hence limiting the input to parafoveal information and information from the periphery, makes reading close to impossible (Rayner and Bertera, 1979). The *parafovea* is a region in the visual field extending 2–5° from the centre of the visual field. However, in the context of reading it is more appropriate to define the crucial regions in terms of number of letters instead of visual angle. The number of letters traversed by saccades is relatively invariant when identical text is read at different distances, with a mean saccade size of 7–9 letter spaces being typical in alphabetic languages (Morrison and Rayner, 1981; for a review see Rayner, 1998). Because letters, and by extension words, are the appropriate metric (see also McDonald, 2006a), the convention is to refer to the word on the right of the currently fixated word as the parafoveal word, even though the word to the right of fixation may not always begin exactly 2° away from the fixation. Another convention often encountered in articles is to refer to the currently fixated word as word *n* and the next word as word *n*+1.

An important question with regards to eye movements in reading is how much information a reader processes during a fixation. Or put differently, how far into the upcoming text to the right of fixation do the eyes pick up useful information? A lot of the basic findings on the size of the perceptual span were obtained using the moving window paradigm (McConkie and Rayner, 1975). In this paradigm, the presented text is altered making it nonsensical except for an experimenter-defined window surrounding the point of fixation. Where the reader is looking, the text is visible, while outside of the window area the text is jumbled. Whenever the reader makes a saccade, a new window of text is presented normally around fixation and all the text outside of the new window region is perturbed. By varying the size of the window and searching for the smallest window that allows the reader to read in a way indistinguishable from normal reading, researchers using this paradigm were able to establish the size of the perceptual span (see also Rayner and Bertera, 1979; Rayner et al., 1980). The results of these studies were quite consistent in showing that the span in an alphabetical language such as English extends from 3–4 letters to the left of fixation and 14–15 letters to the right of fixation. However, word length information is acquired further to the right of fixation than letter information. The area from which letters can be identified during a fixation usually does not exceed 7–8 letter spaces to the right.

Taking into account both the size of the perceptual span and the location of the parafovea, it should be clear by now that readers are able to pick up information from the parafoveal word. And indeed, one of the most robust findings in eye movements during reading is the *parafoveal preview benefit* that can be most clearly observed using a method called the boundary paradigm (Rayner, 1975). In this paradigm, prior to fixating a target word the reader is presented with either a valid or an invalid preview of it. The moment the reader's eyes cross an invisible boundary location, usually the space in front of the word, the incorrect preview switches to the actual target word (see Figure 46.1). The fact that information from the parafoveal word is extracted and used during reading is apparent from the shorter fixation time on the target when the letters of the word were visible during the prior fixation than when the letters were masked or replaced by other letters (e.g. Blanchard et al., 1989; Rayner, 1975; Rayner et al., 1982). This effect is typically in the order of 20–50 ms. From

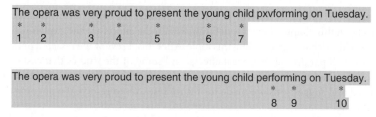

Fig. 46.1 An example of a boundary change experiment. In this example, the target word is *performing*. However, when the participant begins reading the sentence, the second and the third letter of the target word are replaced with visually similar letters (so that *pxvforming* is initially present). When the reader's eye movement crosses an invisible boundary at the end of the word preceding the target word, *pxvforming* changes to *performing*. The asterisks represent the location of each fixation (with the numbers indicating the sequence of fixations).

observations such as these it is clear that the processing of parafoveal information plays an important role during normal reading. There is, however, much controversy over the question of the extent to which information from the parafoveal word (word $n+1$) can influence the fixation duration on and related processing of the currently fixated word (word n). Applied to the scenario just described this would mean that the fixation duration on the foveal word (i.e. the word located before the boundary) can be different as a function of which preview is presented in the parafovea. This latter possibility is referred to as *parafoveal-on-foveal effects* where lexical or sub-lexical information acquired from the parafoveal word has a direct effect on the fixation durations on the foveal word. Note that para-foveally acquired information of a purely visual nature (e.g. word $n+1$ flickering rapidly and brightly) affecting the fixation time on word n has traditionally not been regarded as a parafoveal-on-foveal effect. And this chapter will exclusively focus on effects due to parafoveal processing of lexical or sub-lexical information. Before reviewing those studies that have suggested such effects, I will first briefly outline the theoretical importance of parafoveal-on-foveal effects.

The theoretical importance of parafoveal-on-foveal effects

In the Introduction a number of studies are mentioned which established, in addition to the quintes-sential foveal processing, the existence and importance of parafoveal processing during reading. One of the major questions in eye movements in reading research concerns the time course of these two types of processing (Starr and Rayner, 2001). Does parafoveal processing only kick in when foveal processing has been concluded or do both types of processing occur simultaneously? In other words, do readers process lexical information from more than one word at a time? Whereas nobody doubts that the letters within a word are processed in parallel when they are all located in the fovea (e.g. Rayner and Johnson, 2005), the issue is more controversial when it comes to words.

According to the highly influential E-Z Reader model of eye movement control in reading (Pollatsek et al., 2003, 2006; Rayner et al., 1998a, 2000, 2005; Reichle et al., 1998, 1999, 2003, 2007; see also Reichle, Chapter 42, this volume), words are typically processed only one at a time. Word recognition is considered to be a serial process under the control of an attentional beam. The idea is that attention is allocated serially and sequentially during reading because readers need to keep word order straight (Pollatsek and Rayner, 1999; Pollatsek et al., 2006; Reichle et al., 2009a). So, the word within the attentional beam is the only word that is processed lexically. It is important to note that the use of the term 'serial' with regards to the E-Z Reader model is restricted to lexical processing, as the model does include a parallel scan of the upcoming material (e.g. for determining the saccade target).

The E-Z Reader model (for the most recent version see Reichle et al., 2009b) is a quantitative model in which the core assumption is that cognitive processes associated with encoding the fixated word are the engine behind moving the eyes forward in the text. Two phases of word recognition are distinguished. The termination of the first phase (L1) cues the oculomotor system to start program-ming a saccade to the next word. In its most recent conceptualization, L1 corresponds to a sense of word familiarity, a point at which the system—from prior experience—has learned that recognition of the word should be imminent (Reichle et al., 2007). The termination of the second phase (i.e. L2: full lexical identification) causes the attentional beam to shift to the next word. This shift will usually happen before the eyes move to the next word and during the time that the attentional beam is on the parafoveal word but the eyes are still on the previous word, parafoveal processing occurs.

As is apparent from the architecture of the E-Z Reader model described above, the model upholds a serial view on the time course of foveal and parafoveal processing. In recent years this serial assump-tion has been questioned by studies reporting parafoveal-on-foveal effects. As mentioned earlier, parafoveal-on-foveal effects refer to the possibility that characteristics of the word to the right of the fixation influence the fixation duration on the currently fixated word. It is generally assumed that the existence of such effects would be very damaging to the serial assumption of the E-Z Reader model. After all, in the E-Z Reader model parafoveal processing at the lexical level only begins after foveal processing has been concluded and the programming of the saccade towards the next word has started.

How could parafoveal processing influence foveal processing in this framework if it is the termination of foveal lexical processing that cues the shift of the attentional beam and subsequently results in the start of parafoveal lexical processing?

The 'discovery' of parafoveal-on-foveal effects, which will be discussed in detail in the next sections, has been accompanied by the development of models of eye movement control embracing a parallel view on the time course of foveal and parafoveal word processing. The *SWIFT* model (Engbert et al., 2002, 2005; Kliegl and Engbert, 2003; see also Engbert and Kliegl, Chapter 43, this volume) for instance, while adopting quite a few of the architectural features of the E-Z Reader model, departs from it by assuming that lexical processing is spatially distributed across words and that a competition for processing resources between the different words is constantly going on; for example, a difficult word will use the majority of the resources leaving few resources for the processing of the other words. In SWIFT saccades are directed towards words that have the highest level of excitation, which occurs at intermediate amounts of lexical processing. This is quite different from E-Z Reader where the default saccade target will always be the next unidentified word in the sentence. Other parallel models of eye movement control in reading have been proposed such as the Glenmore model (Reilly and Radach, 2003, 2006; for a comparison of the different models see Reichle, et al., 2003), but suffice it to say that at this point whereas parafoveal-on-foveal effects seem to be incompatible with a serial model, this type of effect flows almost naturally from a model with a parallel architecture of lexical processing during reading. As a result, the hunt for parafoveal-on-foveal effects has recently been considered one of the pre-eminent ways for resolving the serial versus parallel issue of lexical processing in eye movements during reading.

Early reports of parafoveal-on-foveal effects in reading-like tasks

A number of studies have indicated that the foveal viewing time can indeed be altered by the lexical or sub-lexical characteristics of the words presented in the parafovea (e.g. Kennedy, 1998, 2000; Kennedy et al., 2002, 2004; Murray, 1998; Murray and Rowan, 1998; Schroyens et al., 1999; Vitu et al., 2004). In the Kennedy (1998) study, for instance, participants were presented with three words. The first word was either the word '*looks*' or the word '*means*'. In the first case the task for the participants was to decide whether the following two words were physically identical, in the second case they had to decide whether the adjacent words were synonyms. Among the findings of this study, a reduced gaze duration[1] on the first word was reported in the case of a long parafoveal word. This observation was taken as evidence for a parallel processing account in which the system is sensitive to the rate at which sub-lexical parafoveal information can be acquired; a difficult second word (e.g. a long word) would attract an early saccade from the prior word.

However, there are methodological problems associated with quite a number of the earlier studies. More specifically, those studies reporting parafoveal-on-foveal effects quite often used tasks that closely resemble reading, but doubts can be raised whether these tasks require the full range of psycholinguistic processes that occur during normal reading (for a discussion on the generalizability of these tasks, see Rayner et al. (2003)). Criticisms of the look/means task and other such reading-like tasks (e.g. the clothing search task in which a participant has to indicate whether one of the words

---

[1] The most frequently reported fixation times in reading are: The *gaze duration*, which is the sum of the fixations from the moment the eyes land on the word/region of interest until the moment they move off again. If the gaze duration encompasses exactly one fixation it is also called the *single fixation duration*. The *first fixation duration*, which is the duration of the first fixation during first pass independent of the number of fixations that were made on the word/region. Finally, the *go-past time* is the sum of all fixations from first fixating a word/region during first pass reading until the last one before leaving it to the right, including regressive fixations.

presented on the screen is an article of clothing, Schroyens et al., 1999) usually state that the task employed resembles something of a variant of a visual search task than normal reading. This is a serious criticism as research has shown that even the ubiquitous frequency effect on eye movements during reading (i.e. a rare word is looked upon for a longer time than a common word) disappears during visual search (Rayner and Fischer, 1996, Rayner and Raney, 1996), indicating fundamental differences between these two tasks. For this reason, I will focus for the remainder of this chapter on studies in which participants were asked to read for comprehension and occasionally had to answer a question with regard to the material they've just read. There is a wide consensus among researchers that this task requires natural reading.

And indeed, limiting the discussion to studies using 'normal' reading tasks can resolve some of the inconsistencies in parafoveal-on-foveal studies: Underwood et al. (2000) reported longer fixations on the foveal word during normal reading when the parafoveal word had an informative initial trigram, whereas Kennedy (1998, 2000) reported shorter fixations in these circumstances. Kennedy used a reading-like task in these studies but later replicated the longer foveal fixation prior to an informative parafoveal trigram using a normal reading task (Kennedy, 2008; Kennedy and Pynte, 2005). It is reasonable to assume that different task demands could at least be partially responsible for the different results obtained in these studies.

Types of parafoveal-on-foveal effects in reading experiments

Turning to those studies that did require reading for comprehension, distinctions have to be made both on grounds of the type of parafoveal-on-foveal effect observed and on grounds of the methodology used in the research. That is whether or not an effect was observed in a carefully controlled experiment, or in a corpus study in which large amounts of text are read and inferences are drawn from correlational analyses of those data.

Starting with the type of parafoveal-on-foveal effect, I would like to single out two types of parafoveal-on-foveal effects that hold something of a special position for the current discussion, for the simple reason that both serial and parallel models can account for them. The first effect is related to word skipping. A word is skipped when there is no fixation on the word during first-pass reading. This is far from being a rare phenomenon; on average about one-third of the words in a text are skipped (Rayner, 1998). One of the most conspicuous findings in word skipping is that it occurs more frequently with short words than with long words (Brysbaert et al., 2005; Rayner and McConkie, 1976). Evidence seems to suggest that the fixation duration on the prior word is affected when a word is skipped. If so, this would, of course, constitute a parafoveal-on-foveal effect. Pollatsek et al. (1986) observed an inflated fixation duration prior to skipping (as compared to when the word was not skipped). And this effect was also reported in a number of other studies (e.g. Drieghe et al., 2005a; Rayner et al., 2004a).

However, it is somewhat controversial in the sense that other studies did not find such an inflated fixation duration prior to skipping (e.g. Drieghe et al., 2004; Radach and Heller, 2000). The most comprehensive study on this topic so far was carried by Kliegl and Engbert (2005). In a corpus study, they observed shorter fixation durations prior to skipping short and easy words and inflated fixation durations prior to skipping long and difficult words. As already mentioned, the reason why I will not go further into the details with regards to this specific phenomenon is because both serial and parallel models can accommodate it. In the E-Z Reader model, word $n+1$ is skipped because during the time that the attentional beam has shifted to it while it was in the parafovea, the word was recognized sufficiently fast to cue the system to replace the programming of the saccade towards it, by a saccade to word $n+2$. This idea that a word is skipped because it is recognized is backed up by findings indicating that a word that is predictable from the preceding context is skipped more often than a word that is not (Balota et al., 1985; Ehrlich and Rayner, 1981; Rayner and Well, 1996). Moreover, changing a single letter in the preview of a predictable word (turning it into an illegal non-word, e.g. *cahe* as a preview for *cake*), reduces the skipping probability to that of any other non-word preview (e.g. *nohm*; Drieghe et al., 2005a), indicating that the preview was identified quite accurately when the system decided to skip it. Because E-Z Reader is a serial model, cancelling a planned saccade and replacing it by a saccade landing a word further downstream in the sentence, is thought to be time consuming, hence it predicts an inflated fixation duration prior to skipping. For parallel models, an increased fixation duration prior to skipping is not difficult to explain either; a longer fixation time on word *n* will result in word *n*+1 being in the perceptual span for a longer time. This will allow more processing of word *n*+1 to occur, resulting in a higher chance that it will be skipped.

The second effect that arguably can be singled out, is that of parafoveal word length. In a corpus analysis of four participants reading a German translation of the first two parts of the novel *Gulliver's Travels*, Radach (1996, see Kennedy, 1998 for a discussion of these data) observed a reduced fixation duration on the foveal word when the parafoveal word was 7–10 letters long as compared to when the parafoveal word was 4 letters long. This reduction was 24 ms when the foveal word was either a 3- or 4-letter word. However, a subsequent study examining this effect in an experiment allowing more control of the stimuli, found only a (significant) 4 ms reduction in single fixation duration on a 5-letter word when the next word was 8 letters long as compared to when it was 4 letters long (Drieghe et al., 2005b). Taking into account the size of this effect, this is likely due to a very limited number of occasions when the system made a decision to skip the long word—accompanied by an inflated fixation duration—but fell short in the execution of the saccade, resulting in the saccade actually landing on the word. Others studies have also failed to show an influence of parafoveal word length (Henderson and Ferreira, 1993). A thorough discussion of the implications of errors on the execution of saccades is presented in the section on mislocated fixations.

Having identified two effects which cannot be considered to distinguish between serial and parallel models of eye movements in reading, this allows the field of interest to be narrowed to what is the main focus of this chapter: influences of either lexical (e.g. frequency) or sub-lexical (e.g. informativeness of the initial trigram) properties of the parafoveal word on the fixation duration observed on the foveal word when the parafoveal word is subsequently fixated (i.e. not skipped).

Parafoveal-on-foveal effects in controlled experiments

Using normal reading tasks that require reading for comprehension, a number of studies have shown parafoveal-on-foveal effects. Some of these were done in the context of experiments allowing tight control over the stimuli (Hyönä and Bertram, 2004; Inhoff et al., 2000a, 2000b; Pynte et al., 2004; Rayner et al., 2004b; Starr and Inhoff, 2004), others collected a large corpus of eye movement data of people reading large amounts of text (Kennedy and Pynte, 2005; Kliegl et al., 2006). Before examining the corpus studies, I will briefly discuss the experiments as a function of the type of parafoveal-on-foveal effect reported.

Starting with a potential effect of parafoveal frequency on foveal fixation durations, whereas this effect has been reported in reading-like tasks (Kennedy, 1998; Kennedy et al., 2002), it has not been replicated in experiments in which reading for comprehension was examined (e.g. Inhoff et al., 2000b; White, 2008). And there are also a number of other studies that, quite often in the context of other research questions, examined this issue and did not find an effect of parafoveal word frequency on foveal viewing times (e.g. Carpenter and Just, 1983; Henderson and Ferreira, 1993; Kennison and Clifton, 1995; Rayner et al., 1998b). So, failures to replicate this type of effect are not uncommon, and sometimes even occur within the same study: Hyönä and Bertram (2004, experiment 2) report target words preceding compounds with a high frequency first constituent to be gazed upon for less time than those preceding compounds with a low-frequency first constituent. However, in the same study they did not replicate this finding when the whole-word frequency of the parafoveal word was manipulated (Hyönä and Bertram, 2004, experiment 4).

A somewhat different picture emerges when the parafoveal preview presented to the readers consists of an orthographically illegal non-word (e.g. *pxvforming* which is replaced by *performing* when the eyes cross the invisible boundary). Using such a manipulation, Inhoff et al. (2000b) observed longer fixation durations on the foveal word when the next word consisted of jumbled letters compared to when a normal word was presented in the parafovea. This finding has also been replicated by Starr and Inhoff (2004). However, the first study to examine the effects of having a non-word in the parafovea was Rayner (1975; for a discussion of these data see Rayner et al., 2003). Although there were no overall effects of the parafoveal preview of the non-word on foveal fixation durations, an analysis as a function of fixation location did show an increased fixation duration in the non-word preview condition when the eyes were on word n and only 1–3 character spaces away from word $n+1$. A re-analysis of the Kambe data (2004) showed the same effect, also limited to fixations on the final three character positions of the foveal word (and see also Drieghe, Rayner and Pollatsek, 2005a; 2008a). However, again there are studies that did not observe this effect (e.g. Altaribba et al., 2001; White and Liversedge, 2004) and Pynte, et al. (2004) even reported a shortening of the foveal fixation duration when there was a typo in word $n+2$ and word $n+1$ was very short.[2] Finally, White (2008) did find an effect of a different orthographic, sublexical factor, that of parafoveal orthographic familiarity. She reported a small parafoveal-on-foveal effect (6 ms) such that fixation durations on word n were longer when word $n+1$ was orthographically unfamiliar compared to when is was familiar. At this point, it is important to note that the suggestion has also been made that it is not inconceivable that orthographic information from the parafoveal word—as opposed to lexical information—might be processed in a manner that does not require attention. Early pre-attentive processes (such as in the E-Z Reader architecture), that are used, for instance, to obtain word length information of the ensuing words, may also be able to pick up unusual orthographic combinations, such as misspellings (e.g. see Pollatsek et al., 2006), although again the evidence is mixed that these types of effects actually occur (e.g. White and Liversedge, 2004).

The observation that a reported parafoveal-on-foveal effect is quite often restricted to those instances when the eyes are very close to the parafoveal preview (i.e. the last letters of the foveal word) is crucial for understanding the presence or absence of parafoveal-on-foveal effects in studies. Indeed, questions can be raised as to whether the absence of an analysis restricted exclusively to those fixation positions can at least account for some of the discrepancies between those studies that do and those that do not find parafoveal-on-foveal effects. From a parallel perspective on lexical processing during reading, this restriction in fixation locations makes sense due to the reduced acuity of vision further into the parafovea. Only when the eyes are close enough to the preview is acuity good enough to allow processing sufficient to reach the threshold for statistically significant effects on fixation times on the foveal word. However, parafoveal-on-foveal effects restricted to the last letters of the foveal word are not necessarily inconsistent with a serial lexical processing model such as the E-Z Reader model because the model assumes that not all executed saccades land on the intended word. In this view, which has been called the *mislocated fixations account*, saccades sometimes fall short of their intended target resulting in a fixation on word n while attention and presumably lexical processing is actually located on word $n+1$. As a result that specific fixation duration is affected by the processing of word $n+1$. I defer thorough discussion of this account and its potential implications until later in this chapter.

---

[2] As already mentioned, the current chapter focuses almost exclusively on parafoveal-of-foveal effects from word $n+1$ on word n when word $n+1$ is subsequently fixated or is at least long enough to be skipped only rarely. The reason for this restriction is that these observations are the least likely to be affected by potentially inflated or deflated fixation durations associated with the skipping of word $n+1$. The second reason is that, regardless of theoretical framework, the numerically strongest effects are predicted for word $n+1$ manipulations on the fixation times on word n as compared to word $n+2$ manipulations. However, quite a number of studies have examined the issue of preview benefits of word $n+2$ (e.g. McDonald, 2005, 2006b; Rayner et al. 2007a) and whether manipulations of the preview of word $n+2$ can cause parafoveal-on-foveal effects on word n. Again, some studies do not report these parafoveal-on-foveal effects (e.g. Angele et al., 2008; Rayner et al., 2007), whereas others do (e.g. Kliegl et al., 2007). Apparently, the crucial factor is the size of word $n+1$ with observations of parafoveal-on-foveal effects being restricted to studies using a 3-letter word $n+1$, which disappears when word $n+1$ is a 4-letter word or longer.

A different type of parafoveal-on-foveal effect, also restricted to the final characters of the foveal word, was reported by Rayner et al. (2004b; see also Clifton and Staub, Chapter 49, and Rayner and Liversedge, Chapter 41, this volume). In this experiment readers were presented with sentences featuring a target word such as 'carrot' and the plausibility of this target word was manipulated. Consider this example from their materials:

a) John used a knife to chop the large carrots for dinner. (Plausible)

b) John used an axe to chop the large carrots for dinner. (Implausible)

c) John used a pump to inflate the large carrots for dinner. (Anomalous)

Their results showed that the implausible condition resulted in longer fixation times on the target word but only in later measures (i.e. go-past time). The anomalous condition resulted in an earlier effect, yielding longer gaze durations on the target word itself. Crucial to the current discussion is that an increased fixation duration was observed on the pre-target word (*large* in the example) in the anomalous condition as compared to the other two conditions but again, only when the analysis was restricted to the fixations on the final three characters of the pre-target word. There was no difference on the pre-target word between the plausible and implausible condition (see also Joseph et al., 2008; Staub et al., 2007). A somewhat related experiment was carried out by Inhoff et al. (2000a, experiment 1). They manipulated the semantic association between two consecutive words. An example of their stimuli:

a) Did you see the picture of her mother's mother at the meeting? (Repetition)

b) Did you see the picture of her mother's father at the meeting? (Associated)

c) Did you see the picture of her mother's garden at the meeting? (Unassociated)

Inhoff et al. observed shorter fixation times on 'mother's' in the repetition and associated conditions as compared to the unassociated condition. Interestingly, they did carry out an analysis as a function of fixation location and were able to show that this effect was not restricted to those instances when the eyes were at the very end of 'mother's'. However, their analysis also showed slightly more skipping of the second word of the word pair in the Repetition and Associated condition as compared to the Unassociated condition. Taking the Kliegl and Engbert (2005) findings into account in which they observed a shorter fixation duration prior to skipping an easy word, the observation of the shorter fixation times on 'mother's' in the repetition and associated condition could be related to differences in the subsequent skipping behaviour. As already mentioned this type of parafoveal-on-foveal effect can be accounted for by both serial and parallel models, reducing its relevance for the current discussion. A replication of this experiment with a longer second word to prevent word skipping could resolve this issue and establish whether this parafoveal-on-foveal effect is indeed not restricted to fixations on the final three characters of word n.

To briefly summarize, those experiments that used a task that required participants to read for comprehension, resulted in what has to be described as a rather messy picture. There are failures to replicate and even inconsistent results in terms of the directions of effects. The clearest evidence for the existence of parafoveal-on-foveal effects comes from those studies that have carried out analyses restricted to fixation locations very close to the parafoveal preview. More consistent results have been obtained in corpus studies.

Parafoveal-on-foveal effects in corpus studies

Kennedy and Pynte (2005) collected a corpus of eye movement data from 10 English and 10 French participants, each reading a considerable amount of text (i.e. each participant reading about 50,000 words) in their native language. Their results in terms of reported parafoveal-on-foveal effects differed as a function of the length of the foveal word. When word n was short (5–6 letters long), significant effects of the frequency of word $n+1$ were obtained: a low-frequency word $n+1$ in the parafovea induced a 12-ms longer gaze duration on word n compared to when a high-frequency word was in the parafovea. This finding did not hold when word n was long (8–12 letters long); for these words an influence of a sublexical factor was observed, namely, the informativeness of the initial trigram of word $n+1$. The gaze duration on word n was 21 ms longer when the initial trigram of word $n+1$ was informative (i.e. helpful in constraining the identity of the entire word) as compared to when the trigram was not informative. Pynte and Kennedy posed that when word n was long, word $n+1$ extended too far into the parafovea for the frequency of the entire word to affect the foveal fixation duration. However, subsequent analyses on this corpus showed that only the English speakers showed an effect of parafoveal frequency and only the French speakers showed an effect of parafoveal initial trigram informativeness. For a discussion and potential explanation of this discrepancy between languages in terms of the distribution of information across the letters of given words in the different languages, see Pynte and Kennedy (2006).

Kliegl et al. (2006) reported analyses of an impressive corpus of eye movements collected on 222 persons reading 144 sentences. In their analyses they simultaneously tested the influence of 12 factors: the frequency, predictability, and length of the currently fixated word, the preceding, and the next word, and the amplitude of the incoming and outgoing saccades, as well as the position of the fixation within the currently fixated word. Focusing on parafoveal-on-foveal effects in the single fixation duration data, Kliegl et al. reported an 8-ms shorter fixation duration on word n when word $n+1$ was a high-frequency word as compared to when word $n+1$ was a low-frequency word. Consistent with the Pynte and Kennedy (2005) findings this was only true when word n was a short word (6 letters or fewer). There was no effect of parafoveal frequency when word n was longer than 6 letters (a nonsignificant 1 ms). Unexpectedly there was also an effect of the predictability of word $n+1$ on the single fixation time on word n: Low predictability of word $n+1$ was associated with shorter fixation durations on word n and this effect was stronger when word n was longer (3 ms on short words versus 9 ms on long words). Kliegl et al. suggested that the eyes move on quickly only if the next word cannot be guessed from the preceding context. The data on gaze duration showed a different picture: numerically stronger effects of parafoveal frequency and predictability were observed for long than for short words and moreover, the effect of parafoveal predictability changed its direction: Low predictability of word $n+1$ was associated with longer gaze durations on word n.

So in both of the corpus studies, reliable indications of parafoveal-on-foveal effects were observed but they were numerically small (especially in the Kliegl et al. paper), often unexpected and they strongly depended on foveal word length.

Intermediate summary

At this point, I believe it to be a fair summary to say that the corpus studies have done a great deal to move the dispute with regards to the existence of parafoveal-on-foveal effects a large step further. They are the strongest evidence for the existence of such effects so far, but they have also clearly shown the limitations of such effects: parafoveal-on-foveal effects, in terms of effect size, are quite small and only appear in well-defined situations (i.e. when short foveal words are fixated). Returning to the findings of the experiments with well-controlled stimuli, and with a task demanding reading for comprehension, the most conspicuous observation is that those studies that do report parafoveal-on-foveal effects tend to have analyses restricted to fixations falling on the final characters of the foveal word.

When observations of parafoveal-on-foveal effects first started to appear, they very quickly acquired the status of a potential 'game changer' for the dispute between serial and parallel models of eye movements during reading. They were regarded as intrinsically inconsistent with any serial architecture of a model of lexical processing during reading. And indeed, if these effects had turned out to be sizeable and easily replicable, they most definitely would have played that role. In view of the studies discussed so far, I will make two claims: first of all, that for parafoveal-on-foveal effects to still play their role as a game changer, they will minimally need to pass the test of appearing in an experiment with well-controlled stimuli that are experimentally manipulated, with a strong a priori prediction, and which can be replicated. The reason for this statement is because an experiment allows for a higher level of control of the stimuli and a stronger position in terms of causality for interpreting results. This will deal with some of the inherent difficulties associated with the corpus approach (see the next section).

The second claim is that there are a number of phenomena that can also cause apparent para-foveal-on-foveal effects but are not related to parallel lexical processing. These are the influences of mislocated fixations, machine error, and binocular disparity, which will be dealt with subsequently. Contrary to the issue of serial versus parallel lexical processing, these influences are fairly uncontroversial in their existence. The big question is: are they numerically strong enough to account for the entire phenomenon of the parafoveal-on-foveal effects observed so far? This is a claim I will make based on the small effect sizes observed in, for instance, the Kliegl et al. corpus study (2006). In other words, I want to put forward the idea that in order to accept parafoveal-on-foveal effects as evidence for parallel lexical processing, the burden of proof is still on those claiming that these effects exist above and beyond effects caused by the three other phenomena mentioned, which can cause apparent parafoveal-on-foveal effects without being linked to parallel lexical processing.

Limitations of the correlational approach

There is a great deal of value in the approach of collecting a large amount of eye tracking data in a corpus and running different types of correlational analyses on them. The sheer amount of data allows one to do statistical analyses that would not be possible in regular experiments due to a lack of statistical power. The number of variables that were examined simultaneously in the Kliegl et al. (2006) paper is an impressive example of that. For a number of phenomena, they also allow for the highest level of experimental control possible. Taking, for example, the corpus study examining the issue of the fixation duration prior to skipping by Kliegl and Engbert (2005). Regardless of the amount of control over the stimuli, an experimenter can never experimentally control whether the participant decides to skip or not. As such, observations of fixation durations prior to skipping will always have a correlational nature (i.e. skipping cannot be manipulated as an independent variable in an experimental design) and a corpus study at least has the advantage of having a large amount of statistical power.

However, some limitations have to be acknowledged with regards to this approach. In correlational analyses relevant variables can be quite confounded and thus be virtually impossible to examine in an unconfounded way with these analyses. Moreover, controlled experiments allow for stronger inferences about causality (for a discussion see Rayner et al., 2007b). Returning for instance to the inflated fixation duration prior to skipping example, something of a chicken or egg argument can be construed: do readers skip more often because the preceding fixation was long or was the preceding fixation long because they skipped the next word? Some of the corpus studies have adopted an approach closely resembling experiments by embedding target words selected on length and frequency in the sentences that make up the corpus (e.g. The Potsdam Sentence Corpus; Kliegl et al. 2006). Whereas this approach will allow for more stringent control on the properties of the items, it will still lack the power in terms of assigning causality compared to an experiment whereby all variables are kept identical and the impact of one change in a variable is asserted.

These comments should not be taken as downplaying the importance of the corpus approach, but they do reinforce the call for replication in a controlled experiment, particularly of small effects (i.e. potentially due to confounds between variables) and especially unexpected results (e.g. an effect of parafoveal predictability).

The mislocated fixations account

One phenomenon that in all likelihood can cause apparent parafoveal-on-foveal effects is the occurrence of mislocated fixations. As already mentioned, a considerable amount of evidence has been collected showing that there is a margin of error on the execution of saccades and that the eyes quite often do not land exactly on their target (Engbert et al., 2007; McConkie et al., 1988; Nuthmann et al., 2007). Presumably, it is not that rare for a saccade to fall short of its targeted word so that word n is fixated even though word $n+1$ was the intended target and is presumably the word that is actually being processed during that fixation. The problem with the mislocated fixations account is, of course, that there is no way to experimentally determine whether a saccade has been accurately executed.

However, there do exist a few potential markers for the presence of such mislocated fixations. Drieghe et al. (2008a) carried out a boundary change experiment to look for such markers in the context of parafoveal-on-foveal effects. Here is an example of their stimuli. The invisible boundary was always located before the space preceding the word *performing* and if there was an incorrect parafoveal preview (*pxvforming*), this was replaced by the correct target word when the eyes crossed the boundary.

a) The opera was very proud to present the young child performing on Tuesday.

b) The opera was very proud to present the young child pxvforming on Tuesday.

c) The opera was very proud to present the young tenor performing on Tuesday.

d) The opera was very proud to present the young tenor pxvforming on Tuesday.

Besides this preview manipulation on word $n+1$, the frequency of word n was also manipulated: it was either a high-frequency (e.g. *child*) or a low-frequency 5-letter word (e.g. *tenor*). This resulted in four conditions; a) high-frequency word n—normal preview, b) high-frequency word n—incorrect preview, c) low-frequency word n—normal preview and d) low-frequency word n—incorrect preview. Based on the prior research already discussed, a parafoveal-on-foveal effect was predicted on word n in the form of a longer fixation duration when the preview of word $n+1$ was orthographically illegal.

Drieghe et al. (2008) stated that three predictions could be derived from the assumption that (at least a sizeable portion of) this parafoveal-on-foveal effect could be attributed to mislocated fixations. First of all, the observations of the effect would be limited to those instances when the eyes landed on the final letters of word n. If the eyes undershot the intended target word $n+1$, they would of course miss it by a very small number of character spaces. This prediction is also consistent with a parallel view of lexical processing, but it is important to test it because it can falsify the mislocated fixations account if it is not observed. A parafoveal-on-foveal effect was observed in the predicted direction but an analysis as a function of fixation position showed that this effect was completely due to fixations landing on the very last letter.

The second prediction had to do with the frequency manipulation of word n. A parallel model which incorporates limited processing capabilities would assume that a high-frequency word n would allow more processing resources to be attributed to the processing of word $n+1$, resulting in a bigger parafoveal-on-foveal effect. A serial model attributing the parafoveal-on-foveal effect to mislocated fixations would not make this prediction as within this view it is the non-fixated word $n+1$ which is processed, not word n. This prediction was also confirmed, as there was not the slightest hint of an interaction between foveal frequency and the preview manipulation.

Finally, the third prediction was derived from McConkie et al. (1988). They observed that the error between the intended and actual landing position had a systematic component. The oculomotor control system has a tendency to overshoot nearby targets and undershoot far targets. The mislocated fixations account states that the observed parafoveal-on-foveal effect would be due to undershoots of word $n+1$, so this would happen more often following a long prior saccade. This final prediction was also confirmed because there was a significant correlation between the length of the incoming saccade and the fixation duration on the final letters of word n, but only when the preview was incorrect. There was no correlation when the preview was correct.

The Drieghe et al. (2008) study is a very strong indication that at least some of the observed parafoveal-on-foveal effects are due to mislocated fixations. It is also important to note that estimations of how often mislocated fixations can result in landing on the wrong word, indicate that they are far from being rare, especially for short words (Engbert et al., 2007).

Machine error and inadequate calibration

Inadequate calibration and/or machine error can cause an eye tracker to wrongfully indicate that the eye is or that the eyes are fixating on word n while they are actually fixating on word $n+1$. There is, of course, no way to check for this, but suffice it to say that the assumption of perfect eye tracking is unrealistic and that calibration inaccuracies can lead to inaccuracies in assigning actual fixation locations. Even though this cannot be a strong influence it can become of some importance when running an analysis restricted to fixations landing on a limited amount of letters (i.e. the final characters of word *n*) while looking for an influence of the immediately adjacent region (i.e. word *n* +1). And again, given an adequate amount of data, this can turn into a statistically significant influence. Moreover, it is reasonable to assume that inadequate calibration will often play a bigger role in corpus studies, at least those where the frequency of recalibrating the eye tracker is considerably lower than typically employed in experiments with a limited amount of experimental sentences to be read. This would have an effect on the average accuracy of the calibration.

Kliegl et al. (2006) tried to control for this potential confound as much as possible by only taking those instances into the analyses when the tracker assigned the fixation locations for both eyes to the same word. Although this would get rid of some of the machine error, it would appear that the assumption that both eyes are always on the same word when there is no machine error is incorrect during reading (see next section on how fixation disparity is routinely larger than one character) and as such, that fixation disparity may not be a very reliable marker for machine error.

Binocular disparity

The vast majority of reading research has involved recording the movement of one of the two eyes, as there has been an implicit assumption that the two eyes move together and fixate the same letter of a word when we read. However, this assumption turned out to not always be correct as shown by a binocular eye tracking experiment by Liversedge et al. (2006a; see also Liversedge et al., 2006b) of normal readers reading single sentences. Whereas a thorough discussion of binocular disparity during reading is beyond the scope of the current chapter (for a thorough review see Kirkby et al., 2008 and Kirkby et al., Chapter 44, this volume), some of these findings can have repercussions for the observation of parafoveal-on-foveal effects. Liversedge et al. (2006b) found that across all fixations, the fixation positions of the two eyes were on average 1.1 character spaces apart during reading. On 53% of fixations the eyes were aligned to within one character space, but on 47% of fixations the positions of the two eyes were more than one character space apart (disparate fixations). Within the 47% of disparate fixations, the majority were uncrossed with the left eye fixating to the left of the right eye. Only 8% of all the fixations were crossed, such that the fixation position of the right eye was to the left of the left eye. Other researchers have reported other proportions of crossed and uncrossed fixations with higher proportions of crossed fixations (e.g. Nuthmann and Kliegl, 2009). Recent evidence points in the direction of these differences being due to the specific viewing conditions used in the different labs (Blythe et al., 2009).

Although crossed binocular disparity may be rare, very occasionally it will result in the right eye—which is typically the monitored eye during monocular research—being on word *n* while the left eye is on word *n* +1. In this scenario, doubts can be raised whether it is accurate to consider the fixation of the right eye at the very end of word *n* as being on word *n* or on word *n* +1. Moreover, research has shown that binocular disparity tends to be larger following a large saccade (Collewijn et al., 1988). Again, this ties in with the observation that parafoveal-on-foveal effects are somewhat correlated with a large incoming saccade length (Drieghe et al., 2008) and can come into play given large amounts of data.

Future research

I will conclude this chapter by pointing to a few promising directions for future research in terms of: 1) parafoveal-on-foveal effects and 2) the serial versus parallel lexical processing issue.

The first suggestion for pushing the debate forward is the thorough implementation of the mislocated fixations account into the E-Z Reader model. At this moment it is still unclear how often mislocated fixations occur in this framework and whether implementing them would disrupt the model's fit of experimental data for other phenomena during reading. Such an endeavour would also give a stronger indication of whether mislocated fixations can exclusively account for observed parafoveal-on-foveal effects.

Another interesting direction for future research is looking into individual differences (e.g. see Radach et al., 2008). The data from reading-like studies show parafoveal-on-foveal effects. Could it be that as the task gets easier in terms of required processing depth, and/or the more proficient the reader is, then parafoveal-on-foveal effects numerically increase, or for some type of effects, even appear?

The discussion between the serial and parallel view on lexical processing during reading has been translated up until this point into the question of whether a reader processes one or multiple words at a time. However, there is some middle ground for this issue in that two or more words that are strongly associated make up a word group that could be processed as a single unit. In other words, a serial framework but the processing of a single unit could sometimes mean that two words were processed as one whole. Candidates for such a grouping are, for instance, spaced compounds. Juhasz et al. (2009) observed parafoveal preview benefits on the second constituent of a spaced compound considerably larger in size than typically observed between two words. This can be an indication for the special relationship between the two constituents even though there is a space in between them making it arguably a between-word observation (see also Drieghe et al., 2008b and Radach, 1996 for a discussion of a potential article-noun grouping).[3] And related to this latter suggestion, if word by word processing occurs during reading, how does this work for languages where there are no spaces between the words to assist this segmentation, such as Chinese which is unspaced, dense and word segmentation can be ambiguous. A number of studies have already examined this issue (e.g. Bai et al., 2008; Yang et al., 2009; Yen et al., 2009) and for a thorough discussion of the impact of a lack of visual cues for word boundaries for the presence or absence of parafoveal-on-foveal effects in Chinese I refer to Chapter 53, by Zang and colleagues in this book.

Finally, the influence of binocular disparity on the observation of parafoveal-on-foveal effects can be directly tested. Do parafoveal-on-foveal effects sometimes co-occur with binocular disparity causing the assignment of one eye to the foveal word and the other eye to the parafoveal word?

Conclusions

In this chapter I have reviewed a representative section of the literature on parafoveal-on-foveal effects. Early studies that reported parafoveal-on-foveal effects, used reading-like tasks of which the generalizability to reading for comprehension has been questioned. Those experiments that did require reading for comprehension show a rather messy picture of failures to replicate and inconsistencies in the direction of effects. The clearest indication of the existence of these types of effect comes from experiments restricting their analyses to fixation locations on the foveal word which are very close to the parafoveal word and from corpus studies showing numerically quite small but reliable effects.

I have made the case that in relation to the validity of these effects for demonstrating parallel lexical processing during reading, the jury is still out. The appearance of such effects can also be predicted on the basis of mislocated fixations, machine error, and binocular disparity. Whereas it should be completely clear that these three influences cannot account for strong parafoveal-on-foveal effects, a case can be made that they can account for those numerically small effects that have been observed.

---

[3] Interestingly, for unspaced compounds (e.g. bathroom) there are strong indications that the lexical processing of the individual constituents are also processed in a more serial fashion as compared to the letters in a monomorphemic word (e.g. fountain) of equal word length. Drieghe, Pollatsek, Juhasz and Rayner (2010) observed a within-word parafoveal-on-foveal effect on the first letters of a monomorphemic word when there was a misspelling in the final letters of a monomorphemic word, but this effect was not present in fixation durations on the corresponding letters of the first constituent in an unspaced compound when there was misspelling in the 2nd constituent.

Moreover, whereas the issue of parafoveal-on-foveal effects during reading is still highly controversial, a (limited) influence of those three factors is quite likely.

Acknowledgements

I would like to thank Keith Rayner, Barbara Juhasz, and Simon Liversedge for comments on an earlier version of this chapter.

References

Altarriba, J., Kambe, G., Pollatsek, A., and Rayner, K. (2001). Semantic codes are not used in integrating information across eye fixations in reading: Evidence from fluent Spanish-English bilinguals. *Perception & Psychophysics*, **63**, 875–890.

Angele, B, Slattery, T.J., Yang, J.M., Kliegl, R., and Rayner, K. (2008). Parafoveal processing in reading: Manipulating n+1 and n+2 previews simultaneously. *Visual Cognition*, **16**, 697–707.

Bai, X., Yan, G., Liversedge, S.P., Zang, C., and Rayner, K. (2008). Reading spaced and unspaced Chinese text: Evidence from eye movements. *Journal of Experimental Psychology: Human Perception and Performance*, **34**, 1277–1287.

Balota, D.A., Pollatsek, A., and Rayner, K. (1985). The interaction of contextual constraints and parafoveal visual information in reading. *Cognitive Psychology*, **17**, 364–390.

Blanchard, H.E., Pollatsek, A., and Rayner, K. (1989). The acquisition of parafoveal word information in reading. *Perception and Psychophysics*, **46**, 85–94.

Blythe, H.I., Kirkby, J.A., Drieghe, D., and Liversedge, S.P. (2009). Are uncrossed fixation disparities more common than crossed fixation disparities? Lecture held at the XVth European Conference on Eye Movements, August 23–27, Southampton, UK.

Brysbaert, M., Drieghe, D., and Vitu, F. (2005). Word skipping: Implications for theories of eye movement control in reading. In G. Underwood (ed.) *Cognitive Processes in Eye Guidance* (pp. 53–78). Oxford: Oxford University Press.

Carpenter, P.A. and Just, M.A. (1983). What your eyes do while your mind is reading. In: K. Rayner (ed.), *Eye Movements in Reading: Perceptual and Language Processes* (pp. 275–307). New York: Academic Press.

Collewijn, H., Erkelens, C.J. and Steinman, R.M. (1988). Binocular co-ordination of human horizontal saccadic eye movements. *Journal of Physiology*, **404**, 157–182.

Drieghe, D., Rayner, K., and Pollatsek, A. (2005a). Word skipping during reading revisited. *Journal of Experimental Psychology: Human Perception and Performance*, **31**, 954–969.

Drieghe, D., Brysbaert, M., and Desmet, T. (2005b). Parafoveal-on-foveal effects on eye movements in text reading: Does an extra space make a difference? *Vision Research*, **45**, 1693–1706.

Drieghe, D., Rayner, K., and Pollatsek, A. (2008a). Mislocated fixations can account for parafoveal-on-foveal effects during reading. *Quarterly Journal of Experimental Psychology*, **61**, 1239–1249.

Drieghe, D., Brysbaert, M., Desmet, T., and Debaecke, C. (2004). Word skipping in reading: On the interplay of linguistic and visual factors. *European Journal of Cognitive Psychology*, **16**, 79–103.

Drieghe, D., Pollatsek, A., Staub, A., and Rayner, K. (2008b). The word grouping hypothesis and eye movements during reading. *Journal of Experimental Psychology: Learning, Memory and Cognition*, **34**, 1552–1560.

Drieghe, D., Pollatsek, A., Juhasz, B.J., and Rayner, K. (2010). Parafoveal processing during reading is reduced across a morphological boundary. *Cognition*, **116**, 136–142.

Ehrlich, S.F. and Rayner, K. (1981). Contextual effects on word perception and eye movements during reading. *Journal of Verbal Learning and Verbal Behavior*, **20**, 641–655.

Engbert, R., Longtin, A., and Kliegl, R. (2002). A dynamical model of saccade generation in reading based on spatially distributed lexical processing. *Vision Research*, **42**, 621–636.

Engbert, R., Nuthmann, A., and Kliegl, R. (2007). An iterative algorithm for the estimation of the distribution of mislocated fixations during reading. In R.P.G. Van Gompel, M.F. Fischer, W.S. Murray, and R.L. Hill (eds.) *Eye movements: A window on mind and brain* (pp. 319–337). Oxford: Elsevier.

Engbert, R., Nuthmann, A., Richter, E., and Kliegl, R. (2005). SWIFT: A dynamical model of saccade generation during reading. *Psychological Review*, **112**, 777–813.

Henderson, J.M. and Ferreira, F. (1993). Eye movement control during reading: Fixation measures reflect foveal but not parafoveal processing difficulty. *Canadian Journal of Experimental Psychology*, **47**, 201–221.

Hyönä, J. and Bertram, R. (2004). Do frequency characteristics of nonfixated words influence the processing of fixated words during reading? *European Journal of Cognitive Psychology*, **16**, 104–127.

Inhoff, A.W., Starr, M., and Shindler, K.L. (2000b). Is the processing of words during eye fixations in reading strictly serial? *Perception and Psychophysics*, **62**, 1474–1484.

Inhoff, A.W., Radach, R., Starr, M., and Greenberg, S. (2000a). Allocation of visuo-spatial attention and saccade computation during eye fixations in reading. In A. Kennedy, R. Radach, D. Heller, and J. Pynte (eds.) *Reading as a perceptual process* (pp. 221–246). Oxford: Elsevier.

Joseph, H.S.S.L., Liversedge, S.P., Blythe, H.I., White, S.J., Gathercole, S.E., and Rayner, K. (2008). Children's and adults' processing of anomaly and implausibility during reading: Evidence from eye movements. *Quarterly Journal of Experimental Psychology*, **61**, 708–723.

Juhasz, B.J., Pollatsek, A., Hyönä, J., Drieghe, D., and Rayner, K. (2009). Parafoveal processing within and between words. *Quarterly Journal of Experimental Psychology*, **62**, 1356–1376.

Kambe, G. (2004). Parafoveal processing of prefixed words during eye fixations in reading: Evidence against morphological influences on parafoveal preprocessing. *Perception and Psychophysics*, **66**, 279–292.

Kennedy, A. (1998). The influence of parafoveal words on foveal inspection time: Evidence for a processing trade-off. In G. Underwood (ed.) *Eye Guidance in Reading and Scene Perception* (pp. 149–179). Oxford: Elsevier.

Kennedy, A. (2000). Parafoveal processing in word recognition. *Quarterly Journal of Experimental Psychology*, **53A**, 429–455.

Kennedy, A. (2008). Parafoveal-on-foveal effects are not an artifact of mislocated fixations. *Journal of Eye Movement Research*, **2**, 1–10.

Kennedy, A. and Pynte, J. (2005). Parafoveal-on-foveal effects in normal reading. *Vision Research*, **45**, 153–168.

Kennedy, A., Pynte, J., and Ducrot, S. (2002). Parafoveal-on-foveal interactions in word recognition. *Quarterly Journal of Experimental Psychology*, **55A**, 1307–1337.

Kennedy, A., Murray, W.S., and Boissiere, C. (2004). Parafoveal pragmatics revisited. *European Journal of Cognitive Psychology*, **16**, 128–153.

Kennison, S.M., and Clifton, C.C. (1995). Determinants of parafoveal preview benefit in high and low working memory capacity readers: Implications for eye movement control. *Journal of Experimental Psychology: Learning, Memory, and Cognition*, **21**, 68–81.

Kirkby, J.A., Webster, L.A.D., Blythe, H.I., and Liversedge, S.P. (2008). Binocular coordination during reading and non-reading tasks. *Psychological Bulletin*, **134**, 742–763.

Kliegl, R. and Engbert, R. (2003). SWIFT explorations. In Hyönä, J., Radach, R., and Deubel, H. (ed.) *Cognitive and Applied Aspects of Eye Movement Research* (pp. 391–411). Amsterdam: Elsevier.

Kliegl, R. and Engbert, R. (2005). Fixation durations before word skipping in reading. *Psychonomic Bulletin and Review*, **12**, 132–138.

Kliegl, R., Nuthmann, A., and Engbert, R. (2006). Tracking the mind during reading: The influence of past, present, and future words on fixation durations. *Journal of Experimental Psychology: General*, **135**, 12–35.

Kliegl, R., Risse, S., and Laubrock, J. (2007). Preview benefits and parafoveal-on-foveal effects from word n+2. *Journal of Experimental Psychology: Human Perception and Performance*, **33**, 1250–1255.

Liversedge, S.P., White, S.J., Findlay, J.M., and Rayner, K. (2006a). Binocular coordination of eye movements during reading. *Vision Research*, **46**, 2363–2374.

Liversedge, S.P., Rayner, K., White, S.J., Findlay, J.M., and McSorley, E. (2006b). Binocular coordination of the eyes during reading. *Current Biology*, **16**, 1726–1729.

McConkie, G.W. and Rayner, K. (1975). Span of effective stimulus during a fixation in reading. *Perception and Psychophysics*, **17**, 578–586.

McConkie, G.W., Kerr, P.W., Reddix, M.D., and Zola, D. (1988). Eye movement control during reading: I.The location of initial eye fixations on words. *Vision Research*, **28**, 1107–1118.

McDonald, S.A. (2005). Parafoveal preview benefit in reading is not cumulative across multiple saccades. *Vision Research*, **45**, 1829–1834.

McDonald, S.A. (2006a). Effects of number-of-letters on eye movements during reading are independent from effects of spatial word length. *Visual Cognition*, **13**, 89–98.

McDonald. S.A. (2006b). Parafoveal preview benefit in reading is only obtained from the saccade goal. *Vision Research*, **46**, 4416–4424.

Morrison, R.E. and Rayner, K. (1981). Saccade size in reading depends upon character spaces and not visual angle. *Perception and Psychophysics*, **30**, 395–396.

Murray, W.S. (1998). Parafoveal pragmatics. In G. Underwood (ed.) *Eye Guidance in Reading and Scene Perception* (pp. 181–200). Oxford: Elsevier.

Murray, W.S. and Rowan, M. (1998). Early, mandatory, pragmatic processing. *Journal of Psycholinguistic Research*, **27**, 1–22.

Nuthmann, A. and Kliegl, R. (2009). An examination of binocular reading fixations based on sentence corpus data. *Journal of Vision*, **9**, 1–28.

Nuthmann, A., Engbert, R., and Kliegl, R. (2007). The IOVP effect in mindless reading: Experiment and modelling. *Vision Research*, **47**, 990–1002.

Pollatsek, A. and Rayner, K. (1999). Is covert attention really unnecessary? *Behavioral and Brain Sciences*, **22**, 695.

Pollatsek, A., Rayner, K., and Balota, D.A. (1986). Inferences about eye-movement control from the perceptual span in reading. *Perception and Psychophysics*, **40**, 123–130.

Pollatsek, A., Reichle, E.D., and Rayner, K. (2003). Modeling eye movements in reading: Extensions of the E-Z Reader model. In J. Hyönä, R., Radach, and H. Deubel (eds.) *The Mind's Eye: Cognitive and Applied aspects of Eye Movement Research* (pp. 361–390). Oxford: Elsevier.

Pollatsek, A., Reichle, E.D., and Rayner, K. (2006). Tests of the E-Z Reader model: Exploring the interface between cognition and eye-movement control. *Cognitive Psychology*, **52**, 1–56.

Pynte, J. and Kennedy, A. (2006). An influence over eye movements in reading exerted from beyond the level of the word: Evidence from reading English and French. *Vision Research*, **46**, 3786–3801.

Pynte, J., Kennedy, A., and Ducrot, S. (2004). The influence of parafoveal typographical errors on eye movements in reading. *European Journal of Cognitive Psychology*, **16**, 178–202.

Radach, R. (1996). *Blickbewegungen beim Lesen: Psychologische Aspekte der Determination von Fixationspositionen* (Eye Movements in Reading). Münster/New York: Waxmann.

Radach, R. and Heller, D. (2000). Relations between spatial and temporal aspects of eye movement control. In A. Kennedy, R. Radach, D. Heller, and J. Pynte (eds.) *Reading as a perceptual process.* (pp. 165–191). Oxford: Elsevier.

Radach, R., Huestegge, and Reilly, R. (2008). The role of global top-down factors in eye-movement control in reading. *Psychological Research*, **72**, 675–688.

Rayner, K. (1975). Perceptual span and peripheral cues in reading. *Cognitive Psychology*, **7**, 65–81.

Rayner, K. (1998). Eye movements in reading and information processing: 20 years of research. *Psychological Bulletin*, **124**, 372–422.

Rayner, K. and Bertera, J.H. (1979). Reading without a fovea. *Science*, **206**, 468–469.

Rayner, K. and Fischer, M.H. (1996). Mindless reading revisited: Eye movements during reading and scanning are different. *Perception and Psychophysics*, **58**, 734–747.

Rayner, K., and Johnson, R.L. (2005). Letter-by-letter acquired dyslexia is due to the serial encoding of letters. *Psychological Science*, **16**, 530–534.

Rayner, K. and McConkie, G.W. (1976). What guides a readers eye-movements. *Vision Research*, **16**, 829–837.

Rayner, K. and Raney, G.E. (1996). Eye movement control in visual search: Effects of word frequency. *Psychonomic Bulletin and Review*, **3**, 238–244.

Rayner, K. and Well, A.D. (1996). Effects of contextual constraint on eye movements in reading: A further examination. *Psychonomic Bulletin and Review*, **3**, 504–509.

Rayner, K., Well, A.D., and Pollatsek, A. (1980). Asymmetry of the effective visual-field in reading. *Perception and Psychophysics*, **27**, 537–544.

Rayner, K., Reichle, E.D., and Pollatsek, A. (1998a). Eye movement control in reading: An overview and model. In G. Underwood (ed.) *Eye Guidance in Reading and Scene Perception* (pp. 243–268). Oxford: Elsevier.

Rayner, K., Fischer, M.H., and Pollatsek, A. (1998b). Unspaced text interferes with both word identification and eye movement control. *Vision Research*, **38**, 1129–1144.

Rayner, K., Reichle, E.D., and Pollatsek, A. (2000). Eye movement control in reading: Updating the E-Z Reader model to account for initial fixation locations and refixations. In A. Kennedy, R. Radach, D. Heller, and J. Pynte (eds.) *Reading as a perceptual process.* (pp. 701–719). Oxford, UK: Elsevier.

Rayner, K., Reichle, E. and Pollatsek, A. (2005). Eye movement control in reading and the E-Z Reader model. In G. Underwood (ed.) *Eye Guidance and Cognitive Processes.* Oxford: Oxford University Press, in press.

Rayner, K., Juhasz, B.J., and Brown, S.J. (2007a). Do readers obtain preview benefit from word n+2? A test of serial attention shift versus distributed lexical processing models of eye movement control in reading. *Journal of Experimental Psychology: Human Perception and Performance*, **33**, 230–245.

Rayner, K., Well, A.D., Pollatsek, A., and Bertera, J.H. (1982). The availability of useful information to the right of fixation in reading. *Perception and Psychophysics*, **31**, 537–550.

Rayner, K., Ashby, J., Pollatsek, A., and Reichle, E.D. (2004a). The effects of frequency and predictability on eye fixations in reading: Implications for the E-Z Reader model. *Journal of Experimental Psychology: Human Perception and Performance*, **30**, 720–732.

Rayner, K., Warren, T., Juhasz, B.J., and Liversedge, S.P. (2004b). The effect of plausibility on eye movements during reading. *Journal of Experimental Psychology: Learning, Memory, and Cognition*, **30**, 1290–1301.

Rayner, K., White, S.J., Kambe, G., Miller, B., and Liversedge, S.P. (2003). On the processing of meaning from parafoveal vision during eye fixations in reading. In Hyönä, J., Radach, R., and Deubel, H. (ed.) *Cognitive and Applied Aspects of Eye Movement Research* (pp. 213–234), Amsterdam: Elsevier.

Rayner, K., Pollatsek, A., Drieghe, D., Slattery, T.J., and Reichle, E.D. (2007b). Tracking the mind during reading via eye movements: Comments on Kliegl, Nuthmann, and Engbert (2006). *Journal of Experimental Psychology: General*, **136**, 520–529.

Reichle, E.D., Rayner, K., and Pollatsek, A. (1999). Eye movement control in reading: accounting for initial fixation locations and refixations within the E-Z Reader model. *Vision Research*, **39**, 4403–4411.

Reichle, E.D., Rayner, K., and Pollatsek, A. (2003). The E-Z Reader model of eye movement control in reading: comparisons to other models. *Behavioral and Brain Sciences*, **26**, 445–526.

Reichle, E., Pollatsek, A., and Rayner, K. (2007). Modeling the effects of lexical ambiguity on eye movements during reading. In R.P.G. Van Gompel, M.F. Fischer, W.S. Murray, and R.L. Hill (eds.) *Eye movements: A window on mind and brain* (pp. 271–292). Oxford: Elsevier.

Reichle, E.D, Warren, T. and McConnell, K. (2009b). Using E-Z Reader to model the effects of higher level language processing on eye movements during reading. *Psychonomic Bulletin and Review*, **16**, 1–21.

Reichle, E.D., Pollatsek, A., Fisher, D.L., and Rayner, K. (1998). Toward a model of eye movement control in reading. *Psychological Review*, **105**, 125–157.

Reichle, E.D., Liversedge, S.P., Pollatsek, A., and Rayner, K. (2009a). Encoding multiple words simultaneously in reading is implausible. *Trends in Cognitive Sciences*, **13**, 115–119.

Reilly, R.G. and Radach, R. (2003). Foundations of an interactive model of eye movement control in reading. In Hyönä, J., Radach, R., and Deubel, H. (ed.) *Cognitive and Applied Aspects of Eye Movement Research* (pp. 429–455). Amsterdam: Elsevier.

Reilly, R. and Radach, R. (2006). Some empirical tests of an interactive model of eye movement control in reading. *Cognitive Systems Research*, **7**, 34–55.

Staub, A., Rayner, K., Pollatsek, A., Hyönä, J., and Majewski, H. (2007). The time course of plausibility effects on eye movements in reading: Evidence from noun-noun compounds. *Journal of Experimental Psychology: Learning, Memory, and Cognition*, **33**, 1162–1169.

Schroyens, W., Vitu, F., Brysbaert, M, and d'Ydewalle, G. (1999). Eye movements during reading: Foveal load and parafoveal processing. *Quarterly Journal of Experimental Psychology*, **52A**, 1021–1046.

Starr, M. and Inhoff, A.W. (2004) Allocation of attention during eye fixations in reading. Use of orthographic information from multiple word locations. *European Journal of Cognitive Psychology*, **16**, 203–225.

Starr, M.S. and Rayner, K. (2001). Eye movements during reading: Some current controversies. *Trends in Cognitive Sciences*, **5**, 156–163.

Underwood, G., Binns, A., and Walker, S. (2000). Attentional demands on the processing of neighbouring words. In A. Kennedy, R. Radach, D. Heller, and J. Pynte (eds.) *Reading as a perceptual process* (pp. 247–268). Oxford: Elsevier.

Vitu, F., Brysbaert, M., and Lancelin, D. (2004). A test of parafoveal-on-foveal effects with pairs of orthographically related words. *European Journal of Cognitive Psychology*, **16**, 154–177.

White, S.J. (2008). Eye movement control during reading: Effects of word frequency and orthographic familiarity. *Journal of Experimental Psychology: Human Perception and Performance*, **34**, 205–223.

White, S.J. and Liversedge, S.P. (2004). Orthographic familiarity influences initial eye fixation positions in reading. *European Journal of Cognitive Psychology*, **16**, 52–78.

Yang, J., Wang, S., Xu, Y., and Rayner, K. (2009). Do Chinese readers obtain preview benefit from word n+2? Evidence from eye movements. *Journal of Experimental Psychology: Human Perception and Performance*, **35**, 1192–1204.

Yen, M-H., Radach, R., Tzeng, O. J.-L., Hung, D.L., and Tsai, J-L (2009). Early parafoveal processing in reading Chinese sentences. *Acta Psychologica*, **131**, 24–33.

CHAPTER 47

Eye movements and concurrent event-related potentials: Eye fixation-related potential investigations in reading

Thierry Baccino

Abstract

The eye-fixation related potential (EFRP) technique is based on electroencephalogram (EEG) measurements of electrical brain activity in response to eye fixations. EFRPs are extracted from the EEG by means of signal averaging but in contrast to conventional event-related potential (ERP) technique the averaged waveforms are time-locked to the onset and offset of eye fixation, not to the onset of stimulus events. EFRPs have shown to be a useful technique, in addition to eye movement recordings, to investigate early lexical processes and for establishing a timeline of these processes during reading. Moreover, the technique permits one to analyse the EEGs in a natural condition allowing the investigation of complex visual stimuli such as visual scenes or three-dimensional images. However, some challenges remain to be solved. Among them, we discuss the saccadic contamination and the overlap effects that may distort the findings and we propose some suggestions that might improve these issues. EFRPs may also represent a point of interest for many applications involving tools for disabled people, video games, or brain–computer interfaces.

Introduction

In the last 20 years computers and other electronic equipment have become remarkably important for vision research and cognitive psychology in general. While offline techniques such as questionnaires and recall tests were primarily used in experimental psychology during the 1960s and 1970s, the progress in computer science and electronics has allowed development of very accurate equipment for tracking cognitive processes online. Among these techniques, two methods, eye tracking and event-related potentials (ERPs), have become very popular and widely used in laboratories. Both of these techniques hold the potential to give a precise timeline description of processes over time and this temporal accuracy helps to refine the cognitive modelling. However, both techniques also have severe limitations. In this chapter, we start by reviewing the advantages and limitations of these techniques in order to show how their combination can provide a better understanding of cognitive operations. Indeed, seeking a convergence between different techniques has become an actual challenge for many laboratories in brain research and cognitive psychology. There are several attempts to combine EEG and functional magnetic resonance imaging (fMRI) (Rossell et al., 2003), magnetoencephalography (MEG) and fMRI (Sato et al., 2008), and fMRI and eye tracking (Brown et al., 2008) with the aim to find the best cognitive measurement. We will describe here how it is possible and relevant to combine ERP and eye tracking recordings (the so-called eye fixation-related potential (EFRP) technique) and how this EFRP technique can provide valuable information about cognitive processes underlying reading. Finally, we will review a number of challenges to be addressed in the future for improving this technique and to succeed in establishing a reliable technique for investigating cognition.

ERPs and eye movements are complementary techniques

ERPs are widely used in cognitive neuroscience to capture cognitive processes and their time-course with a high temporal resolution (Hillyard and Kutas, 1983). ERPs reflect electrical brain activity (primarily summed postsynaptic potentials of pyramidal cells in the neocortex) that is associated with sensory or cognitive events. ERPs emerge after averaging continuous electroencephalogram (EEG) recorded during many presentations of stimuli. These time-locked average waveforms show several positive (such as P1, P300, etc.) or negative (such as N1, N400, Contingent Negative Variation, etc.) components within a certain latency range after an event onset. Each component has a characteristic scalp distribution, some differences in polarity (positivity or negativity), amplitude, or latency that permit us to correlate them to particular cognitive processes (for a review, see Rugg and Coles, 1995). This technique has been used to investigate mechanisms of sensory memory (for review, see Näätänen, 1990 and Näätänen et al., 1978), semantics of language (for a review, see Kutas and Federmeier, 2000; Kutas and Hillyard, 1980), and visual perception (for a review, see Hegdé, 2008).

However, the ERP signal is contaminated by saccades and cannot be recorded with cognitive activities requiring a free visual inspection (i.e. with sequences of saccades). This limitation strongly constrains the use of this technique in a natural environment. Although several techniques such as multisource component analysis (Berg and Scherg, 1994) and regression-based methods (Wallstrom et al., 2004) have been developed to cope with these ocular artefacts, researchers usually reject the contaminated EEG segments resulting in data loss (Jung et al., 2000). In order to avoid such ocular artefacts caused by excessive saccadic eye movements (blinks, saccades), stimuli are therefore presented in isolation and subjects are asked to maintain their eyes fixated on the display and instructed to avoid any eye movements. This, however, creates difficulties, especially when reading, visual scene perception, or object recognition are under investigation.

Another serious difficulty with the ERP paradigm is that these isolated stimuli are displayed with unnaturally long intervals between them (>500 ms or 1000 ms). These long delays are intended to prevent the overlap between cognitive processes (Dambacher and Kliegl, 2007). They might also explain why rather late components such P300 and N400 have been investigated for studying cognition. For example, in reading studies, the presentation of words isolated with long interstimulus interval (ISIs) (as in Hillyard et al., 1983) prevents the study of any anticipatory or overlapping processes (spillover effects) which occur normally during text comprehension. This situation is far from a natural reading process and the ecological validity of the experimental results is questionable. In real life, most cognitive activities which involve a sequence of visual fixations to inspect the environment have a great majority of fixations lasting less than 300 ms. In reading once again, typical fixation lasts around 200 or 250 ms and during this time period all perceptual and cognitive operations are realized. In reality, studying the typical late ERP components in reading, such as P300 and N400, means that the eyes have already moved to the next word when the peak of these components appears.

Eye movement measurements provide a complementary method to capture cognitive processes with a high resolution. The eye tracking technique provides data about the positions and timing of eye fixations with a high spatial (<0.5° visual angle) and temporal accuracy (>1 kHz). It also allows one to distinguish between early and late processing by comparing first-pass fixations (fixations occurring in a certain region of interest for the first time) with second-pass fixations in the same region in order to capture the processes associated with reprocessing or verification. The eye tracking technique has been used widely during reading, scene viewing, and visual search tasks but also to investigate attentional effects during spoken language comprehension (Tanenhaus et al., 1995). Eye movement variables (such as fixation duration, timing, and saccadic path) provide a robust measure of underlying cognitive processes. In reading studies, for example, it has been shown that fixation duration to a lexically frequent word is shorter than to a non-frequent word (Rayner 1998) or that the length of scanpath can provide a good index of ergonomic difficulty on an interface (Goldberg and Kotval, 1998).

One of the major difficulties in interpreting the eye movements is to determine whether a fixation represents rather deep processing (i.e. semantic processing) or more superficial processing. The researcher can only rely on temporal variables (gaze duration, 1st pass fixation duration, etc.) obtained in certain experimental conditions for interpreting the meaning of these fixations. However, even in this case, the interpretation is not still ensured due to the large variability (between and within-subjects, tasks, etc.) on fixation durations and it would be beneficial to have other indices that might confirm or invalidate it.

Combining measures of ERPs and eye movements: EFRP technique

In our view, ERPs and eye movements provide complementary measures to capture cognitive processes providing the possibility to find out precisely when and in which order (in a text or visual scene) different cognitive operations occur. This approach has been used by measuring ERPs and electro-oculogram (EOG) simultaneously (Yagi et al., 1998; see also the literature on saccade-related potentials), or by measuring eye movements with an eye tracker and ERPs in separate sessions (Sereno et al., 1998), or by measuring ERPs and eye movements by an eye tracker simultaneously (Baccino and Manunta, 2005; Hutzler et al., 2007). Each of these approaches has, however, some limitations and further development is needed to understand the underlying cognitive processes during single eye fixations. In the following section these approaches are briefly described and the synchronized measuring technique is explained in detail.

EOG-based EFRPs

As early as 1964, the analysis of eye movements recorded concurrently with ERPs was used to investigate the neural processes associated with saccades (Gaarder et al., 1964). The so-called saccade-related potentials used EOGs that were measured simultaneously with EEG by electrodes placed on the scalp and around the eyes—horizontal and vertical EOGs, respectively. The EEG signals were time-locked to the onset of the saccades. These neurophysiological investigations were not focused on cognitive processes occurring during a fixation (on a meaningful stimulus) but rather by the topography (frontal or parietal areas) and temporality of human brain potentials *preceding* saccades (visually triggered or self-initiated). In particular, they widely used the well-known pro- and antisaccade task (Brickett et al., 1984; Evdokimidis et al., 1991, 1996; Everling and Fischer, 1998; Everling et al., 1997; Kurtzberg and Vaughan, 1982; Moster and Goldberg, 1990). The pro- and antisaccade terms refer to saccades that are performed towards a target (Pro-) or to the opposite side (Anti-). The overall scope was to determine whether a reflexive response (prosaccade) might be suppressed by a voluntary motor act (antisaccade). In particular, the task served to investigate pathophysiological mechanisms of several disorders of the central nervous system and has been used as a diagnostic tool.

The term EFRP was first introduced by Yagi and colleagues (Joyce et al., 2002; Yagi and Ogata, 1995; Yagi et al., 1998). EFRPs consisted of time-locking the EEG signals to the offset of saccadic eye movements and not at the onset of stimulus events, as in the conventional ERP studies and averaged them to obtain EFRPs for single eye fixations. The most prominent component of the EFRP is called the lambda response, which is a positive component with a latency of about 80 ms from the offset of saccades (Kazai and Yagi, 2003). The lambda response has been shown to exhibit changes with properties of the visual stimulus (e.g. Kazai and Yagi, 1999) and attention (Yagi, 1981). The purpose of these EFRP experiments has been to focus the interest on early ERP components showing that even at these short latencies cognitive signals might be extracted (and not only visual-evoked potentials). However, EFRP technique based on measuring EOG does not provide an accurate measurement of fixation location since the eye position is not tracked directly but recalculated from calibrated positions. Furthermore, the EOG method is sensitive to changes in luminance and the ability to accurately identify the amplitudes for small saccades is not very precise. EOG literature is replete with examples showing the limits of such a practice to determine the spatial accuracy of a fixation (Marton and Szirtes, 1988a, b). For a wide applicability of the EFRP technique, the exact determination of a subject's gaze position by means of an eye tracker is inevitable.

Infrared eye tracking-based EFRPs in two separate sessions

In some other studies, the analyses of eye movements concurrently to ERPs have been made by running two experiments in parallel: one using eye tracking and the other ERPs, but with *different* subjects (Dambacher et al., 2007; Sereno and Rayner, 2003; Sereno et al., 1998). Trying to establish a timeline of lexical processing, Sereno et al. (2003) showed interesting findings on early components (P1, N1, P2) appearing during a single fixation. ERPs appeared to be sensitive to lexical processing as early as 100 ms and to context effects as early as 132 ms (132–192 ms) after stimulus presentation. However, due to parallel and not simultaneous measures of ERPs and eye movements, the results are not confirmative because they come from different experiments increasing the variability of data.

Infrared eye tracking-based EFRPs

The EFRP technique has been recently improved by synchronizing the measures from an infrared eye tracker with an EEG permitting the recording of data simultaneously (Baccino et al., 2005; Hutzler et al., 2007; Simola et al., 2009). The setup of an EFRP experimental platform is based on two computers generally connected through their parallel ports (Fig. 47.1).

While one computer (A) is devoted to stimulus presentation and eye movement (EM) acquisition, the other one (B) collects the EEG signals. The coupling of the two systems is achieved by sending a synchronization signal (TTL Trigger) as soon as the stimulus (words, images, etc.) is presented on the display (stimulus onset). The synchronization signal enables the EM and EEG data to be recorded simultaneously and to get an accurate timestamp for offline data matching. Therefore, one important thing is to ensure that both signals are sampled at the same rate. A sampling rate around 1 KHz is, at present, possible with many EEG and eye trackers and this frequency appears preferable to detect fine processes occurring within a fixation. EFRPs will emerge with segmentation of the continuous EEG signal with reference markers such as fixation onset and offset detected during eye movement analysis. As in ERP studies, EFRPs are obtained by averaging the EEG epochs for every fixation on a specific stimulus but are shorter in time than ERPs.

The EFRP technique has several advantages when compared with previously techniques using EOG or recording eye movements and ERPs in separate sessions.

- *Same subject, same stimulus:* one of the most important advantages is to directly correlate the eye fixations with the EEGs for the same subject, the same stimulus, and within the same region of interest. This procedure decreases the data variability observed in comparing eye movements and ERPs in separate sessions and ensures better interpretation of the underlying cognitive processes.

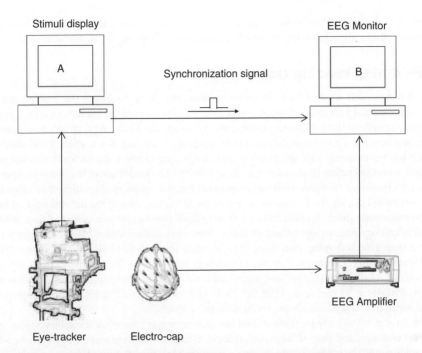

Fig. 47.1 Experimental set-up for recording EFRPs. A TTL trigger synchronizes two computers, one (A) dedicated to presentation of stimuli and eye tracking, and the other one (B) monitoring and recording the EEG.

- *Precise time line:* combined with an eye tracker at high temporal resolution (≥1 KHz) and high accuracy (<1° visual angle), EFRP technique allows one to establish a precise time course of the activation/inhibition sequence of EEG waveforms underlying any fixation. Thus, it is possible to know what EEG components are correlated to a fixation on a specific stimulus and this can be fruitful for cognitive interpretation and modelling. In this sense, the EFRP technique acts as a zoom into a fixation and permits to investigate the role of early components in cognitive activity rather than late components which have been extensively studied by the conventional ERP paradigm. However, some challenges have to be solved as the overlap problem associated to short stimuli presentation (Dambacher et al., 2007) and some suggestions will be given in the next section.

- *Natural context:* another major advantage of the EFRP technique is the ability to capture ERPs in a natural context. As we have seen, the artificial presentation of stimuli during a conventional ERP paradigm requiring a steady gaze during one or more seconds is no longer employed with EFRPs. This artificial presentation could sometimes be the cause of severe restrictions especially for studying spillover effects[1] or integrative processes (as in text comprehension). With the EFRP technique, experimental settings allowing for a strong ecological validity can be used since the technique allows one to move the gaze freely onto any complex stimuli (text, visual scenes, etc.).

- *Categorizing fixations:* recently, Unema et al. (2005) have shown by crossing fixation duration with the amplitude of the following saccade that fixations, at least during free viewing, can be categorized as ambient or focal fixations. EFRP analyses should be able to improve this categorization process by analysing the corresponding EEGs components and detect whether some attentional/semantic component can be associated to the fixation. Separating these components with statistical procedures (see next section) but also the localization of the activation (on which

---

[1] Effects coming from the previous word and spread out on the next word.

electrode) may be highly informative for labelling fixations. These findings will contribute greatly to interpreting scanpaths and fixations on some region of interests in real life activities.

EFRPs during reading tasks

One of the most well-studied ERP components associated with reading is the N400 component which occurs several hundreds of milliseconds after word presentation. There is extensive evidence that the occurrence of the N400 component is related to semantic priming that indicates a semantic relationship between a word and the context in which it occurs (e.g. Kutas et al., 1980, 2000). In a typical N400 experiment, a subject reads a sentence having either a semantically incongruent or congruent sentence ending (Federmeier and Kutas, 1999). The amplitude of the N400 component is smaller for congruent compared with incongruent sentence endings suggesting that more lexical search is required during the incongruent condition. However, during the natural reading process the eye fixations are short (around 200 to 250 ms) which constrains the amount of time for lexical processing and oculomotor operations (Rayner, 1998). As a consequence, ERP components occurring later than 250 ms overlap with those in response to the next word (Dambacher et al., 2007). It seems therefore important to examine the early components and to find out about their role in lexical processing. Only a few studies have examined early components by comparing eye movements and early ERPs (e.g. Sereno et al., 1998, 2003). In both of these studies, ERPs and eye movements were recorded in two separate sessions with different subjects.

In Sereno et al. (1998), eye movements and the ERPs were recorded while the subjects were reading single-line sentences and performing a lexical decision task for words presented in isolation, whereas in the other study, the subjects were reading sentences. However, the words were presented word-by-word, and the target word was always at the end of the sentence (Sereno et al., 2003). High- and low-frequency regular words were compared with high- and low-frequency non-regular words. ERP outcomes showed that a lexical effect emerges around 100 ms post-stimulus as reflected by P1 component, followed by N1 and P2 components associated with word frequency and regularity, respectively (Sereno et al., 1998). On the other hand, Raney and Rayner (1993) studied mechanisms of rereading by recording eye movements and ERPs also in two separate sessions. Eye movement recordings showed that reading speed increased during the second reading, that is, forward fixation durations were shorter, the number of forward fixations decreased, and forward saccade lengths increased. The ERP results showed that the amplitude of N1–P2 complex increased during the second reading, suggesting that during the second reading 'lower level' demands such as initial perceptual and comprehension processes decreased and this facilitation is reflected in the magnitude of N1–P2 responses. As mentioned previously, all of these comparative studies between ERPs and eye movements did not use real EFRPs since both measures have been made with different subjects in separate sessions.

In a first study on reading using a real EFRPs technique, Baccino et al. (2005) recorded EEGs and eye movements simultaneously during a priming task. The prime and the target words were presented simultaneously and subjects were asked to make a judgement about semantic relatedness after reading the two words. The aim of the work was to study parafoveal-on-foveal effect, that is, whether the processing of the next word (word on the right) affects the processing of the fixated word in order to test whether parallel or sequential processing occurs during reading and whether semantic processing occurs in the parafoveal field during early lexical processing. The results showed that even first-pass fixation duration (summed fixation duration before the eyes moved to the second word) did not show any evidence for semantic processing during parafoveal processing, the early EFRPs in response to prime words were sensitive to lexical processing of the target word, especially at occipital O1 electrode (Fig. 47.2). A marginally stronger effect was found for the amplitude of N1 component at around 120 ms post-stimulus. Similarly, a stronger effect was found for non-associated than for non-words for a positive component appearing around at 140 ms post-stimulus at the central and frontal recording sites. These results suggest that these early ERP effects are due to sensitivity to word form in parafoveal area and preventing semantic access of illegal form for further processing. Semantic effects were observed in the P2 component (peaking around 215 ms) which was more pronounced

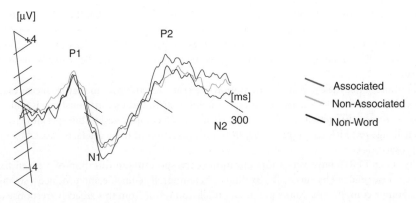

Fig. 47.2 Grand-averaged EFRP waveforms recorded at the left occipital electrode (O1) during three conditions: associated, non-associated and non-word prime-target word pairs.

during processing of prime words followed by associated other than non-associated target words suggesting that semantic processing occurs parafoveally during early lexical processing.

However, in all previous ERP studies, the reading process was mimicked by presenting the words in isolation (Sereno et al., 1998), word-by-word (Sereno et al., 2003), or presenting only two words simultaneously (Baccino et al., 2005). It is questionable whether these paradigms are suitable enough to study the mechanisms of reading or whether they instead capture processes related to single word processing. As a consequence further investigations are needed in order to understand the mechanisms underlying reading sentences but also to find out whether the EFRP technique brings added value in comparison to conventional ERP studies in this area.

In a recent study, Hutzler et al. (2007) attempted to validate the EFRP technique by comparing it with the conventional ERP technique on a very known effect in visual word recognition: the old/new effect (Rugg and Nagy, 1989). This effect is characterized by a positive component peaking around 250 ms for correctly recognized old words. Subjects were instructed to read a sentence with five words presented concomitantly in a row. After correcting the EOG artefacts with an independent component analysis (ICA), similar results were acquired using both techniques. Brain potentials associated with old words were more positive at the right than the left recording sites and in anterior and central regions as reported earlier by Rugg et al. (1989). This positivity occurred in a time window from 250 to 600 ms after reading the last word in a sentence. With this striking similarity of effects, the authors conclude that EFRPs are as reliable indicators of word processing as conventional ERPs.

Challenges in EFRP research

While the EFRPs seem to have a promising future in the cognitive toolbox, some challenges remain to be solved for rendering this technique efficient and reliable. In particular, further investigations are needed to understand which factors have a prominent contribution to EFRP waveforms by removing the effects of previous saccadic amplitude and microsaccades within the fixation and by analysing the effects of overlap processes. These questions cannot be only processed by psychologists but require the contribution of more formal sciences such as mathematics, statistics and signal processing. This renders this technique highly interdisciplinary and very challenging.

EEG source separation: overlap responses, saccade and microsaccade artefacts

During a conventional ERP paradigm, the EEG signal is contaminated by saccadic eye movements. While in the EFRP paradigm, theoretically only the EEG segments occurring during a visual fixation are analysed (and so eye movements are filtered out), it is still possible that these EEG segments are contaminated by saccadic eye movements that precede or follow fixations. A number of ocular corrections algorithms (Schwind and Dormann, 1986; Vigário, 1997; Wallstrom et al., 2004) have been applied to EEG analyses and one challenge would be to test whether they can also be applied to EFRP data.

Furthermore, since the eye is always in motion even during a fixation, miniature saccades (microsaccades, drifts, tremors) are actively generated involuntarily and unconsciously. It is still possible that this microsaccadic[2] activity represents an artefact which complicates the interpretation of EFRPs. A real challenge in EFRP technique is therefore the correction of these artefacts caused by saccades and microsaccades.

Finally, since EFRPs have very short duration (corresponding to duration of a given fixation) neural responses elicited by successive fixations can temporally coincide and produce a strong overlap of cognitive components. Many potential pitfalls can result from this adjacent-response overlap and it can distort the EFRPs averages. A challenge would be to solve this overlap problem.

All these potentials problems (saccades, microsaccades, and overlap) are related to the fact that the EFRP waveforms are complex and difficult to interpret. So, the question for the future, which is also the case for classical ERP studies, would be to dissociate this complex signal into a set of simpler signals in order to determine more clearly the underlying cognitive processes correlated with them. This question has received a lot of consideration in the past mainly by using several decomposition methods.

Saccades artefacts and ocular corrections

As stated above, the EEG signals are contaminated by extracerebral artefacts of biological origin, originating outside the brain, but still recordable from the scalp (Gratton, 1998; Schwind et al., 1986; Vigário, 1997). These extracerebral signals come mainly from tongue, facial, jaw, and neck muscles which generate a persistent low-voltage high-frequency signals (>20 Hz) with focused spatial distribution and rapidly decaying autocorrelation function (Whitham et al., 2007). Since, these artefacts have characteristic signatures in space, time, and frequency, definitely distinct from EEG spontaneous activity (Picton et al., 2000), a number of valuable statistical techniques have been developed to handle these ocular artefacts in the EEG signals and to remove them. The best known methodology for doing this is blind source separation (BSS) based on second-order statistics (such as autocorrelation) or based on higher-order statistics such as principal component analysis (PCA) or independent component analysis (ICA) (Congedo et al., 2008). The principle of BSS is the separation of a set of signals from a set of mixed signals, without the aid of any information (or with little information) about the source signals or the mixing process. BSS can be applied only if source signals does not correlate with each other and thus the separation is realized such that the regularity of each resulting signal is maximized, and the regularity between the signals is minimized (i.e. statistical independence is maximized). BSS methods have proven their usefulness in the removal of eye blinks from the EEG signals because of their high energy (Jung et al., 1998, 2000) and recently to identify the signal of cognitive load in pupillary responses (Jainta and Baccino, 2010). But eye movements, both volitional movements, saccades and microsaccades, generate smaller brain potentials than do blinks and the question is whether these BSS methods can also be applied here. This has been suggested in a comparative study testing different BSS methods (Wallstrom et al., 2004). Other approaches have been introduced using Bayesian techniques (Roberts, 1998) or incorporating a model of brain activity to detect already known brain components (Berg et al., 1994). The research on EEG source separation is still in constant evolution and the challenge for EFRP studies will be to investigate which of the different ocular correction algorithms have to be chosen or developed for having the most reliable EFRPs possible.

---

[2] Here, the term microsaccade will be used generically.

Microsaccades artefacts

Microsaccades (Engbert 2006; Martinez-Conde et al., 2004, see also Martinez-Conde and Macknick, Chapter 6, this volume) are small saccades (mostly <0.5°) occurring involuntarily during fixation. Their role seems to neutralize the natural perceptual fading caused by retinal adaptation during fixation. Even under stabilized conditions of visual stimulus presentation as used with a conventional ERP paradigm, the micro-saccadic activity can be a source of artefacts, specifically an induced enhancement of power in the gamma band (30–70 Hz) around 200–300 ms following stimulus onset. Usually, this gamma-band activity is widely assumed to reflect synchronous neural oscillation associated with perceptual binding (i.e. binding of visual elements into unitary percepts) (Tallon-Baudry et al., 1996), recognition of object category and familiarity (Tallon-Baudry et al., 1997), attention (Kaiser and Lutzenberger, 2005), and consciousness (Summerfield et al., 2002). Recently, it has been suggested that this synchronization reflects rather the outcome of ocular muscle spike potentials generated by microsaccades (Yuval-Greenberg et al., 2008). Most of the classical ERP studies do not control microsaccades although they can represent a serious source of artefacts and consequently for EFRPs analyses. However, due to their weak electrical activity generated, microsaccades cannot be removed automatically by BSS techniques as for saccades previously. Consequently, one challenge is to devise new methods capable of identifying the electrical signature of microsaccades in EFRPs signal according to their characteristics.

Overlap processes occurring during short EFRPs

EFRPs are obtained by signal-averaging EEG epochs which are time-locked to eye fixations. However, as EFRPs are especially short in time around 200–300 ms—which is the delay for fixation duration on average in reading—they can overlap in time because of successive fixations. This overlap can distort the EFRPs averages mostly in the earliest components (P1, N1). A future challenge in EFRP research will be to analyse the distortion of these EFRP averages provoked by the adjacent-response overlap in order to isolate the different components and permit their interpretation. Various methods may be employed to deal with this overlap.

A promising approach seems to be those employed by Woldorff (1993) with a set of algorithms (ADJAR for Adjacent Response Technique) that might be applied to dissociate the effects coming from successive fixations (Talsma and Woldorff, 2005). At the origin, this method has been devised to cope with the overlap problem occurring in the ERPs recorded at high stimulus presentation rates (i.e. short ISIs). Indeed, at short ISIs, the ERP responses to successive stimuli may overlap and distort the ERP averages. The case is similar for eye fixations. The procedure works in two steps: first, by subtracting out the differential distortion from previous fixation overlap and secondly by using an iterative algorithm trying to converge toward the best estimates of the waveform (i.e. by removing distortions resulting from overlap by both previous and subsequent fixation). The method has been employed successfully for dissociating attentional components (Fu et al., 2005) or removing overlap from scalp-recorded activity (Hopfinger and Maxwell, 2005).

Another approach would be to employ a statistical decomposition method already known for removing ocular artefacts and which also may be used to dissociate the different subcomponents which occur during EFRPs data. PCA and ICA are of course popular methods that can be used for this purpose (see also the description of BSS methods given earlier) and are used to create space/time decompositions of the EEG signal. All of them attempt to decompose an array of data into sets of component scores and loadings (Shaw, 2003) using eigenvalue decomposition to derive the components of EEG signals. While PCA supposes that EEG sources are spatially orthogonal to one another (i.e. independent of each other), ICA segregates these EEG sources using non-orthogonal (oblique) factors. A priori, there is no reason to believe that distinct EEG sources are spatially orthogonal and this explains why ICA is generally preferred to PCA (Jung et al., 1998, 2000) for this objective. The ICA approach is better for the study of cortical sources of ERP because ICA components tend to result in single components that are a result of single cortical sources, whereas PCA components often result in single components that are linear combinations of multiple underlying sources and must be modelled with multiple-dipole source models (Richards, 2004). Actually, the problem with these statistical techniques lies in the interpretation of the different isolated components, namely how to associate components to cognitive processes–attention, semantic. . . . One way would be to go beyond the two-way data used in PCA/ICA and overcome the typical time-frequency decomposition of single channels. Such methods are called multi-way methods (Miwakeichi et al., 2004; Mørup et al., 2006) and permit to add more variables into the analysis such as channels, subjects, conditions, etc. One of these multiway methods is the Parallel Factor Analysis (PARAFAC) used in several papers for separating multiple potential components in the EEGs (Mørup et al., 2006, 2007). We assume that PARAFAC may be also well adapted to separate different components elicited by successive fixations (as EFRPs) in entering them into the analysis. This operation should cope with the overlap difficulty inherent to EFRPs and this type of work should be carrying out in the future.

Categorizing fixations and ecological impact

One of the most difficult exercises for any scientific experimenter is to interpret different measures recorded during an experiment. Measurement is usually very variable according to subject variability or task characteristics. As we seen in previous sections, the problem is also obvious for both eye tracking and ERP techniques. For example, how is it possible to compare two fixations apart from their duration or from the orientation of the previous saccade (backward vs. forward saccade) and to be able to interpret the underlying processes occurring during this fixation? One of the major advances of the EFRPs should be to succeed in categorizing or describing more accurately eye movements (fixations and saccades) as a function of the concurrent EEG measures. However, as in any fixation several components overlap, a challenge in the development of the technique would be to index some specific brainwaves that might correlate closely to some cognitive processes (attention, perception, etc.) as the N400 is an index of semantic incongruity. This challenge certainly needs the development of appropriate signal processing analyses as shown above and also to test on simple tasks dedicated to one component the characteristics of the associated EFRPs. Once these questions are addressed, it would be possible to improve the interpretation process by generating some interpretation maps which consists of visualizing the attentional/perceptual/semantic components coupled with gaze positions. Until now, these maps can only represent the position or duration of fixations but with the adjunct of EFRP analyses, it would be possible to categorize fixations from their principal component. For example, in the Unemà experiment (2005) which aims to disentangle between ambient or focal fixations by crossing two different variables (saccade extent and fixation duration), EFRPs will surely bring better information about the characteristics of EFRPs associated with each fixation and would facilitate the cognitive labelling of these fixations. Furthermore, the activation/inhibition phases can be spatially localized on the scalp and this spatial information can provide some information about the type of processing involved. Let's take an illustration from the distinction between ambient/focal fixations during the perception of visual scenes (Velichkovsky, 2002). As the author pointed out, there is a possibility that during the ambient processing (pre-attentive mode) the neural substrates in the 'dorsal visual pathway' guide the eye movements and locate the regions of interest for further examination. In contrast, during focal processing (attentive mode), the neuronal network in the 'ventral visual pathway' is thought to be recruited for further analysis of object shape, colour, and texture. If these claims are true, electrodes attached to the dorsal region should be more activated during ambient fixations and electrodes attached to ventral region more activated during focal fixations. In both cases, EFRPs should reflect these two modes of visual processing and may help in classifying fixations as ambient or focal.

An applied perspective of EFRPs: brain–computer interfaces

BCIs is an emergent field of human–computer interfaces (HCIs) which aims to utilize neurophysiological signals (such as EEG or any brain imagery techniques) originating in the brain to control external devices or computers. Of course, the application of BCIs is obvious for impaired people but can have also many other applications in video-game, remote system control (robot, camera, etc.) and any adaptive interfaces in real or virtual environments. However, nowadays, BCI control capabilities are still not comparable to other HCI peripherals such as joysticks or a computer mouse and the technique remains focused on impairments. Most investigated paradigms include motor commands that are either real or imaginary; virtual spellers or object selectors based on the monitoring of the subject's oriented attention, either auditory or visual (Birbaumer et al., 2006). EFRPs and BCI techniques are very close in essence, they represent the two sides of a same principle: how to interpret an EEG signal either to understand cognitive processes in context (EFRPs) or to work out an action by controlling a device in real-time (BCIs). As a consequence, the same questions need to be solved: how to process the EEG (EFRP) signal, what waves patterns can be picked up as detectable cognitive activity and for BCI how to translate them into control devices.

Conclusion and future studies

The EFRP technique has proven to be a useful approach to investigate cognitive processes during reading by simultaneously measuring eye movements and concurrent ERPs. In comparison with conventional ERP technique, it provides a better tool to investigate these processes in a more natural experimental setting, allowing eye movements to occur naturally during reading or viewing. Moreover, EFRP can have a large number of applications with BCIs in adding the eye position information to the recorded continuous EEGs and allowing a more precise knowledge of the underlying cognitive activity. These applicative forms may be useful for the development of assistive technologies for disabled people. However, as with every new methodology, some challenges need to be resolved, particularly the problem of overlapping processes. Decomposition methods seem to be suitable for disentangling the complex brain waves into simpler and interpretable components. Furthermore, more experimental studies are needed to ascertain the role of factors that influence the EFRP components. Despite some methodological drawbacks, coupling of eye movement and ERP recording techniques (that might be called augmented eye movements) provides a valuable tool to explore the neural, cognitive and behavioural mechanisms and their time course during reading or any other cognitive tasks involving visual inputs such as object recognition (Rämä and Baccino, 2010).

Acknowledgements

This work was supported by a contract from the ANR (Research National Agency) of France given to the project Gaze&EEG under the White Program n°09-0330. Portions of this paper were presented at the ECEM'09 (Southampton, August 2009). I thank Stefan Everling and one anonymous reviewer for their insightful comments.

References

Baccino, T. and Manunta, Y. (2005). Eye-fixation-related potentials: insight into parafoveal processing. *Journal of Psychophysiology*, **19**(3), 204–215.

Berg, P. and Scherg, M. (1994). A multiple source approach to the correction of eye artifacts. *Electroencephalography and Clinical Neurophysiology*, **90**(3), 229–241.

Birbaumer, N., Weber, C., Neuper, C., Buch, E., Haapen, K., and Cohen, L. (2006). Physiological regulation of thinking: brain-computer interface (BCI) research. *Progress in Brain Research*, **159**: 369–391.

Brickett, P.A., Weinberg, H., and Davis, C.M. (1984). Cerebral potentials preceding visually triggered saccades. *Annals of the New York Academy of Sciences*, **425**: 429–433.

Brown, M.R.G., Vilis, T., and Everling, S. (2008). Isolation of saccade inhibition processes: Rapid event-related fMRI of saccades and nogo trials. *NeuroImage*, **39**(2), 793–804.

Congedo, M., Gouy-Pailler, C., and Jutten, C. (2008). On the blind source separation of human electroencephalogram by approximate joint diagonalization of second order statistics. *Clinical Neurophysiology*, **119**(12), 2677–2686.

Dambacher, M., and Kliegl, R. (2007). Synchronizing timelines: Relations between fixation durations and N400 amplitudes during sentence reading. *Brain Research*, **1155**, 147–162.

Engbert, R. (2006). Microsaccades: a microcosm for research on oculomotor control, attention, and visual perception. In Martinez-Conde, S., Macknik, S.L., Martinez, L.M., Alonso, J.-M., and Tse, P.U. (eds.) *Progress in Brain Research* (pp. 177–192). Amsterdam: Elsevier.

Evdokimidis, I., Liakopoulos, D., and Papageorgiou, C. (1991). Cortical potentials preceding centrifugal and centripetal self-paced horizontal saccades. *Electroencephalography and Clinical Neurophysiology*, **79**, 503–505.

Evdokimidis, I., Liakopoulos, D., Constantinidis, T.S., and Papageorgiou, C. (1996). Cortical potentials with antisaccades. *Electroencephalography and Clinical Neurophysiology*, **98**, 377–384.

Everling, S. and Fischer, B. (1998). The antisaccade: a review of basic research and clinical studies. *Neuropsychologia*, **36**(9), 885–899.

Everling, S., Krappmann, P., and Flohr, H. (1997). Cortical potentials preceding pro- and antisaccades in man. *Electroencephalography and Clinical Neurophysiology*, **102**(4), 356–362.

Federmeier, K.D. and Kutas, M. (1999). A rose by any other name: Long-term memory structure and sentence processing. *Journal of Memory & Language*, **41**(4), 469–495.

Fu, S., Caggiano, D.M., Greenwood, P.M., and Parasuraman, R. (2005). Event-related potentials reveal dissociable mechanisms for orienting and focusing visuospatial attention. *Brain research. Cognitive Brain Research*, **23**(2–3), 341–353.

Gaarder, K., Krauskopf, J., Graf, V., Kropfl, W., and Armington, J.C. (1964). Averaged brain activity following saccadic eye movement. *Science*, **146**, 1481–1483.

Goldberg, J. and Kotval, X.P. (1998). Computer interface evaluation using eye movements: methods and constructs. *International Journal of Industrial Ergonomics*, **24**, 631–645.

Gratton, G. (1998). Dealing with artifacts: The EOG contamination of the event-related brain potential. *Behavior Research Methods, Instruments & Computers*, **30**(1), 44–53.

Hegdé, J. (2008). Time course of visual perception: coarse-to-fine processing and beyond. *Progress in Neurobiology*, **84**(4), 405–439.

Hillyard, S.A., and Kutas, M. (1983). Electrophysiology of cognitive processing. *Annual Review of Psychology* **34**, 33–61.

Hopfinger, J.B., and Maxwell, J.S. (2005). Appearing and disappearing stimuli trigger a reflexive modulation of visual cortical activity. *Cognitive Brain Research*, **25**(1), 48–56.

Hutzler, F., Braun, M., Võ, M.L.-H., Engl, V., Hofmann, M., Dambacher, M., *et al.* (2007). Welcome to the real world: Validating fixation-related brain potentials for ecologically valid settings. *Brain Research*, **1172**: 124–129.

Jainta, S. and Baccino, T. (2010). Analyzing the pupil response due to increased cognitive demand: An independent component analysis study. *International Journal of Psychophysiology*, **77**, 1–7.

Joyce, C., Gorodnitsky, I., King, J., and Kutas, M. (2002). Tracking eye fixations with electroocular and electroencephalographic recordings. *Psychophysiology*, **39**(5), 607–618.

Jung, T.P., Humphries, C., Lee, T.W., Makeig, S., McKeown, M.J., Iragui, V., *et al.* (1998). Removing Electroencephalographic Artifacts : Comparison between ICA and PCA. *Neural Networks for Signal Processing*, **VIII**, 63–72.

Jung, T.P., Makeig, S., Humphries, C., Lee, T.W., McKeown, M.J., Iragui, V., *et al.* (2000). Removing electroencephalographic artifacts by blind source separation. *Psychophysiology*, **37**(2), 163–178.

Kaiser, J. and Lutzenberger, W. (2005). Human gamma-band activity: a window to cognitive processing. *Neuroreport*, **16**(3), 207–211.

Kazai, K. and Yagi, A. (1999). Integrated effect of stimulation at fixation points on EFRP (Eye-fixation related brain potentials). *International Journal of Psychophysiology*, **32**, 193–203.

Kazai, K. and Yagi, A. (2003). Comparison between the lambda response of eye-fixation-related potentials and the P100 component of pattern-reversal visual evoked potentials. *Cognitive, Affective & Behavioral Neuroscience*, **3**(1), 46–56.

Kurtzberg, D. and Vaughan, J.H.G. (1982). Topographic analysis of human cortical potentials preceding self-initiated and visually triggered saccades. *Brain Research*, **243**(1), 1–9.

Kutas, M. and Hillyard, S.A. (1980). Reading senseless sentences: brain potentials reflect semantic incongruity. *Science*, **207**, 203–205.

Kutas, M. and Federmeier, K.D. (2000). Electrophysiology reveals semantic memory use in language comprehension. *Trends in Cognitive Science*, **4**, 463–470.

Martinez-Conde, S., Macknik, S.L., and Hubel, D.H. (2004). The role of fixational eye movements in visual perception. *Nature Reviews Neuroscience*, **5**(3), 229–240.

Marton, M. and Szirtes, J. (1988a). Context effects on saccade-related brain potentials to words during reading. *Neuropsychologia*, **26**(3), 453–463.

Marton, M. and Szirtes, J. (1988b). Saccade-related brain potentials during reading correct and incorrect versions of proverbs. *International Journal of Psychophysiology*, **6**(4), 273–280.

Miwakeichi, F., Martínez-Montes, E., Valdés-Sosa, P.A., Nishiyama, N., Mizuhara, H., and Yamaguchi, Y. (2004). Decomposing EEG data into space-time-frequency components using parallel factor analysis. *NeuroImage*, **22**(3), 1035–1045.

Mørup, M., Hansen, L.K., and Arnfred, S.M. (2007). ERPWAVELAB a toolbox for multi-channel analysis of time-frequency transformed event related potentials. *Journal of Neuroscience Methods* **161**(2), 361–368.

Mørup, M., Hansen, L.K., Herrmann, C.S., Parnas, J., and Arnfred, S.M. (2006). Parallel factor analysis as an exploratory tool for wavelet transformed event-related EEG. *NeuroImage*, **29**(3), 938–947.

Moster, M.L. and Goldberg, G. (1990). Topography of scalp potentials preceding self-initiated saccades. *Neurology*, **40**(4), 644–648.

Näätänen, R. (1990). The role of attention in auditory information processing as revealed by event-related potentials and other brain measures of cognitive function. *Behavioral and Brain Sciences*, **13**, 201–288.

Näätänen, R. Gaillard, A.W.K. and Mäntysalo, S. (1978). Early selective-attention effect on evoked potential reinterpreted. *Acta Psychologica*, **42**, 313–329.

Picton, T.W., Bentin, S., Berg, P., Donchin, E., Hillyard, S.A., Johnson, R., Jr, *et al.* (2000). Guidelines for using human event-related potentials to study cognition: recording standards and publication criteria. *Psychophysiology*, **37**(2), 127–152.

Rämä, P. & Baccino, T. (2010). Eye-fixation related potentials (EFRPs) during object identification. *Visual Neuroscience*, **27**, 187–192.

Raney, G.E. and Rayner, K. (1993). Event-related brain potentials, eye movements, and reading. *Psychological Science*, **4**(5), 283–286.

Rayner, K. (1998). Eye movements in reading and information processing: 20 years of research. *Psychological Bulletin*, **124**(3), 372–422.

Richards, J.E. (2004). Recovering dipole sources from scalp-recorded event-related-potentials using component analysis: principal component analysis and independent component analysis. *International Journal of Psychophysiology*, **54**(3), 201–220.

Roberts, S.J. (1998). Independent component analysis: source assessment and separation, a Bayesian approach. *Vision, Image and Signal Processing, IEE Proceedings*, **145**(3), 149–153.

Rossell, S.L., Price, C.J., and Nobre, A.C. (2003). The anatomy and time course of semantic priming investigated by fMRI and ERPs. *Neuropsychologia*, **41**(5), 550–564.

Rugg, M.D., and Coles, M.G.H. (1995). The ERP and cognitive psychology: Conceptual issues. In M.D. Rugg, and M.G.H. Coles (eds.) *Electrophysiology of Mind* (pp. 27–39). London: Oxford University Press.

Rugg, M.D., and Nagy, M.E. (1989). Event-related potentials and recognition memory for words. *Electroencephalography and Clinical Neurophysiology*, **72**(5), 395–406.

Sato, W., Kochiyama, T., Uono, S., and Yoshikawa, S. (2008). Time course of superior temporal sulcus activity in response to eye gaze: a combined fMRI and MEG study. *Social Cognitive and Affective Neuroscience*, **3**(3), 224–232.

Schwind, J., and Dormann, W.-U. (1986). Off-line removal of ocular artifacts from event-related potentials using a multiple linear regression model. *International Journal of Psychophysiology*, **4**(3), 203–208.

Sereno, S. and Rayner, K. (2003). Measuring word recognition in reading: eye movements and event-related potentials. *Trends in Cognitive Sciences*, **7**(11), 489–493.

Sereno, S., Rayner, K., and Posner, M.I. (1998). Establishing a time-line of word recognition: evidence from eye movements and event-related potentials. *Neuroreport*, **9**, 2195–2200.

Shaw, P.J. (2003). *Multivariate Statistics for the Environmental Sciences.* New York: Oxford University Press.

Simola, J., Holmqvist, K., and Lindgren, M. (2009). Right visual field advantage in parafoveal processing: Evidence from eye-fixation-related potentials. *Brain and Language*, **111**(2), 101–113.

Summerfield, C., Jack, A.I., and Burgess, A.P. (2002). Induced gamma activity is associated with conscious awareness of pattern masked nouns. *International journal of psychophysiology*, **44**(2), 93–100.

Tallon-Baudry, C., Bertrand, O., Delpuech, C., and Pernier, J. (1996). Stimulus specificity of phase locked and non-phase-locked 40 Hz visual responses in human. *Journal of Neuroscience Methods*, **16**, 4240–4249.

Tallon-Baudry, C., Bertrand, O., Delpuech, C., and Pernier, J. (1997). Oscillatory gamma-band (30–70 Hz) activity induced by a visual search task in humans. *Journal of Neuroscience Methods*, **17**, 722–734.

Talsma, D., and Woldorff, M.G. (2005). Methods for the Estimation and Removal of Artifacts and Overlap in ERP Waveforms. In T.C. Handy (ed.) *Event-Related Potentials: A Methods Handbook* (pp. 115–148). Cambridge, MA: The MIT Press.

Tanenhaus, M.K., Spivey-Knowlton, M.J., Eberhard, K.M., and Sedivy, J.C. (1995). Integration of visual and linguistic information in spoken language comprehension. *Science*, **268**(5217), 1632–1634.

Unema, P.J.A., Pannasch, S., Joos, M., and Velichkovsky, B.M. (2005). Time course of information processing during scene perception: The relationship between saccade amplitude and fixation duration. *Visual Cognition*, **12**(3), 473–494.

Velichkovsky, B.M. (2002). Heterarchy of cognition: The depths and the highs of a framework for memory research. *Memory*, **10**(5), 405–419.

Vigário, R.N. (1997). Extraction of ocular artefacts from EEG using independent component analysis. *Electroencephalography and clinical neurophysiology*, **103**(3), 395–404.

Wallstrom, G.L., Kass, R.E., Miller, A., Cohn, J.F., and Fox, N.A. (2004). Automatic correction of ocular artifacts in the EEG: a comparison of regression-based and component-based methods. *International Journal of Psychophysiology*, **53**(2), 105–119.

Whitham, E.M., Pope, K.J., Fitzgibbon, S.P., Lewis, T., Clark, C.R., Loveless, S., *et al.* (2007). Scalp electrical recording during paralysis: quantitative evidence that EEG frequencies above 20 Hz are contaminated by EMG. *Clinical Neurophysiology*, **118**(8), 1877–1888.

Woldorff, M.G. (1993). Distortion of ERP averages due to overlap from temporally adjacent ERPs: Analysis and correction. *Psychophysiology*, **30**(1), 98–119.

Yagi, A. (1981). Visual signal detection and lambda responses, *Electroencephalography and Clinical Neurophysiology*, **52**, 604–610.

Yagi, A., and Ogata, M. (1995). Measurement of work load using brain potentials during VDT tasks. In Y. Anzai, K. Ogawa, and H. Mori (eds.) *Symbiosis of Human and Artifact* (pp. 823–826). Hyogo: Elsevier.

Yagi, A., Imanishi, S., Konishi, H., Akashi, Y., and Kanaya, S. (1998). Brain potentials associated with eye fixations during visual tasks under different lighting systems. *Ergonomics*, **41**(5), 670–677.

Yuval-Greenberg, S., Tomer, O., Keren, A.S., Nelken, I., and Deouell, L.Y. (2008). Transient Induced Gamma-Band Response in EEG as a Manifestation of Miniature Saccades. *Neuron*, **58**(3), 429–441.

PART 7

Language processing and eye movements

CHAPTER 48

Lexical influences on eye movements in reading

Barbara J. Juhasz and Alexander Pollatsek

Abstract

In this chapter, we review experiments in which people read text (often single sentences) while properties of individual target words were manipulated. These properties include the frequency of a word
in the language, as well as its orthographic, phonological, morphological, and semantic properties.
We also briefly review contingent display change experiments in which properties of a word seen
only in the parafovea are manipulated. The findings from these experiments indicate that many
aspects related to the structure of a fixated word influence fixation times on that word. It is thus
apparent that lexical processing is having quite an immediate effect on the progress of the eyes
through the text. In the concluding section, we describe how these data are consistent with the E-Z
Reader model (see also Reichle, Chapter 42, this volume), which posits that only one word is attended
to at a time (although more than one word is often processed on a fixation). We also highlight issues
related to lexical processing which are currently not addressed by models of eye movements in
reading.

Introduction

Investigating visual word recognition has been a productive area of research in cognitive psychology.
Sophisticated models of visual word recognition have been created on the basis of experimental
work. These models include the Dual-Route Cascaded model (Coltheart et al., 2001) and the family
of 'triangle' parallel distributed processing models (e.g. Harm and Seidenberg, 2004; Plaut et al.,
1996). Even though these models differ in their general architecture, they share the idea that words
are represented at three different levels within the reader's mind: orthographic, phonological, and
semantic. The orthographic properties of a word include the identities of individual graphemes and
their sequencing. Similarly, the phonological properties consist of individual phonemes and higher-
level units, while the semantic properties of a printed word consist of its meaning(s). However, recent
research suggests that the morphological complexity of visual words is also a determining factor in
the organization of the mental lexicon (see, e.g. Frost et al., 2005).

The technique of using eye movements is particularly informative for investigating word recognition processes during reading. That is, readers can be asked to read sentences or short passages for
meaning while their eye movements are recorded. This limits extraneous task demands that are typical of other types of experimental paradigms such as the lexical decision task, naming words in isolation, or categorizing words based on given semantic categories. While each of these tasks can provide
insight into aspects of visual word recognition, they all require overt responses that are not typical of

Table 48.1 Dependent measures typically reported in eye movement studies examining word recognition processes. Early processing measures are often referred to as *first-pass measures*

Early processing measures	Definition
First fixation duration	The duration of the very first fixation on the target word during the first pass, irrespective of number of fixations
Single fixation duration	The duration of the first fixation on the target word if it only received one fixation during the first pass
Gaze duration	The sum of all first pass fixations on the target word
Skipping rates	The percentage of cases in which the target word is not fixated on the first pass
Later processing measures	
Spillover duration	The duration of the next fixation after a reader moves their eyes off a target word (usually excluding regressions from the target word)
Regression rates	The percentage of regressions into a target word (**regressions in**) or out of a target word (**regressions out**)
Second pass duration	The amount of time spent re-reading a target word after first pass reading
Total fixation duration	The total time spent reading a target word (a sum of gaze duration and second pass duration)

normal silent reading and may involve mental processes that are typically not involved in understanding either written or spoken discourse.

Eye movement researchers who are interested in word recognition often manipulate a single word in text and record the durations of fixations on that word. *First-pass* measures (i.e. those prior to any regressions back to the word) are particularly informative for examining variables that are likely to have an impact on the initial access to representations of a word's orthography, phonology, or meaning. These first-pass measures include *first fixation duration, single fixation duration*, and *gaze duration*. The means of these measures are computed only for those trials on which the word is fixated on the first pass (i.e. not skipped initially). Whether a word is initially skipped during the first-pass is also an informative early measure. Additional measures such as *spillover duration, regression rates, second pass durations*, and *total fixation duration* can be informative for examining whether the manipulated variable has an impact on later processing. These measures are defined in Table 48.1.

The purpose of this chapter is to review research that has informed our knowledge of word recognition through the use of eye movement recording. The first section of the chapter focuses on research in which a trial consists of the participant reading a single sentence. These sentences, typically contain a 'frame' that has a target location in which one of two (or more) alternative target words can be inserted; these target words usually vary on a single attribute (e.g. word frequency) with other variables controlled (e.g. word length). This is illustrated in Fig. 48.1. The second section reviews studies that employ gaze-contingent display techniques that examine lexical influences on parafoveal processing. The last section, briefly discusses a model of eye movement control in reading that explains how the above measures can be good indicators of ongoing lexical processing in reading.

The word frequency effect

One of the most common findings in the word recognition literature is the word frequency effect. Words that occur more frequently are processed faster than words that occur less frequently in a given language. Eye movement studies have indicated that words with high frequency receive shorter fixation durations (e.g. Inhoff and Rayner, 1986; Juhasz and Rayner, 2003, 2006; Juhasz et al., 2006; Kennison and Clifton, 1995; Kliegl et al., 2004, 2006; Rayner and Duffy, 1986; Rayner and Fischer,

Sentence frames identical:

Deb did not read the **chapter** when I told her what was in it.

Deb did not read the **tabloid** when I told her what was in it.

Sentence frames consistent through post-target word:

Becky admired the **congresswoman** who had proposed the new bill.

Becky admired the **cheerleader** who had done an impressive split.

Fig. 48.1 An illustration of two ways sentence frames can be created for word recognition experiments. In the first example, the entire sentence frame is identical and the critical target word (in bold) is manipulated on word frequency (from Juhasz et al., 2006). While identical sentence frames are ideal, they are not always possible. In the second example, the frame is identical through a post-target region. After this, the sentences form a meaningful completion. In the second example, the first lexeme frequency of the compounds in manipulated (Juhasz, 2008). In both examples, it is important for researchers to control how well the two words fit in the sentence frames as well as the predictability of the two words given the beginning sentence context.

1996; Rayner et al., 1996, 2004a; Schilling et al., 1998; Yan et al., 2006). The word frequency effect is often used as a 'benchmark' experimental finding which all models of eye movements in reading must simulate.

The effect of word frequency is unlikely to be localized at one level of the mental lexicon. Instead, it is a general word recognition variable that is likely to influence access to many levels of a word's representation. How often a reader encounters a given word form can potentially influence how quickly the orthographic or phonological representations are activated once the word form is encountered in text. This, in turn, will affect the speed of access to semantic representations. In fact, the relative frequency of the two meanings of an ambiguous word has a large impact on fixation durations (see the 'Semantic influences' section below).

Word frequency is typically measured by counting how often a word occurs in a corpus of text. Research suggests that both the current word frequency, as measured by how often a word is encountered as an adult, and the cumulative lifespan frequency, or how often a word has been encountered since it was initially learned, influence fixation durations (see Juhasz and Rayner, 2003). However, word frequency corpora may not adequately measure actual frequency of occurrence for a given individual. This is especially true at the low-frequency end of the scale (see, e.g. Gernsbacher, 1984). More recent word frequency measures have been developed which take into consideration popular usage of words by the use of subtitles in television shows (e.g. Brysbaert and New, 2009). In addition, a subjective measure of word frequency, or a rating of word familiarity, may provide a good index of the actual word frequency for a given population of readers. The regression analyses of Juhasz and Rayner (2003) demonstrated that rated familiarity accounts for a significant amount of additional variance in fixation durations when either adult word frequency (measured by Francis and Kučera, 1982) or cumulative frequency (measured by Zeno et al., 1995) was included in the analysis. In two experiments where word frequency and word familiarity were factorially manipulated, Williams and Morris (2004) showed an effect of rated familiarity on first fixation duration and gaze durations for low-frequency words. However, they found no standard word frequency effect for words with a high familiarity rating. This may indicate that rated word frequency is a better measurement of actual frequency of occurrence compared to standard published corpora such as Francis and Kučera (1982).

Word frequency, however, is confounded with the frequency of the letter sequences within a word. A study by White (2008) attempted to disentangle these frequencies by independently manipulating the frequency of the whole word (measured by CELEX word frequencies; Baayen et al., 1995) and the *orthographic familiarity* of the letter sequences within the words (which was a manipulation of the summed monogram, bigram, and trigram frequencies within a word). Word frequency had a significant effect on first fixation duration, single fixation duration, and gaze duration even when orthographic familiarity was controlled indicating that a word frequency effect is not merely an artefact of the parts of the word being more familiar. However, there was also a smaller effect of orthographic familiarity for low-frequency words which was only fully reliable in single fixation duration.

A recent study by Staub et al. (2010) further examined the role of word frequency in reading. Staub et al. conducted distributional analyses on the fixation duration results of two recent eye movement experiments examining word frequency effects: Drieghe et al. (2008) and White (2008). The results demonstrated that reading low-frequency words both: 1) shifted the distribution of fixation durations (indexed by the μ component of the Ex-Gaussian distribution) and 2) produced a lengthening of the tail of the distribution (as indexed by τ). The first effect is theoretically important, as it argues against a view that lexical variables such as word frequency only exert an influence on infrequent very long fixations (e.g. Yang, 2006; Yang and McConkie, 2001).

Orthographic influences

The experimental findings of White (2008) suggest that orthographic familiarity has an influence on eye movement behaviour. Two other lines of research also suggest that orthographic properties of words influence word recognition during reading. In the first, the orthographic similarity of a target word to other words in the lexicon is manipulated to examine whether measures of the similarity of a word to other words have an impact on reading. In the second, changes are made to the orthographic structure of a word (notably changing the order of the letters) to examine the influence this has on eye movements.

Orthographic similarity

Much research converges in suggesting that words are organized in terms of orthographic similarity in the mental lexicon (see Andrews, 1997). One way in which orthographic similarity is measured is by examining the size of a word's orthographic neighbourhood (N) and the frequency of those neighbours (e.g. Andrews, 1997; Coltheart et al., 1977). An *orthographic neighbour* is typically defined as a word that differs from a target word (e.g. *house*) by a single letter (e.g. *mouse, horse*). Although recent research (e.g. Davis and Taft, 2005) suggests that this definition of lexical similarity should be broadened (e.g. to include deletion neighbours such as *hose* for *house*), the following discussion will assume the former definition of neighbour.

While the majority of the research on orthographic neighbourhoods has been conducted with standard laboratory tasks, eye movement studies investigating orthographic similarity can provide details about its role during sentence reading. In fact, the results from recording eye movements in reading diverge from the typical results observed with standard word recognition tasks such as lexical decision and word naming. The review of Andrews (1997) indicates that the majority of studies using naming and lexical decision observe a facilitative effect of having a large orthographic neighbourhood. Pollatsek et al. (1999) also observed this facilitative effect in a lexical decision task. However, when the same target words with large and small orthographic neighbourhoods were embedded into sentences, there were significant inhibition effects from having a large orthographic neighbourhood. In addition, Perea and Pollatsek (1998) observed inhibition effects when the presence of a higher-frequency neighbour was manipulated with the number of lower-frequency neighbours controlled. In this experiment, words with at least one higher-frequency neighbour (e.g. *plate* with the higher-frequency neighbour *place*) were compared to words with no higher-frequency neighbours (e.g. *spoon*) embedded in the identical sentence frame. Although one of the three relevant sentence reading experiments (Pollatsek et al., 1999, experiment 2) observed a significant inhibitory effect on gaze duration, the bulk of the inhibitory effect was on 'spillover' effects—notably on the number of regressions back to the target word. The most parsimonious interpretation of this finding is that readers sometimes misidentify the target word as its neighbour, especially a high-frequency neighbour and then regress back to it when subsequent context makes that identification untenable.

Sears et al. (2006) failed to replicate the effect reported by Perea and Pollatsek (1998); however, their study was compromised by the fact that many of the target words were near the beginnings and ends of the line and there is quite a bit of variability in fixation durations in these regions. The Perea and Pollatsek result was subsequently replicated by Slattery (2009). Moreover, Slattery showed that the inhibitory effect of a higher frequency neighbour was eliminated when the higher frequency neighbour was anomalous with prior sentence context. Thus, it appears that prior context can influence the selection process among lexical competitors.

The inhibitory role of orthographic neighbours in sentence reading was further examined by Paterson et al. (2009). In this study, two neighbour words were embedded in sentences (e.g. house, mouse). One neighbour acted as the target word and was preceded in the sentence by either its neighbour or a frequency matched control, which acted as an intrasentential prime. First fixation durations and gaze durations on the target were significantly lengthened when the prime word was an orthographic neighbour. This finding is interpreted as indicating that an earlier encounter of an orthographic neighbour can introduce lexical competition with the target during early word recognition processes. Interestingly, a follow-up study indicated that when there was a morphological relationship between the prime word and the target word (e.g. *creamy-cream*), first fixation durations and gaze durations were significantly shorter on the target word than when a control prime was presented earlier in the sentence (Paterson et al., 2011) These studies thus converge in demonstrating that orthographically similar words affect word processing in normal reading by inhibiting the correct identification of a currently fixated word when there is no morphological relationship between the neighbour words.

This leaves open the question of why there were facilitative effects of having neighbourhoods in the lexical decision task. The most plausible explanation has been captured in a model by Grainger and Jacobs (1996) that attempted to explain such effects. In this model, the decision to respond *yes* (i.e. that the stimulus is a word) is not only due to excitation from the lexical entry of the word that was actually presented, but also to the summed excitation from all lexical entries. Thus, if a word has many neighbours, these will add to this general excitation level. This indicates that lexical decision time should be viewed with caution as an index of how long it takes to identify a word. That is, the excitation of neighbours could speed lexical decision times but, at the same time, interfere with actually identifying the word.

Changes to orthography

A popular email, circulated for over 5 years, has claimed that when the letters within words are transposed, the message can still be easily read (see Rayner et al., 2006a). This has helped encourage the belief that misspelling a word has little or no effect on word identification. Rayner et al. (2006a), however, showed that although readers could comprehend the meaning of sentences when letters were transposed in the words, the reading times on these sentences increased. The most dramatic increase in reading rate occurred when the beginning letters within a word were transposed. This work was followed-up by White and colleagues (White et al., 2008) who provided more detailed analysis of a critical target word within the sentences. In each of the sentences, a target word was embedded, which was either low or high frequency, and was either spelled normally or with two letters transposed. Readers had longer first fixation durations and gaze durations on the target words when a transposition of letters was made compared to when the word was correctly spelled. Moreover, transposition did not interact with word frequency on early fixation duration measures. However, transposition created more interference for low-frequency target words than for high-frequency target words on the total fixation duration measure. In addition, there was a bigger transposition interference effect when the transposition included the beginning and ending letters—especially when it included the beginning letter—than when it was between two internal letters. These findings suggest that the beginning letter sequences are crucially important for word identification (an interpretation that is supported by many parafoveal processing experiments, some of which are summarized below).

Phonological influences

There has been a debate in the word recognition literature for decades regarding whether a direct route exists from orthography to semantics for skilled readers or whether phonological information is obligatorily activated prior to word meaning (see e.g. Frost, 2005). Recording eye movements in reading has provided valuable insight into this debate. Most researchers would agree that phonological information is activated during skilled silent reading. This was demonstrated by classic studies which have shown that tongue twisters are read more slowly than control sentences (e.g. McCutchen and Perfetti, 1982). What is debated is the role of the activated phonology. Some argue that the phonological codes for words are activated prior to semantic representations and are in fact critical to accessing those representations (see e.g. Morris and Folk, 2000). Others argue that phonology is primarily used after semantic representations are activated and may serve to aid error detection (Daneman and Reingold, 2000).

The evidence against the importance of phonological coding in reading comes from a paradigm in which participants read text containing errors (Daneman et al., 1995; Daneman and Reingold, 1993). Some were homophone errors (e.g. meat for meet) and some were (orthographic) control errors (moat for meet). Both of these conditions were compared to correctly spelled target words. Fixation durations were longer on both the homophone and control errors than when the correct word was in the same location; however, there was no difference between the homophone and control conditions. Daneman et al. (1995) interpreted their findings as indicating that orthographic representations rather than phonological representations are used to access word meaning. However, Rayner et al. (1998) did find a greater interference effect for the control errors than for the homophone errors, which indicated that the correct sound for the homophones was helping processing.

In contrast, large effects in reading due to phonological processing have been shown employing words which are both phonologically and semantically ambiguous (such as bows). Folk and Morris (1995) embedded these words in neutral sentence frames and found that fixation durations on these words were significantly longer than on control words that had only one possible phonological representation and meaning. This effect was very large: 40 ms on first fixation duration and 81 ms on gaze duration. This is not the pattern typically seen with semantically ambiguous words where no phonological ambiguity exists (see the 'Semantic influences' section below). This result indicates that phonological representations are being activated early in processing and that the activation of multiple phonological representations for the ambiguous words impeded processing of those words. When the sentence context preceding the phonologically ambiguous words biased the words to their less frequent sound/meaning, the effect was smaller than in a neutral context. However, the effect was still greater than the effect observed for semantically ambiguous words with only one phonological representation (Folk and Morris, 1995). Folk (1999) investigated the time-course of the influence of phonological information through the use of heterographic homophones which have two orthographic representations, one phonological representation, and two meanings (e.g. soul/sole). When the initial sentence context supported the less frequent version of the homophone, gaze durations on the homophone were significantly longer than on an unambiguous control word. This indicates that the phonological representation of the less frequent spelling activated both meanings associated with that phonological representation.

There is also evidence for the importance of phonology in silent reading from examinations of the spelling-to-sound regularity effect. Both Inhoff and Topolski (1994) and Sereno and Rayner (2000)[1]

---

[1] We are only considering the full parafoveal preview condition in Sereno and Rayner (2000). Lexical influences on parafoveal processing will be considered in a later section.

found that phonologically irregular words such as *pint* were fixated longer than phonologically regular words such as *dark*. This phonological regularity effect occurred early in the eye movement record, as it was observed on first fixation durations in both studies. Sereno and Rayner (2000) also observed the regularity effect in gaze durations and found some evidence for an interaction between regularity and word frequency such that there was a larger effect of regularity for low-frequency words. This interaction between regularity and word frequency mirrors what is typically observed in lexical decision tasks (e.g. Seidenberg et al., 1984).

If phonological codes are used to access semantic representations, then the creation of phonological codes must be a relatively fast process as the average fixation duration in reading is roughly 250 ms and many words receive only a single fixation (see Rayner, 1998 for a review of basic characteristics of eye movements in reading). Thus, within this 250 ms access to orthography, phonology, and semantics must occur. One explanation for the time-course issue is that the phonological representation used to activate semantic representations in silent reading contains minimal information (Frost, 1998) and is therefore not a rich phonological representation containing prosodic information such as syllable information and stress. However, as we will indicate in a later section, one reason that phonological information can influence fixation durations on a word is that phonological codes are extracted even before a word is fixated. This means that lexical processing of a word, including processing of its phonology, can occur prior to fixation on the word. In addition, a recent study by Ashby and Clifton (2005) indicates that prosodic information is accessed during reading. In this study, high- and low-frequency words with either one or two stressed syllables were embedded in sentences. Gaze durations were longer on words with two stressed syllables, suggesting that readers are computing stress during silent reading.

Morphological influences

In addition to the orthographic, phonological, and semantic levels of representation in the mental lexicon, research suggests that words are also represented at a morphological level. A morpheme is defined as the smallest unit of meaning in a word, and classic theories of where morphology is situated in the mental lexicon view morphemes as a link between form and meaning (e.g. Marslen-Wilson et al., 1994). Current research, on the other hand, suggests that morphology may also play an earlier role in the mental lexicon; namely at the level of orthographic representations (e.g. Rastle and Davis, 2008).

Irrespective of the localization of morphological processing within the mental lexicon, many eye movement studies converge in demonstrating that morphemes do influence fixation durations in reading. This research has been conducted with compound words (e.g. *deadline*), composed of two or more morphemes that are words on their own (and will henceforth be referred to as lexemes) as well as suffixed words (e.g. *restless*) and prefixed words (e.g. *redo*). Morphological decomposition is usually explored in these studies by taking advantage of the word frequency effect described above. The frequency of the roots within a morphologically complex word can be manipulated independently of the word's overall word frequency. For example, both of the prefixed words 'unkind' and 'untidy' have a frequency of 1 per million as measured by Zeno et al. (1995). However, the root 'kind' has a much higher frequency (420 per million) compared to 'tidy' (3 per million). If complex words are being decomposed during their processing, then the frequency of their morphemes should affect processing time.

Research conducted with Finnish compound words has demonstrated that the frequencies of both lexemes influence fixation durations. First lexeme frequency influences the first fixation on the compound as well as subsequent fixations (Hyönä and Pollatsek, 1998; Pollatsek, and Hyönä, 2005). Second lexeme frequency influences gaze duration as does the overall word frequency of the compound word for long Finnish compounds (Pollatsek et al., 2000a). This pattern of results led Pollatsek et al. (2000) to propose a dual-route model of compound word recognition. In this model, compounds are decomposed into their two lexemes, with access to the first lexeme preceding access to the second lexeme. In parallel with this decomposition process, the full form of the compound is also accessed, and these two routes race against each other. A further study with Finnish demonstrated that the long Finnish compounds are processed primarily through decomposition while shorter Finnish compounds are processed primarily through the whole-word route (Bertram and Hyönä, 2003). Bertram and Hyönä suggest that this is due to visual acuity limitations. For short Finnish compounds, the majority of the compound is available in foveal vision, thus increasing the likelihood the whole-word route will win the 'race'.

The research with English compound words has paralleled the results with Finnish in many respects but has also differed in some details. These differences may be due to factors related to the nature of compounding in the two languages. In English, spatially concatenated compound words are less common than they are in Finnish. This is due to the fact that many compound words in English are written with spaces between the lexemes (e.g. *front door*), whereas virtually all compounds in Finnish do not have spaces between them. Initial research with English spatially unified compound words has supported the view that the beginning lexeme frequency influences early fixation duration measures (Andrews et al., 2004; Juhasz, 2007; Juhasz et al., 2003). However, whether the beginning lexeme frequency influences subsequent fixations on the compound has varied in the studies. Also, similar to the Finnish compound results, the ending lexeme frequency effect in English has been observed on later processing measures (Andrews et al., 2004; Juhasz, 2007; Juhasz et al., 2003). Juhasz (2008) also observed that the rated word frequency of whole English compounds influences processing of those compounds. However, the study failed to find that only long English compounds are decomposed. Instead, this study observed beginning lexeme frequency effects only for *short* English compounds. Thus, Juhasz (2008) suggested that there must be another factor, not word length, yet to be identified, modulating the role of the beginning lexeme frequency effect in English.

Compound words can also differ in whether the meaning of the two lexemes relates to the meaning of the entire compound expression. Words in which the two lexemes contribute to the meaning of the entire compound word are referred to as transparent (e.g. *blackbird*), while compounds where the two lexemes are not related to the meaning of the compound expression are referred to as semantically opaque (e.g. *deadline*). Research examining the role of semantic transparency of compounds has been mixed. One study with Finnish compound words of 12–15 characters failed to find any influence of semantic transparency on reading time (Pollatsek and Hyönä, 2005). This study also demonstrated that both transparent and opaque compounds are decomposed during processing. This study is consistent with the results of Frisson et al. (2006), who did not find an effect of semantic transparency for English unspaced compound words. In contrast to this, both Juhasz (2007) and Underwood et al. (1990) reported main effects of semantic transparency in gaze durations for English compound words, such that transparent compounds were processed more quickly than opaque ones. In Juhasz (2007), the main effect of transparency was 24 ms in gaze durations. Recently, an experiment by Inhoff et al. (2008) examined the relative influence of lexeme frequency for compounds where the majority of the meaning was contained in the first lexeme (referred to as headed compounds) compared to the ending lexeme (referred to as tailed compounds). They observed larger lexeme frequency effects when the meaning location lexeme was varied. Headed compounds, such as '*deathbed*', displayed large beginning lexeme frequency effects in both first fixation duration and gaze duration and small ending lexeme frequency effects, whereas the reverse pattern was observed for tailed compounds such as '*armchair*'.

Research with prefixed and suffixed words has generally been consistent with the compound words studies in demonstrating decomposition for morphologically complex words. Niswander et al. (2000) found effects of root frequencies on first fixation duration for derived suffixed words in English. The results were more complex for inflected suffixed words and suggested that only inflected nouns were decomposed. The results for prefixed words (Niswander-Klement and Pollatsek, 2006), on the other hand mirrored the results for Finnish compounds. That is, for shorter prefixed words, the frequency of the whole word had the dominant effect on measures such as gaze duration, but for longer prefixed words, the frequency of the root had the dominant effect.

These results suggest that if the whole word is either easy to process or about as easy to process as the parts, the whole word route should play the dominant role, whereas if the components are significantly easier to process than the whole word, then a compositional process should dominate the identification process. Pollatsek et al. (2008) attempted to test this hypothesis by comparing root frequency effects for lexicalized prefixed words (e.g. *overload*) with those for prefixed words that were novel (e.g. *overmelt*). (Note that all the prefixes were semantically unambiguous, so that the meaning of the novel words could be computed from the prefix and root morpheme.) Given the above hypothesis, one would predict that the root frequency effect should be substantially larger for the novel prefixed words as there is no 'whole-word' route for accessing their meaning. However, this is not what was found. Even though the novel words were substantially more difficult to process (gaze durations were about 100 ms longer for the novel words), if anything, there was a slightly smaller root frequency effect for the novel prefixed words. These data indicate that the process of identification of morphemically complex words is complex and is likely to involve an interaction of the direct (whole-word) route and a route that constructs the meaning of the word from its component morphemes.

Semantic influences

Reading is a process of deriving meaning from print. It is thus not surprising that fixation durations are sensitive to a number of manipulations related to extraction of the meaning of a word while reading the text. These manipulations fall into two broad categories: 1) manipulation of the sentence context in which the word occurs (usually the context prior to the target word); 2) the semantic properties of the target word.

Sentence context manipulations

Predictability manipulations

Word recognition processes can be influenced by the meaning of the surrounding sentence context. For example, words that are predictable from the beginning sentence context are processed faster than words presented in a neutral context. These predictability effects have also been used as a benchmark for models of eye movements in reading (see Reichle, Chapter 42, and Engbert and Kliegl, Chapter 43, this volume). The effects of predictability on fixation durations and skipping rates have been observed consistently in the literature (see e.g. Altarriba et al., 1996; Ehrlich and Rayner, 1981; Kliegl et al., 2004; Rayner et al., 2004). In one study, Rayner and Well (1996) included low-predictability, medium-predictability, and high-predictability words in sentences. For first fixation duration and gaze duration, there was a main effect of contextual constraint (although it was only marginally significant for first fixation duration). Initial processing was faster on both the high- and medium-constraint words than on the low-constraint words. High- and medium-predictable words did not differ from each other. Rayner and Well (1996) also demonstrated that a contextual constraint manipulation must be large to influence word skipping. In their experiment, high-constraint target words were skipped significantly more than either medium-constraint or low-constraint words, which did not differ in their skipping rates.

Predictability effects have also been examined in Chinese, which uses a logographic script very different from the alphabetic scripts examined in the studies cited above. Rayner et al. (2005) found that medium- and high-predicable Chinese words receive shorter gaze durations compared to low-predictable words. The same pattern emerged for word skipping in Chinese. Thus Chinese readers were more likely to skip over both high- and medium-predictable words compared to words that are not predictable. This pattern differs from the English results reported by Rayner and Well (1996) described above.

In addition to the standard predictability effects described above, McDonald and Shillcock (2003a, 2003b) have observed an effect from a different type of predictability on fixation durations: transitional probability. Forward transitional probability is measured from corpora that provide information on how often two words appear together in written text and can be thought of as the predictability of one word given the preceding word. McDonald and Shillcock (2003a) had participants read sections of newspapers and performed a regression analysis on their fixation durations. When the previous saccade was launched from a near position (less than eight characters away) forward transitional probability significantly predicted first fixation durations, gaze durations, and single fixation durations. In a sentence reading experiment, McDonald and Shillcock (2003b) observed significantly shorter first fixation durations and marginally shorter gaze durations for nouns with a high transitional probability of following the immediately preceding verb. However, Frisson et al. (2005) noted that the predictability of the target word from the preceding sentence context was somewhat confounded with transitional probability in McDonald and Shillcock's (2003a) experiment (nouns with a higher transitional probability also had a higher level of predictability from the beginning sentence context according to cloze probabilities). In an experiment where they unconfounded the two variables and factorially varied sentence predictability and the transitional probability of a target noun, Frisson et al. (2005) observed a significant effect of sentence predictability on gaze duration but no effect of transitional probability and no interaction between the two.

One might want to argue that the above predictability manipulations are not necessarily indices of semantic processing. That is, although it is plausible that these predictability effects arise from constructing the meaning of the prior sentence context and deciding what word is likely to follow, it is possible that one can predict an upcoming target word from a lower-level mechanism that simply is reflecting co-occurrences in language. This alternative hypothesis, however, is made less plausible by the Frisson et al. (2005) data and is also not a parsimonious explanation of effects on fixation times produced by the semantic implausibility of a word in context.

Plausibility manipulations

Rayner et al. (2004b) showed that the plausibility of the word given the prior context had immediate influences on eye movement behaviour, but only when the word was actually anomalous given the prior context. They examined reading times on a word (e.g. *cheese*) when the context preceding the word was plausible (Bill used the knife to cut the hard *cheese* . . .), implausible (Bill used the scissors to cut the hard *cheese* . . .) or anomalous (Bill used the calculator to compute the hard *cheese* . . .). The anomalous condition produced lengthened gaze durations on the target word compared to both the plausible and implausible conditions. However, although differences between the plausible and implausible conditions began to emerge in later processing measures, such as total fixation time on the target word, none of the differences between these two conditions reached standard levels of significance by both participants and items.

A follow-up experiment by Warren and McConnell (2007) examined the nature of these prior contexts more thoroughly. They noted that the original anomalous items used by Rayner et al. (2004) included a mixture of sentences where the context created a situation that was possible but extremely implausible and sentences where the described event was impossible given the semantic restrictions of the verb (the anomalous sentence used above is an example of the latter). In order to further examine the time-course of implausibility effects, Warren and McConnell created three sentence contexts for a given target word: 1) the event described was possible and plausible; 2) the event described was possible but implausible; and 3) the event was both impossible and implausible. Contexts with impossible events influenced early fixation durations on the word: first fixation and single fixation duration. There were no implausibility effects on the early fixation duration measures. On the other hand, total fixation durations differed significantly for both impossible events and implausible events compared to the control context. Combined, the results of Rayner et al. (2004) and Warren and McConnell (2007) suggest that extremely implausible sentence contexts exert an immediate effect on word recognition processes but that the effect is earlier when the sentence context represents an impossible situation (please see Warren, Chapter 50, for a more thorough discussion of semantic plausibility effects and Blythe and Joseph, Chapter 36, this volume for a discussion of similar effects in children's reading).

Semantic ambiguity research

Another line of research that demonstrates that fixation times on words are affected by the extraction of meaning (as opposed to simply recognizing the word form or phonological representation) employs semantically ambiguous words. The words employed in this research have two meanings that are totally unrelated (such as *bank* which can mean a financial institution or a river bank) as opposed to a word that has different shades of meaning (such as *ball* which can mean a physical object used to play a game with, or the game itself). A key variable in this research is the relative frequency of the two meanings of the word; *balanced* ambiguous words are those in which the two meanings are approximately equally frequent (e.g. *quack:* a duck sound or a charlatan), and *biased* ambiguous words are those where one meaning is considerably more frequent than the other (e.g. *port:* a place where ships can dock or a type of wine). With biased ambiguous words, the higher-frequency meaning is referred to as the dominant meaning and the lower-frequency meaning is referred to as the subordinate meaning. The typical experiment studying semantic ambiguity places a semantically ambiguous word in a sentence context and compares this condition to a control word (i.e. one which is not semantically ambiguous) in the same context. The ambiguous and control words are matched on the length and frequency of the word (i.e. the orthographic word) and the sentences are matched so that the words fit equally well with the context.

The following general pattern of results has emerged from eye movement experiments. When the prior context is neutral (i.e. either meaning of the word is plausible given that context), readers have longer fixation durations on a balanced ambiguous word than on a control word with only a single meaning (e.g. Duffy et al., 1988; Rayner and Duffy, 1986), but fixation durations on biased ambiguous words are about the same as on the control words (e.g. Duffy et al., 1988). The latter pattern is almost certainly due to the fact that the dominant meaning is being accessed when the prior context is neutral. The pattern changes however, when the prior context favours the less frequent meaning (e.g. Duffy et al., 1988; Rayner et al., 1994, 2006b; Sereno et al., 2006). This has been termed 'the subordinate bias effect'. For biased ambiguous words, when the beginning sentence context suggests that the subordinate meaning of the biased word is the correct meaning, readers' fixation durations are significantly longer than on a control word, but for balanced ambiguous words, the prior context actually helps to speed up fixation times on the (slightly) less frequent meaning compared to where the prior context is neutral. The pattern of eye movements after the target word has been left is striking. In cases where the prior context was neutral and the context after the target word supports the less frequent meaning of the ambiguous word, there is subsequent disruption in reading, notably many more regressions back to the ambiguous target word. Moreover, this disruption is much bigger for the biased ambiguous words. This pattern supports the hypothesis above that, in neutral contexts, the ambiguous word is usually taken as the more frequent meaning and when posterior context indicates that this is the wrong meaning, the misinterpretation needs to be corrected.

The subordinate bias effect can be explained in terms of the reordered access model (Duffy et al., 1988), which is an extension of the ordered search model of Hogaboam and Perfetti (1978). According to the ordered search model, one meaning of an ambiguous word is always checked first, regardless of context. All other meanings are then checked, until one that fits with the context is found. The order with which the meanings are checked depends on their frequency, and once a meaning that fits with the context is found, no other meanings need to be accessed.

According to the reordered access model (Duffy et al., 1988), disambiguating information prior to the ambiguous word can affect the order of search to a limited degree. If the ambiguous word is balanced and is preceded by context, the contextually appropriate meaning will become active earlier than the contextually inappropriate meaning (and the balanced word will behave like a biased word in a neutral context). If on the other hand, the prior context biases a subordinate meaning of a biased word, the subordinate meaning will become active earlier than usual, possibly at the same time as the dominant meaning, resulting in the biased word acting like a balanced word does in neutral context. Thus, in a neutral context, the frequency of the more frequent meaning of the biased ambiguous word is virtually equal to that of the control word and there is no difference between them, whereas when prior context disambiguates the word in favour of the less frequent meaning, the frequency of the less frequent meaning is substantially less than the control word. The one finding that the model doesn't fully explain is why prior context actually reduces fixation durations on balanced ambiguous words. This would seem to require the idea that there is competition between the two meanings when there is neutral prior context and that this competition essentially disappears when the prior context disambiguates the two. This phenomenon has been successfully modelled by Reichle et al. (2007) using the E-Z Reader model.

Semantic properties of words

Although there are many studies examining aspects of a word's semantic representation in standard word recognition tasks, there are only a handful of published studies which have attempted to generalize these results to eye movement measures. Juhasz and Rayner (2003) found that words which refer to concrete entities receive shorter gaze durations than words which refer to abstract concepts. Dunabeitia et al. (2008) found that the number of semantic associates a word has influences fixation durations: gaze durations were shorter on words with a large number of semantic associates than words with a small number of semantic associates. This is interpreted as resulting from greater spreading activation of words with many associates in the semantic lexicon. Whether the concrete-abstract difference can be explained by differing numbers of semantic associates is yet to be determined.

Age of acquisition (AoA) is another variable that has been found to influence fixation durations in reading (Juhasz and Rayner, 2003; 2006). Words that are learned early in life receive shorter fixation durations than words which are learned later in life. This AoA effect is strongest in single fixation duration and gaze duration and persists even when measures of word frequency, familiarity, and concreteness are controlled. Juhasz and Rayner (2006) interpreted this effect as potentially being semantic in nature. This view is supported by studies which demonstrate a role of AoA in various semantic tasks including object recognition (e.g. Holmes and Ellis, 2006; Moore et al., 2004), word categorization (Brysbaert et al., 2000), a paired associate semantic memory task (Gullick and Juhasz, 2008), and a semantic 'Simon' task (Ghyselinck et al., 2004). See Juhasz (2005) for a review of AoA effects and theories.

What information is extracted from a word before it is fixated?

During reading, information about the upcoming word is obtained prior to fixating it. A great deal of research has focused on what kinds of information are obtained from a word prior to it being fixated for the first time. This research typically uses the *boundary technique* (Rayner, 1975) to measure the extent of parafoveal processing. In this technique, prior to fixating on a target word, a preview of it is given in the parafovea (see Fig. 48.2). During a saccade to the target word, the preview is replaced by the correct target. Due to saccadic suppression, this display change is usually not noticed by the participant. However, fixation times on the target word are influenced by the relationship between the preview word and the target word. The difference between fixation times when a useful preview of a word is given compared to a control preview (usually with no overlap in orthographic, phonological, or semantic information with the target) is a measure of *preview benefit*.

```
Janice went to the restaurant to meet her friout for a nice dinner.
                                            *
Janice went to the restaurant to meet her friout for a nice dinner.
                                                *
Janice went to the restaurant to meet her friend for a nice dinner.
                                                *
```

Fig. 48.2 An illustration of the boundary paradigm in reading (developed from Rayner, 1975). The asterisk indicates the reader's eye position. Prior to fixating on the target word (*friend* in this example), a parafoveal preview of it (*friout*) is provided. Once the reader's eye crosses the invisible boundary between the pre-target and target word, the preview is replaced by the target word. Note that courier font is used so that the spatial locations of the letters in the preview match those of the target word.

Research measuring preview benefit has consistently demonstrated that orthographic information about upcoming words is processed prior to fixation on that word (see Rayner, 1998 for a review of many studies demonstrating this fact). It has been hypothesized that this orthographic information that is obtained from the parafovea is in the form of abstract letter codes, since changing the case of letters on alternating fixations does not disrupt reading significantly (McConkie and Zola, 1979). Recent research conducted by Johnson et al. (2007) indicates that target words are processed more slowly when a preview of the word with letter transpositions in the middle of it is provided compared to a completely correct parafoveal preview. However, previews with transpositions result in faster processing than previews in which the same letters are replaced with visually similar letters. This suggests that while letter identity is processed in the parafovea, the coding of exact letter position is not precise. In addition, Juhasz et al. (2008) found that when a single letter is changed in the para- foveal preview of a long word (average word length = 8.3 letters), this does not influence fixation times on the target word. This stands in contrast to studies which have shown that changes to a single letter in the first few letters of an upcoming word dramatically increase processing time (Drieghe et al., 2005; Pynte et al., 2004; White and Liversedge, 2006).

Parafoveal preview research has consistently demonstrated that phonological information is obtained prior to fixation during reading (e.g. Henderson et al., 1995; Miellet and Sparrow, 2004; Pollatsek et al., 1992). To test this, Pollatsek et al., (1992) used a paradigm that compares the preview benefit of a homophone (e.g. *beach*) of the target word (e.g. *beech*) to the preview benefit of a non- homophone matched with the homophone on its graphemic similarity to the target word (e.g. *bench*). Parafoveal phonological preview information is obtained even in Chinese (Pollatsek et al., 2000b, Liu et al., 2002) although the effects of the preview in Chinese appear somewhat delayed compared to the effects in English. This finding supports the view discussed above that phonological representations are used in reading to access word meaning. In support of this, Chace et al. (2005) found that less skilled college readers were less likely to access phonological information from a parafoveal preview than more skilled college readers. This suggests that as readers become more skilled in reading, they are better able to utilize parafoveal phonological information to aid in word recognition. Research conducted by Ashby (2006; Ashby and Rayner, 2004; Ashby et al., 2004) has shown that college readers extract quite complex phonological information from the parafovea including infor- mation about syllable structure as well as the phonological representation of vowels embedded within parafoveal words.

In English, information about the morphological complexity of an upcoming word does not appear to be extracted from the parafovea (e.g. Juhasz et al., 2008; Kambe, 2004; Lima, 1987). This is also true of the Finnish language (Bertram and Hyona, 2007), which is more morphologically complex than English. However, readers of Hebrew do, in fact, extract morphological information from the parafovea (Deutsch et al., 2003, 2005). This may represent a qualitative difference in the way the languages are processed, as morphemes in Hebrew are not generally prefixes or suffixes, but instead are 'infixes' (and thus not a consecutive sequence of letters).

Not all words are directly fixated during reading. Up to 20% of words are skipped. These words are usually thought to be identified during the fixation prior to the skip (see Drieghe, 2008 for a discus- sion). Thus, semantic information can be obtained from words in the parafovea. However, Rayner et al. (1986) showed that partial semantic information from a parafoveal word provides no subse- quent benefit. That is, providing a semantically related word in the parafovea did not shorten fixa- tion duration on the target word once it is directly fixated. Similarly, a preview of a translation of a word provided no benefit for Spanish–English bilinguals (Altarriba et al., 2001).

Word recognition processes in models of eye movements in reading

There is currently a great debate about whether lexical processing in reading is done word-by-word in a serial fashion or whether the default process for the reader is to process multiple words in parallel (e.g. see Reichle et al., 2009a). In the limited space available in this chapter, we cannot provide a full discussion of these issues. Instead, we will outline the serial process view (see Reichle, Chapter 42, this volume) and argue that it is at least a good approximation to what we will term 'the default process' in reading and argue that there are no serious problems with this view. Our purpose in presenting this view is to describe how some benchmark lexical processes detailed in the review can be incorporated into a model of eye movements in reading and also to highlight issues of lexical processing which are currently not addressed by current models of eye movements in reading. We are not trying to argue that a model that assumes that more than one word is processed in parallel cannot be constructed to fit the data (see, e.g. Engbert et al., 2005, see also Engbert and Kliegl, Chapter 43, this volume); however, whether there are data that seriously compel one to add the extra layers of complexity that are necessitated by a model that posits that multiple words can be processed in parallel is still an open question. Also, we need to be clear on one assumption before proceeding. The model we are describing assumes that all the letters *within* a word are usually processed in parallel. The issue is whether this parallel processing extends over more than one *word*.

To begin, we have to clarify what we mean by 'the default process' in reading. That is, a key assumption of the serial model we will describe, E-Z Reader (Pollatsek et al., 2006; Rayner et al., 2004; Reichle et al., 1998, 2003; Reichle, Chapter 42, this volume), is that the trigger to move the eyes forward is that the currently attended word has been processed sufficiently to move on to the next word. This stage of lexical processing is termed 'the familiarity check'. The tacit assumption is that 'higher-order' processes such as constructing syntactic and discourse structures generally lag behind and only interrupt the forward progress of the eyes when it is detected that there is a problem (e.g. in syntactic 'garden-path' sentences; Frazier and Rayner, 1982). Although more recent versions of the model (Reichle et al., 2009b; Reichle, Chapter 42, this volume) have modelled some types of regressions, we will not discuss them further as our focus is on the relation between eye movement measures and lexical processing.

The details of the E-Z Reader model are discussed in Reichle (Chapter 42, this volume). For our present purposes, the key assumptions are as follows. First, as indicated above, a stage of lexical access called the *familiarity check* is the trigger for an eye movement to be made to the next word, but a later stage of (full) *lexical access* is the trigger to shift covert attention to the next word and begin lexical processing of it. Second, eye movements can be cancelled if the programme is in an early stage. Thus, if the word to the right of the fixated word is easy to process because it is short, very frequent, or predictable from prior context, the 'familiarity check' of the word to the right of the fixated word (word $n+1$) can trigger a saccade to the next word (word $n+2$) and word $n+1$ will be skipped. Another important assumption is that the duration of both the familiarity check stage and the lexical access stage are strongly influenced by variables discussed in our review above such as the frequency of a word, its length, and how predictable it is from prior context.

To quickly summarize, a key assumption of the model is that there is a covert attentional mechanism that attends to one word at a time. Although this covert attentional mechanism is highly correlated with where the eye is fixated, the model posits that shifts of covert attention and signals to move the eye to a new fixation location are separate decisions. A crucial aspect of the model is that the attention shift triggered by the lexical access of the attended word almost always occurs before the saccade to the next word (word $n+1$) occurs due to the latency in programming and executing saccades. Thus, although the model posits that words are processed sequentially, it does not predict that only one word is processed on a fixation; instead, it predicts that typically more than one word will be processed on a fixation and, specifically, that the reader will get benefit from having a preview of a word before it is fixated.

Another important point needs to be made, however. The model also posits that there are both systematic and random errors in where the eyes actually land. That is, although the middle of a word is always the target of the saccade that is programmed either to a new word or to the same word (in case of a refixation), the eyes do not always land there. Thus, the word that was intended to be fixated is not always the word that is actually fixated. (We will return to this issue below.) This is particularly true for shorter words, where they can be skipped simply because intended short saccades tend to be 'overshot' (McConkie et al., 1988). Another important point is that the model obviously has to posit that lower level information (such as word boundaries) has to be processed to guide shifts of attention and saccades before that information is attended to; however, lexical processing only begins when attention shifts to a word.

The model has no 'deep' theory about how variables such as word frequency and predictability influence the speed of lexical processing—they are simply posited to do so. In the case of word frequency, the duration of both the familiarity check and full lexical access are posited to be a linear function of the log of the frequency of a word. In contrast, the reason that word length influences the speed of word processing is not due to a separate postulate of the model; this property falls out of the assumptions relating the speed of visual processing to the distance of a letter from the fovea.

The model does a good job of accounting for the basic phenomena in reading. It accounts for fixation duration measures and the probability of skipping a word both for sentence corpuses and for selected target words in these sentences. This includes predicting first fixation duration and gaze duration on target words as well as spillover measures such as gaze duration on the subsequent word. Moreover, the model gives a good general account of the size of preview benefits (see Reichle, Chapter 42, this volume). However, as the model does not have a detailed model of word identification, it is not equipped at present to give an account of some of the fine details of word recognition which we discussed above such as homophonic effects, transposed letter effects, etc. In broad outline, we see only one problematic aspect to the model related to lexical processing (besides the fact that it doesn't have a detailed model of word processing and doesn't attempt to explain how syntactic and discourse processing work). That is, the model tacitly assumes that the word unit (i.e. what can be attended to at a given moment) is the series of letters between the spaces. However, the patterns of data we have discussed above on long polymorphemic words imply that subword units such as morphemes are driving the system to some extent. In addition, with languages like Chinese that don't have spaces between words (and there is some disagreement about what words are), one may have to come up with a more sophisticated view of what is attended to at an instant. (However, a variant of E-Z Reader has given a good account of eye movements in Chinese assuming that readers define a word to be the same as a consensus of expert Chinese readers; Rayner et al., 2007.)

The E-Z Reader is a simple account of reading. Thus, if it is even only a good approximation to the truth, eye movement measures become fairly easy to relate to ongoing lexical processing. A word of caution is in order, however. Although the model posits that there is quite a close link between where the eyes are and what is being processed, it does not posit that the relationship is completely transparent. That is, the model does not posit that gaze duration is equal either to the time to reach the familiarity check stage or the lexical access time. Nonetheless, the model predicts that gaze duration on a word is a reasonable approximation to how long it took to identify the word, and we think there are experiments that buttress the claim that, for the most part, fixation time on a word is indexing processing of that word. This implies that the serial lexical processing assumption of E-Z Reader is a good approximation to reality.

One paradigm that dramatically shows that the lexical properties of the fixated word are the primary influence on fixation time and strongly suggests that attention at the beginning of a fixation is on the fixated word and not on the one to the right was developed by Rayner et al. (2003). In this paradigm, either a target word (word n) or the following word (word $n+1$) disappeared or was masked 60 ms after the target word was fixated. Many prior experiments with individual words have indicated that words that are visible (and presumably attended to) can be processed with little or no loss in accuracy. What Rayner et al. (2003) found was that this was true when it was the target word that disappeared; moreover, the effect of word frequency was about the same as when the target word was not masked. However, there was a much bigger disruption in reading when word $n+1$ was masked. This is what would be predicted by a serial lexical processing model such as the E-Z Reader model as attention is originally directed to word n and is unlikely to switch over to word $n+1$ in the first 60 ms that word n is fixated.

A second type of study that provides support for the lexical processing distinctions posited in the E-Z Reader model was conducted by Reingold and Rayner (2006). In this study, the primary manipulation was degradation of a target word. When the degradation was of a purely physical nature (e.g. a faint font), they found that the degradation only affected fixation times on the target word and had no 'spillover' effects. This is again predicted by E-Z Reader as the degradation plausibly affects only early stages of lexical processing and hence the duration of the familiarity check stage.

We are not claiming that it is logically impossible for parallel models to predict these effects; however, they do not flow naturally from the architecture of these models. In fact, it should be clear from what we have said that there are many people who favour a view in which several words are processed in parallel. We think the major piece of evidence that people claim supports such models is what are termed *parafoveal-on-foveal effects*. What is meant by this term is that lexical properties of a word not yet fixated (usually word $n+1$) would affect fixation times on word n (see Drieghe, Chapter 46, this volume for a review of these effects). Although it is logically possible for a model like E-Z Reader to predict such effects, it would be difficult, and if such effects were robust, it would indeed be evidence against a model such as E-Z Reader. That is, in the architecture of E-Z Reader, as the decision to fixate word $n+1$ is dictated by completion of the familiarity check stage of word n, it would be hard to see how the speed of processing of word $n+1$ could affect the time spent fixating word n.

One problem with parafoveal-on-foveal effects is that they are not reliably found in alphabetic languages, and indeed they sometimes go one way and sometimes the other way (e.g. Hyönä and Bertram, 2004). Moreover, the most reliable of these effects are not directly observed with lexical properties of word $n+1$ such as its frequency, but instead occur when word $n+1$ is 'strange' in some kind of way (e.g. having very weird letter sequences) and generally occur only when the fixations on word $n+1$ are quite close to word n. Moreover, the problematic nature of parafoveal-on-foveal effects for a serial processing model such as E-Z Reader rests on a crucial assumption: when word n is fixated, it is the word that the reader intended to fixate. However, as we indicated above, E-Z Reader (and, we would argue, any realistic model of reading) posits that there are errors in targeting saccades, such that the probability is definitely less than 1 that the fixated word is the word that was intended to be fixated. If so, parafoveal-on-foveal effects could merely be due to those occasions when the reader intended to fixate word $n+1$ but fixated word n. In these cases, E-Z Reader would predict that characteristics of word $n+1$ would have an effect on fixation times. Moreover, these cases would be most likely to occur when fixations on word n were close to word $n+1$. In addition, we might add that another problem with demonstrating theoretically significant parafoveal-on-foveal effects is that the demonstration implicitly assumes that the recorded position of the eye is perfectly accurate, whereas there can be a character or two error in most eye movement recording systems.[2]

In sum, we think that the preponderance of the evidence indicates that reading usually involves processing one word at a time, with the provision that longer and more morphemically complex words may not be processed as a whole, but instead, the parts may be processed, to some extent, in series (Drieghe et al., 2010). Because this latter phenomenon indicates that what is processed in parallel may not always magically be 'the thing between the spaces', we think it is not unreasonable that some short very frequent combinations of words (e.g. *of the*) could be processed as single units although this possibility needs to be validated experimentally.

Conclusions

The last section on modelling indicates how far we are from having a definitive model of how words are encoded in reading. Our review of the literature, however, indicates that a lot has been learned

---

[2] There is some recent evidence for parafoveal-on-foveal effects in Chinese (Yan et al., 2009; Yang et al., 2009). However, it is far from clear that these bear on whether such effects also occur in European alphabetic languages. Most notably, there are no spaces between characters in Chinese, so that it is far from clear how Chinese readers target their saccades. Moreover, although there is some agreement about what a word is in Chinese (characters are morphemes), the concept of 'word' in Chinese is far less clear than in European languages.

about the process of word encoding in reading. Let us try to summarize how far we have come and what lessons have been learned.

A point that we hope has been clearly made throughout this chapter is that there is quite a tight link between lexical encoding and eye movement measures (see also Rayner and Liversedge, Chapter 41, this volume). In particular, most of the effects we have discussed have had their primary effects on fixation times on the target word, most notably gaze duration. This means, first of all, that these measures can be taken seriously as being closely related to word encoding time. Second, it provides a good backdrop for studying higher-order effects. That is, if higher-order variables, such as predictability or which meaning of an ambiguous word is consistent with prior context, affect these immediate measures, then it is a pretty clear indication that there is an interaction between the processors that are computing these aspects of sentence context and the word identification system. On the other hand, in situations in which context effects only appear later, there is the suggestion that the processors are not interactive, but instead the word identification system is feeding the information into the higher-level system and then the higher-level system is directly intervening to control the eye movement system. We wish to make clear that this argument is a hypothesis and not meant as a logical conclusion. More generally, because eye movement methodology has the potential for sorting out the time-course of effects, it allows us to move forward in understanding how words are encoded in reading. Our chapter has indicated that graphemic, phonological, and morphological codes are all involved in reading. However, we still need to understand a lot more about how these processes interact and the time-course of these interactions.

References

Altarriba, J., Kroll, J.F., Scholl, A., Rayner, K. (1996). The influence of lexical and conceptual constraints on reading mixed language sentences: Evidence from eye fixation and naming times. *Memory and Cognition*, 24, 477–492.

Altarriba, J., Kambe, G., Pollatsek, A., and Rayner, K. (2001). Semantic codes are not used in integrating information across eye fixations in reading: Evidence from Spanish -English bilinguals. *Perception and Psychophysics*, 63, 875–890.

Andrews, S. (1997). The effect of orthographic similarity on lexical retrieval: resolving neighborhood conflicts. *Psychonomic Bulletin and Review*, 4, 439–461.

Andrews, S., Miller, B., and Rayner, K. (2004). Eye movements and morphological segmentation of compound words: There is a mouse in mousetrap. *European Journal of Cognitive Psychology*, 16, 285–311.

Ashby, J. (2006). Prosody in skilled silent reading: Evidence from eye movements. *Journal of Research in Reading*, 29, 318–333.

Ashby, J. and Clifton, C. Jr (2005). The prosodic property of lexical stress affects eye movements during silent reading. *Cognition*, 96, B89–B100.

Ashby, J. and Rayner, K. (2004). Representing syllable information during silent reading: Evidence from eye movements. *Language and Cognitive Processes*, 19, 391–426.

Ashby, J., Treiman, R., Kessler, B., and Rayner, K. (2004). Vowel processing during silent reading: Evidence during eye movements. *Journal of Experimental Psychology: Learning, Memory, and Cognition*, 32, 416–424.

Baayen, R.H., Piepenbrock, R.and Gulikers, L. (1995). *The CELEX Lexical Database [CD-ROM]*. Philadelphia, PA: University of Pennsylvania, Linguistic Data Consortium.

Bertram, R. and Hyönä, J. (2003). The length of a complex word modifies the role of morphological structure: Evidence from eye movements when reading short and long Finnish compounds. *Journal of Memory and Language*, 48, 615–634.

Bertram, R. and Hyönä, J. (2007). The interplay between parafoveal preview and morphological processing in reading. In R. van Gompel, M. Fischer, W. Murray, and R. Hill (eds.) *Eye Movements: A Window on Mind and Brain* (pp 391–407). New York: Elsevier.

Brysbaert, M. and New, B. (2009). Moving beyond Kučera and Francis: A critical evaluation of current word frequency norms and the introduction of a new and improves word frequency measure for American English. *Behavior Research Methods*, 41, 488–496.

Brysbaert, M., Van Wijnendaele, I., and De Deyne, S. (2000). Age-of-acquisition effects in semantic processing tasks. *Acta Psychologica*, 104, 215–226.

Chace, K.H., Rayner, K., and Well A.D. (2005). Eye movements and phonological parafoveal preview: Effects of reading skill. *Canadian Journal of Experimental Psychology*, 59, 209–217.

Coltheart, M., Davelaar, E., Jonasson, J.F., and Besner, D. (1977). Access to the internal lexicon. In S. Dorni (ed.) *Attention and Performance VI* (pp. 535–555). Hillsdale, NJ: Erlbaum.

Coltheart, M., Rastle, K., Perry, C., Langdon, R., and Ziegler, J. (2001). DRC: A dual route cascaded model of visual word recognition and reading aloud. *Psychological Review*, 108, 204–256.

Daneman, M. and Reingold, E.M. (1993). What eye fixations tell us about phonological recoding during reading. *Canadian Journal of Experimental Psychology*, **42A**, 153–178.

Daneman, M. and Reingold, E.M. (2000). Do readers use phonological codes to activate word meanings? Evidence from eye movements. In A. Kennedy, R. Radach, D. Heller. and J. Pynte (eds.) *Reading as a Perceptual Process* (pp. 447–473). Amsterdam: Elsevier Science Ltd.

Daneman, M., Reingold, E.M., and Davidson, M. (1995). Time course of phonological activation during reading: Evidence from eye fixations. *Journal of Experimental Psychology: Learning, Memory, and Cognition*, **21**, 884–898.

Davis, C.J. and Taft, M. (2005). More words in the neighborhood: Interferences in lexical decision due to deletion neighbors. *Psychonomic Bulletin and Review*, **12**, 904–910.

Deutsch, A., Frost, R., Pollatsek, A., and Rayner, K. (2005). Morphological parafoveal preview benefit effects in reading: Evidence from Hebrew. *Language and Cognitive Processes*, **20**, 341–371.

Deutsch, A., Frost, R., Pelleg, S., Pollatsek, A., and Rayner, K. (2003). Early morphological effects in reading: Evidence from parafoveal preview benefit in Hebrew. *Psychonomic Bulletin and Review*, **10**, 415–422.

Drieghe, D. (2008). Foveal processing and word skipping during reading. *Psychonomic Bulletin and Review*, **15**, 856–860.

Drieghe, D., Rayner, K., and Pollatsek, A. (2005). Eye movements and word skipping during reading revisited. *Journal of Experimental Psychology: Human Perception and Performance*, **31**, 954–959.

Drieghe, D., Rayner, K., and Pollatsek, A. (2008). Mislocated fixations can account for parafoveal-on-foveal effects in eye movements during reading. *Quarterly Journal of Experimental Psychology*, **61**, 1239–1249.

Drieghe, D., Pollatsek, A., Juhasz, B.J., and Rayner, K. (2010). Parafoveal processing during reading is reduced across a morphological boundary. *Cognition*, **116**, 136–142.

Duffy, S.A., Morris, R.K., and Rayner, K. (1988). Lexical ambiguity and fixation times in reading. *Journal of Memory and Language*, **27**, 429–446.

Dunabeitia, J.A., Aviles, A., and Carreiras, M. (2008). NoA's ark: Influence of the number of associates in visual word recognition. *Psychonomic Bulletin and Review*, **15**, 1072–1077.

Ehrlich, S.F. and Rayner, K. (1981). Contextual effects on word perception and eye movements during reading. *Journal of Verbal Learning and Verbal Behavior*, **20**, 641–655.

Engbert, R., Nuthmann, A., Richter, E.M., and Kliegl, R. (2005). SWIFT: A dynamical model of saccade generation during reading. *Psychological Review*, **112**, 777–813.

Folk, J.R. (1999). Phonological codes are used to access the lexicon during silent reading. *Journal of Experimental Psychology: Learning, Memory, and Cognition*, **25**, 892–906.

Folk, J.R. and Morris, R.K. (1995). The use of multiple lexical codes in reading: Evidence from eye movements, naming time, and oral reading. *Journal of Experimental Psychology: Learning, Memory, and Cognition*, **21**, 1412–1429.

Francis, W.N. and Kučera, H. (1982). *Frequency Analysis of English Usage: Lexicon and Grammar*. Boston: Houghton Mifflin.

Frazier, L. and Rayner, K. (1982). Making and correcting errors during sentence comprehension: Eye movements in the analysis of structurally ambiguous sentences. *Cognitive Psychology*, **14**, 178–210.

Frisson, S., Rayner, K., and Pickering, M.J. (2005). Effects of contextual predictability and transitional probability on eye movements during reading. *Journal of Experimental Psychology: Learning, Memory, and Cognition*, **31**, 862–877.

Frisson, S., Niswander-Klement, E., and Pollatsek, A. (2006). The role of semantic transparency in the processing of English compound words. *British Journal of Psychology*, **99**, 87–107.

Frost, R. (1998). Toward a strong phonological model of reading: True issues and false trails. *Psychological Bulletin*, **123**, 71–99.

Frost, R. (2005). Orthographic systems and skilled word recognition processes in reading. In M.J. Snowling and C. Hulme (eds.) *The Science of Reading: A Handbook* (pp. 272–295). Oxford: Blackwell.

Frost, R., Grainger, J., and Rastle, K. (2005). Current issues in morphological processing: An introduction. *Language and Cognitive Processes*, **20**, 1–5.

Gernsbacher, M.A. (1984). Resolving 20 years of inconsistent interactions between lexical familiarity, orthography, concreteness, and polysemy. *Journal of Experimental Psychology: General*, **113**, 256–281.

Ghyselinck, M., Custers, R., and Brysbaert, M. (2004). The effect of age of acquisition in visual word processing. Further evidence for the semantic hypothesis. *Journal of Experimental Psychology: Learning, Memory, and Cognition*, **30**, 550–554.

Grainger, J. and Jacobs, A.M. (1996). Orthographic processing in visual word recognition: A multiple read-out model. *Psychological Review*, **103**, 518–565.

Gullick, M. and Juhasz, B.J. (2008). Age of acquisition's effect on memory for semantically associated word pairs. *Quarterly Journal of Experimental Psychology*, **61**, 1177–1185.

Harm, M.W. and Seidenberg, M.S. (2004). Computing the meaning of words in reading: Cooperative division of labor between visual and phonological processes. *Psychological Review*, **111**, 662–720.

Henderson, J.M., Dixon, P., Peterson, A., Twilley, L.C., and Ferreira, F. (1995). Evidence for the use of phonological representations during transaccadic word recognition. *Journal of Experimental Psychology: Human Perception and Performance*, **21**, 82–97.

Hogaboam, T.W. and Perfetti, C.A. (1978). Reading skill and the role of verbal experience in decoding. *Journal of Educational Psychology*, **70**, 717–729.

Holmes, S.J. and Ellis, A.W. (2006). Age of acquisition and typicality effects in three object processing tasks. *Visual Cognition*, **13**, 884–910.

Hyönä, J. and Pollatsek, A. (1998). The role of component morphemes on eye fixations when reading Finnish compound words. *Journal of Experimental Psychology: Human Perception and Performance*, **24**, 1612–1627.

Hyönä, J. and Bertram, R. (2004). Do frequency characteristics of nonfixated words influence the processing of fixated words during reading? *European Journal of Cognitive Psychology*, **16**, 104–127.

Inhoff, A.W. and Rayner, K. (1986). Parafoveal word processing during eye fixations in reading: Effects of word frequency. *Perception and Psychophysics*, **40**, 431–439.

Inhoff, A.W. and Topolski, R. (1994). Use of phonological codes during eye fixations in reading and in on-line and delayed naming tasks. *Journal of Memory and Language*, **33**, 689–713.

Inhoff, A.W., Starr, M.S., Solomon, M., and Placke, L. (2008). Eye movements during the reading of compound words and the influence of lexeme meaning. *Memory and Cognition*, **36**, 675–687.

Johnson, R.L., Perea, M., and Rayner, K. (2007). Transposed-letter effects in reading: Evidence from eye movements and parafoveal preview. *Journal of Experimental Psychology: Human Perception and Performance*, **33**, 209–229.

Juhasz, B.J (2005). Age-of-acquisition effects in word and picture processing. *Psychological Bulletin*, **131**, 684–712.

Juhasz, B.J. (2007). The influence of semantic transparency on eye movements during English compound word recognition. In R. van Gompel, M. Fischer, W. Murray, and R. Hill (eds.) *Eye Movements: A Window on Mind and Brain* (pp. 373–389). New York: Elsevier.

Juhasz, B.J. (2008). The processing of compound words in English: Effects of word length on eye movements during reading. *Language and Cognitive Processes*, **23**, 1057–1088.

Juhasz, B.J. and Rayner, K. (2003). Investigating the effects of a set of intercorrelated variables on eye fixation durations in reading. *Journal of Experimental Psychology: Learning, Memory and Cognition*, **29**, 1312–1318.

Juhasz, B.J. and Rayner, K (2006). The role of age-of-acquisition and word frequency in reading: Evidence from eye fixation durations. *Visual Cognition*, **13**, 846–863.

Juhasz, B.J., Starr, M., Inhoff, A.W., and Placke, L. (2003). The effects of morphology on the processing of compound words: Evidence from naming, lexical decisions and eye fixations. *British Journal of Psychology*, **94**, 223–244.

Juhasz, B.J., Liversedge, S.P., White, B.J., and Rayner, K. (2006). Binocular coordination of the eyes during reading: Word frequency and case alternation affect fixation duration but not binocular disparity. *Quarterly Journal of Experimental Psychology*, **59**, 1614–1625.

Juhasz, B.J. White, S.J., Liversedge, S.P., and Rayner, K. (2008). Eye movements and the use of parafoveal word length information in reading. *Journal of Experimental Psychology: Human Perception and Performance*, **34**, 1560–1579.

Kambe, G. (2004). Parafoveal processing of prefixed words during eye fixations in reading: Evidence against morphological influences on parafoveal processing. *Perception and Psychophysics*, **66**, 279–292.

Kennison, S.M. and Clifton, C. (1995). Determinants of parafoveal preview benefit in high and low working memory capacity readers: Implications for eye movement control. *Journal of Experimental Psychology: Learning, Memory, and Cognition*, **21**, 68–81.

Kliegl, R., Nuthmann, A., and Engbert, R. (2006). Tracking the mind during reading: The influence of past, present, and future words on fixation durations. *Journal of Experimental Psychology: General*, **135**, 12–35.

Kliegl, R., Grabner, E., Rolfs, M., and Engbert, R. (2004). Length, frequency, and predictability effects of words on eye movements in reading. *European Journal of Cognitive Psychology*, **16**, 262–284.

Lima, S.D. (1987). Morphological analysis in sentence reading. *Journal of Memory and Language*, **26**, 84–99.

Liu, W., Inhoff, A.W., Ye, Y., and Wu, C. (2002). Use of parafoveally visible characters during the reading of Chinese sentences. *Journal of Experimental Psychology: Human Perception and Performance*, **28**, 1213–1227.

Marslen-Wilson, W.D., Tyler, L.K., Waksler, R., and Older, L. (1994). Morphology and meaning in the English mental lexicon. *Psychological Review*, **101**, 3–33.

McConkie, G.W. and Zola, D. (1979). Is visual information integrated across successive fixations during reading? *Perception and Psychophysics*, **25**, 221–224.

McConkie, G.W., Kerr, P.W., Reddix, M.D., and Zola, D. (1988). Eye movement control during reading: I. The location of initial eye fixations in words. *Vision Research*, **28**, 1107–1118.

McCutchen, D. and Perfetti, C.A. (1982). The visual tongue-twister effect: Phonological activation in silent reading. *Journal of Verbal Learning and Verbal Behavior*, **21**, 672–687.

McDonald, S.A. and Shillcock, R.C. (2003a). Eye movements reveal the on-line computation of lexical probabilities during reading. *Psychological Science*, **14**, 648–652.

McDonald, S.A. and Shillcock, R.C. (2003b). Low-level predictive inference in reading: The influence of transitional probabilities on eye movements. *Vision Research*, **43**, 1735–1751.

Miellet, S. and Sparrow, L. (2004). Phonological codes are assembled before word fixation: Evidence from boundary paradigm in sentence reading. *Brain and Language*, **90**, 299–310.

Moore, V., Smith-Spark, J.H., and Valentine, T. (2004). The effects of age of acquisition on object perception. *European Journal of Cognitive Psychology*, **16**, 417–439.

Morris, R.K. and Folk, J.R. (2000). Phonology is used to access word meaning during silent reading: Evidence from lexical ambiguity resolution. In A. Kennedy, R. Radach, D. Heller. and J. Pynte (eds.) *Reading as a Perceptual Process* (pp. 427–446). Amsterdam: Elsevier Science Ltd.

Niswander-Klement, E. and Pollatsek, A. (2006). The effects of root frequency, word frequency, and length on the processing of prefixed words during reading. *Memory and Cognition*, **34**, 685–702.

Niswander, E., Pollatsek, A., and Rayner, K. (2000). The processing of derived and inflected words during reading. *Language and Cognitive Processes*, **15**, 389–420.

Paterson, K.B., Alcock, A., and Liversedge, S.P. (2011). Morphological priming during reading: Evidence from eye movements. *Language and Cognitive Processes*, **26**, 600–623.

Paterson, K.B., Liversedge, S.P., and Davis, C.J. (2009). Inhibitory neighbor priming effects in eye movements during reading. *Psychonomic Bulletin and Review*, **16**, 43–50.

Perea, M. and Pollatsek, A. (1998). The effects of neighborhood frequency in reading and lexical decision. *Journal of Experimental Psychology: Human Perception and Performance*, **24**, 767–779.

Plaut, D.C., McClelland, J.L., Seidenberg, M.S., and Patterson, K. (1996). Understanding normal and impaired word reading: Computational principles in quasi-regular domains. *Psychological Review*, **103**, 56–115.

Pollatsek, A. and Hyönä, J. (2005). The role of semantic transparency in the processing of Finnish compound words. *Language and Cognitive Processes*, **20**, 261–290.

Pollatsek, A., Perea, M., and Binder, K. (1999). The effects of neighborhood size in reading and lexical decision. *Journal of Experimental Psychology: Human Perception and Performance*, **25**, 1142–1158.

Pollatsek, A., Hyönä, J., and Bertram, R. (2000a). The role of morphological constituents in reading Finnish compound words. *Journal of Experimental Psychology: Human Perception and Performance*, **26**, 820–833.

Pollatsek, A., Tan, L.H., and Rayner, K. (2000b). The role of phonological codes in integrating information across saccadic eye movements in Chinese character identification. *Journal of Experimental Psychology: Human Perception and Performance*, **26**, 607–633.

Pollatsek, A., Reichle, E.D., and Rayner, K. (2006). Serial processing is consistent with the time course of linguistics information extraction from consecutive words during eye fixations in reading: A Response to Inhoff, Eiter, and Radach (2005). *Journal of Experimental Psychology: Human Perception and Performance*, **32**, 1485–1489.

Pollatsek, A.P., Slattery, T, and Juhasz, B.J. (2008). The processing of novel and lexicalised prefixed words in reading. *Language and Cognitive Processes*, **23**, 1133–1158.

Pollatsek, A., Lesch, M., Morris, R., and Rayner, K. (1992). Phonological codes are used in integrating information across saccades in word identification and reading. *Journal of Experimental Psychology: Human Perception and Performance*, **18**, 148–162.

Pynte, J., Kennedy, A., and Ducrot, S. (2004). The influence of parafoveal typographical errors on eye movements in reading. *European Journal of Cognitive Psychology*, **16**, 178–202.

Rastle, K. and Davis, M.H. (2008). Morphological decomposition based on the analysis of orthography. *Language and Cognitive Processes*, **23**, 942–971.

Rayner, K. (1975). Parafoveal identification during a fixation in reading. *Acta Psychologica*, **39**, 271–282.

Rayner, K. (1998). Eye movements in reading and information processing: 20 years of research. *Psychological Bulletin*, **124**, 372–422.

Rayner, K. and Duffy, S.A. (1986). Lexical complexity and fixation times in reading: Effects of word frequency, verb complexity, and lexical ambiguity. *Memory and Cognition*, **14**, 191–201.

Rayner, K. and Fischer, M.H. (1996). Mindless reading revisited: Eye movements during reading and scanning are different. *Perception and Psychophysics*, **58**, 734–747.

Rayner, K. and Well, A.D. (1996). Effects of contextual constraint on eye movements in reading: A further examination. *Psychonomic Bulletin and Review*, **3**, 504–509.

Rayner, K. Balota, D.A., and Pollatsek, A. (1986). Against parafoveal semantic preprocessing during eye fixations in reading. *Canadian Journal of Psychology*, **40**, 473–483.

Rayner, K., Pacht, J.M., and Duffy, S.A. (1994). Effects of prior encounter and global discourse bias on the processing of lexically ambiguous words: Evidence from eye fixations. *Journal of Memory and Language*, **33**, 527–544.

Rayner, K., Sereno, S.C., and Raney, G.E. (1996). Eye movement control in reading: A comparison of two types of models. *Journal of Experimental Psychology: Human Perception and Performance*, **22**, 1188–1200.

Rayner, K., Pollatsek, A., and Binder, K.S. (1998). Phonological codes and eye movements in reading. *Journal of Experimental Psychology: Learning, Memory and Cognition*, **24**, 476–497.

Rayner, K., Li, X., and Pollatsek, A. (2007). Extending the E-Z Reader model of eye movement control to Chinese readers. *Cognitive Science*, **31**, 1021–1034.

Rayner, K., Liversedge, S.P., White, S.J., and Vergilino-Perez, D. (2003). Reading disappearing text: Cognitive control of eye movements. *Psychological Science*, **14**, 385–389.

Rayner, K., Ashby, J., Pollatsek, A., and Reichle, E.D. (2004). The effects of frequency and predictability on eye fixations in reading: Implications for the E-Z Reader model. *Journal of Experimental Psychology: Human Perception and Performance*, **30**, 720–732.

Rayner, K., Warren, T., Juhasz, B.J., and Liversedge, S.P. (2004). The effects of plausibility on eye movements in reading. *Journal of Experimental Psychology: Learning, Memory and Cognition*, **30**, 1290–1301.

Rayner, K., Li, X., Juhasz, B.J., and Yan, G. (2005). The effect of word predictability on the eye movements of Chinese readers. *Psychonomic Bulletin and Review*, **12**, 1089–1093.

Rayner, K., White, S.J., Johnson, R.L., and Liversedge, S.P. (2006a). Raeding wrods with jubmled lettres: There's a cost. *Psychological Science*, **17**, 192–193.

Rayner, K., Cook, A.E., Juhasz, B.J., and Frazier, L. (2006b). Immediate disambiguation of lexically ambiguous words during reading: Evidence from eye movements. *British Journal of Psychology, 97*, 467–482.

Reichle, E.D., Rayner, K., and Pollatsek, A. (2003). The E-Z Reader model of eye movement control in reading: Comparisons to other models. *Behavioral and Brain Sciences, 26*, 445–476.

Reichle, E.D., Pollatsek, A., and Rayner, K. (2007). Modeling the effects of lexical ambiguity on eye movements during reading. In R. van Gompel, M. Fischer, W. Murray, and R. Hill (eds.) *Eye Movements: A Window on Mind and Brain* (pp. 271–292). New York: Elsevier.

Reichle, E.D., Warren, T., and McConnell, K. (2009b). Using E-Z Reader to model the effects of higher level language processing on eye movements during reading. *Psychonomic Bulletin and Review, 16*, 1–21.

Reichle, E., Pollatsek, A., Fisher, D.L., and Rayner, K. (1998). Toward a model of eye movement control in reading. *Psychological Review, 105*, 125–157.

Reichle, E.D., Liversedge, S.P., Pollatsek, A., and Rayner, K. (2009a). Encoding multiple words simultaneously in reading is implausible. *Trends in Cognitive Sciences, 13*, 115–119.

Reingold, E.M. and Rayner, K. (2006). Examining the word identification stages hypothesized by E-Z Reader. *Psychological Science, 17*, 742–746.

Schilling, H.E., Rayner, K., and Chumbley, J.I. (1998). Comparing naming, lexical decision, and eye fixation times: Word frequency effects and individual differences. *Memory and Cognition, 26*, 1270–1281.

Sears, C.R., Campbell, C.R., and Lupker, S.J. (2006). Is there a neighborhood frequency effect in English? Evidence from reading and lexical decision. *Journal of Experimental Psychology: Human Perception and Performance, 32*, 1040–1062.

Seidenberg, M.S., Waters, G.S., Barnes, M.A., and Tanenhaus, M.K. (1984). When does irregular spelling or pronunciation influence word recognition. *Journal of Verbal Learning and Verbal Behavior, 23*, 383–404.

Sereno, S.C. and Rayner, K. (2000). Spelling-sound regularity effects on eye fixations in reading. *Perception and Psychophysics, 62*, 402–409.

Sereno, S.C., O'Donnell, P.J., and Rayner, K. (2006). Eye movements and lexical ambiguity resolution: Investigating the subordinate-bias effect. *Journal of Experimental Psychology: Human Perception and Performance, 32*, 335–350.

Slattery, T.J. (2009). Word misperception, the neighbor frequency effect, and the role of sentence context: Evidence form eye movements. *Journal of Experimental Psychology: Human Perception and Performance, 35*, 1969–1975.

Staub, A., White, S.J., Drieghe, D., Hollway, E.C. and Rayner, K. (2010). Distributional effects of word frequency on eye fixation durations. *Journal of Experimental Psychology: Human Perception and Performance, 36*, 1280–1293.

Underwood, G., Petley, K., and Clews, S. (1990). Searching for information during sentence comprehension. In R. Groner, G. d'Ydewalle, and R. Parham (eds.) *From eye to mind: Information acquisition in perception, search, and reading.* (pp. 191–203). Oxford: North-Holland.

Warren, T. and McConnell, K. (2007). Investigating effects of selectional restriction violations and plausibility violation severity on eye movements in reading. *Psychonomic Bulletin and Review, 14*, 770–775.

Williams, R.S. and Morris, R.K. (2004). Eye movements, word familiarity, and vocabulary acquisition. *European Journal of Cognitive Psychology, 16*, 312–339.

White, S.J. (2008). Eye movement control during reading: Effects of word frequency and orthographic familiarity. *Journal of Experimental Psychology: Human Perception and Performance, 34*, 205–223.

White, S.J. and Liversedge, S.P. (2006). Foveal processing difficulty does not modulate non-foveal orthographic influences on fixation positions. *Vision Research, 46*, 426–437.

White, S.J., Johnson, R.L., Liversedge, S.P. and Rayner, K. (2008). Eye movements when reading transposed text: The importance of word-beginning letters. *Journal of Experimental Psychology: Human Perception and Performance, 34*, 1261–1276.

Yan, M., Richter, E.M., Shu H., and Kliegl, R. (2009). Readers of Chinese extract semantic information from parafoveal words. *Psychonomic Bulletin and Review, 16*, 561–566.

Yan, G., Tian, H., Bai, X., and Rayner, K. (2006). The effect of word and character frequency on the eye movements of Chinese readers. *British Journal of Psychology, 97*. 259–268.

Yang, S.-N. (2006). An oculomotor-based model of eye movements in reading: The competition/interaction model. *Cognitive Systems Research, 7*, 56–69.

Yang, S.-N., and McConkie, G.W. (2001). Eye movements during reading: A theory of saccade initiation time. *Vision Research, 41*, 3567–3585.

Yang, J., Wang, S., Xu Y., and Rayner, K. (2009).Do Chinese readers obtain preview benefit from word n+2? Evidence from eye movements. *Journal of Experimental Psychology: Human Perception and Performance, 35*, 1192–1204.

Zeno, S.M., Ivens, S.H., Hillard, R.T., and Duvvuri, R. (1995). *The educator's word frequency guide.* Brewster, NJ: Touchstone Applied Science Associates.

CHAPTER 49

Syntactic influences on eye movements during reading

Charles Clifton, Jr and Adrian Staub

Abstract

Measuring where the eyes fixate, and for how long, has arguably been the most valuable way of exploring the time-course of comprehending written sentences. This chapter reviews some of the history of the method's use as well as some recent developments. It provides an extensive review of what eye movement measurement has told us about the syntactic processing of sentences, covering topics such as syntactic ambiguity, syntactic ambiguity resolution, retrieval from memory, syntactic prediction, and syntactic complexity. Alternative models for how syntactic and extra-syntactic information sources are integrated are discussed. The chapter then turns to a discussion of what the eyes actually do in response to syntactic processing complexity, and provides a brief review of models of eye movement control. It concludes by comparing eye movement measurement with other methods of measuring online sentence comprehension processes.

Overview

The use of eye movement monitoring to study sentence processing dates back to nearly the beginning of cognitive psychology. In 1967, Mehler et al. used a Mackworth camera to study where readers fixated when they read ambiguous sentences whose syntactic structures differed depending on the context that they appeared in. Consider the ambiguous sentence *They gave her dog candies*. When this occurred in a context about a girl who liked dog candies, the words *dog* and *candies* must be analysed together as a phrase (or constituent), *dog candies*. When the same sentence occurred in a context about a girl's dog, the words *her* and *dog* have to be analysed as a constituent, *her dog*. Mehler et al. (1967) found more frequent fixations on *dog* in the former case than in the latter case, which they interpreted to mean that readers tend to fixate a word more often when it begins a syntactic constituent than when it terminates one.

The work that made eye tracking the 'gold standard' for studying visual sentence processing, however, appeared a decade and a half later. Frazier and Rayner (1982) used more modern equipment (a SRI dual-Purkinje tracker) that recorded fixation duration as well as position, and tested predictions of an explicit parsing theory (Frazier, 1978). They introduced the 'garden-path' theory of parsing, with the concepts of 'late closure' and 'minimal attachment'. This theory claims that readers and listeners use their implicit knowledge of phrase structure rules to build a syntactic tree. They apply these rules in a parallel race, so that the first sequence of rules that succeeds in attaching an incoming word into the current tree wins. This generally means that the simplest attachment, if there is one, is created (minimal attachment), and if there is no most-simple attachment, then the winner is the one that attaches the new material into the most available material, i.e. material currently being processed (late closure). Frazier and Rayner were able to show that reading was disrupted when these strategies led these readers 'down the garden path,' namely, when a temporary syntactic ambiguity was followed by material that indicated that the minimal or late-closure attachment was incorrect. For instance, readers showed long fixations and frequent regressions when a sentence fragment like *The girl knew the answer* continued *was wrong*. Readers apparently took *the answer* to be the direct object and theme of *know* (the syntactically minimal analysis) and were disrupted when they had to reanalyse it as the subject of a complement sentence, *the answer was wrong*.

The Frazier and Rayner paper led to an outpouring of studies using eye tracking to study parsing and sentence interpretation (see Clifton et al., 2007, for a review of 100 such studies). These studies examined topics such as the effects of plausibility and discourse and referential context on syntactic parsing, the detailed time course of parsing, and the fundamental architecture of the human sentence processing mechanism.

Recent years have seen the development of innovative ways of using eye movements to study sentence comprehension. Most early studies used sentences created for the purpose of testing specific theoretical hypotheses, providing tight experimental control over important variables. Many research-ers continue to create and study such sentences. However, some researchers have turned to measuring eye movements while people read natural texts (e.g. Boston et al., 2008; Kennedy and Pynte, 2005). There are clear costs and benefits to both the experimental and the 'corpus-based' approaches. The latter approach certainly engages more normal comprehension processes, but at the cost of experi-mental control of many factors known to affect eye movements (not the least of them, length and frequency of words). One could hope that the two approaches will triangulate on the fundamental processes underlying eye movements and sentence processing, but that hasn't happened yet (cf. the diverging evidence on whether the content of words in the parafovea affects the duration of the current fixation; Drieghe et al., 2008; Kennedy and Pynte, 2005; see also Drieghe, Chapter 46, this volume).

Another new development is the construction of explicit models of eye movement control (Engbert et al., 2005; Pollatsek et al., 2006; Reichle et al., 1998, among others; see also Reichle, Chapter 42, and Engbert and Kliegl, Chapter 43, this volume). These have greatly sharpened claims about the relation between word recognition and eye movements, even if the disputes among competing claims have not yet been resolved. However, extension of these models to questions of sentence parsing and interpretation is still in its infancy; below we discuss the first, quite recent, attempt to account for how the eyes respond to sentence processing difficulty within the framework of a lower-level model of eye movement control (Reichle et al., 2009).

A third development that has had a great impact on language processing work is the measurement of eye movements while one is listening to spoken language (Tanenhaus et al 1995; cf. Cooper, 1974). Cooper's early work indicated that people tended to look at things that were being talked about, and that the eye movements were quite closely timelocked to speech. Tanenhaus et al. used this phenom-enon to study the time course of word identification and sentence interpretation, and others have used it to study a variety of topics in ambiguity resolution, anticipation of referents, and pragmatic constraints on interpretation (Tanenhaus, 2007; see Henderson and Ferreira, 2004, for a collection of overview chapters). In the remainder of this chapter, we will focus exclusively on the use of eye tracking in read-ing; but cf. Altmann's chapter in this volume (Chapter 54) for a survey of this 'visual world' research.

Syntactic factors that affect eye movements in reading

Ambiguity effects

A great many eye tracking studies have investigated processing of sentences that are temporarily or permanently ambiguous. Ambiguity is interesting in itself: it is pervasive in normal language use, but nonetheless seems to cause little difficulty in communication. Somehow, readers are able to 'see through' the ambiguity and determine the writer's message. Presumably, they use discourse context, knowledge of the writer (and of the writer's knowledge), plausibility, and a great many other factors in resolving ambiguity, seldom violating syntactic constraints (but cf. Ferreira, 2003; Sanford and Sturt, 2002, for some evidence that people aren't quite perfect).

One specific question that has attracted substantial attention is whether a reader entertains multiple interpretations of an ambiguous sentence at one time, and if so, is there a cost to doing so. Although existing theories take sharply different positions on the former question (e.g. Frazier and Rayner, 1982; MacDonald et al., 1995), truly convincing evidence is lacking. However, the evidence about the latter question is fairly clear: there does not seem to be an extra processing cost in the ambiguous region when material is syntactically ambiguous (but see discussion of later costs when the wrong analysis is made of the ambiguous region).

This answer is surprising, given the clear evidence that there is an extra cost in processing a lexically ambiguous item like *bark* than an unambiguous item, reflected in eye tracking measures during reading (Duffy et al., 1988; cf. Juhasz and Pollatsek, Chapter 48, this volume). This extra cost can plausibly be attributed to a time-consuming process of resolving the competition between the dog sense and the tree sense of *bark*. However, there is essentially zero evidence that reading a syntactically ambiguous phrase is slower than reading an unambiguous one, when other factors are controlled (see Clifton and Staub, 2008, for a thorough discussion). In fact, some ambiguous phrases are actually read faster than their disambiguated counterparts (Traxler et al., 1998; van Gompel et al., 2005). This fact can be taken as evidence against the claim that a reader chooses among multiple interpretations of a sentence by activating them all and letting them compete for dominance (which can be taken as an argument against the competitive multiple-analysis models to be discussed in the next section). But it does not convincingly show that only a single interpretation is considered at a time, since it is possible that multiple analyses are considered in a non-competitive, cost-free, manner, perhaps in a 'race' to finding a single acceptable interpretation.

Garden-pathing

One line of evidence that a reader considers only a single interpretation at a time comes from studies following up the original Frazier and Rayner (1982) garden-pathing findings. Frazier and Rayner were interested in temporarily ambiguous sentences not just because of their ambiguity, but because they argued that such sentences could be used to identify the decision processes a reader (or listener) uses in understanding all kinds of sentences. When reading a sentence, a reader must decide how each word fits into its sentence. The reader must build and interpret a mental representation of the relations among words, and a great deal of evidence indicates that this takes place very quickly, often even while the eyes are fixating on a word (Just and Carpenter, 1980; Rayner et al., 2004; cf. Marslen-Wilson, 1973, for comparable evidence about listening).

The 'garden-path' model proposed by Frazier and Rayner was motivated by the assumption that a reader had to have a representation of the structural relations among words in a sentence in order to interpret it (*He gave her the dog candies* and *He gave her dog the candies* mean very different things, which are dependent on the different syntactic structures of the two sentences). Sentences are interpreted nearly without delay, but their interpretation depends on a potentially-vast range of information. If Frazier and Rayner are correct that sentences are not word salad, and that sentence interpretations depend on how words are structurally related in a sentence, it would be very advantageous for a reader or listener to build a syntactic structure as quickly as possible. Frazier and Rayner favoured a model that claimed readers provisionally accept the very first structure they can build, generally the simplest possible structure, so they quickly have *some* structure to interpret. Frazier and Rayner's eye tracking data showed disruptions of processing when material later in a sentence was syntactically inconsistent with the simplest and most quickly built analysis of material earlier in the sentence (and Rayner et al. (1983) showed similar effects when the later material was semantically inconsistent with this structure). When a single word provides the disconfirmation, the disruption can appear on the very first fixation on that word, as well as appearing as lengthened gaze durations and increased frequency of regressions. When a multi-word region provides the disambiguation, the latter two measures (and others, such as go-past time or regression path duration) generally reflect the disruption (see Clifton et al., 2007, for discussion of how disruption appears in later published research).

The early Frazier and Rayner work did have some notable shortcomings. For instance, their test of minimal attachment ('accept the simplest and therefore most quickly-built analysis') compared sentences like (1a) and (1b):

1a. The lawyers think his second wife will claim the inheritance.

1b. The second wife will claim the inheritance belongs to her.

They found that reading was disrupted on *belongs* in (1b) compared to earlier regions of the sentence (presumably because readers took *the inheritance* to be the direct object of *claim*, not the subject of a complement clause—a more complex, non-minimal, analysis). Clearly this is not an ideal comparison: different words are being compared in different sentence contexts. Still, the basic Frazier and Rayner findings have stood up (cf. Clifton et al., 2007, for a review). For instance, reading of *belongs* is still disrupted in (1b) if it is compared to *The second wife will claim that the inheritance belongs to her*, where *that* blocks the normally-preferred attachment (Rayner and Frazier, 1987).

Frazier and Rayner's serial, single analysis, model provides an elegant account of their data, but it nonetheless stimulated the development of several competing models. These models take issue with the garden-path models on several major points: they propose that multiple syntactic analyses are considered at once, not just a single analysis; they generally claim that semantic and pragmatic factors, not just speed of construction, can affect which syntactic analysis is initially considered; and some propose that these syntactic analyses are not built, following phrase structure rules, but instead are activated from pre-existing structures in a mental store (see MacDonald et al., 1994; McRae et al., 1998, for two of the most influential models). All these models are able to account for the basic garden-pathing effects. All of them are able to account for the observation (e.g. Rayner et al., 1983) that semantic effects can appear quite early in the eye tracking record. There have been lively disputes about whether lexical or semantic or pragmatic factors can affect the initial choice of a syntactic analysis or just the reanalysis of an initial, inappropriate analysis—two lines of research where the advantage seems to shift from one side, to the other, and back again, can be found in Ferreira and Henderson (1990), followed by Trueswell et al. (1993), then by Kennison (2001); and in Ferreira and Clifton (1986), followed by Trueswell et al. (1994), and then by Clifton et al. (2003).

It may turn out that convincing evidence can be provided showing that semantic or contextual information can guide the parser's initial choices, at least in the face of weak syntactic biases (Altmann et al., 1998, and Britt, 1994, are apparent instances). But it may take other experimental paradigms to answer the question of whether sentence comprehension is best thought of as a process of constructing a syntactic analysis of a sentence and then using a wide range of semantic and contextual information to interpret and correct this analysis, or a process of allowing this unconstrained range of information to activate multiple possible analyses and eventually settle on a single one (cf. Frazier, 1995, for discussion). From our admittedly-biased perspective, the current authors think that it will be difficult to build a model that deals with the recovery from a garden path and the processing of an ambiguity in the same competitive manner, given that the former disrupts reading while the latter does not; but we acknowledge that not all the facts are in yet.

Memory effects

There is more to sentence processing than ambiguity resolution. The very earliest psycholinguists recognized that difficulty in understanding sentences should be attributed to memory or processing resources being overloaded (Miller, 1962). It's hard to understand *The rat that the cat that the dog worried chased ate the malt*, perhaps because one has forgotten the first subject by the time one reaches the final verb (or perhaps because processing too many subject–verb relations at once overloads the system). Theorists have incorporated memory considerations into their processing theories in various ways. Just and Carpenter (1980) proposed a model of language comprehension and eye movements that made critical appeal to both short- and long-term memory processes in a production model, and in later work (Just and Carpenter, 1992) focused on how individual differences in working memory capacity affected eye movements in reading. Many researchers have examined people with varying working memory spans, often measured using 'reading span' (Daneman and Carpenter, 1980) They have found evidence that (e.g.) low-span readers use contextual or pragmatic information less efficiently than high-span readers (Just and Carpenter, 1992; MacDonald et al., 1992; Pearlmutter and MacDonald, 1995) (but cf. Waters and Caplan, 1996, for a critique of some of this research).

Other researchers have concentrated on trying to develop explicit process models for how memory might play a role in understanding sentences. Work by Gibson and his colleagues and students (Gibson, 2000; Warren and Gibson, 2002) has been very influential. Although it has not yet resulted in published studies of eye tracking during reading, its claim that the distance between dependent elements (perhaps measured in terms of the number of new discourse entities introduced between the elements) affects speed of comprehension has clear implications for eye tracking measures. McElree and his colleagues (e.g. McElree et al., 2003) have developed models in which a content-addressable memory search is involved in comprehending some sentence structures, but as in the case of Gibson's work, most of their research has used techniques other than eye tracking (but cf. Martin and McElree, 2008, for an example of eye tracking research guided by considerations of memory retrieval).

Perhaps the most complete and explicit theory of the roles that memory plays in sentence under-standing is that of Lewis (cf. Lewis et al., 2006, for an accessible introduction). Once again, this approach has not yet been tested extensively in eye tracking studies. However, some of its premises have been supported in eye tracking research conducted by Gordon and colleagues (e.g. Gordon et al., 2006). For example, these researchers argued that the difficulty of understanding an object relative clause sentence like *The banker that the barber praised climbed the mountain just outside of town* was due, at least in part, to interference from *barber* in retrieving the object of *praised*, namely, *the banker*. Comparing these sentences to subject relative clause sentences (*The banker that praised the barber . . .*), they found more regressive rereading after reaching the relative clause in sentences like these than in sentences where the intervening noun phrase was a proper name (*. . . that Sophie praised . . .*). Presumably, a proper name does not interfere as much with retrieval of the required definite description, *the banker*, as another definite description would.

Syntactic prediction

Several recent sentence processing models propose that the difficulty of incremental processing of word-by-word input is a function of how predictable this input is, or more precisely, the probability of the input given the sentence so far (Hale, 2001; Levy, 2008). These models assume that what matters is not only the predictability of specific lexical items (as has been shown to affect eye move-ments; Ehrlich and Rayner, 1981; Rayner et al., 2004; Rayner and Well, 1996), but also the predicta-bility of syntactic structure. There is, in fact, eye movement evidence suggesting that material is read more quickly in a context in which syntactic structure is highly predictable. For example, Staub and Clifton (2006) demonstrated that when a disjunction is preceded by the word *either*, the material just after the word *or* is read faster than when the word *either* is absent. Staub et al. (2006) also showed that the direct object in a so-called 'heavy NP shift' structure (e.g. *Jack watched from the stands his daughter's attempt to shoot a basket.*) is read more quickly when the verb is obligatorily transitive, which licenses a prediction of a shifted object (*Jack praised from the stands his daughter's attempt to shoot a basket*). Recently, Demberg and Keller (2009) and Boston et al. (2008) have shown, using correlational methods, that a significant proportion of word-by-word reading time variance in English and German eye movement corpora is explained by a surprisal metric based on the work of Levy (2008) and Hale (2001). Finally, Staub (2010) has recently demonstrated that readers make many regressive eye movements out of the subject of an object relative clause (e.g. *the fireman* in *The employees that the fireman noticed hurried across the open field.*), which is claimed by the Hale/Levy framework to be a point at which structural expectations are violated.

Another set of findings that may also be interpreted as reflecting syntactic prediction comes from studies of the resolution of long-distance dependencies. It has been proposed that when the parser encounters a constituent prior to the site of its interpretation (as in questions such as *Which puppy did the girl buy?* and relative clauses such as *The puppy that the girl bought was a golden retriever.*) it actively anticipates that this interpretation site will appear in the first grammatically licensed location (De Vincenzi, 1991; Frazier and Flores D'Arcais, 1989). Several eye movement studies (Pickering and Traxler, 2001, 2003; Staub, 2007; Traxler and Pickering, 1996) have contributed to a literature confirming this principle. These studies have shown increased reading time when the first grammatically licensed location turns out not to be correct, either because of an implausible verb-argument relation (e.g. increased fixation durations on *landed* in *That's the truck that the pilot landed carefully behind.*) or because this location turns out to be occupied by other material (e.g. increased reading time on *a few pupils* in *That's the diver that the coach persuaded a few pupils to watch.*; cf. Stowe, 1986).

Syntactic complexity

The findings reviewed to this point make it clear that some grammatical structures are more complex than others to process in the sense of resulting in slower reading. Structures that result in garden paths (i.e. disambiguated structures that require a reader to choose a normally-dispreferred analysis), structures that place excessive demands on memory, structures that violate agreement or disconfirm expectations—these are complex to process in this sense.

For present purposes, though, let us restrict 'syntactic complexity' to refer to some measure of the complexity of linguistic structure or its derivational history (i.e. the series of underlying representations from which a surface form is thought to arise, on generative approaches to syntax). Returning to the origins of psycholinguistics, the 'Derivational Theory of Complexity' claimed that increasing the number of transformations involved in the derivation of a sentence (e.g. the transformation from active to passive, or the transformation from an affirmative sentence to a negative one; Chomsky, 1957) increased its processing difficulty. This theory garnered some support (see Fodor et al., 1974, for a review), for example from the fact that passive or negative sentences were harder to remember than simple actives. However, linguistic theory itself soon adopted a conception of a sentence's derivation that did not involve transformations in Chomsky's (1957) sense, and it soon became clear that other explanations were available for the processing difficulty of transformationally-complex sentences.

Perhaps complexity should, instead, be measured by number or density of syntactic nodes in the kind of tree structure that syntacticians working within a generative grammar framework have been using, in one form or another, since Chomsky (1957). Are structures that have greater syntactic complexity, in this specific sense, read more slowly than structures with less complexity? Some processing perspectives say they should be. If a reader builds up a tree structure by applying linguistic rules or principles to the words in a sentence, and does so in a serial manner, one would expect that more complex trees should result in slower reading time.

Indeed, there have been some sophisticated and promising analyses of the possible effects of syntactic complexity (e.g. Frazier's, 1985, suggestion that complexity should be measured by how many intermediate syntactic nodes have to be postulated essentially at once (e.g. within a window of no more than three words)). However, there is precious little evidence from eye tracking or any other technique that syntactic complexity slows reading. One source of evidence is Frazier and Rayner (1988), who showed that eye tracking was disrupted in sentences that began with a sentential subject (e.g. *That both of the Siamese twins survived the operation is remarkable*). Sentences like this require a large amount of syntactic structure to be built up at the beginning of the subject (*That both...*), which may be the source of their difficulty. However, they are also infrequent and they have an ambiguity (whether *that* is a complementizer or a demonstrative) that lasts for only one word. At the present time, it does not appear that there is clear evidence from eye tracking or elsewhere that increasing syntactic complexity, without introducing additional parsing choices (temporary ambiguity) or memory load, actually increases processing difficulty.

Syntactic violations

Using the event-related potential (ERP) paradigm, researchers have learned a great deal about how the brain responds to syntactic violations (see Kutas et al., 2006, for a recent review). It is perhaps surprising that the use of violations has been relatively rare in the eye movement literature, until one considers that one of the great attractions of the eye movement paradigm has always been its ability to capture language processing under natural conditions. Nevertheless, there are a few studies that have examined how the eyes respond when they encounter either a phrase structure violation or an agreement violation (Braze et al., 2002; Deutsch and Bentin, 2001; Ni et al., 1998; Pearlmutter et al., 1999). These studies vary in when the effect of anomaly first appears in the eye movement record, with two of the studies (Ni et al., 1998, Pearlmutter et al., 1999) failing to find first pass reading time effects on the critical word. Clearly, more work is required in this area.

What do the eyes do when there are syntactic processing problems?

How quickly do syntactic processing problems appear in the eye movement record?

Important properties of lexical items, such as their frequency of occurrence and their predictability in context, affect the time taken to read them in a rather uniform fashion (see Staub and Rayner, 2007, for a review). The effects of these properties consistently appear in such measures as first fixation duration and gaze duration. Some exceptions do exist—e.g. less-skilled readers, upon encountering an infrequent and unpredicted word in a context that strongly predicts a different and more common word, do tend to fixate it relatively briefly, perhaps not even encoding the word (Ashby et al., 2005)—but they are exceptions.

In contrast, effects of syntactic processing difficulty can show up at various points in the eye tracking record. In the original Frazier and Rayner (1982) study, disruption appeared as an apparent lengthening of the very first fixation on the region that disambiguated a sentence to its unpreferred syntactic analysis. Other studies (e.g. Staub, 2007) have also shown first fixation effects. But effects of syntactic processing often do not appear this quickly. In many cases, the disambiguating information is spread out over a multi-word region, and in these cases, one could not expect a first fixation effect. But although effects quite often show up as increases in first pass reading times, they sometimes only show up as an increased frequency of regressions, or as an increased go-past/cumulative region reading time, or even only as an increased time in the following (spillover) region or as increased second pass time. Clifton et al. (2007) listed studies showing each of these patterns of effects, but were unable to pinpoint factors that determined which pattern would appear. Some potentially contributing factors might be the type of ambiguity or syntactic difficulty, or how it is disambiguated, or the reading goals of a subject, or the subject's reading skill, or other factors not yet identified. While there is a substantial amount of work investigating the factors that influence the amount of syntactic processing difficulty that appears in the eye movement record, and there is interesting work on the process of how a syntactic misanalysis is reanalysed (see Fodor and Ferreira, 1998, for a useful overview), very little work has been done investigating how various factors influence the precise timing at which syntactic difficulty first appears in the eye movement record. As pointed out by, e.g. Bornkessel and Schlesewsky (2006), the very existence of first fixation effects of syntactic processing difficulty is superficially inconsistent with the fact that such effects tend to show up later in the electroencephalography (EEG) record, but this may turn out to be a limitation of existing analyses of EEG (cf. Sereno and Rayner, 2003).

The tradeoff problem and distributional effects

One interesting empirical question that has been addressed is whether there is a tradeoff between fixating a longer time on a region (e.g. a disambiguating region) and regressing to an earlier part of the sentence. A series of exchanges between Altmann and his colleagues, on the one hand, and Rayner and Sereno, on the other, is illuminating if less than conclusive (Altmann, 1994; Altmann et al., 1992; Rayner and Sereno 1994a, 1994b). Altmann observed that fixations made prior to a regression out of a word were, for the most part, shorter than fixations made prior to a forward saccade.[1] When a garden-path sentence (a reduced relative clause sentence) was presented by itself, the disruption observed in first pass time in the disambiguating region was at least as large when a fixation in this region was followed by a forward saccade as when it was followed by a regression. But interestingly, he found that when the temporarily ambiguous sentence was presented with a preceding context that biased toward the relative clause reading (by introducing two possible referents named by the same word, so that modification was needed to avoid referential failure), garden-path disruption of first pass time appeared only on trials on which there was a regression out of the disambiguating region. This does not suggest a tradeoff between regressions and lengthened fixations, but instead, suggests that reading time was affected only on those trials where comprehension was disrupted so much that a regression was made.

Rayner and Sereno, in contrast, analysed data in which a discourse context appeared to have only delayed, not immediate, effects on comprehension difficulty. They found a numerically larger effect of garden-pathing when there was no regression out of the disambiguating region than when there was a regression. This pattern, which Rayner and Sereno appeared to believe is typical of eye tracking data (and was true of data for sentences without preceding contexts presented by Altmann et al., 1992), suggests that there may in fact be a tradeoff between longer fixations and regressions. However, it is not yet clear when this tradeoff occurs or what factors govern the choice (stay or look back) that is made.

A related issue, and one which is critical for distinguishing between parsing theories, is whether syntactic processing difficulty is manifested as an all-or-none phenomenon. According to serial accounts like the garden-path theory (Frazier, 1987; Frazier and Rayner, 1982) and the unrestricted race model (van Gompel et al., 2005), reading times at a potential point of difficulty should be bimodally distributed: if the reader was maintaining the correct parse at the point of encountering the critical input, no difficulty should be evident, but if the reader was maintaining an incorrect parse, rather extreme difficulty associated with syntactic revision should appear. On the other hand, a spate of both older (McRae et al., 1998) and more recent (Levy, 2008) parsing models predict that syntactic processing difficulty should be graded, with the amount of difficulty reflecting the amount of required updating of activation levels associated with multiple candidate analyses. Thus, these models would not seem to predict bimodality. We believe that the distributions of fixation durations under different experimental conditions deserve close examination. A promising beginning (limited to lexical variables) can be seen in Staub et al. (2010), who recently carried out formal analyses of distributions of fixation durations, focusing on the distributional effects of word frequency. Staub et al. showed that fixations are longer on essentially all trials when a word is low in frequency (a shift effect), but that the longest fixations were especially lengthened (a skew effect). However, Staub (2011) has recently found that a lexical predictability manipulation results in a shift effect, but no skew effect. This suggests that word frequency and predictability affect fixation durations via different mechanisms.

---

[1] We note that Mitchell and Shen (in press) have recently replicated this observation, and have shown how it is actually predicted by the latest iteration of the E-Z Reader model (Reichle et al., 2009).

Similar analyses of the effects of syntactic and other high-level variables may well shed light on their mechanisms.

Targeting of regressions

When a regression is made, what controls its target? Most regressions are, in all likelihood, simply corrections of misplaced landing positions, and therefore cover only a short distance and do not provide information about parsing (see Mitchell et al., 2008, for relevant discussion). However, it is possible that some regressions can shed light on the process of sentence comprehension.

Frazier and Rayner (1982) analysed regressions, and reported that they frequently went from the disambiguating region to the earlier point of ambiguity. However, as Mitchell et al. have pointed out, the point of ambiguity was often only one or two words before the disambiguation. While it is informative that regressions did not often return to the start of the sentence, suggesting starting over from scratch after a garden-path, the Frazier and Rayner data need not be taken as clear evidence for intelligently-directed regressions.

A report by Meseguer et al. (2002) provides more convincing data. Their Spanish readers were likely to regress from the verb of an adverbial phrase when the form of this verb (indicative vs. subjunctive mood) forced the adverbial phrase to be attached high, modifying the first verb of the sentence, and prevented the normally-preferred low-attachment analysis. More critically, the relative frequency with which a regression from this sentence-final verb landed specifically on the first verb was greater when the sentence was disambiguated toward the normally-unpreferred than the normally-preferred analysis. This does suggest intelligent guidance of regressions. However, the differential frequency of such verb-directed regressions was quite small, only a few percentage points, and (as Mitchell et al., 2008, suggest), it may matter that the regressions were launched from the last word in the sentence, given that regressions from a sentence-final word are quite frequent in any event.

Mitchell et al. (2008) present the most extensive available analysis of the targeting of regressions. They examined regressions out of the disambiguating region of English late closure sentences similar to those studied by Frazier and Rayner (1982) (e.g. . . .*while the men hunted the moose that was sturdy and nimble hurried into the woods*. . .). They found relatively few immediate regressions directly to the ambiguous region (the initial verb *hunted* and its apparent direct object *the moose*). However, they did find a substantial number of returns to this region in the first few regressive saccades after the disambiguating region. This suggests that regressive eye movements may be guided intelligently, perhaps a bit sluggishly or (following Inhoff and Weger, 2005) perhaps guided by an imperfect memory for the position of the ambiguity.

Models of eye movement control and models of sentence processing

Models of eye movement control in reading have achieved a very high degree of sophistication, with the E-Z Reader (Pollatsek et al., 2006; Reichle, Chapter 42, this volume) and SWIFT (Engbert et al., 2005; Engbert and Kliegl, Chapter 43, this volume) models each accounting for a wide range of findings regarding factors that influence the duration and location of readers' eye fixations. In both models, perceptual processing, attentional factors, lexical processing, and oculomotor factors combine (in different ways in the two models) to produce the observed pattern of eye movement behaviour. However, a widely acknowledged shortcoming of these models is that they do not model the effects of linguistic processing above the level of the word. For example, until recently E-Z Reader made no attempt at all to explain inter-word regressions, and while SWIFT does allow for such regressions, it explains them on the basis of incomplete lexical processing of a word that the eyes have already left. Neither model was designed to deal with the fact that difficult syntactic processing inflates reading times and/or causes an increase in the likelihood of a regressive eye movement.

Recently, however, Reichle et al. (2009) have attempted to remedy this situation by modifying the architecture of E-Z Reader. The critical addition is a 'post-lexical integration' stage of processing of word *n* that runs concurrently with the shift of attention to word *n*+1, and then with processing of that word. If integration of word *n* fails rapidly enough, the forward saccade to word *n*+1 is cancelled, resulting in an increased fixation duration on word *n*, a refixation of word *n*, or a regression. If integration of word *n* fails more slowly, and the eyes have already moved to word *n*+1, a regressive eye movement ensues. There are various details in Reichle et al.'s (2009) proposal that are open to debate, such as the assumption of strictly serial lexical and syntactic processing, and the assumption that syntactic processing only intrudes on the normal sequence of eye movements when a parsing breakdown has occurred. Nevertheless, we think that the integration stage in the Reichle et al. model is a major step forward, for it is the first serious attempt to integrate several decades of research on the effects of syntactic processing on eye movements into an implemented model of eye movement control in reading that also takes serious account of lower-level factors.

There have also been some attempts to make explicit the mapping between processing stages and eye movement measures that have started from a detailed parsing model rather than from a detailed model of eye movement control. In these cases, theorists have asked whether the kinds of processing operations proposed by a parsing model (e.g. attaching a word into the phrase marker, checking agreement, checking binding relations, retrieving a head or dependent from memory) can be mapped onto specific eye movement measures. For example, Boland (2004) has claimed that 'the eyes do not leave a word until it has been structurally integrated. Therefore, constraints that control structure-building influence first-pass reading time' (p. 60). An obvious problem with this proposal is the presence of spillover effects where difficulty associated with attaching a word or phrase appears only downstream of the word or phrase itself (see Clifton et al., 2007, for examples). More recently, Vasishth et al. (2008) have suggested that the time needed for memory retrieval in the course of sentence processing is reflected most closely in rereading time (i.e. second-pass time), which is the sum of fixations on a word or phrase after the word or phrase is first exited. While Vasishth et al. demonstrate an impressively tight link between the predictions of their memory retrieval model and empirical rereading times, their analysis faces a serious conceptual problem, as their re-reading time measure was based only on trials on which rereading actually occurred (usually a minority of trials), while the model was designed to predict memory retrieval time in general. Clearly, more work remains to be done in this domain.

Eye tracking, self-paced reading, and event-related potentials: comparison and contrast

In this section, we consider how eye tracking compares to the other dominant paradigms for studying on-line syntactic processing: self-paced reading (SPR) and ERPs. There are important practical issues involved in the choice between these paradigms, with eye tracking falling somewhere between the other two methods in terms of cost and in terms of complexity of the data analysis process. Here, however, we focus on a more substantive issue: what kind of inferences about 'normal' syntactic processing is it possible to draw based on results from the three paradigms?

In the SPR paradigm (Just et al., 1982; cf. Mitchell, 2004), a sentence is revealed on a computer screen one word, or phrase, at a time. The rate at which the sentence is revealed is under the control of the experimental subject, who repeatedly presses a key to reveal each word or phrase. While 'cumulative' versions of this paradigm have been used (Just et al., 1982), it is by far more common to use a 'non-cumulative' version, in which only one word or phrase is visible, with preceding regions being masked when a new region is displayed. The dependent measure in SPR is the latency of button-pressing; it is assumed that as processing becomes difficult, subjects will slow down their rate of button-pressing, in a manner analogous to the way in which, in normal reading, the eyes tend to rest longer before moving past a difficult-to-process word or region.

An enormous amount of sentence processing research has been carried out using SPR (see Mitchell, 2004, for a review), and even more strikingly, implemented computational models of syntactic processing have often been tested against SPR data (Levy, 2008; McRae et al., 1998; Tabor and

Hutchins, 2004.). In our view, this state of affairs is rather problematic. Our main reason for worry is that little is known about how three critical aspects of the SPR task might affect patterns of experimental results.

First, SPR tends to be quite slow compared to normal reading: In the word-by-word variant of SPR, readers may spend up to twice as long on a word as they would in normal reading (though there is a great deal of variability in SPR times obtained in different experiments, and in different labs). Thus, readers have a substantial amount of 'unallocated' time (i.e. time not used in the service of word recognition or eye movement control) in which to process the input material. This time may be used to entertain competing syntactic analyses, make predictions, etc. We do not think it is safe to assume that syntactic processing during slowed-down reading is similar in all relevant respects to syntactic processing during normal reading. Second, in the non-cumulative version of SPR (which is by far the dominant version) readers cannot look back at earlier regions of the sentence. Thus, the 'external memory' that the text provides is not available, and again, it is difficult to say how this might affect processing strategies. (It could be argued that SPR mimics auditory language processing in terms of the lack of a continuously existing external representation of the sentence.) Finally, and perhaps most importantly, SPR substitutes a consciously-controlled, newly-learned method of progressing through a sentence for the relatively automatic, highly-practised skill of moving one's eyes. Again, it is impossible to know how this substitution might affect data patterns. Models of eye movement control in reading have made great progress in accounting for variance in fixation durations and saccade landing positions based on the assumption that readers' eye movements are triggered by a combination of low-level oculomotor routines and ongoing lexical processing. While higher-level linguistic processing, such as syntactic processing, clearly does affect patterns of eye movements, it appears to do so in a relatively circumscribed manner. Indeed, the initial E-Z Reader model adopted the assumption that 'higher-order processes intervene in eye-movement control only when "something is wrong" and either send a signal to stop moving forward or a signal to execute a regression' (Reichle et al., 1998, p. 450). However, when a reader must make a conscious decision to press a button to receive the next input word, a very different balance of factors may be at work; it is within the reader's conscious control (as opposed to the control of highly automatized processing system) to decide what criteria to use for pressing the spacebar. In sum, we think that the time has come for the field to undertake a serious analysis of SPR as a task, to investigate how its demands do (or more happily, do not) modulate normal processing.

In ERP research (see Kutas et al., 2006, for an overview), electrophysiological activity at the scalp is measured, time-locked to the presentation of a visual or auditory stimulus. In the majority of ERP experiments on sentence processing, sentences are presented visually, one word at a time, using the rapid visual serial presentation (RSVP) paradigm, and the response to a critical word is measured. Often, the critical word is the last word of the stimulus, and as noted above, this word often constitutes a violation of some sort (i.e. either semantic or syntactic).

In our view, ERP research provides a very useful complement to eye tracking, as the two paradigms provide distinct types of information. ERP research has distinguished qualitatively distinct electrophysiological responses to different types of linguistic violations, with different latencies, different scalp locations, and different polarities. For example, syntactic and semantic violations have different ERP signatures. Encountering a semantically anomalous but syntactically licensed word in a sentence leads to an increase in the amplitude of a negative electrical potential that peaks about 400 ms after word onset (the N400). In contrast, syntactic violations, depending on their type, may lead either to a left-lateralized negativity in the same time range (the left anterior negativity, or LAN) or to modulation of a later, positive component (the P600); see, e.g. Bornkessel-Schlesewsky and Schlesewsky, 2009). However, these effects are indeed qualitatively distinct, so it is difficult to draw conclusions about the relative amount of difficulty induced by different manipulations. Moreover, it is notoriously problematic to draw conclusions about cognitive timing based on the latency of ERP effects. With eye tracking data, on the other hand, it is more straightforward to assess the relative amount of difficulty induced by an experimental manipulation, and timing is relatively (though not completely) transparent. But with eye tracking data, it is more difficult to tell different kinds of processing apart: all difficulty appears in the form of a slowdown and/or an increase in the likelihood of a regressive eye movement.

As with SPR, one drawback of ERP is artificial stimulus presentation. Recently, a few labs have begun recording EEG during normal reading, with the ultimate goal of establishing correspondence between eye movement behaviour and events in the electrophysiological record (e.g. Dimigen et al., 2007; Kretzschmar, 2010). This is technically very challenging, not least because eye movements and blinks induce artefacts in the EEG record, but we think that this is a very promising line of future research. And, somewhat as compensation, it is possible to time-lock the EEG signal to the onset of auditory words, so ERPs can be used to directly investigate the similarities and differences between auditory and visual processing of linguistic input.

In sum, we think that the artificial modes of stimulus presentation used in ERP and SPR need to be taken into account in interpreting reading data from these paradigms. We think that the ability of the ERP paradigm to elucidate qualitative distinctions between brain responses, and to enable comparisons between visual and auditory processing, are clear advantages of this paradigm. We are somewhat less certain whether there are advantages to SPR studies, especially now that eye tracking technology has become relatively inexpensive and user-friendly, though we do acknowledge that many very important contributions to the study of sentence processing (e.g. the work of Gibson, 2000, and his colleagues, as well as earlier work reviewed by Mitchell, 2004) have been made by SPR studies.

Summary and conclusions

In this chapter, we have attempted to provide an overview of the kinds of questions about syntactic processing that eye movement research has been used to answer, and to provide a general sense of some of the answers to these questions. Obviously, we have only scratched the surface, and the interested reader is directed to the literature cited here. Looking at things the 'other way around,' we have also tried to point out some of the unresolved questions about how the eyes respond to syntactic processing difficulty, and about how syntactic processing should be integrated into full models of eye movement control in reading. We hope the reader takes away from this an appreciation both of how much has been learned from eye movement studies of syntactic processing, and of how much remains to be done.

Acknowledgements

Please send correspondence to Charles Clifton (cec@psych.umass.edu) or Adrian Staub (astaub@psych.umass.edu). We would like to thank Lyn Frazier and Keith Rayner for their comments on an earlier version of this manuscript. Preparation of the manuscript was supported in part by Grant HD-18708 from the National Institute for Child Health and Human Development. The content is solely the responsibility of the authors and does not necessarily represent the official views of the National Institute for Child Health and Human Development or the National Institutes of Health.

References

Altmann, G.T.M. (1994). Regression-contingent analyses of eye movements during sentence processing: Reply to Rayner and Sereno. *Memory and Cognition*, **22**, 286–290.

Altmann, G.T.M., Garnham, A., and Dennis, Y. (1992). Avoiding the garden path: Eye movements in context. *Journal of Memory and Language*, **31**, 685–712.

Altmann, G.T.M., van Nice, K.Y., Garnham, A., and Henstra, J.-A. (1998). Late closure in context. *Journal of Memory and Language*, **38**, 459–484.

Ashby, J., Rayner, K., and Clifton, C.J. (2005). Eye movements of highly skilled and average readers: Differential effects of frequency and predictability. *Quarterly Journal of Experimental Psychology,* **58A**, 1065–1086.

Boland, J. (2004). Linking eye movements to sentence comprehension in reading and listening. In M. Carreiras and C. Clifton Jr (eds.) *The on-line study of sentence comprehension* (pp. 51–76). New York: Psychology Press.

Bornkessel, I. and Schlesewski, M. (2006). The extended argument dependency model: A neurocognitive approach to sentence comprehension across languages. *Psychological Review*, 113, 787–821.

Bornkessel-Schlesewsky, I. and Schlesewsky, M. (2009). *Processing syntax and morphology*. Oxford: Oxford University Press.

Boston, M.F., Hale, J., Kliegl, R., Patil, U., and Vasishth, S. (2008). Parsing costs as predictors of reading difficulty: An evaluation using the Potsdam Sentence Corpus. *Journal of Eye Movement Research*, 2, 1–192.

Britt, M.A. (1994). The interaction of referential ambiguity and argument structure in the parsing of prepositional phrases. *Journal of Memory and Language,* 33, 251–283.

Braze, D., Shankweiler, D., Ni, W., and Palumbo, L.C. (2002). Readers' eye movements distinguish anomalies of form and content. *Journal of Psycholinguistic Research*, 31, 25–45.

Chomsky, N. (1957). *Syntactic structures*. The Hague: Mouton.

Clifton, C. Jr. and Staub, A. (2008). Parallelism and competition in syntactic ambiguity resolution. *Language and Linguistics Compass*, 2, 234–250.

Clifton, C. Jr, Staub, A., and Rayner, K. (2007). Eye movements in reading words and sentences. In R.V. Gompel and M. Fisher and W. Murray and R.L. Hill (eds.) *Eye movement research: Insights into mind and brain* (pp. 341–371). New York: Elsevier.

Clifton, C. Jr., Traxler, M., Mohamed, M.T., Williams, R.S., Morris, R.K., and Rayner, K. (2003). The use of thematic role information in parsing: Syntactic processing autonomy revisited. *Journal of Memory and Language*, 49, 317–334.

Cooper, R.M. (1974). The control of eye fixation by the meaning of spoken language: A new methodology for the real-time investigation of speech perception, memory, and language processing. *Cognitive Psychology*, 6, 84–107.

Daneman, M. and Carpenter, P. (1980). Individual differences in working memory and reading. *Journal of Verbal Learning and Verbal Behavior*, 19, 450–466.

Demberg, V. and Keller, F. (2009). Data from eye-tracking corpora as evidence for theories of syntactic processing complexity. *Cognition*, 109, 193–210.

Deutsch, A. and Bentin, S. (2001). Syntactic and semantic factors in processing gender agreement in Hebrew: Evidence from ERPs and eye movement. *Journal of Memory and Language*, 45, 200–224.

DeVincenzi, M. (1991). *Syntactic parsing strategies in Italian*. Dordrecht: Kluwer Academic Publishers.

Dimigen, O., Sommer, W., Dambacher, M., and Kliegl, R. (2007). Co-registration of eye movements and event-related brain potentials: A new tool to investigate eye movement control in reading. Paper presented at the 14th European Conference on Eye Movements, Potsdam, Germany.

Drieghe, D., Rayner, K., and Pollatsek, A. (2008). Mislocated fixations can account for parafoveal-on-foveal effects in eye movements in reading. *Quarterly Journal of Experimental Psychology*, 61, 1239–1249.

Duffy, S.A., Morris, R.K., and Rayner, K. (1988). Lexical ambiguity and fixation times in reading. *Journal of Memory and Language*, 27, 429–446.

Ehrlich, S.F. and Rayner, K. (1981). Contextual effects on word perception and eye movements during reading. *Journal of verbal Learning and verbal Behavior*, 20, 641–655.

Engbert, R., Nuthmann, A., Richter, E.M., and Kliegl, R. (2005). SWIFT: A dynamical model of saccade generation during reading. *Psychological Review*, 112, 777–813.

Ferreira, F. (2003). The misinterpretation of noncanonical sentences. *Cognitive Psychology*, 47, 164–203.

Ferreira, F. and Clifton, C., Jr (1986). The independence of syntactic processing. *Journal of Memory and Language*, 25(3), 348–368.

Ferreira, F. and Henderson, J. (1990). The use of verb information in syntactic parsing: Evidence from eye movements and word-by-word self-paced reading. *Journal of Experimental Psychology: Learning, Memory, and Cognition*, 16, 555–568.

Fodor, J.D. and Ferreira, F. (Eds). (1998). *Sentence reanalysis*. Dordrecht: Kluwer Academic Publishers.

Fodor, J.A., Bever, T.G., and Garrett, M.F. (1974). *The psychology of language: An introduction to psycholinguistics and generative grammar*. New York: McGraw-Hill.

Frazier, L. (1985). Syntactic complexity. In D. Dowty and L. Kartunnen and A. Zwicky (eds.) *Natural language parsing* (pp. 129–189). Cambridge: Cambridge University Press.

Frazier, L. (1978). On comprehending sentences: Syntactic parsing strategies. Unpublished doctoral dissertation, University of Connecticut.

Frazier, L. (1987). Sentence processing: A tutorial review. In M. Coltheart (ed.) *Attention and performance* (pp. 559–586). Hillsdale, NJ: Lawrence Erlbaum Associates.

Frazier, L. (1995). Constraint satisfaction as a theory of sentence processing. *Journal of Psycholinguistic Research*, 24, 437–468.

Frazier, L. and Rayner, K. (1982). Making and correcting errors during sentence comprehension: Eye movements in the analysis of structurally ambiguous sentences. *Cognitive Psychology*, 14, 178–210.

Frazier, L. and Rayner, K. (1988). Parameterizing the language processing system: Left- vs. right-branching within and across languages. In J.A. Hawkins (ed.) *Explaining Language Universals* (pp. 247–279). Oxford: Basil Blackwell.

Frazier, L., and Flores d'Arcais, G.B. (1989). Filler driven parsing: A study of gap filling in Dutch. *Journal of Memory and Language*, 28, 331–344.

Gibson, E. (2000). The dependency-locality theory: A distance-based theory of linguistic complexity. In Y. Miyashita and A.P. Marantz and W. O'Neill (eds.) *Image, Language, Brain*. Cambridge, MA: MIT Press.

Gordon, P.C., Hendrick, R., Johnson, M., and Lee, Y. (2006). Similarity-based interference during language comprehension: Evidence from eye-tracking. *Journal of Experimental Psychology: Learning, Memory and Cognition*, **32**, 1304–1321.

Hale, J. (2001). A probabilistic Earley parser as a psycholinguistic model. *Proceedings of NAACL*, **2**, 159–166.

Henderson, J.M. and Ferreira, F. (eds.) (2004). *The interface of language, vision, and action: Eye movements and the visual world*. New York: Psychology Press.

Inhoff, A.W. and Weger, U.W. (2005). Memory for word location during reading: Eye movements to previously read words are spatially selective but not precise. *Memory and Cognition*, **33**, 447–461.

Just, M.A. and Carpenter, P. (1980). A theory of reading: From eye fixations to comprehension. *Psychological Review*, **85**, 109–130.

Just, M.A. and Carpenter, P.A. (1992). A capacity theory of comprehension: Individual differences in working memory. *Psychological Review*, **99**, 122–149.

Just, M.A., Carpenter, P.A., and Woolley, J.D. (1982). Paradigms and processes in reading comprehension. *Journal of Experimental Psychology: General*, **111**, 228–238.

Kennedy, A. and Pynte, J. (2005). Parafoveal-on-foveal effects in normal reading. *Vision Research*, **45**, 153–168.

Kennison, S.M. (2001). Limitations on the use of verb information during sentence comprehension. *Psychonomic Bulletin and Review*, **8**, 132–137.

Kretzschmar, F. (2010). The electrophysiological reality of parafoveal processing: On the validity of language-related ERPs in natural reading. Unpublished Doctoral Dissertation, University of Mainz.

Kutas, M., Van Petten, C., and Kluender, R. (2006). Psycholinguistics electrified II (1994–2005). In M.A. Gernsbacher and M. Traxler (eds.) *Handbook of psycholinguistics* (2nd edn.) (pp. 655–720). New York: Elsevier.

Levy, R. (2008). Expectation-based syntactic comprehension. *Cognition*, **106**, 1126–1177.

Lewis, R.L., Vasishth, S., and Van Dyke, J.A. (2006). Computational principles of working memory in sentence comprehension. *Trends in Cognitive Sciences*, **10**, 447–454.

Martin, A. and McElree, B. (2008). A content-addressable pointer mechanism underlies comprehension of verb phrase ellipsis. *Journal of Memory and Language*, **58**, 879–906.

McElree, B., Foraker, S., and Dyer, L. (2003). Memory structures that subserve sentence comprehension. *Journal of Memory and Language*, **48**, 67–91.

MacDonald, M.D., Just, M.A., and Carpenter, P.A. (1992). Working memory constraints on the processing of syntactic ambiguity. *Cognitive Psychology*, **24**, 56–98.

MacDonald, M.C., Pearlmutter, N.J., and Seidenberg, M.S. (1994). The lexical nature of syntactic ambiguity resolution. *Psychological Review*, **101**, 676–703.

Marslen-Wilson, W.D. (1973). Linguistic structure and speech shadowing at very short latencies. *Nature*, **244**, 522–523.

McRae, K., Spivey-Knowlton, M.J., and Tanenhaus, M.K. (1998). Modeling the influence of thematic fit (and other constraints) in on-line sentence comprehension. *Journal of Memory and Language*, **38**, 283–312.

Mehler, J., Bever, T.G., and Carey, P. (1967). What we look at when we read. *Perception and Psychophysics*, **2**, 213–218.

Meseguer, E., Carreiras, M., and Clifton, C., Jr (2002). Overt reanalysis strategies and eye movements during the reading of mild garden path sentences. *Memory and Cognition*, **30**, 551–562.

Miller, G.A. (1962). Some psychological studies of grammar. *American Psychologist*, **17**, 748–762.

Mitchell, D.C. (2004). On-line methods in language processing: Introduction and historical review. In M. Carreiras and C.J. Clifton (eds.) *The on-line study of sentence comprehension: Eyetracking, ERPs, and beyond*. Brighton: Psychology Press.

Mitchell, D.C. and Shen, X. (in press). The timing and control of regressive saccades in reading. *Cognition*.

Mitchell, D.C., Shen, X., Green, M.J., and Hodgson, T.L. (2008). Accounting for regressive eye-movements in models of sentence processing: A reappraisal of the selective reanalysis hypothesis. *Journal of Memory and Language*, **59**, 266–293.

Ni, W., Fodor, J.D., Crain, S., and Shankweiler, D. (1998). Anomaly detection: Eye movement patterns. *Journal of Psycholinguistic Research*, **27**, 515–540.

Pearlmutter, N.J., Garnsey, S.M., and Bock, K. (1999). Agreement processes in sentence comprehension. *Journal of Memory and Language*, **41**, 427–456.

Pearlmutter, N.J. and MacDonald, M.C. (1995). Individual differences and probabilistic constraints in syntactic ambiguity resolution. *Journal of Memory and Language*, **34**, 521–542.

Pickering, M.J. and Traxler, M. (2001). Strategies for processing unbounded dependencies: Lexical information and verb-argument assignment. *Journal of Experimental Psychology: Learning, Memory and Cognition*, **27**, 1401–1411.

Pickering, M. and Traxler, M. (2003). Evidence against the use of subcategorisation frequency in processing unbounded dependencies. *Language and Cognitive Processes*, **18**, 469–503.

Pollatsek, A., Reichle, E., and Rayner, K. (2006). Tests of the E-Z Reader model: Exploring the interface between cognition and eye-movement control. *Cognitive Psychology*, **52**, 1–56.

Rayner, K. and Frazier, L. (1987). Parsing temporarily ambiguous complements. *Quarterly Journal of Experimental Psychology*, **39A**, 657–673.

Rayner, K. and Sereno, S.C. (1994a). Regressive eye movements and sentence parsing: On the use of regression-contingent analyses. *Memory and Cognition*, **22**, 281–285.

Rayner, K. and Sereno, S.C. (1994b). Regression-contingent analyses: A reply to Altmann. *Memory and Cognition*, 22, 291–292.

Rayner, K., Carlson, M., and Frazier, L. (1983). The interaction of syntax and semantics during sentence processing:Eye movements in the analysis of semantically biased sentences. *Journal of verbal Learning and verbal Behavior*, 22, 358–374.

Rayner, K., Warren, T., Juhasz, B.J., and Liversedge, S.P. (2004). The effect of plausibility on eye movements in reading. *Journal of Experimental Psychology: Learning, Memory and Cognition*, 30, 1290–1301.

Reichle, E., Warren, T., and McConnell, K. (2009). Using E-Z Reader to model the effects of higer-level language processing on eye movements during reading. *Psychonomic Bulletin and Review*, 16, 1–21.

Reichle, E.D., Pollatsek, A., Fisher, D.F., and Rayner, K. (1998). Toward a model of eye movement control in reading. *Psychological Review*, 105(1), 125–156.

Rayner, K., and Well, A.D. (1996). Effects of contextual constraint on eye movements in reading: A further examination. *Psychonomic Bulletin and Review*, 3, 504–509.

Rayner, K., Ashby, J., Pollatsek, A, and Reichle, E.D. (2004). The effects of frequency and predictability on eye fixations in reading: Implications for the E-Z Reader model. *Journal of Experimental Psychology: Human Perception and Performance*, 30, 720–732.

Sanford, A. and Sturt, P. (2002). Depth of processing in language comprehension: Not noticing the evidence. *Trends in Cognitive Sciences*, 6, 382–386.

Sereno, S. and Rayner, K. (2003). Measuring word recognition in reading: Eye movements and event-related potentials. *Trends in Cognitive Sciences*, 7, 489–493.

Staub, A. (2007). The parser doesn't ignore intransitivity, after all. *Journal of Experimental Psychology: Learning, Memory and Cognition*, 33, 550–569.

Staub, A. (2010). Eye movements and processing difficulty in object relative clauses. *Cognition*, 116, 71–86.

Staub, A. (2011). The lexical predictability effect: Distributional analysis of fixation durations. *Psychonomic Bulletin & Review*, 18, 371–376.

Staub, A. and Clifton, C. Jr (2006). Syntactic prediction in language comprehension: Evidence from either . . . or. *Journal of Experimental Psychology: Learning, Memory and Cognition*, 32, 425–436.

Staub, A. and Rayner, K. (2007). Eye movements and on-line comprehension processes. In G. Gaskell (ed.) *Oxford Handbook of Psycholinguistics* (pp. 327–342). Oxford: Oxford University Press.

Staub, A., Clifton, C., Jr, and Frazier, L. (2006). Heavy NP shift is the parser's last resort: Evidence from eye movements. *Journal of Memory and Language*, 54, 389–406.

Staub, A., White, S.J., Drieghe, D., Hollway, E.C., and Rayner, K. (2010). Distributional effects of word frequency on eye fixation durations. *Journal of Experimental Psychology: Human Perception and Performance*, 36, 1280–1293.

Stowe, L. (1986). Parsing wh-constructions: Evidence for on-line gap location. *Language and Cognitive Processes*, 1, 227–246.

Tabor, W. and Hutchins, S. (2004). Evidence for self-organized sentence processing: Digging-in effects. *Journal of Experimental Psychology: Learning, Memory and Cognition*, 30, 431–450.

Tanenhaus, M.K., Spivey-Knowlton, M.J., Eberhard, K.M., and Sedivy, J.C. (1995). Integration of visual and linguistic information in spoken language comprehension. *Science*, 268, 1632–1634.

Tanenhaus, M. (2007). Eye movements and spoken language processing. In R.P.G. v. Gompel and M.H. Fischer and W.S. Murray and R.L.Hill (eds.) *Eye movements: A window on mind and brain* (pp. 444–469). Oxford: Elsevier.

Traxler, M.J. and Pickering, M.J. (1996). Plausibility and the processing of unbounded dependencies: An eye-tracking study. *Journal of Memory and Language*, 35, 454–475.

Traxler, M., Pickering, M., and Clifton, C., Jr (1998). Adjunct attachment is not a form of lexical ambiguity resolution. *Journal of Memory and Language*, 39, 558–592.

Trueswell, J.C., Tanenhaus, M.K., and Kello, C. (1993). Verb-specific constraints in sentence processing: Separating effects of lexical preference from garden-paths. *Journal of Experimental Psychology: Learning, Memory, and Cognition*, 19, 528–553.

Trueswell, J.C., Tanenhaus, M.K., and Garnsey, S.M. (1994). Semantic influences on parsing: Use of thematic role information in syntactic disambiguation. *Journal of Memory and Language*, 33, 285–318.

Van Gompel, R.P.G., Pickering, M., Pearson, J., and Liversedge, S.P. (2005). Evidence against competition during syntactic ambiguity resolution. *Journal of Memory and Language*, 52, 284–307.

Vasishth, S., Bruessow, S., Lewis, R.L., and Drenhaus, H. (2008). Processing polarity: How the ungrammatical intrudes on the grammatical. *Cognitive Science*, 32, 685–712.

Warren, T. and Gibson, E. (2002). The influence of referential processing on sentence complexity. *Cognition*, 85, 79–112.

Waters, G.S. and Caplan, D. (1996). The capacity theory of sentence comprehension: Critique of Just and Carpenter. *Psychological Review*, 103, 761–772.

CHAPTER 50

The influence of implausibility and anomaly on eye movements during reading

Tessa Warren

Abstract

This chapter reviews findings investigating the ways the following factors influence eye movements when readers encounter an anomaly or implausibility: 1) the kind of information cueing the anomaly, 2) the severity of the anomaly, 3) the semantic and syntactic context in which the anomaly occurs, and 4) text-external factors like reader-specific characteristics or the orthography of the language being read. The relation of these results to theories of language comprehension is then discussed. The chapter concludes with some ideas about how a new version of the E-Z Reader model of eye movement control during reading (Reichle et al., 2009) might help us understand eye movement reactions to semantic anomalies and how studying those eye movement reactions might help improve the model.

Readers sometimes encounter information that violates their knowledge or expectations. This can happen as a result of a reader's misunderstanding or a writer's mistake, but sometimes a writer intends to communicate something anomalous or implausible. Understanding what readers do in these situations is important for any complete theory of reading and language processing, given that one of language's most important characteristics is its utility for communicating unexpected information. For example, it might be possible to understand the sentence 'dog bites man' simply by activating the concepts dog, man, and bites, and relating them via expectations based on world knowledge. But it would be impossible to understand the sentence 'man bites dog' without language (Pinker, 1994). Additionally, experiments manipulating anomaly and implausibility have been instrumental in advancing our understanding of eye movement control during reading, the architecture of the language comprehension system, and the time course over which readers bring different kinds of knowledge to bear during reading comprehension.

The current chapter will focus on a relatively new body of work using eye tracking to investigate the processing of semantic violations in unambiguous sentences. However, the question of how the language comprehension system responds to anomalies has been an important one in psycholinguistics for some time now (for some early work, see Forster and Olbrei, 1974; Forster and Ryder, 1971).

Hundreds of studies using the event related potential (ERP) methodology, in which changes in the brain's electrical activity are measured on the scalp, have used responses to anomalies as benchmark data (for recent reviews see Kuperberg, 2007; Kutas et al., 2006). The fact that syntactic and semantic anomalies are usually associated with different ERPs has had a strong influence on psycholinguists' conceptualizations of the language processing system (Kuperberg, 2007). Within the eye tracking literature, there are a few lines of work investigating anomalies. Researchers are just beginning to investigate how semantic implausibility affects comprehenders' eye movements across displays of images (e.g. Boland, 2005). But there has been considerable work relying on readers' detection of anomalies to shed light on how they process ambiguous sentences (e.g. Rayner et al., 1983; Ferreira and Clifton, 1986; Trueswell et al., 1994; Pickering and Traxler, 1998). In these experiments, a reader's perception of a syntactic anomaly indicates that he or she has chosen the wrong interpretation for the sentence. Some of these studies also manipulate the presence of semantic anomalies to investigate how semantic factors influence syntactic processing. These bodies of work, using ERPs and eye movements, have significantly advanced our understanding of both anomaly processing and language processing more generally. However, the current chapter will focus on a recent body of work that uses eye movements to investigate the processing of semantic or pragmatic implausibility and anomaly in unambiguous sentences and texts. Surprisingly, there was little work in this area as of 15 years ago. But a recent flurry of activity has created a rapidly growing and promising literature.

The aim of this chapter is to provide an overview of recent work investigating how readers' eye movements are affected by semantic violations in unambiguous sentences, and to describe the unique contributions that this research makes to our understanding of language processing and eye movement control in reading. It will begin by reviewing basic findings related to the influence of the following factors on eye movements associated with anomaly and implausibility: 1) the kind of information cueing the anomaly, 2) the severity of the anomaly, 3) the semantic and syntactic context in which the anomaly occurs, and 4) text-external factors like reader-specific characteristics or the orthography of the language being read. This general overview will conclude with some generalizations about what the eye movement data indicate about the process of language comprehension and how these conclusions fit with current language processing theories. After this, the chapter will turn to questions and issues that eye movement responses to semantic anomalies are uniquely useful for answering; for example, whether readers routinely detect upcoming semantic anomalies prior to looking at the word at which the anomaly occurs (Drieghe, Chapter 46 and Hyönä, Chapter 45, this volume). This question is part of a larger debate about the way that lexical processing and attention are allocated during reading (Reichle, Chapter 42, and Engbert and Kliegl, Chapter 43, this volume). The chapter will conclude with some ideas about how a new model of eye movement control during reading (Reichle et al., 2009), which includes a stage for post-lexical processing, might help us understand the patterns of eye movement reactions to semantic anomalies and how studying eye movement reactions to semantic anomalies might help us improve the model.

In order to understand the results of the experiments described in this chapter, it will be important to be familiar with the most frequently used eye movement measures and how they are calculated. The *first-fixation* measure indexes the duration of the initial fixation (in milliseconds) on a word during first-pass reading, and is usually considered an indicator of very early processing. *Gaze duration* or *first-pass time* is the sum of all fixations on a word or region from when the eyes first land on it during first-pass reading until they first leave it. *First-pass regressions out* is the percentage of trials on which the reader leaves a region during first-pass reading with a regressive eye movement. *Go-past* time or *regression-path duration* is the duration of all fixations from entering a word or region during first-pass reading until progressing past that region. It is therefore equal to gaze duration in regions that were not regressed from during first-pass reading. However, if there was a first-pass regression from a region, go-past will include gaze duration, all fixations across previously processed material, and any subsequent refixations on the region before it is exited to the right (in English). All of these measures are generally considered to index first-pass processing; some researchers in fact report go-past times instead of gaze duration/first-pass times (e.g. Murray, 2006). The reason for this is that there is evidence that fixations preceding regressive saccades are shorter than fixations preceding progressive saccades (Altmann et al., 1992; Mitchell et al., 2008; but cf. Rayner et al., 2003a). If this is true, then difficulty could be evidenced as longer gaze durations in trials in which a region was exited with a progressive saccade, but as shorter gaze durations in trials in which it was exited with a regressive saccade. Go-past avoids this potential issue, but is influenced by re-reading. *Second-pass time* is the sum of all fixations on a region subsequent to first-pass reading. It generally is assumed to reflect relatively late processing. *Total time* is the sum of all fixations on a region and reflects the total amount of processing a word receives.

Perhaps the most important basic issue with respect to eye movements and anomaly is when, or how early, anomalies affect eye movements. This question is important for multiple reasons; it has potential ramifications for debates over issues ranging from the architecture of the language comprehension system (Fodor et al., 1996), to the way attention is allocated during reading (Murray and Rowan, 1998; Rayner et al., 2004), to the impetus behind eye movements in models of eye movement control in reading (Reichle et al., 2003). However, the answer to this question varies greatly across studies. Some report very early effects that occur even before the anomalous or implausible word is read (Kennedy et al., 2004; Murray, 2006; Murray and Rowan, 1998). Other studies find effects on the target word itself (Cook and Myers, 2004; Rayner et al., 2004; Staub et al., 2007; Wang et al., 2008; Warren and McConnell, 2007; Warren et al., 2008), while yet others report effects only after the target word (Boland and Blodgett, 2001; Filik, 2008; Garrod and Terras, 2000; Traxler et al., 1998). The wide variation among these results suggests that many factors likely influence when anomalies are reflected in the eye movement record.

Syntactic versus semantic knowledge

One factor that might be expected to influence an anomaly's effect on the eye movement record is the kind of knowledge that cues it. Some theories of sentence comprehension assume that syntactic information is processed prior to world knowledge, leading to the prediction that syntactic anomalies will be detected before world-knowledge based anomalies (Fodor et al., 1996). Ni et al. (1996) tested this prediction by comparing eye movements to sentences with a syntactic violation (1a), a world knowledge violation (1b), or no violation (1c).

(**1a**) It seems that the cats won't usually <u>eating</u> the food we put on the porch. (Syntax)

(**1b**) It seems that the cats won't usually <u>bake</u> the food we put on the porch. (Knowledge)

(**1c**) It seems that the cats won't usually <u>eat</u> the food we put on the porch. (Baseline)

They found no reliable differences in first-pass reading times on the critical region, made up of the main verb (e.g. *eating*, *bake*, or *eat*) plus the following word. (Region reading times were statistically corrected for length differences between the conditions.) Examination of subsequent regions indicated that there was a tendency for world-knowledge violations to inspire longer first-pass times as compared to baseline, but no such tendency was evident in the syntactic violation conditions as compared to baseline. In contrast to the pattern in the reading time measures, the likelihood of making a regression during first-pass reading was relatively quickly affected by anomaly. Readers were more likely to regress from the critical region in the anomalous conditions, with an initial tendency for more regressions in the syntactic anomaly condition than in the world-knowledge anomaly condition. However, by the final region there were more regressions in the world-knowledge anomaly condition. These results suggest that anomalies arising from syntactic violations and world-knowledge violations are associated with different eye movement profiles, but there is no evidence that one kind of violation is detected earlier than another. Braze et al. (2002) found similar results in a study with the same manipulation but longer post-target regions and closer investigation of regressive eye movement patterns. Similar to Ni et al.'s findings, syntactic violations led to an immediate increase in regressive eye movements. In this experiment, world-knowledge violations led to an immediate increase in fixation times, rather than a slightly delayed one. Interestingly, regressions inspired by world-knowledge violations were likely to land closer to the beginning of the sentence, whereas regressions inspired by syntactic violations were likely to land more locally, suggesting that these regressions reflected different strategies for attempting to resolve the anomaly.

Severity

The severity of an anomaly or plausibility violation might also be expected to influence how quickly it is detected and what patterns of eye movements it induces. Rayner et al. (2004) manipulated plausibility violation severity, testing readers' eye movements across plausible sentences, moderately implausible sentences, and anomalous sentences. One of their experimental items is given below:

(**2a**) John used a knife to chop the large carrots for dinner. (Baseline)

(**2b**) John used an axe to chop the large carrots for dinner. (Implausible)

(**2c**) John used a pump to inflate the large carrots for dinner. (Anomalous)

Rayner et al. found that readers showed earlier and longer-lasting eye movement disruption to the target word *carrots* in the anomalous condition than in the other two conditions. Gaze duration on this target word was longer for the anomalous condition, but did not differ between the baseline and implausible conditions. However, all three conditions differed in the go-past measure, with longest go-past times for the anomalous condition, shorter go-past times for the implausible condition, and shortest go-past times for the baseline condition. In the post-target region, *for dinner* above, the anomalous condition showed more disruption than the other two conditions in every measure.

These results indicate that a plausibility violation's severity influences when disruption becomes apparent in the eye movement record. Whereas strong violations were evident in measures like first-pass reading, more moderate violations appeared only in measures including regressions, like go-past. Severity also influences the duration of disruption. A follow up to the Rayner et al. (2004) study by Warren and McConnell (2007) confirmed these findings. Warren and McConnell delved deeper into the relation between plausibility violation severity and eye movement disruption. Their experiment compared sentences describing events that had been rated as similarly unlikely, but which were possible in one condition and impossible in another condition. If disruption were related to event unlikelihood, then disruption should have been similar across both of these conditions as compared to a baseline condition. However, this was not the case. Warren and McConnell found effects of impossibility as early as the duration of the first fixation on the target word creating the anomaly, but effects of extreme implausibility only in measures indexing regressions, like the proportion of first-pass regressions out of the target word and go-past time on the target word. Disruption to impossibility also lasted longer than disruption to extreme implausibility.

Context

The previously described experiments tested eye movements to anomaly or implausibility in single sentences in a null context. But context can have a strong influence on whether a described event or state is implausible or anomalous. For example, an anvil falling out of the sky and smashing a coyote is a highly implausible event in the real world, but is quite plausible in the context of a Roadrunner cartoon. A few recent eye movement studies have addressed the question of how quickly contextual support can moderate the processing disruption associated with an event that would have been implausible or anomalous without that support. These studies differ in when they show contextual effects, suggesting that context's effects may be mediated by other factors.

Filik (2008) found contextual effects in a 2×2 experiment manipulating context (fictional or non-fictional) and event type (anomalous in the real world or non-anomalous in the real world). Eye movements were recorded over sentences like *He glared at/picked up the lorry and carried on down the road* in contexts where *he* either referred to the Incredible Hulk or to a man named Terry. Filik found no eye movement effects at the critical word (*lorry* in this example), but on the following region (*and carried*), first-fixation duration and first-pass reading showed an interaction such that fixations were longer in the condition in which Terry picked up a lorry than any other condition. The fact that there was no evidence of disruption in the condition in which the Hulk picked up a lorry as compared to the conditions in which either individual glared at a lorry suggests that readers took context into account at the initial stages of processing the anomaly.

Warren et al. (2008) reported a similar experiment with the same design but a different result. In their experiment, readers read sentences describing events like slicing bread or teaching bread in either real world or fantasy contexts. First-pass reading times showed a main effect of event type: reading times were longer on the target word *bread* in sentences describing teaching bread rather than slicing bread, even in a fantasy context in which the event of teaching bread had been judged similarly plausible as the event of slicing bread in a real world context. However, this difficulty associated with the anomalous event in the fantasy context was not apparent in go-past times or any later measures on the target word. This pattern of data suggests that there may be an early stage of processing during which context is not taken into account, but that after this initial stage contextual information quickly modulates both processing difficulty and the eye movements associated with it. Although this finding seems incompatible with Filik (2008), the difference in results could be related to the severity of the violations used in the two experiments. The anomalies in Filik's experiment were generally less severe than those in Warren et al.'s. If less severe anomalies are detected more slowly (Rayner et al., 2004; Warren and McConnell, 2007), then context may have more time to come into play and moderate responses to anomalies. This explanation is consistent with results from Kreiner et al. (2008), who found that context could eliminate eye movement disruption associated with gender mismatches on the initial encounter with nouns whose gender was assigned by world knowledge (e.g. *plumber*, a female plumber being unexpected; see also Duffy and Keir, 2004), but not on the initial encounter with nouns whose gender was part of their lexical representation (e.g. *king*, a female king being impossible).

Although the studies just described have demonstrated that a supportive context can either immediately or relatively quickly eliminate disruption to what would otherwise be a plausibility violation, there are also cases in which context eliminates disruption at initial processing stages, but not at later stages. Cook and Myers (2004) compared short texts in which a character played an unexpected or expected role (e.g. a busboy took an order/cleared the dishes) in a text that did or did not provide a justification for the unexpected role (e.g. the restaurant was very short-staffed). They found that first-pass reading times on the critical character description (e.g. *busboy*) in the justified unexpected role condition were similar to both expected role conditions. Disruption only appeared in the unjustified unexpected role condition. However, in later measures and on following words, eye movement disruption appeared for both unexpected role conditions, regardless of justification. This finding, along with results from Garrod and Terras (2000), Stewart et al. (2004), and many of the studies previously discussed, is consistent with theories from the text processing literature (e.g. Myers and O'Brien, 1998; Sanford and Garrod, 2005) that assert that semantic processing develops over time, with initial processing being most sensitive to relatively coarse-grained, focused, or central aspects of lexical meaning that are quickly activated by low-level automatic retrieval processes, but later processing also being affected by more peripheral aspects of meaning and more complex contextual relations. Given evidence that comprehenders are always predicting upcoming words (e.g. Federmeier, 2007), another potential way to think about this kind of unfolding semantic interpretation process is that the most highly activated semantic features initially might be those that are shared between a predicted word and an encountered word, and only later might shift to be more strongly determined by the encountered word, and potentially even later by slow reasoning processes. Under these kinds of accounts, processing disruption occurs when newly activated semantic features are in conflict with the current semantic context. Therefore, an implausible or anomalous word that shares at least some features with an expected word might be expected to generate later-developing disruption, whereas an implausible or anomalous word that shares no features with an expected word would generate immediate disruption.

Structural factors

The local structural context is one of the few factors that does not seem to affect the latency of eye movement disruption to semantic anomalies. Speer and Clifton (1998) showed that readers reacted similarly to semantic violations in argument and adjunct positions. Patson and Warren (2010) investigated whether the distance and the presence of a theta-assigning relation between the words cueing a violation affect eye movements, using sentences like those in (3) below.

(**3a**) Bryan used a bottle to feed the hungry infant yesterday morning.

(**3b**) Bryan used a bottle to <u>fight off</u> the hungry <u>infant</u> yesterday morning.

(**3c**) Bryan used a <u>trough</u> to feed the hungry <u>infant</u> yesterday morning.

If readers are quicker to detect conflicts between words that are closer together or that share a theta-relation (like verbs and their objects do), then violations resulting from a conflict between a verb and its patient (*fight off* and *infant* in 3b) should be detected more quickly than violations resulting from a conflict between an instrument and a patient (*trough* and *infant* in 3c). However, Patson and Warren found that these manipulations did not affect the latency of eye movement reactions to semantic violations. There was evidence of increased later difficulty in conditions in which the violation occurred between a verb and its object rather than between an instrument and object of the same verb. Patson and Warren hypothesized that this was because it might be easier to imagine a justification and create a consistent discourse model for the use of an unusual instrument in an event (e.g. using a trough to feed a baby) than for an unusual event (e.g. fighting off a baby).

Text-external factors

One important question that has received relatively little investigation is how text-external factors like individual differences among readers, stimulus list characteristics, and the reading task affect eye movements to semantic anomalies. Most eye movement experiments testing anomaly have required readers to read sentences or short passages and answer questions about some proportion of them. Within these experiments, readers necessarily have multiple encounters with anomalies or implausibilities. It is an open question how the proportion of anomalies encountered or the need to answer questions about anomalous sentences affects eye movement reactions to anomalies. There is a concern among some researchers that requiring participants to carefully read many sentences with plausibility violations could make them more likely to use unusual strategies to remember who was doing what to whom in any given sentence, in which case the results of such experiments would not reflect natural reading.[1] For these reasons, some researchers limit anomalies to a relatively small proportion of the encountered sentences and do not ask comprehension questions about anomalous or implausible sentences (e.g. Rayner et al, 2004; Warren and McConnell, 2007). Other researchers attempt to avoid concerns about strategies by changing the task. For example, instead of requiring participants to read for comprehension, Murray and Rowan (1998) had them engage in a sentence-matching task in which they had to judge whether two sentences were identical. Eye movement measures were gathered over participants' encoding of the first sentence. Although this task can be performed at a purely perceptual level, experiments show that readers' eye movements are sensitive to semantic anomalies in the sentences (Kennedy et al., 2004; Murray, 2006; Murray and Rowan, 1998). Murray and colleagues argue that this task reduces the likelihood that readers will strategically

---

[1] This is not to say that the implementation of strategies and the eye movements associated with them are not interesting, or that strategy-free reading exists. However, models of eye movement control in reading have been designed to capture the situation in which reading proceeds automatically so researchers looking to use reactions to anomalies to inform models of eye movement control have a vested interest in minimizing non-automatic strategizing.

engage more deeply than usual in a text, but it is also possible that it might allow readers to strategically engage less deeply than usual.

Related to this debate, there is evidence suggesting that the early eye movement disruption sometimes observed to anomalies is not driven by a strategy related to reading multiple nonsensical sentences. Immediate eye movement disruption to anomalies can be found in the absence of any globally anomalous sentences. Staub et al. (2007) had participants read sentences containing noun-noun compounds, in which the first noun was either plausible or implausible given the previous context, but in which the full compound was always plausible. Staub et al. found that the duration of readers' first fixations on the first noun of the compound were inflated when that noun created a local anomaly, even though the following word always resolved the anomaly.

Staub et al.'s (2007) results suggest that in English, semantic interpretation is highly incremental and takes place word by word. However, researchers have hypothesized this may not be the case for all languages. For example, some have argued that in languages like Chinese in which the orthography is character-based and word boundaries are not marked, it would be a better strategy for comprehension to progress at a delay, so that local ambiguities about word boundaries and character meanings can be resolved (Aaronson and Ferres, 1986). Wang et al. (2008) tested this hypothesis in an eye tracking study investigating semantic anomalies in Chinese. They found that readers fixated a target character longer during first-pass reading when it introduced an anomaly than when it didn't. This finding indicates that readers of Chinese build incremental semantic interpretations character by character, and is consistent with the possibility that immediate incremental semantic interpretation can occur in any language, with any orthography. However, given how few experiments there are investigating semantic anomaly detection in non-alphabetic non-European languages, this is a very tentative claim.

Although this review has focused on eye movements when readers detect anomalies, it is well documented that readers sometimes fail to notice anomalies (see Sanford, 2002 for a review). Rayner et al. (2006) found that readers were less likely to detect an anomaly between an anaphor and antecedent (e.g. referring to carrots as celery later in a paragraph) when there were more sentences between the anaphor and antecedent. Their evidence of lower detection rates was a decrease in the proportion of regressive eye movements at the point of the anomaly. Two experiments have investigated whether readers who fail to report the presence of an anomaly in a passage, or who fail to take an anomaly into account when answering a comprehension question related to the anomaly, show any eye movement disruption to that anomaly. Daneman et al. (2007) and Bohan and Sanford (2008) both found no evidence of eye movement disruption to undetected anomalies, suggesting that participants' eye movement systems do not register these anomalies at a subconscious level. Interestingly, Daneman et al. included a manipulation of reading skill (as measured by performance on the Nelson-Denny reading comprehension test) in their experiment. They found that less-skilled readers were less likely to detect anomalies than more-skilled readers, particularly when the anomaly was local (internal to a noun phrase; e.g. *tranquilizing stimulants*) rather than caused by a mismatch between events earlier in the text and a subsequent noun phrase (e.g. in a paragraph about a plane crash, asking participants to figure out where to bury the surviving injured). However, they found no effects of reading skill on eye movement disruption to detected anomalies.

One final investigation of the effect of reader characteristics on the detection of anomalies was carried out by Joseph et al. (2008), who tested children on the items from Rayner et al.'s (2004) study with the aim of determining whether child readers process implausibility and anomaly in the same way as adult readers. Joseph et al.'s results with adult readers replicated Rayner et al.'s findings, but with child readers they found a slightly different pattern. Although children showed immediate effects of anomaly like adults, their implausibility effects were delayed relative to those of the adults. This suggests that children may take longer to distinguish smaller variations in the likelihood of events than adults.

The body of work reviewed thus far establishes that in unambiguous sentences, if a reader detects a semantic anomaly or implausibility, his or her fixations will lengthen and probability of regressing to prior regions of the sentence and re-reading will increase. This holds for adults and children, more-skilled and less-skilled readers, languages as diverse as English and Chinese, and experiments with many or no global anomalies. The latency of these eye movement effects varies between experiments, but in general, stronger semantic violations tend to have effects that are evident earlier and longer lasting in the eye movement record (Kreiner et al., 2008; Rayner et al., 2004; Warren and McConnell, 2007). A violation's relation to context also affects eye movements to it. Placing what would normally be a semantic violation into a fully supportive context can entirely (Filik, 2008) or partially (Ferguson and Sanford, 2008; Warren et al., 2008) eliminate disruption to it. On the other hand, providing mild contextual support to a word causing a violation or allowing the word to share semantic features with an appropriate word can delay disruption to it (Cook and Myers, 2004; Stewart et al., 2004). These findings are consistent with an account of language processing in which early automatic or associative processes determine initial semantic fits, continued processing refines those fits [sometimes finding that they are better than they initially seemed (Warren et al., 2008) and sometimes finding that they are worse (Cook and Myers, 2004)], and late processing attempts to reconcile or repair poor fits. This general framework is consistent with a number of proposals, some of which are based on findings from other methodologies like self-paced reading and ERPs (e.g. Garrod and Sanford, 2005; Kuperberg, 2007; Myers and O'Brien, 1998).

Eye movements are just one of a number of sources of evidence that can shed light on how language comprehension works. They have some advantages over other sources of evidence, but in general, eye movement studies of semantic anomaly have complemented the more extensive work on anomalies in the self-paced reading and ERP literatures. However, there are some important questions related to the process of reading for which eye movement studies of semantic violations have provided crucial evidence. The remainder of this chapter will focus on two such areas. It will first address the way eye movement studies of semantic violations have informed a debate about how readers allocate their attention across words as they read. Then it will conclude with a discussion of a new version of the E-Z Reader model of eye movement control in reading (Reichle et al., 2009) that hypothesizes a framework for how lexical and post-lexical processing jointly affect eye movements in reading. Because this model includes a role for post-lexical processing, it can simulate effects of semantic anomalies on eye movements in reading. This makes the model a potentially valuable tool for improving our understanding of such effects and makes simulating experiments with semantic anomalies an important means for testing and furthering the model.

The debate about parafoveal anomaly processing

Models of eye movement control in reading can be categorized into two kinds: those that assume that attention is allocated serially, to only one word at a time (Reichle et al., 2003; Reichle, Chapter 42, this volume), and those that assume attention is allocated as a gradient, to multiple words at a time (Engbert et al., 2005; Engbert and Kliegl, Chapter 43, this volume). These assumptions about attention allocation lead to differing predictions about the time course of lexical processing during reading. According to attention gradient models, readers attend to and process multiple words at a time. If this is the case, then the processing of upcoming words that have been attended but not yet fixated should be able to influence processing on the currently fixated word. This would be referred to as a parafoveal-on-foveal effect, because information being processed in the parafovea (the area surrounding the two degrees of central vision) is affecting the processing of information in the fovea (the two degrees of central vision) (Drieghe, Chapter 46, and Hyönä, Chapter 45, this volume). According to serial attention models, words are attended only one at a time. Because under this view, lexical processing on one word must finish before processing on the next word begins, there is no way that lexical processing of an upcoming word can affect lexical processing on the currently fixated word. Serial models thus predict that parafoveal-on-foveal effects should never be observed.

There is some debate over whether parafoveal-on-foveal effects have been found in experiments testing plausibility violations. Murray and colleagues have reported what they argue to be parafoveal-on-foveal effects of semantic implausibility (Kennedy et al, 2004; Murray 2006; Murray and Rowan, 1998), but others have questioned this evidence and suggested that the observed effects might have alternative explanations (Rayner et al., 2003b, 2004). Most experiments reporting purported parafoveal-on-foveal effects of plausibility have taken the following form. The methodology is delayed sentence matching, meaning that participants read a sentence and then push a button to make a second sentence appear immediately under the first. Participants then must judge whether the two sentences are identical or not. Eye movement measures are analysed across the reading of only the initial sentence. The stimuli cross plausibility (plausible versus moderately implausible) with syntactic relation (subject-verb or verb-object), as in this example from Murray and Rowan (1998):

1) The savages smacked the child. (Plausible/Plausible)

2) The savages smacked the money. (Plausible/Implausible)

3) The uranium smacked the child. (Implausible/Plausible)

4) The uranium smacked the money. (Implausible/Implausible)

Although experiment-specific differences exist, with some experiments showing no early effects (e.g. Murray, 2006 experiment 1), for the most part these experiments find longer go-past times on the initial noun when it serves as an implausible agent of the following verb than when it serves as a plausible agent of the following verb. In Murray and Rowan (1998) this effect was driven by inflated fixations at the end of the noun, right before the verb. In Experiment 2 of Murray (2006), the effect appeared on a prepositional phrase intervening between the initial noun and verb, and was driven by an increased likelihood of regressing to the initial noun.

There is debate about whether this evidence truly reflects parafoveal-on-foveal effects of plausibility. First, there is some concern about the sentences used in these experiments. Rayner et al. (2004) questioned the success of the plausibility manipulations in Murray and Rowan (1998)'s sentences, based on the outcome of a new plausibility questionnaire on their items, and Murray's (2006) Experiment 2 had a plausibility confound at the point at which early effects were detected, although a statistical analysis suggested the confound was not likely to be responsible for the effect. More importantly, not every early effect is a parafoveal-on-foveal effect. There are alternative ways that early effects can arise. Rayner et al. (2004) found an early implausibility effect, namely inflated fixation times on the last three characters of the word preceding the target word in their anomalous condition, but argued that this finding, and others like it, likely reflected mislocated fixations rather than a parafoveal-on-foveal effect. According to this account, readers targeted a saccade to the target word, but on some proportion of trials the saccade was too short, either because of random motor error or a systematic tendency towards undershooting (McConkie et al., 1988, 1991; Rayner et al., 1996). This would result in a situation with the eyes fixated on the end of the pre-target word but attention focused on the target word. If lexical processing and attention are coupled, as all models of eye movement control in reading assume (Reichle et al., 2003), then lexical processing on the target word could have occurred while the eyes were fixated on the pre-target word. This account can therefore explain any early effects of implausibility localized to fixations occurring just before the target word.

This debate about the existence of parafoveal-on-foveal effects of plausibility remains unresolved. The fact that some experiments show parafoveal effects of plausibility (e.g. Murray and Rowan, 1998; Rayner et al., 2004; Experiment 2 of Murray, 2006), but other very similar experiments don't (e.g. Rayner et al., 2003; Warren and McConnell, 2007; Experiment 1 of Murray, 2006), could be taken to favor the possibility that these effects result from mislocated fixations rather than the hypothesis that they are a consequence of concurrent lexical processing. This is because mislocated fixations tend to be observed only in infrequent circumstances occurring as the result of stochastic processes (Drieghe et al., 2008). Thus experiments might be expected to vary in whether enough mislocated fixations occur to cause a reliable effect. If readers almost always attended to and processed multiple words at a time (Engbert et al., 2005), one would expect these kinds of early effects to appear much more consistently. Regardless of which account of early anomaly effects is correct, and which kind of eye movement model finds more support in these data, the bringing together of models of eye movement control in reading with eye movement data from semantic anomalies has the potential to significantly advance both fields.

Modeling eye movements to semantic violations

Recently, evidence about eye movement reactions to implausibility and anomaly has begun to impact the field of eye movement control in reading in a new way. Although almost all models of eye movement control in reading account for effects of lexical processing on eye movements, until very recently almost none have addressed effects of higher-level language processing on eye movements (cf. Just and Carpenter, 1980). Given that words (or more correctly their referents) are only implausible or anomalous with respect to a given context, effects of implausibility or anomaly must come about during the integration of a word into context. This means that most models of eye movement control do not account for effects of anomalies on eye movements.

The most recent version of the E-Z Reader model of eye movement control in reading (E-Z Reader 10: Reichle et al., 2009; Reichle, Chapter 42, this volume), redresses this limitation and provides a hypothesis about the way that post-lexical interpretation, lexical processing, attention, and the oculomotor system interact to generate the patterns of eye movements observed during reading. E-Z Reader 10 proposes two mechanisms by which difficulty integrating a word into context can affect eye movements (see Reichle, Chapter 42, this volume, for a more detailed description of these mechanisms and the model). The first mechanism comes into play when the fit between a word and context is so poor that a violation is detected and integration fails before lexical processing on the following word is completed. Any saccades in the labile stage when this failure occurs are cancelled, and a regression is programmed instead. This cancellation and restarting of saccadic programming causes the initial fixation on the problematic word to be longer than it otherwise would have been, allowing the model to capture post-lexical effects on first fixation durations. The second mechanism accounts for cases in which integration may not fail, but is difficult and therefore slow. If word n is not satisfactorily integrated into context by the time lexical processing on word $n+1$ completes, then lexical processing halts, attention shifts back to the locus of processing difficulty, and a regression is programmed. With these two mechanisms, E-Z Reader 10 can account for longer fixations on and more regressions from words that are difficult to integrate into a higher-level representation for a sentence or text. However, E-Z Reader 10 was not designed to include a full account of re-reading. In the model, regressions move the eyes back only one or two words, and re-reading involves re-doing lexical access on the word where difficulty was encountered. To avoid infinite loops, lexical and post-lexical processing are assumed to always succeed on this second pass.

E-Z Reader 10 assumes that when post-lexical processing is proceeding normally, it has little effect on eye movements. However, when post-lexical processing becomes difficult, it can stop the forward progression of the eyes and cause regressions. Therefore, E-Z Reader 10 provides a useful framework for explaining eye movement reactions to the post-lexical processing difficulty associated with semantic anomaly and implausibility. Effects of violation severity would seem to map straightforwardly onto E-Z Reader 10's two mechanisms, with stronger violations causing earlier integration failure and less strong violations causing slowed integration. In fact, Reichle et al. (2009) successfully used E-Z Reader 10 to simulate the results of Warren and McConnell's (2007) experiment comparing eye movements to anomalies versus severe implausibilities in exactly this way. Other findings could likely be simulated in similar ways. For example, Cook and Myers (2004)'s finding of inflated first-pass reading times on the target word in a condition in which the target word referred to an implausible actor participating in an event without justification could be simulated by increasing the duration of post-lexical processing on the target word in this condition. Their findings of inflated first-pass reading times on the post-target region and more re-reading in the target region whenever the target was an implausible actor, regardless of justification, could likely be simulated by assuming that post-lexical processing was slowed on the post-target word in both of these contexts.

However, E-Z Reader 10 has clear limitations; it is only a first attempt at describing the interaction between post-lexical processing difficulty and other factors influencing eye movement control in reading. Its account of the events following a regression seems plausible as an explanation for what might happen if a reader misperceives or initially accesses the wrong meaning for a word but then reprocesses it and quickly resolves any difficulty. But E-Z Reader 10 was not developed to account for extended re-reading or continued processing difficulty on a re-read word. This means its predictions for go-past times are generally poor. Further experimental investigation of eye movements to semantic violations, specifically focusing on elucidating factors influencing the length and targets of regressions and the patterns of re-reading, would be very useful in providing data to drive further development of the model.

E-Z Reader 10 simulations of eye movement patterns associated with semantic violations have the potential to advance our understanding of the variability associated with eye movements to violations. One of the most striking characteristics of eye movement reactions to semantic violations is their variability across experiments. This variability is evident in the latency of the onset of eye movement disruption across experiments, as well as in the overall amount of disruption. Simulations with E-Z Reader 10 provide a hint as to why disruption might be so variable. Complex interactions between lexical processing, saccadic programming, and post-lexical processing mechanisms lead to considerable variability from simulation to simulation in whether a saccadic program for a regression that was initiated as a result of post-lexical processing difficulty is actually executed or whether it is overridden by a subsequent saccadic program set up as a result of some other process. Even when E-Z Reader 10's post-lexical processing parameters are set to generate regressive saccadic programs 100% of the time, many progressive saccades result (see Figure 4 of Reichle et al., 2009). This relatively high likelihood of canceling a regressive saccadic program will likely decrease if the model's simplifying assumptions of no re-processing difficulty are made more realistic, but the high degree of stochasticity in the system will remain. The complexity of the interactions between multiple stochastic processes likely underlies at least some of the variance observed in eye movement responses to semantic violations and other post-lexical processing manipulations (for a review of such responses not limited to semantic anomalies, see Clifton et al., 2007).

However, there are other important sources of variance influencing eye movements to semantic anomalies. Some of these sources of variance are related to post-lexical processing itself and will remain outside of E-Z Reader 10's scope until the model's post-lexical processing 'black box' is replaced with a fully articulated theory. This more fully articulated theory of post-lexical processing will likely be built in large part on evidence from experiments testing semantic violations, like those reviewed at the beginning of this chapter, and take the form of a dynamic process proceeding from initial coarse-grained and/or automatic activations through more fine-grained and accurate representations to attempts to reconcile or repair inconsistent or incoherent discourse models (e.g. Garrod and Sanford, 2005; Kuperberg, 2007; Myers and O'Brien, 1998). Presumably, factors like violation severity or amount of feature overlap between an anomalous word and an expected word would cause differences in when during this processing stream a semantic violation was detected (Garrod and Sanford, 2005; Stewart et al., 2004; Warren and McConnell, 2007), leading to differences in eye movement disruption latency. But even if a theory of post-lexical processing is implemented within E-Z Reader 10, the model will be incomplete without allowing some role for even higher-level influences. For example, the fact that readers sometimes fail to notice semantic anomalies indicates that readers process texts incompletely (Sanford, 2002; Ferreira et al., 2002). If different readers, reading for different purposes, perform post-lexical processing more or less quickly or completely (Daneman et al., 2007; Swets et al., 2008), the precise combination of reader, purpose, and motivation will affect the patterns of eye movements to semantic violations.

Although studying eye movements to semantic violations in unambiguous sentences is still relatively new, such studies have already made important contributions to our understanding of the time course and process of semantic comprehension, the debate about attention allocation in reading, and models of eye movement control in reading. Continued research in this area, especially coupled with continued modeling work, has the potential to significantly advance our understanding of the time course of semantic processing and our understanding of how such processing interfaces with other processes during reading.

Acknowledgements

During the preparation of this chapter, T. Warren was supported by grants HD053639 and HD048990. Thanks to Erik Reichle, Natasha Tokowicz, and Michael Walsh Dickey for comments on early drafts.

References

Aaronson, D., and Ferres, S. (1986). Sentence processing in Chinese-American bilinguals. *Journal of Memory and Language,* **25**, 136–162.

Altmann, G.T.M, Garnham, A., and Dennis, Y. (1992). Avoiding the garden path: Eye movements in context. *Journal of Memory and Language,* **31**, 685–712.

Bohan, J. and Sanford, A.J. (2008). Semantic anomalies at the borderline of consciousness: An eye-tracking investigation. *Quarterly Journal of Experimental Psychology,* **61**, 232–239.

Boland. J. (2005). Visual arguments. *Cognition,* **95**, 237–274.

Boland, J.E., and Blodgett, A. (2001). Understanding the constraints on syntactic generation: Lexical bias and discourse congruency effects on eye movements. *Journal of Memory and Language,* **45**, 391–411.

Braze, D., Shankweiler, D., Ni, W., and Palumbo, L.C. (2002). Readers' eye movements distinguish anomalies of form and content. *Journal of Psycholinguistic Research,* **31**, 25–44.

Clifton, C., Staub, A., and Rayner, K. (2007). Eye movements in reading words and sentences. In R.P.G. van Gompel, M.H. Fischer, W.S. Murray, and R.L. Hill (eds.) *Eye movements: A window on mind and brain* (pp. 341–371). New York: Elsevier.

Cook, A. and Myers, J.L. (2004). Processing discourse roles in scripted narratives: The influences of context and world knowledge. *Journal of Memory and Language,* **50**, 268–288.

Daneman, M., Lennertz, T., and Hannon, B. (2007). Shallow semantic processing of text: Evidence from eye movements. *Language and Cognitive Processes,* **22**, 83–105.

Drieghe, D., Rayner, K., and Pollatsek, A. (2008). Mislocated fixations can account for parafoveal-on-foveal effects in eye movements during reading. *Quarterly Journal of Experimental Psychology,* **61**, 1239–1249.

Duffy, S.A., and Keir, J.A. (2004). Violating stereotypes: Eye movements and comprehension processes when text conflicts with world knowledge. *Memory and Cognition,* **32**, 551–559.

Engbert, R., Nuthmann, A., Richter, E., and Kliegl, R. (2005). SWIFT: A dynamical model of saccade generation during reading. *Psychological Review,* **112**, 777–813.

Federmeier, K.D. (2007). Thinking ahead: The role and roots of prediction in language comprehension. *Psychophysiology,* **44**, 491–505.

Ferguson, H.J. and Sanford, A.J. (2008). Anomalies in real and counterfactual worlds: An eye-movement investigation. *Journal of Memory and Language,* **58**, 609–626.

Ferreira, F. and Clifton, C. (1986). The independence of syntactic processing. *Journal of Memory and Language,* **25**, 348–368.

Ferreira, F., Bailey, K.G.D., and Ferraro, V. (2002). Good-enough representations in language comprehension. *Current Directions in Psychological Science,* **11**, 11–15.

Filik, R. (2008). Contextual override of pragmatic anomalies: Evidence from eye movements. *Cognition,* **106**, 1038–1046.

Fodor, J.D., Ni, W.J., Crain, S., and Shankweiler, D. (1996). Tasks and timing in the perception of linguistic anomaly. *Journal of Psycholinguistic Research,* **25**, 25–57.

Forster, K.I. and Olbrei, I. (1974). Semantic heuristics and semantic analysis. *Cognition,* **2**, 319–347.

Forster, K.I. and Ryder, L. (1971). Perceiving the structure and meaning of sentences. *Journal of Verbal Learning and Verbal Behavior,* **10**, 285–296.

Garrod, S. and Terras, M. (2000). The contribution of lexical and situational knowledge to resolving discourse roles: Bonding and resolution. *Journal of Memory and Language,* **42**, 526–544.

Joseph, H.S.S.L., Liversedge, S.P., Blythe, H.I., White, S.J., Gathercole, S.E., and Rayner, K. (2008). Childrens' and adults' processing of anomaly and implausibility during reading: Evidence from eye movements. *Quarterly Journal of Experimental Psychology,* **61**, 708–723.

Just, M.A. and Carpenter, P.A. (1980). A theory of reading: From eye fixations to comprehension. *Psychological Review,* **87**, 329–354.

Kennedy, A., Murray, W.S., and Boissiere, C. (2004). Parafoveal pragmatics revisited. *European Journal of Cognitive Psychology,* **16**, 128–153.

Kreiner, H., Sturt, P., and Garrod, S. (2008). Processing definitional and stereotypical gender in reference resolution: Evidence from eye-movements. *Journal of Memory and Language,* **58**, 239–261.

Kuperberg, G. (2007). Neural mechanisms of language comprehension: Challenges to syntax. *Brain Research,* **1146**, 23–49.

Kutas, M., Van Petten, C., and Kluender, R. (2006). Psycholinguistics electrified II: 1994–2005. In M. Traxler and M.A. Gernsbacher (eds.) *Handbook of Psycholinguistics, 2nd Edition* (pp. 659–724). New York, NY: Elsevier.

McConkie, G.W., Kerr, P.W., Reddix, M.D., and Zola, D. (1988). Eye movement control during reading: I. The location of the initial eye fixations on words. *Vision Research, 28*, 1107–1118.

McConkie, G.W., Zola, D., Grimes, J., Kerr, P.W., Bryant, N.R., and Wolff, P.M. (1991). Children's eye movements during reading. In J.F. Stein, *Vision and visual dyslexia* (pp. 251–262). London, England: Macmillian Press.

Mitchell, D.C., Shen, X., Green, M.J., and Hodgson, T.L. (2008). Accounting for regressive eye-movements in models of sentence processing: A reappraisal of the selective reanalysis hypothesis. *Journal of Memory and Language, 59*, 266–293.

Murray, W.S. (2006). The nature and time course of pragmatic plausibility effects. *Journal of Psycholinguistic Research, 35*, 79–99.

Murray, W.S. and Rowan, M. (1998). Early, mandatory, pragmatic processing. *Journal of Psycholinguistic Research, 27*, 1–22.

Myers, J.L. and O'Brien, E.J. (1998). Accessing the discourse representation during reading. *Discourse Processes, 26*, 131–157.

Ni, W.J., Fodor, J.D., Crain, S., and Shankweiler, D. (1996). Anomaly detection: Eye movement patterns. *Journal of Psycholinguistic Research, 27*, 515–537.

Patson, N.D. and Warren, T. (2010). Eye movements when reading implausible sentences: Investigating potential structural influences on semantic integration. *Quarterly Journal of Experimental Psychology, 63*, 1516–1532.

Pickering, M.J. and Traxler, M.J. (1998). Plausibility and recovery from garden paths: An eye-tracking study. *Journal of Experimental Psychology: Learning, Memory and Cognition, 24*, 940–961.

Pinker, S. (1994). *The Language Instinct.* New York: W. Morrow and Co.

Rayner, K., Carlson, M.A., and Frazier, L. (1983). The interaction of syntax and semantics during sentence processing: Eye movements in the analysis of semantically biased sentences. *Journal of Verbal Learning and Verbal Behavior, 22*, 358–374.

Rayner, K., Sereno, S.C., and Raney, G.E. (1996). Eye movement control in reading: a comparison of two types of models. *Journal of Experimental Psychology: Human Perception and Performance, 22*, 1188–1200.

Rayner, K. Juhasz, B.J., Ashby, J., and Clifton, C. (2003a). Inhibition of saccade return in reading. *Vision Research, 43*, 1027–1034.

Rayner, K., Warren, T., Juhasz, B., and Liversedge, S. (2004). The effects of plausibility on eye movements in reading. *Journal of Experimental Psychology: Learning, Memory and Cognition, 30*, 1290–1301.

Rayner, K., Chase, K.H., Slattery, T.J., and Ashby J. (2006). Eye movements as reflections of comprehension processes in reading. *Scientific Studies of Reading, 10*, 241–255.

Rayner, K., White, S.J., Kambe, G., Miller, B., and Liversedge, S.P. (2003b). On the processing of meaning from parafoveal vision during eye fixations in reading. In J. Hyönä, R. Radach, and H. Deubel (eds.) *The mind's eye: Cognitive and applied aspects of eye movement research* (pp. 213–234). Oxford, England: Elsevier.

Reichle, E.D., Rayner, K., and Pollatsek, A. (2003). The E-Z Reader model of eye movement control in reading: Comparisons to other models. *Behavioral and Brain Sciences, 26*, 445–476.

Reichle, E.D., Warren, T., and McConnell, K. (2009). Using E-Z Reader to model effects of higher level language processing on eye-movements in reading. *Psychonomic Bulletin and Review, 16*, 1–20.

Reichle, E.D., Pollatsek, A., Fisher, D.L., and Rayner, K. (1998). Toward a model of eye movement control in reading. *Psychological Review, 105*, 125–157.

Sanford, A. (2002). Context, attention and depth of processing during interpretation. *Mind and Language, 17*, 188–206.

Sanford, A. and Garrod, S. (2005). Memory-based approaches and beyond. *Discourse Processes, 39*, 205–224.

Speer, S.R., and Clifton, C. (1998). Plausibility and argument structure in sentence comprehension. *Memory and Cognition, 26*, 965–978.

Staub, A., Rayner, R., Pollatsek, A., Hyönä, J., and Majewski, H. (2007). The time course of plausibility effects on eye movements in reading: Evidence from noun-noun compounds. *Journal of Experimental Psychology: Learning, Memory and Cognition, 33*, 1162–1169.

Stewart, A.J., Pickering, M.J., and Sturt, P. (2004). Using eye movements during reading as an implicit measure of the acceptability of brand extensions. *Applied Cognitive Psychology, 18*, 697–709.

Swets, B., Desmet, T., Clifton, C., and Ferreira, F. (2008). Underspecification of syntactic ambiguities: Evidence from self-paced reading. *Memory and Cognition, 36*, 201–216.

Traxler, M.J., Pickering, M.J., and Clifton, C. (1998). Adjunct attachment is not a form of lexical ambiguity resolution. *Journal of Memory and Language, 39*, 558–592.

Trueswell, J.C., Tanenhaus, M.K., and Garnsey, S.M. (1994). Semantic influences on parsing: Use of thematic role information in syntactic ambiguity resolution. *Journal of Memory and Language, 33*, 285–318.

Wang, S., Chen, H-C., Yang, J., and Mo, L. (2008). Immediacy of integration in discourse comprehension: Evidence from Chinese readers' eye movements. *Language and Cognitive Processes, 23*, 241–257.

Warren, T. and McConnell, K. (2007). Investigating effects of selectional restriction violations and plausibility violation severity on eye-movements in reading. *Psychonomic Bulletin and Review, 14*, 770–775.

Warren, T., McConnell, K., and Rayner, K. (2008). Effects of context on eye movements when reading about plausible and impossible events. *Journal of Experimental Psychology: Learning, Memory and Cognition, 34*, 1001–1010.

CHAPTER 51

The influence of focus on eye movements during reading

Ruth Filik, Kevin B. Paterson, and Antje Sauermann

Abstract

In this chapter, we review research investigating the influence of linguistic focus on eye movements during reading. Focus is the assignment of prominence by phonological or syntactic means, which either marks new information or indicates that a contrast should be made between the focused information and some alternatives to it. We show that focus has a wide ranging influence on reading, from the processing of individual words, to the processing of sentence structure, the computation of reference, and the nature of the mental representation constructed by a reader. We conclude that eye movement research has been successful in revealing readers' sensitivity to focus during language comprehension, and its influence on higher-order language processing during the reading and understanding of text.

What is focus and what does it do?

The term *focus* has been used in many different ways. For example, in the literature on discourse processing, focus can refer to a salient individual in the discourse, such as the first character to be mentioned (Gernsbacher and Hargreaves, 1988). However, here we will use *focus* as a general term for the characteristic assignment of prominence by phonological or syntactic means, which serves the function of either marking new information, or contrasting the focused element(s) with a set of alternatives, which can be either explicit or implicit (Chomsky, 1971; Halliday, 1967; Jackendoff, 1972; Kiss, 1998; Rochemont and Culicover 1990; Rooth, 1992, 1996; Selkirk, 1995).

The following examples (where capital letters indicate the placement of phonological stress) illustrate the way in which the alternatives invoked by focus can be either explicit or implicit. For instance, both *Mary* and *Susan* are focused expressions in (1):

1. John kissed MARY, and not SUSAN.

In (1), an explicit contrast is made between *Mary* and *Susan*. However, sentences such as (2) show that the contrast in question does not have to be explicit:

2. John kissed only MARY.

In (2), focus is assigned to *Mary*, and readers will understand the sentence as asserting that John kissed *Mary*, rather than some alternative. The alternatives to *Mary* are implicit and must be inferred by the reader. In principle, anything that belongs to the same semantic category as the focused element (in this case another person, or more specifically, anything that can be kissed) could be considered an alternative, but realistically this set of possible alternatives is restricted by our knowledge of the situation.

Example (2) uses the focus-sensitive particle *only* (discussed in more detail later) along with prosodic cues to indicate which element is in focus. There are a number of other ways in which focus can be established. One syntactic focusing technique is the use of cleft or pseudo-cleft sentence constructions (e.g. Kiss, 1998). Clefted sentences (e.g. (3)) usually begin with the word *it*, followed by the element to be focused and then the rest of the statement, and are argued to increase prominence by placing focus, or contrast, on the fronted item (Carpenter and Just, 1977; Rochemont and Culicover, 1990). Pseudo-cleft sentences (e.g. (4)) contain a *wh*-cleft on the subject or complement.

3. It was Alice who made a cake. (Focus on Alice)

4. What Alice made was a cake. (Focus on cake)

Von Stechow (1991) argued that the semantics of questions is very important for a theory of focus. Specifically, a *wh*-question sets the background for an answer, which, in turn, determines the focus of the answer. For example, the implicit question answered by (3) is '*Who made a cake?*', whereas the implicit question answered by (4) is '*What did Alice make?*'. Now consider a question like (5):

5. Is it JOHN who writes poetry?

Intuitively, (6) is a *natural* response to this, but (7) is not.

6. No, it is BILL who writes poetry.

7. No, it is JOHN who writes short stories.

To explain this intuition, Jackendoff (1972) introduced the notions of *focus* and *presupposition*. He used the term *focus* to denote the information in the sentence that is assumed by the speaker <u>not</u> to be shared by him/her and the hearer, whereas *presupposition* denotes the information in the sentence that the speaker assumes <u>is</u> shared by him/her and the hearer. In (5) the presupposition is that someone writes poetry. *John* is the focus, that is, the information assumed by the speaker to be known by the hearer, but not known to the speaker, or else they wouldn't be asking the question. In (6) the presupposition is also that someone writes poetry, and *Bill* is the focus, that is, the new information being conveyed. In (7), however, the presupposition is that someone writes short stories.

The advantages of focus

There are a number of processing benefits associated with focused items. Focus preferentially directs the reader's or listener's attention to the focused entity (Carpenter and Just, 1977; Engelkamp and Zimmer, 1982; Klin et al., 2004; Zimmer and Engelkamp, 1981). Furthermore, it has been found that listeners perceive focused information more easily than non-focused information (Cutler and Fodor, 1979; Hornby, 1974), and that memory for focused words is enhanced (Birch et al., 2000; Birch and Garnsey, 1995; Malt, 1985; Osaka et al., 2002; Singer, 1976). Speech comprehension is easier when focused information is marked using prosody than when it is not (Birch and Clifton, 1995, 2002; Bock and Mazzella, 1983; Noteboom and Kruyt, 1987; Terken and Noteboom, 1987), and using prosody to assign focus can influence how ambiguous sentences are interpreted (Carlson et al., 2009; Schafer et al., 2000). In a corpus study, Arnold (1998) demonstrated that clefted elements were referred to more often than other referents in the same sentence. Gergely (1992) found that focusing relevant information facilitates inference. Moreover, readers are more likely to detect a semantic anomaly when it occurs as part of the sentence focus (Bredart and Modolo, 1988), and are more likely to detect that a word has changed to a semantically similar word when the changed word is in focus, during a text change-detection task (Sturt et al., 2004). Thus, it should be clear that focus plays an important role in language understanding. The question addressed in this review is what influence it has on the actual reading process and on readers' eye movement behaviour.

Chapter outline

In the remainder of this chapter we will review research which has examined the influence that focus has on eye movements during reading. We will demonstrate that focus has a wide ranging influence on reading, from influencing processing at the level of the individual word, to the processing of reference, and to the processes involved in computing the structure and meaning of a sentence. A particular aim in conducting this review is to assess what effects of focus have been observed in various experiments and when these effects emerge in the reader's eye movement record. In common with other researchers in this area, we will draw a distinction between effects that manifest in early eye movements for a critical word or phrase (such as gaze durations or first-pass reading times) and those effects that are delayed and appear either further downstream in the sentence or in later measures of eye movements (e.g. total reading times). Such information can reveal whether focus affects the initial or early processing of a critical word or phrase or only exerts an influence during later stages in the reading process.

This issue is of particular relevance to an emerging debate about the influence of higher-order language processing on eye movements during reading (Clifton et al., 2007; Reichle et al., 2009; see also Mitchell et al., 2008). A starting point for this debate is the observation that although current models of eye movement control (e.g. Engbert et al., 2005; Reichle et al., 1998; Reilly and Radach, 2006, see also Engbert and Kliegl, Chapter 43, and Reichle, Chapter 42, this volume) provide comprehensive accounts of the influence of visual and lexical factors on eye movements during reading, these models are relatively silent about how higher-order processes associated with language comprehension might influence this behaviour (apart from predictability effects). Recent research has addressed this issue by systematically examining how different aspects of higher-order language processing are manifest in eye movement behaviour (Clifton et al., 2007) and how these processes might be incorporated within a model of eye movement control (Reichle et al., 2009).

The model that Reichle et al. (2009, see also Warren, Chapter 50, this volume) proposed is a revised version of the E-Z Reader model (e.g. Reichle et al., 1998) that retains the assumption that the progression of the eyes through a sentence is determined primarily by visual factors and the lexical processing of words. However, the revised model also incorporates a post-lexical integration stage of language processing in which a word is integrated into the higher level representations that are constructed during reading. This post-lexical stage is not intended as a theory of higher-order language processing, but instead provides an account of how this processing might interact with eye movement control. The model makes two key assumptions about this interaction. The first is that post-lexical integration takes time to complete. The second is that its interruption or failure can cause both the eyes and attention to be halted, or even directed back towards the source of integration difficulty. Thus, while ongoing comprehension processes might not be apparent in eye movement behaviour, disruption to these processes or their failure may well be evident in the pattern of pauses and regressions made during reading. The model has already been used to simulate a variety of phenomena related to higher-order language processing (see Reichle et al., 2009, and Reichle, Chapter 42, this volume), including 'wrap-up' effects observed when readers pause at the ends of clauses and sentences (Warren et al., 2009), effects that occur when readers encounter violations in verb selectional restrictions (Warren and McConnell, 2007), and effects that occur when readers misanalyse sentence structure (e.g. Frazier and Rayner, 1982). However, a comprehensive account of the influence of post-lexical language processing on readers' eye movements must account for an even greater variety of higher-order language processes, including the processing of linguistic focus. Our aim in conducting the present review is to provide a comprehensive account of the influence of focus on eye movements during reading, in order to reveal how this aspect of higher-order language processing is manifest in readers' eye movement behaviour.

Focus effects at the level of the focused word

Several eye movement studies have assessed the influence of focus on the processing of individual words (Birch and Rayner, 1997, 2010; Morris and Folk, 1998; Ward and Sturt, 2007). Much of this work was conducted in the context of research showing that prior sentence context can influence early stages of word processing associated with the retrieval of information about a word (e.g. Binder and Morris, 1995; Morris, 1994). The question addressed in focus research was what effect including a focusing device in the prior sentence or discourse has on word processing. These studies used syntactic focusing devices or interrogative contexts to investigate the influence of focus on eye movements while participants were reading words that were focused or non-focused (see also Breen and Clifton, 2008, for recent work on lexical stress effects in silent reading).

For instance, Birch and Rayner (1997) examined the effect of syntactic focus and *wh*-phrase questions on readers' eye movements. In one experiment, they manipulated syntactic focus using *it*-clefts or *there*-insertion devices in sentences such as:

8. It was the suburb that received the most damage from the ice storm.

9. Workers in the suburb hurried to restore power after the ice storm.

These devices were used to focus on a single word (in this case, the word *suburb*). The results indicated that this manipulation did not influence either the number of first-pass fixations or gaze duration for words. However, an effect was observed in later eye movement measures. Birch and Rayner (1997) found that participants were more likely to make a regression to the critical word and to spend more time re-reading that word in focused (e.g. (8)) than non-focused conditions (e.g. (9)). As these effects emerged relatively late in the eye movement record, Birch and Rayner concluded that using syntactic focus to highlight a word had not influenced early word processing but had led to additional processing after the reader had identified the word and started to integrate it with context.

A second experiment used *wh*-phrases in interrogative contexts to focus on different parts of a following sentence in texts like (10) and (11):

10. Where were the soldiers? The soldiers in the underground bunker were playing cards to relieve their boredom.

11. What were the soldiers playing? The soldiers in the underground bunker were playing cards to relieve their boredom.

The answer to the question in (10) is found at the phrase *in the underground bunker* in the following sentence but in (11) the answer is found at the word *cards*. As in their earlier experiment, Birch and Rayner (1997) observed no first-pass effects of focus but found that readers made more regressions and spent longer reprocessing focused than unfocused regions of the sentence. Thus, the results of both experiments showed that while readers are sensitive to manipulations of focus, effects are not observed during the first-pass processing of a word or phrase, and emerge only during the reprocessing of that text. These findings led Birch and Rayner to suggest that focus influences relatively late stages of sentence processing associated with the integration of information within the reader's discourse model and that focusing devices, such as clefts or interrogatives, cause readers to perform additional processing of focused words as part of this integrative stage of processing. Birch and Rayner suggested that this additional processing may result in a memory encoding benefit for focused information, which may explain some of the processing advantages observed for focused information (discussed above).

Subsequent research by Morris and Folk (1998) also used *it*-cleft sentences to investigate the impact of syntactic focus on readers' eye movements. Like Birch and Rayner (1997), they observed no effects of this manipulation on gaze durations for the critical word and concluded that using syntactic focusing devices to highlight a word in a text does not affect the early processing of that word. However, in contrast to findings reported by Birch and Rayner, Morris and Folk found that total reading times were actually shorter for focused than for non-focused words. They argued that this was due to focused information in their experiment being easier to integrate into the discourse model than non-focused information, and that this enhanced integration of focused information might lead to more detailed memory representations.

Neither of the above studies revealed effects of syntactic focus in early eye movements for the critical word or phrase. However, the studies produced conflicting effects of focus on the reprocessing of words. Ward and Sturt (2007) wanted to further investigate these apparently conflicting results, and so conducted an experiment that employed eye movement recording in conjunction with a text-change detection manipulation used in an earlier study by Sturt et al. (2004). In this study, Sturt et al. had used a text change-detection paradigm to investigate the influence of focus on the process of encoding words. This was achieved by having participants read two successive displays of a passage of text with an interposing blank screen. A word was changed between these displays, either to a semantically related word (e.g. *hat* changed to *cap*) or an unrelated word (e.g. *hat* changed to *dog*). In addition, the word that was changed was either focused or unfocused, and focus was manipulated using either cleft constructions or *wh*-phrase questions in the prior context.

The results showed that when the word changed to a semantically related word, detection rates were higher for words that were in focus, but there was no difference between focused and non-focused conditions when the word changed to an unrelated word. Sturt et al. (2004) interpreted these results in terms of the level of granularity at which a word is represented, arguing that focus increases the level of specificity at which a word is represented. Thus, a change from *hat* to *cap* was noticed more often in the focus condition, because the relevant semantic information had been represented at a finer grain. In contrast, when the word was not in focus, a less specific representation of its meaning led to a lower level of change detection.

It was not possible on the basis of this study to reach conclusions about the underlying processes responsible for the focus benefit, so Ward and Sturt (2007) conducted their follow-up study to assess the influence of focus on eye movements during performance of the text change-detection task. Focus was manipulated using context, and the critical word was changed to another semantically-related word. An analysis of eye movements during the first display of the text showed no differences for the focused word. However, change-detection results showed that participants were more successful at detecting a change when the word was in focus (replicating the findings of Sturt et al., 2004). Additionally, during the second display of the text, there were more fixations and longer reading times (in both early and late eye movement measures) on a changed than an unchanged word, but only when the word was in focus. Taking account of eye movement behaviour during both the first and second displays of the text, Ward and Sturt suggested that although linguistic focus may lead to more detailed lexical-semantic representations, these do not necessarily result from more effortful encoding of information.

Findings from recent experiments by Birch and Rayner (2010) that revisited the effects of syntactic prominence on word processing add further to this debate. Birch and Rayner considered whether differences in findings produced by previous studies are due to confounding factors. In particular, they investigated whether differences between focused and unfocused conditions in these studies, in addition to the presence or absence of a focusing device, are responsible for the observed effects. For instance, Birch and Rayner note that in their original (1997) experiment, the non-focused condition consisted of sentences that not only lacked the *it*-cleft or *there*-insertion present in the focused condition, but also relocated the target word to a less prominent syntactic position (see, e.g. McKoon et al., 1993; Wilson and Sperber, 1979). Specifically, the target word *suburb* in the focused condition in (8) appears without the *it*-cleft but also appears in a subordinate syntactic position in the non-focused condition in (9). Birch and Rayner argue that this additional shift in syntactic position will have affected processing and may have contributed to the difference in word processing between focused and non-focused conditions observed in their experiment. They also argued that similar confounds exist in Morris and Folk's (1998) experiment, where the non-focused condition involved not only the removal of the *it*-cleft preceding the target word, but the addition of a subordinate clause and an *it*-cleft preceding an alternative word. Also, experiments that have used questions to manipulate focus (Birch and Rayner, 1997, Ward and Sturt, 2007) do not examine the effects of removing focus but of focusing on different constituents within a sentence. Therefore, in order to eliminate these potentially confounding factors and gain a clearer indication of the effects of focus on word processing, Birch and Rayner re-examined the effects of syntactic focus on words in short discourses that included a critical sentence that differed only in the presence or absence of a focusing device (e.g. the sentences in 12 and 13, where *landlady* is the target word).

12. It was the landlady who confronted the woman who lived there.

13. The landlady confronted the woman who lived there.

Using similar discourses, Birch et al. (2000) had observed enhanced accessibility of and memory for target words in the focused compared to the non-focused condition, as measured by sentence continuation and delayed probe recognition tasks. The results from Birch and Rayner's (2010) eye movement experiment showed that focus did not lead to increased processing of target words (as Birch and Rayner, 1997, had previously argued) and that targets words actually received shorter initial fixations when focused. Birch and Rayner attributed this difference in findings in their experiments to the nature of the non-focused conditions used, and argued that shorter reading times for focused target words in their more recent experiment indicate (contrary to their previous claims) that syntactically prominent constituents are encoded and/or accessed more quickly during reading. The effect they observed emerged much earlier in the eye movement record (in first fixation durations for target words) than in previous experiments, and so also re-opens the possibility that focus can influence early stages of word processing associated with the encoding of a word.

In summary, it is evident that focus can influence eye movements at the level of the individual word during reading. However, effects differ between studies. Birch and Rayner (1997) found increased total reading times for focused than for non-focused words, and argued that syntactic focus caused readers to reprocess focused words to a greater extent than non-focused words (and see Price, 2008, for recent work on the influence of focus on eye movements in younger and older readers that shows similar effects). By contrast, Morris and Folk (1998) found that focus led to shortened total reading times on a word, and Ward and Sturt (2007) found no differences in reading behaviour on focused compared to non-focused words during either first-pass processing or reprocessing of text. More recently, Birch and Rayner (2010) have suggested that these differences in findings may be due to the control conditions used in the various experiments and showed that when possible confounding factors are controlled for, target words receive shorter fixations when focused. As the effect in this experiment emerged early in the eye movement record, in measures usually associated with early word processing, it re-opens the possibility that focus can affect the encoding of words and not just later stages of text processing.

From this it is clear that there are many processing benefits associated with material that is in focus, and that readers are sensitive to manipulations of focus. However, it is also clear that there are a limited number of eye movement studies which have investigated the underlying processes responsible for these focus benefits, and results from these studies are mixed in terms of how these benefits map on to observable differences in eye movement behaviour. Further investigations of the effects of syntactic focus on word processing evidently must also take care to manipulate only the presence or absence of a focusing device so as to avoid contaminating the findings with the influences from other factors that affect word processing, such as differences in the syntactic prominence of words.

Focus and referential processing

Other research has used measures of eye movements during reading to investigate the effects of focus on the processing of a subsequent anaphor. Again, here we will concentrate on focus induced by syntactic means, but see also Moxey et al. (2009) and Paterson et al. (1998) for research on the influence of quantifier focus on eye movements during the processing of a subsequent anaphor (and for more general accounts of quantifier focus, see Moxey and Sanford, 1993; Paterson et al., 2009; and Sanford et al., 2007).

Studies of the influence of clefting on the ease of subsequent anaphoric reference have provided relatively clear results. Almor (1999) used self-paced reading to investigate the influence of clefting and found that a noun-phrase that co-referred with a clefted antecedent was easier to resolve than one that co-referred with an unclefted antecedent (see also Almor and Eimas, 2008, for recent work on the influence of focus on repeated and non-repeated NP anaphors in lexical decision and cued recall tasks). Foraker (2004) found a similar clefting advantage during pronoun co-reference. Specifically, self-paced reading times on the word following a pronoun were shorter when the pronoun's antecedent was clefted, suggesting that clefted antecedents had more prominent representations.

Foraker and McElree (2007, Experiment 2) further investigated this issue by monitoring participants' eye movements as they read sentences such as (14) and (15):

14. It was the cheerful waitress who made the decaffeinated coffee.

15. What the cheerful waitress made was the decaffeinated coffee.

   a) Reassuringly, she gossiped behind the counter of the diner.

   b) Reassuringly, it brewed behind the counter of the diner.

The study focused on the effect that clefting had on eye movements on the region of text containing the pronoun (e.g. *she gossiped/it brewed*) and the following region (e.g. *behind*) for pronouns that referred to either clefted or unclefted antecedents. In (14), the word *waitress* is placed in focus, whereas in (15) the words *decaffeinated coffee* are in focus. The waitress is subsequently referred to by *she* in (a), and the coffee is subsequently referred to by *it* in (b). The results of this experiment showed that clefting did not influence early eye movements for the regions of analysis and so did not affect the early processing of the pronoun. Instead, Foraker and McElree (2007) observed an advantage for clefted antecedent conditions in several late eye movement measures; namely, second-pass reading times and regression rates (i.e. second-pass reading times were shorter and there were fewer regressions in the focused condition). Foraker and McElree argued that these findings indicated that although clefting did not aid the early processing of the anaphor, the effects that emerged in later eye movement behaviour showed that clefting had nevertheless helped the reader to resolve the meaning of the pronoun and to integrate it within their discourse model.

That clefting might aid integration without influencing early word processing is generally consistent with previous studies of cleft constructions (Birch and Rayner, 1997; Morris and Folk, 1998). In terms of how the antecedent of the pronoun is represented, Foraker and McElree (2007) concluded that rather than increasing the accessibility of an antecedent representation through active maintenance (e.g. Gundel, 1999), clefting simply served to make the antecedent more prominent by amplifying the strength of the representation in the reader's discourse model, and so increasing its availability for on-going operations such as reference resolution and integration. Such an account is consistent with findings from other studies showing that clefted constituents have stronger memory representations than non-clefted controls (e.g. Birch et al., 2000; Birch and Garnsey, 1995). Thus, the results of this research, like the findings from research examining the effects of focus on individual words, suggest that focus has a relatively late influence on sentence processing, and affects the integration and consolidation of information within the reader's discourse model.

The influence of focus-sensitive particles on eye movements during reading

So far we have examined the manipulation of focus by syntactic means. Another way in which linguistic focus can be introduced in a sentence is through the use of words such as *only, just, also, too,* and *even*. These function words are known as focus-sensitive particles (focus operators, or focusing adverbs) because of their tendency to *associate* with a focused constituent in a sentence, with the range over which they exert their effect being known as their 'scope' (e.g. Jackendoff, 1972; König, 1991). Focus-sensitive particles signal that a contrast is to be made between the referent of a sentential constituent and some alternatives to it, although the precise nature of this contrast depends on the lexical characteristics of the particular particle. In the following sections, we will review research that has used measures of eye movements during reading to assess the influence of focus-sensitive particles on processes involved in computing the structure and meaning of a sentence.

Focus-sensitive particles and syntactic processing

Much of the existing research in this area has concentrated on the influence of the word *only* on the processing of structural ambiguities. In particular, this research has been concerned with whether the choice of focus in a sentence can guide the processing of these ambiguities (following Ni et al., 1996, see also Clifton et al., 2000; Filik et al., 2005; Kemper et al., 2004; Liversedge et al., 2002; and Paterson et al., 1999; furthermore, see Sedivy, 2002 for related research using self-paced reading). Earlier research into structure processing has shown that the disruption to comprehension that occurs when a temporarily syntactically ambiguous sentence is mis-analysed (i.e. a so-called 'garden path' effect; e.g. Frazier and Rayner, 1982) is detectable early in the processing of a disambiguating word. Research into the influence of focus on structure processing has examined whether using the particle *only* to indicate contrastive focus can eliminate the comprehension difficulty that otherwise would occur during the reading of temporarily ambiguous sentences like (17):

16. The businessmen loaned money at low interest were told to record their expenses.

17. Only businessmen loaned money at low interest were told to record their expenses.

In (16) and (17), the phrase *loaned money at low interest* is ambiguous between a main clause analysis (stating *what* the businessmen did) and a reduced relative clause analysis (that provides additional modifying information, i.e. that the businessmen had been loaned money at low interest). This phrase is disambiguated as being a reduced relative clause at the phrase *were told*. In sentences like (16), which do not include a focus particle, readers typically initially assign a main clause analysis to such an ambiguity, and as a result experience difficulty when the sentence is disambiguated as a reduced relative clause construction (e.g. Frazier and Rayner, 1982).

Ni et al. (1996) proposed that including *only* can eliminate such difficulty. They argued that on encountering the phrase *only businessmen* in (17) there are two things that readers may do. Firstly, readers might construct a discourse model that contrasts a focus set denoted by the head noun with another set of entities (e.g. contrasts businessmen with lawyers). Alternatively they might construct a model that contrasts subsets of the head noun (e.g. two sets of businessmen). In this case, they would then anticipate additional information specifying the difference between the two sets of businessmen. This additional information may be supplied by the relative clause analysis of the ambiguity (e.g. that the focus set of businessmen were loaned money at low interest, whereas the contrast set were not). Ni et al. argued that readers preferentially contrast subsets of the head noun (e.g. two sets of businessmen) as this avoids referential presuppositions about entities that are not made explicit in the text (e.g. lawyers, see also Altmann and Steedman, 1988; Crain and Steedman, 1985). Thus, in summary, the account predicts that on encountering the phrase *only businessmen* in (17), readers will contrast two sets of businessmen and anticipate modifying information that disambiguates the focus set, thereby predisposing readers to adopt a relative clause analysis of the ambiguity.

In line with this account, Ni et al. (1996) found that *only* eliminated comprehension difficulty for the disambiguating phrase of ambiguous sentences (e.g. *were told* in (17)). However, including an adjective (e.g. only *wealthy* businessmen) reintroduced that difficulty, as in this case the need for modifying information was satisfied by the adjective, and so the readers no longer anticipated modifying information in the form of a relative clause. Thus, according to Ni et al., referential processing demands associated with contrastive focus can predispose readers to adopting the relative clause analysis of an ambiguity, and thus influence readers' eye movements during the processing of such an ambiguity. A subsequent eye movement experiment by Kemper et al. (2004) using the same stimuli showed that such effects were found only for readers who had a high working memory span. By contrast, readers who had a lower working memory span appeared to be unable to make use of this information when reading structurally ambiguous sentences and had difficulty in processing these sentences even when a focus particle was present.

One criticism of the Ni et al. (1996) research (and also the Kemper et al., 2004, study), has focused on their use of stimuli that consisted of a variety of constructions, including some where an active transitive analysis was initially available, and some where it was not (Paterson et al., 1999). An active transitive analysis is one in which a *noun-phrase, verb, noun-phrase* sequence can be processed as *noun, verb, direct object.* This was seen as important, as research suggests that readers are strongly predisposed to adopt the active transitive analysis of a syntactic ambiguity whenever it is available (MacDonald, 1994; Townsend and Bever, 2001), and that the preference cannot be over-ridden by prior referential context (Britt et al., 1992; Ferreira and Clifton, 1986; Murray and Liversedge, 1994). Thus, the heterogeneous nature of the constructions examined by Ni et al. prevented a clear assessment of whether garden path effects had been eliminated by the inclusion of the focus particle even for constructions that permit an active transitive analysis of the ambiguity and for which structure processing has previously been shown to be impervious to context effects. Paterson et al. (1999) investigated this issue by examining the influence of *only* for sentences such as (18) that temporarily permit an active transitive analysis with the second noun-phrase being analysed as a direct object (e.g. *Only teenagers allowed a party in the evening*).

18. Only teenagers allowed a party invited a juggler straightaway.

Paterson et al. (1999) also noted that Ni et al. (1996) had used a large disambiguating region for many stimuli, often comprising two words (e.g. *were told* in (16) and (17)), and argued that reading times at this region might include fixations made during reanalysis as well as during initial processing. Consequently, the effects they obtained might have been due to *only* aiding recovery from a misanalysis rather than actually guiding processing decisions. To address this possibility, Paterson et al. used stimuli that were disambiguated at a single word (e.g. *invited* in (18)).

Paterson et al. (1999) compared ambiguous sentences with unambiguous counterparts that were created by adding the phrase *who were* after the head noun (e.g. *Only teenagers who were allowed a party...*). There was clear evidence that readers had difficulty due to initially misanalysing the ambiguity, with longer gaze durations at the critical verb (e.g. *invited*) of ambiguous sentences, and no modulating effect of *only*. However, the inclusion of *only* did affect other aspects of sentence processing. More time was spent reprocessing text following the disambiguation of sentences without *only*, which Paterson et al. took as evidence that *only* had facilitated the reanalysis of ambiguous sentences when they were disambiguated as reduced relative clause constructions. Therefore, it appeared that using the particle *only* to evoke contrastive focus had a relatively late influence on the processing of this form of ambiguity.

A follow-up eye movement study by Liversedge et al. (2002) examined the processing of sentences such as (19):

19. Only motorists stopped in the car park received a warning about their outdated permits.

These included a prepositional phrase (e.g. *in the car park*) that ruled out the possibility of an active transitive analysis, and they were temporarily ambiguous between an intransitive analysis (in which the ambiguity describes what the referent of the head noun did, e.g. the motorists stopped in the car park) and a reduced relative clause analysis (in which the ambiguity provides modifying information). With the most strongly preferred analysis ruled out, readers must select between two relatively dis-preferred analyses. Under these circumstances structure processing might be susceptible to extrasyntactic factors, such as contrastive focus. Liversedge et al. (2002) observed no effects in first-pass reading times but found that readers made fewer regressive saccades and spent less time reprocessing text following disambiguation for sentences with than without *only*. Readers also took longer to complete reading the remainder of the ambiguous sentences irrespective of whether they included *only*. Thus, although there was an effect of *only* at disambiguation, it did not fully eliminate comprehension difficulty.

Finally, Filik et al. (2005) conducted two eye movement experiments that examined the processing of temporarily ambiguous sentences with *only* in *wh*-phrase interrogative contexts that either did or did not support a contrast between subsets of a referent. In Experiment 1, Filik et al. examined the processing of sentences used by Paterson et al. (1999) in *wh*-phrase contexts which either further supported a relative clause reading of the ambiguity by emphasizing that a contrast was to be made between subsets of the same type (e.g. *Tom wondered which teenagers invited a juggler*) or were neutral (e.g. *Tom wondered who invited a juggler*). Experiment 2 examined the processing of sentences used by Liversedge et al. (2002) placed in *wh*-phrase contexts which either further supported a relative clause analysis of the ambiguity by indicating that the contrast was between sets of the same type (e.g. *Tom wondered which motorists received a warning*) or supported a main clause analysis by specifying that the contrast was between different sets (e.g. *Tom wondered whether the motorists or the pedestrians received a warning*). Filik et al.'s findings supported those of Paterson et al. and Liversedge et al. in that focusing effects due to *only* and a *wh*-phrase context only influenced initial parsing decisions when a transitive main clause analysis of the ambiguity was unavailable. Crucially, when both *only* and context supported a relative clause analysis of the ambiguity in these sentences, this eliminated comprehension difficulty.

In summary, eye movement studies subsequent to Ni et al. (1996) demonstrate that the timing of the influence of *only* on eye movement behaviour during the processing of structurally ambiguous sentences depends on which analyses are available to the parser. When there is a strong predisposition to adopt a particular analysis, focus has a relatively late effect on processing, and has been argued to facilitate reanalysis. However, when the parser is not strongly predisposed to adopt a particular analysis, and the nature of the contrast that is to be represented is clearly specified (e.g. by a combination of discourse context and the use of a focus particle), contrastive focus can immediately influence structural decision-making.

Focus-sensitive particles and semantic interpretation

There is a growing interest in fundamental questions concerning the processing of focus structure (e.g. Arnold, 2008; Carlson, 2004; Carlson et al., 2005; Gennari et al., 2004; Ito and Speer, 2008; Sedivy et al., 1995; Stolterfoht et al., 2007; Weber et al., 2006), and again, we concentrate on studies which have examined the effects on eye movements during reading.

As stated above, it has been argued that particles such as *only* 'associate with focus' (e.g. Jackendoff, 1972), meaning that they are often, but not always, interpreted as specifying a contrast between the referent of a focused syntactic constituent and its alternatives. Jackendoff proposed that grammatical constraints govern the range (or scope) over which a focus-sensitive particle can exert its influence, such that it associates with a focused constituent within its scope. Jackendoff defined these constraints in terms of the constituents that the particle dominates in the syntactic structure, and other researchers, such as Reinhart (1999), have proposed that *only* ranges over constituents that it c-commands. C-command refers to a syntactic relation between a constituent (in our case *only*) and other constituents in the syntactic parse tree that places important grammatical constraints on how sentences are interpreted (for a definition of c-command see e.g. Radford, 1997, p. 99). Because many focus-sensitive particles, including *only*, occur fairly freely in different syntactic positions in a sentence, the flexibility in their placement affords a means of evaluating grammatical influences on their interpretation.

Paterson et al. (2007) reported three eye movement experiments that investigated the influence of grammatical cues supplied by the surface position of a focus-sensitive particle on focus assignment during normal sentence comprehension. Specifically, the study examined whether locating *only* in different surface positions can modulate the assignment of focus in a sentence. Their experimental stimuli included a ditransitive verb that permitted dative alternation, as shown in examples (20) and (21) below (where square brackets indicate the alternative locations of the particle).

20. At dinner, Jane passed [only] the salt to [only] her mother but not (the pepper/her father) as well because she couldn't reach.

21. At dinner, Jane passed [only] her mother [only] the salt but not (the pepper/her father) as well because she couldn't reach.

For dative sentences (e.g. (20), which were studied in Experiment 1), the indirect object (e.g. *her mother*) followed the direct object (e.g. *the salt*). This constituent order was reversed for double object sentences (e.g. 921), used in Experiment 2). Each sentence was continued by a replacive construction (e.g. either *but not pepper as well* or *but not her father as well*) that served to supply an explicit, congruous contrast for either the direct or the indirect object. Experiment 3 examined processing of the same sentences without *only*. The assumption followed was that syntactic constraints would require *only* to associate with the immediately adjacent constituent (to the right) that is within its scope and so assign focus to that constituent. It was also assumed that readers would find it easier to process the replacive when it supplied a contrast that was congruous with the focused constituent. In line with this logic, it was predicted that if the sentences were interpreted with *only* associating with the indirect object (e.g. *her mother*) then readers should have difficulty with replacives supplying a contrast that is incongruous with this constituent (e.g. *but not the pepper*) as compared with congruous replacives (e.g. *but not her father*). Conversely, if *only* associated with the direct object (e.g. *the salt*) then readers should have difficulty for incongruous replacives (e.g. *but not her father*) but not for congruous replacives (e.g. *but not the pepper*). Paterson et al. (2007) considered that key issues concerned whether focus was assigned during the processing of a sentence (i.e. whether congruity effects were observed at all), and whether these effects emerged during the early processing of the replacive or later during sentence processing.

The results revealed that focus was computed during sentence comprehension and that effects of replacive congruency influenced eye movement behaviour. However, these effects were not observed during the early processing of the replacive, and emerged only in reading times for a post-replacive region in Experiments 1 and 2 (e.g. the words *as well because*), where readers had difficulty when the replacive was incongruous with the constituent that *only* adjoined (the earliest indications of an incongruency effect occurred in regression path reading times for the post-replacive region in Experiment 1, and first-pass reading times for the post-replace region in Experiment 2). No such effects were observed for sentences that omitted the focus particle (Experiment 3), indicating that it was the presence of *only* that caused the effects in the other experiments. Paterson et al. (2007) suggested that the lateness of the effect they observed was due to time-consuming inferential processes necessary to evaluate the congruency of the supplied contrast. Despite the incongruency effect being delayed, the effects it had on eye movement behaviour indicated nevertheless that contrastive focus is computed during sentence comprehension and sufficiently rapidly for its referential consequences to affect sentence processing.

Other experiments have examined the influence of *wh*-phrase contexts on focus assignment (Paterson et al., 2006; Sauermann et al., 2009). The aim of these experiments was to determine if discourse context can modulate focus assignment and to determine how rapidly these context effects occur. The experiments used the same dative sentence constructions as Paterson et al. (2007), in which *only* followed the main verb and a replacive continuation supplied a congruous contrast for either the direct or indirect object, but placed these in contexts where they followed an interrogative containing either a *who*-phrase (e.g. (22)) or a *what*-phrase (e.g. (23)).

22. Her sister wondered who Jane would pass the salt at dinner. At dinner, Jane passed only the salt to her mother but not (the pepper/her father) as well because she couldn't reach.

23. Her sister wondered what Jane would pass her mother at dinner. At dinner, Jane passed the salt to only her mother but not (the pepper/her father) as well because she couldn't reach.

The results showed that the *wh*-phrase context affected processing of the replacive in examples like (22) but not (23). First consider the findings for examples like (22) where *only* precedes both grammatical objects. These showed that when the context included a *who*-phrase, readers had difficulty when the replacive (e.g. *the pepper*) was incongruous with the indirect object (e.g. *her mother*). Therefore, it appeared that the interrogative context could over-ride the preference for *only* to associate with the direct object (e.g. *the salt*), which is the adjacent constituent in this sentence. By contrast, when context included a *what*-phrase, and so focused on the direct object, readers had difficulty when the replacive was incongruous with this constituent. The situation was quite different when *only* was located between the direct and indirect objects (e.g. '. . . *the salt to only her mother* . . .') in examples like (23) so that the direct object (e.g. *the salt*) was no longer within its scope. In this case, readers had difficulty when the replacive supplied an incongruous contrast for the direct object regardless of which *wh*-phrase was used. These effects were observed in first-pass and regression path reading times for the replacive region itself, and so emerged earlier in the eye movement record in this experiment than in the Paterson et al. (2007) studies, suggesting that the interrogative contexts facilitated the processing of focus. However, the effects of context were mediated by syntactic constraints, as the results indicate that although context <u>can</u> over-ride a preference for associating a focus particle with an immediately adjacent constituent, it <u>cannot</u> over-ride syntactic constraints on focus assignment. Moreover, the fact that these effects were observed in eye movement behaviour for sentences read normally provided further evidence that focus structure is computed during normal sentence comprehension.

Finally in this section, we consider a recent study by Filik et al. (2009) that examined the influence of *only* and *even* on on-line sentence interpretation. We have already reviewed several studies showing that including *only* in a sentence has marked effects on the processing of sentence structure and the assignment of focus. However, to our knowledge, no studies have examined the processing of other focus-sensitive particles during reading, even though the various particles that exist in English differ in their lexical characteristics. One important distinction concerns the nature of the contrast that different particles specify. For example, *only* is classed as an exclusive focus particle (e.g. Kadmon, 2001; König, 1991), as it specifies a contrast such that a property of the referent does not also belong to its alternatives. That is, readers will understand a sentence such as '*Only MARY kissed John*', (where capital letters indicate the placement of phonological stress), to mean that Mary alone kissed John. *Even*, on the other hand, is an *inclusive* particle (as are *also* and *too*) and indicates that the focus set and alternative sets share the properties mentioned in the sentence (e.g. Kadmon, 2001; König, 1991). Thus, readers will understand the sentence '*Even MARY kissed John*' as asserting that as well as Mary kissing John, others kissed John too. An additional function served by *even*, which is not shared by *also* and *too*, is that these alternatives are ranked on a scale (Horn, 1989; Kay, 1990). It has been argued that this scale can be viewed in terms of likelihood, with the focused element (e.g. *Mary*) being ranked at the lower end of the scale (cf. Kartunnen and Peters, 1979; see also Bennett, 1982; Fauconnier, 1975; Giannakidou, 2007; and Lycan, 1991, for discussions of the semantics of *even*). Thus, in the case of the current example, the felicitousness of the sentence depends upon the focused element (*Mary*) being less likely than some contextually defined alternatives; that is, the other people that had kissed John. As a consequence, the focused element is characterized as an unexpected or surprising one in relation to the event described in the sentence (e.g. Francescotti, 1995). Filik et al. (2009) wanted to compare the processing of sentences containing either *only* or *even* in light of the differences in their function. They used sentences like the following:

24. Only students taught by the best teacher passed the examination in the summer.

25. Only students taught by the worst teacher passed the examination in the summer.

Passing an examination may be considered more likely for students taught by the best teacher than for those taught by the worst teacher. Thus, events described in (24) may be perceived as being more felicitous, in relation to the reader's knowledge of the world, than those described in (25). Specifically, the information conveyed by (24) is congruous with the contrast set up by *only*. In the absence of context, if we were told that any one group of students passed an exam (to the exclusion of other groups) then the group of students who were taught by the best teacher would be a highly likely set, given our knowledge of the world. By contrast, in the absence of any explanatory context, (25) sounds somewhat less likely. Given what we know about the semantic properties of *even*, consider examples (26) and (27):

26. Even students taught by the best teacher passed the examination in the summer.

27. Even students taught by the worst teacher passed the examination in the summer.

With the minimal change of *even* being substituted for *only*, the felicity of the sentences is reversed. Since *even* signals an unexpected event, it now becomes felicitous to state that students taught by the worst teacher passed the exam, as this event may be somewhat unexpected, or surprising, and thus fits with the use of *even*. On the other hand, (26) is now incongruous, as the information it conveys is not surprising and so does not justify the use of *even*. Thus, one way to investigate how different particles influence sentence processing is to examine what happens when the lexical properties of the particles are congruous or incongruous with information supplied by subsequent text.

Filik et al. (2009, Experiment 1) found that this reversal in felicity for sentences containing *only* and *even* was reflected in readers' eye movement behaviour, with shorter reading times when information supplied by the text was congruous with the particle. The eye movement data also revealed a difference in how rapidly these effects emerge. For sentences with *only*, the incongruence would appear to be calculated fairly quickly, and effects were observed in first-pass reading times on the critical region (e.g. *passed the examination*), which is the earliest point in the sentence at which the incongruity could become apparent. By contrast, effects for sentences with *even* appeared to emerge more slowly, and were observed only in first-pass reading times on the post-critical region (e.g. *in the summer*). Readers were also more likely to make a regression back to the region of text containing the focus particle when sentences with *even* described a normally likely set of events (e.g. (26)). Filik et al. suggested that this may reflect the influence of higher-order language processing on the control of regressions. Specifically, as *even* signals the appearance of unexpected information, the subsequent description of relatively *likely* circumstances is incongruous with its use. Thus, the subject of the sentence might need to be re-evaluated in relation to expectations in order to achieve a felicitous interpretation (see Mitchell et al., 2008, for discussion of factors involved in guiding regressive eye movements). The absence of similar reading time or regression effects for sentences without *only* or *even* (Experiment 2) indicated that the effects were indeed due to the inclusion of a focus particle. Thus, this final study shows that highly complex semantic-pragmatic information associated with different focus-sensitive particles has a significant influence on the comprehension of sentences that are read normally. Moreover, these effects are revealed in the patterns of eye movements made during reading.

Conclusions and future directions

It should be clear from this review that focus has a wide-ranging influence on reading, from influencing processing at the level of the individual word, to the processing of reference, and to the computation of the structure and meaning of a sentence. Readers' eye movements are clearly sensitive to these effects, as effects of focus have been readily observed in eye movement behaviour at each of these levels of language processing. The research has also addressed the question of *when* focus exerts an influence on eye movement behaviour. Studies of the effects of focus at the level of the individual word dispute whether focus effects emerge relatively early in the eye movement record, and so influence the encoding of words, or only exert their influence at a later stage in text processing. Other research investigating the influence of focus on the processing of the structure and meaning of sentences has shown that that focus can exert a relatively rapid influence on eye movement behaviour when comprehension is disrupted. This research suggests that there is a complex interplay between different levels of linguistic information during the processing of structural ambiguities and sentence interpretation, and so makes a valuable contribution to understanding how higher-order language processing affects the reading and understanding of text.

Possible avenues for future research include further investigation of factors affecting the time-course of the influence of focus effects on eye movements during reading. For example, a key issue concerns whether recent findings reported by Birch and Rayner (2010) revealing an effect of focus in eye movement measures usually associated with early stages of word processing can be shown more generally. Birch and Rayner suggest that the much earlier appearance of an effect in their study as compared to previous studies may be due to differences between the unfocused conditions used in their experiments compared to other experiments. However, this remains to be demonstrated conclusively. Other factors may also be important and are worthy of further research. For instance, studies of focus at the level of the individual word have largely investigated cases where the contrast set was implicit and must be inferred by the reader, and it is possible that making the contrast set explicit would produce more pervasive and/or earlier effects in processing. In addition, given the relationship between focus and the allocation of cognitive resources, possible research directions include further investigation of the relationship between focus and eye movements during reading throughout the lifespan, or under different cognitive load conditions (see e.g. Price, 2008, for initial work on focus and eye movements during reading in older adults). Furthermore, it is apparent from this review that there is currently a paucity of research investigating eye movements and focus in languages other than English. It seems likely that interesting questions related to focus may be addressed in other languages and even cross-linguistically. Finally, the challenge remains to integrate these findings within contemporary models of eye movement behaviour.

References

Altmann, G.T.M., and Steedman, M. (1988). Interaction with context during human sentence processing. *Cognition*, **30**, 191–238.

Almor, A. (1999). Noun–phrase anaphora and focus: the informational load hypothesis. *Psychological Review*, **106**, 748–765.

Almor, A. and Eimas, P.D. (2008). Focus and noun-phrase anaphors in spoken language comprehension. *Language and Cognitive Processes*, **23**, 201–225.

Arnold, J.E. (1998). Reference form and discourse patterns. Unpublished doctoral dissertation, Stanford University, California.

Arnold, J.E. (2008). THE BACON not the bacon: How children and adults understand accented and unaccented noun phrases. *Cognition*, **108**, 69–99.

Bennett, J. (1982). Even if. *Linguistics and Philosophy*, **5**, 403–418.

Binder, K.S., and Morris, R.K. (1995). Eye movements and lexical ambiguity resolution: Effects of prior encounter and discourse topic. *Journal of Experimental Psychology: Learning, Memory, and Cognition*, **21**, 1–11.

Birch, S.L., Albrecht, J.E., and Myers, J.L. (2000). Syntactic focusing structures influence discourse processing. *Discourse Processes*, **30**, 285–304.

Birch, S. and Clifton, C. (1995). Focus, accent, and argument structure: Effects on language comprehension. *Language and Speech*, **38**, 365–391.

Birch, S. and Clifton, C. (2002). Effects of varying focus and accenting adjuncts on the comprehension of utterances. *Journal of Memory and Language*, **47**, 571–588.

Birch, S.L. and Garnsey, S.M. (1995). The effect of focus on memory for words in sentences. *Journal of Memory and Language*, **34**, 232–267.

Birch, S.L. and Rayner, K. (1997). Linguistic focus affects eye movements during reading. *Memory and Cognition*, **25**, 653–660.

Birch, S.L. and Rayner, K. (2010). Effects of syntactic prominence on eye movements during reading. *Memory and Cognition*, **38**, 740–752.

Bock, J.K. and Mazzella, J.R. (1983). Intonational marking of given and new information: Some consequences for comprehension. *Memory and Cognition*, **11**, 64–76.

Bredart, S. and Modolo, K. (1988). Moses strikes again: Focalization effect on a semantic illusion. *Acta Psychologica*, **67**, 135–144.

Breen, M. and Clifton, C. (2008, November). Lexical stress effects in silent reading. Poster presented at the 49th Annual Meeting of the Psychonomic Society, Chicago, USA.

Britt, M.A., Perfetti, C.A., Garrod, S., and Rayner, K. (1992). Parsing in discourse: Context effects and their limits. *Journal of Memory and Language*, **31**, 293–314.

Carlson, K. (2004, September). Only in context. Paper presented at the Architectures and Mechanisms for Language Processing conference, Aix-en-Provence, France.

Carlson, K., Frazier, L., Clifton, C., and Dickey, M.W. (2005, March/April). How contrastive is contrastive focus? Paper presented at the 18th Annual CUNY Sentence Processing Conference, Tucson, AZ.

Carlson, K., Dickey, M.W. Frazier, L., and Clifton, C., Jr. (2009). Information structure in sentence comprehension. *Quarterly Journal of Experimental Psychology*, **62**, 114–139.

Carpenter, P.A. and Just, M.A. (1977). Reading comprehension as eyes see it. In M. A. Just and P. A. Carpenter (eds.) *Cognitive processes in comprehension* (pp. 100–139). Hillsdale, NJ: Erlbaum.

Chomsky, N. (1971). Deep structure, surface structure, and semantic interpretation. In D. Steinberg and L. Jakobovits (eds.) *Semantics: An interdisciplinary reader in philosophy, linguistics, and philosophy* (pp. 183–216). New York: Cambridge University Press.

Clifton, C., Bock, J., and Rado, J. (2000). Effects of the focus particle only and intrinsic contrast on comprehension of reduced relative clauses. In A. Kennedy, R. Radach, D. Heller and J. Pynte (eds.) *Reading as a Perceptual Process* (pp. 591–619). Amsterdam: Elsevier.

Clifton, C., Jr, Staub, A., and Rayner, K. (2007). Eye movements in reading words and sentences. In R.P.G. van Gompel, M.H. Fischer, W.S. Murray, and R.L. Hill (eds.) *Eye movements: A window on mind and brain* (pp. 341–371). Amsterdam: Elsevier, North-Holland.

Crain, S. and Steedman, M. (1985). On not being led up the garden path: The use of context by the psychological syntax processor. In D. R. Dowty, L. Kartunnen, and A. M. Zwicky (eds.) *Natural language parsing: Psychological, computational, and theoretical perspectives* (pp. 320–358). Cambridge: Cambridge University Press.

Cutler, A. and Fodor, J. A. (1979). Semantic focus and sentence comprehension. *Cognition*, 7, 49–59.

Engbert, R., Nuthmann, A., Richter, E., and Kliegl, R. (2005). SWIFT: A dynamical model of saccade generation during reading. *Psychological Review*, 112, 777–813.

Engelkamp, J. and Zimmer, H. D. (1982). The interaction of subjectivization and concept placement in the processing of cleft sentences. *Quarterly Journal of Experimental Psychology*, 34A, 463–478.

Fauconnier, G. (1975). Pragmatic scales and logical structure. *Linguistic Inquiry*, 6, 353–375.

Ferreira, F. and Clifton, C. (1986). The independence of syntactic processing. *Journal of Memory and Language*, 25, 348–368.

Filik, R., Paterson, K.B., and Liversedge, S.P. (2005). Parsing with focus particles in context: Evidence from eye movements in reading. *Journal of Memory and Language*, 53, 473–495.

Filik, R., Paterson, K.B., and Liversedge, S.P. (2009). The influence of *only* and *even* on on-line semantic interpretation. *Psychonomic Bulletin and Review*, 16, 678–683.

Foraker, S. (2004). The mechanisms involved in the prominence of referent representations during pronoun coreference. Doctoral dissertation, New York University. (UMI ProQuest Digital Dissertations.)

Foraker, S. and McElree, B. (2007). The role of prominence in pronoun resolution: Availability versus accessibility. *Journal of Memory and Language*, 56, 357–383.

Francescotti, R.M. (1995). *Even*: The conventional implicature approach reconsidered. *Linguistics and Philosophy*, 18, 153–173.

Frazier, L. and Rayner, K. (1982). Making and correcting errors during sentence comprehension: Eye movements in the analysis of structurally ambiguous sentences. *Cognitive Psychology*, 14, 178–210.

Gennari, S. Meroni, L., and Crain, S. (2004). Rapid relief of stress in dealing with ambiguity. In J. C. Trueswell and M. K. Tanenhaus (eds.) *Approaches to studying world-situated language use: Bridging the language-as-product and language-as-action traditions* (pp. 245–260). Cambridge, MA: MIT Press.

Gergely, G. (1992). Focus-based inferences in sentence comprehension. In I. A. Sag and A. Szabolcsi (eds.) *Lexical matters* (pp. 47–65). Stanford: Stanford Center for the Study of Language and Information.

Gernsbacher, M. A. and Hargreaves, D. (1988). Accessing sentence participants: The advantage of first mention. *Journal of Memory and Language*, 27, 699–717.

Giannakidou, A. (2007). The landscape of EVEN. *Natural Language and Linguistic Theory*, 25, 39–81.

Gundel, J.K. (1999). On different kinds of focus. In P. Bosch and R. van der Sandt (eds.) *Focus: Linguistic, cognitive, and computational perspectives* (pp. 293–305). Cambridge: Cambridge University Press.

Halliday, M.A.K. (1967). Notes on transitivity and theme in English, Part 2. *Journal of Linguistics*, 3, 199–244.

Horn, L.R. (1989). *A natural history of negation*. Chicago, IL: Chicago University Press.

Hornby, P.A. (1974). Surface structure and presupposition. *Journal of Verbal Learning and Verbal Behavior*, 13, 530–538.

Ito, K. and Speer, S.R. (2008). Anticipatory effects of intonation: Eye movements during instructed visual search. *Journal of Memory and Language*, 58, 541–573.

Jackendoff, R.S. (1972). *Semantic interpretation in generative grammar*. Cambridge, MA: MIT Press.

Kadmon, N. (2001). *Formal pragmatics*. London: Wiley-Blackwell.

Kartunnen, L. and Peters, S. (1979). Conventional implicatures. In C. Oh and D. Dinneen (eds.) *Syntax and semantics II: Presuppositions* (pp.1–56). New York: Academic Press.

Kay, P. (1990). Even. *Linguistics and Philosophy*, 13, 59–111.

Kemper, S., Crow, A., and Kemtes, K. (2004). Eye fixation patterns of high and low span young and older adults: Down the garden path and back again. *Psychology and Aging*, 19, 157–170.

Kiss, K.É. (1998). Identificational focus versus information focus. *Language*, 74, 245–273.

Klin, C.M., Weingartner, K.M., Guzmán, A.E., and Levine, W.H. (2004). Readers' sensitivity to linguistic cues in narratives: How salience influences anaphor resolution? *Memory and Cognition*, 32, 511–522.

König, E. (1991). *The meaning of focus particles*. London: Routledge.

Liversedge, S.P., Paterson, K.B., and Clayes, E.L. (2002). The influence of *only* on syntactic processing of 'long' relative clause sentences. *Quarterly Journal of Experimental Psychology*, 55A, 225–240.

Lycan, W. (1991). Even and even if. *Linguistics and Philosophy*, 14, 115–150.

MacDonald, M.C. (1994). Probabilistic constraints and syntactic ambiguity resolution. *Language and Cognitive Processes*, 9, 157–201.

Malt, B. (1985). The role of discourse structure in understanding anaphora. *Journal of Memory and Language*, 24, 271–289.

McKoon, G., Ratcliff, R., Ward, G., and Sproat, R. (1993). Syntactic prominence effects on discourse processes. *Journal of Memory and Language*, 32, 593–607.

Mitchell, D.C., Shen, X., Green, M.J., and Hodgson, T.L. (2008). Accounting for regressive eye-movements in models of sentence processing: A reappraisal of the Selective Reanalysis hypothesis. *Journal of Memory and Language*, 59, 266–293.

Morris, R.K. (1994). Lexical and message-level sentence context effects on fixation times in reading. *Journal of Experimental Psychology: Learning, Memory, and Cognition*, 20, 92–103.

Morris, R.K. and Folk, J.R. (1998). Focus as a contextual priming mechanism in reading. *Memory and Cognition*, **26**, 1313–1322.

Moxey, L.M. and Sanford, A.J. (1993) *Communicating quantities: A psychological perspective*. Hillsdale, NJ; Lawrence Erlbaum Associates.

Moxey, L.M., Filik, R., and Paterson K.B. (2009). On-line effects of what is expected on the resolution of plural pronouns. *Language and Cognitive Processes*, **24**, 843–875.

Murray, W.S. and Liversedge, S.P. (1994). Referential context effects on syntactic processing. In C. Clifton Jr, L. Frazier, and K. Rayner (eds.) *Perspectives on sentence processing* (pp. 359–388). Hillsdale, NJ: Lawrence Erlbaum Associates.

Ni, W., Crain, S., and Shankweiler, D. (1996). Sidestepping garden paths: The contribution of syntax, semantics and plausibility in resolving ambiguities. *Language and Cognitive Processes*, **11**, 283–334.

Noteboom, S.G. and Kruyt, J.G. (1987). Accent, focus distribution, and perceived distribution of given and new information: An experiment. *Journal of the Acoustic Society of America*, **82**, 1512–1524.

Osaka, M., Nishizaki, Y., Komori, M., and Osaka, N. (2002). Effect of focus on verbal working memory: Critical role of the focus word in reading. *Memory and Cognition*, **30**, 562–571.

Paterson, K.B., Liversedge, S.P., and Underwood, G. (1999). The influence of focus operators on syntactic processing of 'short' relative clause sentences. *Quarterly Journal of Experimental Psychology*, **52A**, 717–737.

Paterson, K.B., Liversedge, S.P., and Filik, R. (2006, March). Focus assignment in reading. Poster presented at the 19th Annual CUNY Sentence Processing Conference, New York.

Paterson, K.B., Sanford, A.J., Moxey, L.M., and Dawydiak, E. (1998). Quantifier polarity and referential focus during reading. *Journal of Memory and Language*, **39**, 290–306.

Paterson, K.B., Filik, R., and Moxey, L.M. (2009). Quantifiers and discourse processing. *Linguistics and Language Compass*, **3**, 1390–1402.

Paterson, K.B., Liversedge, S.P., Filik, R., Juhasz, B. J., White, S. J., and Rayner, K. (2007). Focus identification during sentence comprehension: Evidence from eye movements. *Quarterly Journal of Experimental Psychology*, **60**, 1423–1445.

Pollatsek, A., Reichle, E.D., and Rayner, K. (2006). Tests of the E-Z Reader model: Exploring the interface between cognition and eye-movement control. *Cognitive Psychology*, **52**, 1–56.

Price, J.M. (2008). The use of focus cues in healthy aging. Unpublished doctoral thesis, University of Glasgow, UK.

Radford, A. (1997). *Syntactic theory and the structure of English*. Cambridge: Cambridge University Press.

Rayner, K. (1998). Eye movements in reading and information processing: 20 years of research. *Psychological Bulletin*, **124**, 372–422.

Rayner, K. and Duffy, S.A. (1986). Lexical complexity and fixation times in reading: Effects of word frequency, verb complexity, and lexical ambiguity. *Memory and Cognition*, **14**, 191–201.

Reichle, E.D., Pollatsek, A., Fisher, D.L., and Rayner, K. (1998). Toward a model of eye movement control in reading. *Psychological Review*, **105**, 125–157.

Reichle, E.D., Rayner, K., and Pollatsek, A. (2003). The E-Z Reader model of eye-movement control in reading: Comparisons to other models. *Behavioral and Brain Sciences*, **26**, 445–526

Reichle, E.D., Warren, T., and McConnell, K. (2009). Using E-Z Reader to model the effects of higher level language processing on eye movements during reading. *Psychonomic Bulletin and Review*, **16**, 1–21.

Reinhart, T. (1999). The processing cost of reference-set computation: Guess patterns in acquisition *OTS working papers in linguistics*. Utrecht: Utrecht University.

Reilly, R. and Radach, R. (2006). Some empirical tests of an interactive activation model of eye movement control in reading. *Cognitive Systems Research*, **7**, 34–55.

Rochemont, M.S. and Culicover, P.W. (1990). *English focus constructions and the theory of grammar*. New York: Cambridge University Press.

Rooth, M. (1992). A theory of focus interpretation. *Natural Language Semantics*, **1**, 75–116.

Rooth, M. (1996). Focus. In S. Lappin (ed.) *The handbook of contemporary semantic theory* (pp. 271–298). Oxford: Blackwell.

Sanford, A.J. (2002). Context, attention, and depth of processing during interpretation. *Mind and Language*, **17**, 188–206.

Sanford, A.J. and Sturt, P. (2002). Depth of processing in language comprehension: Not noticing the evidence. *Trends in Cognitive Sciences*, **6**, 382–386.

Sanford, A.J. Dawydiak, E., and Moxey, L. M. (2007). A unified account of quantifier perspective effects in discourse. *Discourse Processes*, **44**, 1–32.

Sauermann, A., Paterson, K. B., and Filik, R. (2009, September). Context influences association with focus in reading. Poster presented at the Architectures and Mechanisms for Language Processing Conference, Barcelona, Spain.

Schafer, A., Carlson, K., Clifton, C., and Frazier, L. (2000). Focus and the interpretation of pitch accent: Disambiguating embedded questions. *Language and Speech*, **43**, 75–105.

Sedivy, J.C. (2002). Invoking discourse-based contrast sets and resolving syntactic ambiguities. *Journal of Memory and Language*, **46**, 341–370.

Sedivy, J.C., Tanenhaus, M., Eberhard, K., Spivey-Knowlton, M., and Carlson, G. (1995). Using intonationally-marked presuppositional information to study spoken- language comprehension: Evidence from eye movements to a visual model. *Proceedings of the 17th Annual Conference of the Cognitive Science Society* (pp. 375–380). Hillsdale, NJ: Erlbaum.

Selkirk, E.O. (1995). Sentence prosody: Intonation, stress and phrasing. In J. Goldsmith (ed.) *Handbook of phonological theory* (pp. 550–569). London: Blackwell.

Singer, M. (1976). Thematic structure and the integration of linguistic information. *Journal of Verbal Learning and Verbal Behaviour,* **15**, 549–558.

Stolterfoht, B., Friederici, A.D., Alter, K., and Steube, A. (2007). Processing focus structure and implicit prosody during reading: Differential ERP effects. *Cognition,* **104**, 365–390.

Sturt, P., Sanford, A.J., Stewart, A., and Dawydiak, E. (2004). Linguistic focus and good-enough representations: An application of the change-detection paradigm. *Psychonomic Bulletin and Review,* **11**, 882–888.

Terken, J. and Noteboom, S.G. (1987). Opposite effects of accentuation and deaccentuation on verification latencies for given and new information. *Language and Cognitive Processes,* **2**, 145–163.

Townsend, D.J. and Bever, T.G. (2001). *Sentence Comprehension: The integration of habits and rules.* London: MIT.

Von Stechow, A. (1991). Focusing and background operators. In A. Werner (ed.) *Discourse particles: Pragmatics and beyond* (pp. 37–84). Amsterdam: Benjamins.

Ward, P. and Sturt, P. (2007). Linguistic focus and memory: An eye movement study. *Memory and Cognition,* **35**, 73–86.

Weber, A., Braun, B., and Crocker, M.W. (2006). Finding referents in time: Eye-tracking evidence for the role of contrastive accents. *Language and Speech,* **49**, 367–392.

Warren, T., and McConnell, K. (2007). Investigating effects of selectional restriction violations and plausibility violation severity on eye-movements in reading. *Psychonomic Bulletin and Review,* **14**, 770–775.

Warren, T., White, S.J., and Reichle, E.D. (2009). Wrap up effects can be independent of interpretative processing: Evidence from eye movements. *Cognition,* **111**, 132–137.

Wilson, D. and Sperber, D. (1979). Ordered entailments: An alternative to presuppositional theories. *Syntax and Semantics,* **11**, 299–323.

Zimmer, H.D. and Engelkamp, J. (1981). The given–new structure of cleft sentences and their influence on picture viewing. *Psychological Research,* **43**, 375–389.

CHAPTER 52

Eye movements in dialogue

Helene Kreysa and Martin J. Pickering

Abstract

Owing to their availability as easily measurable indicators of attention in the visual surroundings, eye movements can inform the study of dialogue in several different ways. This chapter provides an overview of three strands of dialogue-related research that have employed eye movements, summarizing the theoretical questions which have been addressed, the technical challenges involved, and promising areas for future research. First, eye movements have proved particularly useful as dependent measures in examining the role of common ground for reference resolution in temporally ambiguous utterances. A completely different use of eye movements has been made when comparing patterns of fixations between interlocutors: Here, they indicate the extent of coordinated attention. Finally, recent investigations into the role played by an interlocutor's gaze in comprehension and interaction draw on eye movements as an independent variable.

Why study eye movements in dialogue?

Eye movements have played an important role in psycholinguistics for many years, in particular as dependent variables in reading-based studies of sentence processing (Clifton et al., 2007; Rayner, 1998). More recently, innovations in eye tracking technology have reduced the need to constrain participants' head and body movements (Land, 2007). This makes it possible to record fixation behaviour during more interactive and world-situated language use (for a summary see Henderson and Ferreira, 2004).

In particular, the popular visual-world paradigm (Cooper, 1974; see also Altmann, Chapter 54, this volume) uses fixations in a pre-defined visual context as online indicators of how sentences are interpreted during auditory comprehension (Altmann and Kamide, 1999; Tanenhaus et al., 1995). Similarly, eye movements on a to-be-described image have also proved exceedingly useful for investigating the planning and formulation required for object naming and sentence production (Griffin and Bock, 2000; Meyer et al., 1998). In language production, the most pervasive finding has been the tight link between gazes and referring expressions: Generally, speakers consistently look at the object they are going to mention until just before they actually do so (Bock et al., 2003; Griffin, 2001). During comprehension, listeners show an equally strong tendency to fixate the objects that are being referred to, but the temporal relationship between fixation of an object and its mention is less fixed than in production. Thus, whether eye movements during comprehension follow (e.g. Allopenna et al., 1998) or precede referring expressions (e.g. Altmann and Kamide, 1999; Knoeferle and Crocker, 2006) depends in part on how well the representation which the listener has constructed so far corresponds to what they see around them, as well as on word frequency and other factors.

In addition, visual-world studies of comprehension have found consistent effects of the visual context on the earliest moments of syntactic processing (Knoeferle et al., 2005; Spivey et al., 2002; Tanenhaus et al., 1995). For instance, listeners' assessment of how a temporarily ambiguous instruction such as 'pour the egg in the bowl over the flour' could be carried out given real-world constraints (in this case, whether one or two eggs could be poured) influenced their syntactic analysis of the sentence as it unfolded (Chambers et al., 2004). In contrast, although reading experiments (e.g. Trueswell et al., 1994) also sometimes find very early context effects, in other studies they are quite delayed (e.g. Ferreira and Clifton, 1986), and the conditions that lead to immediate effects remain unclear and controversial (see Pickering and van Gompel, 2006). This raises the possibility that sentence processing may actually be more interactive in auditory contexts referring to matters at hand than in the reading tasks on which most traditional parsing models are based.

Yet the majority of experiments conducted in the psychology of language suffer from a critical limitation in this regard: They investigate language processing only in a monologue setting (see Pickering and Garrod, 2004). One reason for the lack of interest in dialogue is that most psycholinguistic theories are derived from formal linguistics, which has also focused almost entirely on monologue. Perhaps even more importantly, the controlled study of dialogue often appears too difficult, especially if the goal is to explicate mental representations and processes. Unlike a static stimulus presented in a neutral experimental booth, it is hard enough to control what one person says and when (Bock, 1996), let alone how their interlocutor responds. Hence, there can be good reasons for limiting an individual experiment to the monologue study of comprehension or production.

At the same time, key differences between language use in monologue and dialogue may limit the generalizability of potential findings. For instance, Tanenhaus and Trueswell (2005) pointed out that language which interlocutors generate and understand in interactive conversations can differ radically from the controlled and well-formed sentences used in studies of monologue and reading. As we shall see, dialogue is often characterized by fragments of utterances crossing speaker boundaries, ellipsis, repetitions, false starts, overlapping speech, and referential terms specific to that conversation and its context. In addition, dialogue is opportunistic and spontaneous. Thus, interlocutors often comprehend an utterance and simultaneously plan their own response, which they may subsequently need to modify again online. Finally, dialogue requires constant task-switching between the roles of speaker and listener. Considering these characteristics, holding a conversation is surprisingly easy—often easier than monologue activities such as giving a speech or writing a paper (Garrod and Pickering, 2004). In addition, conversation requires no formal training, as this is the form in which a child acquires language in the first place. Face-to-face conversation can therefore be seen as the primary and most basic form of language use (Clark, 1996; Fillmore, 1981; Garrod and Pickering, 2004). In its most typical form, dialogue is immediate. It is produced spontaneously and simultaneously by both interlocutors, and is inherently transient (Clark and Brennan, 1991). Indeed, Clark (1996) argued that forms of interaction which lack any of these basic dialogue features are experienced as more costly and difficult than simple conversation. This consideration has profound implications for many classic psycholinguistic research paradigms, where comprehenders are treated as overhearers rather than as addressees (Schober and Clark, 1989).

Accordingly, there are compelling reasons to try to overcome the theoretical and practical difficulties in studying dialogue, with the prospect that our knowledge of how people use language will be much enriched by such endeavours. Recording participants' eye movements during real-time interactions would seem to be a method well-suited to such investigations. One basis for our optimism in this regard is the substantial contribution of the visual-world paradigm towards our understanding of language comprehension and production—both of which obviously form an integral part of dialogue. In addition, modern recording systems have become fairly unobtrusive and are thus ideal for studying spontaneous and ongoing interactions between interlocutors (Tanenhaus and Trueswell, 2005).

The aim of this chapter is to provide an overview of the research conducted in this emerging field to date, as well as an introduction to the theoretical questions underlying these studies. To this end, we will review research in three separate, only loosely related areas, beginning with the debate on the observance of common ground versus more egocentric strategies of language processing. Next we will ask whether and how interlocutors coordinate their eye movements in dialogue, and how such coordination might relate to the ways in which their linguistic representations become aligned during a conversation. We will conclude by discussing how a partner's overt gaze can be exploited to facilitate comprehension.

The chapter will also highlight the methodological challenges that must be overcome to record and interpret eye movement behaviour in dialogue contexts. In fact, observant readers will notice that very few of the studies we cite have actually recorded eye movements from two (or more) participants in unscripted conversation, the most basic form of dialogue. To some extent, this is surely due to technical constraints, but also perhaps because researchers are still working out how to balance spontaneity with experimental control, as well as developing appropriate methods for analysing the data (see Carletta et al., 2010). At the same time, we believe that the scarcity of 'true' dialogue studies does not constitute a critical problem, since dialogue and monologue are not two dichotomous modes of language use. Instead, language is employed in many diverse ways, including casual conversation, formal interactions, and narratives. The issue is that traditional studies of monologue investigate one extreme of this continuum, whereas the research reviewed below is situated at different positions along its course, thus providing insights into more spontaneous language in different types of interactive settings.

Dialogue as joint action: the importance of common ground in reference resolution

Despite being instructed at school not to write as you would speak, most people don't realize just how far removed interactive dialogue is from formal prose. The following transcript reveals some of its characteristic features; it is part of a conversation between two students (A and B) in a joint *spot-the-difference* task, comparing photographs of a cluttered kitchen. (Note: square brackets indicate overlapping speech, with their position indicating roughly where it occurred.)

1. A: . . . and then two pots, maybe for sugar, I don't know, two white pots . . .

2. B: . . . are yours spotty?

3. A: No, they're just plain white.

4. B: Oh, I've got spotty ones.

5. A: OK. And then directly above the pots there should be a plug socket, and the orange light's on.

6. A: OK, to the right of the pots there should be Fairy [washing-up liquid] and a scrubbing brush . . .

7. B: Yeah, a blue scrubbing brush?

8. A: . . .   [uh . . .]

9. B: [well, blue-black,] looks like.

10. A: Yeah.

11. B: And green   [Fairy]

12. A: [Yeah.]

13. B: and then the sink

14. A: Mhm, with a white tray inside it

15. B: Yeah, and a chopping board just behind the sink

16. A: Yes. Yeah, we're going good here!

17. A: So, above the Fairy, on the window sill, I can see two wine bottles in a wine rack?

18. B: Yeah. Are they on the upper . . . [ones?]

19. A: [No, they're on the lower . . .]

20. B: Oh, mine are on the upper!

21. A: ok. Yeah,   [and they've got red . . . tops.]

22. B: [. . . and they're pointing down, yeah?]

Although their task is comparatively straightforward, these two interlocutors regularly produce elliptical and fragmentary utterances that would make little sense on their own (e.g. 9, 11, 13, 14, 20). The excerpt also features interruptions (2, 19, 22), overlapping speech (11/12, 21/22), and disfluencies (1, 8, 18), and it is generally quite repetitive. Yet the interlocutors appear satisfied with the conversation (16); they seem to understand each other—as do non-participants such as ourselves—and indeed they are successful in their task of discovering differences between the photographs they are looking at.

Clark (1996) argued that dialogue is generally successful because interlocutors collaborate in generating their conversation and achieving mutual understanding. He viewed it as a joint activity such as ballroom dancing, playing tennis, or completing a commercial transaction—coordinated actions of two or more participants advancing step by step towards a common goal (for a more recent review of research on joint action, see Galantucci and Sebanz, 2009). A successful interaction of this type does not mean that participants perform the same moves at the same time; rather, their moves must be carefully coordinated to complement each other. In conversation, this means that each utterance should be appropriate for the addressee at that particular point, which in turn requires the speaker to pay constant attention to any feedback (e.g. indicating whether a particular term has been understood). For example, A's hesitation at (8) caused B to modify and reformulate her potentially misleading description of the scrubbing brush. Hence, both participants were responsible for reaching the understanding signalled in (10): B was trying to produce an adequate description for A, but in order for her to accommodate his needs, he let her know when he encountered difficulties, and when they were resolved.

As in the example, most contributions to a conversation consist of two phases: a so-called *presentation* by a speaker, and its *acceptance* by the listener (Clark and Schaefer, 1989; Clark and Wilkes-Gibbs, 1986). Acceptance can be immediate, as when the listener takes or allows the next turn (e.g. 13/14/15, and 5/6, respectively), or responds appropriately to a question (e.g. 2/3). Alternatively, and in particular if there is a problem, he or she may first signal a need for clarification (e.g. 7/8). The contribution is only concluded when both participants are satisfied that the listener has reached a sufficient understanding for the present purposes. In this way, even an extensive conversation can be viewed as 'a chain of paired actions' (Clark and Bly, 1995, p. 385), consisting of many such individual contributions negotiated between the interlocutors.

One of the critical points speakers and listeners need to reach understanding on is which objects or events they are actually referring to. The problem of reference ambiguity and its resolution has been the subject of most of the studies to date which have recorded eye movements in interactive communication tasks. From a practical viewpoint, referring expressions are particularly suited to investigations using the visual-world paradigm, as they can be investigated by presenting participants with a limited number of easily identifiable objects, either as images on a computer screen or set out in grid fashion. This facilitates experimental control of the materials, as well as allowing a simple analysis of fixations to the regions of interest surrounding each object (though see Tanenhaus et al., 2000, and Henderson and Ferreira, 2004, on the limitations of such 'closed sets' and 'ersatz scenes', respectively). In addition, such displays can be combined with fairly natural experimental tasks: Typically, participants follow or provide instructions to move, manipulate, or click on pre-defined objects, either in response to recorded instructions or in interactive conversation. Eye movement measures in these studies are generally concerned with the amount of fixations on the target object relative to fixations on a depicted competitor. Although the statistical basis for this type of analysis is

under debate (e.g. Barr, 2008; Mirman et al., 2008), the most common practice is to compare proportions of saccades or fixations to the depicted objects within a specific time-window, generally defined
through the on- or offsets of critical words in the speech stream (see also Altmann, Chapter 54, this
volume). The rationale behind this analysis is that language users tend to look at whatever visible
entity best corresponds to the referent under discussion; thus the fixated entity can throw light on a
comprehender's current interpretation of the sentence, or, in production, on what the speaker is
going to mention next.

In monologue, some of the first applications of the visual-world paradigm found that listeners
fixated a named referent (e.g. *beaker*) within 400 ms of its linguistic disambiguation from any visible
cohort competitors (e.g. *beetle*) (Allopenna et al., 1998). More interestingly, instructions such as
'touch the plain red square' (in a context where two out of four available blocks were red and one of
these was marked with a square) seem to be processed incrementally; participants used each new
word to narrow down the potential referents, again fixating the correct object within 500 ms of the
final disambiguating word, in this case *square* (Eberhard et al., 1995). Further experiments showed
that vague referring expressions such as *the tall glass* are rapidly interpreted with regard to the available contrast set (i.e. whether other glasses are visible, and their relative size; Chambers et al., 2002;
Sedivy et al., 1999).

Reference ambiguity and its resolution is theoretically interesting for dialogue research because it
allows an insight into the extent to which speakers and addressees take each other's perspectives into
account when formulating and interpreting utterances. Definite references such as *the tall glass*, or
indeed pronouns such as *he* or *she*, are generally only felicitous when the referent can be uniquely
identified in the current context. But how far do addressees search for potential referents? What
constitutes the domain of reference has been hotly debated between supporters of an optimal design
account—which states that speakers design their utterances to be understood from the addressee's
perspective—and those who hold that production and comprehension are primarily egocentric, and
that knowledge about the interlocutor plays only a secondary role. We will summarize the two positions in the following, and relate them to the empirical evidence.

Common ground and optimal design

Clark and Wilkes-Gibbs (1986) observed that, over the course of a conversation, pairs of interlocutors tend to develop idiosyncratic expressions to refer to objects and concepts (e.g. using the term
ice-skater for an ambiguous tangram picture). They argued that accepting the initial contribution
containing this referring expression 'grounds' the term and makes it available for the interlocutors.
Consequently, it can be reused in subsequent turns without further specification, because both of
them now understand it as referring to that particular figure (for more detail, see Brennan and Clark,
1996). In Clark and colleagues' terminology, the expression has become part of '*common ground*': if
I am an interlocutor, this means I know that my partner knows the term, and that he or she knows
that I know this, and so on. The form of common ground described so far, which develops out of the
collaborative process of grounding contributions, is based on the linguistic copresence of the expressions in question (Clark and Marshall, 1981). *Linguistic copresence* here refers to the fact that, in the
course of their conversation, the interlocutors have together experienced the use of a particular
expression to refer to a specific object or concept. Another kind of common ground particularly
relevant to visual-world studies is *physical copresence*: Objects that all interlocutors know are visible
to everyone else, and that can therefore be referred to easily. Finally, common ground can be based
on *community membership*; for instance, we can assume that someone who has lived in Edinburgh
knows what 'Arthur's Seat' refers to, or that readers of this book will not require further explanation
of the term 'saccade'.

Importantly, Clark (1996) postulated that interlocutors adhere to the principle of *optimal design*,
producing and comprehending utterances that are consistent with common ground. On the one hand,
this implies that speakers formulate their utterances in such a way that the available common ground
limits the scope of possible interpretations to a single—correct—meaning. Conversely, addressees can

assume that the speaker will provide any information required to generate an appropriate and unambiguous parse, for instance when there are several potential referents. Optimal design thus predicts that only entities which are in common ground are considered as potential referents of formally ambiguous utterances.

Arguments for egocentric processing

However, it is also possible that interlocutors are more egocentric, interpreting and formulating references from their own perspective, rather than considering which facts are shared. They may make use of common ground only when time and resources allow, or perhaps during later but not initial processing.

For instance, Keysar and colleagues (Horton and Keysar, 1996; Keysar et al., 1998, 2000; Kronmüller and Barr, 2007) proposed a two-stage account in which addressees initially conduct a fast, unrestricted search for any suitable referent. Common ground is used only during later monitoring, and serves to correct errors of interpretation. Because it involves knowledge about knowledge, this is a cognitively demanding and relatively slow process. However, in dialogue, one's own knowledge is often a good proxy for relevant common ground (Bard et al., 2000; Pickering and Garrod, 2004). The speed and efficiency benefits of using an egocentric heuristic may therefore often outweigh the risks of occasional misinterpretation, particularly in an ongoing conversation.

To determine whether comprehenders behave egocentrically, many experiments provide the comprehender with a piece of information that he or she knows the speaker does not know. This item is *privileged* information for the comprehender, as opposed to the shared items in common ground. In one of the first published studies using eye tracking in dialogue, Keysar et al. (1998) used a version of the referential communication task (Krauss and Weinheimer, 1966) to investigate the comprehension of demonstrative reference. Participants were presented with a set of four pictures in a square array (e.g. a plane, a purse, some bowls, and a bird). They were asked to instruct an 'artist'—who was actually a confederate of the experimenter—how to colour an incomplete outline of one of these pictures (e.g. the plane). Simultaneously, they also heard instructions such as 'look at the bird' from the experimenter, allegedly for calibration purposes. These were presented via headphones, so the participants presumably assumed that the artist was not aware of them. But immediately following such a calibration instruction, the artist would sometimes ask a question related to a feature shared by the bird and the plane (e.g. 'Its wings, what colour are they?'). In this condition, participants were 180 ms slower to launch a saccade back to the plane than if they had been looking at an object without the critical feature (e.g. the purse). This indicated that they initially considered the bird's wings as referents, which were not in common ground, rather than the mutually available plane.

To test their perspective-adjustment account with regard to adjectival modification, Keysar et al. (2000) monitored the eye movements of an addressee who was following instructions from a confederate director to move everyday objects. These were positioned in a vertical lattice between the interlocutors, but the addressee could see that some slots were occluded from the director's view (see Fig. 52.1). In this example, a critical instruction would be 'Move the small candle beside the bottle'. If the addressee initially interpreted this instruction egocentrically, she would be expected to fixate the smallest candle on the bottom row, considering it as a potential referent. In contrast, if she immediately used common ground to restrict the potential referents, she should ignore this occluded candle, which was not physically copresent for her interlocutor, and consider only the middle-sized candle, which was the smallest one he could be aware of. Keysar and colleagues found that addressees in this test condition fixated the hidden object earlier and for longer than in the control case, where the smallest candle was replaced with a small monkey. In fact, on about a fifth of trials, they actually reached for or even picked up the critical object. Thus, despite being aware of the different status of shared and hidden objects, their eyes were still drawn to the hidden distractor, in accord with the perspective-adjustment account.

However, Hanna et al. (2003) pointed out that the critical hidden object was always the best perceptual match for the referring expression. Thus, the term *the small candle* fits the smallest candle

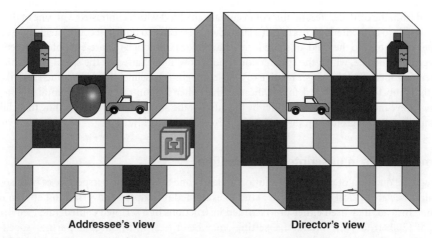

Addressee's view   **Director's view**

Fig. 52.1 Black slots were visible to the addressee but occluded for the director. The critical hidden object is the small occluded candle on the bottom row, visible only to the addressee. From B. Keysar, D.J. Barr, J.A. Balin, and J.S. Brauner, *Psychological Science*, **11**(1), p. 33, copyright (c) 2000 by Sage Publications. Reprinted by Permission of SAGE Publications.

of the three better than the middle-sized one, even if this is also small compared to the large one. It is therefore possible that addressees simply found it easier to look at the most typical referent. Hanna and colleagues also noted that the referents were not jointly entered into common ground, and that common ground was based on physical copresence only. In their own experiment, the speaker (again, a confederate) instructed the addressee to arrange shapes on a board. This ensured that critical referents were grounded via linguistic copresence, in that they had already been mentioned in the previous discourse. Each trial began with the addressee placing a 'secret shape' on the board. In the test condition, this 'secret shape' was identical to a referent the speaker would refer to in the critical utterance, for instance a red triangle in 'Now put the blue triangle on the red one'. The visual context for this utterance could thus include either one or two red triangles, of which one could be 'secret' or both shared. The critical question was whether a same-colour competitor would compete with the target as strongly when it was privileged information as when it was in common ground. This was not the case: Two competing shapes in common ground led to frequent shifts of fixation between the two, and participants often asked for clarification. In contrast, when one red triangle was shared and one secret, initial looks were more often directed to the (shared) target than to the (secret) competitor, and the proportion of looks to the target was consistently higher than to the competitor.

Two conclusions can be drawn from this result: On the one hand, the competing referent in privileged ground was not wholly ignored, so common ground did not completely restrict the domain of reference. At the same time, there was no evidence for an initially egocentric stage of processing, as argued by Keysar and colleagues; common ground contributed to reference resolution from the earliest moments of processing. Hanna et al. (2003) therefore suggested that alternative referential interpretations are assessed in parallel and based on multiple cues (see also Brown-Schmidt, 2009b). In this view, common ground is just one kind of contextual constraint, the strength of which depends on various factors. Using an innovative real-world design where the participant helped a confederate to bake cup-cakes, Hanna and Tanenhaus (2004) subsequently showed that affordances of the task can constitute another such constraint: Participants looked at different sets of objects depending on whether the cook's hands were full or empty when she uttered an ambiguous instruction.

Finally, Nadig and Sedivy (2002) showed that even five- and six-year-olds can make rapid use of common ground in reference resolution, as well as when producing instructions themselves (Experiment 1). In their comprehension study (Experiment 2), a confederate instructed children to move objects in a lattice. This was essentially a 2×2 version of the lattice used by Keysar et al. (2000): One slot was clearly occluded from the confederate, and this could contain an object which contrasted with one of the three objects visible to both interlocutors (e.g. if a large glass was visible to both, a second, smaller glass could be either visible only to the child, or shared with the speaker). Although the presence of a competitor in privileged ground (i.e. which the speaker could not know about) affected the speed with which the children first identified the target relative to a no-competitor baseline, they were much less likely to fixate the competitor object or ask for clarification than when the contrast was in common ground. The patterns of eye movements began to differ by the offset of the ambiguous noun, revealing that children can employ common ground for disambiguation exceedingly quickly.

Eye movements in unscripted conversation

Although the question of reference resolution is clearly one to which the perspective of both speaker and addressee are critical, none of these studies examined unscripted conversation between interlocutors. Instead, they used either pre-recorded instructions or a scripted confederate (see Brown-Schmidt (2009a) for why interactive settings may be critical to findings of partner-specificity; Kronmüller and Barr (2007) for arguments in support of pre-recorded instructions; Lockridge and Brennan (2002) for a discussion of the risks of using confederates). As an alternative, Brown-Schmidt and Tanenhaus (2008; Brown-Schmidt et al., 2008) have recently used *targeted language-games* to study referential communication. These are designed to elicit high proportions of the kind of utterance under examination (e.g. *wh*-questions), while allowing pairs of naïve participants to interact with each other naturally and to focus on the collaborative task they are performing.

In one study, pairs of participants described complementary patterns of blocks to each other, which were arranged in different subsections of large display boards (Brown-Schmidt and Tanenhaus, 2008). Both participants had the tasks of replacing stickers with blocks, and of ensuring that their interlocutor placed the same kind of block in the equivalent position on their board. In some cases, the pictures stuck to the blocks began with the same phonemes (e.g. *cloud* and *clown*). In monologue, such a situation would lead to competition, with listeners often looking at the wrong block until it was linguistically disambiguated (Allopenna et al., 1998). Indeed, this was exactly what was found in a control condition in which the experimenter named the blocks, allegedly for calibration. By contrast, the results in the interactive setting differed in an interesting way: Addressees looked at the correct picture (e.g. the cloud) well before their partner reached the point of disambiguation.

A second experiment helped to explain this finding. It confirmed that while speakers quite frequently produced ambiguous descriptions (e.g. *the green piece* when there was more than one green block on the board), addressees usually seemed to know which block was meant, fixating only the correct target. It seems that speakers considered only certain areas of the board as belonging to the referential domain, therefore specifying their descriptions only when the two conflicting blocks were actually within the same sub-area—and the fact that addressees were usually not troubled by the ambiguity shows that they had narrowed their referential domain in the same way. This result can be interpreted as a strong effect of common ground on both formulation and interpretation, but it also presents striking evidence for the alignment of the interlocutors' perspectives, in a way which could not be shown in monologue studies.

Brown-Schmidt et al. (2008) compared such a targeted language-game, involving pairs of naïve participants manipulating cards with animal pictures in a large lattice, with a more controlled version of the same task, where similar items were presented in a 3×3 array on a computer display, and the experimenter's utterances were scripted. Eye movements were recorded during both comprehension and production of *wh*-questions, such as 'What's above the cow with the shoes?'. The authors reasoned that if interlocutors shared a joint goal requiring the exchange of information, it would actually be appropriate (rather than egocentric) to consider privileged information when responding—after all, in a realistic setting, it is unlikely that the speaker would ask a question if he already knew the answer. Indeed, almost all unscripted *wh*-questions referred to information which was available only to the addressee. In both experiments, addressees' eye movements showed immediate sensitivity to common ground: On hearing a question which contained a temporarily ambiguous referent (for instance if the display contained both a cow with shoes and a cow with a hat), they directed their attention to the privileged information (e.g. a slot above one of the two cows which was occluded from their interlocutor) well before the point of linguistic disambiguation. Thus, Brown-Schmidt et al. (2008) concluded that there is no simple distinction between the strategies of egocentric processing or considering common ground. Instead—at least in situations where interlocutors share joint goals and can exchange information freely—whether and when addressees attend to privileged information or to common ground will depend on the circumstances, including the visual and linguistic context, as well as the task at hand (see also Brown-Schmidt, 2009a, 2009b).

In sum, common ground exerts an early effect on reference resolution, but numerous studies have also shown that interlocutors are by no means limited to optimal design considerations. As this section has illustrated, reference resolution is an area where findings and methods from monologue studies, in particular the visual-world paradigm, have been successfully transferred to more interactive contexts. These, in turn, have revealed just how finely tuned the coordination between interlocutors in the joint activity of dialogue can become.

Yet such studies employ eye movements only as indicators of what the speaker or listener is currently attending to. The next section considers the processes which produce this coordination between interlocutors. In this context, the study of eye movements serves a different purpose: Rather than considering how soon a particular object is fixated depending on the experimental condition, comparisons of the pattern of looks between interlocutors are used to examine the extent of their coordination. Research here is only just beginning, but we present some promising paradigms and future directions.

Coordination in dialogue

The interactive-alignment model

To provide a theoretical basis for the study of dialogue, Pickering and Garrod (2004) presented a model of collaborative and interactive language use, based on what they call *interactive alignment*. According to this account, dialogue is successful to the extent that interlocutors end up with aligned situation models (Johnson-Laird, 1983; Zwaan and Radvansky, 1998). This occurs if they generate similar representations of those aspects of the world which are relevant to their conversation: information about the individuals under discussion, the time, place, and so on. Pickering and Garrod proposed that interlocutors' situation models become aligned primarily as a consequence of automatic and non-conscious imitation or *priming* both within and between linguistic levels of representation. An example of within-level priming is the tendency for interlocutors to repeat each other's syntactic choices (Branigan et al., 2000). An example of between-level priming is the finding that such syntactic priming is enhanced if lexical expressions are also repeated or semantically related: More participants produce 'the sheep that's red' (rather than 'the red sheep') after hearing 'the sheep that's red' or 'the goat that's red' than after 'the book that's red' (Cleland and Pickering, 2003). On this account, priming provides an explanation for much of the repetitiveness of dialogue, as illustrated in the frequent recurrence of referring expressions in the transcript above (see also Garrod and Pickering, 2004, 2009). Accordingly, alignment at one level leads to alignment at other levels, with alignment at the highest level of representation, the situation models, resulting from alignment at lower levels. This means that interlocutors do not need to model each other's perspective extensively. Instead of maintaining separate representations of one's own and one's partner's knowledge of a situation—which is extremely resource-intensive to do—each interlocutor can rely on his or her own knowledge state as a proxy for their interlocutor's. If they are well-aligned, this will not lead to misunderstandings.

Visual coordination and alignment

Since eye movements in production and comprehension are in general tightly linked to the utterance being produced or understood, it seems plausible that the coordination of linguistic moves and the alignment of representations between interlocutors might also be reflected in their eye movements. Exploring this possibility requires the ability to quantify the overlap of visual attention between individuals. Richardson and Dale (2005) recorded the eye movements of speakers talking about familiar TV characters, which were depicted on-screen. Using cross-recurrence analysis (Eckmann et al., 1987; Zbilut et al., 1998), speakers' gaze recordings were subsequently compared with the eye movements of listeners who heard the description while looking at the same display. Cross-recurrence analysis determines the number of occasions on which their fixations fall on the same object, either simultaneously or across different time lags between speaker and listener. Richardson and Dale found that listeners' patterns of fixation most resembled the fixations speakers had made about two seconds earlier, suggesting that listeners were indeed likely to repeat the speaker's gaze behaviour.

In fact, in a subsequent study where two interlocutors sat in different eye tracking labs and communicated via telephone, Richardson et al. (2007) found the greatest overlap of fixations without any lag at all. They suggest that this is because participants in dialogue take turns to speak and listen; correspondingly, their eye movements switch between leading and following their partner's, creating an average lag of zero. An alternative explanation, in line with Brown-Schmidt and Tanenhaus's (2008) data, is that precisely because participants are interacting in real-time, they are able to restrict their referential domains and coordinate more closely.

However, recent data from syntactic priming experiments in which participants' eye movements were monitored suggests that this global similarity between interlocutors' gazes does not apply to individual fixations while comprehending and producing similar sentences. Arai et al. (2011) found that even when interlocutors were syntactically aligned (i.e. when participants repeated a previously-heard sentence structure) the timing of gazes to the relevant entities differed between comprehension and production. In their experiments, participants and scripted confederates took turns describing simple line-drawings of transitive and ditransitive actions to each other (see Branigan et al., 2000). In line with previous research on monologue comprehension and production, fixations during production were tightly linked to upcoming sentence content, with the target structure exerting the strongest influence (Griffin and Bock, 2000; Meyer et al., 1998): Speakers tended to fixate each entity roughly one second before mentioning it. In contrast, although the structure of the sentence as a determinant of fixations increased in importance as it unfolded, fixations during comprehension were influenced by a variety of other factors as well, such as event roles (agents were particularly likely to attract fixations, especially at the onset of the sentence) and the layout of the display. In addition, some gazes in comprehension were confirmatory (i.e. fixating the entity after its mention; Allopenna et al., 1998), and others were anticipatory (predicting what would be mentioned next; Altmann and Kamide, 1999). This meant that while mentioned entities were generally fixated at some stage during both comprehension and production, the time-course of these gazes could differ quite radically between the two tasks.

The conclusions of Richardson and colleagues (Richardson and Dale, 2005; Richardson et al., 2007) and Arai et al. (2011) are based on very different tasks and analyses. The cross-recurrence analyses employed by Richardson and colleagues reflect the emergence of overall patterns of similar behaviour (i.e. fixations to the same object) between interlocutors (see also Bard et al., 2009; Richardson et al., 2009). In contrast, the more traditional visual-world analyses of Arai et al. are time-locked to critical linguistic events, and thus allow more fine-grained conclusions with regard to how language processing affects visual attention, depending on the interlocutor's current task. Taken together, the studies reported in this section suggest that, on the one hand, globally similar patterns of fixations can reflect understanding between interlocutors. On the other hand, at a more fine-grained level, the different determinants of and motivations for gazes in comprehension and production make it unlikely that precise alignment of visual attention plays a critical role in communicative interactions. Instead, it makes sense for comprehenders to integrate all available forms of information into their ongoing interpretation of the utterance, including the currently available visual context. Nonetheless, the situations that do lead to overlapping patterns of attention clearly merit further investigation, especially since other forms of movement and posture coordination are well-documented between interlocutors (Chartrand and Bargh, 1999; Shockley et al., 2009). Recording eye movements during interaction can serve two distinct purposes in such studies: Most obviously, they provide easily measurable indices of the extent to which interlocutors have become aligned, and are thus useful for exploring factors affecting alignment. In addition, coordination of eye movements causes the focus of attention to overlap between interlocutors. Such instances of shared attention in turn seem likely to improve the quality of the interaction itself (Richardson et al., 2007), an intriguing possibility which is certainly worth further exploration (see also Spivey and Dale, Chapter 30, this volume). In a similar vein, the final section of this chapter summarizes research on how interlocutors make use of each other's eye gaze to facilitate reference resolution and other instances of disambiguation, thus exploiting an additional clue to the content of the unfolding linguistic utterance.

The importance of gaze in interaction

We have already pointed out that there is a close link between eye movements and what is being said, both in production and in comprehension. Consequently, eye movements are informative about upcoming speech content, as well as about the extent to which an utterance has been understood correctly. This is particularly relevant in view of the fact that perceiving another person's gaze direction generates a strong incentive to follow their line of regard (Emery, 2000; Langton et al., 2000). But what information can be gleaned from an interlocutor's eye movements, and how can this be useful in interactive tasks?

Feedback for the speaker

Although dialogue involves contributions by both (or all) participants, at any point in time only one interlocutor tends to 'hold the floor' (e.g. Sacks et al., 1974). At the same time, we have already noted that addressees are generally not passive, and contribute in many ways—acknowledging with 'okay' or a head nod, querying with 'eh?' or 'who?', expressing surprise with 'oh!' or raised eyebrows. The availability of such backchannel responses and other forms of feedback has been shown to affect the nature and quality of speakers' narratives and descriptions quite dramatically (e.g. Bavelas et al., 2000). In fact, during face-to-face interaction, speakers actively recruit such information by looking at the listener at critical points, such as at possible turn-transitions (Bavelas et al., 2002).

Disambiguation for the addressee

From the point of view of the addressee, seeing where the speaker is looking is particularly useful for clarifying what he or she is talking about, since speakers show a strong tendency to fixate what they will mention next. For instance, Hanna and Brennan (2007) set up an unscripted referential communication task such that naïve pairs of participants were able to see each other's faces, but not their partner's view of the display. The director instructed the matcher to move coloured shapes arranged in a row between them, but in some cases the presence of a competitor shape (e.g. *a blue circle with five dots on it*) made the description temporarily ambiguous. In this case, matchers' eye movements showed that they successfully used the director's gaze to select the correct shape well before linguistic disambiguation, unless the competitor and target objects were positioned very close to each other (see Staudte, 2010; Staudte and Crocker, 2008, for a similar demonstration using robot gaze).

The advantages of face-to-face availability of the speaker's gaze are not always this clear, particularly if it is hard to work out where he or she is looking (Clark and Krych, 2004; Whittaker, 2003). Nevertheless, gaze as a component of the conversational context frequently provides an easily accessible clue to the utterance meaning and for resolving ambiguous reference terms, as well as reflecting the pragmatics of the interaction itself. Incidentally, another area where establishing reference on the basis of a speaker's gaze plays an important role is language acquisition, where it allows the child to determine the correct mapping between object and name (Baldwin, 1993; Bloom, 2000; Butterworth, 1995). Yet, because recruiting such gaze information generally requires at least two separate fixations (to the interlocutor's eyes, and to what they are looking at), we argue that the success of the dialogue does not depend on interlocutors exhibiting aligned patterns of eye movements, in the sense of following the same path of fixations. Thus, error-free comprehension may often be more likely to result from multiple rapid fixations of both the speaker's face and the larger visual context, than from inflexibly echoing the speaker's fixation pattern.

Gaze projection paradigms

Recently, a number of studies have used a projected cursor to study how knowledge of what one's interlocutor is attending to can be exploited in a joint task, whether this be referential communication, visual search, or collaborative construction. The focus of one or both participants' gaze is projected onto the workspace or into the visual world in form of a moving dot (e.g. Carletta et al., 2010; Velichkovsky, 1995). Processing such a cursor is clearly not the same as estimating an interlocutor's focus of attention by looking at his or her eye and head direction. In a sense however, the cursor may even be more likely to lead to coordinated patterns of attention than the availability of 'real' gaze, because one participant's gaze tends to be drawn to the cursor, which is based on the other participant's gaze. Thus, while it remains debateable how the processing of a gaze cursor compares to that of real gaze, such artificial cues do provide researchers with a means of investigating the importance of overlapping attention for language understanding. In fact, an additional advantage of this kind of stimulus is that it does not even require speaker and addressee to be physically or temporally copresent.

To our knowledge, the first report of projecting interlocutors' eye movements onto an experimental display in this way comes from Velichkovsky (1995). To explore the influence of shared attention on a cooperative problem-solving task, he asked experts, who had received previous practice, to provide verbal advice to novices solving computerized puzzles. Two conditions of additional visual feedback were compared to the baseline of unscripted conversation: A cursor on the novice's screen reflected either where the expert was looking or the position of the expert's computer mouse. A second experiment reversed the direction of the manipulation by projecting the novice's gaze to the expert's screen (for a similar design, see also Bard et al., 2008, 2009). Experts and novices both adapted readily to the novel forms of information, frequently using them deliberately as pointing devices. For instance, experts' instructions often took the form of: '*Take this (marked by eye or mouse), place it there (again marked)*' (Velichkovsky, 1995, p. 208). This supports the conclusion that the additional modality created a situation resembling direct physical copresence, which facilitated reference and grounding, and benefited understanding and task success (Clark and Brennan, 1991).

In Velichkovsky's (1995) experiments, the gaze cursor was useful in both directions: While the experts whose gaze was projected used it deliberately as a pointer, they also benefited from the feedback contained in the novice's gaze. This contrasts with findings by Bard and colleagues (Bard et al., 2007), who used a map task to study speakers' sensitivity to information indicating that their addressee had misunderstood them. Speakers described a path between landmarks on a fictitious map, allegedly for an addressee to follow. The feedback provided could be visual (in the form of a simulated cursor representing the addressee's gaze) or verbal (produced by a confederate addressee). Overall, when providing instructions in order to bring an erring addressee back on track, speakers tended not to exploit the location information provided by the gaze cursor; yet they responded to utterances that signalled problems by rephrasing their instructions, even when the cursor suggested that all was well.

In contrast, Brennan et al. (2008) reported an experiment where success depended precisely on being able to avoid following the gaze cursor. Pairs of participants performed a collaborative visual search task, looking for a letter O in an array of Qs. The availability of the partner's (real) gaze in the form of an on-screen cursor led to substantial reductions in the time required to complete the task; strikingly, even a condition which allowed both verbal and visual feedback delayed task completion compared to seeing only the gaze cursor, though this may be an effect of the specific task. One of the most interesting aspects of this study is that although participants' eye movements must primarily have been driven by the search task rather than any intention to communicate with their partner, they clearly monitored for the moving cursor and interpreted it as exactly what it was: their partner's gaze.

At the same time, the usefulness of the gaze cursor in this task cannot be simply explained through bottom-up attraction of attention to the moving cue: If participants only followed the cursor instead of searching independent regions of the screen they would not have been faster to locate the target than a single participant searching alone.

Finally, one of the most convincing applications of a gaze cursor comes from Yu et al. (2005) and is reported as part of a larger investigation into how language acquisition is affected by so-called 'embodied intentions' (i.e. body movements relating to language). In their study, eye movements were recorded from a Mandarin Chinese speaker as he related a children's picture-book in his own words. The narrative was played to monolingual adult Americans, who were subsequently tested on Mandarin word segmentation and semantics. Those who had heard only the audio recording were no better than chance at these tasks, but the two groups who had seen a video as well had learnt a considerable amount of Mandarin. This was particularly the case for participants who had seen a cursor reflecting the speaker's eye movements, as opposed to those who just saw a video of the book. Yu et al. proposed that the gaze cursor is more effective than the simple video because it maintains the tight time-lock between speech and body movements, which they claim is essential for filtering meaningful word-object pairings out of a continuous speech and gaze stream.

However, recent data from a series of experiments suggests that the precise time-lock is not critical for profiting from a speaker's gaze cursor while searching for objects described in a familiar language (Kreysa, 2009). An unscripted speaker's verbal descriptions of photographs of cluttered rooms were recorded, together with his eye gaze. Listeners heard these descriptions and were asked to click on the described objects as quickly as possible. They also saw a gaze cursor, but its connection with the speech utterance was sometimes manipulated both spatially and temporally. For instance, the cursor could be shifted ahead or delayed in time relative to the speech with which the corresponding fixation would naturally have co-occurred. In general, listeners integrated the visual and verbal information, and benefited substantially from the availability of any gaze cursor that was roughly consistent with the utterance. This was apparent both in earlier first fixations to the target objects, and earlier mouse-clicks identifying them. The precise lag between cursor and speech made little difference, as long as they were clearly linked. At the same time, if the cursor conflicted with the speech utterance or did not provide additional information (e.g. if it was substantially delayed relative to speech), listeners were also quite successful at ignoring the gaze cue.

Without a doubt then, speaker gaze provides listeners with useful information regarding the identity of objects that are being mentioned. This seems to be the case irrespective of whether gaze direction is extracted in a face-to-face situation (e.g. Hanna and Brennan, 2007) or is projected to the screen in form of a gaze cursor (e.g. Yu et al., 2005). In some situations, it seems likely that speakers will also benefit from seeing a projection of their addressee's gaze, at least in the sense that it allows them to modify their utterances in accordance with the addressee's current needs.

Conclusions and outlook

In summary, eye movements have been employed in studies of interactive language use for at least three different purposes: as a fine-grained measure for assessing interlocutors' consideration of common ground, as a more global estimate of coordination between interlocutors, and as a means of conveying conversationally relevant information in the form of gaze. We have summarized the most important paradigms and findings in the three sections of this chapter.

Research in this area is only just taking off and has a highly exploratory character, at least in the two latter areas; many conclusions must therefore remain tentative at present. In fact, the three strands of research summarized here are by no means exclusive, and it seems likely that eye movements can prove useful as measures of attention in many other ways. In addition to the research mentioned above, one area they seem eminently suited to investigating is the study of spatial perspective-taking (e.g. Tversky and Hard, 2009). The fact that the technical requirements for recording eye movements are rapidly becoming both cheaper and easier to implement also opens up considerable potential for exploiting them in applied contexts, as does the availability of high-powered computers to deal with the resulting quantities of data in innovative ways. The use of gaze projection in remote learning and tuition settings (cf. Yu et al., 2005) or for error-detection and problem-solving (e.g. Stein and Brennan, 2004) are just two examples of interesting applications.

Yet the diversity of the studies reviewed in this chapter has also shown that there is no single eye movement measure that adequately reflects all the factors affecting language production and comprehension, let alone the development of a conversation over time. Instead, the selection of a suitable measure (e.g. fixation proportions, saccade latencies, durations, target detection rates, cross-recurrence patterns, scan paths, and probably others as well) will depend on the research question, the available equipment, and the type of interaction examined. More generally, studies of dialogue are also faced with the difficulty of taking into account the spontaneous nature of interactive language, while maintaining sufficient control over experimental conditions. This requirement will hopefully lead to the development of creative new experimental designs and novel methods of analysis (for recent examples, see Carletta et al., 2010; Koesling et al., in press; Nappa and Arnold, 2009), as will technological progress in this area. Thus, current state-of-the-art eye trackers show vast improvements in accuracy, flexibility, and simplicity of use, and even value for money, compared to their predecessors of just a few years ago. At the same time, these exciting advances urgently require the development of more specific theoretical models of the link between fixation behaviour and speech processing in interactive contexts than are currently available.

In addition, we must bear in mind that one of the prime motivations for using language at all—both in monologue and in dialogue—is to communicate about things that are *not* physically co-present. The extent to which eye movements can be used in the study of more abstract language remains to be seen, though initial findings seem surprisingly promising. For example, changes in fixation patterns have been reported due to imagined changes to a scene (Altmann and Kamide, 2009), while Richardson et al. (2009) reported coordination of eye movements affected by beliefs about what an interlocutor can see. Despite undeniable challenges, we hope therefore to have shown that eye movements are extremely well-suited to investigating quite diverse aspects of processing in dialogue, and expect to see many interesting research questions addressed in this way in the coming years.

Acknowledgements

This chapter and our thoughts on the issues we discuss here have benefited substantially from fruitful discussions with many different people. Among these, we would particularly like to thank Sarah Haywood, Manabu Arai, Ellen Bard, Holly Branigan, and Gerry Altmann for their comments and contributions.

References

Allopenna, P.D., Magnuson, J.S., and Tanenhaus, M.K. (1998). Tracking the time course of spoken word recognition using eye movements: Evidence for continuous mapping models. *Journal of Memory and Language*, 38, 419–439.

Altmann, G.T.M. and Kamide, Y. (1999). Incremental interpretation at verbs: Restricting the domain of subsequent reference. *Cognition*, 73, 247–264.

Altmann, G.T.M. and Kamide, Y. (2009). Discourse-mediation of the mapping between language and the visual world: Eye movements and mental representation. *Cognition*, 111, 55–71.

Arai, M., Kreysa, H., Haywood, S.L., and Pickering, M.J. (2011). How language mediates between mind and eye in comprehension and production. Unpublished manuscript.

Baldwin, D.A. (1993). Infants' ability to consult the speaker for clues to word reference. *Journal of Child Language*, 20, 395–418.

Bard, E.G., Hill, R.L., and Arai, M. (2009). Referring and gaze alignment: Accessibility is alive and well in situated dialogue. Paper presented at the 31st Annual Conference of the Cognitive Science Society, Amsterdam, NL.

Bard, E.G., Hill, R.L., and Foster, M.E. (2008). What tunes accessibility of referring expressions in task-related dialogue? Paper presented at the 30th Annual Conference of the Cognitive Science Society, Washington, D.C.

Bard, E.G., Anderson, A.H., Sotillo, C., Aylett, M.P., Doherty-Sneddon, G., and Newlands, A. (2000). Controlling the intelligibility of referring expressions in dialogue. *Journal of Memory and Language*, 42, 1–22.

Bard, E.G., Anderson, A.H., Chen, Y., Nicholson, H.B.M., Havard, C., and Dalzel-Job, S. (2007). Let's you do that: Sharing the cognitive burdens of dialogue. *Journal of Memory and Language*, **57**, 616–641.

Barr, D.J. (2008). Analyzing 'visual world' eyetracking data using multilevel logistic regression. *Journal of Memory and Language*, **59**, 457–474.

Bavelas, J.B., Coates, L., and Johnson, T. (2000). Listeners as co-narrators. *Journal of Personality and Social Psychology*, **79**, 941–952.

Bavelas, J.B., Coates, L., and Johnson, T. (2002). Listener responses as a collaborative process: The role of gaze. *Journal of Communication*, **52**, 566–580.

Bloom, P. (2000). *How Children Learn the Meanings of Words*. Cambridge, MA: MIT Press.

Bock, K. (1996). Language production: Methods and methodologies. *Psychonomic Bulletin and Review*, **3**, 395–421.

Bock, K., Irwin, D.E., Davidson, D.J., and Levelt, W.J.M. (2003). Minding the clock. *Journal of Memory and Language*, **48**, 653–685.

Branigan, H.P., Pickering, M.J., and Cleland, A.A. (2000). Syntactic co-ordination in dialogue. *Cognition*, **75**, B13–25.

Brennan, S.E., and Clark, H.H. (1996). Conceptual pacts and lexical choice in conversation. *Journal of Experimental Psychology: Learning, Memory, and Cognition*, **22**, 1482–1493.

Brennan, S.E., Chen, X., Dickinson, C.A., Neider, M.B., and Zelinsky, G.J. (2008). Coordinating cognition: The costs and benefits of shared gaze during collaborative search. *Cognition*, **106**, 1465–1477.

Brown-Schmidt, S. (2009a). Partner-specific interpretation of maintained referential precedents during interactive dialog. *Journal of Memory and Language*, **61**, 171–190.

Brown-Schmidt, S. (2009b). The role of executive function in perspective taking during online language comprehension. *Psychonomic Bulletin and Review*, **16**, 893–900.

Brown-Schmidt, S. and Tanenhaus, M.K. (2008). Real-time investigation of referential domains in unscripted conversation: A targeted language game approach. *Cognitive Science*, **32**, 643–684.

Brown-Schmidt, S., Gunlogson, C., and Tanenhaus, M.K. (2008). Addressees distinguish shared from private information when interpreting questions during interactive conversation. *Cognition*, **107**, 1122–1134.

Butterworth, G. (1995). Origins of mind in perception and action. In C. Moore and P.J. Dunham (eds.) *Joint Attention. Its Origins and Role in Development* (pp. 29–40). Hillsdale, NJ: LEA.

Carletta, J., Hill, R.L., Nicol, C., Taylor, T., de Ruiter, J.P., and Bard, E.G. (2010). Eyetracking for two-person tasks with manipulation of a virtual world. *Behavior Research Methods, Instruments, & Computers*, **42**, 254–265.

Chambers, C.G., Tanenhaus, M.K., and Magnuson, J.S. (2004). Actions and affordances in syntactic ambiguity resolution. *Journal of Experimental Psychology: Learning, Memory, and Cognition*, **30**, 687–696.

Chambers, C.G., Tanenhaus, M.K., Eberhard, K.M., Filip, H., and Carlson, G.N. (2002). Circumscribing referential domains during real-time language comprehension. *Journal of Memory and Language*, **47**, 30–49.

Chartrand, T.L. and Bargh, J.A. (1999). The chameleon effect: The perception-behavior link and social interaction. *Journal of Personality and Social Psychology*, **76**, 893–910.

Clark, H.H. (1996). *Using Language*. Cambridge: Cambridge University Press.

Clark, H.H. and Bly, B. (1995). Pragmatics and discourse. In J.L. Miller and P.D. Eimas (eds.) *Speech, Language, and Communication* 2nd edn. (pp. 371–410). San Diego, CA: Academic.

Clark, H.H. and Brennan, S.E. (1991). Grounding in communication. In L.B. Resnick, J.M. Levine and S.D. Teasley (eds.) *Perspectives on Socially Shared Cognition* (pp. 127–149). Washington, DC: APA.

Clark, H.H. and Krych, M.A. (2004). Speaking while monitoring addressees for understanding. *Journal of Memory and Language*, **50**, 62–81.

Clark, H.H. and Marshall, C.R. (1981). Definite reference and mutual knowledge. In A.K. Joshi, B.L. Webber and I.A. Sag (eds.) *Elements of Discourse Understanding* (pp. 10–63). Cambridge: Cambridge University Press.

Clark, H.H. and Schaefer, E.F. (1989). Contributing to discourse. *Cognitive Science*, **13**, 259–294.

Clark, H.H. and Wilkes-Gibbs, D. (1986). Referring as a collaborative process. *Cognition*, **22**, 1–39.

Cleland, A.A., and Pickering, M.J. (2003). The use of lexical information in language production: Evidence from the priming of noun-phrase structure. *Journal of Memory and Language*, **49**, 214–230.

Clifton, C., Jr, Staub, A., and Rayner, K. (2007). Eye movements in reading words and sentences. In R.P.G. van Gompel, M.H. Fischer, W.S. Murray and R.L. Hill (eds.) *Eye Movements: A Window on Mind and Brain* (pp. 341–371). Amsterdam: Elsevier.

Cooper, R.M. (1974). The control of eye fixation by the meaning of spoken language: A new methodology for the real-time investigation of speech perception, memory, and language processing. *Cognitive Psychology*, **6**, 84–107.

Eberhard, K.M., Spivey-Knowlton, M.J., Sedivy, J.C., and Tanenhaus, M.K. (1995). Eye movements as a window into real-time spoken language comprehension in natural contexts. *Journal of Psycholinguistic Research*, **24**, 409–436.

Eckmann, J.-P., Oliffson Kamphorst, S., and Ruelle, D. (1987). Recurrence plots of dynamical systems. *Europhysics Letters*, **4**, 973–977.

Emery, N.J. (2000). The eyes have it: The neuroethology, function and evolution of social gaze. *Neuroscience and Biobehavioral Reviews*, **24**, 581–604.

Ferreira, F. and Clifton, C., Jr (1986). The independence of syntactic processing. *Journal of Memory and Language*, **25**, 348–368.

Fillmore, C. (1981). Pragmatics and the description of discourse. In P. Cole (ed.) *Radical Pragmatics* (pp. 143–166). New York: Academic.

Galantucci, B. and Sebanz, N. (2009). Joint action: Current perspectives. *Topics in Cognitive Science*, 1, 255–259.

Garrod, S. and Pickering, M.J. (2004). Why is conversation so easy? *Trends in Cognitive Sciences*, 8, 8–11.

Garrod, S. and Pickering, M.J. (2009). Joint action, interactive alignment, and dialog. *Topics in Cognitive Science*, 1, 292–304.

Griffin, Z.M. (2001). Gaze durations during speech reflect word selection and phonological encoding. *Cognition*, 82, B1-B14.

Griffin, Z.M. and Bock, K. (2000). What the eyes say about speaking. *Psychological Science*, 11, 274–279.

Hanna, J.E. and Brennan, S.E. (2007). Speakers' eye gaze disambiguates referring expressions early during face-to-face conversation. *Journal of Memory and Language*, 57, 596–615.

Hanna, J.E. and Tanenhaus, M.K. (2004). Pragmatic effects on reference resolution in a collaborative task: Evidence from eye movements. *Cognitive Science*, 28, 105–115.

Hanna, J.E., Tanenhaus, M.K., and Trueswell, J.C. (2003). The effects of common ground and perspective on domains of referential interpretation. *Journal of Memory and Language*, 49, 43–61.

Henderson, J.M., and Ferreira, F. (2004). Scene perception for psycholinguists. In J.M. Henderson and F. Ferreira (eds.) *The Interface of Language, Vision, and Action: Eye Movements and the Visual World* (pp. 1–58). New York: Psychology Press.

Horton, W.S. and Keysar, B. (1996). When do speakers take into account common ground? *Cognition*, 59, 91–117.

Johnson-Laird, P.N. (1983). *Mental Models. Towards a Cognitive Science of Language, Inference, and Consciousness* (Vol. 6). Cambridge, MA: Harvard University Press.

Keysar, B., Barr, D.J., Balin, J.A., and Paek, T.S. (1998). Definite reference and mutual knowledge: Process models of common ground in comprehension. *Journal of Memory and Language*, 39, 1–20.

Keysar, B., Barr, D.J., Balin, J.A., and Brauner, J.S. (2000). Taking perspective in conversation: The role of mutual knowledge in comprehension. *Psychological Science*, 11, 32–38.

Knoeferle, P. and Crocker, M.W. (2006). The coordinated interplay of scene, utterance, and world knowledge: Evidence from eye tracking. *Cognitive Science*, 30, 481–529.

Knoeferle, P., Crocker, M.W., Scheepers, C., and Pickering, M.J. (2005). The influence of the immediate visual context on incremental thematic role-assignment: Evidence from eye-movements in depicted events. *Cognition*, 95, 95–127.

Koesling, H., Sichelschmidt, L., and Ritter, H. (in press). Search strategies and mult-modal alignment in collaborative change detection. *Journal of Eye Movement Research*.

Krauss, R.M. and Weinheimer, S. (1966). Concurrent feedback, confirmation, and the encoding of referents in verbal communication. *Journal of Personality and Social Psychology*, 4, 343–346.

Kreysa, H. (2009). Coordinating speech-related eye movements between comprehension and production. *Doctoral Dissertation*, The University of Edinburgh.

Kronmüller, E. and Barr, D.J. (2007). Perspective-free pragmatics: Broken precedents and the recovery-from-preemption hypothesis. *Journal of Memory and Language*, 56, 436–455.

Land, M.F. (2007). Fixation strategies during active behaviour: A brief history. In R.P.G. van Gompel, M.H. Fischer, W.S. Murray and R.L. Hill (eds.) *Eye Movements: A Window on Mind and Brain* (pp. 75–95). Amsterdam: Elsevier.

Langton, S.R.H., Watt, R.J., and Bruce, V. (2000). Do the eyes have it? Cues to the direction of social attention. *Trends in Cognitive Sciences*, 4, 50–59.

Lockridge, C. and Brennan, S.E. (2002). Addressees' needs influence speakers' early syntactic choices. *Psychonomic Bulletin & Review*, 9, 550–557.

Meyer, A.S., Sleiderink, A.M., and Levelt, W.J.M. (1998). Viewing and naming objects: Eye movements during noun phrase production. *Cognition*, 66, B25–B33.

Mirman, D., Dixon, J.A., and Magnuson, J.S. (2008). Statistical and computational models of the visual world paradigm: Growth curves and individual differences. *Journal of Memory and Language*, 59, 475–494.

Nadig, A.S. and Sedivy, J.C. (2002). Evidence for perspective-taking constraints in children's online reference resolution. *Psychological Science*, 13, 329–336.

Nappa, R. and Arnold, J. (2009). Paying attention to intention: Effects of intention (but not egocentric attention) on pronoun resolution. Poster presented at the 22nd Annual CUNY Conference on Human Sentence Processing, Davis, CA.

Pickering, M.J. and Garrod, S. (2004). Toward a mechanistic psychology of dialogue. *Behavioral and Brain Sciences*, 27, 169–226.

Pickering, M.J. and van Gompel, R.P.G. (2006). Syntactic parsing. In M.A. Gernsbacher and M.J. Traxler (eds.) *Handbook of Psycholinguistics*, 2nd ed. (pp. 455–503). San Diego, CA: Academic.

Rayner, K. (1998). Eye movements in reading and information processing: 20 years of research. *Psychological Bulletin*, 124, 372–422.

Richardson, D.C. and Dale, R. (2005). Looking to understand: The coupling between speakers' and listeners' eye movements and its relationship to discourse comprehension. *Cognitive Science*, 29, 1045–1060.

Richardson, D.C., Dale, R., and Kirkham, N.Z. (2007). The art of conversation is coordination: Common ground and the coupling of eye movements during dialogue. *Psychological Science*, 18, 407–413.

Richardson, D.C., Dale, R., and Tomlinson, J.M., Jr (2009). Conversation, gaze coordination, and beliefs about visual context. *Cognitive Science*, **33**, 1468–1482.

Sacks, H., Schegloff, E.A., and Jefferson, G. (1974). A simplest systematics for the organization of turn-taking for conversation. *Language*, **50**, 696–734.

Schober, M.F. and Clark, H.H. (1989). Understanding by addressees and overhearers. *Cognitive Psychology*, **21**, 211–232.

Sedivy, J.C., Tanenhaus, M.K., Chambers, C.G., and Carlson, G.N. (1999). Achieving incremental semantic interpretation through contextual representation. *Cognition*, **71**, 109–147.

Shockley, K., Richardson, D.C., and Dale, R. (2009). Conversation and coordinative structures. *Topics in Cognitive Science*, **1**, 305–319.

Spivey, M.J., Tanenhaus, M.K., Eberhard, K.M., and Sedivy, J.C. (2002). Eye movements and spoken language comprehension: Effect of visual context on syntactic ambiguity resolution. *Cognitive Psychology*, **45**, 447–481.

Staudte, M. (2010). Joint Attention in Spoken Human-Robot Interaction. *Doctoral Dissertation*, Saarland University. Available at: http://scidok.sulb.uni-saarland.de/volltexte/2010/XYZ.

Staudte, M. and Crocker, M. (2008). The utility of gaze in spoken human-robot interaction. Paper presented at the HRI Workshop on Metrics for Human-Robot Interaction, Amsterdam.

Stein, R. and Brennan, S.E. (2004). Another person's eye gaze as a cue in solving programming problems. Paper presented at the ICMI 2004, Sixth International Conference on Multimodal Interfaces, Penn State University, State College, PA.

Tanenhaus, M.K. and Trueswell, J.C. (2005). Eye movements as a tool for bridging the language-as-product and language-as-action traditions. In J.C. Trueswell and M.K. Tanenhaus (eds.) *Approaches to Studying World-Situated Language Use: Bridging the Language-as-Product and Language-as-Action-Traditions* (pp. 3–37). Cambridge, MA: MIT press.

Tanenhaus, M.K., Spivey-Knowlton, M.J., Eberhard, K.M., and Sedivy, J.C. (1995). Integration of visual and linguistic information in spoken language comprehension. *Science*, **268**, 1632–1634.

Tanenhaus, M.K., Magnuson, J.S., Dahan, D., and Chambers, C. (2000). Eye movements and lexical access in spoken-language comprehension: Evaluating a linking hypothesis between fixations and linguistic processing. *Journal of Psycholinguistic Research*, **29**, 557–580.

Trueswell, J.C., Tanenhaus, M.K., and Garnsey, S.M. (1994). Semantic influences on parsing: Use of thematic role information in syntactic ambiguity resolution. *Journal of Memory and Language*, **33**, 285–318.

Tversky, B. and Hard, B.M. (2009). Embodied and disembodied cognition: Spatial perspective-taking. *Cognition*, **110**, 124–129.

Velichkovsky, B.M. (1995). Communicating attention: Gaze position transfer in cooperative problem solving. *Pragmatics and Cognition*, **3**, 199–223.

Whittaker, S. (2003). Things to talk about when talking about things. *Human-Computer Interaction*, **18**, 149–170.

Yu, C., Ballard, D.H., and Aslin, R.N. (2005). The role of embodied intention in early lexical acquisition. *Cognitive Science*, **29**, 961–1005.

Zbilut, J.P., Giuliani, A., and Webber, C.L. (1998). Detecting deterministic signals in exceptionally noisy environments using cross-recurrence quantification. *Physics Letters A*, **246**, 122–128.

Zwaan, R.A. and Radvansky, G.A. (1998). Situation models in language comprehension and memory. *Psychological Bulletin*, **123**, 162–185.

CHAPTER 53

Eye movements during Chinese reading

Chuanli Zang, Simon P. Liversedge, Xuejun Bai, and Guoli Yan

Abstract

Research on eye movements during Chinese reading is reviewed. We begin by briefly describing the basic characteristics of the Chinese writing system, and then address five main topics: 1) basic characteristics of eye movements during Chinese reading; 2) the influence of the intrinsic characteristics of Chinese orthography on eye movements (e.g. stroke complexity, frequency, predictability, and neighbourhood size); 3) selection of saccade targets during Chinese reading; 4) parafoveal effects (perceptual span, parafoveal preview effects, and parafoveal-on-foveal effects); and 5) developmental changes in eye movements during Chinese reading. Finally, some important theoretical issues associated with Chinese reading are discussed.

Overview

Eye movements have been extensively examined as an effective indicator of human visual information processing and cognition. They provide a valuable tool in revealing important aspects of online cognitive processing (Liversedge and Findlay, 2000; Rayner, 1998, 2009). During the past few decades a tremendous amount of research has investigated the characteristics of eye movements in reading. However, these investigations have mainly studied reading in alphabetic language scripts (see reviews by Rayner, 1998, 2009). In contrast, comparatively little research has explored eye movements during non-alphabetic scripts, even though these languages are widely used (Chinese, Japanese, Arabic, etc). This chapter focuses on reading of Chinese, a language that is used by one-fifth of the world's population. To our knowledge, the earliest eye movement study investigating Chinese reading was carried out by Miles and Shen in 1925 at Stanford University. They used photographic equipment to record readers' eye movements in the reading of Chinese text presented vertically and horizontally (Miles and Shen, 1925; E. Shen, 1927). Recently, more and more researchers who have endeavoured to understand the nature of Chinese written language comprehension have turned to the use of eye movement methodology. Research in this area has so far been largely empirical and some important aspects of eye movement behaviour during Chinese reading have now been established. There have even been preliminary attempts at computationally modelling eye movement control during Chinese reading (e.g. see Reichle, Chapter 42, this volume). In this chapter, we begin by briefly describing the basic characteristics of the Chinese writing system relative to the alphabetic writing system.

Basic characteristics of the Chinese writing system

Chinese characters

Unlike English (and other alphabetic writing systems), written Chinese is generally considered to be a logographic language comprised of characters, each of which occupies a square unit of space, but differs in their visual and linguistic complexity. Chinese characters are comprised of a variety of strokes with some simple features such as dots, lines, and curves. Different characters may vary in the number of strokes (e.g. one stroke as in '一' meaning *one*, up to 36 strokes as in '齉' meaning *sniffling*). The number of strokes in the characters of the Chinese language ranges from 1–36 for the 7000 most frequently used characters (Modern Chinese Commonly Used Character Stroke Order Standard, 1997).

It should be noted that there are two versions of Chinese characters: simplified and traditional characters. Traditional Chinese characters are more complex and are often comprised of many strokes. In 1956 the Chinese government published a 'Scheme for Simplifying Chinese Characters' specifying that Chinese characters should be changed to be visually simpler in order to promote literacy development. More recently in 1964 and 1986, the State Language Commission provided additional modifications to the list of simplified characters in an attempt to establish definite norms and clarify any confusion over the forms of Chinese characters. Thus, during this period the nature of Chinese characters was changed formally (see Yin and Rohsenow, 1994). Simplified Chinese characters are now used throughout mainland China, whilst traditional Chinese characters are mainly used in Taiwan and Hong Kong.

Chinese characters are comprised of a series of individual strokes; moreover, those strokes are often combined to form subcharacters termed 'radicals' (Taft et al., 1999). Radicals can be arranged in different positions to form the structure of characters. According to the *Dictionary of Chinese Character Information* (1988), Chinese characters may generally be classified into five categories on the basis of their structural form. A small proportion of characters can be taken as whole units called single-element characters (4%, like '人' meaning *person*). The majority of characters are compound characters with a left-right radical structure (65%, like '好' meaning *good*). Then there are top-bottom characters (21%, like '忘' meaning *forget*), enclosed characters (9%, like '闭' meaning *close*), and finally nested structure characters (1%, like '乘' meaning *multiply*) (see also Yin and Rohsenow, 1994).

Radicals often provide linguistic information concerning semantic and phonological properties of a character. About 90% of Chinese characters are compounds with semantic and phonetic radicals (Hoosain, 1991). For horizontally structured characters, the left-hand radicals are usually the *semantic* radicals, providing information concerning the meaning of the character (e.g. 女 means *female*, and 妈 means *mother*), whereas the right-hand radicals are usually the *phonetic* radicals, providing information concerning the pronunciation of the character (e.g. 马 is pronounced mǎ, and 妈 is pronounced mā). However, the relationship between characters and their radicals is not always so transparent or systematic for vertically structured characters (Taft and Zhu, 1997; Taft et al, 1999).

Generally, Chinese characters are most analogous to morphemes in alphabetic languages, though in very rare cases, a character may not be a morpheme on its own and is required to combine with another character, which is also not a morpheme on its own. For example, 葡萄 (means *grape*) in which the constituents 葡 and 萄 do not carry any meaning on their own and may serve to represent a syllable. Finally, as Chinese written language was developed from pictographs, a Chinese character often has a quite direct connection between its shape and its meaning. However, the correspondence between the shape and its pronunciation is relatively weak. Also, graphemically similar characters may have different pronunciations, and it is possible to come up with a set of Chinese homophonic characters that share no orthographic components (Feng et al., 2001; Inhoff et al., 1999; Sun and Feng, 1999).

Chinese words

Words in Chinese are comprised of one or more characters (on average 1.5 characters, see Sun et al., 1985). According to the *Modern Chinese Frequency Dictionary* (1986), a small proportion of Chinese words are formed by a single character (approximately 20%), while the majority are comprised of two characters (approximately 70%), and the remainder consist of three or more characters (approximately 10%). Thus, the majority of Chinese characters are actually constituents of compound words rather than being individual words in their own right.

In contrast to alphabetic languages, the notion of a word in written Chinese language is not completely unambiguous. There are no spaces (or other forms of demarcation) between words in Chinese text (the width of the space between words is identical to that between characters within a word). Furthermore, Chinese words do not have explicit physical or linguistic markers that specify their grammatical categories, nor inflectional indicators of number, gender, tense and other aspects (e.g. Bai et al., 2008; Chen, 1992, 1999; Chen et al., 2003; Wang et al., 2008). In fact, there can often be ambiguity concerning the lexical status of a character, that is, whether it constitutes a word or comprises part of a word (Hoosain, 1991, 1992). However, there is currently no evidence indicating that this ambiguity disrupts reading performance of Chinese readers (e.g. Bai et al., 2008; Inhoff et al., 1997).

There are some properties of Chinese words that affect eye movement behaviour in reading (Yang and McConkie, 1999; G. Yan et al., 2006). First, Chinese words vary in their visual complexity in terms of their constituent characters. For example, a two-character word may have high or low visual complexity for its first and second constituents. Second, Chinese words may vary in their frequency of use in the language. Also, the two individual characters of a two-character word may each be high or low frequency. Third, Chinese words may vary in the distribution of meaning across their constituents. As each Chinese character conveys meaning by itself, in some cases, each constituent character contributes equally to the meaning of the whole word (e.g. 城镇 meaning *urban area*, 城 means *city*, and 镇 means *town*), whereas in other cases, one of the constituents conveys more of the meaning than does the other (e.g. 石油 meaning *petroleum*, 石 means *stone*, and 油 means *oil*). Fourth, for a compound word, the meanings of the constituent characters may be transparent or opaque to the word meaning. Transparent words are those whose meaning is relatively obvious from the meanings of their constituent characters (e.g. the characters for '电' meaning *electricity*, '脑' meaning *brain*, combine to form the word '电脑' meaning *computer*), whereas for the opaque words, the meaning is not so apparent from the meanings of its constituent characters (e.g. the characters for '马' meaning *horse*, '虎' meaning *tiger*, combine to form the word '马虎' meaning *careless*). Finally, there are some special Chinese compound word pairs that are composed of the same two characters, but differ only in the order of their constituent characters, that is, AB-BA words, as one gets a legitimate word by reading either from left to right or from right to left. However, sometimes transposition of the constituent characters does not change the meaning of the compound words, e.g. '相互' (mutual) vs. '互相' (mutual), but sometimes the meaning of the compound words are changed completely after the transposition, e.g. '结巴' (stammer) vs. '巴结' (toady). Such words exist in English as well, for example, *dog* and *god* contain the same letters but in a reversed order.

Overall, Chinese written language is character based, with several intrinsically unique characteristics that are often quite different to those of alphabetic languages. Therefore, issues related to reading in Chinese are of particular interest. Furthermore, research with different languages is crucial in order to establish which aspects of eye movement behaviour during reading apply to a wide range of languages, which apply to certain kinds of languages, and which are language-specific.

Basic patterns of eye movements during Chinese reading

When we read, we continually make a series of short and rapid movements, called saccades, to bring new text into the centre of vision (Rayner, 1998, 2009; Reichle et al., 2003). Between saccades, our eyes remain relatively still for a brief period of time, called fixations, and during fixations the new information is processed (Rayner, 1998, 2009; Reichle et al., 2003). In alphabetic languages, the mean fixation duration is typically 200–300 ms, and the mean forward saccade (saccades that move forwards in the text) length is 7–9 character spaces. Regressions (saccades that move backwards in the text) occur about 10–15% of the time in skilled readers. However, it should be noted that there is considerable variability in these measures, depending upon the ease or difficulty involved in processing the currently fixated text, reading skill of readers, and characteristics of the writing system (Rayner, 1998, 2009 for a review).

Sun and Feng (1999) directly compared eye movements during the reading of Chinese and semantically equivalent English text. Their results showed that the mean fixation duration of Chinese participants who read Chinese text amounted to 257 ms, mean saccade length was 2.6 character spaces (ranging from 2.0–3.0 characters), equivalent to 1.7 words. Reading rate was 580 characters per minute, the equivalent of 386 words per minute. The mean fixation duration of native English speakers who read English text with the same content amounted to 265 ms, mean saccade length was 1.8 words, and reading rate was 382 words per minute (c.f., Chen et al., 2003; Gary, 1956; Inhoff and Liu, 1998; Miles and Shen, 1925; Sun et al., 1985). This suggests that although the visual format of Chinese and English are strikingly different (i.e. Chinese is logographic but English is alphabetic), the gross characteristics of readers' eye movements are very similar. It appears that the basic encoding of the linguistic information in Chinese reading is as efficient as in reading of English text regardless of the visual form of the particular language (see also Tsang and Chen, 2008).

Furthermore, Sun et al. (1985) recorded the eye movements of readers when reading vertical Chinese text. It should be pointed out that written Chinese text can be arranged either vertically from top to bottom within a column, or horizontally as in English. Vertical Chinese text was very common in China until the second quarter of 20th century, and although it can still be seen on some occasions (e.g. calligraphies, drawings, or paintings), or in certain regions (e.g. Taiwan), horizontal Chinese text is more prevalent at present, especially in mainland China. Sun et al. found for vertical Chinese text that the average saccade length (approximately 1.2 characters) was only about half that for horizontal Chinese text (approximately 2.6 characters), mean fixation duration was longer for vertical Chinese text (approximately 290 ms) than for horizontal Chinese text (approximately 260 ms), and consequently, reading rate was slower for vertical Chinese text (approximately 260 characters per minute, 170 equivalent words per minute) than for horizontal Chinese text (approximately 580 characters per minute, 390 equivalent words per minute). The vertical text was clearly read more slowly, and this was probably due to participants' increased skill in reading horizontal compared to vertical text.

Overall, the basic characteristics of Chinese readers' eye movements tend to be similar to those of English readers, despite the two writing systems differing in terms of their visual format. However, other aspects of eye movement behaviour during reading of Chinese (perhaps similar to other logographic languages) have been shown to be quite different to that during reading of alphabetic languages. Researchers have endeavoured to explore some fundamental issues concerning how readers target saccades and how words are recognized in reading unspaced Chinese text, how much information can be obtained in a given eye fixation, what kind of information can be extracted from a Chinese word before it is fixated, as well as whether readers process information from more than one word at a time during Chinese reading. We will consider these issues in the following section.

The influence of the intrinsic characteristics of Chinese orthography on eye movements during reading

Word boundary information and eye movements

In alphabetic writing systems, like English, words are perceptually salient because spaces between them provide a strong visual cue to demarcate the word beginning and ending. Word spacing has been demonstrated to be vital for efficient word identification and eye movement control in alphabetic languages (see Rayner and Pollatsek, 1996; Rayner et al., 1998). When spacing information is removed from English sentences, reading speed is dramatically reduced, fixations durations are increased (e.g. Malt and Seamon, 1978; Morris et al., 1990; Pollatsek and Rayner, 1982; Rayner and Pollatsek, 1996; Rayner et al., 1998; Spragins et al., 1976; Perea and Acha, 2009) and saccades become shorter (Rayner et al., 1998). Of course, as mentioned earlier, Chinese text does not contain salient word boundaries, and therefore, the strings of characters that comprise the words are not as immediately visually apparent as is the case in spaced languages such as English. Thus, it is intriguing to consider how Chinese readers target saccades and recognize words during unspaced Chinese reading.

Inhoff et al. (1997) examined how inserting spaces between words in Chinese influenced reading. They required participants to read the sentences in three presentation conditions: normal unspaced text, word spaced text in which a space appeared between each Chinese word, and non-word spaced text in which a space was inserted randomly between characters such that the resulting groups of Chinese characters formed non-words. Their results did not show any reliable differences in total reading times, mean fixation durations, and mean saccade lengths for any of the presentation conditions. The null results are somewhat surprising (particularly given that a non-word spacing condition was included in the experiment), and probably occurred due to the comparatively low spatial resolution of the eye tracker that was used, or relatively weak spacing manipulations (the spaces that were inserted were half the size of one character).

Bai et al. (2008) employed an eye tracker with high spatial and temporal accuracy, along with a more robust spacing manipulation to further examine the role of word boundary information in Chinese reading. In the first of the two experiments they reported, sentences were constructed with four types of spacing information: normal unspaced text, text with spaces between every character, text with spaces between words, and text with spaces between characters that yielded non-words. In their second experiment, highlighting was used to create analogous conditions whilst controlling the spatial layout of sentences. Both experiments showed consistent effects. Character and non-word spaced (or highlighted) text produced disruption to reading. Word spaced text (or highlighting) did not facilitate reading Chinese, but did not interfere with reading. Participants read word spaced text as quickly as normal unspaced text, even though this format is very visually unfamiliar. Bai et al. argued that facilitatory and inhibitory factors traded off against each other when words were clearly marked (in contrast to normal unspaced text). Normal unspaced text is extremely visually familiar for adults, but word identification may be hindered due to poor word demarcation. In contrast, word spaced text is visually unfamiliar but word identification may be facilitated due to good word demarcation.

In contrast to skilled adult readers, beginning Chinese readers have less experience in reading text without spaces. Consequently, the familiarity of this format is comparatively limited. On the basis of the findings from Bai et al. (2008), we (Zang et al., 2011) directly compared the effect of interword spacing on children's (8–9 years) and adults' eye movement behaviour to examine whether word spaced text might have a greater facilitatory effect for Chinese beginning readers than was obtained for skilled adult readers. The results showed a reliable effect of word spacing for first fixation, single fixation, and gaze duration on Chinese words, with shorter reading times for word spaced than for normal unspaced text. Furthermore, a reliable interaction occurred for gaze duration (but not on first fixation or single fixation durations). Further analysis showed that children and adults had longer gaze durations for unspaced than word spaced text, but this difference was much greater for the children (52 ms) than for the adults (28 ms). These results indicate that during the earliest stages of lexical identification, spacing had a similar influence on eye movement behaviour in both children and adults. However, adults were less likely to require a second fixation on a word prior to leaving it than were children. Note, however, that when total sentence reading times were computed, word spaced and normal unspaced text did not differ, a finding that is entirely consistent with the results of Bai et al. (2008). These findings indicate that word spacing facilitates early segmentation of the text, but the unusual visual appearance of the word spaced text also causes some disruption. The results also reveal that by the age of 8 years, children are as familiar with the visual layout of text in their native language as are adults. As a consequence of this, children show the same tradeoff between visual familiarity and word boundary demarcation as do skilled adult readers. In addition, this study also investigated the saccadic targeting in reading spaced and unspaced Chinese text which we will cover later.

In a second follow-up line of research, D. Shen et al. (2011) investigated the effect of word segmentation on Chinese reading for non-native Chinese readers who were learning Chinese as a second language. Participants' native languages were different in terms of their basic characteristics being either spaced (English and Korean) or unspaced (Japanese and Thai), and either alphabetic (English, Thai, and Korean) or character based (Japanese). D. Shen et al. investigated whether any spacing effects that we might observe were modulated by native language characteristics. For second language learners, eye movement measures showed least disruption to reading for word spaced text, and longer reading times for unspaced and character spaced text, with non-word spaced text yielding the longest times. These effects were uninfluenced by native language characteristics. Thus, word spacing can be useful to readers when they are learning a new language, irrespective of whether this spacing leads to a visually familiar or unfamiliar layout.

Apart from the spaces being a segmentation cue, a comma can provide additional space as well and serve as a visual segmentation cue in Chinese text. Ren and Yang (2010) investigated whether a comma influenced the reading of Chinese sentences comprised of different types of syntactic constituents such as words, phrases and clauses. Participants were required to read Chinese sentences that did or did not include a comma at the end of a syntactic constituent. The results showed that fixation times were shorter for target words followed by a comma than for those followed by no comma. The same pattern of fixation times appeared for target words in three types of syntactic constituents. These data suggest that a comma after a word facilitated the lexical identification of that word during Chinese reading.

Overall, these experiments indicate that clear word boundary information demarcated by spaces or highlighting in Chinese text can facilitate word identification (at least to some degree) during reading of Chinese, especially for the non-native Chinese speakers when learning Chinese as their second language. These findings provide some evidence for word-based processing in Chinese reading, and perhaps, have some promising practical implications for educational practice in relation to both learning Chinese as a native and as a second language.

Lexical influences on eye movements

Although Chinese word boundaries are not demarcated, it is the case that properties of words (complexity, frequency, etc.) influence readers' eye movement behaviour. Chinese words do play an important role in lexical processing and text comprehension more generally (e.g. Chen et al., 2003; Rayner et al., 2005; Tsai et al., 2006; G. Yan et al., 2006, 2011; Yang and McConkie, 1999). We will consider some of these in the next section.

Character and word complexity

Chinese characters vary in the number, type and configuration of internal features they contain. The visual complexity of Chinese characters (or words) is usually indexed by the number of strokes that they (or their constituent characters) contain. Just and Carpenter (1987) recorded the eye movements of native Chinese readers as they read Chinese text, and found the Chinese readers spent more time on characters that contained more strokes. Furthermore, the average gaze duration increased reliably by 4.6 ms for each additional stroke. Yang and McConkie (1999) manipulated the frequency of a word and the complexity of its constituent characters in a two-character word. The results showed that both the complexity of characters and words influenced the skipping rate, refixation probability and gaze duration. Specifically, more complex words are less likely to be skipped, but more likely to receive a refixation and take longer to identify. Yang and McConkie assumed for the more complex words, readers need more time to decompose a character into its components, or to process the different components entering into the lexical identification system. Furthermore, more complex words may not be processed efficiently in the parafovea, which probably accounts for the effect of complexity on skipping rates and refixation probabilities.

It is clear that the number of strokes provides a reasonable measure of visual complexity influencing character and word identification during Chinese reading. However, the number of strokes is not a perfect indicator, since it ignores configural properties of Chinese characters. Recently, G. Yan et al. (2011) examined the role of stroke encoding in Chinese character identification by removing strokes either from the beginning or from the end of the character construction sequence. G. Yan et al. also included a condition in which strokes were removed such that the overall configuration of the character was retained. Furthermore, in order to quantify the influence of stroke removal, the proportion of strokes that were removed from Chinese characters (15%, 30%, and 50%) was manipulated. Readers' eye movements were recorded when they read sentences comprised of characters with different types and proportions of stroke removal. Reading times, number of fixations and regression measures all showed that Chinese characters with 15% of strokes removed were as easy to read as Chinese characters without any strokes removed, reflecting some redundancy in relation to stroke complexity within simplified Chinese characters. Moreover, when 30% or more of a character's strokes were removed, characters with their configuration retained were the easiest to read, characters with ending strokes removed were more difficult, whilst characters with their beginning strokes removed were the most difficult to read. These findings suggest that not all strokes within a character have equal status during character identification, and a flexible stroke encoding system must underlie successful character identification during Chinese reading.

Character and word frequency

Apart from visual complexity, Chinese characters and words differ in the frequency of their occurrence in the language. G. Yan et al. (2006) investigated how word and character frequency influenced the eye movements of Chinese readers. They orthogonally manipulated word frequency (high/low), initial character frequency (high/low), and second character frequency (high/low). The eight word types were balanced in terms of the number of strokes and radicals of characters. The results showed a robust effect of word frequency on fixation times on a target word, that is, Chinese readers looked longer at low frequency words than high frequency words (see also Chen et al., 2003; Inhoff et al., 1999; Just and Carpenter, 1987; Yang and McConkie, 1999). Furthermore, they also found that character frequency influenced fixation times on the two-character words and the effect of the initial character was more pronounced than that of the second. Specifically, fixations were longer on words with a low frequency initial character than with a high frequency initial character. However, more importantly, this effect was modulated by word frequency. That is, the effect of character frequency was attenuated for high frequency words while it was quite apparent for low frequency words. G. Yan et al. assumed that a two-character word with high frequency may be accessed as a single entity in the Chinese mental lexicon, whereas a word with low frequency may be accessed via the characters (and hence an effect of character frequency emerges).

Word predictability

Word predictability refers to the extent to which readers can predict the upcoming words from the preceding context. Rayner et al. (2005) recorded eye movements of Chinese readers as they read sentences containing target words whose predictability from the preceding context was high, medium, or low. Target word frequency, character frequency, and character complexity were controlled. They found a robust predictability effect. Specifically, Chinese readers fixated less time on high- and medium-predictable target words than on low-predictable target words, and were more likely to fixate on low-predictable target words than on high- or medium-predictable target words. The results were highly similar to those observed from readers of English by Rayner and Well (1996), indicating that Chinese readers use contextual constraint/predictability factors in the same way as English readers do.

Recently, Wang et al. (2010) employed two computational methods, latent semantic analysis and transitional probability, which capture co-occurrences in relation to lexical semantic representations within large text corpora. In this way they examined the effects of word predictability in Chinese reading. They found influences of transitional probability on first fixation duration and gaze duration and of latent semantic analysis on total time. In sum, their findings were consistent with

Rayner et al. (2005), demonstrating that how predictable a word is influences how long readers fixate them during Chinese reading.

Neighbourhood size

Research in alphabetic languages has shown that processing time for identifying a word is influenced by other words within its neighbourhood. A word's neighbours are those words that are the same length and share all but one letter with it (Coltheart et al., 1977; see also eye movement studies by Perea and Pollatsek, 1998; Pollatsek et al., 1999). Neighbourhood effects might also be linked to 'morphological neighbourhoods' or 'family size' (see the discussion at the end of Juhasz, 2008). Neighbourhood effects indicate that when identifying a word, not only can the target word's representation be activated, but also orthographically similar words (e.g. Andrews, 1997). Tsai et al. (2006) defined the neighbourhood size of a Chinese word as the number of two-character words sharing the same initial constituent character. They manipulated the neighbourhood size (small/large) of the initial characters, but controlled the neighbourhood size of the second constituent character of a two-character word. The results showed a facilitative effect of neighbourhood size. Specifically, Chinese words with more neighbours produced higher skipping rates and shorter first fixations and gaze durations than words with fewer neighbours. This indicates that representations of neighbour words are partially activated and play a role in the early stage of lexical access.

Overall, although some clear differences between Chinese and English exist in terms of the fact that there are no spaces between words and the fact that the information is more densely packed in Chinese text, the findings reviewed above in Chinese reading are comparable to those typically found with readers of English. Clearly, effects of word frequency, predictability and neighbourhood etc during Chinese reading are very similar to these effects in alphabetic language reading. However, effects of character complexity perhaps are more specific to logographic languages. Therefore, reading processes and lexical influences appear to have similarities but also differences in different languages.

Selection of saccade targets during Chinese reading

As can be seen from the literature we reviewed above, some basic properties of Chinese words influence word identification. Furthermore, the research on word spacing (e.g. Bai et al., 2008) provides evidence for the psychological reality of words during Chinese reading. Thus, it might be expected that the word unit plays as a central role not only in word identification and text comprehension but also in eye movement control for Chinese readers. In other words, it might be expected that eye guidance in Chinese reading is word based as in reading of alphabetic language scripts.

One source of evidence that has been used to argue that saccades are directed to words in reading of alphabetic language scripts is the observation of the preferred viewing location (PVL, Rayner, 1979). That is, the eyes most often fixate a position slightly to the left of the centre of a word (McConkie et al., 1988; Rayner, 1979). If initial fixations in Chinese were centred on characters or words, then this would help inform the debate as to whether characters or words in Chinese are the unit of saccadic target selection. The initial evidence indicated that there was no clear PVL effect in Chinese reading, and the PVL curves that were obtained for both Chinese characters and words were almost flat (Yang and McConkie, 1999; Tsai and McConkie, 2003). Given this finding, Tsai et al. argued that Chinese readers do not select words as the saccadic target, but left open the possibility of character-based saccadic targeting.

However more recently, M. Yan et al. (2010a) required participants to read sentences in which the word boundaries were completely unambiguous (as determined by a segmentation pretest). They found readers exhibited a strong tendency to fixate at the word centre in single fixation cases, indicating that Chinese readers can segment parafoveal character strings into word units (at least to some extent) and select the word centre as the saccadic target. They also found when readers made multiple fixations they were more likely to fixate at the word beginning. M. Yan et al. argued that Chinese readers dynamically select the beginning or centre of words as saccadic targets depending on failure or success with word segmentation of parafoveal character strings.

Li et al. (2011) examined landing positions for a four-character word and a four-character region comprised of a two-character word and two following characters. Their results replicated Yan et al.'s (M. Yan et al., 2010a) findings that readers' eyes landed at the word centre when they made only a single fixation on a word, and that they landed at the word beginning when they made more than one fixation on a word. Furthermore, the PVL curve was similar for the four-character word and two-character word conditions. However, when all the forward fixations (including initial fixations and refixations within a word) were considered, the distribution changed such that it was flat. Li et al. provided an alternative account of these data, namely, that readers made fixed length saccades during Chinese reading, and their simulations suggested that a constant distance model could predict the different PVL curves in single and multiple fixation cases.

A further study has examined saccadic targeting in reading word spaced and normal unspaced text (Zang et al., 2011). Previous studies (e.g. Rayner et al., 1998) suggest that spaces between words facilitate saccadic targeting in English readers, and when spaces are removed from English text in the parafovea, saccadic targeting becomes more difficult, with initial landing positions on words substantially shifted towards their beginning. Zang et al. examined whether readers could use space information to guide the eyes in Chinese reading. Their results showed that mean initial landing positions (regardless of the number of fixations on a word) were closer to the word centre for spaced than unspaced text. However, detailed analysis of the landing position data showed differential effects for single and multiple fixation situations. For single fixations, where readers apparently identified the word efficiently, there were clear preferred viewing position effects across the word, and mean landing positions were identical in spaced and unspaced conditions. For multiple fixation situations, where readers presumably found word identification more difficult, landing positions were closer to the preferred viewing position for spaced than unspaced text, suggesting that demarcated word boundaries facilitated parafoveal processing of words and saccadic targeting.

To summarize, quite an amount of evidence supports the view that words are important in relation to lexical processing and eye movement control during Chinese reading. Indeed, Rayner et al. (2007) successfully simulated the eye movement behaviour of Chinese readers in the context of the E-Z Reader model, by maintaining the basic assumptions associated with word based processing in reading of alphabetic language scripts. However, it is important to note that Chinese characters are also, obviously, very important, and at some level their identification is an intrinsic part of successful word identification in Chinese. Suffice it to say that further work is required to better understand the role of characters and words as units of analysis in relation to saccadic targeting during Chinese reading.

How much information is extracted during a fixation?

The perceptual span in Chinese reading

Perceptual span refers to the area of effective vision from which useful information can be obtained during a fixation in reading (McConkie and Rayner, 1975; Rayner and Pollatsek, 1989; D. Shen et al., 2008). To determine the size of the perceptual span, the classic gaze-contingent moving-window technique was developed (McConkie and Rayner, 1975). In this technique, the text outside a predefined window around the point of fixation is masked by Xs or scrambled letters. Thus, wherever the reader looks, the text is visible within the window, but outside the window the text is disrupted in some way. By varying the size of the window systematically, the researcher can determine the effective visual field by observing under which condition of window size reading performance is identical to the normal text reading. Research using this technique (as well as a recent variant– parafoveal magnification, Miellet et al., 2009) has demonstrated that skilled adult readers of English and other alphabetic writing systems obtain useful information from an asymmetric region extending roughly 3–4 character spaces to the left of fixation to about 14–15 character spaces to the right of fixation (e.g. McConkie and Rayner, 1976; Rayner and Bertera, 1979; Rayner et al., 1980; see also Rayner, 1998, 2009 for a review).

Similarly, Inhoff and Liu (1998) used the moving-window technique to examine the perceptual span during reading of Chinese sentences. Eleven viewing conditions were created, including two baseline conditions, in which readers either saw the full line of text during each fixation (normal sentence), or only the fixated character, i.e. all text to the right and left of the character was masked by dissimilar characters. The visibility of text to the right and left of the fixated character was manipulated respectively. In seven right-directed preview conditions, one to seven characters of text were shown to the right of the fixated character, and in two left-directed preview conditions, an additional one or two characters were shown to the left of fixation. The window of legible text moved with the eyes in all conditions. The results revealed an asymmetric perceptual span during Chinese reading that extended one character to the left of the fixated character and up to three characters to its right (see also Chen and Tang, 1998; Gray, 1956; Sun and Feng, 1999). Furthermore, Inhoff et al. found that successive perceptual spans slightly overlap, that is, the forward saccade length is shorter than the perceptual span. This suggests that Chinese readers usually fixate an area that has already been partially processed in the previous fixation. In addition, Inhoff et al. examined the size of a forward saccade from a fixated character as a function of the length of the next word in the text, and they found the forward saccades were not influenced by the length of the next word. However, linguistic properties of to-be-fixated text did determine saccade length, as readers made larger saccades to a parafoveally visible context-consistent character than to an inconsistent character (the mask). This suggests that Chinese readers may rely more on linguistic information rather than on pure visual cues to determine the next saccadic target during Chinese reading.

Overall, the perceptual span in Chinese appears to be smaller than in English, probably due to the increased complexity of Chinese characters, higher density of information in Chinese, and lack of word boundary information in the parafovea compared with English. However, Inhoff et al. argued that the difference in span sizes between English and Chinese appears less dramatic when the span was measured in word units. Since the majority of Chinese words contain two character constituents, readers of Chinese thus obtain useful information from the fixated word and from the next few words in the text. Correspondingly, the mean word length in English is six to seven letters, also implying that readers of English obtain useful information from the fixated word and from one or two, words to its right.

Parafoveal preview effect

Research on the perceptual span has clearly demonstrated that parafoveal vision is very important in reading Chinese (as well as other languages), such that readers can begin to process the next (parafoveal) word in the text. To determine what kind of information can be extracted from a word before it is fixated, the gaze-contingent boundary technique was developed (Rayner, 1975). In this technique, an invisible boundary is just to the left of a target word, and before readers cross the boundary, the preview of the following target word is either correct or incorrect. When the eyes cross the boundary, the preview is always replaced by the correct version of the target word. Readers do not notice the display change because it occurs during a saccade. If the preview shares some information with the target, viewing durations on the target word are shortened. The facilitation in viewing durations is termed 'preview benefit' (Rayner, 1975). A large number of studies using this paradigm have revealed that readers of English and other alphabetic languages can obtain the information about letter position, orthographic and phonological codes from the parafovea, but not morphological (except for readers of Hebrew), or semantic information (Rayner, 1998, 2009, for a review).

Given that information is more densely packed in Chinese than English, more information may be available from characters to the right of fixation during reading of Chinese than of English text. Several studies using the boundary technique have investigated the acquisition of parafoveal word information in Chinese (e.g. Liu et al., 2002; Pollatsek et al., 2000; M. Yan et al., 2009; Yen et al., 2008, 2009; Tsai et al., 2004). These studies will be discussed in the following sections.

The acquisition of phonological and orthographic information from the parafovea

Pollatsek et al. (2000) investigated the extraction of parafoveal phonological information using a variation of the boundary technique. In this technique, participants fixate a central point until a character appears in the parafovea. Then they execute a saccade to the parafoveal character ('the preview'), and the preview is replaced by a target character during the saccade. Participants name the target character as quickly and accurately as possible. In Experiment 1, the preview of the target was either: 1) identical, 2) orthographically similar homophonic, 3) orthographically dissimilar homophonic, 4) synonymous (without orthographic overlap with targets), or 5) an unrelated control. The results showed that naming latencies of target characters were shorter for homophonic previews than for unrelated control previews, regardless of whether homophones were orthographically similar to targets or not. In contrast, a preview synonymous to the target did not have any effect on naming. This indicated that phonological but not semantic information from the parafovea, facilitated character identification. Experiments 2 and 3 further examined whether the phonological information at the phonetic radical level was accessed prior to fixation. In Experiment 2, the preview of the target was either: 1) identical, 2) homophonic and sharing a phonetic radical with the target, 3) non-homophonic and sharing a phonetic radical with the target, 4) orthographically dissimilar homophonic, or 5) an unrelated control. The phonological regularity of target characters was also manipulated. The results of Experiment 2 replicated the main findings of Experiment 1—previews that were homophonic provided preview benefit (relative to the unrelated control condition). Moreover, the naming times were longer and more naming errors appeared for phonetically irregular targets than regular targets, indicating phonological representations of the radicals could be activated. Orthographic information was also extracted parafoveally as there was a significant preview benefit from non-homophones sharing a phonetic radical. Experiment 3 added an onset control condition (a non-homophone sharing an initial phoneme), in order to rule out one possible account of the effects from homophonic previews, that is, whether programming of articulatory responses might be easier in the homophonic condition than in the control condition. However, the data did not show any difference in the initial phoneme condition compared to the unrelated control condition, and thus the findings obtained in Experiment 1 and 2 were not due to the programming of articulatory responses. Overall these data suggested that both lexical and sublexical phonological codes, as well as the orthographic information of Chinese characters were extracted prior to fixation and integrated across saccades.

One may assume, however, the naming response employed in Pollatsek et al.'s (2000) study might require participants to focus particularly on the use of phonological information. Therefore, subsequent research (e.g. Liu et al., 2002; Tsai et al., 2004) used the gaze-contingent boundary technique to further examine these issues during Chinese reading, and to determine the time course of phonological and orthographic processing in the parafovea. Specifically, Tsai et al. (2004) orthogonally manipulated the phonological and orthographic similarity of preview and target characters (Experiment 1), as well as the consistency of target characters (Experiment 2), which was defined as the relative ratio of homophonic characters within a given set of characters sharing the same phonetic radical. Consistent with the findings of Pollatsek et al. (2000), Tsai et al. found an early and rapid parafoveal phonological activation at both character and radical levels.

Liu et al. (2002), in contrast, manipulated the previews which were identical, or graphemically similar, homophonic, or dissimilar to the targets (Experiment 1). The results revealed a robust preview benefit from graphemically similar previews in all viewing durations, but the homophonic preview benefit occurred only in gaze and total fixation time, but not in first fixation duration. Furthermore, to systematically scrutinize the possible source of the graphemic preview benefit, Liu et al. created four previews according to whether the target and its preview shared semantic or phonetic radicals, and a stroke overlap condition in which neither the phonetic nor the semantic radicals were shared but a substantial number of strokes overlapped (Experiment 2). The results showed parafoveal preview of graphemically similar characters yielded benefits primarily when they shared the phonetic radical with their targets. The previews with stroke overlap or with the same semantic radical as the targets produced relatively small benefits that were not significant during first-pass reading. Thus, the orthography of phonetic radicals played a major role in the early stage of character identification. In other words, Chinese character identification initially involves the extraction of orthographic information, and thereby, activation of the character's phonological form (see also Feng et al., 2001; Inhoff et al., 1999; Wong and Chen, 1999, for similar effects using other paradigms).

The acquisition of semantic information

It has been demonstrated that phonological and orthographic information can be obtained from the parafovea during Chinese reading. Another related question is whether semantic information can be extracted from Chinese characters in the parafovea. Recall, previous research investigating reading of alphabetic languages suggests that semantic information is not obtained prior to fixation (e.g. Rayner et al., 1986, 2003). However, given that Chinese characters have a close connection between meaning and visual form, and that information is more densely packed in Chinese text than in English text, one may expect that semantic information could be extracted parafoveally during Chinese reading.

M. Yan et al. (2009) manipulated preview characters that were either identical, or unrelated, or orthographically, phonologically, or semantically related to the targets. In order to avoid the confounding from sublexical/radical activation during reading, they selected some visually and structurally simple and relatively common pictographic characters as targets, whose meanings are taken directly from their form (e.g. 门 means *door*). The results showed a significant preview benefit from orthographically- and semantically-related characters on first fixation and gaze durations. The phonological preview was significant on gaze duration but not on first fixation duration. More importantly, they also obtained a significant semantic parafoveal-on-foveal effect for gaze duration; we will discuss this later. Overall, this study suggests that Chinese readers are able to obtain semantic information to some extent from the parafovea during Chinese reading.

The acquisition of lexical properties and its time course

The previous studies have provided evidence that parafoveal preprocessing occurs at the level of the character (in relation to orthography, phonology and semantics), as the target character was often either an independent character (e.g. Pollatsek et al., 2000) or a constituent character of a multiple character word (e.g. Tsai et al., 2004; M. Yan et al., 2009). A further question is whether parafoveal preprocessing operates at the word level. Yen et al. (2008) used the boundary paradigm to examine this question in two experiments. In Experiment 1, the preview was either a real word, or a pseudoword made up of two real characters. The results showed that targets with real word previews, even unrelated and contextually inappropriate ones, were more likely to be skipped than were those with pseudowords (see also Inhoff and Wu, 2005, for a similar finding). In Experiment 2, all of the previews shared the first character (e.g. 戒) with the target word (e.g. 戒烟, *to quit smoking*; 烟, *tobacco*). However, there were three types of previews: a word sharing a common morpheme with the target (e.g. 戒除, *to give up a habit*; 除, *to get rid of*), a word with no morpheme the same as the target (e.g. 戒备, *to guard against*; 备, *to be equipped*), and a pseudoword (e.g. 戒料). Yen et al.'s results showed that targets with the same morpheme previews were fixated for less time than were those with pseudoword previews, indicating that morphological pre-processing of parafoveal words may occur, but not simply due to the orthographic preview of the first character in common with the target. Thus, Yen et al. provided some evidence that information at the level of the word can be extracted parafoveally in Chinese reading.

More recently, Yen et al. (2009) examined the time course of acquisition of lexical information from the parafovea. The visibility of the parafoveal word (the target) was manipulated in two time intervals during the fixation on the pretarget word. That is, the parafoveal word was either visible or masked by a pseudoword during the initial 140 ms or after the initial 140 ms viewing on the pretarget word. Their results showed that the masking effect occurred regardless of the preview time, specifically, viewing durations were longer if the target word was masked parafoveally both before and after

140 ms during a fixation on the pretarget. Therefore, Yen et al. assumed that information about the parafoveal word can be acquired relatively early under conditions of restricted visibility.

Parafoveal preview benefit from word $n+2$

Yang et al. (2009) examined whether Chinese readers could obtain the preview benefit from a more distant word, word $n+2$, as well as word $n+1$. In Experiment 1, the targets were one-character words (note that Yang et al. generally referred to them as characters), the preview of the target was either identical, or dissimilar (i.e. a different character). The results showed readers could obtain preview benefit from character $n+2$ as well as character $n+1$. In Experiment 2, two-character words were used as targets. Furthermore, to determine if readers could discriminate whether a word was presented to the right of their fixation point, a pseudoword (i.e. two characters that did not form a word) preview was added. Their results showed that robust preview benefit from word $n+1$ occurred. There was also marginally significant evidence from gaze duration (but not first fixation duration) suggesting preview effects for word $n+2$ were obtained to some extent, however, Yang et al. suggested this most probably occurred when the words preceding the targets were high frequency function words.

   M. Yan et al. (2010b) investigated whether the preview benefit from word $n+2$ was modulated by the parafoveal processing load with respect to the frequency of word $n+1$ (low frequency word $n+1$ = high load, high frequency word $n+1$ = low load). Furthermore, the type of preview at word $n+2$ was also manipulated to determine the type of parafoveal information that was available from word $n+2$ during Chinese reading. Previews were identical, semantically related, orthographically related, and non-words. The results showed a preview benefit from word $n+2$, but there was also an interaction between the frequency of word $n+1$ and the preview benefit of word $n+2$ such that readers obtained parafoveal benefit from word $n+2$ (identity relative to non-word preview) when word $n+1$ was a high frequency word (low parafoveal load) in comparison to when word $n+1$ was a low frequency word (high parafoveal load). However, neither semantic nor orthographic previews facilitated subsequent processing of word $n+2$ regardless of the processing difficulty of word $n+1$.

   Together all the findings above indicate that readers of Chinese can obtain useful orthographic, phonological, and perhaps to some extent, semantic information from a parafoveally visible character or word during reading. Recall we mentioned earlier, that semantic information is, arguably, not acquired parafoveally in reading of alphabetic languages (e.g. Rayner et al., 1986, 2003). Finally, for readers of Chinese, the availability of information from word $n+2$ is modulated by how easy word $n+1$ is to process.

Parafoveal-on-foveal effects

In contrast to the research about information acquisition from the parafovea, relatively few studies have examined another related measure of preprocessing, that is, whether the lexical characteristics of the word to the right of fixation can influence the processing of the currently fixated word, or whether readers lexically process more than one word at a time. It has been argued that the influence of the characteristics of a parafoveal word on reading times on the fixated foveal word ('parafoveal-on-foveal' (PoF) effects) provide evidence for processing of multiple words in parallel (see Drieghe Chapter 46, this volume). Such effects are currently highly controversial in reading of alphabetic languages, and have become something of a focus in the debate between current computational models of eye movement control, such as the E-Z Reader model (see Reichle, Chapter 42, this volume) and SWIFT (see also Engbert and Kliegl, Chapter 43, this volume). In comparison with parafoveal preview effects, PoF effects appear to be weak (see Rayner, 2009, for a review). There are three reports of PoF effects during Chinese reading. As mentioned earlier, M. Yan et al. (2009) observed a semantic PoF effect during Chinese reading such that gaze durations on pretarget words in the semantic preview condition were significantly shorter than on those followed by unrelated previews. Also, Yang et al. (2009) obtained a PoF effect of the target word on the pretarget word such that the fixation times on the pretarget word were longer when a dissimilar word was the preview than when the target word was the preview, suggesting that readers of Chinese do sometimes obtain some (lexical) information regarding the word to the right of the fixated word, and that this can influence the duration of the current fixation. M. Yan et al. (2010b) also obtained a significant PoF effect from the influence of the frequency of word $n+1$ on word n for first fixation and gaze durations, but no evidence indicated that previews of word $n+2$ influenced the fixation duration on word n.

In our view, these studies report data that should be regarded as preliminary. At this stage, it is extremely difficult to know exactly what constitutes a PoF effect in Chinese reading, and how any such effect is comparable to a PoF effect in an alphabetic language. This is particularly the case given that questions still remain as to exactly what elements within the text the language processing system operates over during any particular fixation, and also what the primary units of information are in Chinese reading. We believe that more work is required to investigate a variety of issues before a clearer picture about the extent and nature of PoF effects emerges. From our perspective, however, it is clear that Chinese is a good candidate language in which to anticipate obtaining PoF effects since it is very visually dense and word boundaries are not clearly demarcated.

Developmental changes in eye movements during Chinese reading

Most of the literature we reviewed above is mainly from eye movement studies of adult readers. Studies on children's eye movement control during reading are comparatively rare. However, several studies have demonstrated that eye movement behaviour gradually develops with age (Rayner, 1998; see also Blythe and Joseph, Chapter 36, this volume). Specifically, as reading skill increases, saccade lengths and perceptual span increase, while fixation durations, the number of fixations, and regressions decrease.

We will now consider the developmental trends of eye movements during Chinese reading. Chen et al. (2003) reported an eye movement data set including second-, fourth-, and sixth-grade children, as well as the undergraduate students. The results showed that second grade children spent about 38% more total time fixating a word than undergraduate students. The proportion of change for gaze duration and first fixation duration on a word from second grade children to undergraduate students were 29% and 21%, respectively. Furthermore, total word reading time still decreased about 10% even from sixth-grade children to undergraduate students, but no such difference occurred for gaze duration and first fixation duration (only 3–4%) reduction. Considering these measures reveal the time course of lexical processing in reading, with first fixation duration being sensitive to the earliest visual encoding and orthographic processing, gaze duration reflecting later processing and total fixation duration reflecting later, but higher level text integration (Liversedge and Findlay, 2000; Rayner, 1998), Chen et al. assumed that basic word identification processes are acquired by sixth-grade children. In contrast, higher levels of language processing, such as text integration take longer to develop. Finally, Chen et al. also report some other eye movement measures such as regression rates and saccade length, which appeared to be more stable across different grades. Chen et al. suggested that this was probably related to the physical layout of Chinese text, which required smaller, and therefore, less variable saccades for effective visual encoding.

More recently, Feng et al. (2009) carried out a cross-language developmental study that compared the developmental trajectories of eye movement behaviour in English- and Chinese-speaking children and adults. In their experiment, third-grade, fifth-grade, and undergraduate students, who were native speakers of either English or Chinese, were required to read age-appropriate texts in their native language. They found changes in fixation duration showed very similar developmental trajectories across age (McConkie et al., 1991) and languages (Sun and Feng, 1999). Specifically, mean fixation duration was approximately 263, 244, and 191 ms for American third-grade, fifth-grade, and adult readers, and 265, 238, and 212 ms for Chinese third-grade, fifth-grade students, and adults, respectively. Mean fixation duration decreased significantly with age, but no significant effect of language, or any interaction occurred. However, more interestingly, differential effects across languages occurred, when the percentage of progressive fixations, regressions, and refixations were analysed based on whether participants fixated on a new word, a word that had already been read, or the current word. Specifically, Chinese readers made significantly more regressions than American readers, but the regression rate remained similar across different grades (McConkie et al., 1991; Chen et al., 2003). However, American children (third grade and fifth grade) made fewer progressive fixations, but were more likely to make refixations compared to Chinese children (third grade and fifth grade), whereas adult readers of both languages did not differ in the two measures. Feng et al. argued that when reading unfamiliar words, English speaking children perhaps are more likely to sound out words, and thus make more refixations. Alternatively, children may have more problems in parsing long English words into morphologically meaningful units. Whatever the reason, in general, the effects that were observed were greater for children than for skilled adult readers.

Finally, as mentioned earlier, Zang et al. (2011) also compared landing positions on target words in children (8–9 years) and adults to examine whether children and adults differ in their saccade targeting strategies during Chinese reading. In addition, Zang et al. manipulated the visual presentation of text either in normal unspaced, or word spaced format, to further examine whether interword spacing may facilitate readers (especially the children) in their selection of appropriate saccadic targets. The results showed basic developmental characteristics in word identification and eye movement control for fixation durations, refixation probabilities and for mean landing positions and refixation locations. Specifically, adults spent less time and made fewer refixations to identify a word. The mean landing position for adults was further into words compared to children (though no difference appeared when only single fixations were made), and the locations of refixations showed that adults' refixations were targeted more systematically in relation to the location of the first fixation on a word than was the case for children. If adults first fixated the word beginning, then they tended to make a refixation towards the end of the word. However, children were less effective in targeting refixations. These differences are likely due to differences in reading proficiency and oculomotor control skills of child and adult readers, in line with other studies in alphabetic languages (e.g. Joseph et al., 2009; Rayner, 1986).

Final remarks

Since the earliest studies by Miles and Shen (1925) who used photographic equipment to record readers' eye movements, there has been a substantial amount of work to investigate eye movements during Chinese reading. As we have reviewed above, many intriguing and important phenomena that have been well established in alphabetic writing systems like English have been shown to occur in reading of Chinese text. Comparisons between two different language scripts provide valuable opportunities to determine universal, as well as language specific aspects of the reading process. There are still many basic issues that need to be investigated in Chinese reading. For example, how Chinese words are segmented and extracted from a series of characters in the fovea and parafovea; whether Chinese words are processed serially or in parallel, etc. Furthermore, the computational models of eye movement behaviour during reading of Chinese might be further developed. It should be clear that much more research is required before we have developed a comprehensive understanding of eye movements during Chinese reading.

Acknowledgements

The first author received a Postgraduate Scholarship from the China Scholarship Council to fund a research visit to the University of Southampton. The second author acknowledges support from ESRC grant (RES 000-22-3398), the third author was supported by a grant from the Natural Science Foundation of China (30870781), and the fourth author was supported by award 2009JJDXLX005 Ministry of Education Project of Key Research Institute of Humanities and Social Sciences in Universities. The authors would like to thank Denis Drieghe and Sarah White for helpful comments on an earlier draft of this paper.

References

Andrews, S. (1997). The role of orthographic similarity in lexical retrieval: Resolving neighborhood conflicts. *Psychonomic Bulletin and Review*, **4**, 439–461.

Bai, X., Yan, G., Liversedge, S.P., Zang, C., and Rayner, K. (2008). Reading spaced and unspaced Chinese text: Evidence from eye movements. *Journal of Experimental Psychology: Human Perception and Performance*, **34**, 1277–1287.

Chen, H.-C. (1992). Reading comprehension in Chinese: Some implications from character reading times. In H.-C. Chen and O. Tzeng (eds.) *Language processing in Chinese* (pp. 175–205). Amsterdam: North-Holland (Elsevier).

Chen, H.-C. (1999). How do readers of Chinese process words during reading for comprehension? In J. Wang, A.W. Inhoff, and H.-C. Chen (eds.) *Reading Chinese Script: A Cognitive analysis* (pp. 257–278). Mahwah, NJ: Erlbaum.

Chen, H.-C. and Tang, C.K. (1998). The effective visual field in reading Chinese. *Reading and Writing*, **10**, 3–5.

Chen, H.-C., Song, H., Lau, W.Y., Wong, K.F.E., Tang, S.L. (2003). Developmental characteristics of eye movements in reading Chinese. In C. McBride-Chang, and H.-C. Chen (eds.) *Reading development in Chinese children* (pp. 157–169). Westport, CT: Praeger Publishers.

Coltheart, M., Davelaar, E., Jonasson, J.T. and Besner, D. (1977). Access to the internal lexicon. In S. Dornic (ed.) *Attention and Performance VI* (pp. 535–555). Hillsdale: NJ Erlbaum.

Dictionary of Chinese Character Information (Hanzi Xinxi Zidian) [in Chinese]. (1988). Beijing: Science Press.

Feng, G., Miller, K., Shu, H., and Zhang, H. (2001). Rowed to recovery: The use of phonological and orthographic information in reading Chinese and English. *Journal of Experimental Psychology: Learning, Memory, and Cognition*, **27**, 1079–1100.

Feng, G., Miller, K., Shu, H., and Zhang, H. (2009). Orthography, and the development of reading processes: An eye-movement study of Chinese and English. *Child Development*, **80**, 720–735.

Gray, W.S. (1956). *The teaching of reading and writing: An international survey*. Chicago, IL: Scott Foresman.

Hoosain, R. (1991). *Psycholinguistic implications for linguistic relativity: A case study of Chinese*. Hillsdale, NJ: Lawrence Erlbaum Associates.

Hoosain, R. (1992). Psychological reality of the word in Chinese. In H.-C. Chen and O. J.L. Tzeng. (eds.) *Language processing in Chinese* (pp. 111–130). Amsterdam: North-Holland.

Inhoff, A.W. and Liu, W. (1998). The perceptual span and oculomotor activity during the reading of Chinese sentences. *Journal of Experimental Psychology: Human Perception and Performance*, **24**, 20–34.

Inhoff, A.W. and Wu, C. (2005). Eye movements and the identification of spatially ambiguous words during Chinese sentence reading. *Memory and Cognition*, **33**, 1345–1356.

Inhoff, A.W., Liu, W., and Tang, Z. (1999). Use of prelexical and lexical information during Chinese sentence reading: Evidence from eye-movement studies. In J. Wang, A.W. Inhoff, and H.-C. Chen (eds.) *Reading Chinese script: A cognitive analysis* (pp. 223–238). Mahwah, NJ: Lawrence Erlbaum.

Inhoff, A.W., Liu, W., Wang, J., and Fu, D.J. (1997). Use of spatial information during the reading of Chinese text. In D. Peng, H. Shu, and H.-C. Chen (eds.) *Cognitive research on Chinese language* (pp. 296–329). Jinan: Shan Dong Educational Publishing.

Joseph, H.S.S.L., Liversedge, S.P., Blythe, H.I., White, S.J., and Rayner, K. (2009). Word length and landing position effects during reading in children and adults. *Vision Research*, **49**, 2078–2086.

Juhasz, B.J. (2008). The processing of compound words in English: Effects of word length on eye movements during reading. *Language and Cognitive Processes*, **23**, 1057–1088.

Just, M.A. and Carpenter, P.A. (eds.) (1987) *The Psychology of reading and language comprehension*. Newton, MA: Allyn and Bacon.

Li, X., Liu, P., and Rayner, K. (2011). Eye movement guidance in Chinese reading: Is there a preferred viewing location? *Vision Research*, **51**, 1146–1156.

Liu, W., Inhoff, A.W., Ye, Y., and Wu, C. (2002). Use of parafoveally visible characters during the reading of Chinese sentences. *Journal of Experimental Psychology: Human Perception and Performance*, **28**, 1213–1227.

Liversedge, S.P. and Findlay, J.M. (2000). Saccadic eye movements and cognition. *Trends in Cognitive Science*, **4**, 6–14.

Malt, B.C. and Seamon, J.G. (1978). Peripheral and cognitive components of eye guidance in filled-space reading. *Perception and Psychophysics*, **23**, 399–402.

McConkie, G.W. and Rayner, K. (1975). The span of the effective stimulus during a fixation in reading. *Perception and Psychophysics*, **17**, 578–586.

McConkie, G.W. and Rayner, K. (1976). Asymmetry of the perceptual span in reading. *Bulletin of the Psychonomic Society*, **8**, 365–368.

McConkie, G.W., Kerr, P.W., Reddix, M.D., and Zola, D. (1988). Eye movement control during reading: I. The location of initial fixations in words. *Vision Research*, **28**, 1107–1118.

McConkie, G.W., Zola, D., Grimes, J., Kerr, P.W., Bryant, N. R., and Wolff, P.M. (1991). Children's eye movements during reading. In J.E. Stein (ed.), *Vision and visual dyslexia* (pp. 251–262). London: Macmillan Press.

Miellet, S., O'Donnell, P.J., and Sereno, S.C. (2009). Parafoveal magnification: Visual acuity does not modulate the perceptual span in reading. *Psychological Science*, **20**, 721–728.

Miles, R.S. and Shen, E. (1925). Photographic recording of eye movements in the reading of Chinese in vertical and horizontal axes: Method and preliminary results. *Journal of Experimental Psychology*, **8**, 344–362.

Modern Chinese Commonly Used Character Stroke Order Standard (Xiandai Hanyu Tongyongzi Bishun Guifan) [In Chinese]. (1997). Beijing: Language and Literature Press.

Modern Chinese Frequency Dictionary (Xiandai Hanyu Pinlv Cidian) [In Chinese]. (1986). Beijing: Beijing Language and Culture University Press.

Morris, R.K., Rayner, K., and Pollatsek, A. (1990). Eye movement guidance in reading. *Journal of Experimental Psychology: Human Perception and Performance*, **16**, 268–281.

Perea, M. and Acha, J. (2009). Space information is important for reading. *Vision Research*, **49**, 1994–2000.

Perea, M. and Pollatsek, A. (1998). The effects of neighborhood frequency in reading and lexical decision. *Journal of Experimental Psychology: Human Perception and Performance*, **24**, 767–779.

Pollatsek, A. and Rayner, K. (1982). Eye movement control in reading: The role of word boundaries. *Journal of Experimental Psychology: Human Perception and Performance*, **8**, 817–833.

Pollatsek, A., Perea, M., and Binder, K.S. (1999). The effects of 'neighborhood size' in reading and lexical decision. *Journal of Experimental Psychology: Human Perception and Performance*, **25**, 1142–1158.

Pollatsek, A., Tan, L., and Rayner, K. (2000). The role of phonological codes in integrating information across saccadic eye movements in Chinese character identification. *Journal of Experimental Psychology: Human Perception and Performance*, **26**, 607–633.

Rayner, K. (1975). The perceptual span and peripheral cues in reading. *Cognitive Psychology*, **7**, 65–81.

Rayner, K. (1979). Eye guidance in reading: Fixation locations within words. *Perception*, **8**, 21–30.

Rayner, K. (1986). Eye movements and the perceptual span in beginning and skilled readers. *Journal of Experimental Child Psychology*, **41**, 211–236.

Rayner, K. (1998). Eye movements in reading and information processing: 20 years of research. *Psychological Bulletin*, **124**, 372–422.

Rayner, K. (2009). The thirty-fifth Sir Frederick Bartlett Lecture: Eye movements and attention in reading, scene perception, and visual search. *Quarterly Journal of Experimental Psychology*, **62**, 1457–1506.

Rayner, K. and Bertera, J.H. (1979). Reading without a fovea. *Science*, **206**, 468–469.

Rayner, K. and Pollatsek, A. (1989). *The psychology of reading*. Englewood Cliffs, NJ: Prentice Hall.

Rayner, K. and Pollatsek, A. (1996). Reading unspaced text is not easy: Comments on the implications of Epelboim et al.'s study for models of eye movement control in reading. *Vision Research*, **36**, 461–465.

Rayner, K. and Well, A.D. (1996). Effects of contextual constraint on eye movements in reading: A further examination. *Psychonomic Bulletin and Review*, **3**, 504–509.

Rayner, K., Well, A.D., and Pollatsek, A. (1980). Asymmetry of the effective visual field in reading. *Perception and Psychophysics*, **27**, 537–544.

Rayner, K., Balota, D.A., and Pollatsek, A. (1986). Against parafoveal semantic preprocessing during eye fixations in reading. *Canadian Journal of Psychology*, **40**, 473–483.

Rayner, K., Fischer, M.H., and Pollatsek, A. (1998). Unspaced text interferes with both word identification and eye movement control. *Vision Research*, **38**, 1129–1144.

Rayner, K., Li, X., and Pollatsek, A. (2007). Extending the E-Z Reader model to Chinese reading. *Cognitive Science*, **31**, 1021–1033.

Rayner, K., Li, X., Juhasz, B.J., and Yan, G. (2005). The effect of word predictability on the eye movements of Chinese readers. *Psychonomic Bulletin and Review*, **12**, 1089–1093.

Rayner, K., White, S.J., Kambe, G., Miller, B., and Liversedge, S.P. (2003). On the processing of meaning from parafoveal vision during eye fixation in reading. In J. Hyönä, R. Radach, and H. Deubel (eds.) *The mind's eye: Cognitive and applied aspects of eye movements* (pp. 213–234). Amsterdam: Elsevier Science.

Reichle, E.D., Rayner, K., and Pollatsek, A. (2003). The E-Z Reader model of eye-movement control in reading: Comparisons to other models. *Behavioral and Brain Sciences*, **26**, 445–476.

Ren, G. and Yang, Y. (2010). Syntactic boundaries and comma placement during silent reading of Chinese text: Evidence from eye movements. *Journal of Research in Reading*, **33**, 168–177.

Shen, D., Bai, X., Yan, G., and Liversedge, S.P. (2008). The perceptual span in Chinese reading. In K. Rayner, D. Shen, X. Bai, and G. Yan (eds.) *Cognitive and cultural influences on eye movements* (pp. 255–276). Tianjin: Tianjin People's Publishing House.

Shen, D., Liversedge, S.P., Tian, J., Zang, C., Cui, L., Bai, X., *et al.* (2011). Eye movements of second language learners when reading spaced and unspaced Chinese text. *Journal of Experimental Psychology: Applied*, under revision.

Shen, E. (1927). An analysis of eye movements in the reading of Chinese. *Journal of Experimental Psychology*, **10**, 158–183.

Spragins, A.B., Lefton, L.A., and Fisher, D.F. (1976). Eye movements while reading and searching spatially transformed text: A developmental examination. *Memory and Cognition*, **4**, 36–42.

Sun, F. and Feng, D. (1999). Eye movements in reading Chinese and English text. In J. Wang and A. W. Inhoff and H.-C. Chen (eds.) *Reading Chinese script: A cognitive analysis* (pp. 189–206). Mahwah, NJ: Lawrence Erlbaum.

Sun, F., Morita, M., and Stark, L.W. (1985). Comparative patterns of reading eye movement in Chinese and English. *Perception and Psychophysics*, **37**, 502–506.

Taft, M. and Zhu, X. (1997). Submorphemic processing in reading Chinese. *Journal of Experimental Psychology: Learning, Memory, and Cognition*, **23**, 761–775.

Taft, M., Zhu, X., and Peng, D. (1999). Positional specificity of radicals in Chinese character recognition. *Journal of Memory and Language, 40*, 498–519.

Tsai, J.L. and McConkie, G.W. (2003). Where do Chinese readers send their eyes? In J. Hyönä, R. Radach, and H. Deubel (eds.) *The mind's eye: Cognitive and applied aspects of eye movement research* (pp. 159–176). Oxford: Elsevier.

Tsai, J.L., Lee, C.Y., Tzeng, O.J.L., Hung, D.L., and Yen, N.S. (2004). Use of phonological codes for Chinese characters: Evidence from processing of parafoveal preview when reading sentences. *Brain and Language, 91*, 235–244.

Tsai, J.L., Lee, C.Y., Lin, Y.C., Tzeng, O.J.L., and Hung, D.L. (2006). Neighborhood size effects of Chinese words in lexical decision and reading. *Language and Linguistics, 7*, 659–675.

Tsang, Y.K. and Chen, H.-C. (2008). Eye movements in reading Chinese. In K. Rayner., D. Shen, X. Bai, and G. Yan (eds.) *Cognitive and cultural influences on eye movements* (pp. 235–254). Tianjin, China, Tianjin People's Publishing House.

Wang, H., Pomplun, M., Chen, M., Ko, H., and Rayner, K. (2010). Estimating the effect of word predicatability on eye movements in Chinese reading using latent semantic analysis and transitional probability. *Quarterly Journal of Experimental Psychology, 63*, 1374–1386.

Wang, S., Yang, J., and Chen, H.-C. (2008). Immediacy of processing intra-sentential and inter-sentential information in reading Chinese. In K. Rayner, D. Shen, X. Bai, and G. Yan (eds.) *Cognitive and cultural influences on eye movements* (pp. 315–341). Tianjin: Tianjin People's Publishing House.

Wong, K.F.E. and Chen, H.-C. (1999). Orthographic and phonological processing in reading Chinese text: Evidence from eye fixations. *Language and Cognitive Processes, 14*, 461–480.

Yan, G., Tian, H., Bai, X., and Rayner, K. (2006). The effect of word and character frequency on the eye movements of Chinese readers. *British Journal of Psychology, 97*, 259–268.

Yan, G., Bai, X., Zang, C., Bian, Q., Cui, L., Qi, W., *et al.* (2011). Using stroke removal to investigate Chinese character identification during reading: Evidence from eye movements. *Reading and Writing*, [Epub ahead of print].

Yan, M., Richter, E.M., Shu, H., and Kliegl, R. (2009). Readers of Chinese extract semantic information from parafoveal words. *Psychonomic Bulletin and Review, 16*, 561–566.

Yan, M., Kliegl, R., Richter, E., Nuthmann, A., and Shu, H. (2010a). Flexible saccade target selection in Chinese reading. *The Quarterly Journal of Experimental Psychology, 63*, 705–725.

Yan, M., Kliegl, R., Shu, H., Pan, J., and Zhou, X. (2010b). Parafoveal load of word n+1 modulates preprocessing effectiveness of word n+2 in Chinese reading. *Journal of Experimental Psychology: Human Perception and Performance, 36*, 1669–1676.

Yang, H.M. and McConkie, G.W. (1999). Reading Chinese: Some basic eye-movement characteristics. In H.-C. Chen (ed.) *Reading Chinese script: A cognitive analysis* (pp. 207–222). Mahwah, NJ: Lawrence Erlbaum Associates, Inc.

Yang, J., Wang, S., Xu, Y., and Rayner, K. (2009). Do Chinese readers obtain preview benefit from word n+2? Evidence from eye movements. *Journal of Experimental Psychology: Human Perception and Performance, 35*, 1192–1204.

Yen, M.H., Tsai, J.L., Tzeng, O.J.L., and Hung, D.L. (2008). Eye movements and parafoveal word processing in reading Chinese. *Memory and Cognition, 36*, 1033–1045.

Yen, M.H., Radach, R., Tzeng, O.J.L., Hung, D.L, and Tsai, J.L. (2009). Early parafoveal processing in reading Chinese sentences. *Acta Psychologica, 131*, 24–33.

Yin, B.Y. and Rohsenow, J.S. (1994). *Modern Chinese Characters*. Beijing: Sinolingua Press.

Zang, C., Liversedge, S.P., Liang, F., Bai, X., and Yan, G. (2011). Interword spacing and landing position effects during Chinese reading in children and adults. *Journal of Experimental Psychology: Human Perception and Performance*, under review.

CHAPTER 54

The mediation of eye movements by spoken language

Gerry T.M. Altmann

Abstract

Many factors can influence eye movements around a visual scene. Here, we consider the influence of spoken language. The first part of the chapter reviews a range of studies which illustrate how eye movements can illuminate aspects of spoken language understanding. The second presents a hypothesis of how spoken language mediates visual attention. The chapter then considers how this mediation might depend on the participant's goals, including consideration of what the timing of these eye movements might, or might not, tell us about their generalizability. Methodological issues, including how to depict the dynamically changing eye movement record, and how to analyse it, are considered next. The chapter concludes with some issues that are likely to dominate the field in future years.

Introduction

L.N. Fowler is perhaps best remembered for his now-ubiquitous bust illustrating the supposed relationship between the shape and size of the human cranium and the mental abilities of the mind housed within. Fowler's Phrenology, dating from around 1865, is of little relevance to contemporary Psychology, except for his bust's left eye, immediately below which is inscribed a mental faculty that, until recently, was rarely associated with the eye—*language*. That language should have any influence on the movement of the eyes is unsurprising; just as pointing can direct attention in one direction or another, or to one location or another, so language can do the same. Of interest, however, is *how* language exerts this influence on eye movement control. With respect to the coordination of eye and *hand* movements, Neggers and Bekkering (2002) concluded that 'ocular gaze is always forced to follow the target intended by a manual arm movement' (p. 365), with Horstmann and Hoffman (2005) concluding further that 'the saccadic system is no longer autonomous during a coordinated, goal-directed movement of eye and arm.' (p. 7) A natural question, then, given this tight coordination between eye and hand, is whether there are situations where referring to an object in the immediate environment might be as constraining of eye movements as reaching towards that object would be.

The chapter proceeds in five sections: 1) an overview of findings from the spoken language processing literature on language-mediated eye movements; 2) an account developed primarily from within that literature of how, and why, spoken language mediates eye movements; 3) consideration of task-dependence and the conditions under which language-mediation of visual attention and concomitant oculomotor control might be considered 'automatic'; 4) a survey of methodological issues that pervade research with language-mediated eye movements; and 5) a (brief) outline of the future directions in which this research is likely to proceed. Throughout, the emphasis is on spoken language; the literature on eye movements during *written* language processing will not be considered here.

Psycholinguistics and the language-mediation of eye movements

Roger Cooper first observed that as participants listen to a sentence referring to objects in a concurrently presented visual scene, the eyes move seemingly automatically to the objects in the scene as expressions referring to those objects are heard (Cooper, 1974). For instance, participants were more likely to fixate the picture of a snake when hearing 'snake' or part of 'snake' than pictures of referents of unrelated control words. Moreover, participants were more likely to fixate pictures showing a snake, a zebra, or a lion when hearing the semantically related word 'Africa' than they were to fixate referents of semantically unrelated control words. These were the first demonstrations that the patterns of eye movements in the context of unfolding language might reflect the online activation of word-level representations and their semantics, and the integration of these representations with the object-representations associated with (or activated by) a concurrent visual scene. It was not until almost 20 years later, however, that this seminal work was followed-up by Michael Tanenhaus and his students (Tanenhaus et al., 1995). Whereas Cooper had demonstrated the range of issues that might be addressed using this new methodology, Tanenhaus and his colleagues 'validated' the methodology by showing not only how classical results found elsewhere in the psycholinguistic literature could be 'replicated' within this new 'visual world paradigm', but also how the paradigm could be applied to the investigation of a broad range of language-related phenomena.

It should be borne in mind, throughout this chapter, that the influence of spoken language on eye movements to visual scenes (or towards regions of space in which a scene had previously been present) is limited; there are many factors *other than the language* which drive the eyes around a scene even as the spoken language unfolds. Throughout, when language is described as *mediating* eye movements, the data in fact show that it merely changes the *bias* to look at a part of space; on occasion, these biases are large and on occasion, small (see 'Task-sensitivity and language-mediated eye movements' and 'Methodological issues' sections). What is remarkable is *when* these biases change, and what is of interest is *why* they change, and what cognitive representations and processes these changes reflect.

The first study that synchronized the eye movement record with the unfolding language on a moment-by-moment basis was reported by Allopenna et al. (Allopenna et al., 1998; neither Cooper (1974) nor Tanenhaus et al. (1995) synchronized against the *moment-by-moment* unfolding of the concurrent language). They applied the technique to what at first blush appears to be a straightforward replication of standard 'competitor' effects first observed in investigation of the cohort model of spoken word recognition (Marslen-Wilson, 1987; Zwitserlood, 1989). They presented participants with a visual display depicting a beaker (the target item), a beetle (the onset of the word 'beetle' overlaps with the onset of 'beaker'), a (loud)speaker (the word 'speaker' rhymes with 'beaker') and a baby carriage ('carriage' is unrelated to any of the other words). At issue is what the eyes would do as participants heard the instruction to 'pick up the beaker' (which they did by clicking with the computer mouse). For the first 400 ms after the onset of 'beaker', the probability of participants fixating the beaker or the beetle rose, with no distinction between the two. After around 400 ms, the probabilities diverged, with the probability of fixation on the beetle dropping toward zero. This point coincided, roughly, with the end of the word 'beaker', and is approximately 200 ms after the point in the word that distinguishes it from 'beetle'. Allopenna et al. thus replicated the competitor effects predicted by the cohort model, although unlike prior demonstrations they were able to show how these effects unfold in real time. Interestingly, looks towards the speaker also increased in those first 400 ms before subsiding as the speech signal became more unambiguously compatible with 'beaker'. This was the first demonstration of *rhyme competitor* effects predicted by the Neighbourhood Activation Model (Luce et al., 1990; but see Marslen-Wilson, 1993 for discussion of such effects within the cohort model), which in turn demonstrated the utility of the visual world paradigm for exploring effects which hitherto had not been found using other techniques.

The 'first wave' of research with this paradigm focused more on language-mediated eye movements as a dependent measure used to study *language processing* rather than on language-mediated eye movements *as an object of study in their own right* (studies that are as relevant to eye movement control as they are to language processing are surveyed in subsequent sections). The survey that follows does not attempt to exhaustively summarize individual findings, nor is it an exhaustive listing—rather it is an indication of the range and breadth of psycholinguistic issues that have been elucidated with this paradigm. The vast majority of the findings support theories of language processing termed 'constraint satisfaction' theories (MacDonald et al., 1994; Trueswell and Tanehaus, 1994). These theories assume that language processing consists of the application of probabilistic constraints, in parallel, as a sentence unfolds, with no single constraint being more or less privileged than any other except in respect of its probabilistic strength. The origins of this constraints-based approach are rooted in the development of the parallel distributed processing (i.e. *connectionist*) models of cognitive representation and process (e.g. Rumelhart and McClelland, 1986). Thus, information that could *in principle* be applied to the task of interpreting a segment of the unfolding language *can be* applied, and at the earliest possible opportunity, subject to whatever other information might also be applied at that time, be it acoustic-phonetic, lexical, prosodic, syntactic, semantic, or pragmatic. There are some notable exceptions, and these are referred to as appropriate below.

◆ *Sensitivity to acoustic-phonetic and prosodic variation*—these studies showed that eye movements are extremely finely time-locked to the unfolding acoustic signal, reflecting graded effects on lexical access of subtle phonetic variation, including coarticulation, in the input. The essential finding is that as a word unfolds in the acoustic input, so the eyes move towards whatever in the visual scene that unfolding word *could* refer to, taking into account the 'goodness of fit' between the acoustic signal and words in the mental lexicon (Dahan et al., 2001; Magnuson et al., 2003a; McMurray et al., 2002; Salverda et al., 2003, 2007).

◆ *Lexical competition, lexical neighbourhood, and frequency effects*—building on Allopenna et al. (1998), these studies used profiles of dynamically changing fixation probabilities to explore the time-course of activation of words differing in frequency (Dahan et al., 2001) or occupying 'dense' or 'sparse' neighbourhoods (Magnuson et al., 2007). They found that eye movements towards objects whose names differed in frequency, or were from differing neighbourhood types, had different dynamic fixation profiles. Thus, the lexical context (the neighbourhood) within which an unfolding word must be processed, as well as its frequency, influences the activation of the corresponding lexical representation (cf. Marslen-Wilson, 1990; Luce et al., 1990), in turn influencing the eye movements towards its referent. Some of these studies employed artificial languages so as to more precisely control word frequency and similarity to other words in the (artificial) lexicon (e.g. Magnuson et al., 2003b).

◆ *The bilingual lexicon*—only a minority of the world's population speak a single language; the majority have to contend with word forms which, depending on the language they are hearing at the time, may mean one thing or another or nothing. Spivey and Marian (1999) used the visual world paradigm to show that hearers do not only activate lexical representations for words in the language being spoken/heard—they also activate competitor (i.e. phonologically overlapping) words from the other language

◆ *Lexical semantics*—whereas the studies described thus far have focused primarily on word *form*, the visual world paradigm has also been applied to individual word *meaning*. Yee and Sedivy (2001) showed that hearing 'piano' not only engenders saccades towards a piano (cf. Allopenna et al., 1998), but also towards a trumpet if present (see Yee and Sedivy, 2006, for the full report). Huettig and Altmann (2005) extended Yee and Sedivy's design to include the case where a trumpet was present without the piano. They also computed a measure of the 'conceptual similarity' between pianos and trumpets (and the other pairings in the study), using semantic feature norms (Cree and McRae, 2003). These similarity scores predicted the probability of launching a saccade during the target word (e.g. 'piano') towards the semantic competitor (e.g. the trumpet). They also predicted the time subsequently spent fixating the semantic competitor. We return later, in the section 'How, and why, language mediates eye movements', to the significance of these data for understanding *why* the eyes move in this paradigm; the Yee and Huettig data prove the key to understanding the *linkage* between language and eye movements. More recently, the paradigm has been used also to explore differences in the lexical representation of concrete vs. abstract words (the distinction between words referring to objects that can be directly perceived vs. words that refer to concepts that cannot be perceived directly, such as 'honesty'; Duñabeitia et al., 2009).

♦ *Syntactic ambiguity resolution, in adults and in children*—moving 'up' into the realm of sentence processing, and building on earlier findings by Crain and Steedman (1985) and Altmann and Steedman (1988), Tanenhaus et al. (1995) and Spivey et al. (2002) reported a study showing how the real-time interpretation of syntactically ambiguous sentences depends on the context within which the sentence is interpreted. They showed participants either one apple or two (with one of the apples on a towel), and told participants to 'put the apple on the towel in the box'. Analyses of the eye and hand movements (i.e. which apple and where it was moved to) indicated that when there were two apples, 'on the towel' was interpreted as indicating which apple (i.e. it was interpreted as a modifier), but when there was just one apple, it was temporarily interpreted as where the apple should be put (i.e. it was interpreted as the goal). Trueswell et al. (1999) repeated a version of this study with children, and found that they do not use such *referential context* in the same way as do adults. Subsequent research with the visual world paradigm, again investigating real-time processing in adults and in children, showed that this is most likely due to children's increased sensitivity (relative to adults) to the particular syntactic contexts in which different verbs are most often found (Snedeker and Trueswell, 2004). Snedeker and Trueswell (2003) described a separate study showing also how speakers and hearers use prosody to disambiguate these kinds of ambiguity, and how this interacts with referential context. Other studies that have used this paradigm to explore effects of prosody and pitch accent, and their interactions with referential and discourse contexts, include Dahan et al. (2002) and Ito and Speer (2008).

♦ *Prediction in sentence comprehension, in adults and in children*—similar to Altmann (1999), who used a word-by-word reading task, Altmann and Kamide (1999) used the visual world paradigm to show how participants anticipate upcoming information in a sentence. They showed participants scenes depicting a person, a single edible object, and other distractor objects, and found that when hearing 'the boy will eat . . .' participants' eyes moved towards that edible object before the subsequent noun phrase was heard (e.g. '. . . the cake'). Similar results have been found using other syntactic structures: Sussman and Sedivy (2003) showed that, on hearing 'what did Jodie squash the spider with?' the eyes anticipated at 'squash' the spider, but at 'the spider' they immediately anticipate a shoe (that had been used for the squashing). Arai et al. (2007) showed also that participants anticipate the *ordering* of referents if there will be more than one, as in 'the boy will give the girl the cake' (for related studies see Scheepers and Crocker, 2004; Thothathiri and Snedeker, 2008). Subsequently, verb-based anticipatory effects have been found in children, whether skilled or less-skilled at comprehension (Nation et al., 2003), and also in infants (Anne Fernald, personal communication). Equivalent results have also been shown using other empirical methods, such as ERP (DeLong et al., 2005; van Berkum et al., 2005). Dahan and Tanenhaus (2004) used the visual world paradigm to show that verb-based constraints such as those used by Altmann and Kamide (1999) exclude from consideration semantically incompatible cohort competitors (thus, a cable would not be entertained during the earliest moments of 'cake' when preceded by 'the boy will eat'). A related result was obtained by Magnuson et al. (2008), using an artificial language; they showed that expectations with respect to the anticipated *form-class* (e.g. noun versus adjective) modulated cohort competitor effects such that a competitor from the 'wrong' form-class was not entertained.

◆ *Morphosyntactic variation and cross-linguistic differences in word order*—building on this last finding that participants can anticipate at the verb what may be referred to next, Kamide et al. (2003a) showed that in German, a language that permits OVS (object–verb–subject) word order rather than just SVO as in English, speakers use case-marking on the individual nouns to drive their predictions: if the first noun is marked in the nominative (indicating it refers to the agent of some event), the eyes anticipate at the verb whatever would be a suitable 'patient' (i.e. the object on which the agent acts); but if the first noun is marked in the accusative (indicating it refers to the patient), the eyes anticipate whatever would be a suitable agent. Related work (focusing on other aspects of grammatical marking or discourse status) has been reported in Finnish (Kaiser and Trueswell, 2004) and in Japanese (Kamide et al., 2003b), with the latter study showing that anticipation need not be verb-driven (Japanese is a verb-final language, so any predictive processing is necessarily triggered by non-verbal constituents).

◆ *Combinatorial semantic processing*—Kamide et al. (2003) followed-up their original observation of anticipatory eye movements with a study in which they showed that it was the semantic combination of the verb with its subject that drove the anticipatory process: it was not simply whatever was edible that would be looked at after 'the boy will eat . . .', but rather what would most plausibly be eaten by the person doing the eating. This result was significant because it showed that it was not simply a form of semantic priming ('eat' causing looks toward anything edible) that drove the original effect, but was in fact the product of the syntactic and semantic processes that combine the verb with its subject, coupled with real-world knowledge of which kinds of event are more likely given the depicted participants in those events. Related data were reported by Knoeferle and colleagues (Knoeferle and Crocker, 2006; Knoeferle et al., 2005). Boland (2005) demonstrated that there are limits on anticipation during sentence processing: In the sentence 'Chris recommended a movie to Kim in the hallway', the movie and Kim are both *arguments* of the verb; the meaning of the verb entails that there is something being recommended and someone to whom the recommendation is made. But 'in the hallway' is an *adjunct*—it is not a part of the core meaning of the verb, and Boland showed that adjuncts are not anticipated to the same extent as arguments. Thus the grammatical status of the objects that might be anticipated does appear to influence the likelihood of their anticipation.

◆ *Resolving pronominal reference during sentence processing*—most of the above studies take advantage of the fact that, as the language refers to something in a concurrent visual scene (or even beforehand), so the eyes look towards it. The paradigm is thus particularly useful for determining when, and what basis, readers or listeners interpret words such as 'he/she/they/himself/etc.' Reading studies, for example, can determine how such words are interpreted only *indirectly* (e.g. through increased reading times in certain circumstances). The visual world paradigm provides a more direct assessment of how pronouns are interpreted as they are encountered: For example, in the following sentence, 'He' is ambiguous: 'Donald is bringing some mail to Mickey while a violent storm is beginning. He's carrying an umbrella'. By observing eye movements at 'He' it is possible to infer which of the two possible characters the hearer attributes as the referent for the pronoun. And by changing 'Mickey' to 'Minnie' it is possible to explore the timing with which gender information (Minnie is a girl) is applied. Of course, and as mentioned at the outset of this chapter, individual participants rarely saccade to a language-relevant target 100% of the time; when they do saccade to it, it is likely that they do so because of that relevance (although there will always be some smaller likelihood that they did so for some other reason), but when they do not, aggregating across subjects and trials allows one to determine at what point relative to the language the *bias* to look towards the target changes. A range of studies have shown the immediacy with which information about accessibility (Donald is more accessible as he was mentioned in subject position) and gender (the Mickey/Minnie alternation) can be applied during pronoun resolution (e.g. Arnold et al., 2000). Interestingly, 3–5-year-old children show immediate use of gender information, but appear relatively insensitive to the order of mention in the first sentence (Arnold et al., 2007a). Other studies have focused on the processing of reflexive pronouns ('himself/herself') in various contexts (e.g. Runner et al., 2003; 2006; Sekerina et al., 2004). And most recently, Arnold and Lao (2009) have used an exogenous attentional capture paradigm (Gleitman et al., 2007) to show how attentional mechanisms (exogenous and endogenous) impact on pronoun comprehension. Distinguishing between such influences will prove crucial to a fuller understanding of how language interpretation (and production; see below) interacts with systems that (also) serve visual processing.

The use of pronouns reflects dynamic changes in the perspectives that both hearer and speaker take as their shared language unfolds: speakers use pronouns when they anticipate that their listeners will be able to interpret them given the context. The studies described thus far have focused on comprehension. Unsurprisingly, the visual world paradigm has been used also to investigate a number of issues relating to language production (see Griffin, 2004b, for review), dialogue, and perspective-taking.

- ◆ *Name retrieval*—the first study to use eye movements to study planning processes during speech production was reported by Antje Meyer and colleagues (Meyer et al., 1998). Participants had to name the objects presented across a screen. This study showed that participants do not look away from a to-be-named object until they have recognized the object and retrieved the phonological form associated with its name. A number of studies, including this one, explored how the ease of retrieving the phonological form modulates gaze durations (see also Griffin, 2001).

- ◆ *Sentence planning*—Griffin and Bock (2000) asked participants to describe simple transitive events depicted by line drawings of e.g. a dog chasing a postman. They found that, irrespective of whether the dog or the postman is about to be named, it is fixated around 900 ms before the articulation of its name. But as in Meyer et al.'s (1998) study, the eyes leave the object around 100–300 ms before articulating it, moving towards the next object to be named. Interestingly, participants fixate objects around 900 ms before articulating even an incorrect name for the object, as in 'gira- uh zebra' (Griffin, 2004a). One important aspect of the Griffin and Bock (2000) study is that they managed to distinguish between event apprehension and utterance formulation by comparing eye movements during the event-description task with eye movements made by a different group of participants whose task was to discern who was acted upon in the event (the postman in the above example). That different patterns of eye movements can be observed as a function of task is something we return to in the section 'Task-sensitivity and language-mediated eye movements'. Gleitman et al. (2007) reported a study which used exogenous attentional capture to direct attention towards one protagonist or another; this influenced their order of mention in a subsequent description (e.g. between 'a dog is chasing a man' vs. 'a man is running from a dog'). This study also found that early *endogenous* shifts in attention during scene apprehension also predicted order of mention, unlike in the Griffin and Bock (2000) study. This difference between the studies may have been due to differences in both the visual and linguistic stimuli used, and it remains unclear whether endogenous shifts in attention during early scene apprehension do indeed influence 'accessibility' of concepts for subsequent linguistic processing (cf. Bock, 1986, 1987). Gleitman et al. (2007) concluded that the on-line construction of descriptive utterances mirrors the on-line apprehension of the events which the utterance describes.

- ◆ *Dialogue: common ground and speaker perspective*—speakers rarely engage in monologue, without due regard for the knowledge, beliefs, and perspectives of their addressee(s). In dialogue, speaker and hearer change turns as they converse about things and ideas that are, or become, common knowledge to both (see Kreysa and Pickering, Chapter 52, this volume). A lasting issue concerns how speaker and hearer keep track of the overlap between what they know and what their interlocutor (i.e. the other) does and does not know; i.e. what is in 'common ground' and what is 'privileged'. Keysar et al. (2000) employed a commonly used technique in production research whereby a 'confederate speaker' (i.e. one of the experimenters) instructed a hearer to manipulate objects arranged in cubbyholes—the speaker sat on one side, and the hearer on the other, looking through the cubbyholes to one another. Most of the objects could therefore be seen jointly by both speaker and hearer. But some of the cubbyholes were blocked off so that the hearer knew that only he/she could see them. Thus, there might be two boxes, one in a cubbyhole seen by both speaker and hearer and the other in a cubbyhole seen only by the hearer (and thus privileged). In this case, where might the hearer look on hearing 'move the box . . .'? If the hearer tracks in real time what is and what is not in common view, eye movements during 'the box' should be directed only to the box in common ground (seen by both), but if the hearer does not track in real time what is common and what is privileged, the expression 'the box' would be ambiguous. Eye movements in fact suggested the latter, with looks toward both objects. This result has proved extremely controversial, with other studies finding that interlocutors do keep track in real time of what is privileged and what is common (e.g. in adults: Hanna et al., 2003; in children: Nadig and Sedivy, 2002. See Barr (2008a), for an example of an attempt to reconcile the different findings).

- *Social referencing and common ground*—Crosby et al. (2008) reported an ingenious version of the common/privileged ground work: participants viewed a screen showing four other individuals. In one condition all four were apparently able to hear what the participant could hear; in the other, only two of the four could hear, and participants knew which. Subsequently, when participants heard one of the four utter something that was potentially offensive to one of the other individuals (for example, a negative remark about affirmative action when one of the other individuals was an African American), participants looked towards that individual only when they supposed that he/she could also hear what the speaker had said. In this case, social referencing (referring to a class of individual, rather than to the specifically depicted individual) directed eye gaze, but only when that individual was in what might be called 'communicative common ground'.

- *Unscripted dialogue*—a number of studies have extended the prior work into the realm of unscripted dialogue, monitoring eye movements either to just one of the interlocutors (e.g. Brown-Schmidt and Tanenhaus, 2006; Brown-Schmidt et al., 2005), or to both (Richardson and Dale, 2005; Richardson et al., 2007). The Richardson and Dale (2005) study involved one participant describing, for example, the characters from the sitcom *Friends* while the other listened. Both were viewing a display showing all six faces of the main characters. Listeners' eye movements closely mirrored the eye movements of the speaker. Of course, whereas the speaker fixated the individual characters in advance of referring to them (cf. Griffin and Bock, 2000; Meyer et al., 1998), listeners' eye movements were delayed until shortly after each was referred to (we return to timing issues later, in the section 'Task-sensitivity and language-mediated eye movements').

- *Interpreting speakers' disfluencies*—unscripted dialogue (and even scripted dialogue) is rarely fluent. Jennifer Arnold and colleagues have used the visual world paradigm to explore how listeners interpret disfluencies such as 'Click on thee uh red . . .' and showed that listeners interpret such disfluencies as indicating that the speaker is having difficulty, which in turn triggers an inference about the likely cause of this difficulty (such as naming something that is new to the domain of discourse (Arnold et al., 2004); or something that is unfamiliar (Arnold et al., 2007b). This work is as important in demonstrating the role of higher-level inferences with regard to speakers' intentions as it is in demonstrating hearer's ability to interpret disfluencies as being informative.

This sensitivity of language-mediated eye movements to speaker intentions, and not just to the *linguistic form* of an utterance (i.e. sensitivity to *pragmatic* knowledge), renders the paradigm particularly useful with respect to determining how pragmatic information is recruited in real time as a sentence unfolds within a concurrent context. We conclude this review of psycholinguistic topics with a range of studies that have demonstrated more pragmatic influences on language-mediated eye movements.

- *Gricean Pragmatics*—Sedivy (2003) reviews a range of eye movement data on interactions between listeners' expectations and the informativity of the expressions produced by the speaker (and what listeners do when the speaker is more informative than might otherwise be assumed necessary to identify a particular referent). For example, Sedivy et al. (1999) monitored eye movements as listeners heard instructions such as 'Pick up the tall glass'. Analysis of eye movements showed that listeners interpret *scalar adjectives* such as 'tall' by explicitly comparing against contrasting objects; a tall glass is identified through its intended contrast with a shorter glass (and in the absence of a contrasting glass would be inappropriately over-informative, just as uttering 'the yellow banana' would be over-informative in some contexts but appropriately informative in others (Grice, 1975)). Interestingly, listeners take account of speaker characteristics when computing such contrastive inferences (i.e. if the speaker uses the expression 'tall glass' it is because there must be a shorter glass available in the domain of reference); listeners did not appear to compute these inferences when they had evidence that the speaker was not adhering to the usual Gricean (cooperative) conversational maxims (Grodner and Sedivy, in press).

◆ *Visual affordances*—so far we have seen that language-mediated eye movements are not simply driven by linguistic form, but also by the communicative goals of the speaker and listener (cf. Sedivy, 2003). Unsurprisingly, they are also driven by the *behavioural* goals of the listener (and we return to this again in the section 'Task-sensitivity and language-mediated eye movements'). These are in turn modulated by the affordances of the objects to which that behaviour is directed. Chambers et al. (2004) showed, for example, that the instrument given to the listener with which to perform an action influenced which objects were entertained as the 'target' of that action; holding a hook would cause eye movements during a referring expression such as 'the whistle' to only those whistles to which were attached loops that could be hooked. Related findings were reported by Chambers et al. (2002). Altmann and Kamide (2007) re-interpreted their earlier findings of anticipatory eye movements as reflecting the goodness-of-fit between the interpretation of the sentence and the affordances of the objects depicted within the scene; they used a tense manipulation ('will drink' vs. 'has drunk') to show how eye movements at the verb were driven towards objects that either would afford drinking in the future (e.g. a full glass of beer) or had afforded drinking in the past (e.g. an empty glass of wine). A similar tense manipulation in the visual world is described by Knoeferle and Crocker (2007). That study was notable also because they showed how language-mediated eye movements were modulated by the interpretation of an event that unfolded across a series of scenes (cf. distinct panels of a comic strip, with earlier panels setting the context for later panels).

◆ *Linguistic relativity*—different languages describe events in different ways, and since Whorf's original observations (Whorf, 1956), researchers have questioned to what extent such differences may influence how people may conceive the world and apprehend events. Slobin (1996) proposed that speakers' utterances as they plan to describe an event may be shaped by the language they will use for that utterance, and this in turn may influence how the event is conceived as its articulation is planned (the 'thinking for speaking' hypothesis). Papafragou et al. (2008) addressed this issue by comparing eye movements of Greek and English speakers as they viewed motion events and prepared to either describe them or remember them. English and Greek differ in respect of how they describe the *manner* and *path* of motion; English tends to encode manner on the verb and not path ('slide', 'skip', but less commonly 'ascend' favouring instead 'go up'), while Greek tends to encode path on the verb and not manner. In support of the 'thinking for speaking' perspective, attention to distinct landmarks (indicating path) or to instruments indicating the kind of motion (e.g. skates) *did* differ as a function of native language. However, in the non-linguistic task in which participants did not have to prepare a description of the unfolding event they were viewing, there was no effect of native language on the manner in which attention was allocated as the events were apprehended. In this study at least, differences with respect to which elements of the language refer to which constituents of an event did not, contra Whorf and others, affect the way in which attention was allocated during the apprehension of the events.

Economies of space preclude a more thorough overview of what has been learned about language processing through the use of the visual world paradigm. A variant of this paradigm, the findings from which are beyond the remit of this survey, is the 'preferential looking' paradigm. This is in common use in developmental psychology. In this paradigm, as applied to language processes, an infant might be sat upon a carer's lap, and different screens (e.g. one to each side of a central fixation light) may show different objects or scenes; the infant's preference to look towards one object/scene or another, as a word or sentence is heard, is then measured. The technique has been used widely and to significant effect. Of course, here the dependent measure is not eye movements per se, as infants will most often move their heads also in this paradigm. Nonetheless, what is common to each paradigm is the language-mediated deployment of visual attention, a phenomenon that pervades the lifespan. In the following section, we consider the mechanism by which language mediates eye movements (and/or visual attention), and the data (only some of which have been previewed in this section) that reveal this mechanism.

How, and why, language mediates eye movements

A number of distinct findings are key to understanding the mechanism by which language may direct eye movements. The fact that it does so at all is not particularly surprising, as mentioned at the outset of this article. More interesting is the *mechanism* by which language fulfils that part of its purpose concerned with making the hearer look one way or another. And as we shall see, the actual act of looking is almost incidental—what language does is not so much direct attention towards objects in the external world, but rather towards objects as represented in an internal mental representation of that external world. This is rendered possible in the visual world paradigm because, typically, the onset of the scene and the objects it contains *precedes* the onset of the language, and thus the objects can be apprehended, and their locations established, before the onset of the language. As will become clear, the visual world paradigm appears to work as it does precisely because, as the language unfolds, the locations of the objects that become relevant to that language are already known (but see Moores et al., 2003, for an example of where the language preceded the scene).

The first finding that bears on the mechanism of language-mediation is simply that as the name of an object unfolds, so the likelihood of moving the eye towards that object rises (Allopenna et al., 1998). These and related data (e.g. Dahan and Tanehaus, 2004) suggest a continuous mapping between the activation of lexical representations through linguistic input and the likelihood of moving the eyes towards the object(s) in the scene that match those lexical representations. But crucially, the match need not be an exact one: Shifts in visual attention (which can be assumed to precede eye movements) are not tied only to direct reference. Thus, hearing 'piano' engenders looks towards a trumpet (Yee and Sedivy, 2006) and does so in proportion to the semantic relatedness of the object referred to by the word and the object depicted in the scene (Huettig and Altmann, 2005). This second set of findings (and other related data; e.g. Myung et al., 2006) suggest that it is the *conceptual overlap* between the word and the object that mediates between language and eye movements. These semantic relatedness data rule out an account based solely on phonological overlap between the unfolding word and the names associated with the objects in the scene.

A third set of findings suggests that it is not even the object itself, as depicted in the concurrent scene, that is the 'target' to which eye movements are directed; a number of studies have demonstrated that even if the scene is removed *prior* to the onset of the linguistic stimulus, the eyes move back to wherever the named, or anticipated, objects *had been located* (Altmann, 2004; see also Hoover and Richardson, 2008; Knoeferle and Crocker, 2007. For related work see Richardson and Spivey (2000), and for eye movements during visual imagery, see Brandt and Stark, 1997; Laeng and Teodorecu, 2002). These 'blank screen' effects demonstrate that the eyes can be directed not towards the object per se (because in the blank screen there is no object), but rather, towards a particular location as indexed by an *episodic representation* of that object (cf. Richardson et al., 2009). A final set of findings demonstrates that this episodic trace is malleable. Altmann and Kamide (2009) described a study using the blank screen paradigm in which the unfolding language described a change in location for one of the objects (e.g. 'the woman will move the glass onto the table'). Subsequent reference to that object (e.g. 'she will pour the wine into the glass') engendered looks during the critical referring expression ('the glass') towards the *new* location of that object, and not to the old location as had actually been seen in the previous scene (in fact, and perhaps surprisingly, the old location was looked at no more than the location of other distractor objects; this location held no residual 'attraction').

Unlike in earlier blank screen studies, the spatial representations that directed the eye movements were not reliant on the objects actually having occupied particular locations within the scene—in the example, the glass had never been seen on the table, and yet the eyes moved there on hearing the sentence-final 'glass'.

These and other related data prompted Altmann and Kamide (2007) to articulate an account of the language mediation of eye movements that is based on the activation, by the scene, of a memory representation of an object—its *episodic trace* (see Richardson and Spivey, 2000, for a precursor of this account). This trace includes information not only about the object's properties but its location also. When a sequence of words is subsequently heard (the assumption being that the activation of these episodic traces precedes the onset of the language), the representations engendered by the unfolding language may overlap with the pre-existing representations activated by the concurrent or prior scene (i.e. those episodic traces). This overlap causes an increase in the activation of those traces (due to the dual support they now receive), and this in turn percolates through to the spatial indices associated with those traces. Altmann and Kamide (2007) view the change in activation of an object's representation as a change in the attentional state of the cognitive system (cf. Cohen et al., 2004), with this change either *constituting*, or *causing*, a shift in covert attention. This shift in covert attention, in turn, is accompanied by an increased likelihood of an overt eye movement (due to the increased activation to the spatial index associated with that trace). Altmann and Kamide (2007) offer one possible explanation, based on Hebbian learning, for why increased activation of the spatial index associated with the episodic trace should lead to an eye movement: Orienting towards an object increases the activation of the mental representation of that object and its encoded location. Successive pairings of this kind during development may result in the opposite pattern, with increases in the activation of a mental representation of an object and its location resulting in the increased likelihood of an orientation response towards that location. This is, of course, both simplistic and speculative. But it does account for why, irrespective of whether the scene is concurrent *or* absent at the time of the unfolding language, the unfolding language can cause eye movements towards objects' current or past locations. What remains to be explained, however, are the 'moved glass' effects reported by Altmann and Kamide (2009). That study showed that the spatial index associated with the episodic trace of an object is not fixed, and is not determined solely by its past perceptual correlates. They proposed that the targeting of saccadic eye movements can be supported by two distinct kinds of representation; those based on perceptual properties of the configuration of objects as directly experienced in the scene, and those based on the conceptual properties of the objects and their configuration, with the latter changing dynamically as a function of the unfolding language and ensuing event representations. Both kinds of representation are required, as otherwise it would not be possible to explain how the eyes can return either to the original location of the glass (as directly perceived previously) or to the new location (as conceptually determined by the language-induced event representation).

Task-sensitivity and language-mediated eye movements

The previous section reviewed an account of the mechanism underlying the language-mediation of eye movements in which such mediation occurs non-consciously. But does this mean that language-mediation of eye movements will occur the same way regardless of the *goals* of the hearer? Certainly, language-mediation of eye movements can be non-conscious in the same way that priming can be (i.e. the recognition of a word or object being facilitated if there has been prior exposure to a related item; for review and an example of priming of picture recognition by unconsciously perceived primes, see Dell'Acqua and Grainger (1999)). Many of the findings reviewed above suggest a non-conscious quality to language-mediated eye movements: the fact that the eyes move at 'piano' to a trumpet, and do so in proportion to their semantic relatedness (Huettig and Altmann, 2005, Yee and Sedivy, 2006). Or the fact that language-mediated eye movements are sensitive to frequency and neighbourhood effects (Dahan et al., 2001, Magnuson et al., 2007). And so on. These effects suggest that participants are not consciously directing their eyes. But this is not the same as saying that participants are not being *strategic*; the mechanism described in the preceding section does not entail *task-independence* (within contemporary views of attention and 'cognitive control', the task is key to modulating the flow of relevant information within the cognitive system (Cohen et al., 2004)). Unsurprisingly, there has been some speculation about the extent to which the patterns of eye movements reviewed above may be specific to the particular tasks employed in each study. However, and as reviewed by Tanenhaus and Trueswell (2006), there is of course no one 'task' that corresponds to 'spoken language comprehension'—how we process and react to language depends on the situation and the communicative and behavioural goals of the interlocutors. But rightly, investigators have questioned the extent to which the results reported using one task or another might generalize to different communicative situations.

Perhaps the majority of tasks employed within the visual world paradigm have involved asking participants to use a mouse to move objects around a visual display, or to click on objects mentioned in the unfolding sentence (a typical instruction might be: 'click on whichever object in the display is the object referred to in the sentence which is acted upon by someone or something else. So if you hear "the girl rode the bicycle", you would click on the bicycle'). Some of the earliest studies involved participants reaching for objects placed in front of them (e.g. Tanenhaus et al., 1995). Eye movements in such cases are in service of a behavioural task which requires the eyes to actively look at the targets of the reaching motion or the mouse movement. One advantage is that the likelihood of fixating the target objects in these cases is very high. On the other hand, a disadvantage is that we cannot be sure that these eye movements would have occurred in the absence of an explicit instruction to target one object or another (with the accompanying eye movements being a necessary precursor to the mouse/hand movements). This is true of both the reaching/clicking tasks but also the sentence-picture verification studies (e.g. Altmann and Kamide, 1999, expt. 1; Sedivy et al., 1999, expt. 3); these do not entail a targeted mouse or hand movement, but they do entail a visual search in service of the verification task. Alternative to these explicit instruction tasks are the 'look-and-listen' tasks in which participants are told only that there will be occasional comprehension questions that may target either the pictures or the sentences. In some instances, a 'cover story' is given to participants to explain why their eyes are being tracked (e.g. 'We are interested in the manner in which different words cause the pupil to dilate or contract as the eyes are engaged, or have been engaged, in normal viewing'—this of course involves an element of deception that may be of concern to local ethics committees!). The look-and-listen task was employed in the more recent blank screen studies of Altmann and Kamide (2009); it has occasionally been referred to as a 'passive listening' task, although this is probably a misnomer; if it were really passive, the eyes would not so actively move. A disadvantage of this task is that the likelihood of fixating the target object(s) can be quite low, and may dynamically rise and fall throughout the unfolding speech as other objects in the scene compete for attention. One concern with the look-and-listen tasks is that participants may adopt different processing strategies as the moment takes them—at one extreme, for example, a participant in such a study may attempt to memorize each scene and its correspondence to the language; at the other, a participant may maintain central fixation without attending at all to the scene or its relationship to the language. It is all the more remarkable, therefore, that in the face of such variance, consistent patterns of eye movements can nonetheless be observed which generalize statistically across participants. Nor is this problem unique to this particular paradigm; reading time studies (and indeed, many others) suffer the same problem—participants may choose to process each sentence to more or less 'depth' as a function of their engagement, alertness, mood, or their perception of the experimenter's goals. The freedom with which participants can strategize is a problem endemic to experimental psychology, not to one paradigm or another. But again, finding consistent patterns in the face of this processing anarchy is usually taken to be indicative of some specific, generalizable, cognitive tendency.

A more serious concern for some has been what Tanenhaus and Trueswell (2006) refer to as the 'closed set problem'—the fact that the visual environment in typical visual world studies is very much more restricted than the usual environment with which we typically interact. Many studies have presented participants with displays containing as few as just four objects (e.g. Allopenna et al., 1998;

Altmann, 2004; and others). It is rare that in everyday life our visual environment contains so few discernable items. The use of displays depicting only a very small set of objects could in principle lead to 'unnatural' processing strategies (e.g. implicit naming of the objects in the scene, although as already pointed out, such a strategy is unlikely to be widespread in view of the semantic relatedness data of Huettig and Altmann (2005), and Yee and Sedivy (2006), discussed earlier). With respect to whether this closed set problem compromises generalizability to language processing more generally, it should be noted that most often interlocutors also restrict themselves to talking about only a small number of discourse entities (most studies of reading introduce fewer entities into the domain of reference than does the typical visual world study). Similarly, observers generally attend within their visual environment to just a few objects. Thus, much (if not most) of our experience is in the context of only a limited number of objects to which we attend/refer. However, while it can be said that the *modus operandi* of natural language is to restrict the domain of reference to a subset of all the things we could possibly know about, natural scenes are rarely restricted in the ways that are typical of visual world studies. But most often, researchers are not intending the scenes they use as surrogates of real visual environments—they are instead artificial 'targets' against which the unfolding language can be 'aimed'. The paradigm is limited in some respects, but liberating in others.

Notwithstanding this last defence of the closed set problem, how we select one object from a smaller or larger set of visual alternatives may reflect quite different visual search strategies. When there are only a handful of objects in view, naming one of those objects will generally cause the eyes to move directly to that object (see the previous section for an account of how this can come about, predicated upon prior knowledge of the identities and locations of the depicted objects). But the same is unlikely upon hearing the name of one of 100 objects in view—rather, a visual search may be initiated around the area in which we conjecture that the object is located.

A further task-related issue concerns the timing of language-mediated eye movements. The timing with which language can mediate eye movements is an important issue because of the manner in which researchers typically synchronize the eye movement record with the unfolding speech (see 'Methodological issues' section for further detail). The standard assumption is that it takes up to 200 ms to program and launch a saccade, with many researchers assuming that any eye movement launched within 200 ms of word onset could not have been influenced by that word. The majority of studies that investigated the delay between stimulus onset and saccadic initiation used visual stimuli as both triggers (i.e. the signal to move) and targets (e.g. Rayner et al., 1983; Saslow, 1967). One oft-cited study, which attempted to measure 'saccadic overhead'—roughly, the time to plan and launch a saccade once the target has been identified—estimated around 100 ms (Matin et al., 1993). It is perhaps curious that this study is often cited by users of the visual world paradigm in the context of the 200 ms figure, especially as this study did not even monitor eye movements! (It required participants to make judgements that either did or did not require saccadic eye movements; button press reaction times were collected and subtracted from one another across the different saccadic conditions.)

To address the lack of any data on language-mediated launch times, Altmann and Kamide (2004) reported a study in which participants were told to move their eyes to a pre-determined location as soon as they heard an auditory cue. In that case, the mean, median, and modal launch times were 254, 181, and 132 ms respectively. This highly skewed distribution (an early peak, in this case at around 130 ms, followed by a long tail) is typical of saccadic launch times (e.g. Carpenter, 1988); thus, the mean launch time in such a distribution is not an appropriate measure of the 'central tendency'. However, in this task, participants knew in advance where they would have to move their eyes, and it is known that such prior knowledge can speed launch times (Saslow, 1967). The Altmann and Kamide (2004) study also included a condition in which participants did not have such prior knowledge; the auditory cue was the name of the target object to which they had to move their eyes. In this case, launch times were much slower, with a median response time (in error-free trials) of 484 ms At first glance, this suggests that the 200 ms assumption is a conservative estimate. However, it needs to be borne in mind that eye movement control is, independently of linguistic mediation, sensitive to task differences: The time to launch a saccade depends on the urgency of the response

(Reddi and Carpenter, 2000), the likelihood of having to saccade to one location or another (Carpenter and Williams, 1995), and the number and positioning of distractor objects (e.g. McSorley and Findlay, 2003; Walker et al., 1997; and references therein). Thus, in the absence of information about the distribution of launch times that would be typical for a given language-mediated task and a given set of visual configurations, it is probably safest to err on the side of caution, and to assume that some number of eye movements which were launched within 200 ms of some word's onset were indeed influenced by that word. More recently, and in a reanalysis of the studies published by Kamide et al. (2003) and by Altmann (2004), Altmann (2010) has provided evidence that language can in fact influence the eye movement record within as little as 100 ms (notwithstanding the look-and-listen task used in these studies). Most likely, these very fast effects are due to language-mediated *cancellation* of already-planned saccades.

A final comment on task: A number of studies that have not utilized the visual world paradigm have also considered the influence of language on visual attention (e.g. Estes et al., 2008; Meteyard et al., 2007). Liu (2009) found that auditory words such as 'ascend' and 'plummet' either facilitated or interfered with eye movements during the *smooth pursuit* of a target dot moving vertically down the screen (the effects were apparent at word offset). These effects were modulated by whether the gaze position of the eye was ahead of, or behind, the dot being tracked; the directionality implied by the verb's semantics (up vs. down) interacted with the direction in which attention had to be deployed (up vs. down) to match the velocity of the dot. This interaction with gaze position relative to the moving dot suggested that the modulatory effects of verb semantics were not under conscious control (participants are not aware that their eye is a few pixels ahead of, or behind, the target). This study is also interesting because all studies to date which have explored the influence of language on eye movements have employed situations in which eye movements are driven towards a target object on the basis of the match between the content conveyed by a word or phrase and the knowledge associated with that target object. In the smooth pursuit task, the language is incidental to the oculomotor task, and neither the semantics of the language, nor indeed the semantics of the visual object (whatever that may be in the case of a moving dot) are, a priori, relevant to the initiation and maintenance of pursuit eye movements.

Methodological issues

The visual world paradigm has engendered interest, in part, because of the very precise synchronization that is possible between the eye movement record and the linguistic input or output. It is possible, for example, to record the number of times the eyes saccade to a target location during a particular word or phrase, whose onset and offset vary on a trial-by-trial basis. *Plotting* such data is not straightforward however.

Plotting the data

Figs. 54.2 and 54.3 illustrate the problem. Both figures show the same data, taken from the 'blank screen' data reported in Altmann (2004).[1] Participants heard 'The man will eat the cake' having *previously* seen an image with just four objects (one in each quadrant): a cake, a newspaper, a woman, and a man (see Fig. 54.1, which also shows the relative sparseness of the stimuli that are sometimes used in such studies—see Henderson and Ferreira, 2004, for discussion). The regions of interest were the quadrants in which each object had been located (see below for further discussion of the choice of region of interest).

---

[1] Only the saccadic analyses, corresponding to Fig. 54.4, were reported in Altmann (2004). The same data set that generated those analyses was used to generate the fixation plots shown in Figs. 54.2, 54.3, and 54.5.

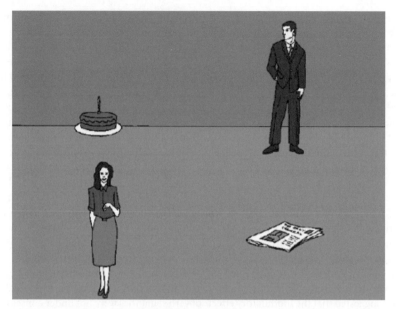

Fig. 54.1 Example scene from Altmann (2004). Reprinted from *Cognition*, **93**(2), Gerry T.M. Altmann, Language-mediated eye movements in the absence of a visual world: the 'blank screen paradigm', pp. B79–B87 © 2004, with permission from Elsevier.

The plots in Figs. 54.2 and 54.3 both show the percentage of trials over time (quantized into successive 50 ms 'slices') on which one of three locations was fixated as the accompanying sentence unfolded. Figure 54.2 synchronizes time from the onset of 'The man . . .'. The first vertical (black) line shows the average offset of 'The man', the second shows the average onset of 'eat' and the third the average onset of 'the cake'. The shaded regions attached to each such line show the range of actual offsets/ onsets, with the leftmost edge marking the earliest, and the rightmost edge marking the latest.

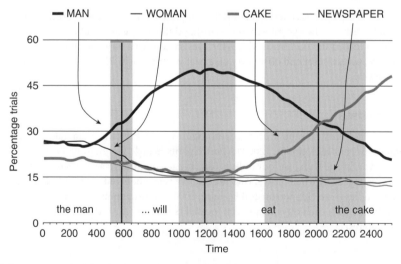

Fig. 54.2 Percentage of trials with fixations across time, synchronized from sentence onset. Reprinted from *Cognition*, **93**(2), Gerry T. M. Altmann, Language-mediated eye movements in the absence of a visual world: the 'blank screen paradigm', pp. B79–B87, Copyright (2004), with permission from Elsevier.

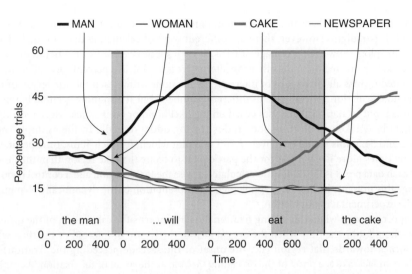

Fig. 54.3 Percentage of trials with fixations across time, resynchronized at each marked interval onset and at sentence offset. Reprinted from *Cognition*, **93**(2), Gerry T. M. Altmann, Language-mediated eye movements in the absence of a visual world: the 'blank screen paradigm', pp. B79–B87, Copyright (2004), with permission from Elsevier.

The problem that such a plot presents (assuming that the shaded regions were not present) is the indeterminacy that results from the progressive *desynchronization* between the eye movement record and the trial-by-trial timings of interest that occur the further into the sentence one goes. For example: the rise in looks to where the cake had been during the verb 'eat', which is of theoretical importance with respect to the demonstration of *anticipatory* eye movements even when viewing a blank screen, appears to occur during the acoustic lifetime of the verb itself. But the shaded regions show that *one half* of the average duration indicated for the verb includes trials in which the verb had already ended and the postverbal noun phrase had begun. Thus, what appear to be anticipatory looks towards the cake may not be anticipatory at all, but may in fact reflect those trials in which acoustic information pertaining to 'cake' had occurred earlier than average. Plotting the data as in Fig. 54.2 (without the shaded regions) would therefore give a misleading impression of what might actually be going on. To avoid this, the data can be plotted as in Fig. 54.3.

In Figure 54.3, the calculation of fixations has been computed separately for each interval of interest (see Altmann and Kamide, 2009, for details). For example, for the verb 'eat', the interval of interest begins at the onset of the verb, calculated on a trial-by-trial basis, and proceeding for 800 ms (the average duration of the verb). The vertical line at the offset of 'eat' in the graph represents the onset of 'the' in 'the cake' (to avoid any coarticulatory influences on the estimation of anticipatory eye movements), and the calculation of fixations during 'the cake' was *resynchronized* to the onset of this interval, again calculated on a trial-by-trial basis (in principle, there could be discontinuities between the curve just before resynchronization and just after; in practice there are few). The grey bars show the 'uncertainty'; that is, for roughly the last 400 ms of 'eat' some of the rise in looks towards where the cake had been may still be due to trials in which the onset of the postverbal noun phrase occurred sooner than 800 ms after the onset of the verb (the corresponding grey bar at sentence offset is not shown in the interests of clarity). However, because the vertical line at the onset of 'the cake' indicates resynchronization, this line (or rather, where the curves cross this line) shows accurately where the eyes were fixating *at this onset* and its equivalent across the different trials. The graph tells us, therefore, that the rise in looks to the cake in advance of the onset of 'the cake' is truly anticipatory. It is noteworthy that the two graphs are very similar; this reflects the fact that the sentences were short, had the same syntactic structure, and were designed to be similar; the greater the variability amongst the sentences, the greater the desynchronization problem.

Plotting fixations is perhaps the most common method for conveying the dynamics of eye movements in this paradigm. However, there are different ways of calculating these plots. In Figs. 54.2 and 54.3, the plots show the percentage of trials, at each successive 50-ms time point, on which the eyes were fixating one region or the other. An alternative is to plot, as a percentage of all fixations that were counted (across all the regions of interest), the fixations within each specific region of interest. This second calculation generally yields different numbers, but it also more accurately reflects the data that is input to statistical analyses based on log likelihood or odds ratios. More recently, some researchers have taken to plotting odds ratios (or log odds) directly. In the example shown in Figs. 54.2 and 54.3, this would effectively result in a plot which, for each 50ms. time point, showed how many times more likely it was for the participant to fixate the cake region than the newspaper region (each data point is the odds ratio calculated across the target region and a control region). The advantage this presents is that the graph is then a representation of the dynamically changing *effect size* of the experimental manipulation.

An important issue when calculating fixational data concerns the calculation of the onset of the fixation: should it be the time when the eyes *landed* in the region of interest, or the time when the eyes *launched* towards that region (i.e. the onset of the saccade preceding the fixation)? Many researchers in fact take the onset of the preceding saccade as the onset of the fixation. As outlined in Altmann (2010) this has the advantage of eliminating the noise that is due to variable saccade duration as a function of where in the scene the eyes were before the critical fixation—fixation onset will be determined by the prior distance of the eye from the new fixation (the further away, the later the fixation onset). Saccade onset is a more accurate estimate of when covert attention switched to the new fixation location.

An alternative to plotting or analysing fixation patterns is to plot/analyse saccades (often calculated as the number of trials on which at least one saccade was launched within some interval of interest, calculated on a trial-by-trial basis, to some region of interest). Although the two dependent measures are related through reflecting different components of the oculomotor response, they can dissociate (see Altmann and Kamide, 2004, for examples). The onset of a saccade is, roughly, the earliest moment at which there is a measurable oculomotor response to some change in cognitive state, and which measure one reports depends, of course, on the specific hypothesis being tested. The saccadic equivalent to the fixation plots shown in Figs. 54.2 and 54.3 is shown in Fig. 54.4. In this

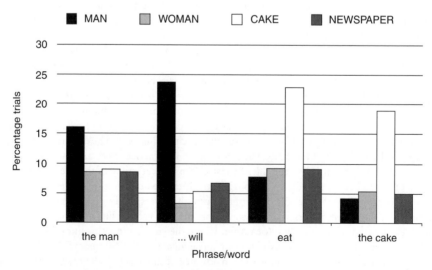

Fig. 54.4 Percentage of trials with saccades launched, during each phrase/word towards the quadrants of interest. Reprinted from *Cognition*, **93**(2), Gerry T. M. Altmann, Language-mediated eye movements in the absence of a visual world: the 'blank screen paradigm', pp. B79–B87, Copyright (2004), with permission from Elsevier.

case, there is no indeterminacy with respect to the relationship between the plot and the trial-by-trial onset/offset of the temporal intervals of interest. Notice the discrepancy at the interval 'eat' between Figs. 54.4 and 54.3: in Fig. 54.3 there are still considerable numbers of fixations on the man, whereas Fig. 54.4 clarifies that there are no more trials on which saccades were launched to the man during 'eat' than there were trials on which saccades were launched towards the other unmentioned objects.

Less common dependent measures derived from the oculomotor response, and which are occasionally used in the visual world paradigm, include saccade launch times and fixation durations—either first fixation duration, gaze duration (the sum of all fixations within the region's boundaries before the eyes first leave that region), or total fixation duration. Less is known about the factors that influence these measures, some of which are unrelated to the relationship between language *per se* and the eye movement response.

Regions of interest, in time and space

Exploring different dependent measures is just one part of analysing 'visual world data'. Equally important is exploring different regions of interest. Unfortunately, the term 'region' has been applied in both the temporal *and* spatial domains. Henceforth, the term 'interval' of interest will refer to regions in time, and 'region' of interest to regions in space. Again, choosing the appropriate intervals of interest depends in large part on the hypotheses to be tested. Studies of word recognition (e.g. Allopenna et al., 1998) tend to focus on an interval that corresponds to the word and some (occasionally arbitrary) period beyond (but see Magnuson et al., 2007, for statistically motivated alternatives such as growth curve analysis). Here, the questions of interest concern when, relative to some part of the word (e.g. onset, uniqueness point, offset, etc.) the eyes can be seen to look more to one region than to another. The analyses of these data often assume that it takes some time from when the cognitive system 'decides' to move the eye to that movement becoming manifest in a saccade being launched, and some period of time is added to the onset and/or offset of the interval of interest to take this time into account (see above, and also Altmann, 2010). Studies of *sentence* processing are often more complex in respect of which intervals to choose; in these case, the intervals of interest will be determined in part by theoretically-driven predictions about which parts of the sentence might be relevant given the goals of the experiment.

For the most part, issues concerned with how to define the (spatial) regions of interest are the same as those encountered when studying eye movements in the absence of concurrent language. The usual caveats in such situations apply: comparisons between eye movements to one object with eye movements towards another object can be contaminated by confounds due to differences in size or the visual saliency of the different objects (e.g. colour, contrast, texture, spatial frequencies and so on). Given that most commonly in the visual world paradigm, it is the language that is manipulated rather than the objects themselves, it is possible to eliminate such confounds by ensuring that the visual scene is held constant while the language is manipulated. In such cases, each object can be its own control—in the example used for Figs. 54.1–54.4, (different) participants in fact heard both 'the man will eat the cake' and 'the woman will read the newspaper'. The plotted data show the *aggregated data* such that looks shown in the graph towards where the cake had been are the sum of looks towards where the cake had been during 'the man will eat the cake' and of looks towards where newspaper had been during 'the woman will read the newspaper'. Comparing the curves for the cake and newspaper in Figs. 54.2 and 54.3 (or the bars in Fig. 54.4) is equivalent, therefore, to comparing looks to the cake during '. . . eat the cake' with looks to the cake during '. . . read the newspaper' (and conversely, of course, for looks to the newspaper); any difference between the cake and the other objects within the same scene that might cause it to attract fewer, or more, looks will therefore cancel out.

Perhaps surprisingly, of less concern is how precise the definition of the (spatial) regions of interest should be. For the case where the scene is concurrent with the language, the majority of fixations on an object will indeed be on that object—that is, the majority will land within a region defined by the external boundary of the object. Defining the region of interest as extending beyond the exact boundary of the object will change the absolute number of fixations that 'count' as landing on the object, but the overall patterns across conditions will be virtually unchanged. Some researchers therefore choose to report 'pixel analyses' (the region's boundary is the object's boundary) or analyses in which fixations landing some arbitrary amount beyond the object's edge are still included (cf. a 'blob' or rectangle drawn around the object to define the region of interest). Neither analysis is intended to make assumptions regarding the resolution of either the human visual system (e.g. how accurately fixations can be targeted) or the eye trackers deployed in such studies (e.g. how accurate the eye tracker is in reporting the actual screen coordinates on which the fixation was located). Some studies (e.g. Allopenna et al., 1998) depicted objects on a grid, and a fixation anywhere within the corresponding cell of the grid counted as a fixation on that object. Other studies (e.g. Huettig and Altmann, 2004) also depicted objects on a virtual grid (e.g. one object in each quadrant), but still the results were based on pixel analyses. There is no reason to suppose that the data patterns would differ at all if one kind of analysis were replaced with another. However, where it *might* matter is in respect of the increasingly used blank screen paradigm—the data shown in Figs. 54.2–54.4 are based on quadrant analyses. But what is the result of increasing the spatial gain and computing a finer-grain analysis of these same data? Figure 54.5 shows the results of increasing the gain to capture rectangular regions of interest as well as pixel analyses. The fixation plots use the unsynchronized variant in which fixations are synchronized to sentence onset (cf. Fig. 54.2). As can be seen, it makes very little difference to the *pattern* of fixations, albeit not to their absolute numbers, if the regions of interest are drawn one way or another. Most striking about these data are that they are from the blank screen paradigm; the fixations plotted in Fig. 54.5 were directed towards empty space that had *previously* been occupied by the depicted objects.

Statistical issues

As with any dependent measure, how to analyse differences in that measure as a function of the experimental manipulation is an issue that warrants careful attention. A variety of methods have been used to test for differences in fixations or saccades at moments of interest (e.g. at the offset of some critical word or phrase) or during intervals of interest. These include traditional ANOVA or t-tests on untransformed proportions (cf. the percentages shown in the plots above). A problem with these tests is that proportions are often skewed, and may therefore violate the assumptions that need to be met for such tests to be appropriate; ANOVA or t-tests on *arcsin transformed* proportions are therefore preferred. Recently, researchers have started to use hierarchical log linear analyses on raw numbers (based on chi-square distributions, and similar in many respects to chi-square except that they allow main effects and interactions to be tested). The first studies employing hierarchical log linear analyses included Huettig and Altmann (2005) and Knoeferle et al. (2005)—see Scheepers, 2003, for discussion of hierarchical log linear analyses more generally, and Altmann and Kamide, 2007 and 2009, for further discussion of their use in visual world analyses. One important difference between the ANOVA and chi-square families of tests is that they assume a different underlying distribution of the data—they are, in effect, different classes of statistical 'model' (see below). Typically, ANOVA is used more with reaction times, and chi-square with frequencies or counts. Even more recently, investigators have started to use mixed effects models. These are equivalent in some respects to log linear analyses but they tend to be used when multiple predictors need to be assessed (when, for example, they cannot be included in a standard factorial design). Mixed effects models are also advantageous as they allow for simultaneous treatment of subjects and items as random effects (see Baayen et al., 2008).

An entirely different class of statistical modelling needs to be carried out for analysing *time-course* data. For example, and with reference to Figs. 54.2 or 54.5, how can one determine that any pair of curves are different from one another? How can one determine where the *peak* is located for any such curve (given that aggregating data for the purposes of such plots hides the true underlying distribution of the data across subjects and trials)? And most importantly, perhaps, how can one model the dynamic changes to fixation proportions across time when successive time points are not independent of one another? This latter question has been addressed most recently using multilevel logistic

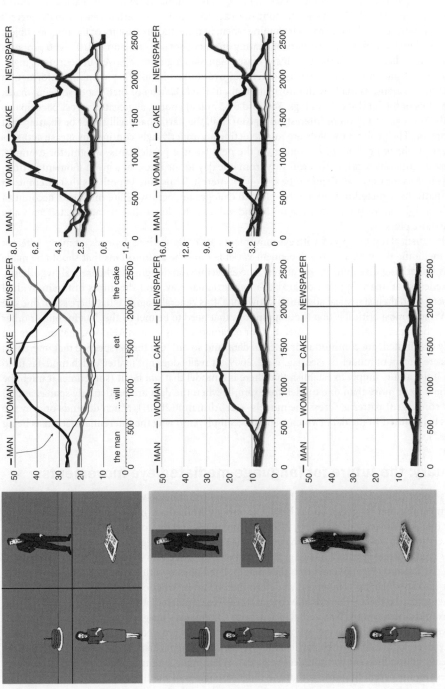

Fig. 54.5 Percentage trials with fixations in each region of interest defined as quadrants (top row), rectangles (middle row), pixels (bottom row). The central column shows the fixation percentages on the same scale. The rightmost column shows the pixel analyses re-scaled to illustrate their similarity to the rectangle and quadrant analyses. Reprinted from *Cognition*, **93**(2), Gerry T. M. Altmann, Language-mediated eye movements in the absence of a visual world: the 'blank screen paradigm', pp. B79–B87, Copyright (2004), with permission from Elsevier.

regression (Barr, 2008b), which simultaneously handles the continuous variable of time and the categorical variable of gaze location. Magnuson et al. (2007) used growth curve analysis to address similar statistical complexities in their time-course data. This technique 'decomposes' each curve into a number of parameters which can then be compared across conditions. Perhaps surprisingly, there is no standard statistical technique for determining when, in time, the probability of fixating one object in the scene *diverges* from the probability of fixating another (but see Altmann (2010), who proposes a simple method based on a variant of cluster-based Gaussian logic as employed in neuroimaging).

A feature of time-course plots that is sometimes overlooked is that they combine information about *when* a response is made with information about the *likelihood* of that response being made. Fixation plots of the kind shown in Figs. 54.2 and 54.3 are, of course, aggregated across participants and trials. For a given region of interest on a given trial, the participant will either be fixating that region or not. The probability plots are not depicting an underlyingly continuous measure that is continuously changing from one moment to the next (unlike participants' weight, for example, which is a continuous measure that can vary from one day to the next); at a given moment in time, the eyes either are or are not fixating the region of interest. Thus, any hypothesis that attempts to link the patterns depicted in time-course plots to changes in cognitive state must take account of the underlyingly discontinuous nature of the individual behaviours that are aggregated across to generate those plots.

Which statistical test to employ with eye movement data of these kinds depends on many different factors, including the nature of the dependent variable (and the assumptions that should be made about its underlying distribution; see above), the experimental design, the theoretical hypotheses, the precedents for analysing particular data in a particular way, and the limits of the individual researchers' (and their statistical advisors') knowledge. It is generally agreed that there is no 'one size fits all'. What is most critical is that the assumptions that need to be met by the data for one or other analysis to be appropriate are indeed met (e.g. for parametric tests such as ANOVA, that the data are normally distributed, are continuous or interval data, and so on). On the perspective that inferential statistics are a form of model-fit (see, e.g. Field, 2009), it really does not matter which model is fit to the data if the aim is simply to establish that there is a model that *can* be fit (sometimes it might be appropriate to fit more than one model, for example when the data are particularly sparse, and to look for convergent patterns across the models—see Altmann (2010)). Much depends on *why* the model is being fitted to the data (which translates, simply, into why the inferential statistic is being computed).

Summary: the future for language-mediated eye movements

Whereas Roger Cooper first observed the tight temporal coupling between language and eye movements (meaning that language could have a seemingly immediate influence on the bias to look towards one part of space or another), Michael Tanenhaus and his colleagues were able to ground that observation in developments in the vision sciences that were beginning to explore eye movements as a goal-directed behaviour (e.g. Ballard et al., 1997; see also Land et al., 1999). Instead of tracking participants' eye movements as they manipulated objects with the goal of connecting pieces together into some larger-scale object as determined by an instructional diagram, Tanenhaus and colleagues tracked participants' eye movements as they manipulated objects with the goal of moving pieces around as determined by a verbal instruction. Tanenhaus's insight was that language-directed eye movements *are* goal-directed eye movements. The goals are determined by the task—either explicitly given, or brought by the participant into the experiment (just as, when speaking, we might dynamically adopt different communicative goals). What made language-mediated eye movements so interesting for psycholinguists is that the indeterminacies of the linguistic signal manifested in uncertainties with respect to what the immediate attentional goals should be (for example, whether to attend to a beaker or to a beetle during the first moments of the word 'beaker', or whether to attend to Mickey or to Donald on hearing 'he'). The field blossomed with epidemic speed (but without the negative connotations usually associated with epidemics), in large part because language is indeterminate at so many different levels of analysis, with its indeterminacies changing dynamically as a word or sentence unfolds. The scope for exploring these indeterminacies, using a new paradigm that is sensitive in close to real time to psychological processes relevant to their resolution, seemed limited only by the number of eye trackers available to the field (undoubtedly, a part of the field's blossoming was due to the availability of ever-cheaper and more user-friendly eye tracking devices, associated software, and analysis tools). As the field has matured, so researchers are beginning to reflect on *why* language has this mediating influence on visual attention (see the earlier section 'How, and why, language mediates eye movements'). But the consideration of language-mediated eye movements not as a psycholinguistic tool, but as reflecting a deeper connection between language, perception, cognition, and action, is still in its infancy. Beyond its continuing development in service of psycholinguistic research, it is in this direction that the field is likely to develop in new ways— borrowing theoretical tools that already exist beyond the confines of psycholinguistics to understand better the relationship between language and cognition. Theoretical frameworks such as those developed in the context of cognitive control and attention—how task-relevant features become more activated than task-irrelevant features (e.g. Cohen et al., 2004)—are likely to provide a bridge between the many disparate features of the paradigm. Such frameworks are likely to lead also to a greater understanding not simply of the mechanisms underlying the linkage between language and eye movements (see 'How, and why, language mediates eye movements' section) but also of the task-specificity of this mediation (see 'Task-sensitivity and language-mediated eye movements' section).

As suggested earlier, the fact that language mediates eye movements at all is not so surprising. What is more surprising is that 'higher-level' cognitive factors can penetrate so deeply into what might be presumed to be 'lower-level' processes controlling oculomotor behaviour (cf. Liu's work on language-mediation of smooth-pursuit eye movements (Liu, 2009)). A natural question to consider, then, is how language interacts, in different task contexts, with other factors that constrain oculomotor control. For example, global and remote distractor effects (see Cruickshank and McSorley, 2009, and references therein), systematic biases favouring eye movements in one direction rather than another (e.g. Tatler and Vincent, 2008), or factors influencing visual salience and its impact on overt and covert attention (e.g. Itti and Koch, 2000; Parkhurst et al., 2002). One may even ask, again, the question posed at the start of this review; how, and under what conditions, do eye movements in service of language differ from those in service of reaching movements? A final question that no doubt will receive attention concerns the neural pathways implicated in the interaction between language and oculomotor control (most likely there will be more than one).

The study of language-mediated eye movements has become a fundamental tool in the study of psycholinguistic process. It is fast becoming a fundamental tool in the study of cognitive processes more generally. The past 15 years have seen extraordinary growth accompanied by real advances in our understanding of the cognitive processes with which language makes contact. The next 15 years will surely be as extraordinary.

Acknowledgements

This review would not have been possible without the original contributions of the authors whose work I refer to. Any omissions do not reflect a value judgement, but most likely reflect a lapse of memory and limited time in which to research the ever-growing field. Thanks are due to Yuki Kamide, Jelena Mirkovic, and Silvia Gennari for encouragement and suggestions, the Economic and Social Research Council (ref. RES-063-27-0138) for funding the time in which this article was written, the editors of this volume for their patience in awaiting the arrival of this manuscript, and two anonymous reviewers for their insightful comments on an earlier version of the manuscript.

References

Allopenna, P.D., Magnuson, J.S., and Tanenhaus, M.K. (1998). Tracking the time course of spoken word recognition using eye movements: Evidence for continuous mapping models. *Journal of Memory and Language*, **38**(4), 419–439.

Altmann, G.T.M. (1999). Thematic role assignment in context. *Journal of Memory and Language*, **41**, 124–145.

Altmann, G.T.M. (2004) Language-mediated eye movements in the absence of a visual world: The 'blank screen paradigm'. *Cognition*, **93**, B79–B87.

Altmann, G.T.M. (2010). Language can mediate eye movement control within 100 milliseconds, regardless of whether there is anything to move the eyes to. *Acta Psychologica.* doi:10.1016/j.actpsy.2010.09.009

Altmann, G.T.M. and Kamide, Y. (1999). Incremental interpretation at verbs: Restricting the domain of subsequent reference. *Cognition*, **73**(3), 247–264.

Altmann, G.T.M. and Kamide, Y. (2004) Now you see it, now you don't: mediating the mapping between language and the visual world. In J. Henderson and F. Ferreira (eds.) *The integration of language, vision and action* (pp. 347–386). Hove: Psychology Press.

Altmann, G.T.M. and Kamide, Y. (2007). The real-time mediation of visual attention by language and world knowledge: Linking anticipatory (and other) eye movements to linguistic processing. *Journal of Memory and Language*, **57**, 502–518.

Altmann, G.T.M. and Kamide, Y. (2009). Discourse-mediation of the mapping between language and the visual world: eye-movements and mental representation. *Cognition*, **111**, 55–71.

Altmann, G.T.M. and Steedman, M.J. (1988). Interaction with context during human sentence processing. *Cognition*, **30**(3), 191–238.

Arai, M., van Gompel, R.P.G., and Scheepers, C. (2007). Priming ditransitive structures in comprehension. *Cognitive Psychology*, **54**, 218–250.

Arnold, J.E., and Lao, S-Y.C., (2009). Effects of non-shared attention on pronoun comprehension. Ms, University of North Carolina at Chapel Hill.

Arnold, J.E., Brown-Schmidt, S., and Trueswell, J.C. (2007a). Children's use of gender and order-of-mention during pronoun comprehension. *Language and Cognitive Processes*, **22**, 527–565.

Arnold, J.E., Hudson-Kam, C., and Tanenhaus, M.K. (2007b). If you say *thee uh-* you're describing something hard: the on-line attribution of disfluency during reference comprehension. *Journal of Experimental Psychology: Learning, Memory, and Cognition*, **33**, 914–930.

Arnold, J.E., Eisenband, J.G., Brown-Schmidt, S., and Trueswell, J.C. (2000). The rapid use of gender information: Evidence of the time course of pronoun resolution from eye tracking. *Cognition*, **76**, B13–B26.

Arnold, J.E., Tanenhaus, M.K., Altmann, R.J., and Fagnano, M. (2004). The old and thee, uh, new: Disfluency and reference resolution. *Psychological Science*, **15**, 578–582.

Baayen, R.H., Davidson, D.J., and Bates, D. (2008). Mixed-effects modeling with crossed random effects for subjects and items. *Journal of Memory and Language*, **59**, 390–412.

Ballard, D.H., Hayhoe, M.M., Pook, P.K., and Rao, R.P.N. (1997). Deictic codes for the embodiment of cognition. *Behavioral and Brain Sciences*, **20**, 723–767.

Barr, D.J. (2008a). Pragmatic expectations and linguistic evidence: Listeners anticipate but do not integrate common ground. *Cognition*, **109**, 18–40.

Barr, D.J. (2008b). Analyzing 'visual world' eyetracking data using multilevel logistic regression. *Journal of Memory and Language*, **59**, 457–474.

Bock, J.K. (1986). Meaning, sound, and syntax: Lexical priming in sentence production. *Journal of Experimental Psychology: Learning, Memory, and Cognition*, **12**, 575–586.

Bock, J.K. (1987). An effect of the accessibility of word forms on sentence structure. *Journal of Memory and Language*, **26**, 119–137.

Boland, J.E. (2005). Visual arguments. *Cognition*, **95**, 237–274.

Brandt, S.A. and Stark, L.W. (1997). Spontaneous eye movements during visual imagery reflect the content of the visual scene. *Journal of Cognitive Neuroscience*, **9**, 27–38.

Brown-Schmidt, S. and Tanenhaus, M.K. (2006). Watching the eyes when talking about size: An investigation of message formulation and utterance planning. *Journal of Memory and Language*, **54**, 592–609.

Brown-Schmidt, S., Campana, E., and Tanenhaus, M.K. (2005). Real-time reference resolution in a referential communication task. In: J.C. Trueswell, and M.K. Tanenhaus (eds.) *Processing world-situated language: Bridging the language-as-action and language-as-product traditions*. Cambridge, MA: MIT Press.

Carpenter, R.H.S. (1988). *Movements of the Eyes* (2nd edn.). London: Pion.

Carpenter, R.H.S. and Williams, M.L.L. (1995). Neural computation of log likelihood in control of saccadic eye movements. *Nature*, **377**, 59–62.

Chambers, C.G., Tanenhaus, M.K., and Magnuson, J.S. (2004). Action-based affordances and syntactic ambiguity resolution. *Journal of Experimental Psychology: Learning, Memory and Cognition*, **30**, 687–696.

Chambers, C.G., Tanenhaus, M.K., Eberhard, K.M., Filip, H., and Carlson, G.N. (2002). Circumscribing referential domains during real-time language comprehension. *Journal of Memory and Language*, **47**, 30–49.

Cohen, J.D., Aston-Jones, G., and Gilzenrat, M.S. (2004). A systems-level perspective on attention and cognitive control: Guided activation, adaptive gating, conflict monitoring, and exploitation vs. exploration. In M.I. Posner (ed.), *Cognitive neuroscience of attention* (pp. 71–90). New York: Guilford Press.

Cooper, R.M. (1974). The control of eye fixation by the meaning of spoken language: A new methodology for the real-time investigation of speech perception, memory, and language processing. *Cognitive Psychology*, **6**, 84–107.

Crain, S. and Steedman, M.J. (1985). On not being led up the garden path: the use of context by the psychological parser. In D. Dowty, L. Karttunen, and A. Zwicky (eds.) *Natural Language Parsing: Psychological, Computational, and Theoretical perspectives* (pp. 320–358) Cambridge: Cambridge University Press.

Cree, G.S. and McRae, K. (2003). Analyzing the factors underlying the structure and computation of the meaning of chipmunk, cherry, chisel, cheese, and cello (and many other such concrete nouns). *Journal of Experimental Psychology: General*, **132**, 163–201.

Crosby, J.R., Monin, B. and Richardson, D.C. (2008). Where do we look during potentially offensive behavior? *Psychological Science*, **19**, 226–228.

Cruickshank, A.G. and McSorley, M. (2009). Involuntary inhibition of movement initiation alters oculomotor competition resolution. *Experimental Brain Research*, **193**, 467–476.

Dahan, D. and Tanenhaus, M.K. (2004). Continuous mapping from sound to meaning in spoken-language comprehension: Evidence from immediate effects of verb-based constraints. *Journal of Experimental Psychology: Learning, Memory and Cognition*, **30**, 498–513.

Dahan, D., Magnuson, J.S., and Tanenhaus, M.K. (2001). Time course of frequency effects in spoken-word recognition: Evidence from eye movements. *Cognitive Psychology*, **42**(4), 317–367.

Dahan, D., Tanenhaus, M.K., and Chambers, C.G. (2002). Accent and reference resolution in spoken-language comprehension. *Journal of Memory and Language*, **47**(2), 292–314.

Dahan, D., Magnuson, J.S., Tanenhaus, M.K., and Hogan, E.M. (2001). Subcategorical mismatches and the time course of lexical access: Evidence for lexical competition. *Language and Cognitive Processes*, **16**, 507–534.

Dell'Acqua, R. and Grainger, J. (1999). Unconscious semantic priming from pictures. *Cognition*, **73**, B1–B15.

DeLong, K.A., Urbach, T.P., and Kutas, M. (2005). Probabilistic word pre-activation during language comprehension inferred from electrical brain activity. *Nature Neuroscience*, **8**, 1117–1121.

Duñabeitia, J.A., Aviles, A., Afonso, O., Scheepers, C., and Carreiras., M. (2009). Qualitative differences in the representation of abstract versus concrete words: Evidence from the visual-world paradigm. *Cognition*, **110**, 284–292.

Estes, Z., Verges, M., and Barsalou, L.W. (2008). Head up, foot down: Object words orient attention to the objects' typical location. *Psychological Science*, **19**, 93–97.

Field, A. (2009). *Discovering statistics using SPSS* (3rd ed.). London: Sage Publications.

Gleitman, L.R., January, D., Nappa, R., and Trueswell, J.C. (2007). On the give and take between event apprehension and utterance formulation. *Journal of Memory and Language*, **57**(4), 544–569.

Grodner, D. and Sedivy, J. (in press). The effect of speaker-specific information on pragmatic inferences. In N. Pearlmutter and E. Gibson (eds.) *The Processing and Acquisition of Reference*. Cambridge, MA: MIT Press.

Grice, H.P. (1975). Logic and conversation. In: P. Cole, and J. Morgan (eds.) Syntax and semantics 3: Speech acts (pp. 41–58). New York: Academic Press.

Griffin, Z.M. (2001). Gaze durations during speech reflect word selection and phonological encoding. *Cognition*, **82**, B1–B14.

Griffin, Z.M. (2004a). The eyes are right when the mouth is wrong. *Psychological Science*, **15**, 814–821.

Griffin, Z.M. (2004b). Why look? Reasons for eye movements related to language production. In J. M. Henderson and F. Ferreira (eds.) *The integration of language, vision, and action: Eye movements and the visual world*. New York: Psychology Press.

Griffin, Z.M. and Bock, J.K. (2000). What they eyes say about speaking. *Psychological Science*, **11**, 274–279.

Hanna, J.E., Tanenhaus, M.K., and Trueswell, J.C. (2003). The effects of common ground and perspective on domains of referential interpretation. *Journal of Memory and Language*, **49**, 43–61.

Henderson, J. and Ferreira, F. (2004). Scene perception for psycholinguists. In J. Henderson and F. Ferreira (eds.) *The integration of language, vision and action* (pp. 1–58). Hove: Psychology Press.

Hoover, M.A. and Richardson, D.C. (2008). When facts go down the rabbit hole: Contrasting features and objecthood as indexes to memory. *Cognition*, **108**, 533–42.

Horstmann, A. and Hoffman, K.P. (2005). Target selection in eye–hand coordination: Do we reach to where we look or do we look to where we reach? *Experimental Brain Research*, **167**(2), 187–189.

Huettig, F., and Altmann, G.T.M. (2005). Word meaning and the control of eye fixation: Semantic competitor effects and the visual world paradigm. *Cognition*, **96**(1), 23–32.

Ito, K. and Speer, S.R. (2008). Anticipatory effects of intonation: Eye movements during instructed visual search. *Journal of Memory and Language*, **58**, 541–573.

Itti, L. and Koch, C. (2000). A saliency-based search mechanism for overt and covert shifts of visual attention. *Vision Research*, **40**, 1489–1506.

Kaiser, E. and Trueswell, J.C. (2004). The role of discourse context in the processing of a flexible word-order language. *Cognition*, **94**, 113–147.

Kamide, Y., Scheepers, C., and Altmann, G.T.M. (2003a) Integration of syntactic and semantic information in predictive processing: A cross-linguistic study in German and English. *Journal of Psycholinguistic Research*, **32**, 37–55.

Kamide, Y., Altmann, G.T.M., and Haywood, S.L. (2003b). The time-course of prediction in incremental sentence processing: Evidence from anticipatory eye movements. *Journal of Memory and Language*, **49**, 133–159.

Keysar, B., Barr, D.J., Balin, J.A., and Brauner, J.S. (2000). Taking perspective in conversation: The role of mutual knowledge in comprehension. *Psychological Science*, **11**, 32–38.

Knoeferle, P. and Crocker, M. (2006). The coordinated interplay of scene, utterance, and world knowledge: Evidence from eye tracking. *Cognitive Science*, **30**, 481–529.

Knoeferle, P. and Crocker, M.W. (2007). The influence of recent scene events on spoken comprehension: Evidence from eye movements. *Journal of Memory and Language*, **57**, 519–543.

Knoeferle, P., Crocker, M.W., Scheepers, C., and Pickering, M.J. (2005). The influence of the immediate visual context on incremental thematic role-assignment: Evidence from eye-movements in the depicted events. *Cognition*, **95**, 95–127.

Laeng, B. and Teodorecu, D. (2002). Eye scan-paths during visual imagery reenact those of perception of the same visual scene. *Cognitive Science*, **26**, 207–231.

Land, M., Mennie, N., and Rusted, J. (1999). Eye movements and the roles of vision in activities of daily living: making a cup of tea. *Perception*, **28**, 1311–1328.

Liu, X. (2009). What can a moving dot tell us about cognition: Language, eye movements and attention. Unpublished PhD Thesis. University of York.

Luce, P.A., Pisoni, D.B., and Goldinger, S.D. (1990). Similarity neighborhoods of spoken words. In G.T.M. Altmann (ed.) *Cognitive models of speech processing: Psycholinguistic and computational perspectives* (pp. 122–147). Cambridge, MA: MIT.

MacDonald, M.C., Pearlmutter, N.J., and Seidenberg, M.S. (1994). The lexical nature of syntactic ambiguity resolution. *Psychological Review*, **101**, 676–703.

Magnuson, J.S., McMurray, B., Tanenhaus, M.K., and Aslin, R.N. (2003a). Lexical effects on compensation for coarticulation: The ghost of Christmash past. *Cognitive Science*, **27**, 285–298.

Magnuson, J.S., Tanenhaus, M.K., Aslin, R.N., and Dahan, D. (2003b). Time course of spoken word learning and recognition: Studies with artificial lexicons. *Journal of Experimental Psychology: General*, **132**, 202–227.

Magnuson, J.S., Dixon, J.A., Tanenhaus, M.K., and Aslin, R.N. (2007). The dynamics of lexical competition during spoken word recognition. *Cognitive Science*, **31**, 133–156.

Magnuson, J.S., Tanenhaus, M.K., and Aslin, R.N. (2008). Immediate effects of form-class constraints on spoken word recognition. *Cognition*, **108**, 866–873.

Marslen-Wilson, W.D. (1987). Functional parallelism in spoken word recognition. *Cognition*, **25**, 71–102.

Marslen-Wilson, W. (1990). Activation, competition, and frequency in lexical access. In G.T.M. Altmann (ed) *Cognitive Models of Speech Processing: Psycholinguistic and Computational Perspectives*. Cambridge, MA: The MIT Press.

Marslen-Wilson, W. (1993). Issues of process and representation in lexical access. In G.T.M. Altmann and R.C. Shillcock (eds.) *Cognitive Models of Speech Processing: The second Sperlonga meeting*. Hove: Lawrence Erlbaum Associates Ltd.

Matin, E., Shao, K., and Boff, K. (1993). Saccadic overhead: information processing time with and without saccades. *Perception and Psychophysics*, **53**, 372–380.

McMurray, B., Tanenhaus, M.K., and Aslin, R.N. (2002). Gradient effects of within-category phonetic variation on lexical access. *Cognition*, **86**(2), B33–B42.

McSorley, E. and Findlay, J.M. (2003). Saccade target selection in visual search. Accuracy improves when more distractors are present. *Journal of Vision*, **3**, 877–892.

Meteyard, L., Bahrami, B., and Vigliocco, G. (2007). Motion detection and motion verbs. *Psychological Science*, **18**, 1007–1013.

Meyer, A.S., Sleiderink, A.M., and Levelt, W.J.M. (1998). Viewing and naming objects: Eye movements during noun phrase production. *Cognition*, **66**, B25–B33.

Moores, E., Laiti, L., and Chelazzi, L. (2003). Associative knowledge controls deployment of visual selective attention. *Nature Neuroscience*, **6**, 182–189.

Myung, J-Y, Blumstein, S.E., and Sedivy, S. (2006). Playing on the typewriter, typing on the piano: Manipulation knowledge of objects. *Cognition*, **98**, 223–243.

Nadig, A. and Sedivy, J. (2002). Evidence for perspective-taking constraints in children's on-line reference resolution. *Psychological Science*, **13**, 329–336.

Nation, K., Marshall, C., and Altmann, G.T.M. (2003) Investigating individual differences in children's real-time sentence comprehension using language-mediated eye movements. *Journal of Experimental Child Psychology*, **86**, 314–329.

Neggers, S.F.W. and Bekkering, H. (2002). Coordinated control of eye and hand movements in dynamic reaching. *Human Movement Science*, **21**, 349–376.

Papafragou, A., Hulbert, J., and Trueswell, J. (2008). Does language guide event perception? Evidence from eye movements. *Cognition*, **108**, 155–184.

Parkhurst, D., Law, K., and Niebur, E. (2002). Modeling the role of salience in the allocation of overt visual attention. *Vision Research*, **42**, 107–123.

Rayner, K., Slowiaczek, M.L., Clifton, C., and Bertera, J.H. (1983). Latency of sequential eye movements: implications for reading. *Journal of Experimental Psychology: Human Perception and Performance*, **9**, 912–922.

Reddi, B.A.J. and Carpenter, R.H.S. (2000). The influence of urgency on decision time. *Nature Neuroscience*, **3**, 827–830.

Richardson, D.C. and Dale, R. (2005). Looking to understand: The coupling between speakers' and listeners' eye movements and its relationship to discourse comprehension. *Cognitive Science*, **29**, 1045–1060.

Richardson, D.C. and Spivey, M.J. (2000). Representation, space and hollywood squares: Looking at things that aren't there anymore. *Cognition*, **76**, 269–295.

Richardson, D.C., Dale, R. and Kirkham, N.Z. (2007) The art of conversation is coordination: Common ground and the coupling of eye movements during dialogue. *Psychological Science*, **18**, 407–413.

Richardson, D.C., Altmann, G.T.M., Spivey, M.J., and Hoover, M.A. (2009). Much ado about eye movements to nothing. *Trends in Cognitive Sciences*, **13**, 235–236.

Rumelhart, D.E. and McClelland, J.L. (eds). (1986). *Parallel distributed processing: Explorations in the microstructure of cognition*. Cambridge, MA: MIT Press.

Runner, J.T., Sussman, R.S., and Tanenhaus, M.K. (2003). Assignment of reference to reflexives and pronouns in picture noun phrases: Evidence from eye movements. *Cognition*, **89**, B1–B13.

Runner, J.T., Sussman, R.S., and Tanenhaus, M.K. (2006). Assigning referents to reflexives and pronouns in picture noun phrases. Experimental tests of binding theory. *Cognitive Science*, **30**, 1–49.

Salverda, A.P., Dahan, D., and McQueen, J.M. (2003). The role of prosodic boundaries in the resolution of lexical embedding in speech comprehension. *Cognition*, **90**, 51–89.

Salverda, A.P., Dahan, D., Tanenhaus, M.K., Crosswhite, K., Masharov, M., and McDonough, J. (2007). Effects of prosodically modulated sub-phonetic variation on lexical competition. *Cognition*, **105**, 466–476.

Saslow, M.G. (1967). Latency for saccadic eye movement. *Journal of the Optical Society of America*, **57**, 1030–1033.

Scheepers, C. (2003). Syntactic priming of relative clause attachments: Persistence of structural configuration in sentence production. *Cognition*, **89**, 179–205.

Scheepers, C. and Crocker, M.W. (2004). Constituent order priming from reading to listening: A visual-world study. In M. Carreiras and C.J. Clifton (eds.) *The On-line study of sentence comprehension: Eyetracking, ERP and beyond* (pp. 167–185). Hove: Psychology Press.

Sedivy, J.C. (2003). Pragmatic versus form-based accounts of referential contrast: Evidence for effects of informativity expectations. *Journal of Psycholinguistic Research*, **32**, 3–23.

Sedivy, J.C., Tanenhaus, M.K., Chambers, C.G., and Carlson, G.N. (1999). Achieving incremental semantic interpretation through contextual representation. *Cognition*, **71**, 109–147.

Sekerina, I.A., Stromswold, K. and Hestvik, A. (2004). How do adults and children process referential ambiguity? *Journal of Child Language*, **31**,123–152.

Slobin, D. (1996). From 'thought and language' to 'thinking for speaking'. In J. Gumperz and S. Levinson (eds.) *Rethinking linguistic relativity* (pp. 70–96). New York: Cambridge University Press.

Snedeker, J. and Trueswell, J. (2003). Using prosody to avoid ambiguity: Effects of speaker awareness and referential context. *Journal of Memory and Language*, **48**,103–130.

Snedeker, J. and Trueswell, J. (2004). The developing constraints on parsing decisions: The role of lexical-biases and referential scenes in child and adult sentence processing. *Cognitive Psychology*, **49**, 238–299.

Spivey, M.J. and Marian, V. (1999). Cross talk between native and second languages: Partial activation of an irrelevant lexicon. *Psychological Science*, **10**, 281–284.

Spivey, M.J., Tanenhaus, M.K., Eberhard, K.M. and Sedivy, J.C. (2002). Eye movements and spoken language comprehension: Effects of visual context on syntactic ambiguity resolution. *Cognitive Psychology*, **45**, 447–481.

Sussman, R. and Sedivy, J. (2003). The time course of processing syntactic dependencies: Evidence from eye movements during spoken narratives. *Language and Cognitive Processes*. **18**, 143–163.

Tanenhaus, M.K., and Trueswell, J.C. (2006). Eye movements and spoken language comprehension. In M. Traxler and M. Gernsbacher (eds.) *Handbook of Psycholinguistics: 2nd Edition* (pp. 863–900). Amsterdam: Elsevier.

Tanenhaus, M.K., Spivey-Knowlton, M.J., Eberhard, K.M., and Sedivy, J.C. (1995). Integration of visual and linguistic information in spoken language comprehension. *Science*, **268**(5217), 1632–1634.

Tatler, B.W. and Vincent, B.T. (2008). Systematic tendencies in scene viewing. *Journal of Eye Movement Research*, **2**, 1–18.

Thothathiri, M. and Snedeker, J. (2008). Give and take: Syntactic priming during spoken language comprehension. *Cognition*, **108**, 51–68.

Trueswell, J.C. and Tanenhaus, M.K. (1994). Towards a lexicalist framework of constraint-based syntactic ambiguity resolution. In C. Clifton, L. Frazier, and K. Rayner (eds.) *Perspectives on Sentence Processing* (pp. 155–179) Hillsdale, NJ: Lawrence Erlbaum.

Trueswell, J.C., Sekerina, I., Hill, N., and Logrip, M. (1999). The kindergarten-path effect: Studying on-line sentence processing in young children. *Cognition*, **73**, 89–134.

Van Berkum, J.J.A., Brown, C.M., Zwitserlood, P., Kooijman, V., and Hagoort, P. (2005). Anticipating upcoming words in discourse: Evidence from ERPs and reading times. *Journal of Experimental Psychology: Learning, Memory, and Cognition*, **31**, 443–467.

Walker, R., Deubel, H. and Findlay, J.M. (1997). The effect of remote distractors on saccade programming: evidence for an extended fixation zone. *Journal of Neurophysiology*, **78**, 1108–1119.

Whorf, B.L. (1956). *Language, thought and reality: Selected writings of Benjamin Lee Whorf* (J. Carroll, ed.) Cambridge, MA: MIT Press.

Yee, E. and Sedivy, J. (2001). Using eye movements to track the spread of semantic activation during spoken word recognition. Paper presented at the 13th annual CUNY sentence processing conference, Philadelphia.

Yee, E. and Sedivy, J. (2006). Eye movements to pictures reveal transient semantic activation during spoken word recognition. *Journal of Experimental Psychology: Learning, Memory and Cognition*, **32**(1), 1–14.

Zwitserlood, P. (1989). The locus of the effects of sentential-semantic context in spoken-word processing. *Cognition*, **32**, 25–64.

Author Index

Page numbers in *italic* indicate figures.

Subject Index

Page numbers in *italic* indicate figures and tables.